MW01593500

Atlas of

PEDIATRIC UROLOGIC SURGERY

Atlas of
PEDIATRIC UROLOGIC SURGERY

FRANK HINMAN, JR, MD
FACS, FAAP, FRCS (ENG) HON
Clinical Professor of Urology,
University of California School of Medicine, San Franciso, California

Illustrated by
PAUL H. STEMPEN, MA, AMI

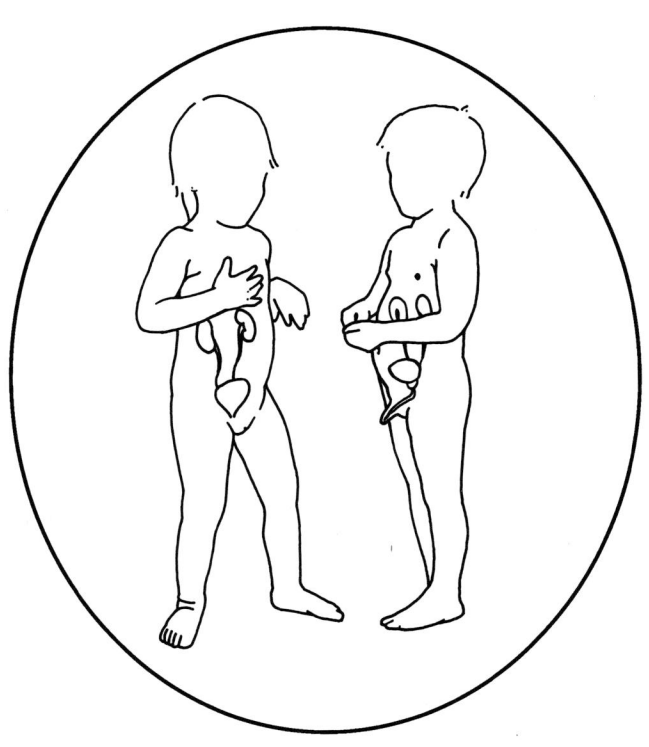

W.B. SAUNDERS COMPANY
A Division of Harcourt Brace & Company
Philadelphia London Toronto Montreal Sydney Tokyo

W.B. SAUNDERS COMPANY
A Division of
Harcourt Brace & Company

The Curtis Center
Independence Square West
Philadelphia, Pennsylvania 19106

Library of Congress Cataloging-in-Publication Data

Hinman, Frank

Atlas of pediatric urologic surgery / by Frank Hinman, Jr;
illustrated by Paul H. Stempen.

    p.   cm.

ISBN 0–7216–4231–4

1. Genitourinary organs—Surgery.   2. Children—Surgery.
   3. Pediatric urology.   I. Title.

[DNLM: 1. Urologic Diseases—in infancy & childhood—
atlases.   2. Urologic Diseases—surgery—atlases.
3. Urogenital Diseases—in infancy & childhood—atlases.
4. Urogenital Diseases—surgery—atlases.   WS 17 H663a
1994]

RD571.H548   1994

617.4′6′0083—dc20

DNLM/DLC   94–4205

Portions of this book including both text and illustrations have appeared previously in the *Atlas of
Urologic Surgery* by Frank Hinman, Jr. published by W.B. Saunders Company, 1989.

Atlas of Pediatric Urologic Surgery   ISBN 0–7216–4231–4

Copyright © 1994 by W.B. Saunders Company

All rights reserved. No part of this publication may be reproduced or transmitted in any form or
by any means, electronic or mechanical, including photocopy, recording, or any information storage
and retrieval system, without permission in writing from the publisher.

Printed in the United States of America

Last digit is the print number: 9   8   7   6   5   4   3   2   1

This atlas is dedicated to the pioneers who developed the procedures of a new subspecialty, practiced them, and then taught them. And to the children who have gained so much from their efforts.

Commentators

TERRY D. ALLEN, MD, FACS, FAAP
Professor of Urology, University of Texas Southwestern Medical School, Dallas, TX
Coronal Repair, 574

JULIAN S. ANSELL, MD, FACS
Professor of Urology, Emeritus, University of Washington Medical School, Seattle, WA
Reconstruction for Vesical Exstrophy, 314

SAMI ARAP, MD
Professor of Urology, Faculdade de Medicina da Universidade de São Paulo, Divisão de Clinica Urológica, Hospital das Clinicas, São Paulo, Brazil
Reconstruction for Vesical Exstrophy, 318

JOHN M. BARRY, MD, FACS
Professor of Surgery and Chairman, Division of Urology and Renal Transplantation, Oregon Health Sciences University, Portland, OR
Renal Transplantation, 151
Shunts, 154

FRANCIS F. BARTONE, MD, FACS
Associate, Pediatric Urology, Geisinger Clinic, Danville, PA
Sutures, 18

LAURENCE S. BASKIN, MD
Assistant Professor, Department of Urology, University of California, San Francisco, San Francisco, CA
Meatal Advancement and Glanuloplasty, 579

STUART B. BAUER, MD, FACS, FAAP
Associate Professor of Surgery (Urology), Harvard Medical School, Senior Associate in Surgery (Urology), Children's Hospital, Boston, MA
Pubovaginal Sling, 281

A. BARRY BELMAN, MD, FAAP, FACS
Professor of Urology and Pediatrics, George Washington University School of Medicine; Chairman, Department of Urology, Children's Hospital, Washington, DC
Varicocele Ligation, 535
Basic Instructions for Hypospadias Repair, 568

ABDELLATIF BENCHEKROUN, MD
Professor of Urology, Head of Urology Department, Rabat-Morocco, Morocco
Ileonipple Conduit, 426

A. BIANCHI, MD, FRCS, FRCS (EDIN)
Consultant Neonatal and Paediatric Surgeon, Royal Manchester Children's Hospital, Manchester, United Kingdom
Microvascular Orchiopexy, 505

DAVID A. BLOOM, MD, FACS, FAAP
Chief, Pediatric Urology, The University of Michigan School of Medicine, Ann Arbor, MI
Meatotomy, 571

GUY A. BOGAERT, MD
Clinical Instructor in Pediatric Urology, University of California, San Francisco, San Francisco, CA
Laparoscopic Methods for Impalpable Testis, 519

VICTOR BRAREN, MD, FACS, FAAP
Associate Clinical Professor of Urology, Assistant Clinical Professor of Pediatrics, Vanderbilt University School of Medicine, Nashville, TN
Suprapubic Cystostomy, 349
Perineal Urethrostomy, 355

WILLIAM A. BROCK, MD, FACS, FAAP
Professor of Urology, Chief, Pediatric Urology, Albert Einstein College of Medicine, New Hyde Park, NY
Pediatric High Ileal Conduit, 392

KEVIN A. BURBIGE, MD, FACS, FAAP
Associate Professor of Urology, College of Physicians and Surgeons, Columbia University, New York, NY
Psoas Hitch Procedure, 239
Bladder Flap Repair, 243
Renal Displacement and Autotransplantation, 245

ANTHONY A. CALDAMONE, MD, FACS, FAAP
Associate Professor of Urology, Brown University School of Medicine, Providence, RI
Excision of the Urachus, 338

BERNARD M. CHURCHILL, MD, FRCS(c), FAAP
Professor of Urology and Chief, Pediatric Urology, University of Toronto and Hospital for Sick Children, Toronto, Ontario
Sigmoid Conduit, 396

LAWRENCE B. COLEN, MD, FACS
Associate Professor of Plastic and Reconstruction Surgery, Eastern Virginia Medical School, Norfolk, VA
Construction of Penis, 666

ARNOLD H. COLODNY, MD, FACS, FAAP
Senior Surgeon and Associate Director, Division of Urology, Children's Hospital, Boston; Clinical Professor of Surgery, Harvard Medical School, Boston, MA
Concealed and Webbed Penis, 609

WILLIAM J. CROMIE, MD, FACS, FAAP
Clinical Professor of Surgery and Pediatrics, Albany Medical College, Albany, NY
Orchiopexy for Abdominal Testis, 511
Laparoscopic Methods for Impalpable Testis, 519

JACOB CUKIER, MD
Professor of Urology, Hospital Necker, Paris, France
Penile and Bulbourethral Strictures, 690

SAKTI DAS, MBBS, FACS, FRCS(c)
Clinical Associate Professor of Urology, University of California, Davis, CA
Lumbotomy Incision, 117

TOM P. V. M. DE JONG, MD
Pediatric Urologist, Pediatric Renal Center, University Children's Hospital, "Het Wilhelmina Kinderziekenhuis," Utrecht, The Netherlands
Lower Midline Extraperitoneal Incision, 266
Lower Abdominal Transverse Incision, 269
Gibson Incision, 271

CHARLES J. DEVINE, JR, MD, FACS
Professor of Urology, Eastern Virginia Medical School; Director, The Devine Center for Genitourinary Reconstruction at Sentara, Norfolk General Hospital, Norfolk, VA
Perimeatal-Based Tube Repair, 587
Concealed and Webbed Penis, 608

JOSEPH D. M. DEVRIES, MD
Associate Professor of Urology and Chief of Pediatric Urology, Department of Urology, University Hospital Nijmegen, St. Radboud, Nijmegen, The Netherlands
Calyceal Diverticulectomy, 188

DAVID A. DIAMOND, MD, FAAP
Associate Professor of Urology and Pediatrics, Director of Pediatric Urology, University of Massachusetts Medical Center, Worcester, MA
Repair of Female Urethra, 671

JOHN W. DUCKETT, MD, FACS, FAAP
Professor of Urology, University of Pennsylvania School of Medicine, Chief of Urology, Philadelphia Children's Hospital, Philadelphia, PA
Cecoileal Reservoir, 418
Meatal Advancement and Glanuloplasty, 578
Transverse Preputial Island Flap, 592

JOSEPH Y. DWOSKIN, MD, FACS, FAAP
Clinical Assistant Professor, State University of New York at Buffalo, Buffalo, NY
Cutaneous Ureterostomy and Pyelostomy, 365
Pediatric Loop Ureterostomy, 369

RICHARD M. EHRLICH, MD, FACS, FAAP
Clinical Professor of Surgery/Urology, University of California, Los Angeles Center for Health Sciences, Los Angeles, CA
Prune Belly Syndrome: Abdominal Repair and Umbilicoplasty, 328

JACK S. ELDER, MD, FACS, FAAP
Associate Professor of Urology and Pediatrics, Case Western Reserve University School of Medicine; Director of Pediatric Urology, Rainbow Babies and Children's Hospital, Cleveland, OH
Repair of Female Urethra, 671
Urethral Diverticulectomy, 678
Excision of Utricular Cyst, 679

BLACKWELL B. EVANS, SR, MD, FAAP*
Sobin Professor of Pediatric Urology, Tulane University School of Medicine, New Orleans, LA
Perimeatal-Based Flap Repair, 582

R. BRUCE FILMER, MB, BS, FACS, FAAP
Associate Professor of Pediatric Urology, Thomas Jefferson University Hospital, Philadelphia, PA; A. I. duPont Institute of the Nemours Foundation, Wilmington, DE
Ileal Bladder Substitution, 477
Ileocecal Bladder Substitution, 479

CASIMIR F. FIRLIT, MD, PhD, FAAP, FACS
Professor of Urology, Northwestern University Medical School; Chief of Pediatric Urology, Children's Memorial Hospital, Chicago, IL
Ileal Ureteral Replacement, 259

---

*Deceased

JOHN P. GEARHART, MD, FACS, FAAP
Director of Pediatric Urology and Associate Professor of Pediatrics, Johns Hopkins University School of Medicine, Baltimore, MD
Vaginal Reconstruction, 659

LOUIS G. GECELTER, MD
Senior Urologist, University of the Witwatersrand, Johannesburg, South Africa
Closure of Rectourethral Fistula, 334

AMILGAR M. GIRON, MD
Associate Professor of Pediatric Urology, Urology Division, Department of Surgery, Hospital das Clinicas, São Paulo, Brazil
Reconstruction for Vesical Exstrophy, 318

KENNETH I. GLASSBERG, MD, FACS, FAAP
Professor of Urology and Director, Division of Pediatric Urology, State University of New York Health Science Center at Brooklyn, Brooklyn, NY
Testis Biopsy, 487
Reduction of Testis Torsion, 527

EDMOND T. GONZALES, JR, MD, FAAP
Professor of Urology, Scott Department of Urology, Baylor College of Medicine; Chief of Pediatric Urology Service, Texas Children's Hospital, Houston, TX
Ileocystoplasty, 443
Microphallus, 605

RICARDO GONZALEZ, MD, FAAP
Professor of Urology, Director of Pediatric Urology, University of Minnesota, Minneapolis, MN
Epispadias Repair, 620

DAVID C. S. GOUGH, FRCS, FRACS, DCH
Consultant Paediatric Urologist, Royal Manchester Children's Hospital, Manchester, England
Repair of Penile and Testicular Injuries, 663

MONEER K. HANNA, MD, FRCS, FACS
Clinical Professor of Urology, New York University Medical Center, New York, NY
Vesicostomy, 359

W. HARDY HENDREN, MD, FAAP, FACS, FRCS, IRE (HON)
Robert E. Gross Professor of Surgery, Harvard Medical School; Chief of Surgery, Children's Hospital, Boston, MA
Ureteroneocystostomy With Tailoring, 224
Female Urethral Construction, 297

TERRY W. HENSLE, MD, FACS, FAAP
Professor of Urology, Director of Pediatric Urology, Columbia Presbyterian Medical Center, New York, NY
Pediatric Heminephrectomy, 167

NORMAN B. HODGSON, MD, FAAP
Clinical Professor of Urology, Medical College of Wisconsin, Wauwatosa, WI
Basic Instructions for Hypospadias Repair, 560
Double-Faced Transverse Island Flap, 595

RUDOLF HOHENFELLNER, MD
Professor of Urology and Chief of Pediatric Urology, Department of Urology, Johannes Gutenberg University School of Medicine, Mainz, Germany
Cecocystoplasty, 458

STUART S. HOWARDS, MD, FACS, FAAP
Professor of Urology, University of Virginia, Charlottesville, VA
Laparoscopic Varicocele Ligation, 537

GERALD H. JORDAN, MD, FACS
Professor of Urology, Eastern Virginia Medical School; Director of Adult Reconstruction, The Devine Center for Genitourinary Reconstruction, Norfolk, VA
Strictures of the Fossa Navicularis, 687

GEORGE W. KAPLAN, MD, MS, FACS, FAAP
Clinical Professor of Surgery and Pediatrics, University of California, San Diego School of Medicine, San Diego, CA
Tube Repair, 597

WILLIAM E. KAPLAN, MD, FAAP
Associate Professor of Urology, Northwestern University School of Medicine; Director, Neurologic Urology, Children's Memorial Hospital, Chicago, IL
Supracostal Incision, 100

EVAN J. KASS, MD, FAAP, FACS
Chief, Division of Pediatric Urology, William Beaumont Hospital, Royal Oak, MI
Ureteroureterostomy, 252
Calycoureterostomy, 254
Ureterolithotomy, 260

ROBERT KAY, MD, FACS, FAAP
Head, Section of Pediatric Urology, The Cleveland Clinic Foundation, Cleveland, OH
Nephrostomy, 142
Ureterostomy, 143
Open Renal Biopsy, 145

PANAYOTIS P. KELALIS, MD, FACS, FAAP
The Anson L. Clark Professor of Pediatric Urology, Mayo Clinic and Mayo Foundation, Rochester, MN and Jacksonville, FL
Surgery of Horseshoe Kidneys, 139

OM P. KHANNA, MD, FACS
Professor and Director, Division of Urology, Department of Surgery, Hahnemann University, Philadelphia, PA
Circumcision, 626

ANTOINE E. KHOURY, MD, FRCSC, FAAP
Assistant Professor, Hospital for Sick Children, Toronto, Ontario
Penile and Bulbourethral Strictures, 691

LOWELL R. KING, MD, FACS, FAAP
Professor of Urology, Head, Section on Pediatric Urology, Duke University Medical Center, Durham, NC
Reconstruction for Vesical Exstrophy, 313
Ureteroileostomy, 387
Ileocecocystoplasty, 466

GEORGE T. KLAUBER, MB, BS, FRCS(C), FACS, FAAP
Professor of Urology and Pediatrics, Tufts University School of Medicine, Boston, MA
Transverse Colostomy and Closure: Loop Ileostomy, 399
Gastrostomy, 400

BARRY A. KOGAN, MD, FACS, FAAP
Associate Professor Urology and Pediatrics, University of California, San Francisco, CA
Splenic Repair, 120
Partial Nephrectomy, 165
Appendectomy, 401
Colocystoplasty and Sigmoidocystoplasty, 451
Meatal Advancement and Glanuloplasty, 580

STANLEY J. KOGAN, MD, FACS, FAAP
Clinical Professor of Urology, New York Medical College; Associate Clinical Professor of Pediatrics, Albert Einstein College of Medicine, Valhalla, NY
Long-Loop Vas Orchiopexy, 496
Vaginoplasty and Clitoriplasty for the Adrenogenital Syndrome, 647

MARTIN A. KOYLE, MD, FACS, FAAP
Associate Professor of Surgery and Chief, Pediatric Urology, The Children's Hospital and University of Colorado, Denver, CO
Excision of Wilms' Tumor, 185

R. LAWRENCE KROOVAND, MD, FACS, FAAP
Professor of Surgery (Pediatric Urology) and Pediatrics; Head, Section on Pediatric, Adolescent, and Reconstructive Urology, The Bowman Gray School of Medicine, Wake Forest University, Winston-Salem, NC
Ureterosigmoidostomy, 435
Basic Instructions for Hypospadias Repair, 559

KENNETH A. KROPP, MD, FACS
Professor of Urology and Pediatrics; Chairman, Department of Urology, Medical College of Ohio, Toledo, OH
Intravesical Urethral Lengthening, 291

GUY W. LEADBETTER, MD, FACS, FAAP
Professor and Chief Emeritus Urology, University of Vermont Medical School, Burlington, VT
Trigonal Tubularization, 284

ELLIOT LEITER, MD, FACS, FRCM
Clinical Professor of Urology, The Mount Sinai School of Medicine, New York, NY
Inguinal Hernia Repair, 523
Preperitoneal Indirect Inguinal Herniorrhaphy, 525

J. KEITH LIGHT, MB, BCH, FCS (SA), FACS
Professor and Chairman, Department of Urology, State University of New York, Syracuse, NY
Insertion of Artificial Sphincter, 294

ANDREW E. MACNEILY, MD, FRCS(C)
Queen's University, Kingston, Ontario, Canada
Supracostal Incision, 100

MAX MAIZELS, MD, FACS, FAAP
Assistant Professor of Urology, The Children's Memorial Hospital and Northwestern Memorial Hospital, Department of Urology, Northwestern University Medical School, Chicago, IL
Pyeloureteroplasty, 133

JAMES MANDELL, MD, FACS, FAAP
Associate Professor of Surgery, Harvard Medical School, Children's Hospital, Boston, MA
Ureteroneocystostomy With Tailoring, 224

FRAY F. MARSHALL, MD, FRCS
Professor of Urology, Director, Division of Adult Urology, The Johns Hopkins Hospital, Baltimore, MD
Simple Nephrectomy, 159
Subcapsular Nephrectomy, 160
Partial Nephrectomy, 164

CHARLOTTE MASSAD, MD
Clinical Assistant Professor, Emory University, Atlanta, GA
Simple Nephrectomy, 159

JACK W. McANINCH, MD, MS, FACS
Professor of Urology, University of California, San Francisco; Chief of Urology, San Francisco General Hospital, San Francisco, CA
Repair of Renal Injuries, 148
Penile and Bulbourethral Strictures, 697

HRAIR-GEORGE J. MESROBIAN, MD
Director of Pediatric Urology, Associate Professor of Surgery and Pediatrics, University of North Carolina School of Medicine, Chapel Hill, NC
Venous Access, 28

DAVID T. MININBERG, MD
Associate Professor of Urology, Director of Pediatric Urology, The New York Hospital, New York, NY
Long-Loop Vas Orchiopexy, 499
Orchiopexy for Abdominal Testis, 511

MICHAEL E. MITCHELL, MD, FACS, FAAP
Professor of Urology and Chief of Pediatric Urology, University of Washington Medical School, Seattle, WA
Cecoileal Reservoir, 416
Colocystoplasty and Sigmoidocystoplasty, 451
Gastrocystoplasty, 473
Gastric Bladder Substitution, 481

PAUL MITROFANOFF, MD
Professor of Pediatric Surgery, Hôpital Charles Nicolle, Centre Hospitalier Universitaire, Rouen, France
Appendicovesicostomy, 424

GEORGE R. NAGAMATSU, MD, FACS
Professor of Urology, New York University School of Medicine, New York, NY
Dorsal Flap Incision, 111

H. NORMAN NOE, MD, FACS, FAAP
Professor of Urology, Chief, Pediatric Urology, University of Tennessee, Memphis; LeBonheur Children's Medical Center, Memphis, TN
Anterior Subcostal Incision, 78
Pediatric Extended Anterior Incision, 80
Anterior Transverse (Chevron) Incision, 82
Excision of Neuroblastoma, 186

ANDREW C. NOVICK, MD, FACS
Chairman, Department of Urology, Cleveland Clinic Foundation, Cleveland, OH
Vena Caval Thrombectomy, 180

JOHN M. PALMER, MD, FACS, FAAP
Professor of Urology and Pediatrics, Chief of Pediatric Urology, University of California, Davis, School of Medicine, Davis, CA
Closure of Female Vesical Neck, 303

HELEN PARKHOUSE, FRCS, FRACS (Urol), FEBU
Consultant Urological Surgeon to Hillingdon Hospital and Mount Vernon Hospital, London, United Kingdom
Cecocystoplasty, 462

THOMAS S. PARROTT, MD, FAAP, FACS
Clinical Associate Professor of Surgery (Urology), Emory University School of Medicine, Atlanta, GA
Nephroureterectomy With Node Dissection, 168
Radical Nephrectomy, 179

GIACOMO PASSERINI-GLAZEL, MD
Professor of Urology, University of Padova School of Medicine, Padova, Italy
Vaginoplasty and Clitoriplasty for the Adrenogenital Syndrome, 647

UMESH B. PATIL, MD, FRCS, FAAP
Professor of Urology, Professor of Pediatrics, SUNY Health Science Center, Syracuse, NY
Penile and Bulbourethral Strictures, 695

ALBERTO PEÑA, MD, FACS
Professor of Surgery, Albert Einstein College of Medicine; Chief Pediatric Surgery, Schneider Children's Hospital, Long Island Jewish Medical Center, New Hyde Park, NY
Closure of Rectourethral fistula, 332

ALAN B. RETIK, MD, FACS, FAAP
Professor of Surgery (Urology), Harvard Medical School; Chief, Division of Urology, Children's Hospital, Boston, MA
Ileal Reservoir, 411
Cecoileal Reservoir, 418

RICHARD C. RINK, MD, FAAP, FACS
Associate Professor of Urology, Chief, Pediatric Urology, James Whitcomb Riley Hospital for Children, Indiana University School of Medicine, Indianapolis, IN
Gastrocystoplasty, 472

RANDALL G. ROWLAND, MD, PhD, FACS
Professor of Urology, Indiana University School of Medicine, Indianapolis, IN
Radical Orchiectomy, 546
Retroperitoneal Lymph Node Dissection, 547

H. GIL RUSHTON, MD, FAAP
Associate Professor Urology and Pediatrics, George Washington University School of Medicine; Vice Chairman, Department of Urology, Children's National Medical Center, Washington, DC
Simple Orchiectomy, 539
Laparoscopic Orchiectomy, 540

ROELOF J. SCHOLTMEIJER, MD
Former Professor of Pediatric Urology, Erasmus University/Sophia Children's Hospital, Rotterdam, The Netherlands
Correction of Hydrocele, 530

CLAUDE C. SCHULMAN, MD, PhD
Professor of Urology, Erasme Hospital, Brussels, Belgium
Operations for Ureteral Duplication, 231
Repair of Ureterocele, 235

AHMED SHAFIK, MB, BCh, DS, MCh, MD
Professor and Chairman, Department of Surgery and Research, Cairo University Faculty of Medicine, Cairo, Egypt
Free Tube Graft and Partial Island Flap, 602

ALLAN M. SHANBERG, MD, FACS, FAAP
Clinical Professor of Surgery (Urology), University of California, Irvine, Irvine, CA
Radical Cystectomy for Rhabdomyosarcoma, 343

STEPHEN R. SHAPIRO, MD, FAAP, FACS
Pediatric Urologist, Sacramento, CA
Open Renal Biopsy, 145
Two-Stage Orchiopexy, 502

E. DURHAM SMITH, MD, MS, FRACS, FACS
Honorary Senior Surgeon, Royal Children's Hospital, Melbourne, Australia
Basic Instructions for Hypospadias Repair, 561

HOWARD McC. SNYDER, III, MD
Professor of Urology, University of Pennsylvania, Children's Hospital of Philadelphia, Philadelphia, PA
Thoracoabdominal Incision, 107

HARRY M. SPENCE, MD, FACS
Clinical Professor of Urology and Former Chairman of Division, University of Texas Southwestern Medical School at Dallas, Dallas, TX
Midline Transperitoneal Incision, 84
Coronal Repair, 574

F. DOUGLAS STEPHENS, MB, MS, FRACS, FAAP (HON)
Professor (Emeritus) of Surgery and Urology, Northwestern University Medical School, Chicago, IL; Senior Honorary Research Fellow, Royal Children's Hospital Research Foundation, Melbourne, Victoria, Australia
Long-Loop Vas Orchiopexy, 498

EMIL A. TANAGHO, MD, MBS, CHB, MCH, FACS
Professor and Chairman, Department of Urology, University of California School of Medicine, San Francisco, CA
Vesical Neck Tubularization, 288

RICHARD TURNER-WARWICK, CBC, BSC, MCH, DM (OXON), DSC (HON), FRCP, FRCS, FRCOG, FACS, FRACS (HON)
Emeritus Surgeon, The Middlesex Hospital and St. Peter's Group Hospitals, London, United Kingdom
Mobilization of the Omentum, 275

JAN D. VAN GOOL, MD, PHD
Pediatric Nephrologist, Pediatric Renal Center, University Children's Hospital, "Het Wilhelmina Kinderziekenhuis," Utrecht, The Netherlands
Lower Midline Extraperitoneal Incision, 266
Lower Abdominal Transverse Incision, 269
Gibson Incision, 271

E. DARRACOTT VAUGHAN, JR, MD, FACS
James J. Colt Professor of Urology, The New York Hospital-Cornell Medical Center, New York, NY
Surgical Approaches to the Adrenal, 197

JONATHAN S. VORDERMARK, II, MD, FACS, FAAP
Associate Professor of Urology and Pediatrics, Texas Tech University, Lubbock, TX
Penile and Bulbourethral Strictures, 688

JEFFREY WACKSMAN, MD, FACS, FAAP
Assistant Professor of Clinical Surgery, University of Cincinnati College of Medicine, Children's Hospital Medical Center, Cincinnati, OH
Retropubic Y-V Plasty, 298

R. DIXON WALKER, III, MD, FACS, FAAP
Professor of Surgery and Pediatrics, University of Florida College of Medicine, Gainesville, FL
Penoscrotal Transposition, 632
Penile Curvature, 634

GEORGE D. WEBSTER, MB, FRCS
Professor of Urology, Duke University Medical Center, Durham, NC
Urethral Strictures: General Considerations, 682
Bulbomembranous Urethral Strictures, 699

SIR DAVID INNES WILLIAMS, KBE, MD, MCHIR, FRCS, FACS (HON)
Consulting Urological Surgeon, The Hospital for Sick Children, London, United Kingdom
Surgery of Horseshoe Kidneys, 139

HOWARD N. WINFIELD, MD, FACS, FRCS(C)
Associate Professor of Urology, University of Iowa College of Medicine, Iowa City, IA
Laparoscopic Varicocele Ligation, 537

JOHN R. WOODARD, MD, FACS, FAAP
Clinical Professor of Surgery (Urology), Director of Pediatric Urology, Emory University School of Medicine, Atlanta, GA
Inguinal Orchiopexy, 495
Two-Stage Orchiopexy, 501

MARK ZAONTZ, MD, FACS, FAAP
Associate Professor of Urology, Robert Wood Johnson Medical School at Camden; Head, Section of Pediatric Urology, Cooper Hospital/University Medical Center, Camden, NJ
Ureteroneocystostomy, 216

Preface

Fewer than 500 urologists worldwide limit their practice to children. However, most other urologists perform some pediatric operations, and an appreciable number cite pediatric urology as a field of special interest. A source of surgical instructions is not currently at hand either for the simpler pediatric procedures performed by the generalist or for the more complicated ones by the subspecialist. Because of the preponderance of the 1989 *Atlas of Urologic Surgery*, which served as a guide for adult operations, it seemed logical to develop a work focusing on the pediatric aspects of urologic surgery.

Many of the procedures and precautions described in this volume were learned while the author was Chief of Urology at the Children's Hospital of San Francisco and San Francisco General Hospital, and many have come from publications, presentations, and discussions with colleagues in the Urology Section of the American Academy of Pediatrics (AAP) and the Society for Pediatric Urology (SPU). The chapters were selected to include all of the common procedures plus many of the new techniques coming into use in children's centers. Each is presented in a step-by-step manner, with an illustration drawn as viewed at the table by a surgically oriented illustrator, Paul H. Stempen. The result is that each operative step has both an illustration and straightforward directions on what to do as well as what not to do.

A preliminary section explains the structural and functional differences between adults and children, with the special problems associated with fluid balance, anesthesia, and intraoperative care. Another describes the special techniques involved in operating on neonates and infants and the problems of postoperative care. The remainder of the volume is divided into sections for each organ, each containing detailed illustrations accompanied by a description of the operation, extending from procedures for the kidney to those for the penis. Most of the new pediatric operations are included, and, in addition, much of the relevant material from our 1989 *Atlas* has been appropriately adapted.

The authority of the book is guaranteed by the inclusion of commentaries for each operation written by prominent pediatric urologists selected from the membership of the SPU and the Urology Section of the AAP. These commentators have reviewed and corrected the text and illustrations, verified the accuracy of the description, and written a critique from the perspective of their own experience.

Although the descriptions of operations in this volume are as accurate as possible, the surgeon cannot put the book on a Mayo stand at the operating table and just follow directions. Pediatric surgery is demanding. It requires special training and special skills, both because of the complexity of the operations and because of the size and delicacy of the tissues in children. For genital operations in particular, training must be gained under the guidance of an accomplished pediatric urologist.

The book should be especially useful for the experienced subspecialist confronted with an operation done infrequently, for the young urologist in training, and for the other urologists who are interested in expanding their pediatric repertoire with new procedures and with new insights into older ones.

FRANK HINMAN, JR
February 15, 1994

Acknowledgments

The author and illustrator appreciate the cooperation of the members of the Department of Urology at the University of California, San Francisco, under Chairman Emil A. Tanagho. They put up with us as we observed their operations and quizzed them on their techniques, especially Dr. Barry A. Kogan and his residents and fellows in the Pediatric Urology group. We also acknowledge the great help from the over 100 pediatric urologists who took the time to review the text and figures of the many chapters and who made important corrections and comments. Without their collaboration, the atlas would have been much less authoritative.

The author composed the volume on his word processor, but thanks are due to Carole Beebe, who transcribed the commentaries and formatted the bibliography, and to the staff at W.B. Saunders Company for their helpful collaboration.

Contents

SECTION 1

Preparation for Pediatric Operations

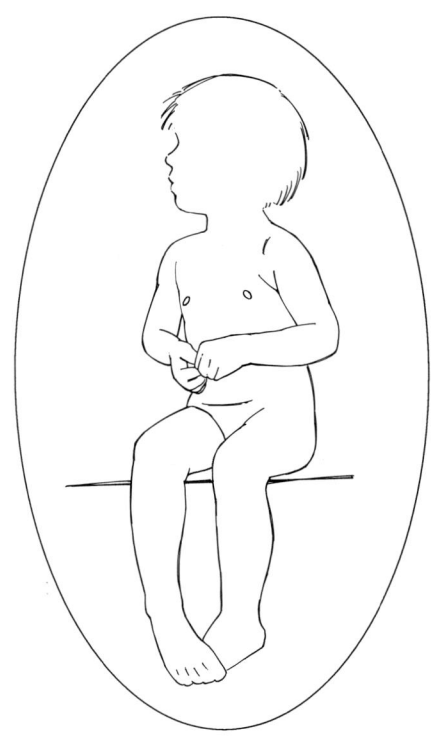

CHAPTER 1

Preoperative Evaluation

The infant is best served if the responsible urologist rather than a resident takes the history and performs the physical examination, which are essential to establish rapport.

For the child who is well, few tests are needed before an operation other than complete blood tests and urinalysis. These may be done within a month of the procedure. An exception is the black child, who needs a sickle cell test.

For the chronically ill child, often with marginal renal function, obtain consultations to look for immunologic or hematologic abnormalities secondary to the disease or to the treatment of it. Correct electrolyte imbalance, especially hyperkalemia (greater than 7 mmol/L) or uncompensated metabolic acidosis (capillary blood pH level less than 7.30) with oral solutions if possible, because intravenous administration is harder to control. Correct any defects in coagulation. Restore blood volume with donor-designated blood, usually from the parents. Blood is replaced with oral sodium chloride unless there is also metabolic acidosis, in which case bicarbonate (Pedialyte) is added. Look for defects in coagulation, detected by platelet count, bleeding time, prothrombin time, and partial thromboplastin time. Check the hemoglobin level, realizing that neonates have a lower normal hemoglobin level. Restore blood volume and give packed cells to obtain a hemoglobin level of 13 or 14 g/dl, although 10 g/dl has been considered a safe lower level for anesthesia. Be sure the protein level is up to 5 g/dl; provide tube feedings if needed to bring the child into positive nitrogen balance. Give supplemental vitamins, especially vitamin C.

Children with reduced renal function may be admitted to the hospital to allow evaluation. In the hospital, the intake and output measurement may be monitored and abnormalities in serum electrolytes corrected.

Collection of urine specimens can be a problem. Midstream samples, which can be obtained from cooperative older children, are best. Bag specimens are less reliable but necessary from infants. After washing and drying the genitalia, apply tincture of benzoin compound to the area. Cut out an opening just large enough to surround the male genitalia and as small as practicable for the female in the adhesive side of the disposable drainage bag and apply it to the perineum. Leave it in place only long enough to collect one voiding and immediately empty it into a sterile container. If culture is not important, wipe the perineum and have the child void in a clean bedpan. From indwelling catheters, clamp the tubing, gingerly wipe the wall with an alcohol sponge, and aspirate a sample with a syringe and fine needle. Avoid disconnection of the sterile pathway.

EVALUATION BY THE ANESTHETIST

Inform the anesthetist about the projected procedure, and transmit any information about the child's status that was gained from your history and physical examination (especially concerning drugs that may cause intraoperative hypotension) and from previous operations (especially hyperpyrexia, drug reactions, and bleeding problems). Do not hesitate to cancel an elective operation if the anesthetist believes that the child has an upper respiratory infection.

Be certain that the child arrives with an empty stomach, having taken nothing by mouth for 2 hours before arrival. Infants will become dehydrated, so they should be scheduled for operation early in the day even when they have been awakened for a 2 AM feeding; otherwise they should have clear liquids to within 2 hours of the operation.

For the older adolescent, if blood loss is anticipated, arrange blood storage prior to the operation to reduce the risk of viral acquisition.

NUTRITION

Enteral Nutrition. Be certain that weight gain has been normal (Table 1–1). Check serum albumin level, which is 2.5 g/dl in infants and 3.5 g/dl in older children. For infants, oral feedings may be started soon after operation, using standard infant formulas, which contain 50 percent fat and 10 to 20 percent

Table 1–1. Normal Weight Gain

Age	Growth Rate, g/kg
8–28 d	10
1–2 mo	6.5
3–4 mo	3.5
1 y	1

Data from Luck SR: Preoperative evaluation and preparation. In: Raffensperger JG (Ed): *Swenson's Pediatric Surgery*, 5th ed. Norwalk, CT, Appleton and Lange, 1990, p. 7.

protein, given at a concentration of 0.67 calories per mililiter. This level may be doubled in malnourished infants and should be supplemented with vitamins and minerals.

Parenteral Nutrition. Chronically ill children coming to operation require restoration of their nutritional deficit to avoid poor wound healing, immunologic deficiencies (total lymphocyte count should be above 1500 mm^3), and organ malfunction. Premature infants have less nutritional reserve.

Total parenteral nutrition is feasible by infusion of glucose, amino acids, emulsified fat, minerals, vita-

mins, and trace elements. For neonates, special formulas are needed that mimic breast milk. Protein and calorie requirements are listed in Table 1–2.

Table 1–2. Protein and Calorie Requirements

Age	Protein, g/kg/d		Calories per kilogram per day	
	Enteral	Parenteral	Enteral	Parenteral
Premature	4–6	2.5–3.5	150	85–130
Neonate	1.8–2.0	2.5	100–110	100–110
1 y	1.5	1.5–2.0	80–135	80–135
Adolescent	0.85–1.0	1.0–1.5	50–60	50–60

CHAPTER 2

Preparation for Surgery

BOWEL PREPARATION

On the day before surgery, admit the child to the hospital and check the electrolytes and determine the weight. Order a clear liquid diet. Start an intravenous (IV) infusion of metoclopramide at noon. The purpose of this drug is to tighten the gastroesophageal junction and stimulate peristalsis, thereby having an antiemetic effect. (This is in contrast with prochlorperazine maleate, which acts centrally to achieve an antiemetic effect but peripherally retards the activity of the entire bowel.) After 30 minutes, insert a nasogastric tube using topical anesthetics. (A nasogastric tube is necessary in children because they cannot be relied on to drink the required amount of fluid.) Begin continuous instillation of a balanced bowel preparation solution (GoLYTELY) starting at a rate of 500 ml/h and increasing to a rate of 1000 ml/h to give a total amount of between 4 and 6 L, depending on the age of the child, the tolerance to the infusion, and the clearness of the return. Electrolytes and body weight will be little affected because GoLYTELY is not exchanged. However, it is best to recheck the electrolytes at 6 PM. It is probably worthwhile to give 1 g each of neomycin and erythromycin base at 1 PM, 2 PM, and 2 AM. Stop oral intake 4 hours before the operation.

For children with *neurogenic bladder* undergoing surgery on the bowel, a different method of preparation is required because of the accompanying impaired bowel motility. Three days before surgery, have the child start a regular liquid diet and undergo an enema in the evening. Two days preoperatively, have the diet changed to clear liquids and repeat the enema. The day before surgery, have the child admitted to the hospital at noon and have an enema given every 2 to 3 hours, as often as needed to obtain a clear return before bedtime. Order the same antibiotic regimen, instillation of balanced bowel preparation solution through the nasogastric tube, and checking of electrolytes before and after the instillation as for children without a neurogenic disorder.

VASCULAR ACCESS

The anesthetist will obtain vascular access by percutaneous methods in 90 percent of cases using local or topical anesthetic. Femoral vein catheterization carries risk of infection. Percutaneous subclavian vein puncture done by the interventional radiologist does not require general anesthesia but does carry a slight risk of pneumothorax or arterial puncture. The pediatric urologist should have knowledge of the methods of vein cannulation described in Chapter 6, which occasionally may be required.

PREOPERATIVE MEDICATION

Sedation is essential for any child separated from parents and entering a strange environment, the exception being infants younger than 9 months of age. It is the child between 9 months and 4 years of age that is the most difficult to prepare for anesthesia. For children older than 4 years, make a judgment on the need for premedication on the initial visit. Give the dose 45 to 60 minutes before the child is called, and atropine may be combined with the narcotic in the same syringe. It is essential that oxygen, suction equipment, and drugs and equipment for airway support and resuscitation be available. For monitoring, the pulse oximeter is ideal. Now that most operations are done without admission to the hospital, avoid a needle stick by having the anesthetist give the atropine IV at the time of induction. Drugs in current use at University of California, San Francisco are listed in Table 2–1. What narcotic agent is best has not been determined. Morphine is an effective tranquilizer but may promote more nausea and vomiting. Pentazocine may be a good substitute. Because needles hurt and rectal drugs are not dependable, drugs may be administered orally. Meperidine (Demerol) 10 mg with scopolamine hydrobromide 0.375 mg in syrup has been shown to be as effective as a comparable parenteral dose (Root and Loveland, 1973). An alternative is diazepam 0.2 mg and scopolamine 0.25 mg per pound of body weight. Dosages are listed in Table 2–2.

Table 2–1. Pediatric Premedication in Current Use at University of California, San Francisco

Agent*	Oral	Intranasal	Rectal	IM
Midazolam maleate	yes	yes	yes	yes
Ketamine	yes		yes	
Combination	yes			
Meperidine hydrochloride				
Benzodiazepine				
Atropine				
Sufentanil		yes		
Methohexital			yes	yes

*The dose of the drug will vary with the dosage form.

Table 2–2. Dosages for Preoperative Medication

Agent	Dosage, mg/kg
Morphine	0.1–0.2
Meperidine hydrochloride	1–1.5
Pentobarbital	2–3 IM or orally
	5 rectally
Pentazocine	1
Diazepam	0.4
Chlorpromazine	0.5
Atropine	0.03 (0.6 maximum)

Data from Luck SR: Preoperative evaluation and preparation. In: Raffensperger JG (Ed). *Swenson's Pediatric Surgery*, 5th ed. Norwalk, CT, Appleton and Lange, 1990, p. 7.

The anesthetist needs vascular access but in children up to 9 years of age usually will induce anesthesia with an inhalation agent (nitrous oxide plus halothane). A topical anesthetic often will be used in addition for placement of the IV needle.

Fluids must be limited before operation. A schedule is shown in Table 2–3.

PERIOPERATIVE INFECTION

The following precepts are accepted:

1. Favor outpatient operations to reduce the chance for cross-infection.
2. Clear infections if present preoperatively.
3. Have the child bathe immediately before operation.
4. Prepare the bowel thoroughly.
5. Provide antibacterial prophylaxis for children undergoing major surgery.

Prophylaxis. Wound infections are placed into three categories depending on the type of wound from which they originate: (1) from clean, uncontaminated wounds; (2) from clean/contaminated wounds; and (3) from frankly contaminated wounds. Postoperative infections are more common in neonates in all three categories, perhaps related to poor immunity and the presence of the contaminated umbilicus. Other factors are undernutrition, diabetes, obesity, and hypoxemia.

For prophylaxis in the absence of bacteriuria or tissue infection, antibacterial agents in sufficient con-

Table 2–3. Preanesthetic Orders

	Age		
	Under 6 mo	*7 mo to 12 y*	*Over 12 y*
Start clear liquids*	4 h before surgery	Midnight or 8 h before surgery	Midnight or 8 h before surgery
Nothing by mouth	2 h before surgery	2 h before surgery	2 h before surgery

*Clear liquids include breast milk (not formula) and clear, filtered juices. If there is doubt about directions, recommend water only.

centrations need to be present in the body only during the actual operation when the wound might become contaminated and during the immediate postoperative period before any introduced bacteria can become established. For *clean* cases, prophylactic antibiotics are unnecessary; the incidence of infection is too low. The exception would be during insertion of prosthetic devices. Their presence in *clean/contaminated* cases at most is needed only at the time of operation and for the subsequent 3 or 4 hours. In *contaminated* cases, antibiotics assume a therapeutic rather than a prophylactic role and are selected by the type of bacteria expected. For abdominal contamination, clindamycin plus gentamicin are effective. One program is to give a dose of a broad-spectrum antibiotic, such as gentamicin, intramuscularly (IM) 1 hour preoperatively and repeat it two times at 8-hour intervals. If an indwelling catheter has been in place, add ampicillin IV to cover any enterococcus species. Trimethoprim with sulfamethoxazole may be given for several days following removal of a catheter. Note that except in certain cases, the value of perioperative antibiotics has yet to be proved.

Specific prophylactic situations include (1) placement of balloon catheter or cystoscopy (give a cephalosporin [cephalexin] 25 mg/kg IV); (2) ventriculoperitoneal shunt or valvular heart disease (for non–urinary tract-related operations give vancomycin IV immediately before surgery and for 2 days following and add gentomycin if the urinary tract is involved); and (3) operations involving bowel (prepare the bowel and give ampicillin, gentamicin, and metronidazole intraoperatively and continue for 3 to 5 days).

PRELIMINARIES TO OPERATION

With present instrumental and imaging techniques, it is almost always possible to define the problem that needs to be corrected before starting any pediatric operation and to plan the appropriate procedure accordingly. Going over the steps of the operation in your mind the night before will guarantee a more precise and quicker procedure. Review the operation from a book or journal and visualize the details of the procedure in your mind's eye, moving step by step, the morning of surgery. This will make the actual operation flow much more easily and accurately.

OUTPATIENT SURGERY

Operations in a "come-and-go" setting are becoming necessities in pediatric urology. Children are the perfect candidates for outpatient surgery. Currently, as many as 85 percent of all pediatric surgical procedures are being performed on an outpatient basis. The advantages are reduced psychologic upset, including minimal disruption of family life; decreased hospital-acquired infection; and potential cost savings. Much depends on the ability of parents or guardians to understand and follow the perioperative instructions and on the procedure itself. Procedures such as inguinal and scrotal surgery, many endoscopic procedures, and distal hypospadias repairs may be done with the expectation of few postoperative hospitalizations and very few complications, either surgical or anesthetic. Prior to the day of surgery, arrange for the child and parents to be interviewed by the anesthetist and, if feasible, by a member of the house staff. Admit the patient to the same-day surgery unit at least 1 hour before the operation. After the operation and the necessary stay in the postanesthesia care unit, the pediatric patient can be transferred to a less supervised room to recover fully before discharge to parents. A subsequent telephone call to them from the unit nurse allows immediate follow-up.

After stopping by the same-day surgery waiting room to reassure the parents, go to the operating room before the child is put to sleep (and there provide more reassurance). Greet the scrub and circulating nurses by name; things will then run much more smoothly. However, avoid noisy talk that disturbs the child. Supervise each step of anesthetization and preparation for which you are responsible. Put the radiographs and scans on the view boxes and check them to refresh your memory. They will help determine the site and level of the incision and will be available for review of the findings during the operation.

PREOPERATIVE CHECKLIST

Table 2–4 is a checklist for the surgeon to review before operation.

LATEX ALLERGY

Children with ventriculoperitoneal shunts, especially those with multiple operations, are at risk for "latex allergy." Therefore, equipment and gloves at surgery that are free of latex should be used (lists are available in the operating room). To avoid prob-

Table 2–4. Preoperative Checklist

Preparation of the child for the operation
Informed consent and permit
Banked blood
Skin preparation
Bowel preparation
Preanesthetic medication
Blood transfusion
Hydration
Medications
Antibiotics

lems preoperatively, administer an H_1 blocker such as diphenhydramine and an H_2 blocker such as ranitidine.

It is a good idea, at the time of the urodynamic study, to ask the nurse to blow up a latex glove and let the child play with it. If the child starts sneezing, suspect latex allergy and arrange for preoperative testing (radioallergosorbent test [RAST] or skin test).

Suspicion of latex allergy should be considered if approximately 30 minutes after the incision is made, the child suddenly starts wheezing and shows a decrease in lung compliance and therefore difficulty in ventilation accompanied by a significant drop in oxygen saturation. Recognition and supportive therapy at this time can be life saving. Give boluses of isotonic saline (5 to 10 ml/kg) with epinephrine (0.5 to 1 μg/kg). In addition, give a corticoid with diphenhydramine and ranitidine. If the patient does not immediately recover, stop the operation.

PROTECTION OF THE CHILD DURING SURGERY

The appropriate position is shown in the atlas for each operation, but the details for protection of the child will vary. Be thorough in placing foam rubber padding over all bony prominences to avoid damage to adjacent nerve trunks, especially to the ulnar nerve. When the child is in the lateral position, place a pad in the axilla to protect the brachial plexus. Avoid positions that put strains on muscles, ligaments, and joints.

SECTION 2

Operating on Neonates, Infants, and Children

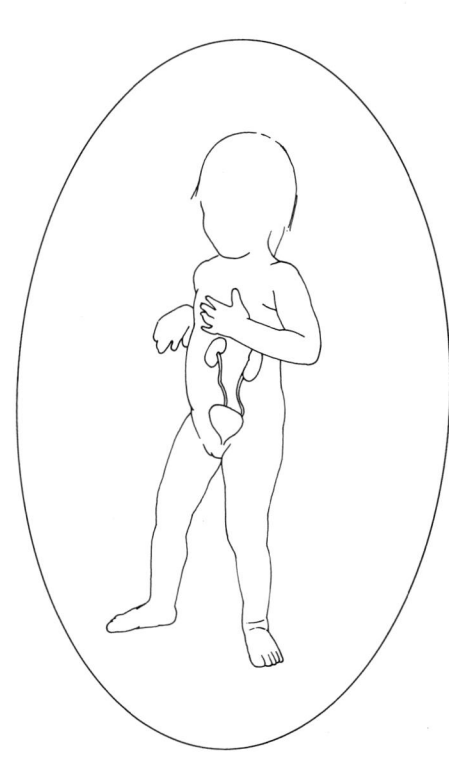

CHAPTER 3

Anesthesia

Accompany the child to the operating room, and brief the anesthetist and operating team on the procedure. Reassure the child and avoid noisy talk. The child may be given a choice between mask or needle, but the surgeon must stand by, both for reassurance and restraint.

The surgeon also must be ready to help if difficulty is encountered in placing an airway or giving drugs to control laryngospasm. Consider placement of a nasogastric tube to prevent vomiting and consequent aspiration postoperatively.

Monitoring of the *cardiovascular system* is achieved by observing vital signs and observing pulse rate, blood pressure, electrocardiogram (EKG), and oxygen saturation. An arm cuff usually is satisfactory for following the blood pressure. For difficult cases, direct arterial cannulation not only is more precise but also allows blood sampling; alternatively, a Doppler ultrasound flowmeter provides direct measurements. It also may be necessary to monitor end-expiratory carbon dioxide (CO_2). A precordial stethoscope allows the heart and breath sounds to be followed.

Body temperature is followed via a rectal (or esophageal) probe. This is important because temperature regulation (especially in neonates) has yet to mature, and the disproportion of surface area to body mass exaggerates surface losses ten times more than in adults. Body temperature will be lowered by radiation and conduction and should be controlled by a warming blanket with a thermostat. Because of the risk of burn, the infant must be separated from the blanket by several layers of sheet.

SKIN PREPARATION

In infants, skin preparation and draping are particularly important. Make the skin prep brief, use warmed solutions, and avoid agents that evaporate on the skin or run under the body. Povidone-iodine applied as a scrub with stick sponges is preferable to soap and water.

Adhesive drapes form a barrier to bacteria and heat. Cover the areas adjacent to the site of the incision with sterile dry towels, and keep them in place with small clips. Try to keep the towels dry. Nonabsorbent, plastic stick-on drapes may reduce contamination but foster bacterial proliferation under them unless porous to vapor. Fold the covering drape on itself to form a lateral pocket to hold instruments.

It is advisable to have an infrared lamp focused on the child during the interval between placement on the table and application of the drapes. For long operations, warm the intravenous (IV) fluids to body temperature. Apply a small grounding plate to minimize heat loss. Wipe your gloves to remove cornstarch that will react in the peritoneum.

FLUID REPLACEMENT

Blood volume must be normal before operation. The blood lost at delivery requires replacement, as does any fluid deficit. A neonate tolerates mild dehydration better than fluid overload because of limitations on water and salt excretion. Look for dry mouth, flabby skin, and some depression of the fontanelles, and replace the loss with 0.25 normal saline containing some potassium. Feed the neonate 4 hours preoperatively, and give oral fluids 2 hours before operation.

Fluids and Electrolytes. Fluid losses increase during surgery because of the warming pad and lights, requiring an infusion of 3 to 4 mg/kg of 0.25 normal saline. Lactated Ringer's solution will replace the third-space losses incurred by the surgery. The state of hydration can be monitored by changes in the blood pressure, although for difficult cases, a central venous pressure (CVP) line is needed.

During surgery, monitor the circulation by blood pressure cuff and central venous and arterial catheters, EKG, a stethoscope on the chest, and a recording thermometer. Ventilation is followed by the continuous measurement of end-expiratory CO_2 and the oxygen saturation of hemoglobin. Catching blood from the wound in a small trap, soaking the sponges, and measuring hemoglobin in the wash allows the following of small losses of blood. Replace with packed red blood cells when a loss of more than 20 percent of blood volume occurs in the neonate whose hematocrit is below 35 percent. If the loss is below 10 percent, use lactated Ringer's solution and use combinations between these levels.

The anesthetist will provide sufficient fluid to replace insensible fluid loss and that lost at the operative site, giving lactated Ringer's solution in 5 percent dextrose in water at a rate of 10 ml/kg/h. You can assist the anesthetist in monitoring blood loss and can advocate replacing it with whole blood or packed cells after you believe 10 percent of the blood volume is lost. It is necessary that the urinary output, serum electrolytes, blood glucose, and hematocrit levels are monitored.

BLOOD SUGAR

Watch for hypoglycemia, a blood sugar level below 45 mg/dl. Supply 3 to 4 ml/h of 10 percent dextrose, but do not allow the level to get above approximately 130 mg/dl for fear of intraventricular bleeding and dehydration-hyponatremia from the resulting diuresis.

BODY TEMPERATURE

Body temperature must be maintained constantly at a normal level by transporting the neonate in incubators, maintenance of a warm operating room, placing the neonate on a warming pad under warming lights, and administering warmed fluids; a newborn is very susceptible to changes in ambient temperature. With cold, the metabolic rate rises, and more oxygen is used. The hypoxia resulting from reduced perfusion of the tissues and increased resistance to flow secondary to the increased viscosity and peripheral vasoconstriction induces metabolic acidosis. Furthermore, the reduced temperature interferes with enzyme systems that metabolize drugs.

LOCAL ANESTHESIA

Anesthesia with lidocaine hydrochloride (Xylocaine) is achieved in 5 minutes and will last from 1½ to 2½ hours. Do not use more than 30 ml of a 1 percent solution, without epinephrine, through a 27-gauge needle as a regional block and as a subcutaneous anesthesia. In children, reduce the amount proportionately. For ilioinguinal and penile block and for caudal block, use 0.5 to 1 ml/kg of 0.25 percent bupivacaine (Marcaine) solution. Suggested maximum doses (with and without epinephrine) are as follows: procaine (Novocain), 14 to 18 mg/kg; lidocaine, 7 to 9 mg/kg; and bupivacaine, 2 to 3 mg/kg. Short-beveled needles are less apt to injure nerves and provide more precise localization of the agent. When walking a needle off bone, place the bevel toward the edge of the bone. The addition of epinephrine 1:200,000 decreases local blood flow and the rate of absorption of the agent, with a resulting prolongation of anesthesia and a 25 percent reduction in blood levels. However, epinephrine can produce systemic side effects and will potentiate infection. Great care must be used when injecting bupivacaine; entry into the venous system may cause irreversible cardiomyopathy with asystole, a sequel that is not dose related. Treat a toxic reaction to a local anesthetic by starting oxygen administra-

tion. Give barbiturates or benzodiazepines IV (eg, diazepam 5 to 10 mg as the initial dose). Make provisions for positive-pressure ventilation (mask or endotracheal tube) whenever large doses of local anesthetics are used.

Even if the child is given a general anesthetic, blocking the site at the end of the procedure with the long-acting agent, bupivacaine, can reduce postoperative pain; this is especially useful when the child is not kept in the hospital. Alternatively, caudal block with 0.5 to 1.0 ml/kg of 0.25 percent bupivacaine given just before making the incision will continue to provide good analgesia to a child after the return home (note precautions described previously). The block affects the sensory nerves more than the motor ones, although loss of motor function can be disturbing to older children. Check motor function before discharge, and alert the parents to any residuum. Drain the bladder; urinary retention may be a problem. Remember that droperidol intraoperatively can decrease nausea and vomiting in children who receive local anesthesia.

GENERAL ANESTHESIA

Premedication. Because infants and children experience greater vagal activity than older children and adults, resulting in hypotension, bradycardia, and laryngospasm, atropine always must be given. For infants, who rarely can cooperate, give a heavy dose of sedative; less is needed in older children who can understand what is going on.

Nasogastric Tube. Because children swallow air when crying, placing a small nasogastric tube (orally in neonates because they breathe exclusively through the nose) that can be aspirated periodically by a nurse prevents gastric distention and can be removed at the end of the procedure unless the operation involved the gastrointestinal tract.

Anesthetic Agent. Whether an inhalation agent such as halothane or one given IV is used depends in part on the preference of the child. Most children 9 to 10 years of age prefer IV induction; for younger children, inhalation of nitrous oxide and halothane without a face mask usually is best. Endotracheal intubation is not necessary in cases that do not require muscular relaxation if the laryngeal mask airway (LMA) is used. The LMA is a combination mask and airway with a conventional silicone tracheal tube that has been cut off diagonally to remove the cuff and an inflatable cuff in the shape of a pediatric face mask attached to the distal end. The anatomic arrangement of the upper airway is quite different, especially in neonates, and the chance of regurgitation is greater than in older children, making tracheal intubation worthwhile, even for brief procedures. It may well be performed before the neonate is anesthetized, because unknown anomalies may be present and the passage is protected at the time by the reflexes associated with normal breathing. The LMA provides a fall-back position should intubation be impossible.

Oxygen Requirements. The requirements for an infant are twice those of an adult, and oxygen is depleted rapidly because of small functional residual capacity and high cardiac output. Even brief periods of apnea or obstruction are harmful. In premature infants having a history of periodic breathing, apnea can be a special problem postoperatively; these infants must be monitored closely the day after surgery. In addition, they are liable to aspiration, infection, and hypothermia.

Blood Sugar. Watch for hypoglycemia at a blood sugar level below 45 mg/dl. Supply 10 percent dextrose at 3 to 4 ml/h but do not allow the blood sugar level to rise above approximately 130 mg/dl for fear of intraventricular bleeding and dehydration-hyponatremia from the resulting diuresis.

MONITORING

Anesthetic deaths in infants result from airway obstruction or cardiovascular depression. Operations under general anesthesia are better done before 6 months of age, or at least before 1 year, because the infant's separation from parents is easier (the nurse is a substitute parent). Also, the infant is less likely to find anesthetic agents objectionable. The disadvantages to anesthesia in infants are that (1) apnea and bradycardia are the usual responses to great physical stress, (2) diaphragmatic breathing is easily compromised, (3) breath control is immature, (4) functional reserve capacity is decreased with less reserve on induction, and (5) increased oxygen concentration is required. Gastroesophageal reflux is not common if the infant has had nothing by mouth for the previous 2 hours, but if abdominal distention is present, regurgitation and aspiration of gastric contents will occur. However, there are psychologic reasons for not deferring operations after 6 months of age: by that age, the child experiences anxiety and is unable to understand the reasons for it; separation from the parents is stressful; and regression is common after discharge.

Careful monitoring of body temperature, EKG, blood pressure, and blood loss is essential. CVP may be added. For major cases, monitoring must be provided for (1) heart rate, (2) EKG, (3) blood pressure (Doppler meter), (4) CVP (indwelling lines), (5) filling pressure, (6) pulse oximeter, and (7) PO_2. Heat loss is reduced by the use of sterile adhesive drapes, radiant heat, heated fluids, warmed anesthetic agents, head coverings, and elevated room temperature (*eg*, 26.6°C for neonates; 25.5°C for children 6 months of age, and 24.4°C for those 6 months to 6 years).

Malignant hyperthermia is a serious complication and may be suggested by change in blood gases and by tachypnea or paralysis, dark blood in the wound, and cardiac arrhythmias. It must be treated immediately (Table 3–1). Because it will not be known which agent may have precipitated it, stop all anesthetic agents and rapidly terminate the procedure.

Hyperventilate the child with 100 percent oxygen at a rate three to five times normal to rid the body of excess CO_2, and give sodium bicarbonate for the acidosis and hyperkalemia (Britt, 1985). Start diuretics and insert a catheter to monitor the urine color and volume. Give dantrolene 1 to 10 mg/kg IV at a rate of 1 mg/kg/min, and repeat the dose in 15 minutes if the response is not adequate. Place the child in an ice pack. Consider cardiopulmonary bypass with heat exchange (Ryan, 1986). Give hypertonic glucose solution for hypoglycemia.

Monitoring blood loss is discussed in Chapter 4.

Table 3–1. Checklist for Malignant Hyperthermia

Action	Dosage or Other Instructions
Remove triggering agent	
Hyperventilate with 100 percent O₂	O₂ requirement 3–5 times normal
Administer bicarbonate	
Administer dantrolene	1–10 mg/kg at 1 mg/kg/min
Apply ice pack	
Administer diuretics	
Insert urethral catheter	Monitor urine color, pH level, volume
Administer procainamide	1 mg/kg
Monitor for elevated serum potassium	Give insulin in 50 percent glucose
Monitor for decreased serum potassium	Replace potassium

CHAPTER 4

Operative Management

PEDIATRIC SURGICAL TECHNIQUE

The techniques and maneuvers in pediatric surgery are much the same as those in adults but are carried out much more precisely because of the size of the patient and the friability of the tissues. The operation must be planned in advance so that it can be completed with the fewest false steps, even if the findings are different from those expected. Keep in mind possible complications so that they may be avoided.

The skin of children is malleable so that incisions may be made to follow Langer's lines (page 42). Choose a transverse incision over a vertical one if the exposure will be the same; there is less chance for dehiscence. For major operations, mark the incision with a pen. If you and your assistant press along the margins of the incision, fewer small vessels will need fulguration, and the skin will become everted to expose the remaining bleeders in the subcutaneous tissue. Divide muscles with the cutting current, and fulgurate the vessels with the coagulating current through a needlepoint stylus. Dissect vessels by opening the scissor parallel to them to avoid tearing and to allow fulguration or ligation before division.

Develop your operative technique for work on children. Make your movements delicate and precise. Do not hurry; pediatric operations naturally take longer than those on adults. Add extra time when you schedule the case so that you will not be hurried by the following surgeon and team. As you work, think ahead to what you will need for the next step; then you will not have to wait for a special instrument or suture because the scrub nurse will have it ready.

The tissue of young children is tenuous, requiring care as each instrument is applied. Depending on antibacterial agents to avoid infection is not the same as handling tissues gently so that healthy cells can resist infection. The tools of the careful surgeon are stay sutures, skin hooks, and delicate forceps. Needle or bipolar electrodes are used for point fulguration. Fine ligatures and sutures are important. Also, keeping the tissues covered with moist gauze protects them.

1 Holding fine forceps inverted using the thumb and second finger keeps the hands from obscuring the view and blocking the light.

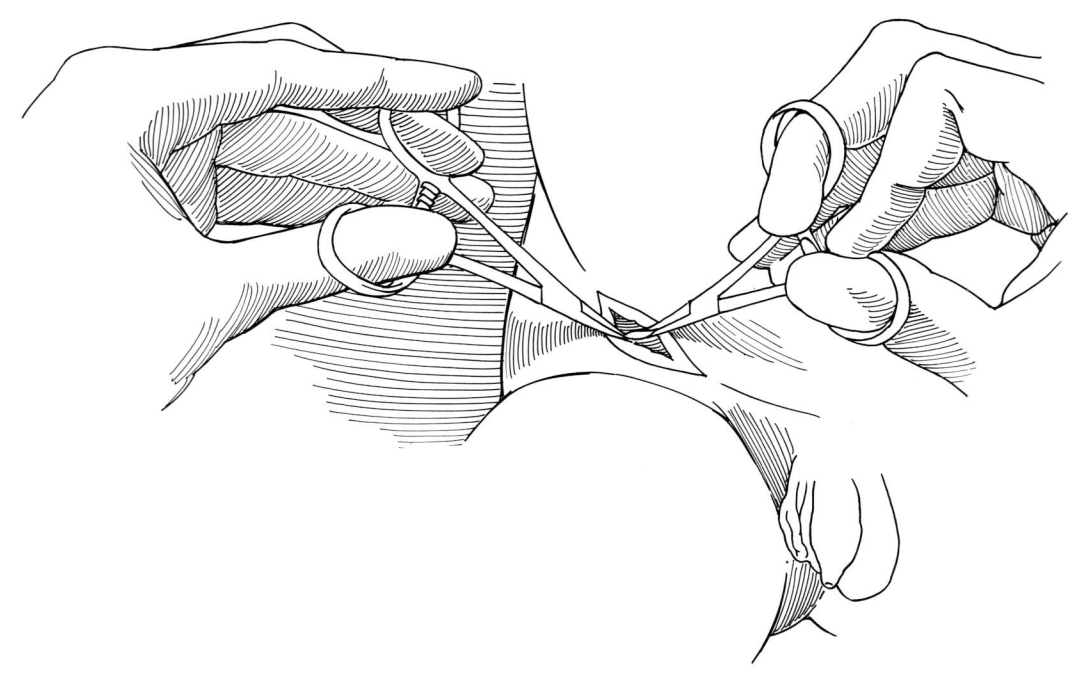

PEDIATRIC SURGICAL INSTRUMENTS

A set of instruments designed for operations on neonates and infants must be organized, with size and weight being the most important features. The needle-point electrosurgical unit divides fascia and muscle with minimal injury and allows immediate control of small vessels by coagulation.

With the help of the operating room nurse or technician, make out a card for each operation you commonly do, listing position of the patient, instruments needed, and sutures to have ready. In this atlas, lists of special instruments are provided for many operations. Keep these instrument cards up to date, and check them with the scrub nurse at the instrument table when you arrive to be sure everything is at hand.

A pediatric "GU cart" is a necessity because of the special needs of children. Set up a five- or six-drawer roll-around cart; outfit it with the required special sutures, stents, and special instruments; and have it in your operating room during the operation.

VISIBILITY

Visual acuity is directly related to the intensity of the light in the wound. At least two light sources are required, with one shining over the surgeon's right shoulder. Focused beams should reach the bottom of the wound without interference from heads. For deep wounds in children, a head lamp will help.

Magnification also increases the ability to see what you are doing and is particularly important for pediatric operations. Every pediatric urologic surgeon needs to have his or her own pair of binocular loupes permanently attached to plain or prescription glasses. Be sure the glasses fit well behind the ears; otherwise they may end up in the wound. For occasional assistants, less expensive industrial-type loupes on plastic headbands can be kept in the operating room to be slipped on when needed.

INCISION

A single stroke through the skin and subcutaneous tissue using a good-sized scalpel does the least damage. Multiple small cuts injure the vulnerable subcutaneous tissue and promote infection. Do not use the cutting current in the subcutaneous tissue; it damages a wider path than does the knife. Select a very sharp knife for the same reason. Let the scalpel float down through the fat until it meets the fascia. You do not need to discard the skin knife unless it is dull; it has been shown that it does not pick up bacteria from the skin.

For incising muscle and fascia, select the undamped cutting current delivered through the smallest available electrode, a needle electrode. A foot pedal leaves the hand free to grasp the handle of the stylus in any position. A laser knife decreases blood loss but greatly increases tissue damage; it may be found useful for massive parenchymal excisions. Realize that the surgical electrode is similar to a ray gun; it does not cut or coagulate through contact but rather through the arc that emanates from its tip. Avoid burrowing under a muscle before dividing it; this only opens more tissue planes. Rather, cut through the muscle progressively with the cutting current, using long strokes while taking care not to go deeply in any one area. The muscle retracts so that its vessels are seen and the next layer is exposed before you cut it. It is therefore not necessary to clamp, cut, and ligate muscles, a process that causes more necrosis than does electrosurgery.

DISSECTION

All forceps cause some injury to tissue. If a forceps grasping your skin can cause you pain, it also will damage tissue. Hemostats held inverted between the thumb and third finger keep the bulk of the hand away from the wound.

HEMOSTASIS

Control vessels less than 2 mm in diameter with pinpoint coagulation using damped current rather than suture ligature, because it produces less local destruction. A special bipolar coagulating forceps operated by the first assistant speeds up the operation and produces minimal damage to delicate tissues. An insulated knife or scissors connected to monopolar current also may reduce time. In any case, do not wave the electrode back and forth but be precise and zap only the bleeding vessel. For small bleeders in retractile muscle, insert the electrode first and then apply the current. For larger vessels, do not fulgurate but clamp first and then divide and ligate. These methods damage less tissue than when the vessel is cut and then clamped. Electrocoagulation, similar to electroincision, increases the chance of infection three-fold; therefore, avoid its use in the skin and subcutaneous tissue. Finally, use only bipolar coagulation on the penis; monopolar current increases the risk of urethral injury and fistula, even at low power.

ASSISTANTS AND ASSISTANCE

Always perform major surgery with an assistant capable of taking over should you become ill. The assistant should have reviewed the operative steps and be familiar with the procedure. Teaching as you operate makes you more aware of anatomic details and is invaluable for the assistant. The main function of an assistant is to provide exposure. This is accomplished not just by retraction, which is really the job of a self-retaining ring retractor or of the second assistant if you have one. A good first assistant, by anticipating the next move and grasping the appropriate tissue layer at the right time and place, can essentially perform the operation, with the surgeon merely following the lead.

PROTECTION OF THE SURGICAL TEAM FROM INFECTION

Whether every child should be tested preoperatively for human immunodeficiency virus (HIV) reaction is unclear, nor is the surgeon's responsibility to operate on those with positive reactions. The assumptions must be made, however, that every surgical patient would test positively and that it is our responsibility to operate on all patients, regardless of their HIV status. The result is that extreme care must be constantly exercised by all the team members as they are exposed to blood or secretions. This means that surgeons, anesthetists, and scrub personnel should wear protective glasses during invasive procedures in the operating room and routinely wear protective boots or impervious shoe coverings. The use of double gloves may need to be routine. Exposed skin surfaces should be washed with detergent immediately after contamination with blood or body fluids. Hands should be washed immediately after gloves are removed at the end of a procedure.

Extreme caution should be exercised with needles and sharp instruments. Meticulous technique is required both in the immediate operative field and the entire operating room to minimize accidental HIV exposure.

Have the scrub nurse place sharp instruments on a tray from which you can pick them up. Although needles are the greater hazard, a scalpel in the hand of the surgeon or the assistant can puncture through two layers of glove. Take extreme care to avoid needle sticks. Needles should not be recapped, bent, or broken. After use, needles and disposable sharp instruments should be immediately placed in puncture-resistant containers for disposal.

Personnel scrubbing in the middle of a case should put on their own gowns and gloves to prevent contamination of the inside of the garments with the patient's blood or bodily fluids, which may be on the scrub nurse's gloves. If a gown becomes contaminated with blood, it should be changed as soon as possible.

SELECTION OF SUTURES

The wounds of infants and children heal faster than those of adults, but only after a lag phase of 5 days

when they are dependent on the holding power of sutures. Major fibrous repair occurs for 2 weeks, followed by a slow increase in strength.

We each have our own preferences for sutures, but two important variables must be considered in their selection: persistence of strength and tissue reactivity. The initial strength is proportional to size, but the rate of loss of strength is a function of the suture material itself. Sutures are absorbed at variable rates, but the strength of the sutures is lost much more rapidly than it is absorbed. Reactivity of the tissue to the foreign body depends on the amount and type of reaction it invokes. The larger the size, the greater the reaction. Natural sutures incite a greater immunologic reaction than synthetic sutures. Also, greater suture size with larger knots creates increased reactivity. (The knots contribute most to the mass for reaction.)

Absorbable and nonabsorbable sutures have different effects. Plain catgut and chromic catgut sutures stimulate a large macrophage response with resultant proteolysis leading to significant tissue reactivity and variable absorption time. Synthetic absorbable sutures, in contrast, are removed by acid hydrolysis and have moderate tissue reactivity and more predictable absorption times. Those made from polyglycolic acid (Dexon, Vicryl) retain only 20 percent of their strength at 14 days, whereas polydioxanone sutures (PDS) retain 50 percent of their strength at 4 weeks. Dexon and Vicryl in the gastrointestinal tract are absorbed in 3 to 4 weeks. Maxon sutures and PDS retain the most strength in infected urine. Nonabsorbable sutures as monofilaments (Maxon) stimulate the least reaction in the tissues and have the least attraction for bacteria; when braided, they handle better and tie more securely. They are unsuitable in the presence of bacteria or urine. Silk and cotton rapidly lose their strength after the second month but probably are useful in the outer layer of an intestinal anastomosis and in the mesentery. Nylon is a polyamide, Dacron is a polyester, and polyethylene and polypropylene are polyolefins; of these, nylon loses its strength first.

In general, polyglycolic acid sutures are preferable to plain or chromic catgut for urologic surgery, except in cases of infected urine and for the skin. Because of expense, as few different sizes and kinds of sutures as possible should be opened in any given case. Although suture selection is an individual matter, certain practical guidelines can be followed. The composition and trade names of the most used sutures are listed in Table 4–1, and their application is described in Table 4–2.

Fascia. Regardless of what suture is used, the immediate strength of the wound is only 40 to 70 percent of the intact structure. With nonabsorbable sutures, this reduced strength persists at least for the 3 months or so that it takes for the wound to heal

Table 4–1. Suture Types

Material	Coated	Name of Suture
Absorbable		
SYNTHETIC BRAIDED		
Polyglactin	Yes	Vicryl*
	No	Dexon "S"†
Polyglycolic acid	Yes	Dexon plus†
SYNTHETIC MONOFILAMENT		
Polyglyconate		Maxon†
Polydioxanone		PDS*
GUT		
Plain gut		Plain gut*†
Chromic glut		Chromic gut*†
Nonabsorbable		
SYNTHETIC BRAIDED		
Polyester	No	Merseline,* Dacron†
Nylon	Yes	Surgilon†
SYNTHETIC MONOFILAMENT		
Nylon		Ethilon,* Dermalon†
Polypropylene		Proline,* Surgilene†

*Manufactured by Ethicon.
†Manufactured by Davis & Geck.
Adapted from Edlich R, Rodeheaver GY, Thacker JG: Considerations in the choice of sutures for wound closure of the genitourinary tract. *J Urol* 137:373, 1987.

completely. For an absorbable suture, the strength initially is the same as that of a nonabsorbable one if an equivalent size is used, but in 1 or 2 weeks, its strength will have declined appreciably. The exceptions are PDS and Maxon, which are still strong at 2 weeks. By this time, however, the wound itself will have gained enough strength to balance the diminished strength derived from the sutures. Thus, it is during the 2nd week that the wound is most vulnerable to separation. For this reason, sutures of nonabsorbable material often are used for closure of wounds subjected to stress, such as those in the abdomen and flank.

In clean wounds, PDS, a monofilament absorbable suture, is absorbed by 26 weeks but maintains adequate strength for 6 weeks. However, it is stiff, and firm knots are hard to tie. Be sure to invert the sutures to avoid bumps on the outside. Monofilament polyglycolic acid suture (Vicryl, Dexon) maintains its strength and is eventually resorbed; it is preferable to PDS because it is easier to handle, and the knots will hold if they consist of a surgeon's knot with a square knot superimposed or four square knots.

For contaminated wounds, the process of absorbing the sutures stimulates macrophage activity, with re-

Table 4–2. Suggested Type and Size of Suture for Various Tissues

Tissue	Adult		Pediatric	
	Type	Size	Type	Size
Skin				
Cosmetic closure	Absorbable	4-0	Absorbable	5-0
Noncosmetic closure	Staples	4-0	Nonabsorbable	5-0
	Nonabsorbable	3-0		4-0
Fascia	PDS	Zero	PDS	3-0
	Maxon silk	1-0	Maxon silk	2-0
Muscle	Absorbable	1-0	Absorbable	3-0
		2-0		3-0
Bladder	Absorbable	3-0	Absorbable	4-0
		2-0		3-0
Ureteropelvic junction	Absorbable	5-0	Absorbable	5-0
		4-0		6-0
Urethra	Absorbable	4-0	Absorbable	5-0
	(Maxon, PDS)	5-0		6-0
Bowel	Staples		Staples	
	Absorbable	3-0	Absorbable	5-0
	(inner layer)	4-0	(inner layer)	4-0
	Nonabsorbable	3-0	Nonabsorbable	4-0
	(outer layer)		(outer layer)	
Vascular	Nonabsorbable	4-0	Nonabsorbable	4-0
		5-0		5-0

Adapted from Foster LS, McAninch JW: Suture material and wound healing; an overview. AUA *Update* Vol. XI, Lesson 11, 1992.

sultant low tissue oxygen tension. This activity also reduces endothelial migration and capillary formation, thus providing a suitable environment for anaerobic bacterial growth. Polyglycolic acid sutures foster the least inflammatory response of absorbable sutures, and the degradation products themselves may be antibacterial. Conversely, nonabsorbable sutures, especially monofilaments, produce the least reaction, but once infected they may stay infected because they remain in the wound. Polypropylene is the best choice in contaminated wounds; it is much better than silk or cotton. For a debilitated patient; in whom poor healing is expected, use either a nonabsorbable suture or the absorbable suture that retains its strength the longest (ie, PDS). Retention suture of heavy nonabsorbable material (polypropylene or wire) may be needed in a debilitated patient, especially if the wound is contaminated. Bolsters cut from a red rubber catheter reduce damage to the skin.

Subcutaneous Tissue. This layer is the site of most wound infections because of the weak defense mechanisms in the fatty areolar tissue. Do not use sutures here unless really necessary, and then use the finest minimally reactive absorbable suture of polyglycolic acid. Avoid plain or chromic catgut.

Skin. Tape is best to approximate skin edges if they are not subjected to too much tension. Staples, if not too tight, are the next best choice, because they do not penetrate the wound, but they cost more and are a nuisance because they require subsequent removal, to the distress of the child. Monofilament nonabsorbable material leaves a better wound but must be removed. Polyglycolic acid sutures subcuticularly can remain until resorbed, at the same time producing little reaction. By using a skin hook, the subcutaneous layer can be pulled forward to aid in placing each stitch. This material is not suitable when placed as interrupted sutures in the skin because it depends on hydrolysis for absorption and so will persist on the dry surface.

Urinary Tract. Urothelium covers the suture line within 5 days. Ureteral and vesical wounds gain strength more rapidly than those in the body wall; normal strength is reached in 21 days. The type of suture material is not as critical here, but absorbable sutures cause less reaction than nonabsorbable ones in the long term. Although more subject to encrustation, absorbable sutures usually are gone before stones can form. PDS lasts too long to be of use in the urinary tract. Polyglycolic acid sutures are less reactive than chromic catgut sutures, and they have a more predictable rate of absorption. Although polyglycolic acid sutures are not completely absorbed before 28 days, they are usually the better choice, with one exception: In the presence of *Proteus* infection, resorption is much too rapid, and catgut should be used.

Intestine. Use interrupted nonabsorbable sutures, reaching well into the submucosa. If a hemostatic layer is desired, place a running absorbable suture in the mucosa. Chromic catgut is suitable for sutures penetrating the lumen; otherwise, use synthetic absorbable sutures. Controlled-release needles speed the process of suturing.

Vascular Sutures. Monofilament synthetic nonabsorbable sutures are strongest and least reactive.

Commentary by Francis F. Bartone

Bladder and Ureter. For bladder and ureter, which regain their strength rapidly (100 percent by 14 days) and are essentially healed by 21 days, the polyglycolic acid sutures (Dexon, Vicryl) can be used. They retain strength within the time required and yet are absorbed quickly enough to avoid calculi forming on them. Even in the presence of infection, the epithelium rapidly grows over the suture, which I believe resists disintegration *in vivo*. If active infection is suspected, I would not hesitate to recommend an inner layer of continuous suture of Dexon or Vicryl and an outer layer of one of the slowly absorbing monofilament absorbables, glycolic acid–trimethylene carbonate (Maxon) or PDS. (PDS was used clinically in the bladder in an unpublished study by Hargraves in 1988.)

Fascia. I still favor a nonabsorbable monofilament suture, such as polypropylene (Prolene), for fascial closure because there is evidence that it retains its strength well beyond the time necessary and still does not need to be removed if infection occurs. Perhaps the slowly absorbable monofilaments Maxon or PDS will be considered the suture of choice for most fascial closures. Prolene knots occasionally cause chronic discomfort when used to suture fascia in patients with little subcutaneous fat, whereas absorbable sutures do not. PDS retains 50 percent of its strength at 4 weeks, even in the presence of infection. PDS retains its strength longer than Maxon, but the handling and knot-tying characteristics are reportedly better with Maxon suture.

Skin. Generally, a subcuticular suture using Dexon or Vicryl is most often used. Healing is excellent, and the advantages of not having to remove the suture postoperatively when the child is fully awake are obvious. This is the rule with skin closure on our service.

Hypospadias. For most procedures, PDS is now being used by a hypospadiologist of renown because it slides through the tissue easily and retains its strength for long periods. It is especially useful in glans approximation where multilayered buried sutures are used.

To prevent suture tracks, there is evidence that a subcuticular closure with PDS is very useful. I would assume that Maxon sutures would be equally useful. The skin also seems to heal more quickly and with less edema. I have used this suture in this situation, but my period of postoperative follow-up is shorter than the quoted authority. In the skin, chromic catgut in small sizes (6-0 or 7-0) must be the suture of choice because it is absorbed quickly and causes less reaction on the surface. It also is used almost exclusively when the urethra is sutured to the glans circumferentially. The polyglycolic acid sutures are absorbed much too slowly, as are PDS and Maxon. These sutures should never be used on the skin surface, because they will be absorbed too slowly.

Vascular Anastomoses. Although the standard suture material for vascular anastomoses is Prolene, there are several excellent papers showing that arterial anastomoses made with Maxon heal better, have wider lumina, and do not form thrombi on the suture. This may be important in the small-size vessels in children.

POSITION AT SURGERY

Decide on which side of the table to stand for each operation. In this atlas, position is shown for right-handed surgeons, and the exposure and procedure also are illustrated from that point of view.

Start with the table at a height that allows your elbows to be flexed at right angles when your hands are resting on the surface of the patient. The operative field is small, so avoid putting your head down; your naked eyes (or with corrective glasses) have a reading distance of greater than 30 cm. A loupe will provide needed magnification. Infants have short legs, so the surgeon and assistants can work best while standing, even when operating on the perineum.

INTRAOPERATIVE BLEEDING

Although screening has been carried out preoperatively, abnormal bleeding may occur intraoperatively. Vitamin K deficiency occurs if the neonate has received only breast milk without prophylactic vitamin K supplement at birth. This deficiency should be picked up by a disproportionately prolonged prothrombin time and is readily treated by giving 1 to 2 mg of vitamin K oxide intravenously (IV). The cause of bleeding may be disseminated intravascular coagulation secondary to hypoxemia, trauma, and infection.

Thrombocytopenia can be improved with IV gamma globulin. Packed red blood cells are a direct answer to intraoperative bleeding given along with fresh frozen plasma, although whole blood is better if the bleeding is rapid.

BLOOD LOSS AND TRANSFUSIONS

Because 7 percent of body weight is blood, a child weighing 10 kg has a circulating blood volume of approximately 700 ml. A loss at operation of up to 15 percent of this volume will not affect blood pressure, pulse pressure, respiration rate, or capillary blanch test results. Unless other fluid losses are occurring, you can count on transcapillary refill and other compensatory mechanisms to restore blood volume.

A volume loss between 15 percent and 30 percent, however, representing 100 to 200 ml of blood in a

child (class II hemorrhage according to trauma surgeons), causes tachycardia, tachypnea, and, most significantly, a decrease in pulse pressure. Realize that the systolic pressure may be fairly well sustained, but the rise in diastolic pressure is ominous. The capillary blanch test results become positive, and the urinary output falls moderately to between 20 and 30 ml/h. Patients with this condition require transfusion.

A volume loss of over 30 percent produces a measurable drop in systolic blood pressure (class III hemorrhage).

Blood loss in the postoperative period can be recognized by clinical signs. Hematocrit determinations are unreliable and inappropriate to estimate acute blood loss. A child who is cool and tachycardic is in shock and needs immediate transfusion. Septic shock produces a wide pulse pressure, an important differentiating point.

Use lactated Ringer's solution for initial replacement, giving a bolus of 20 ml/kg in a child. Observe the response. If the signs are not reversed or are only transiently improved, and if urinary output remains low, give packed red blood cells if already matched, and establish a central venous pressure (CVP) line. Crystalloid replacement is made in a ratio of three volumes for each volume of blood lost. In an emergency, use type-specific or type O blood. Matched whole blood, of course, is best, if it can be obtained.

After 700 ml of blood replacement in a 10-kg child, coagulopathy becomes a problem, mainly because of hemodilution. Should abnormal bleeding appear after replacement, obtain a "clotting screen" and give a platelet pack. If clotting factors are found to be significantly deficient, give at least 400 ml of fresh frozen plasma.

Be concerned about possible fluid overload, even when the CVP has not reached normal levels. Instead of depending on the CVP, watch for return of adequate perfusion by the urinary output, skin color, and return of pulse rate and blood pressure reading toward normal. However, if overload does occur, avoid diuretics because they render measurement of urine output useless as a guide and may precipitate hypovolemia.

FIXATION OF ORGANS AND TISSUES BEFORE CLOSURE

All structures should be restored to a position as near normal as possible. Pull the omentum down and spread it out to separate the intestine from the wound. In the flank, tack Gerota's fascia and the perirenal fat together with fine plain catgut sutures to isolate pelvic and ureteral repairs from the body wall. If the kidney has been freed, it must be repositioned with one or two nephropexy stitches taken into the psoas muscle. After constructions from intestinal segments, be sure to close the proximal edge of the mesentery against the retroperitoneal surface to prevent an internal hernia in the "trap."

OPERATIVE CONTAMINATION AND INFECTION

Washing the fat and tissue debris from the wound with sterile water by repeatedly filling and aspirating the wound bed is good practice. It will effectively reduce the inoculum and allow primary closure in contaminated wounds, because an inoculum must contain at least 10^6 bacteria to cause infection, no matter what the species. If contamination is especially feared, use a solution of bacitracin, 500,000 units, and neomycin, 0.5 g, in 1000 ml of saline as extraperitoneal irrigation. Erythematous infected wounds or those grossly contaminated should be left open, covered with gauze, and then closed secondarily 3 or more days after the operation. For invasive infections, supplement antibiotic therapy with nasal oxygen.

DRAINS

The harmful effects of drainage tubes are usually outweighed by their benefits after urologic operations, especially those that enter the urinary tract. Drains render the tissue more susceptible to bacterial invasion and provide the route for bacterial entry from the skin and external environment, but they do facilitate the exit of potentially contaminated serum and blood, as well as collections of pus. Most important, they allow egress of urine that may leak from the tract. The most common purpose of a drain is prophylaxis, to prevent the accumulation of potentially infected blood, serum, or urine. Any surgical wound is susceptible to infection, and hematomas increase that risk. The indications for drainage are still controversial; neither drains nor antibiotics are substitutes for an atraumatic surgical technique. Make a decision about drainage at the end of the operation based on the pros and cons. For example, after a retroperitoneal operation, a drain allows trapped air and blood to escape; it may be removed the next day. When the urinary tract has been opened, a drain placed extraperitoneally through the fascial layers is especially important to provide an escape route for urinary leakage; remove it 2 or 3 days after you are sure drainage has stopped.

Two types of drains are in current use: (1) passive drains, such as the Penrose, and (2) the more expensive, active-suction drains, such as the closed (Jackson-Pratt or Hemovac) or open (sump) drains. Passive drainage depends on intra-abdominal or wound pressure; active drainage, on suction. Passive drainage is adequate for most urologic wounds, because it permits escape of air and any accumulated blood. If the urinary passages have been opened, it prevents formation of urinomas because urine as a dilute fluid will follow any route of escape through the body wall if such is provided. Stated another way, urine does not require suction for drainage. However, active, closed suction drainage is valuable in more superficial operations, such as inguinal node dissection and, with miniaturization, in certain cases of hypospadias, to obliterate the space beneath the skin flaps. It also may be useful after major pelvic operations to detect postoperative bleeding and reduce the incidence of lymphoceles. It is not effective for urine leaks, because the holes are easily plugged. In fact, if urinary leakage is a good possibility, two Penrose drains exiting through the wound, rather than through a stab wound, will ensure the best drainage.

Be careful to keep the end of the drain away from contact with the site of repair or from an anastomosis, but suture the Penrose drain to an adjacent structure so that it will not be displaced during closure. Use a simple catgut stitch, or better, use the *long suture technique*. First, stitch a 3-0 synthetic absorbable suture through one end of the Penrose drain and tie it to it. Then pass the suture through the adjacent fat or muscle so that the end of the drain lies within 2 or 3 cm of the repair site. Now stitch the suture to the distal end of the drain that will lie outside the body after wound closure and tie it after taking up the slack. To remove the drain, cut the suture flush with the skin; the rest of the suture will now follow the drain as it is withdrawn. In all cases, especially in children, suture the drain to the skin. Pierce it with a safety pin so that it cannot be lost, except in young children for whom the safety pin itself could be a hazard. A drain causes less harm to the wound if brought out through a separate stab wound; however, if significant urinary leakage or gross contamination with leakage is anticipated, it is much more efficient to have it come through the wound itself. In children, stab wounds become unsightly with growth.

CATHETERS AND TUBES

Catheters are placed transurethrally before an operation to empty the bladder to get it out of the way, to fill the bladder preparatory to its incision, to instill antibacterial or antineoplastic agents, or to allow identification of the urethra and vesical neck. For these purposes, an 8 or 10 F catheter is usually satisfactory in children. One made of silicone is preferable, even if it is to remain only a few days. For a given external size, a balloon catheter has a smaller drainage channel than a straight tube or catheter. Intraoperatively, the catheter may be replaced with one of a smaller size, also made of silicone, so that it will be better tolerated by the urethral wall as it is left indwelling. If clots are anticipated, a larger catheter is necessary. In complicated cases, the catheter should be stitched to the glans and taped to the penis and abdomen or leg, because its inadvertent removal could be disastrous.

Waterproof tape applied over tincture of benzoin is required to hold catheters or tubing. Once applied, it must be regularly checked. A good alternative to a balloon catheter for bladder operations, especially in children, is to place a suture in the end of a Robinson catheter with a curved Keith needle, then insert both ends of the suture in the eye of the needle and run them through the bladder and body walls. Tie them together over a bolster. Remember at the end of the operation to attach the drainage tube to the catheter while the patient is still on the table to prevent contamination of the connector.

Suprapubic drainage has several advantages over the transurethral route. It allows cystography with a trial of voiding before removal. This type of drainage is the preferred method in a patient who is expected to have difficulty emptying the bladder postoperatively, as after sling procedures and bladder augmentation. It is less likely than a balloon catheter to fall out, because it is routinely stitched to the skin and may be less likely to introduce infection than one through the urethra. The disadvantages are the need to create a wound in the bladder and body wall and the tendency to irritate the trigone if the tip is not held in the dome of the bladder.

STENTS

Stents are useful for several purposes: to relieve obstruction, to align the ureter and its connections, to facilitate closure of fistulas, and to provide a scaffold for repair. They may be placed retrogradely, antegradely by a percutaneous route, or intraoperatively on a temporary or permanent basis. However, they should not be used without a definite indication, and they do not obviate meticulous surgical technique.

Available stents range from straight silicone rubber tubing to double pigtail stents with fixed curves on either end that are self-retaining. Certain polymers are stiffer than silicone and so can be placed retrogradely or antegradely. By preliminary insertion of guide wires, passage is facilitated. Drainage holes may be located at the proximal end or at both ends. For stent selection, see page 38.

WOUND CLOSURE

Before closing the incision, search for bleeding, and at the same time, look for sponges. Irrigate the wound copiously with water to flush out free tissue and clots. Place drains so that they drain the space without making contact with the site of repair, using the long suture technique described previously after ureteral or ureteropelvic repair.

DRESSINGS

An occlusive dressing is less desirable than one porous enough to allow skin products and wound secretions to move away from the wound.

Apply tincture of benzoin to the skin before placing tape. Montgomery straps are useful if appreciable drainage is expected and abdominal pads are to be applied. Leave the dressing in place for at least 3 days. By that time, the incision will be sealed and no longer susceptible to contamination.

CHAPTER 5

Management After Operation

POSTOPERATIVE CARE OF THE NEONATE

Be sure the newborn is responding, has been extubated before the monitoring equipment is detached, and is placed on one side to go to the postanesthesia care unit (PACU) in a prewarmed incubator. It is better if the child and the surgeon stay in the operating room until improvement is obvious. Take the neonate to the PACU, which should be organized like an intensive care unit, before removing the endotracheal tube. Check on the status of the child and on the orders; do both even when you have a responsible resident. Provide additional oxygen, especially as long as fever, hypothermia, or acidosis exists. Determine blood gases as a guide; oxygen saturation should be maintained between 85 and 95 percent. Neonates with exstrophy or prune-belly syndrome may require assisted ventilation to be continued much longer.

For the next 24 hours, watch for apnea, especially in premature or cold or metabolically unbalanced infants (hypoglycemic, hypocalcemic, or acidotic). Provide additional oxygen, especially as long as fever, hypothermia, or acidosis exists.

Infuse 5 percent dextrose in 0.25 percent normal saline IV at 3 ml/kg/h for the first 2 days of life and 4 ml/kg/hr thereafter. Losses other than insensible ones, as from the gastrointestinal tract or into the third space, need replacement with lactated Ringer's solution. Monitor the blood pressure to detect hypovolemia from dehydration or from concealed blood loss. Look for a urinary output between 1.5 and 2 ml/kg/h. If a central venous pressure (CVP) line is in place, the pressure should be above 5 cm H_2O.

POSTOPERATIVE CARE OF THE INFANT AND CHILD

For the first 24 hours after operation, continue IV fluids to provide daily maintenance and balance losses. Measure both volume and electrolyte concentration of enteric losses and replace them. Caloric requirements are charted in Tables 1–2 and 1–3. It is rare that oral intake is not resumed in 2 to 5 days. After 5 days, if the child cannot ingest adequately nutritious oral fluids, resort to total parenteral nutrition.

RESPIRATORY SUPPORT

After operation, place the child in a lateral position and provide for frequent turning. Have infants cry and force older children to breathe deeply and cough. Prevent drying of the airways by humidification and mist therapy in a tent, hood, or mask, but avoid overhydration from water absorption in the respiratory tract, especially with the endotracheal tube in place.

Children recovering from anesthesia have depressed respiration from anesthetic agents or muscle relaxants. They are subject to hypoxemia, which can be corrected with oxygen supplementation in a tent or hood (not by nasal catheter). Because of the possibility of oxygen toxicity and retrolental fibroplasia, 100 percent oxygen administration should be reduced to 40 percent after 24 hours, unless hypoxia demands a higher level. Respiration may require assistance with a mask and bag or even by endotracheal tube for longer control.

POSTOPERATIVE ORDERS

For most peripheral operations, the only orders needed are to check on vital signs for an hour or so until the child is fully awake. At this time, the child may have clear liquids. If the child is nauseated, delay offering clear liquids for a few hours, then start with small amounts at short intervals, with a solid diet held to the next day. Acute gastric dilatation can occur, evidenced by distention on examination or by gas in the stomach on radiograph. Insert a nasogastric tube. If bile continues to come from the tube in a child with an intestinal anastomosis, suspect obstruction at that site. Maintain nutritional and fluid balance, but if the obstruction persists for 2 or 3 weeks, reoperation may be required. Obstruction appearing later is most likely from intussusception of the small bowel and needs immediate relief.

FLUID REQUIREMENTS

After a major operation, continue IV fluids for the first 24 hours to provide daily maintenance and to balance losses. Measure both volume and electrolyte concentration of enteric losses and replace them.

Watch for apathy, weakness, and orthostatic hypotension, along with tachycardia, weak pulse, dry tongue, poor skin turgor, and weight loss—all evidence of severe volume depletion. The blood urea nitrogen level rises disproportionately to the serum creatinine level. Serum sodium levels may be up or down, depending on the cause of the dehydration. For severe dehydration, monitor CVP and replace half the estimated deficit in 8 hours and the other half in the subsequent 16 hours in addition to maintenance fluids. Use hypotonic solutions in children with elevated sodium levels and isotonic saline solution for the others. Fluid overload of 400 to 700 ml in a 10-kg child results in edema, often with dyspnea, tachycardia, venous engorgement, and pulmonary congestion.

Hypotonic hyponatremia occurs from third-space losses and results in low urine volumes with high osmolarity. Replace the losses with saline solutions. Hypovolemic hypernatremia results from unreplaced renal or gastrointestinal water losses, producing thirst, hypotension, and lethargy. Use 5 percent dextrose in water to return the serum sodium level to normal over 24 hours, measuring it every 6 hours.

POSTOPERATIVE INFECTIONS

Fevers occurring during the 1st or 2nd postoperative day probably originate in the respiratory tract. Enforce coughing and deep breathing; ask the respiratory team for help. After the 2nd day, look for infection in the urinary tract as well as for abscesses and extravasation.

Neonates. Infections are not easy to detect in neonates because the symptoms are so nonspecific. Disseminated infections produce symptoms such as irritability, weakness, and especially difficulty in breathing or convulsions. They even can result in hypoglycemia and hypocalcemia and demand a screen for the source in the wound, urine, blood, and spinal fluid. Treatment with an aminoglycoside and ampicillin must be started at once, rather than waiting for the laboratory results. Then, a cephalosporin may be given instead of the aminoglycoside.

Infants and Children. The infection tends to be more localized. Wound culture, along with blood culture, is enough, and treatment is based on the likely pathogen.

Hospital-acquired infections are a particular problem in children's hospitals. Closed catheter systems are essential.

PAIN

Postoperative pain may be aborted by bupivacaine nerve blocks and wound infiltration to provide enough time for the child to start oral pain medication.

Regional anesthetic techniques are particularly versatile because they can be applied as the entire anesthetic and thus reduce the dose of general anesthetics or as a method of providing postoperative pain relief. Side effects are few, and the benefits are many, including excellent pain relief, decreased analgesic requirements, and decreased nausea and vomiting (all three the most common postoperative complications). All this results in earlier ambulation and discharge and more rapid return to normal activity. Over 95 percent of parents are very satisfied with the use of a regional anesthetic for their child.

For circumcision, hypospadias repair, hernia repair, orchiopexy, and hydrocelectomy, a caudal block is most commonly used, using 0.125 to 0.25 percent bupivacaine (0.5 to 0.75 ml/kg). This block has an excellent safety record.

An ilioinguinal/iliohypogastric block (0.25 to 0.5 percent bupivacaine, up to 2 mg/kg) also may be effective for an inguinal incision.

A caudal block or dorsal nerve block of the penis (1 to 4 ml of 0.25 percent bupivacaine without epinephrine) is appropriate for circumcision or hypospadias repair, although there have been minor complications from dorsal nerve block. Instillation of local anesthetic or topical application can also be useful.

If these measures are inadequate, use IV agents, such as morphine given at a rate of 0.05 mg/kg/h or meperidine hydrochloride (Demerol) given every 2 hours in a dose of 0.5 mg/kg.

If for any reason the child could not have a local anesthetic as postoperative analgesia for severe pain, a narcotic such as fentanyl (up to a dose of 2 μg/kg IV) is appropriate. If the pain is mild, an oral analgesic such as acetaminophen with or without codeine can be given. For pain control at home, elixir of acetaminophen (Tylenol) with codeine can be effective.

POSTOPERATIVE PROGRAM

Plain Film. In older children after extensive intraabdominal procedures, consider exposing a plain film of the operated area on the way to the PACU to be certain sponges and clamps have not been included in the wound.

Checklist. Use a checklist in the PACU to avoid overlooking important orders and to monitor respiratory functions.

Operative Report. Dictate the operative report yourself not only for medical and legal reasons but to make it useful in the follow-up of the child and as a reference for future operations. Residents must be discreet but should include all the pointers that can be helpful next time. These records can provide a valuable education.

Parental Support

Support by parents is valuable. Infants seem to get well faster when their parents are present.

Nursing Care

For urologic cases, the maintenance of urinary drainage is most important. Instruct the nursing staff immediately of the routes of urinary drainage, whether from the urethra or from a tube. Labels and diagrams help in complicated cases. Before the child goes to the general care unit, be sure the catheters are firmly secured to the child, are reasonably child-proof, and are draining. Have the nurse check the adequacy of drainage periodically but do not allow disconnection except under sterile precautions. Milk the tubing instead. Fluid output should be recorded. The nurse needs to reassure the child that the feeling of the need to void is from the presence of tubing, not urine. For bladder spasm, have the nurses give oxybutynin 0.1 mg/kg three times a day. The tubing should not unduly inhibit the child's activity, the exception being after hypospadias repair. Wait 3 days before being concerned about lack of bowel movement.

After the catheter(s) has been removed, check for adequacy of the stream, volume voided, and leaks, either at the exit sites of the tubes or in the repair, before the child is discharged. Explain to the parents what to expect when the child gets home.

MANAGEMENT OF COMPLICATIONS

Problems will occur postoperatively, although many can be prevented with care and anticipation. If you think of all possible untoward events, you can take measures to prevent them. In this atlas, most of the important postoperative problems are described at the end of the surgical protocols. By the end of the operation, it may be too late to prevent them; therefore, be sure to review the possibilities before starting. With equally difficult case loads, the better surgeons will have fewer postoperative complications. *Bleeding* that should have been controlled during the operation can occur soon after operation. Bleeding that appears later comes from disruption of part of a suture line and requires immediate intervention. *Peripheral ischemia* must be watched for postoperatively by checking the femoral, popliteal, or dorsalis pedis pulse, by comparing pedal temperatures, and by inspecting skin color.

Perioperative Techniques

Surgeons specializing in pediatric urology have need for skills and techniques common to all urologists, especially in approximating tissue, anastomosing bowel, and closing wounds. More than these abilities, they occasionally must perform procedures that are not strictly in their field. They may lacerate a spleen or tear a vessel; they may need to create a gastrostomy for feeding during recovery or a transverse colostomy for fecal diversion. Although a pediatric surgical colleague can help, if available, the urologist operating on children should have an adequate repertoire of suitable procedures in general surgery and have the ability to do a few standard general surgical procedures without outside help.

VASCULAR ACCESS

Percutaneous Cannulation

The use of plastic cannulas with an inner metal needle stilet (Medicut) facilitates access to the antecubital vein of the forearm in children and the dorsal surface of the hand in infants. First, place the arm on a padded board held with roller gauze to hyperextend it, and tape the board to the mattress. Apply a Penrose drain tourniquet. Wipe the site and the surgeon's palpating finger with antiseptic solution, then dry the area. Use an 18-gauge needle to make an initial puncture a centimeter distal to the vein, then insert the cannula very slowly with the bevel down, at the same time palpating it and the vein with a finger of the other hand. Slowly advance it toward the vein while aspirating with the syringe. When blood appears in the chamber, aspirate a small amount into the syringe, then reinject it to dilate the vein ahead of the needle, while at the same time advancing the cannula. Withdraw the stilet and advance the cannula until the hub meets the skin. If blood does not flow, slowly withdraw the cannula until it does, then rotate and advance it. Fix the cannula permanently with waterproof tape over tincture of benzoin, and fasten the arm firmly to the arm board so that flexion is not possible. In neonates, the cannula may be placed in a dorsal vein of the hand by grasping the fist to stretch the vein.

Central Venous Catheterization

Placement of a central venous catheter is possible either by cutting down on the basilic vein in the antecubital fossa or—the standard procedure—via the jugular veins in the neck, particularly the deep jugular. A percutaneous technique has been developed but requires considerable experience.

1 With the child under general anesthesia in a 20-degree Trendelenburg position to eliminate the possibility of introducing air, elevate the infant's shoulders, and extend the neck to the left. Prep the neck, chest, and upper arm. Make a 1.5-cm transverse incision above the clavicle over the right external jugular vein (a). If this incision is not adequate, usually because of previous utilization, extend the skin incision medially to expose the internal jugular vein between the heads of the sternocleidomastoid muscle. The anterior facial vein, an excellent alternative, is reached through an incision 1½ cm below the angle of the jaw over the medial border of the sternocleidomastoid. Make a second transverse incision on the chest below (b).

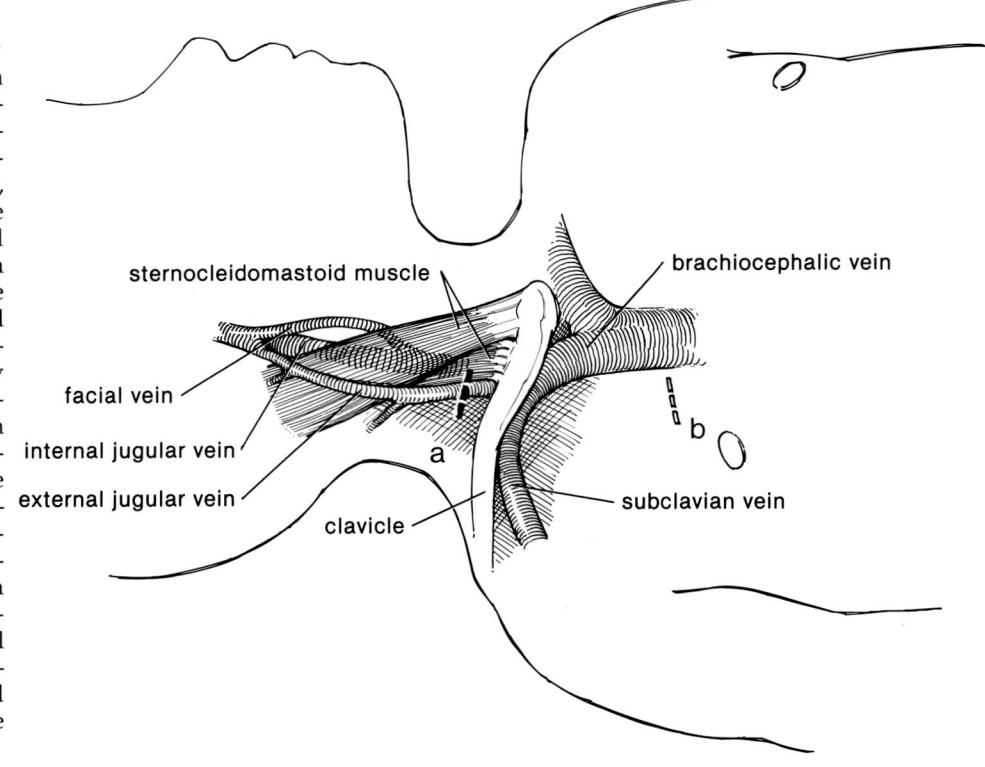

sternocleidomastoid muscle

brachiocephalic vein

facial vein

internal jugular vein

external jugular vein

a

b

clavicle

subclavian vein

2 **A,** Free the vein, and loop it with fine sutures. If the internal jugular vein is used, it is advisable to put a pursestring 5-0 or 6-0 polydioxanone suture at the proposed venotomy site. Alternatively, use the anterior facial vein by making an incision 1.5 cm below the angle of the jaw over the medial border of the sternocleidomastoid. **B,** Select a catheter suitable for the age and weight of the child. The smaller Broviac catheters (beginning at 2.7 F) can be used in newborns and infants; the larger Hickman catheters (up to 9.6 F) can be used in older children. Insert a large hollow (ventricular) needle with a bore equal to the diameter of the venous catheter from the upper to the lower incision, and draw the tip of the catheter up through the tunnel. Position the monofilament knitted polypropylene cuff 2 to 5 cm deep to the site of entry. Trim the catheter to the appropriate length to lie at the junction of the superior vena cava and right atrium. Estimate the length by following the external landmarks.

Elevate the vein, and cut it on a tangent with fine scissors. Flush the catheter with heparinized saline (1 unit per milliliter), and insert the tip of the catheter into the vein (a small vein introducer may facilitate this maneuver).

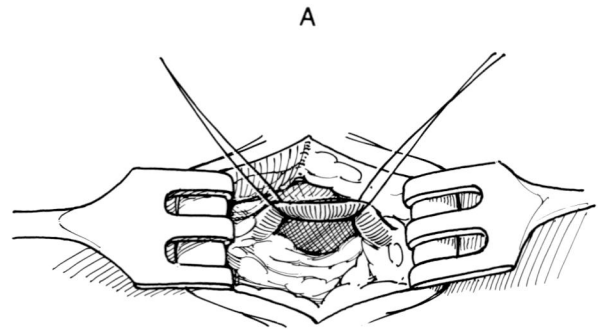

A

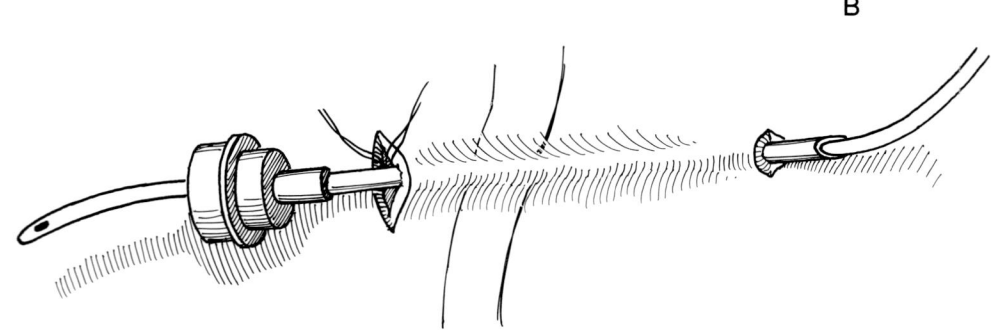

B

3 Advance the catheter into the superior vena cava toward the right atrium. The position of the catheter can be checked fluoroscopically. Be sure the catheter irrigates freely and that blood can be readily withdrawn. Ligate the vein above with the upper suture, and tie the catheter in place with the lower one. Infuse the catheter with heparinized saline solution (100 units per milliliter), and cover the end with the Luer-Lok cap.

4 Suture the catheter to the skin and cover it with sterile strips.

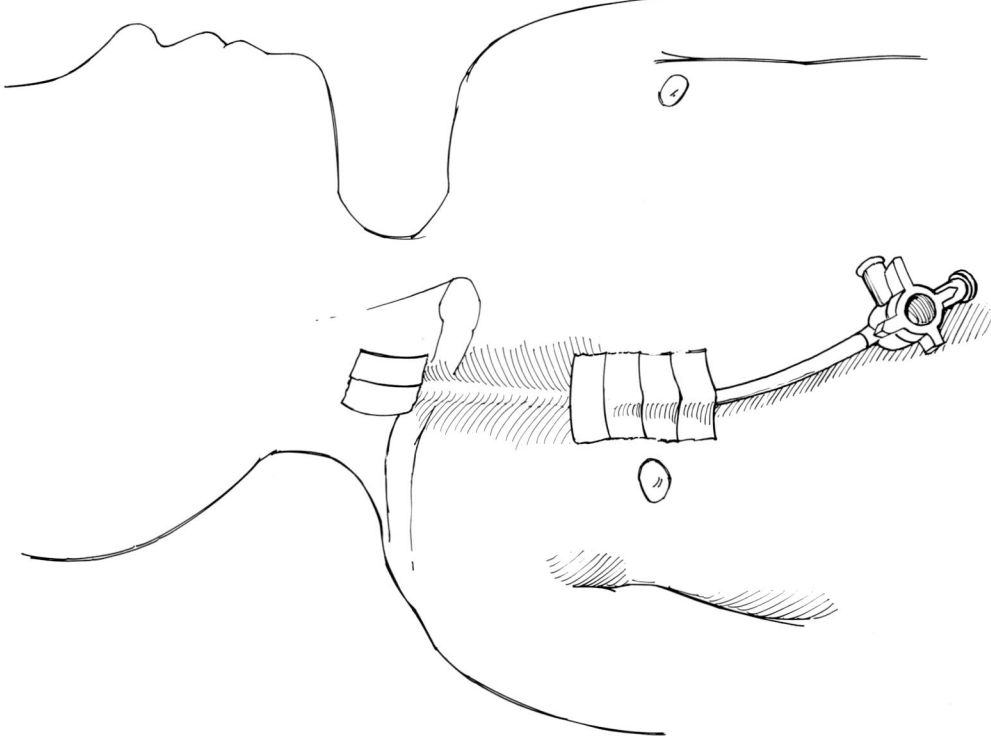

Cutdown Peripheral Vein Catheterization

With the development of percutaneous techniques of venous catheterization, an open procedure rarely is used. However, if other methods fail in older children, cutdown catheterization of the cephalic vein may be required.

5 Sit down to be able to rest your forearms on the table. Place the child's forearm in the prone position, tape it to a padded arm board, and prep it to the elbow. Clip the drapes to the armboard. Place a venous catheter on the drapes attached to a sterile syringe of saline. **A,** Identify the anatomic snuffbox; the cephalic vein will be found crossing the center of the snuffbox and over the styloid process of the radius as it runs up the lateral side of the elbow. Locate it visually or by palpation. If that is not possible, use your knowledge of local anatomy that it lies dorsal and proximal to the radial styloid. **B,** Make a short vertical (not transverse) incision, one that can be extended proximally if the vein becomes injured.

A

B

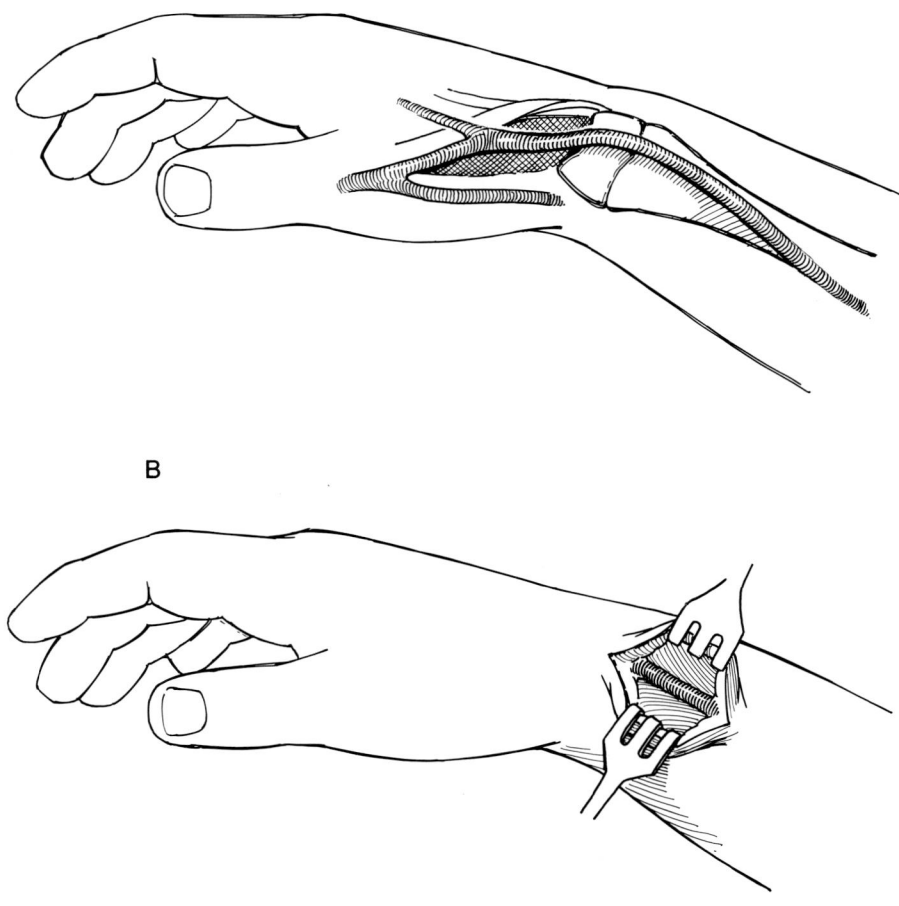

6 **A,** Grasp the vein with a fine forceps, and ligate it with a fine absorbable suture. Encircle it with a second suture proximally to aid in manipulation; it will be used to ligate the vein around the catheter before closure. **B,** Elevate the vein and cut it on a tangent with fine scissors. **C,** Insert the tips of the scissors, or use a plastic catheter introducer if the hole is too small. Grasp and insert the catheter without taking your eyes off the venotomy. Slowly infuse saline as you advance the catheter. Tie the vein over the catheter proximally with the loop suture. Close the incision with a running fine synthetic absorbable suture, and fix the catheter with sterile tape.

An alternative in infants in shock is to use the saphenous vein by prepping the groin, making a transverse incision medial to the femoral triangle and 1 to 2 cm below the inguinal ligament. Enter Scarpa's fascia and elevate the vein.

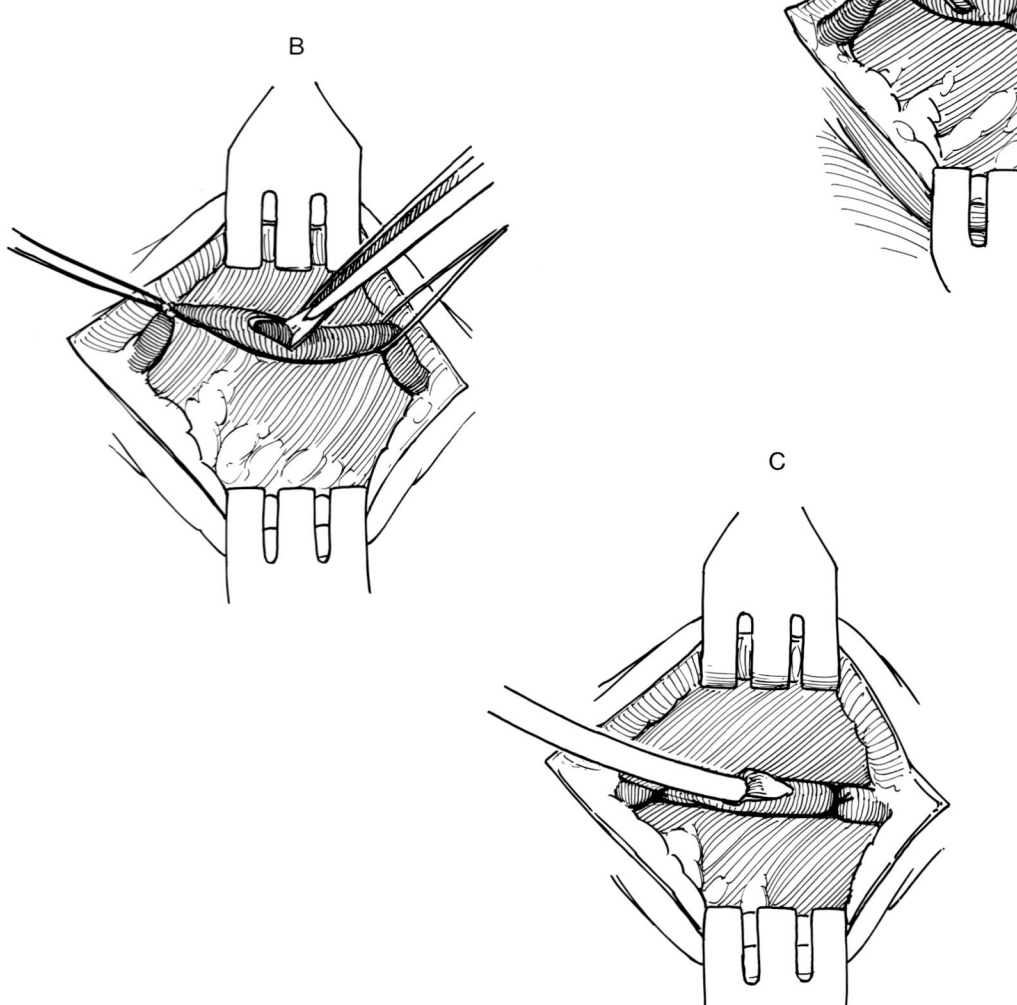

A

B

C

Commentary by Hrair-George J. Mesrobian

After consulting with my pediatric surgical colleagues, I find that we never, at least in children, place a venous catheter in the cephalic vein. Moreover, 90 percent of all central venous access is performed percutaneously. The saphenous vein cutdown is important in the hypotensive child following trauma, but even there it is rarely used.

Our preference for central venous catheter insertion is the external jugular venous system, followed by the anterior facial vein, because they have large lumina, provide a direct route to the right atrium, and are readily accessible.

Alternatives include the subcutaneous port system, which requires multiple needle punctures to reach the reservoir and thus is not easily accepted by infants and children. It is ideally suited for the adolescent who requires intermittent use and is concerned about the cosmetic appearance of an external catheter.

Finally, the percutaneous subclavian vein puncture, which does not require administration of a general anesthetic, can be performed by an interventional radiologist with perhaps a slightly higher risk of pneumothorax or arterial puncture and is an excellent alternative to the cutdown techniques of vein cannulation.

SUTURE TECHNIQUES

The objective of suturing is to approximate the tissues with the least injury to their blood supply. Use the technique most suitable for the tissue, but try to use the smallest size and the fewest different types of sutures. Tie the suture while holding it near its free end; it may thus be used twice, saving suture material and time. Tie synthetic absorbable sutures with three (or better, four) knots and monofilament nonabsorbable sutures with six or seven.

Skin

7 *Subcuticular closure*: Use a 4-0 synthetic absorbable suture (5-0 or 6-0 for children) or a pull-out suture of monofilament nonabsorbable suture material. **A,** Start the stitch with a buried knot at one end. Pull the subcutaneous tissue forward with a fine skin hook, and drive the needle point well into the dermis in a plane parallel to the surface, entering exactly opposite the exit site of the last bite. **B,** Bury the last knot with a deep stitch. Alternatively, apply absorbable interrupted sutures, burying the knots.

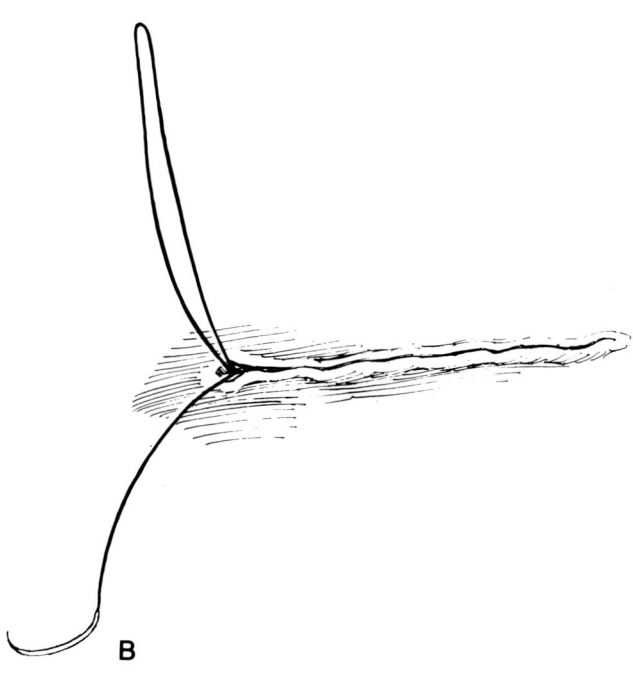

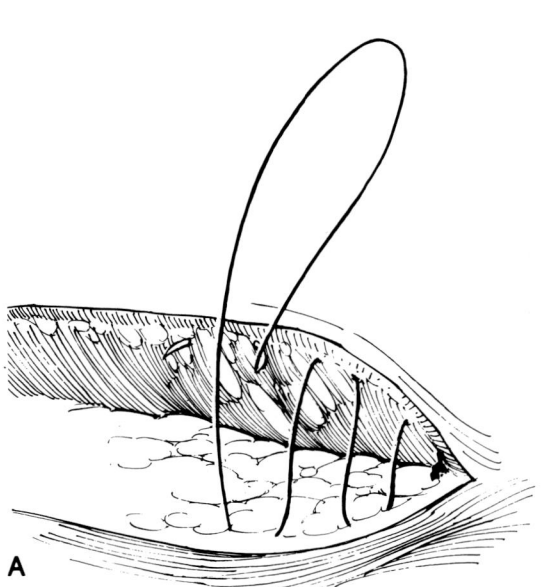

A

8 *Vertical mattress suture*: A double stitch that forms a loop about the tissue on both sides produces eversion of the skin. Use monofilament nonabsorbable sutures and catch only the very edge of the skin in the second bite. Throw four to five knots. Alternatively, use a subcuticular closure, skin staples, or tapes.

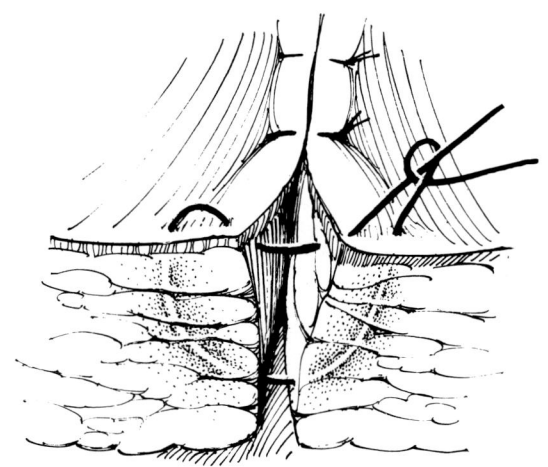

9 **A,** *Everting interrupted suture*: For plastic procedures, penetrate the skin close to the edge of the incision, then encircle a larger amount of tissue beneath. **B,** *Halsted mattress suture*: Inverts the edge.

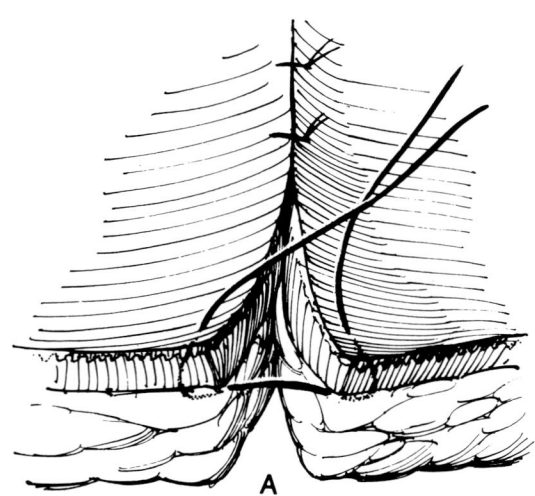

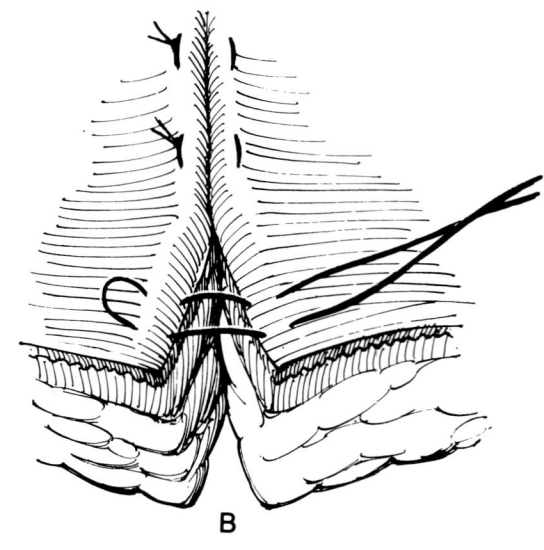

Fascia

10 *Interrupted sutures*: **A,** Place 2-0 synthetic absorbable sutures 1 cm deep and 1 cm apart. **B,** Tie them only tight enough to bring the edges in contact. Throw at least three square knots. An alternative to absorbable sutures is nonabsorbable monofilament sutures made from polypropylene. In thin adolescents and in children, be sure that the knot is buried to avoid wound discomfort.

11 *Far-and-near sutures*: Use 2-0 synthetic absorbable sutures at 1-cm intervals.

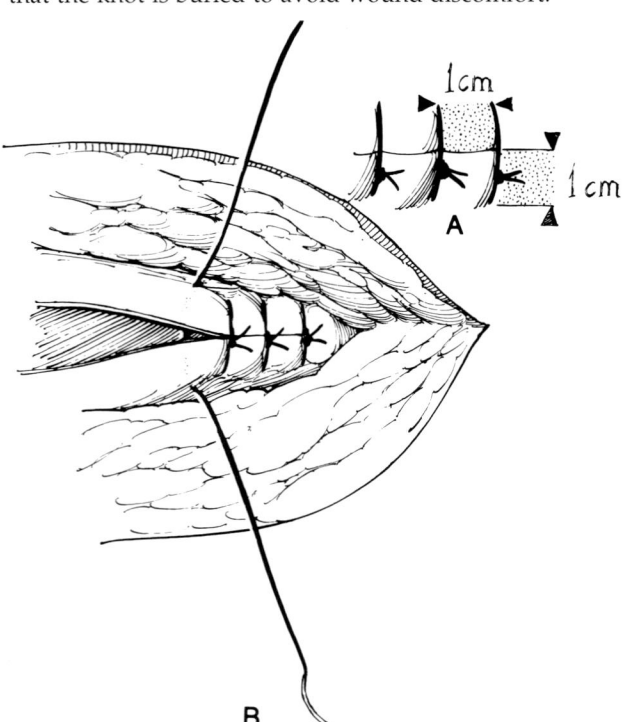

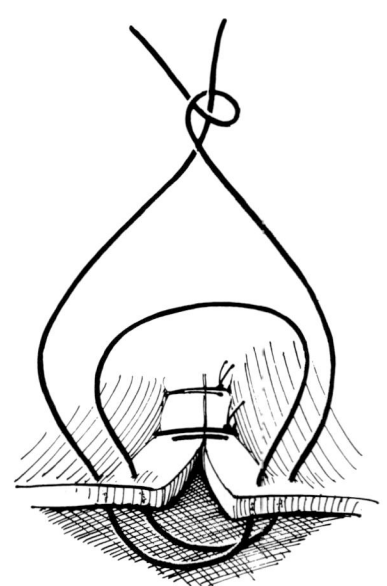

12 *Near-and-far suture for mass closure of the abdomen*: Use #2 nonabsorbable sutures.

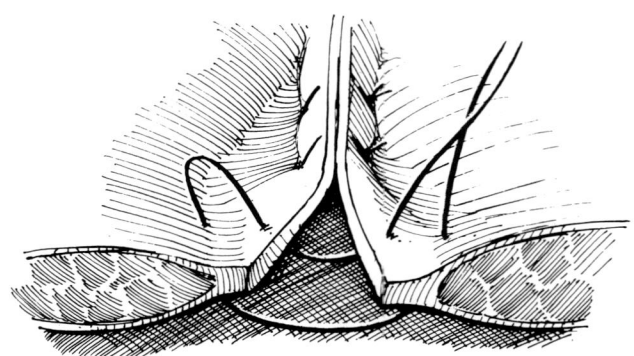

Bowel

13 *Connell suture*: A continuous suture that inverts the inner wall of the intestine. The stitch enters and exits the bowel on each side successively. It may include only the mucosa and submucosa. Use 3-0 synthetic absorbable sutures. It is an especially useful technique for closing the angles of a bowel anastomosis.

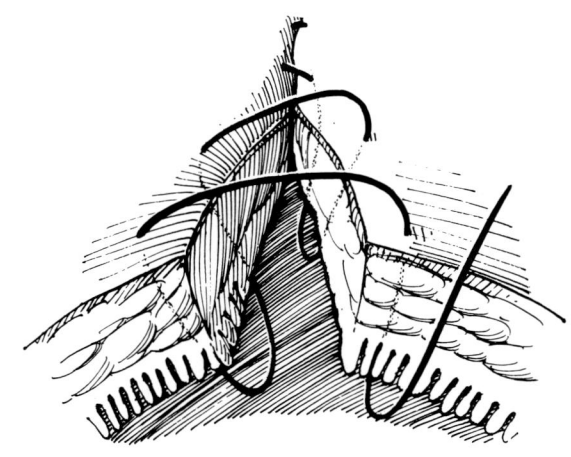

14 *Lembert suture* An inverting suture that produces serosal apposition; it includes the muscular layer. It may be interrupted (**A**) or placed continuously (**B**). It is useful for closing the end of the bowel or to anastomose two ends. Use 4-0 braided nonabsorbable sutures. Each bite should reach into but not through the tough submucosal layer. To close the end of the bowel, use interrupted Lembert sutures over a clamp, starting by placing a traction suture at each end and laying all the sutures (**C**). Remove the clamp carefully and tie each suture successively as the mucosa is inverted. For a one-layer bowel anastomosis, place interrupted Lembert sutures on both sides, then have your assistant gently withdraw the clamps and successively tie each suture, while you take care that the edge is inverted (**D**).

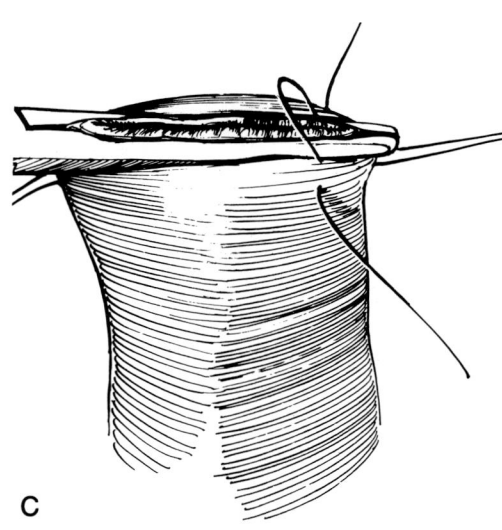

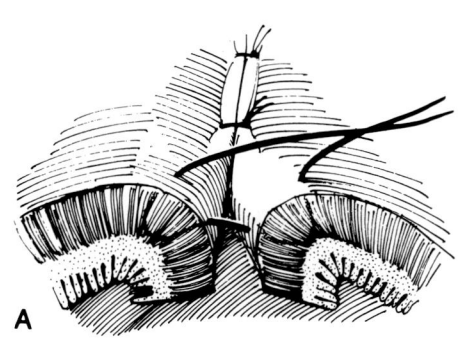

A

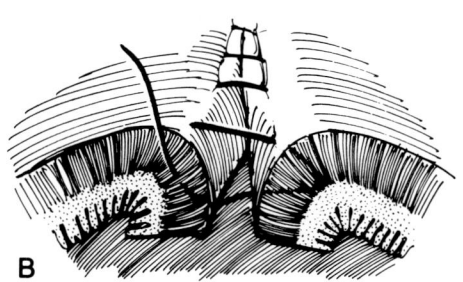

B

C

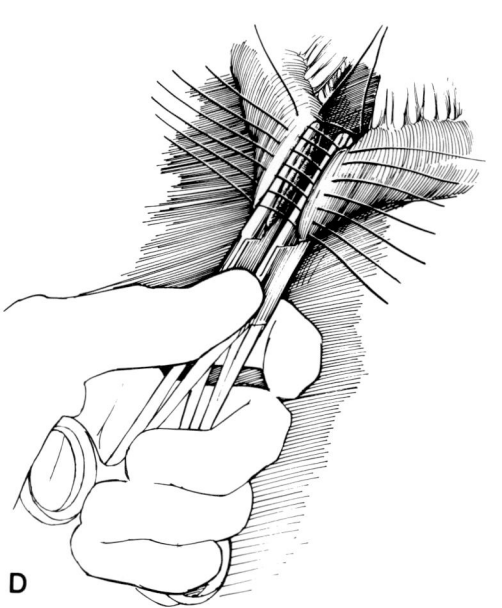

D

15 *Parker-Kerr suture*: An inverting suture that is used to close the end of the intestine. It may be laid continuously or may be interrupted. Use 4-0 nonabsorbable suture with bites taken parallel to the edge rather than across it, as in the Lembert stitch.

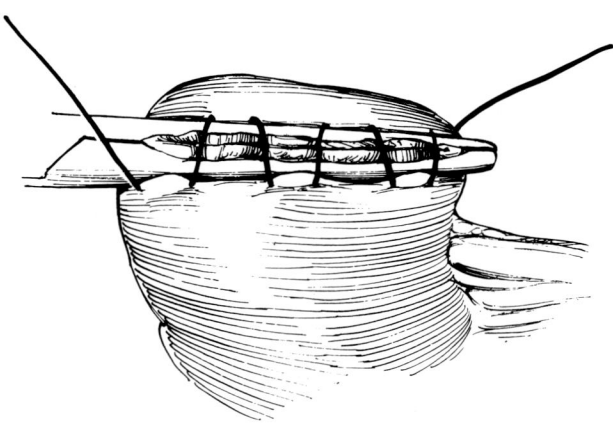

16 *Pursestring suture*: A continuous suture that is placed around a defect for inversion (appendix) or closure (hernia sac).

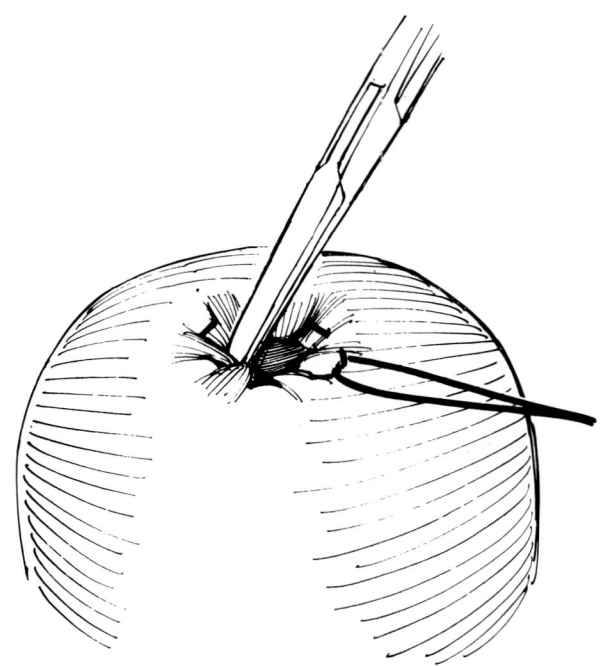

17 *Lock-stitch suture*: A continuous suture used for mucosal edges in which every third or fourth stitch is passed under the previous one. Select it when puckering is to be avoided.

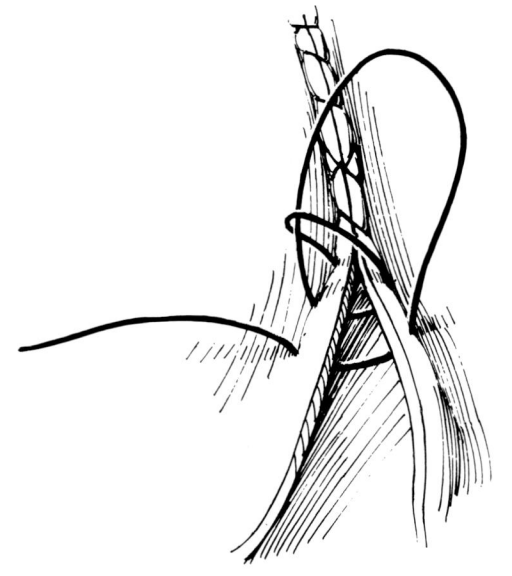

Tissue Sealer. A protein-thrombin solution (Tisseel) that produces stable fibrin on a dry raw tissue surface can be useful for small defects or leaks remaining after suturing, such as in ureteral implantation and hypospadias repair, and for fixation of an ileal intussusception in conjunction with scarification of the opposed surfaces. Two solutions are drawn into two syringes, mixed, and injected through a blunt needle onto the surfaces to be glued together.

BOWEL STAPLING TECHNIQUES

See Section 6 for application of these techniques to noncontinent and continent diversion.

Stapled anastomoses are less likely to leak than sutured ones but are more likely to bleed because they do not devascularize the margins as thoroughly. It is important to check the staple line for bleeding from both the mucosal and serosal sides, although it is not always possible to check the mucosal surface. Placement of a figure-eight stitch of 4-0 synthetic absorbable suture usually will control the bleeding.

Several autostaplers should be available: models TA 55, TA 30, EEA, and GIA.

End-to-End Anastomosis

18 Clear the mesentery from the ends of the bowel for a distance of 1 cm. Place a stay suture through the full thickness at the mesenteric and antimesenteric edges. Grasp and elevate both walls with an Allis clamp. Place the jaws of the TA 55 stapler to include the bowel beneath the Allis clamp and the stay sutures. Approximate the blades by turning the thumb screw until the black lines on them are aligned. Push the pin firmly in place. Release the safety catch and fire the staples.

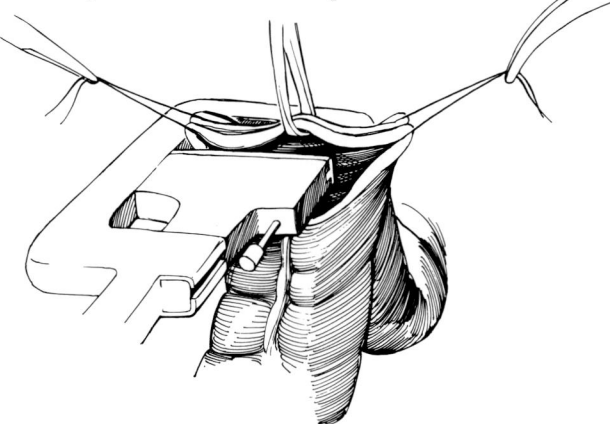

20 Insert everting stay sutures through the midpoint of both edges to triangulate the defects.

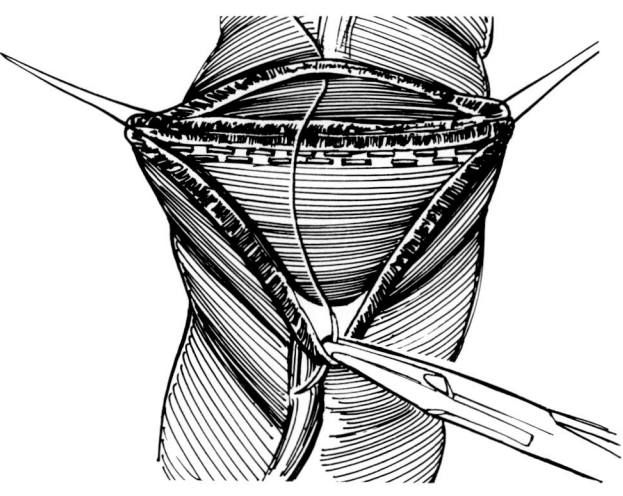

22 Staple the remaining half similarly, being sure that the rows overlap both in the center and at the angle. Shave the excess bowel. Check the anastomosis visually to be certain no gaps remain. Cut the stay sutures and close the mesenteric defect. *Alternatively,* triangulate the bowel with three everting stay sutures, staple the mesenteric border first, and then close the other two sides of the triangle. Take care not to catch the back wall, and be sure to incorporate the end of the previous line of staples. Check the staple line for bleeding, and place a figure-eight stitch, if necessary.

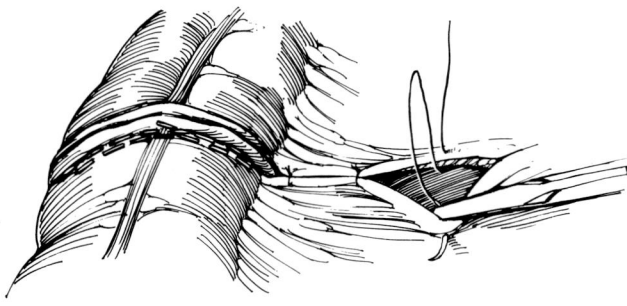

19 Shave off the excess bowel wall with a knife. Cut as close as possible to the anvil and cartridge to prevent retention of necrotic tissue.

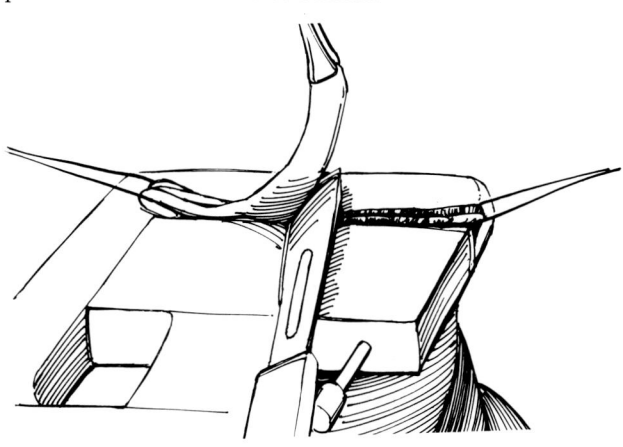

21 Place half the remaining edge in the TA 30 stapler. Be certain to overlap the original row of staples at the angle. Push the pin in place and fire the staples. Trim the excess bowel wall, but preserve the central suture. Reinforce the mucosal edges with figure-eight sutures at any bleeding sites.

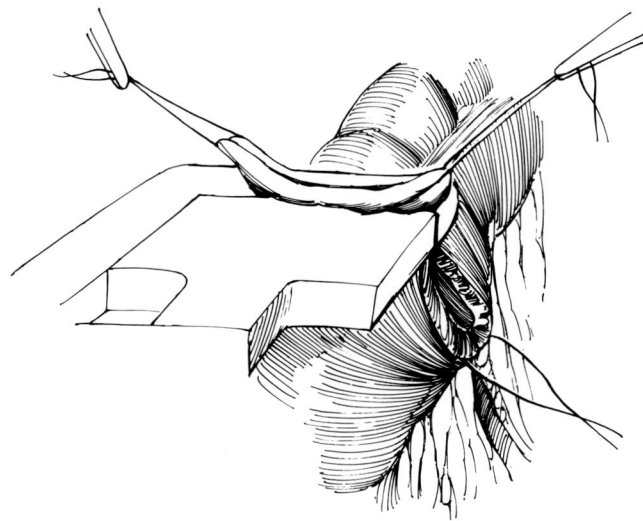

End-to-Side Anastomosis of Ileum to Ascending Colon

23 Make a window in the antimesenteric border of the ascending colon 3 cm from the open end. Through it insert the EEA stapler into the ileum and clamp the stapler. After firing and removing the stapler, check the anvil to be sure the tissue button is complete. Hemostasis only can be checked and sutured with horizontal, inverting mattress suture of 4-0 silk from the serosal side.

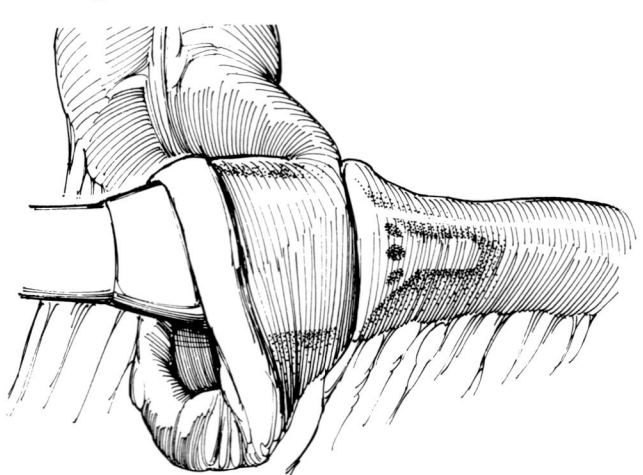

24 To close the end of the colon, place two stay sutures in the mesenteric and antimesenteric borders. Apply the TA 55 stapler proximal to them. Turn the thumbscrew clockwise to approximate the blades so that the black lines are aligned. Release the safety catch and clamp the handles. Trim the excess and close the mesentery. Reinforce the mucosal edges with figure-eight sutures at any bleeding sites. Check for viability because the blood supply may be attenuated here. This same closure technique can be used for the ileum.

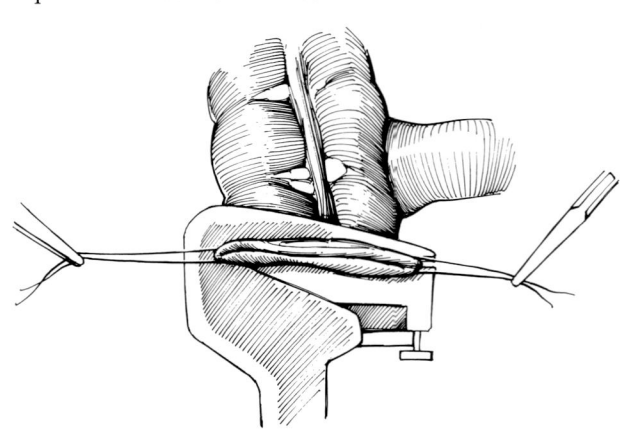

Side-to-Side Anastomosis of Ileum

25 **A,** Clear the mesentery from the distal ends of the bowel for a distance equal to the length of the limbs of the GIA stapler. Place stay sutures in the mesenteric and antimesenteric edges of both ends of the bowel to maintain alignment. Insert the limbs of the GIA stapler so that they lie in line with the mesentery. Lock the stapler together, and push the driver that inserts the staples and activates the knife. **B,** Remove the driver, unlock the limbs, and remove the stapler. Check for viability of the distal mucosa and for hemostasis. Reinforce the serosal edges with horizontal, inverting mattress sutures of 4-0 silk as required.

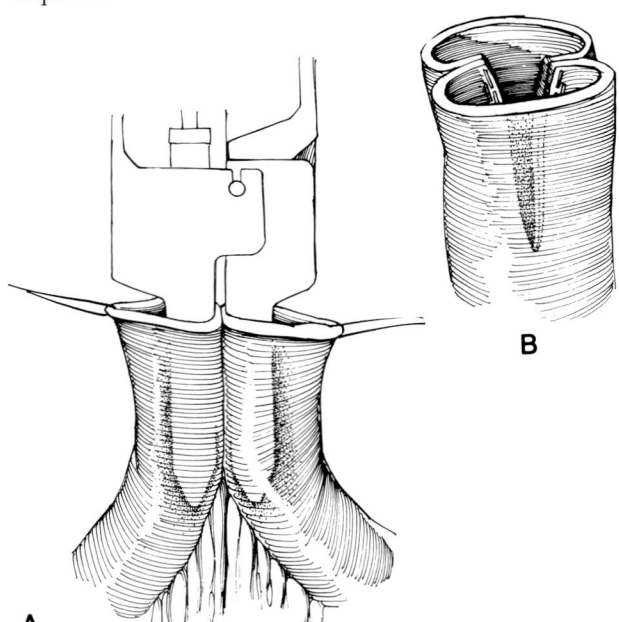

26 Apply the TA 55 stapler to each side of the common opening, as described in "End-to-End Anastomosis." Check for viability, because the blood supply may be attenuated here. Close the mesentery.

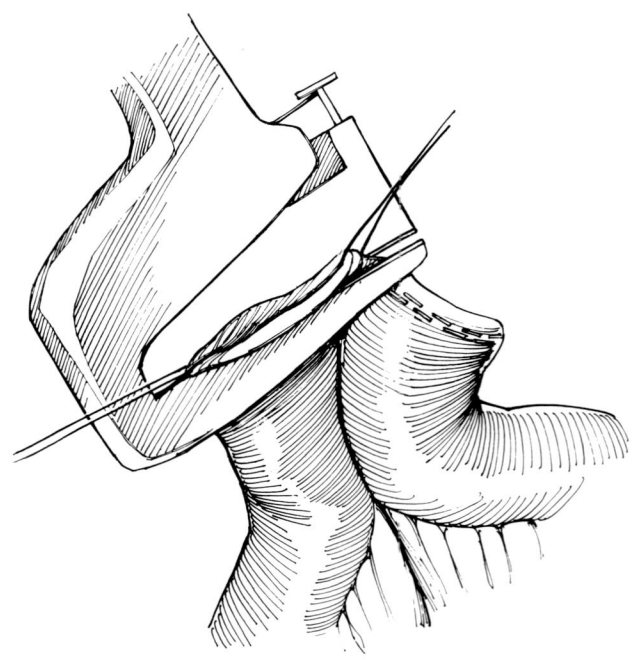

Formation of an Ileal Conduit

27 Select a segment of ileum and divide the mesentery. Place the GIA stapler at the appropriate site and push the lever home, placing two rows of staples and dividing the bowel between. Repeat the procedure at the other side.

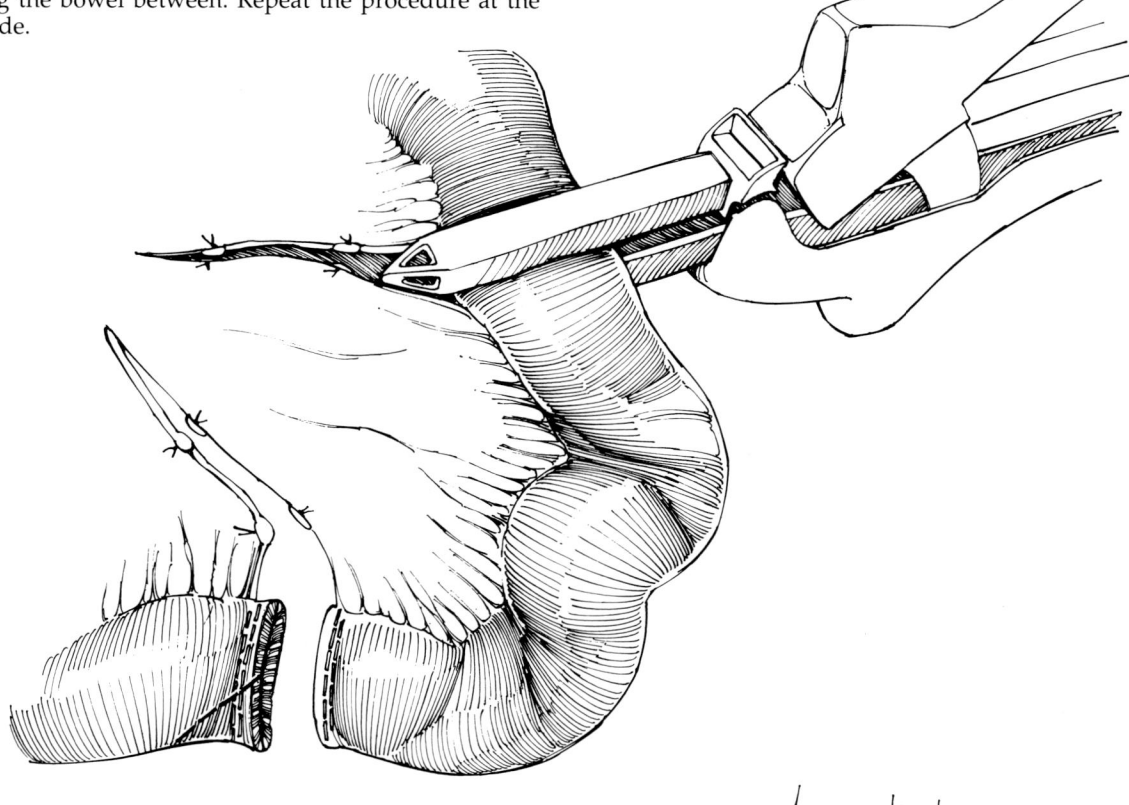

28 For ileal reanastomosis, trim the antimesenteric corner from both staple lines. Rotate the bowel 180 degrees, and insert a blade of the GIA stapler all the way into each lumen. Connect the blade's handles together and push the lever to make two rows of sutures with an opening between. Check the serosal side of the staple lines for hemostasis, and reinforce with horizontal, inverting mattress sutures of 4-0 silk as needed.

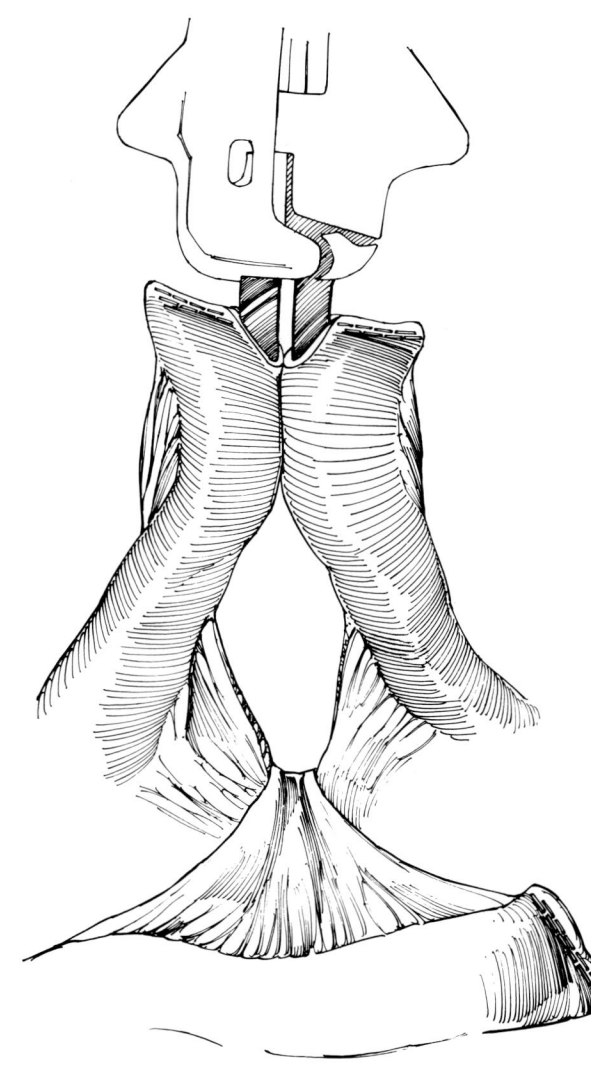

29 Place a stay suture at the end of each row of staples. Then apply the TA 30 stapler over the remaining opening to overlap the original rows of staples; drive in the staples. Close the mesentery.

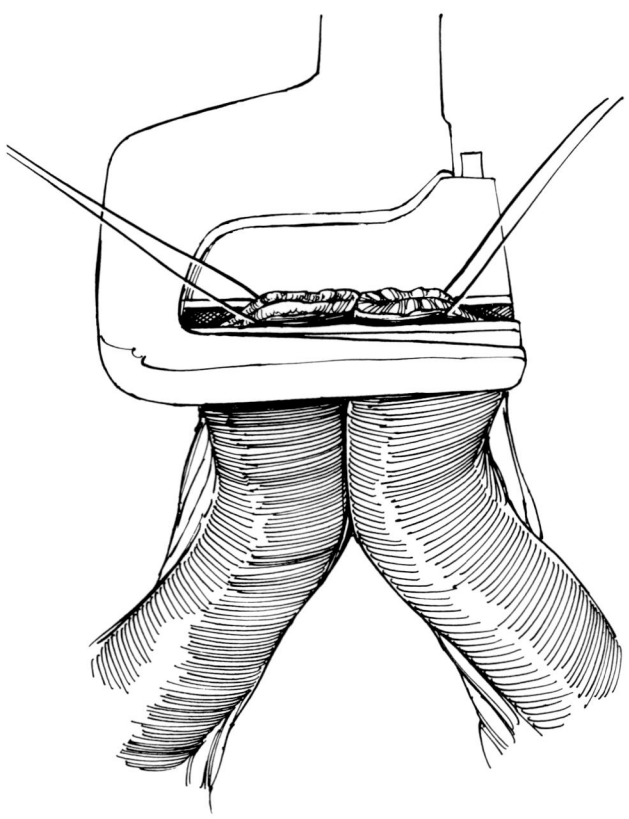

30 Complete the procedure by anastomosing the ureters to the loop, drawing the distal end of the bowel through the abdominal wall, trimming the end proximal to the staples, and suturing the edge to the skin. Check for hemostasis on the serosal surface and reinforce it with horizontal, inverting mattress suture of 4-0 silk.

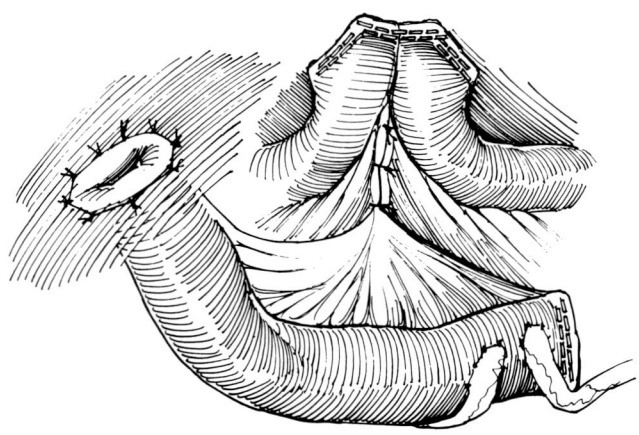

MICROVASCULAR SURGICAL TECHNIQUES

Instruments. Wear a 2.5× surgical loupe in conjunction with a headlight to expose the vessels before using the operating microscope. For sutures, use 10-0 monofilament nylon on a triangular cutting needle. Provide a nonlocking spring-handle needle holder with a curved tip long enough to fit in the hand like a pen, a #5 jeweler's forceps for vascular work (be sure the tips are aligned), both sharp-tipped and blunt-tipped slightly curved scissors, nontraumatic vascular clamps (both straight and curved, which may be mounted on a bar), bipolar coagulator using low power, microsurgical sponges, a suction tip (3 F), a 30-gauge blunt-angled needle for delivery of heparin-saline irrigating solution, and plastic background material.

Arterial Anastomosis

For arteries with diameters less than 2 mm, use the operating room microscope. Have your assistant sitting opposite. For larger vessels, a three-power or four-power loupe is adequate.

Dissect the severed ends of the arteries adequately in both directions. Coagulate any fine branches with the bipolar current, and divide them 1 mm away from the vessel. Place a piece of blue background material behind the vessel. Looking through the microscope or loupe, carefully remove the perivascular connective tissue. Reverse vasospasm with a few drops of 1 percent lidocaine, and then keep the vessel moist with warm saline solution. Apply the fixed arm of the vascular clamp to the less mobile end of the vessel, then move the other arm to grasp the more mobile end, leaving the arms approximately 1 cm apart.

31 Cut the end of the vessel cleanly across. Pick up the adventitia at the cut end and tease it out over the end in several places to form a stocking (circumcision technique). Trim this flush with the end of the vessel. Even a small tag projecting into the lumen can initiate a thrombus. Alternatively, carefully lift the adventitia from the vessel wall, and trim it with the microscissors. Be careful when cleaning the adventitia of small delicate vessels not to be too thorough and injure the vessel. Irrigate the lumen with heparinized saline to clear it of blood.

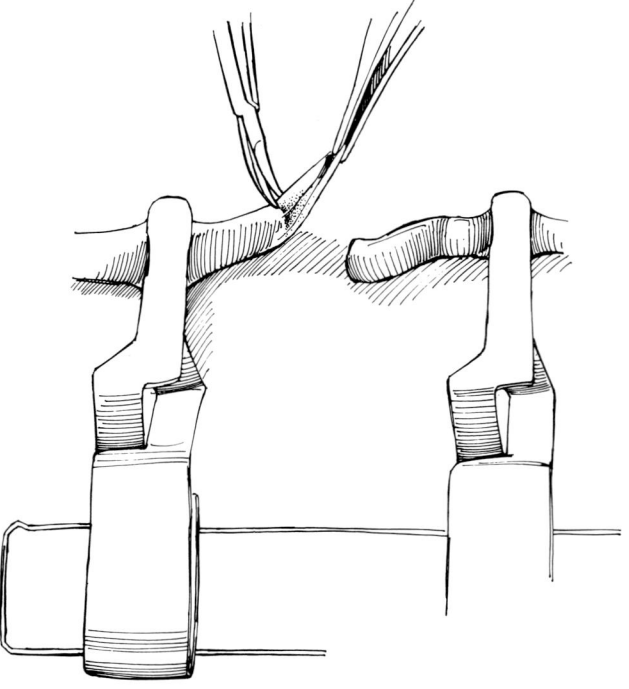

32 Dilate the lumen with a #5 jeweler's forceps. Repeat these steps on the opposite stump, and bring the two ends together to lie approximately one vessel diameter apart by adjusting the movable arm.

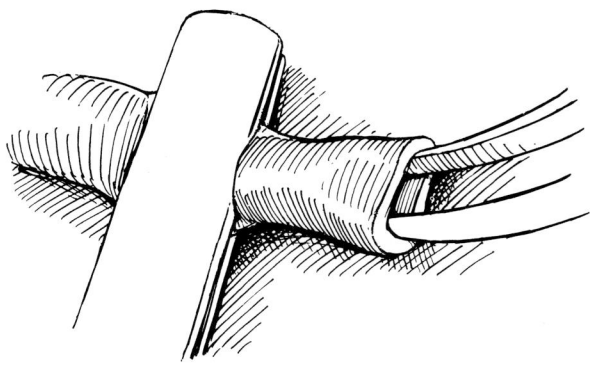

33 Place the first guide suture (G1) of monofilament nylon through the vessel edge on the right at 10 o'clock. Grasp the needle again, pass it through the vessel to the left, and pull it until only 3 or 4 mm remain free. Tie it with a double-throw (surgeon's) knot, then with two square single-throw knots. Cut the short end near the knot, then cut the long end to a length of 1.5 cm. For small vessels, use 25× magnification for placing the sutures and 16× for tying.

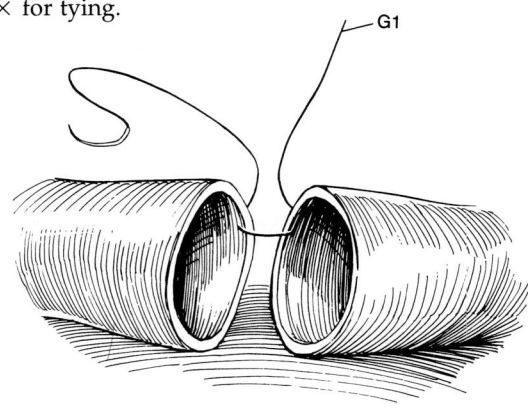

34 Have your assistant put slight traction on the first suture (G1). Place the second guide suture (G2) one third of the way around; tie and cut it in the same way as described in the previous step.

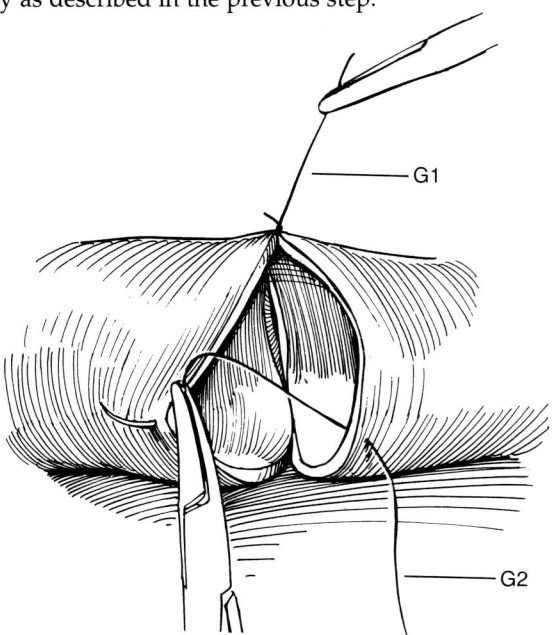

35 Place one or two approximating sutures (A1) between the guide sutures (G1, G2); use a single-throw technique and cut both ends of the suture.

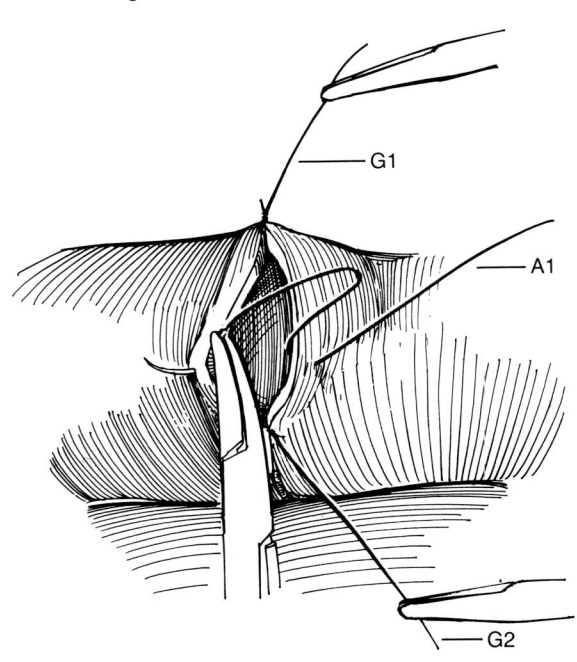

36 Invert the vessel and its holder, and inspect the interior for defects in the anterior suture line. Place the third guide suture (G3) equidistant from the other two (G1, G2).

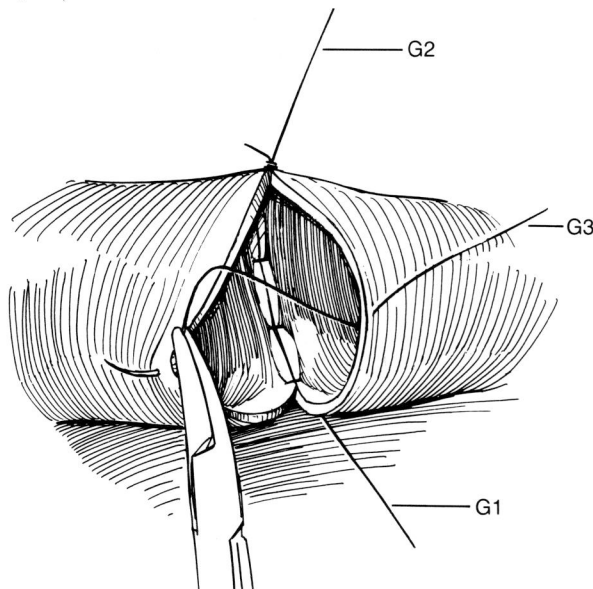

37 Insert one or two approximating sutures between G1 and G3 and between G2 and G3, having the assistant manipulate the guide sutures appropriately.

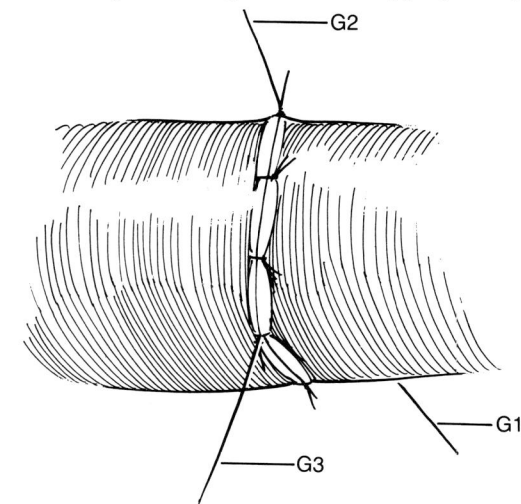

38 Remove the distal clamp first, and be sure that reverse blood flow fills the entire segment immediately; otherwise, the anastomosis must be revised. If it fills slowly, apply papaverine solution to release any factor of spasm. Release the proximal clamp and observe for pulsation beyond the repair. Irrigate away any blood that leaks out to prevent initiation of a thrombus and to avoid spasm. If there is a leak, it is wise to replace the clamps and place a suture at the point to get a watertight seal. Doppler ultrasound may be helpful in assessing flow in doubtful cases.

Pulsation alone does not mean that the anastomosis is open. In very small vessels in which the flow cannot be visualized, perform a patency test 20 minutes after completing the anastomosis by gently pressing the blood from a segment of vessel just below the anastomosis and ascertaining that it rapidly refills when the more proximal forceps is released. Be careful not to injure the intima by too much force. Do not hesitate to do the anastomosis again if you are concerned about a technical detail, because even a small error can result in failure.

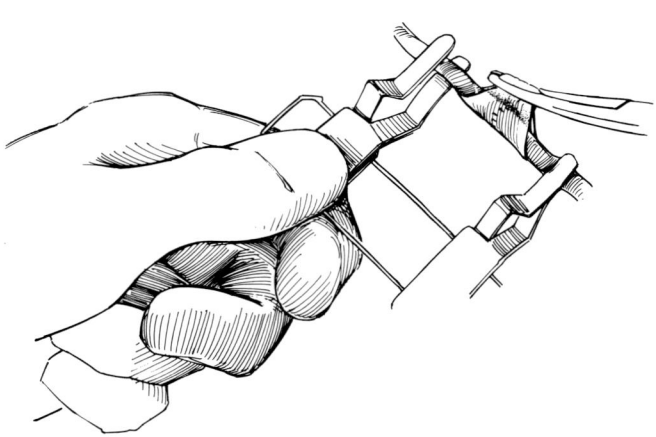

Venous Anastomosis

Dissect a small vein with round-tipped microscissors to avoid damage to the media or inadvertent puncture. Avoid grasping the vein with a forceps. Use maximum illumination. Place the vessel clamp arm on the body side first to avoid overstretching the vein. Clear the periadventitial tissue carefully with two pairs of #5 jeweler's forceps, working longitudinally. To see the lumen, float the walls open with saline irrigation. This must be done with each stitch to keep from catching the opposite wall. The technique of suturing is the same as that for small arteries but requires constant visualization of the vessel wall and the tip of the needle to prevent incorporation of the opposite wall. Wrapping is not necessary. Release the proximal clamp, then the distal clamp, and perform a patency test.

SELECTION OF STENT

39 *Double pigtail*: Select a stent of the proper length and of the largest caliber that will fit easily inside the ureter without stretching it. Provide low-dose antibiotic coverage. For *intraoperative insertion*, length can be determined by passing a calibrated ureteral catheter to the renal pelvis and the bladder, adding the measured lengths together. Aspiration and irrigation may be used to prove that the tip of the catheter is in the pelvic and vesical lumina. To place the stent, cut an extra hole in its midportion or gently enlarge a drainage hole with a mosquito clamp. Insert the guide wire or stilet to straighten the curve. Feed the stent into the renal pelvis and remove the wire. Repeat the process for passage to the bladder.

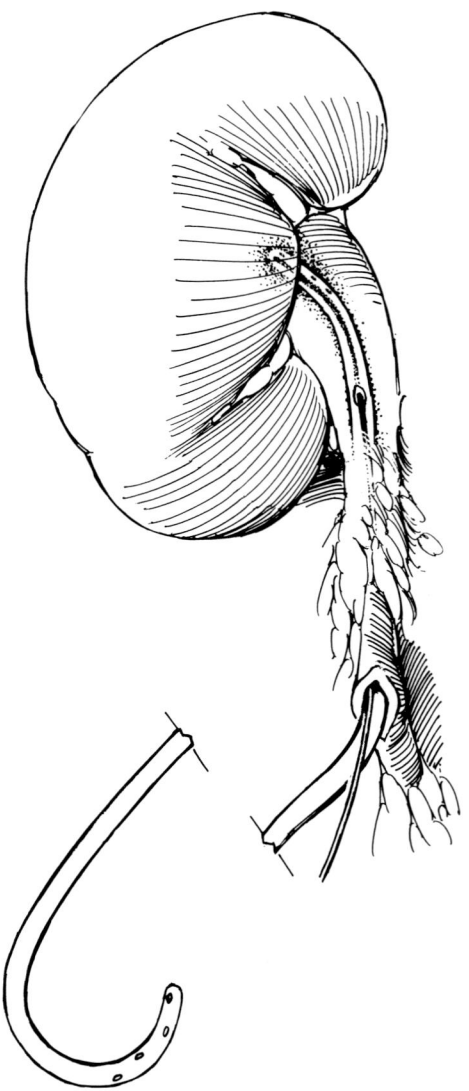

Alternatively, place the stent on two guide wires. Pass one wire into the bladder, and feed the stent over it; do the same for the renal end. For easy early removal in boys, make a small opening in the bladder, grasp the tip of the balloon catheter, and tie the stent to it. Close the cystostomy in two layers. In girls, tie a long suture to the catheter, draw it out of the meatus, and fasten it to the labia. Close the ureterotomy, and drain the area or proceed with ureteral anastomosis if the ureter has been divided.

If the stent is to remain long term, check its position occasionally by roentgenography and follow with regular urine cultures and serum creatinine determinations to detect obstruction. In a child at risk for stone formation, change the stent at least every 6 weeks. When removing a stent, do not try to pull it out with a sharp forceps; it may shear the stent off.

40 *Silicone-rubber T tube*: After measurement, trim the proximal end of the T to the proper length to reach the renal pelvis. Cut several extra holes in the end. Remove a V-shaped segment from the T tube opposite the junction with the stem to aid later removal. Pull on the stem to test its strength. Insert the T tube through a 1.5-cm ureterotomy below the defect, passing one limb up the ureter and the other down. Close the ureterotomy loosely with a single 4-0 synthetic absorbable suture. Bring the stem retroperitoneally, then out through a stab wound. Fasten it to the skin with a 3-0 silk suture.

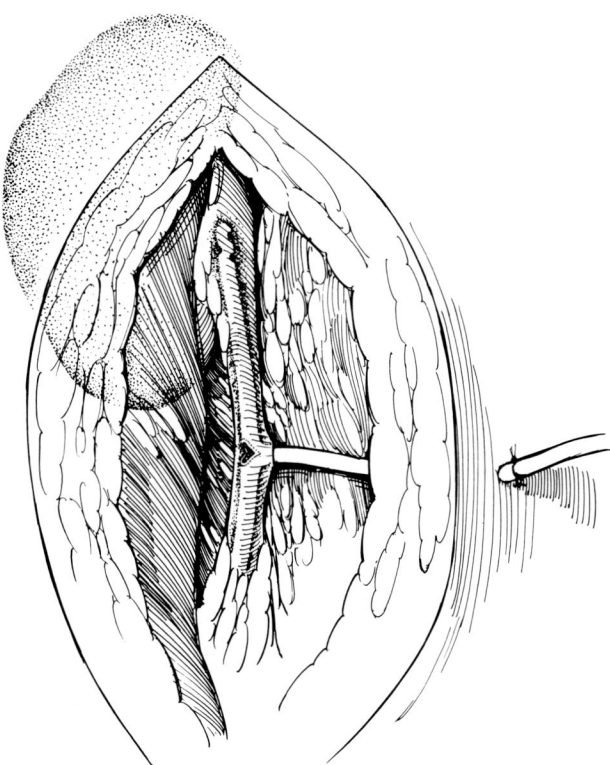

41 *Straight tubing*: Use clear silicone-rubber tubing (5 to 10 F) or an infant feeding tube (5 and 8 F) with extra holes. Silicone-rubber tubing is more pliable, thinner walled, and better utilized in smaller sizes, and it is considerably less expensive than J-shaped stents. Insert the tubing through a short ureterotomy below the site of the defect, and pass one end of the measured distance to the renal pelvis and the other to the bladder. Control displacement with a clamp placed loosely on the stent at the site of entry. Fasten the stent to the ureteral wall. **A,** Run a 5-0 plain catgut suture (for shorter stay) or a 5-0 synthetic absorbable suture (for longer stay) directly through the walls of the ureter and the walls of the stent and tie it loosely on top of the ureter. **B,** Alternatively, use a 2-0 nonabsorbable suture placed as in panel A but bring both ends to the skin over a button. Later, cut the suture flush with the skin, and withdraw both the stent and suture through the bladder.

An alternate technique: Pass the tubing with extra holes through the ureterotomy below the defect and up to the renal pelvis. Tack it to the exit site with a 4-0 absorbable suture through the ureteral edge tied around the tubing. Bring the stent retroperitoneally and out through a stab wound. If a stent is used with a nephrostomy, as in pediatric pyeloplasty, pass a length of fine-caliber silicone rubber tubing through a 10 F Silastic balloon catheter with the tip cut off and fasten them together with a nonabsorbable suture.

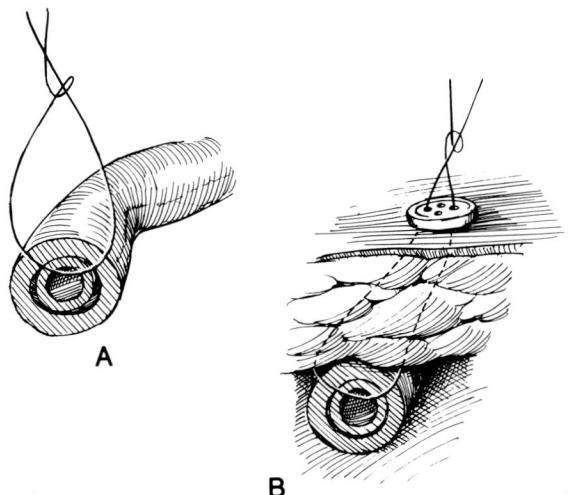

42 *Stents for ureteroureterostomy* (page 247): Place a stent unless the ureters are of good caliber and vascularity with no suspected constriction or tension at the anastomosis. Before completing the anastomosis, select the largest-caliber silicone-rubber tubing, infant feeding tube, or pigtail catheter that will fit loosely in the normal ureter. Measure the distance to the donor pelvis and to the bladder with a 5 F ureteral catheter. If a feeding or silicone-rubber tube is used, cut holes in it at 1-cm intervals and mark it with a removable suture at the length required to reach the pelvis. Cut the other end at the length needed to reach the bladder, but add 3 cm so that it can be retrieved transvesically. Pass it up the donor ureter to the pelvis and down into the bladder. Fix it in place with a 5-0 chromic catgut suture through the edge of the ureteral wall and through the tubing, tied loosely. Complete the anastomosis. If the recipient ureter is large, pass a second stent up and down it, as described previously for the pigtail and straight catheters. Cystoscopic removal of stents can be done utilizing local anesthesia and a flexible nephroscope, through which a ureteral catheter containing a loop of nylon is passed to snare the exposed end of the stent.

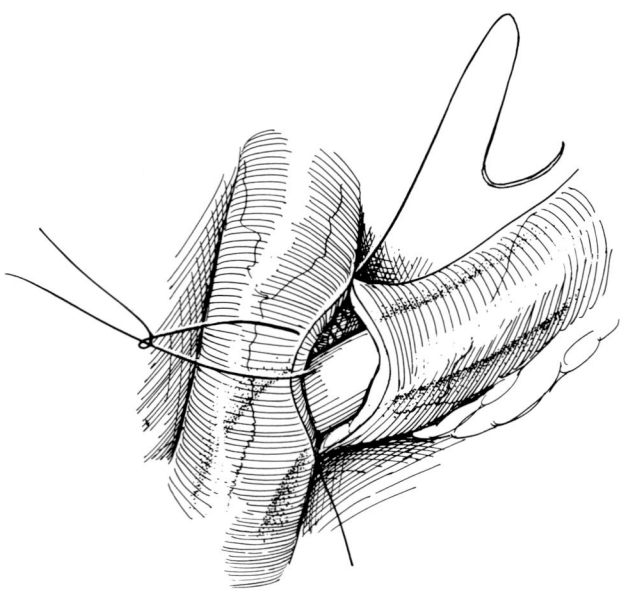

Problems Associated With Stents

Dysuria; urinary frequency, and nocturia are common, especially early after placement. Give antispasmodic drugs and wait for subsidence of the symptoms. *Flank pain* or pain in the lower abdomen is a frequent complaint. *Reflux* sometimes results in flank pain during micturition but is buffered by leakage of urine through the side holes. *Urinary tract infections* may intervene less frequently if prophylactic antibiotics are given, especially in girls, but these carry the risk of selecting for resistant organisms. Check the urine by culture at semimonthly intervals. If results are positive and antibacterial therapy does not eradicate the infection, change the stent and again provide antibiotics.

Severe complications can evolve silently. *Obstruction* is a common and serious sequela, usually occurring 2 months after insertion. Regularly scheduled replacement is a good practice in a child who forms stones. For others, checking every month by roent-genography and serum creatinine level determinations may be adequate. A program of regular replacement every 6 to 8 weeks may be safest, but the interval must be tailored to the conditions of the individual child, who in turn (with the parents) must be kept informed of the need for follow-up. *Stent migration* toward the bladder arises if the initial placement was faulty or if the proximal end of a J stent loses its curvature. *Breakage* of a stent occurs with acute angulation during traction or from cutting the stent with the grasping (biopsy) forceps. If a stent is not easily withdrawn, do not pull on it but try again in 24 hours. Sometimes weak rubber-band traction will withdraw a recalcitrant stent. *Fragmentation* can occur in stents left in place over several months. Both these types of accidents require cystoscopic, ureteroscopic, or percutaneous retrieval.

A *blocked Foley balloon catheter* may be managed by injecting mineral oil or running a wire into the inflation port, by hyperinflation, or by percutaneous puncture.

Management of Intraoperative Injury to the Ureter

Ureteral injury during a difficult abdominal operation is less likely to occur if the ureters are stented at the beginning. A plugged balloon catheter in the bladder will allow detection of hematuria if ureteral catheters are not placed. Cross-clamping the ureter *in situ* for an appreciable length of time should be treated with insertion of a double-J stent for at least 10 days, but if the ureter already has been isolated, resection and anastomosis are advisable, accompanied by insertion of a Penrose drain (page 20). Inadvertent ligation of a ureter, even if recognized immediately, usually warrants ureteral stenting. If the involved segment is obviously ischemic, it is better to excise and anastomose it. Should the ureter be cauterized, inspect it for damage to the adventitial vessels. Such ischemic tissue must be excised. A severed ureter requires spatulation and anastomosis over a stent, but avulsion or extensive damage makes use of a psoas hitch (page 236) or bladder flap (page 240) necessary. Ureteral injury is suspected postoperatively from (1) the presence of flank pain and tenderness in the costovertebral angle, (2) low-grade fever, and (3) ileus. Ultrasonography and urography may reveal the site and extent. Retrograde passage of a double-J stent should be tried first, with or without a guide wire. Percutaneous nephrostomy is an alternative to await the dissolution of obstructing absorbable sutures. If the patient is in good condition, consider immediate surgical correction.

PLASTIC SURGICAL TECHNIQUES

Skin grafts and flaps are viscoelastic. A pull for 10 or 15 minutes will enlarge a flap, because of stress relaxation and creep. However, a compromise must be made between tension and vascularity.

Blood is supplied to the skin through either (1) a longitudinal artery lying deep to the muscle that supplies perforators to the subdermal and dermal plexus in the overlying skin, or (2) longitudinal vessels lying superficial to the muscle that connects directly to the plexus in the skin, beneath the dermis, or in the periadnexal dermis. These channels are extremely delicate and cannot withstand compression in forceps. Skin hooks and stay sutures are essential tools.

Important Grafting Concepts

Grafts for the first 24 hours pick up nutrients from the bed, then during the next 2 days establish vascular connections. Thus, the graft must remain immobilized and closely applied to the bed, which in turn must be well vascularized. Seromas or hematomas block these steps, as do infection and scar tissue. Full-thickness grafts are made up of all skin layers and must be cleared of underlying fatty tissue before application. They contract only 15 to 25 percent and provide durable skin covering. However, because of fewer vessels available for vascularization, they have a greater incidence of failure to take. Split-thickness skin grafts, composed of only part of the dermis along with the epidermis, will take better but do provide a more fragile covering. They contract approximately 50 percent or more in loose areas. Dermal grafts, free of epidermis, are more elastic and can become vascularized on both sides. If skin is not available, grafts of bladder epithelium can be used for urethral construction.

Flaps, in contrast to grafts, bring their own blood supply with them. They also can be attached directly to a new supply by microvascular techniques. They may be peninsular or random flaps, without special orientation of the blood supply; these require a 1:1 ratio between base and flap. An axial flap has an organized, self-contained blood supply and may be used as a free flap with microvascular anastomosis. An island flap is a form of axial flap that has dangling blood vessels. A pedicle flap is actually a misnomer because pedicle and flap mean the same thing. A musculocutaneous flap results from elevating skin and muscle together.

The deep surface of a cutaneous flap is composed of fat; a fasciocutaneous flap, fascia; and a muscle flap, muscle. Flaps are used simply for cover or are used for structure and revascularization (muscle), sensation (fasciocutaneous flaps), and function (muscle).

Choose a flap with size and ability to arc into place, with adequate vasculature, accessibility, and proper composition, and an acceptable donor site remaining. Outline the defect to be grafted with a marking pen, then quickly press a piece of glove-wrap paper against it to obtain a pattern for the graft.

Split-thickness grafts cut with an electrical dermatome may be thin (0.08 to 0.10 in), medium (approximately 0.18 in), or thick (over 0.18 in). For a medium-thickness graft, put two thirds of the bevel of a #15 knife between the blade and the cutting block. Meshing the graft in a cutter will provide greater coverage and allow escape of serum and blood; however, the graft will contract more. These grafts must be placed with good hemostasis, be free of contamination, and be immobilized. Mesh grafts are placed with the slits parallel to the skin line. They can be expected to contract 30 to 60 percent, except on the back of the hand, on the scrotum, and on the penis.

Stretch the graft in place to overcome the elastic fibers in the skin. Secondary contraction occurs with maturation of the scar tissue, lying between the skin graft and its bed, beginning after the 10th day and continuing for 6 months. Thin grafts, flexible beds, and complete take of grafts all reduce the chances for contraction. Skin grafts require good contact with the recipient bed. Tension, fluid beneath, and movement eliminate adherence by preventing capillary revascularization.

Avoid suture marks in the skin that result from tension. Tie the suture just tight enough to approximate the edges and no tighter. Subcutaneous sutures reduce the tension, as does placing the incision parallel to the skin lines. The length of time the sutures remain is also a factor; 6 or 7 days are usually adequate, but allow 10 to 14 days on the back. Small bites of tissue close to the edge are associated with less-apparent skin marks; infection is accompanied by more prominent ones. Of course, a patient prone to keloid formation is at greatest risk.

Slight eversion of the skin edges results in a flat scar; inverted edges leave a depressed scar. In some areas, a vertical mattress suture (page 29) is necessary to stabilize the skin edges. If skin clips are used, they should grasp the skin with equal bites and should be angled so that they slightly evert the skin. Microporous skin tape, used in conjunction with buried sutures, may be placed initially as primary skin closure or applied at the time of suture or clip removal. It helps to wipe the skin with alcohol or acetone before application. Skin tapes have the advantages of quick application and prevention of suture marks, and they do provide better tensile strength. Their disadvantages are that they do not evert the skin edges and may come off prematurely.

Sensation returns to a graft beginning in 3 weeks if dense scarring does not occur. Skin grafts and flaps grow as the patient grows, stimulated by tension from the surrounding skin.

For local anesthesia in adults, use 1 percent lidocaine with 1:200,000 epinephrine; for a child, use 0.5 percent lidocaine with 1:400,000 epinephrine. Hyaluronidase may aid in diffusion of the agents. Inject it slowly while explaining the procedure to the child. Stop for a minute if the injection is causing pain. Regional block often may be better than local infiltration.

43 Use Langer's lines of minimal tension along skin folds by making incisions parallel to them to avoid contracture and formation of keloids.

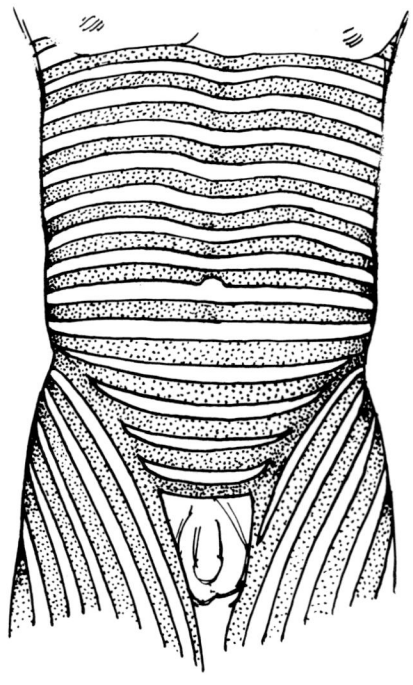

Z-Plasty
(Horner)

44 **A,** Incise along the length of the scar. Make a cut at a 30-, 45-, or 60-degree angle at each end of this incision. The gain in length will be 25 percent, 50 percent, and 75 percent, respectively. The length of these two incisions should be the same as that of the vertical incision, and they should lie along the lines of minimal tension (Langer's lines). **B,** Mobilize the two triangular flaps. **C,** Move one flap (a) down and the other (b) up, and suture them in place. Expect an almost two-fold increase in length.

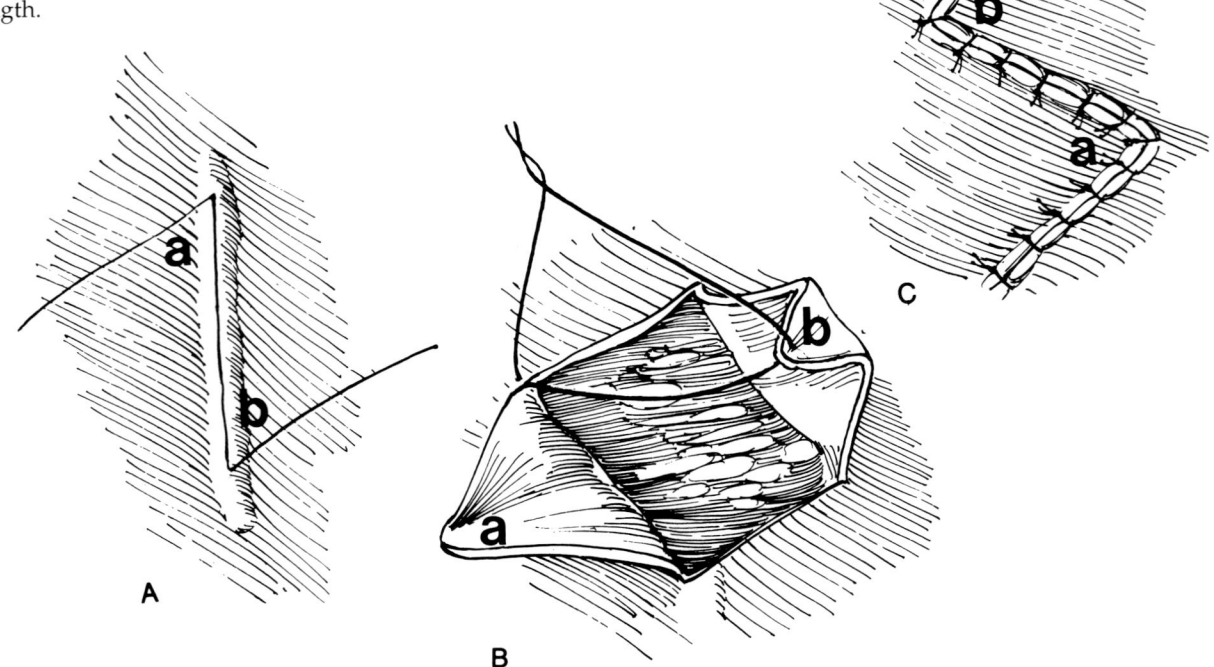

Four-Flap Z-Plasty
(Berger)

45 **A,** Make the usual vertical incision and the two incisions angled at 60 degrees as done for the Z-plasty. Make two more incisions at 60-degree angles in the opposite direction. **B,** Move the two triangular flaps on the left (a and b) down and the two on the right (c and d) up. **C,** Suture them in place.

V-Y Advancement

46 **A,** Mark and cut a V in the line of tension. **B,** Lift the flap. **C,** Close the limb of the Y first.

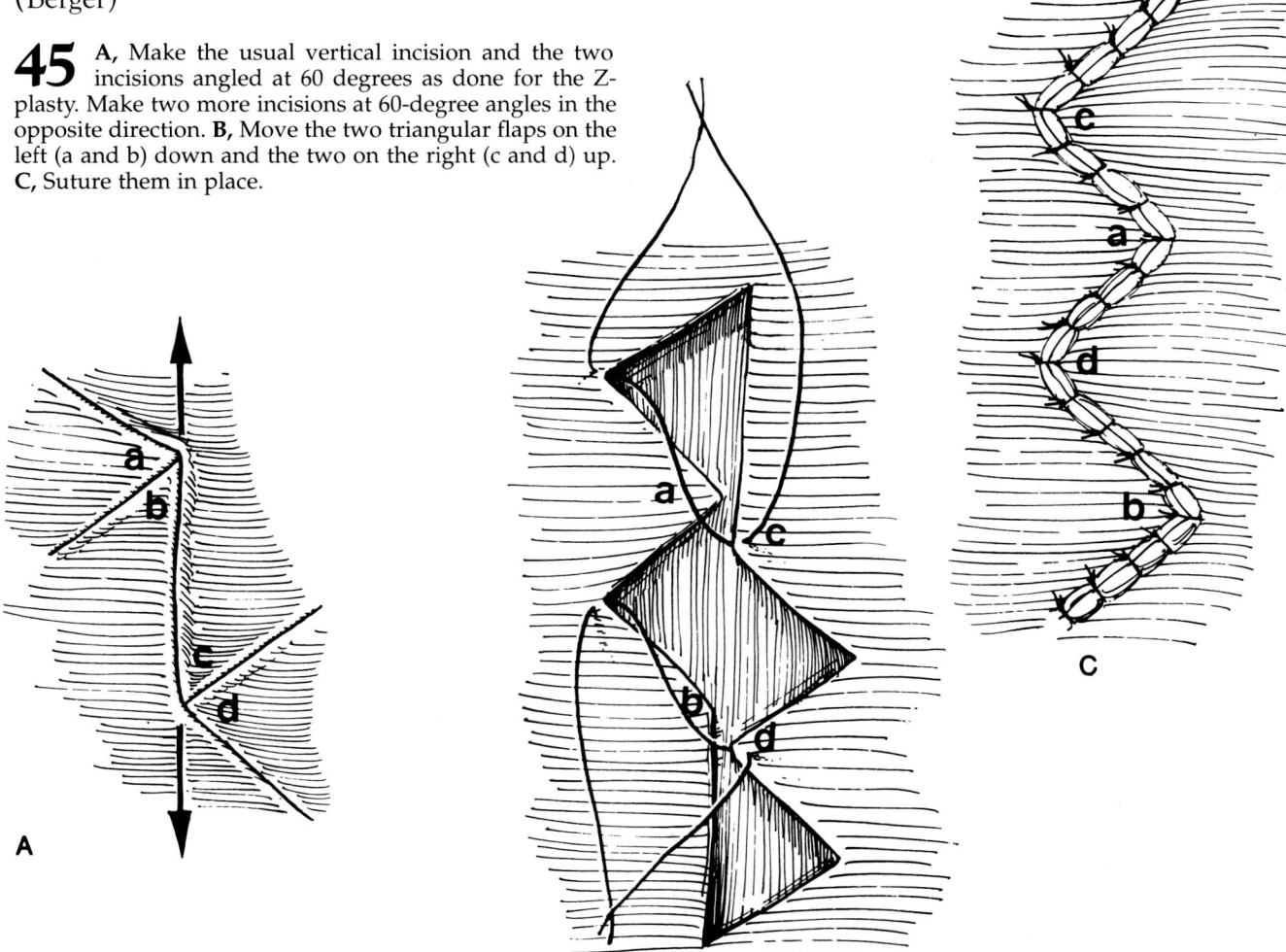

Rhomboid Flap
(Limberg)

47 **A,** Pinch the skin between the thumb and forefinger to determine in which direction the excess skin lies. Draw a 60- to 120-degree angle across this excess skin. Excise the lesion in the rhomboid. Draw a line perpendicular to the long axis of the defect equal to the length of one side of the rhomboid. Draw a second line at a 120-degree angle, making it parallel to a side of the rhomboid. (The other three optional incisions are shown by dotted lines.) **B,** Raise the flap, rotate it, and suture it in position.

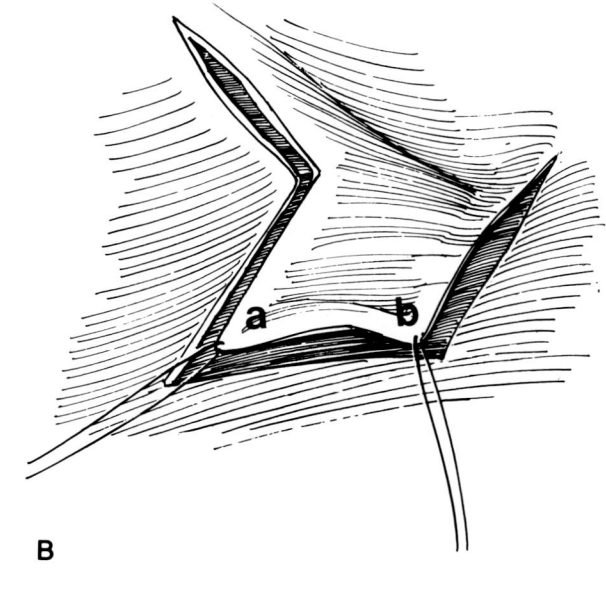

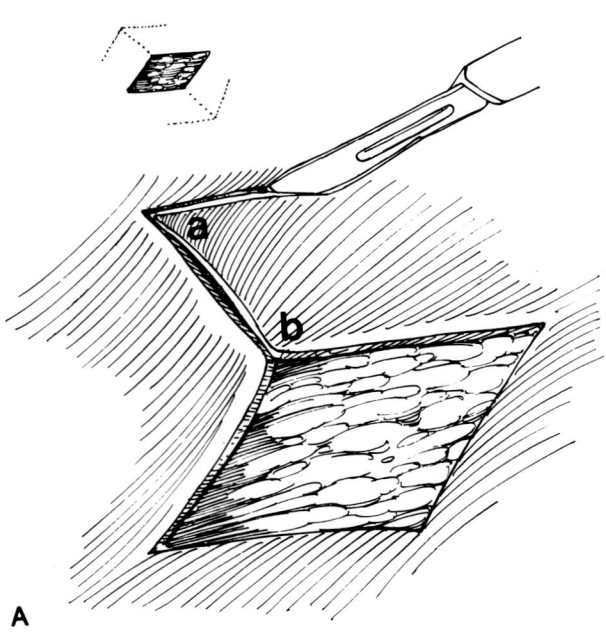

Flap Rotation

48 **A,** Trim a piece of suture paper the size of the defect. Rotate it on the pivot point of the flap (a) to check the arc of rotation of the flap. Mark and incise the skin. Excise a small triangle at the base of the flap on the outside of the arc. **B,** Raise and rotate the flap. *Note:* Cutting paper models of defects often helps the surgeon visualize the needed cuts and rotations.

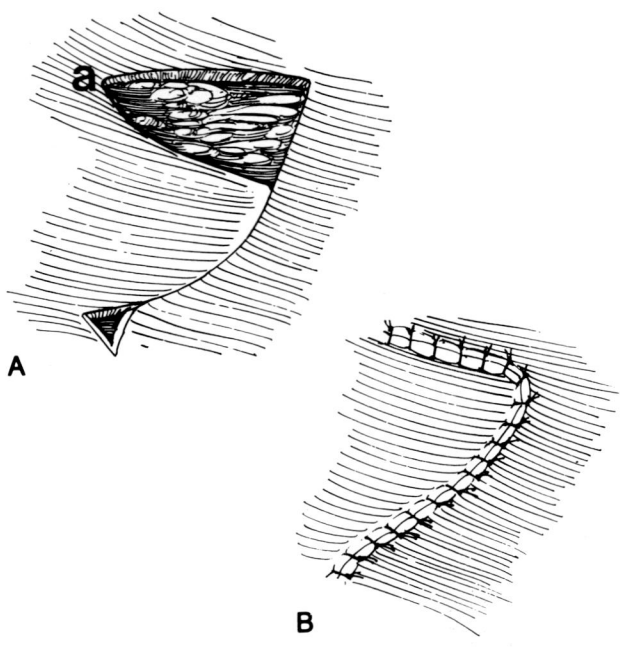

Flap Advancement by Excising Two Burow Triangles

49 **A,** Mark and incise two parallel lines extending from the edges of the defect and two triangles with bases slightly shorter than the length of the defect. Excise the triangles. **B,** Mobilize the flap and secure it over the defect.

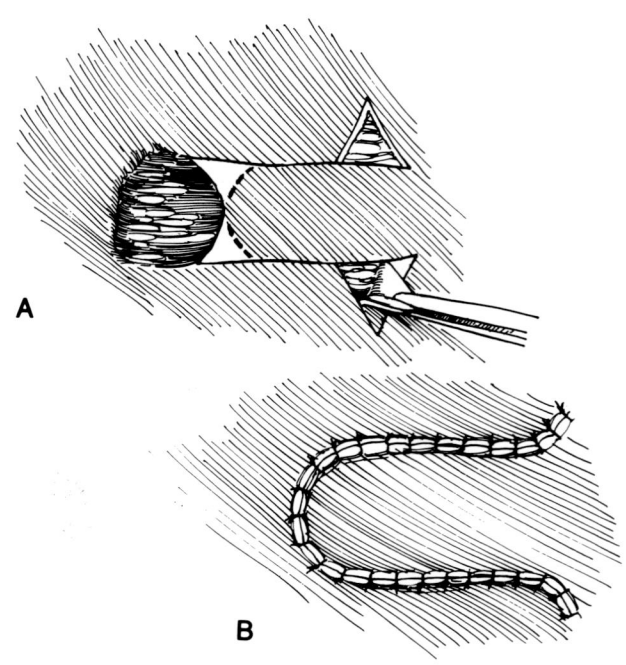

Flap Advancement by Perpendicular Basal Incisions

50 A, Mark and make two incisions obliquely from the defect, with an acute cut medially at the ends at c. **B,** Advance the flap to form triangular defects. **C,** Close the gaps while suturing the flap in place.

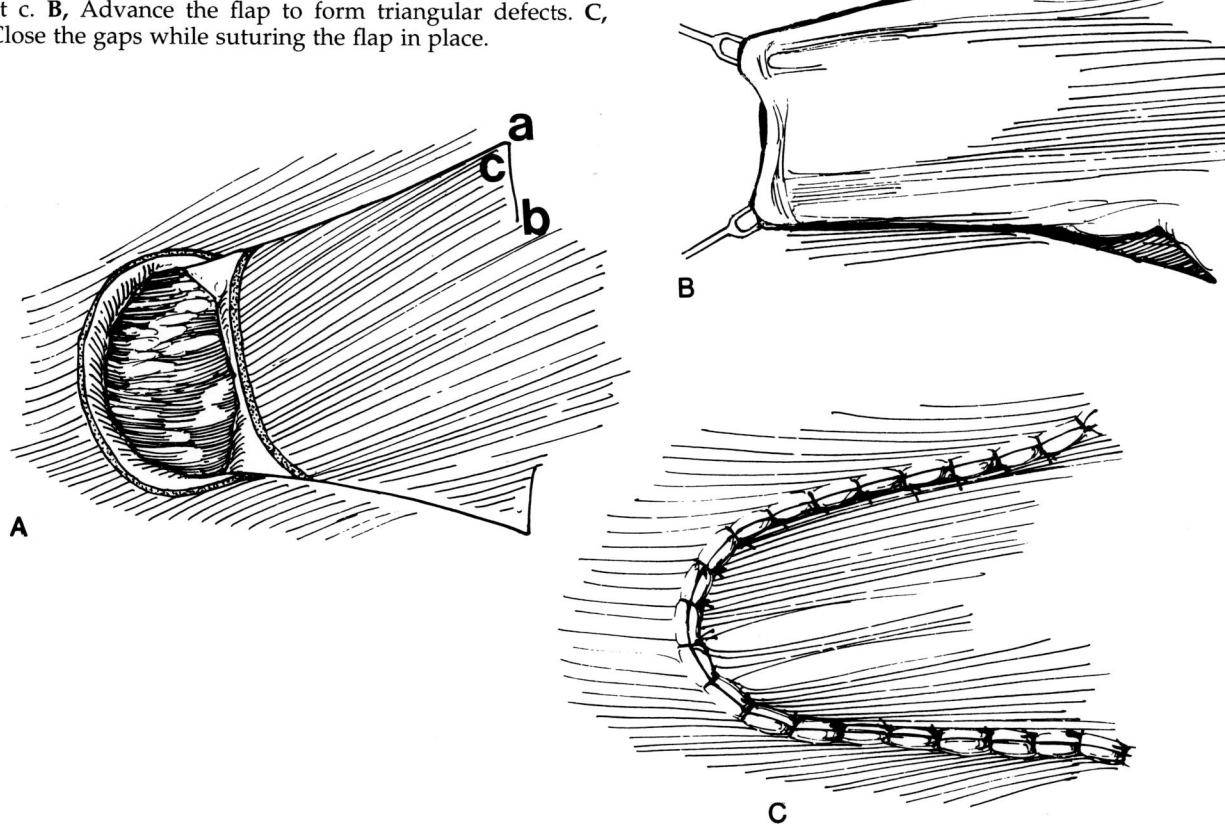

Correction of Dog Ear

51 A, Retract the longer edge from a point that equalizes the length of the two sides of the incision. **B,** Divide the skin on the other side of the line of the incision. **C,** Excise the flap of excess skin. **D,** Close the wound.

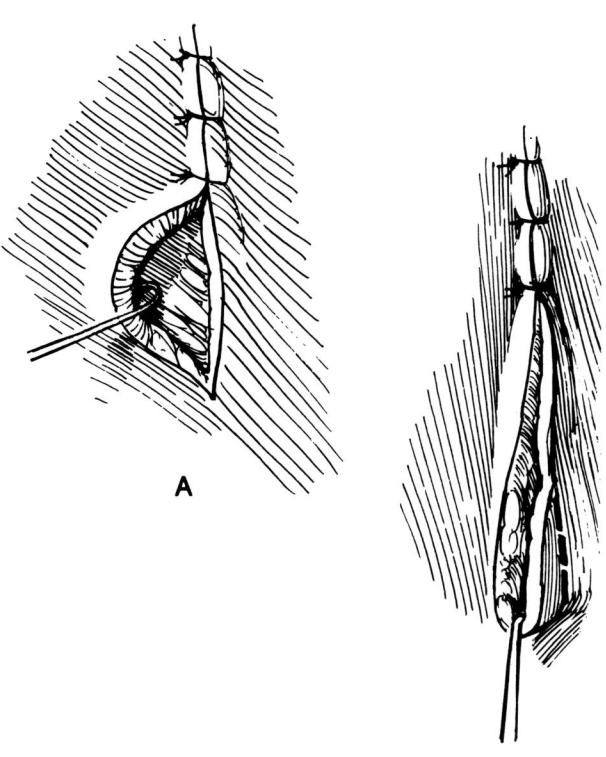

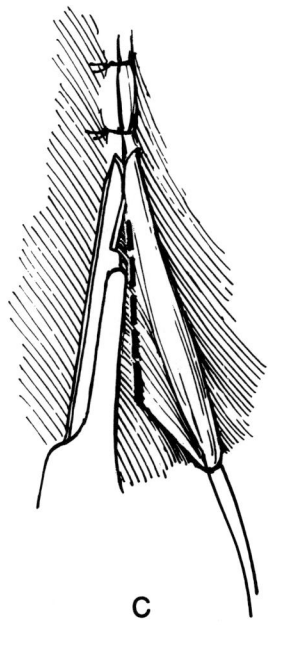

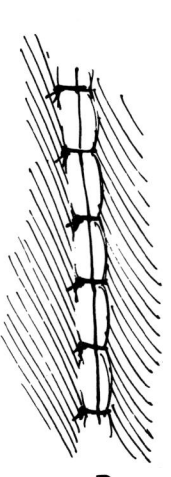

Contracture Release
(Borges)

52 **A to D,** Mark and incise the length of the scar, and make a succession of staggered oblique cuts. Advance the intervening Vs and suture the edges.

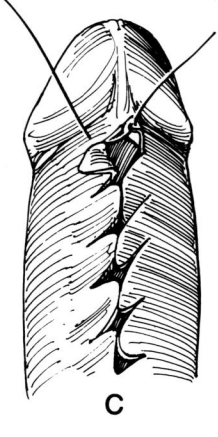

C

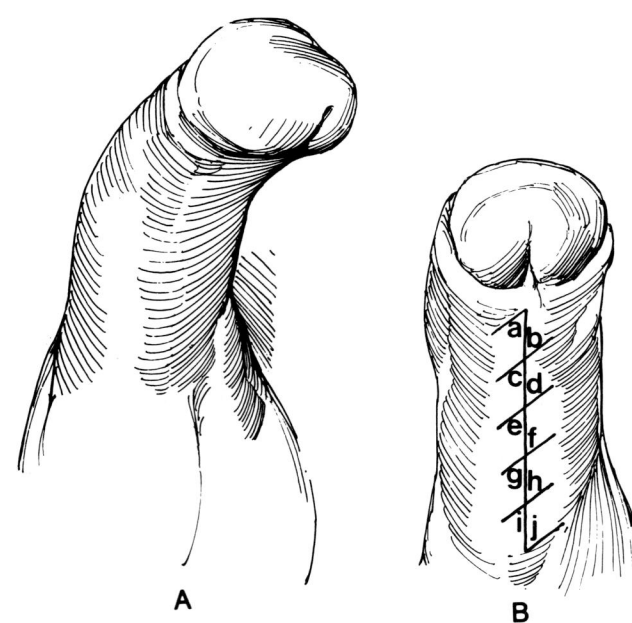

A   B

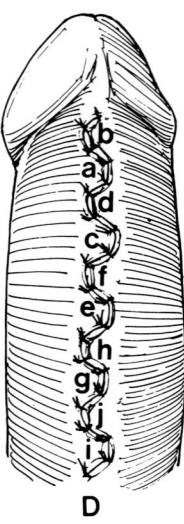

D

Problems After Grafting

Loss of a skin graft results from poor adherence, most often caused by hematoma, but improper immobilization of the graft is next in importance, making perfect hemostasis and proper fixation the keys to success in skin grafting. *Hematomas* can compromise the dermal-subdermal circulation and lead to necrosis not only by pressure but by a direct toxic effect. They indicate a technical error that should be corrected at once. Otherwise, early (within 24 hours) aspiration of the hematoma may salvage the flap. *Fixation* is dependent on the quality of the dressing. *Infection* can arise after bacterial contamination in a poorly vascularized wound. Deficiency in the *size* of the flap is the result of improper selection of the site or design of the flap. Rarely, failure results from putting the graft on upside down.

Ischemia results in necrosis of the flap and can come from direct damage to the blood supply or from overstretching of the skin through failure to use a back cut or a long-enough pedicle. Release a few of the sutures at once. However, it may be necessary to redesign the closure or even replace the flap in its original position, using it at a later time. Inadequate blood supply is the principal cause, mostly from deficient arterial inflow, although poor venous drainage with stasis may be an important factor. Appropriate techniques during the procedure will preserve the blood supply but not completely eliminate the risk of ischemia. *Tension* is harmful when the blood supply is marginal.

Gracilis Musculocutaneous Flap

53 Consider the anatomic relationships of the muscles in the upper leg. The gracilis muscle is the most medial of the superficial muscles when the leg is abducted, lying medial to the adductor longus. It originates on the inferior ramus of the pubis and the ischial ramus and inserts on the medial shaft of the tibia below the medial condyle.

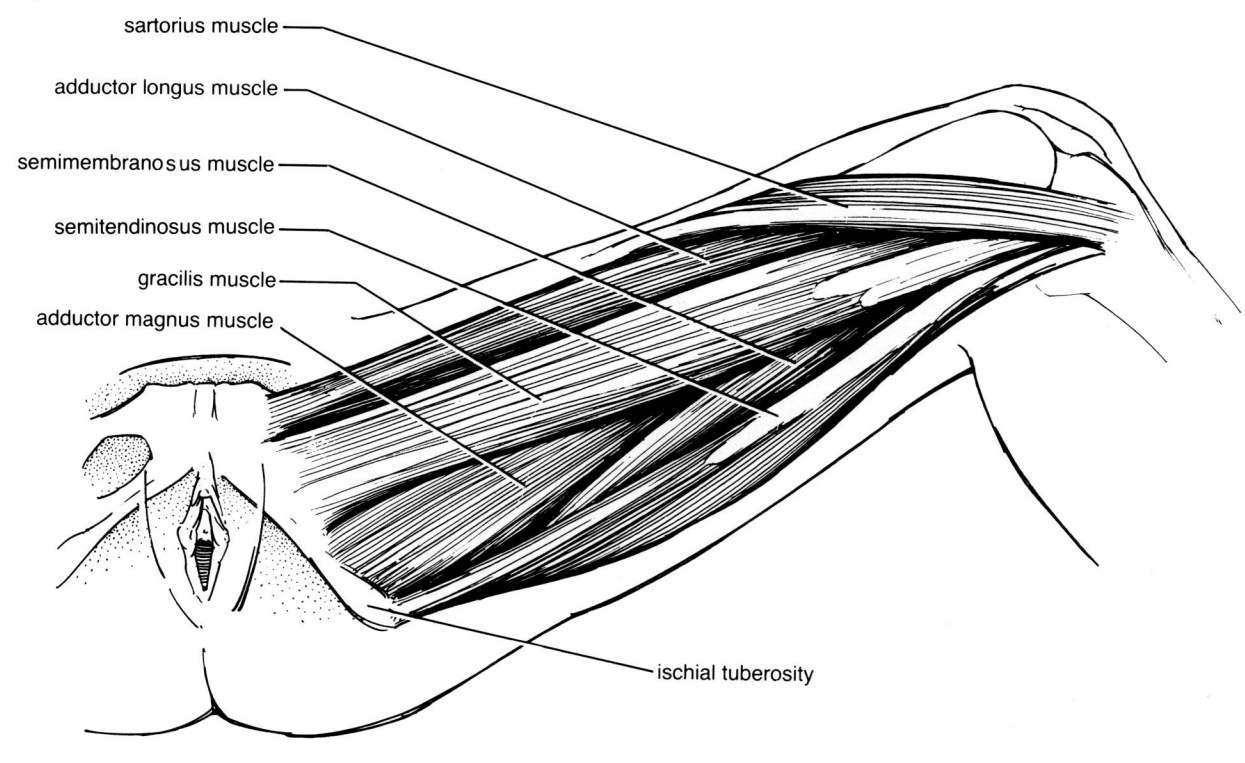

sartorius muscle

adductor longus muscle

semimembranosus muscle

semitendinosus muscle

gracilis muscle

adductor magnus muscle

ischial tuberosity

54 The medial femoral circumflex artery, arising from the deep femoral artery, provides the blood supply to the gracilis.

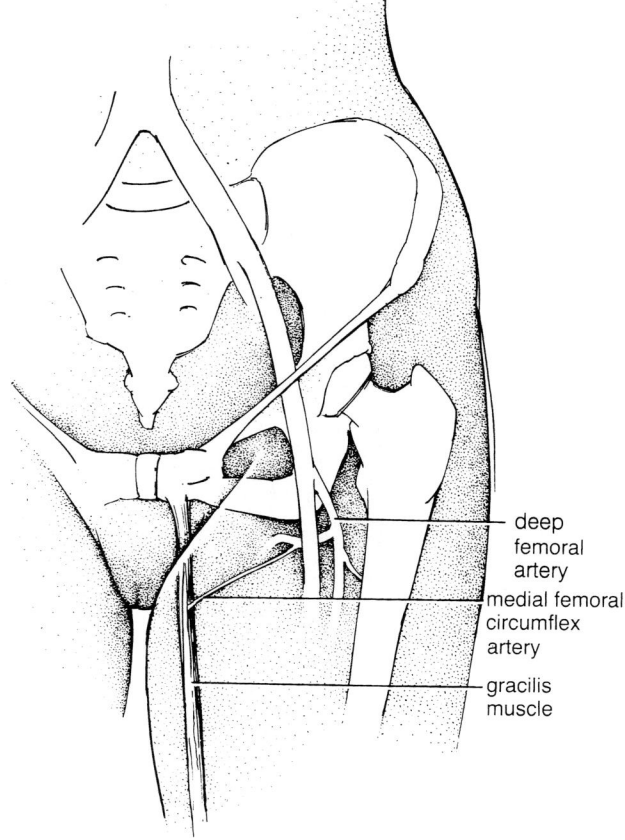

deep femoral artery

medial femoral circumflex artery

gracilis muscle

55 *Position:* Place the child in the dorsal lithotomy position and establish the normal anatomic relationships before abducting the leg. *Incision:* The adductor longus tendon, inserting on the tubercle, is on tension as the leg is abducted; this is the key to locating the gracilis muscle, lying medial to it. Mark the pubic tubercle and the medial condyle at the knee, because the flap will be raised from the skin and muscle below a line between these two structures. Palpate the soft area below the pubic tubercle;

the gracilis muscle originates here. Now mark an ellipse 6 or 7 cm wide—it can be as wide as the 12 cm needed for a neovagina—beginning 10 cm below the tubercle and ending approximately 18 cm distally. The length of this ellipse is made longer than required for the flap to allow provision for a tapering closure of the defect; the ends will be trimmed later. Prepare the left (or right) leg from the lower abdomen to below the knee. Also prepare the vulva and vaginal area. Drape the area appropriately.

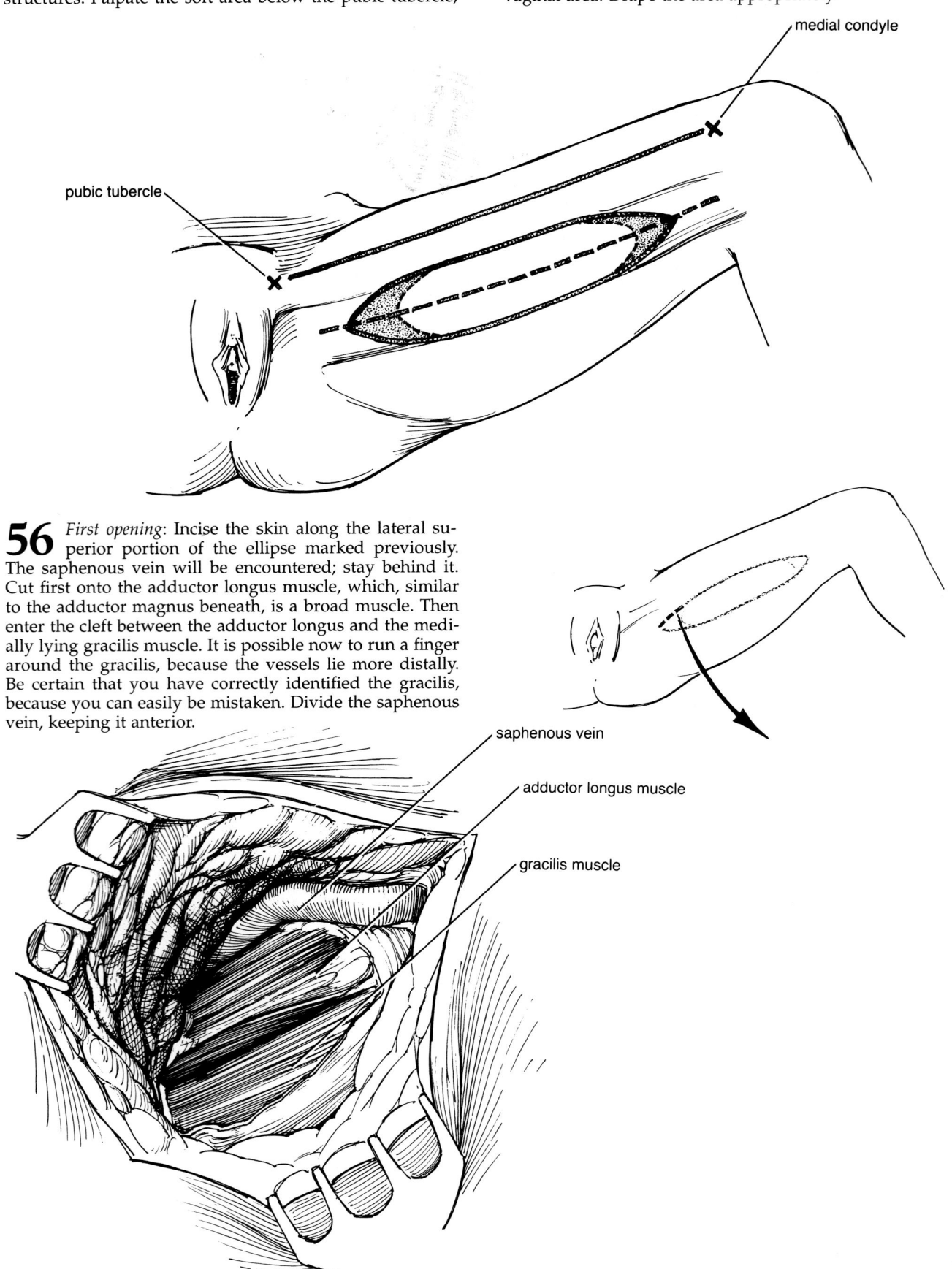

56 *First opening:* Incise the skin along the lateral superior portion of the ellipse marked previously. The saphenous vein will be encountered; stay behind it. Cut first onto the adductor longus muscle, which, similar to the adductor magnus beneath, is a broad muscle. Then enter the cleft between the adductor longus and the medially lying gracilis muscle. It is possible now to run a finger around the gracilis, because the vessels lie more distally. Be certain that you have correctly identified the gracilis, because you can easily be mistaken. Divide the saphenous vein, keeping it anterior.

medial condyle

pubic tubercle

saphenous vein

adductor longus muscle

gracilis muscle

57 *Second opening*: Make this incision along the lateral inferior portion of the ellipse. The sartorius muscle and the saphenous vein will be found lying anterior to the gracilis. Dissect to the deep fascia, and punch through it to pass a finger under the gracilis inferiorly. Note that the sartorius muscle crosses obliquely from below, running in a lateral direction, and that it is composed exclusively of muscle fibers, in contrast with the distal end of the gracilis, which is half muscle and half tendon. You will not confuse the gracilis with the semimembranosus and semitendinosus muscles that lie behind, because they are made up entirely of tendon.

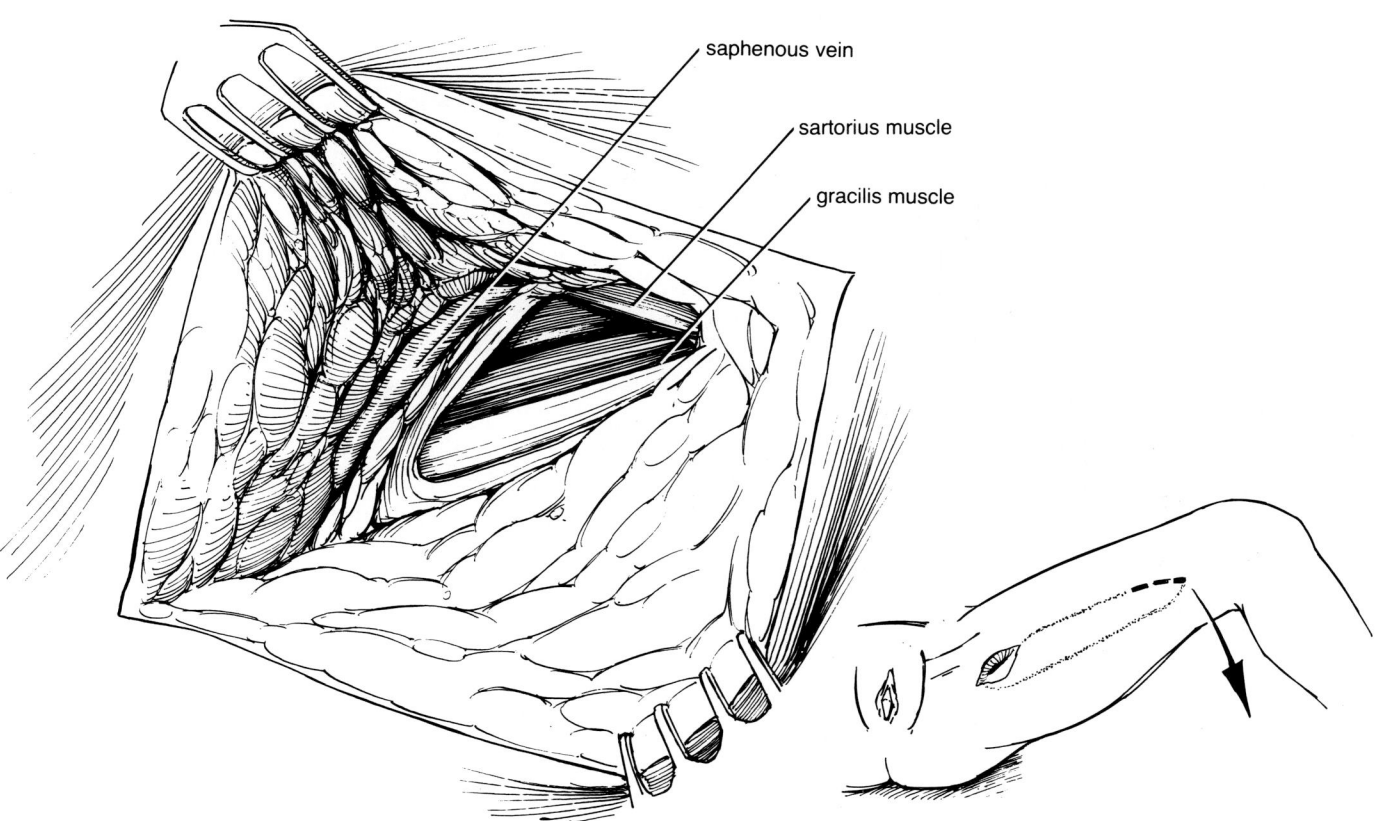

saphenous vein

sartorius muscle

gracilis muscle

58 Dissect against the adductor longus. The branches from the saphenous vein to the gracilis can be divided. Continue cutting on the medial side of the adductor longus, exposing the belly of the gracilis muscle until the vascular pedicle of the gracilis muscle is approached.

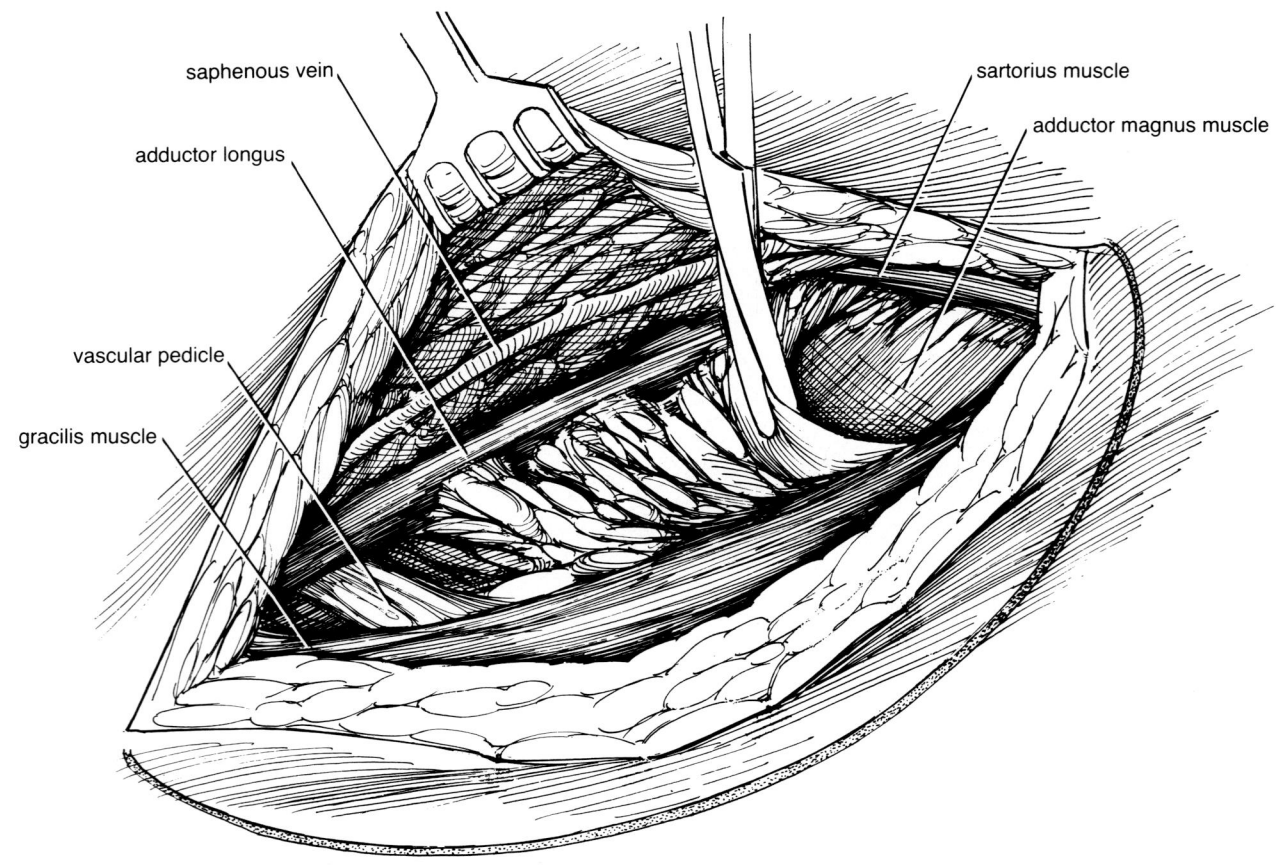

59 Complete the elliptic incision of the skin down the medial border, and cut the deep fascia medial to the gracilis muscle.

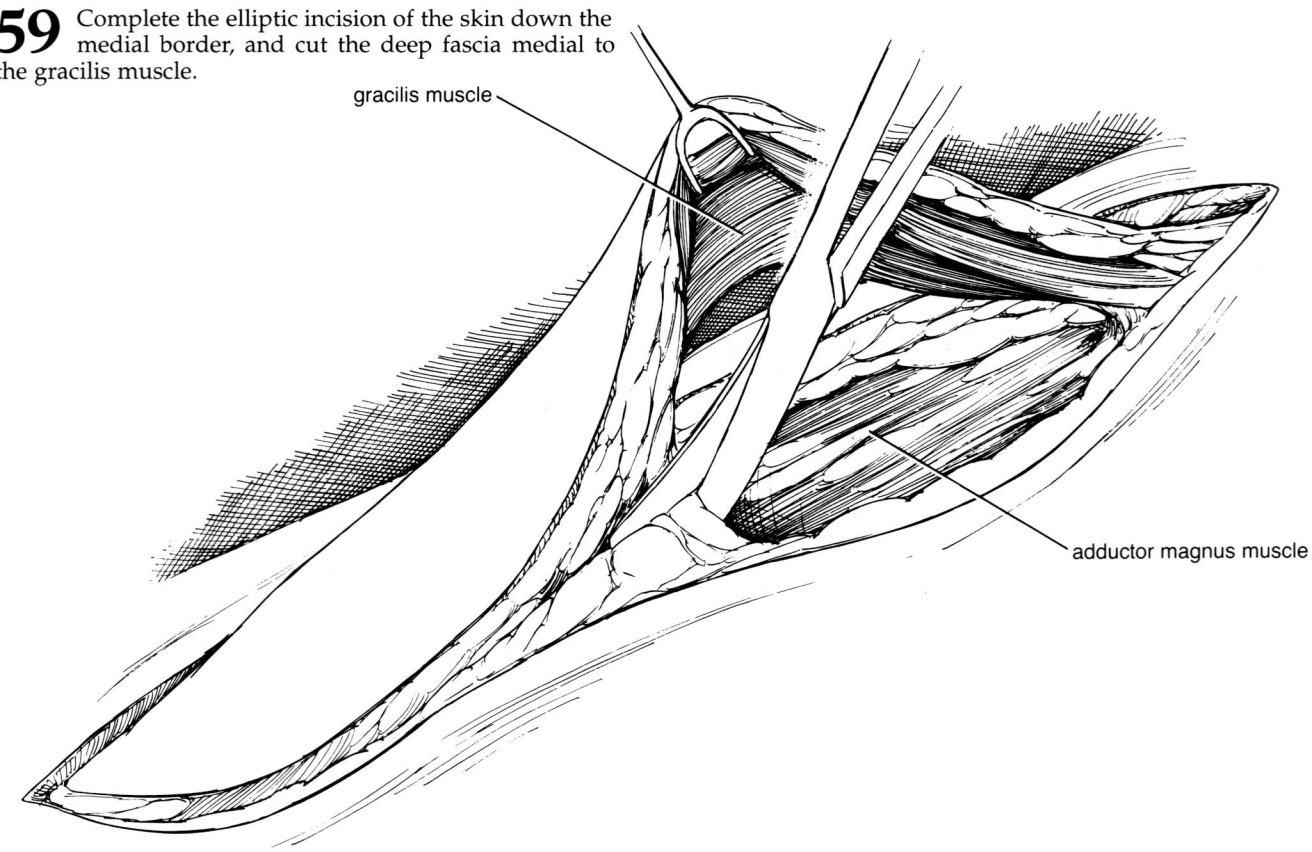

60 Elevate the flap from below after cutting the gracilis muscle on the tendon. Insert a silk suture for traction, but take care not to pull on the flap, which can induce spasm of the entering artery. Tack the skin edges to the muscle. The vascular pedicle will be encountered approximately 9 cm below the pubic tubercle, with the motor (obturator) nerve to the gracilis lying above it. A minor pedicle, arising from the superficial femoral artery, must be divided. This artery is the blood supply to the distal skin, which will be discarded. Use Stevens scissors for this dissection; a loupe is not necessary. Skeletonize the small

vessels lying behind the pedicle and watch out for branches of the obturator nerve. Do not do too much dissecting. Continue freeing the proximal end of the muscle, but leave its origin intact. The flap is now ready for rotation into position to cover perineal defects or for vesicovaginal reconstruction.

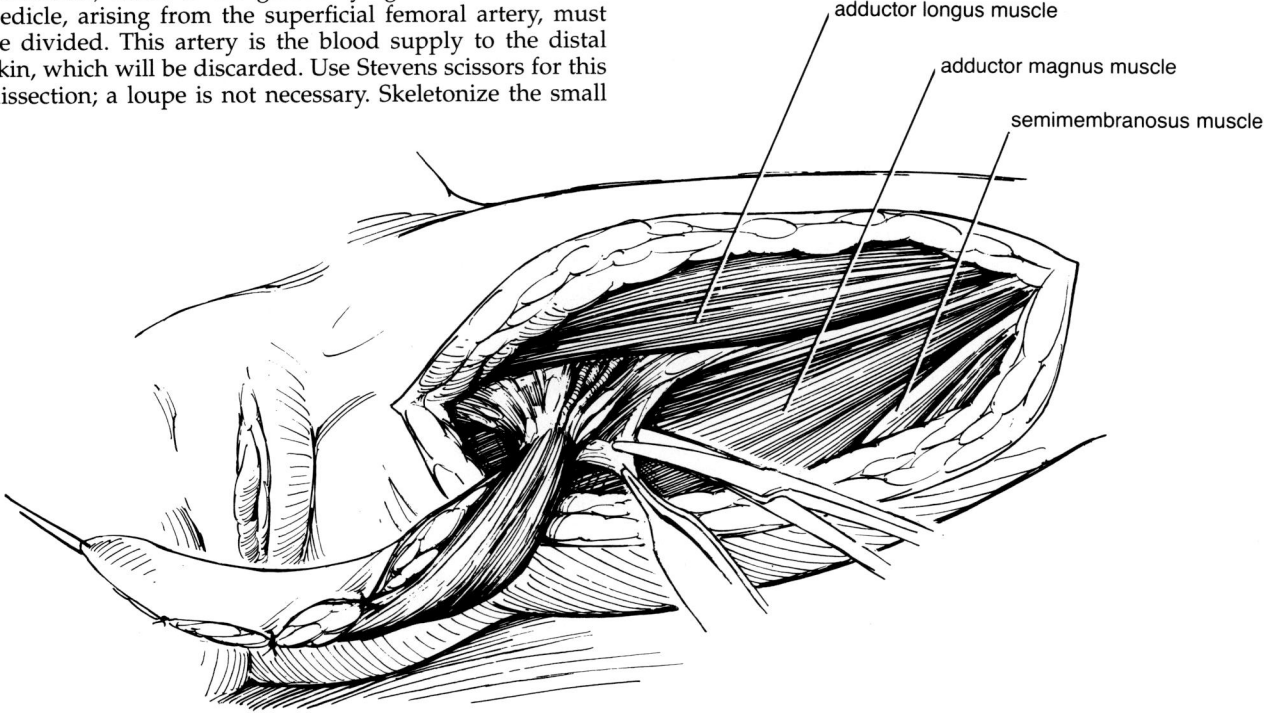

adductor longus muscle
adductor magnus muscle
semimembranosus muscle

61 A, Tunnel (or divide) the bridge of skin and subcutaneous tissue in the groin; rotate the flap clockwise, counterclockwise for the right. B, Suture the muscle in position with 3-0 chromic catgut sutures. Approximate the skin edges with the same suture.

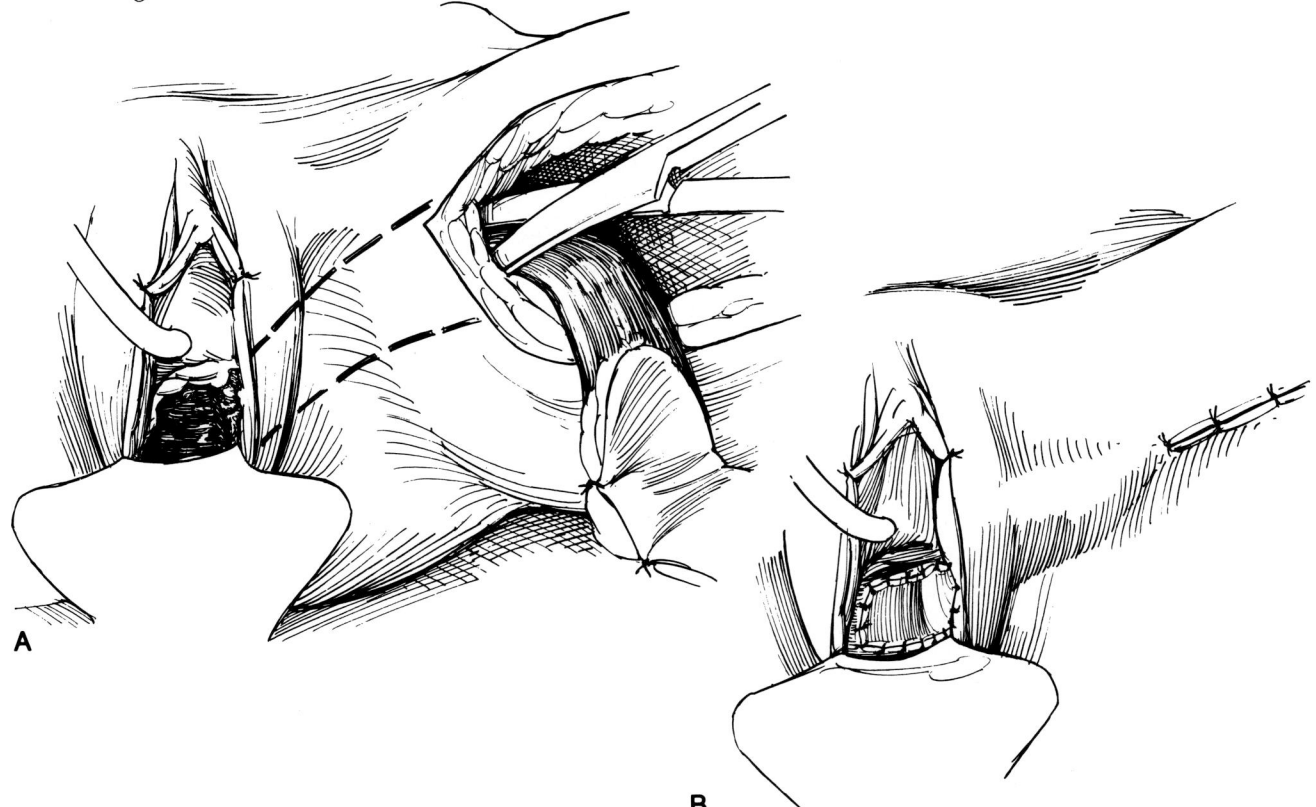

A

B

62 A and **B,** For a muscular flap, raise the gracilis muscle as a flap without overlying skin, as previously described. Adduct the leg, pass the flap through a tunnel, and suture it in place. Fix the base of the flap to the adductor magnus.

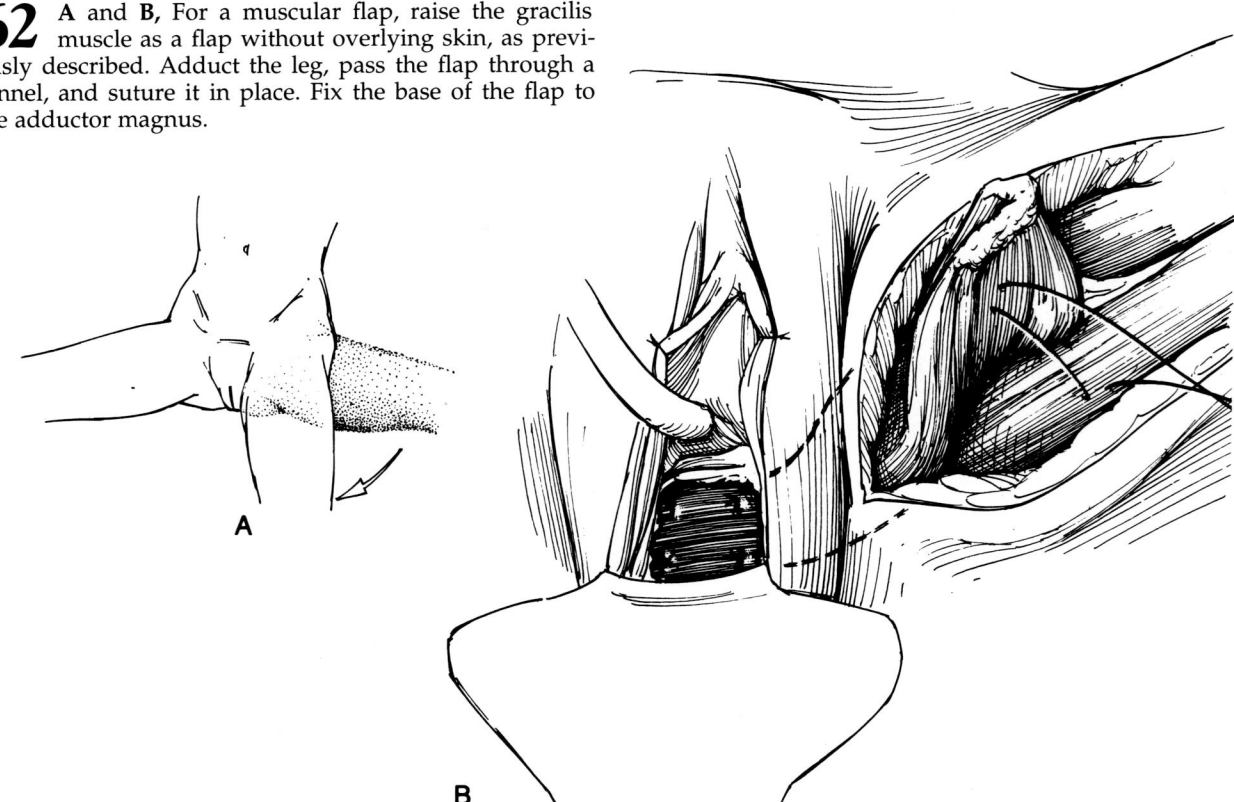

Inferior Rectus Abdominis Flap

This operation is a good selection if the largest possible flap is needed both to fill a defect and to provide a vascularized base if applied free of skin (in contrast to the gracilis flap that should be accompanied by its overlying skin). The donor site is readily closed. Either rectus muscle may be used, depending on the quality of the common femoral artery. The center of rotation of the flap allows placement into the perineum for reconstruction of the vagina and for repair of defects of the base of the bladder.

63 Prepare the recipient site first. If there is any question regarding the integrity of the common femoral artery on one side, use the contralateral rectus muscle. **A,** Outline an asymmetric flap extending well below the umbilicus to include the perforating vessels entering there. The width depends in part on the size needed for coverage of the defect and also on the laxity of the abdominal wall for closure. Incise the skin and subcutaneous tissue down to the rectus sheath. Circumscribe the umbilicus so that it may remain behind, adherent to a part of the rectus sheath. **B,** Alternatively, incise beside the umbilicus for a better cosmetic appearance. **C,** Elevate the skin edges. **D,** Divide the fascia beneath the skin edges, beginning along the lateral border. Leave 1 to 1.5 cm of the anterior sheath laterally for closure.

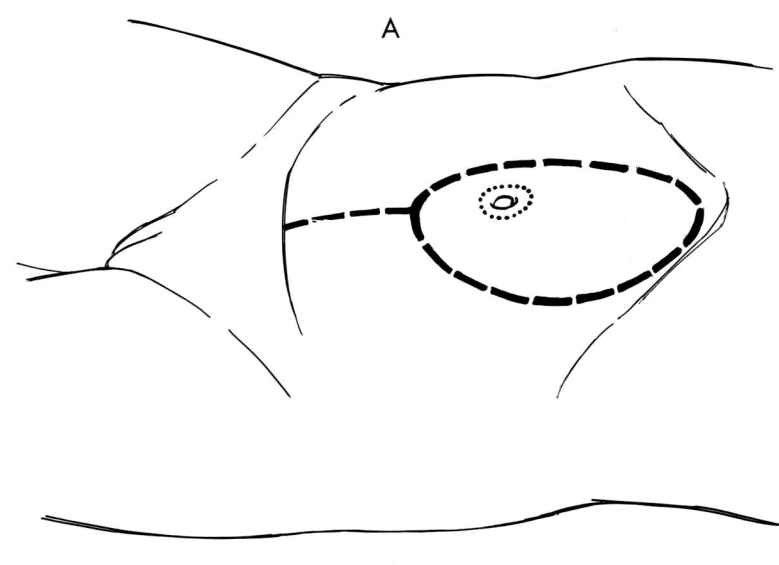

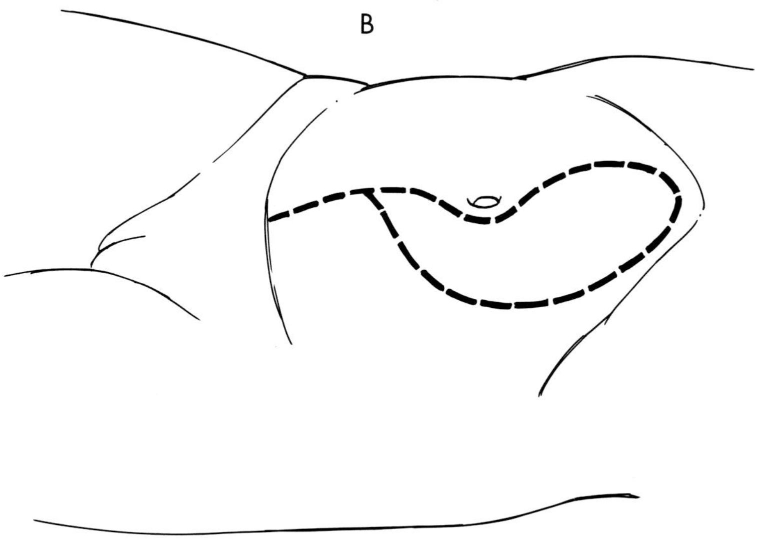

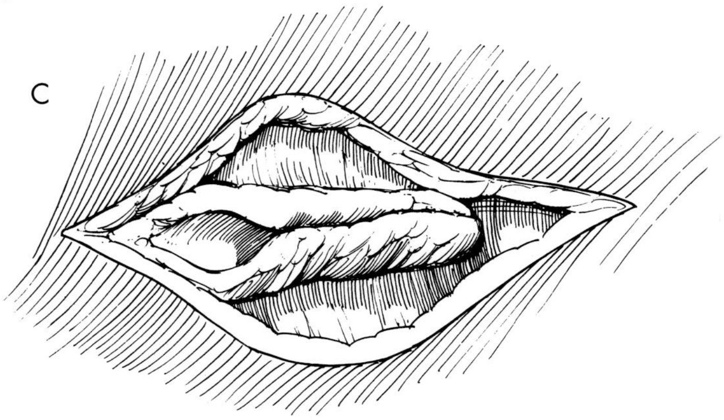

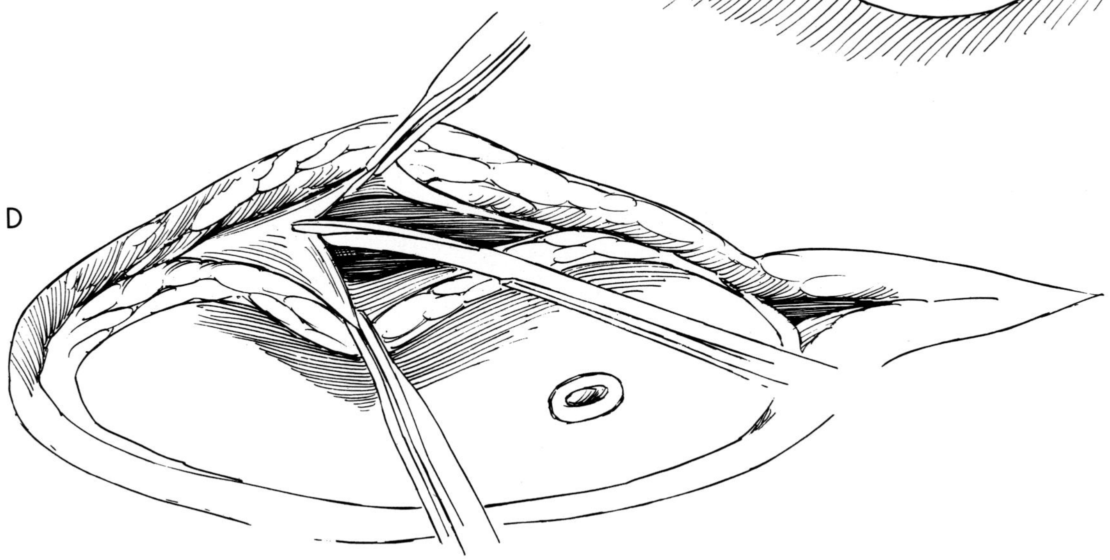

64 Dissect the rectus muscle from its sheath, again starting laterally, freeing its upper half to the midline posteriorly.

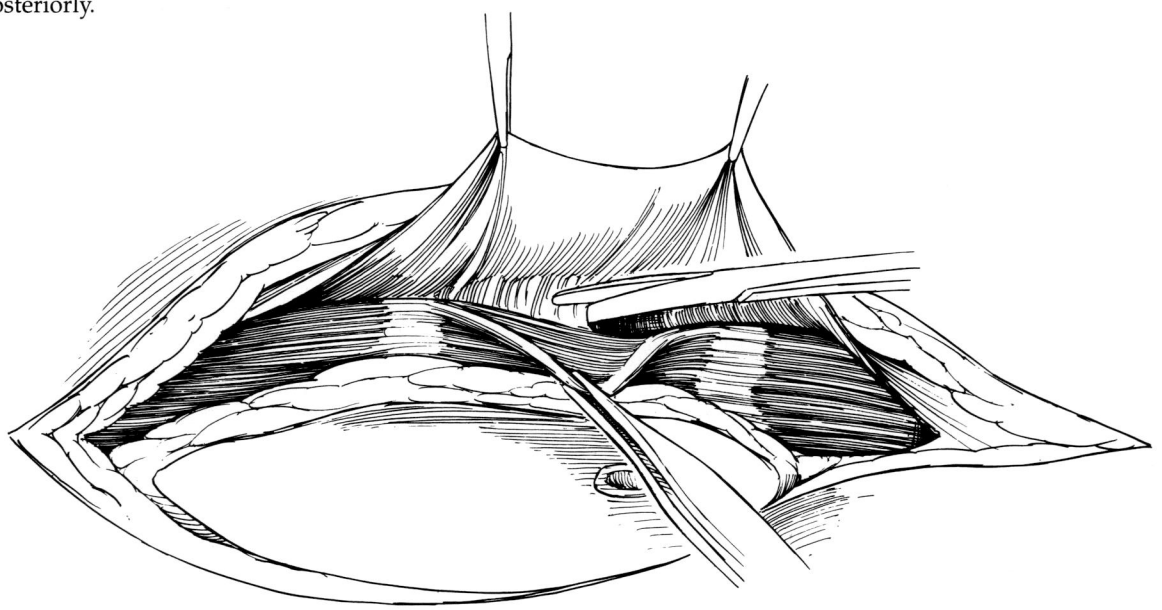

65 First take the anterior and then the posterior sheath off the muscle. Inferiorly below the arcuate line the dissection will be directly on the peritoneum. Leave the major perforating vessels joining fascia to skin. Place silk tacking sutures to hold the skin edges to the muscle. During this dissection, be cautious not to injure the muscle or small vessels, although the separation of muscle from sheath is usually not difficult, except at the tendinous inscriptions.

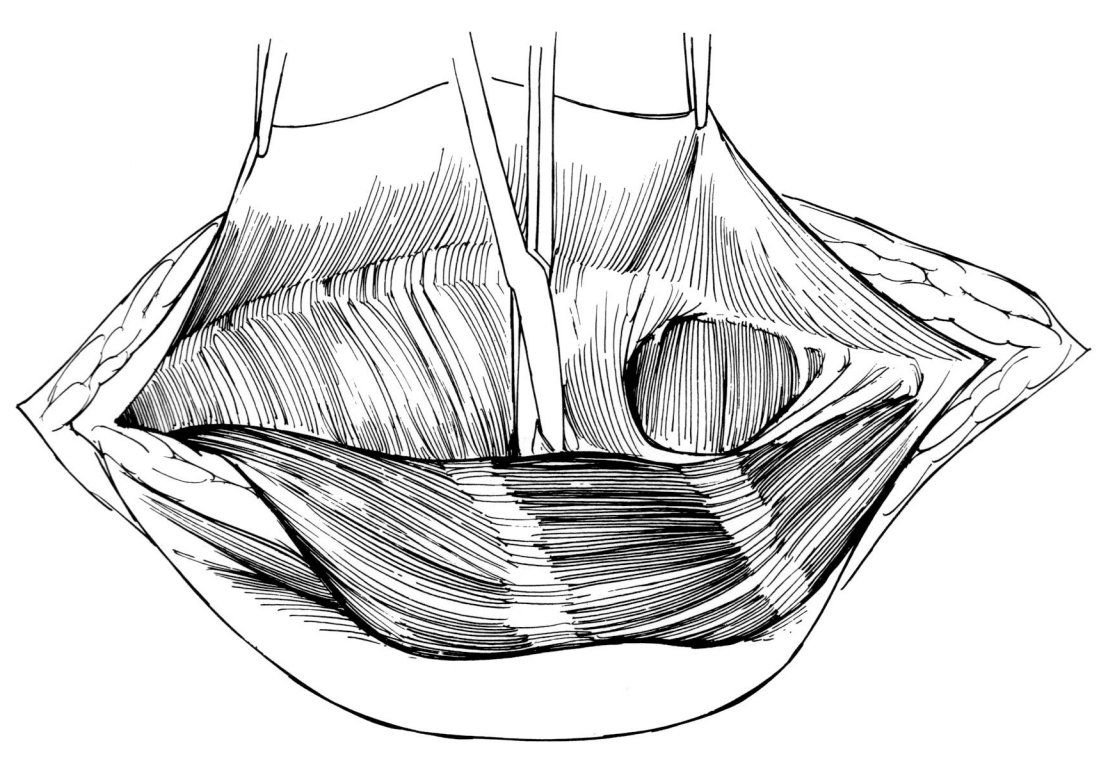

66 Divide the rectus muscle at its attachment at the xiphoid, and secure the superior epigastric artery. Insert a traction suture of 2-0 silk in the end. Continue freeing the muscle posteriorly, while dividing and clipping the segmental motor branches.

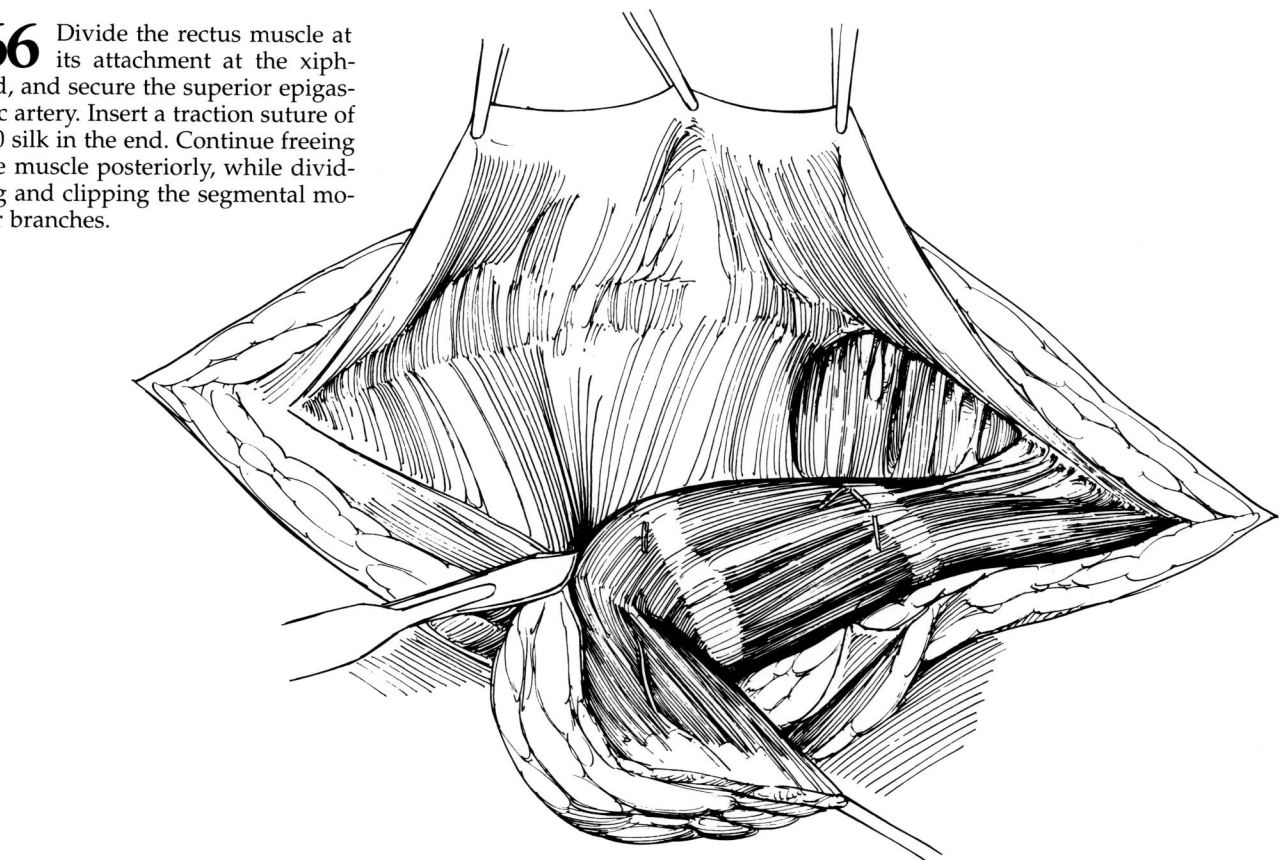

67 Approach the inferior end with care. The inferior epigastric vessels that make up the vascular pedicle arise somewhat laterally to enter into the lower fifth of the rectus muscle. Dissect the vessels and encircle them with a vessel loop. Divide the inferior end of the rectus muscle to allow freer rotation of the flap and to reduce concern that it will be compressed when placed in a tunnel, or leave it intact to provide a margin of safety against harmful traction during placement. If it is divided, insert a stay suture in that end to aid in positioning.

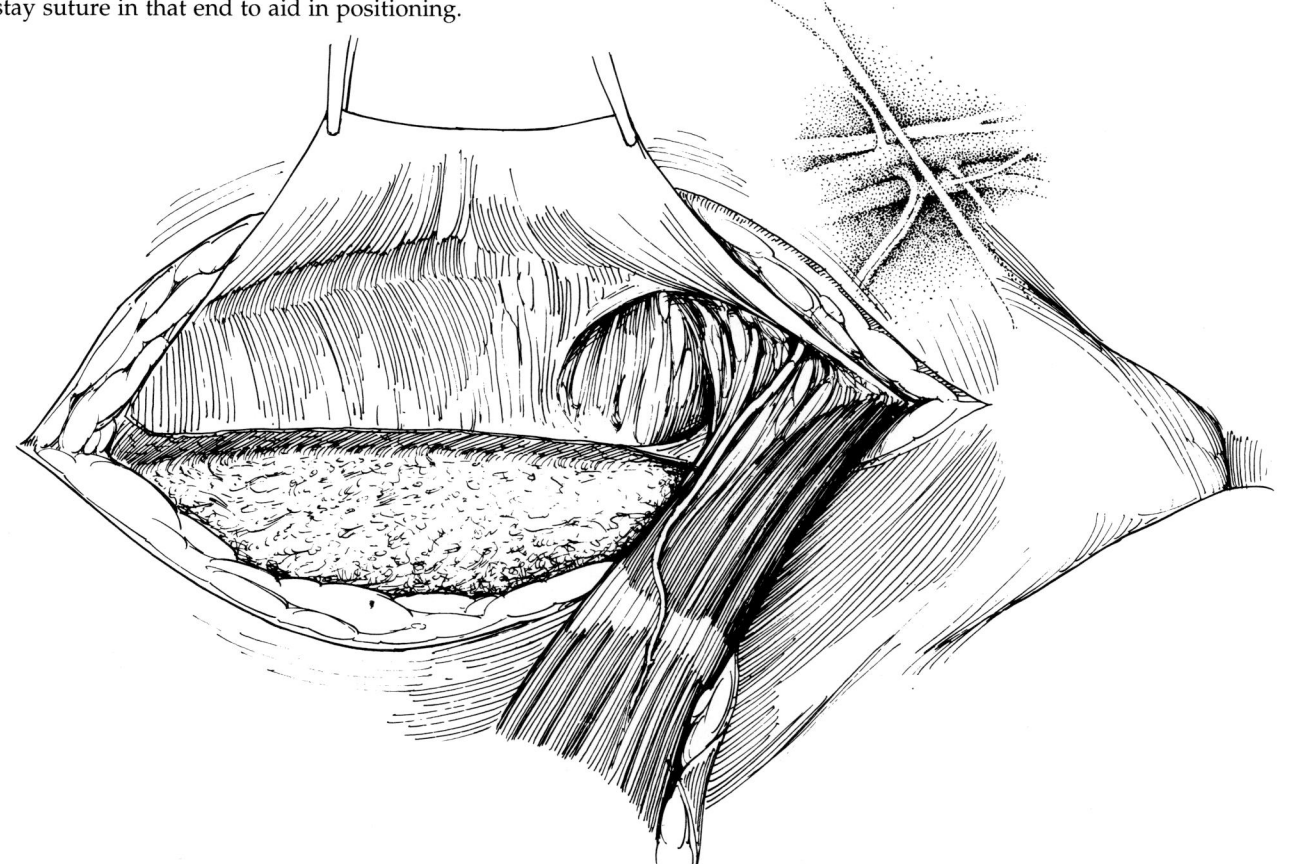

68 Tunnel the flap into position in the perineum or groin, making sure that the pedicle is not kinked or constricted, and fasten it in place with two layers of sutures after inserting a suction drain beneath it. Close the rectus sheath with a running doubled #0 nylon suture. Because the posterior wall is weak in the distal third where the posterior sheath is absent, a sheet of synthetic material (Gore-Tex) may be cut to size and sutured in place with heavy synthetic sutures tied with eight or nine knots. Insert a suction drain within the rectus sheath, because it often communicates with the perineal or groin defect, which may drain lymph. Close the skin of the abdomen with running sutures of 2-0 Vicryl subcutaneously with 4-0 synthetic absorbable suture on PC3 needles intracuticu-larly. Postoperatively, give methylprednisolone (Solu-Medrol) twice to reduce the inflammatory reaction. Provide simethicone to reduce intestinal gas. The child will find it hard to walk but should not be allowed to sit more than a few minutes (*eg*, either stand or lie down, perhaps in an air-cushioned bed).

Other musculocutaneous flaps may be useful in urologic repair: (1) the *rectus femoris* can fill large defects, but terminal knee extension may become limited; (2) the *inferior half of the gluteus maximus muscle* not only can provide filling for closure of a vesicovaginal fistula but also can support the vaginal wall; and (3) a *gluteal thigh flap* also will perform much the same function.

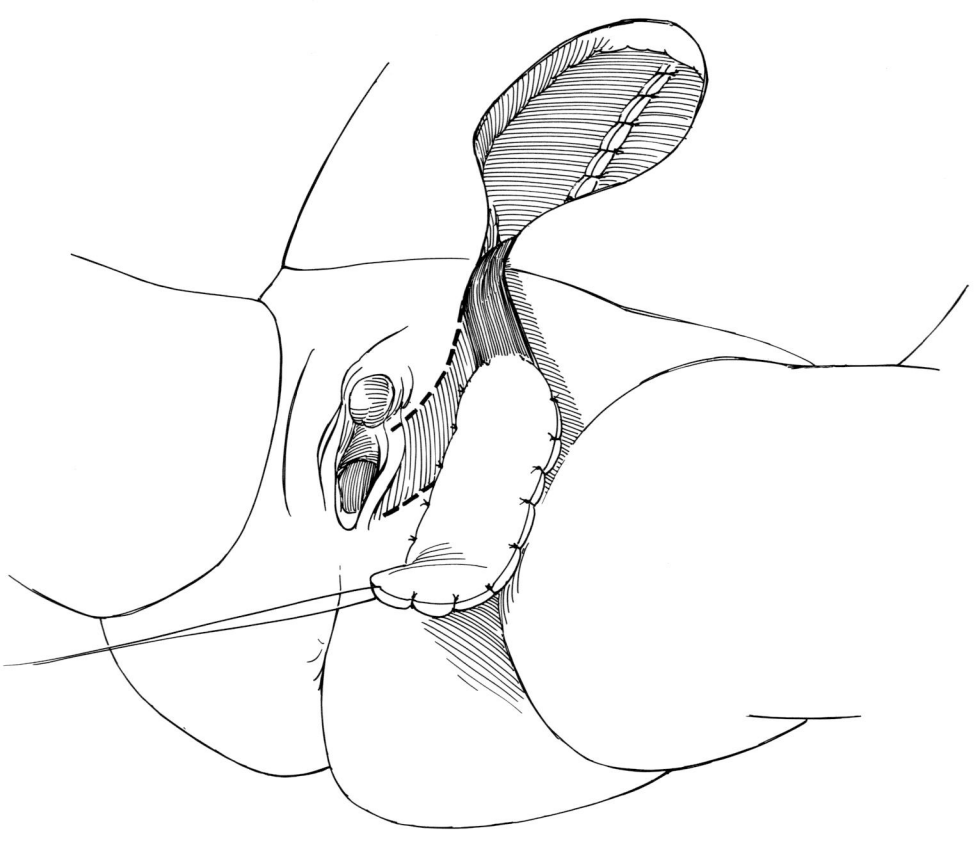

NERVE BLOCK TECHNIQUES

Consider preliminary sedation. Avoid an overdose of the agent as well as inadvertent intravascular injection. When aspirating, allow sufficient time for the blood to become visible. Do it gently so that the vessel wall will not occlude the lumen. Should toxic symptoms appear, it may not be necessary to treat them, as long as respiration and circulation are adequate. Be prepared for reactions to the anesthetic agent, although these are rare. Have at hand a naso-pharyngeal tube for obstructed airway, a bag and mask for assisted breathing, a blood pressure cuff to monitor arterial pressure and pulse, preparations for possible cardiopulmonary resuscitation, diazepam in 2.5-mg doses or intravenous (IV) pentobarbital for convulsions, antihistamines for mild allergic reactions and epinephrine for more severe ones, and 5 to 30 mg of ephedrine for hypotension from cardiovascular depression along with elevation of the legs and IV fluids.

Monitor the child's blood pressure and, when available, the electrocardiogram recording. Observation of color, pulse, respiratory pattern, and incidence of sweating is the most valuable monitor.

Intercostal Nerve Block

69 *Anatomic relationships*: The intercostal nerves run segmentally under the respective ribs external to the endothoracic fascia. After passing the angle of the rib, the nerve continues below the artery and vein in the costal groove between the internal and external intercostal muscles.

Procedure: Place the patient in a lateral position with the ipsilateral arm extended over the head. Palpate the lower margin of the rib just beyond the angle. Insert a fine needle vertically until it touches the lower half of the rib. With the free hand, pull the skin caudally until the needle point slips off the rib. Push it 3 mm deeper until a click is felt. Then angle the needle upward and advance it 2 to 3 cm under the lower edge of the rib. Aspirate for air or blood. Inject 5 ml of anesthetic agent, preferably bupivacaine 0.5 percent with epinephrine. Pneumothorax, even tension pneumothorax, can result if the rib is difficult to palpate and the needle is inserted too deeply.

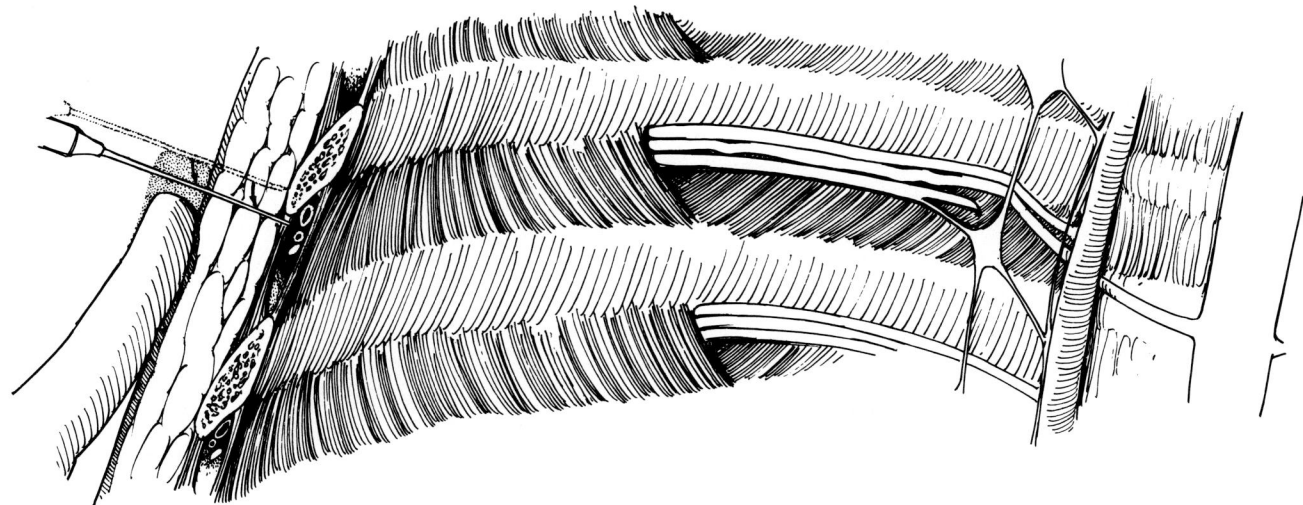

Penile Nerve Block

70 The right and left dorsal nerves of the penis arise from the pudendal nerve, pass under the symphysis, and penetrate the suspensory ligament of the penis to run under the deep (Buck's) fascia.

Procedure: Palpate the symphysis pubis. Insert a short 22-gauge needle to one side of the midline at the 10 o'clock position to reach the caudal border of the symphysis. Withdraw it slightly and move it so that it just misses the bone. Pop it through Buck's fascia. Aspirate and inject 10 ml of 1 percent lidocaine solution. Repeat the procedure at the two o'clock position.

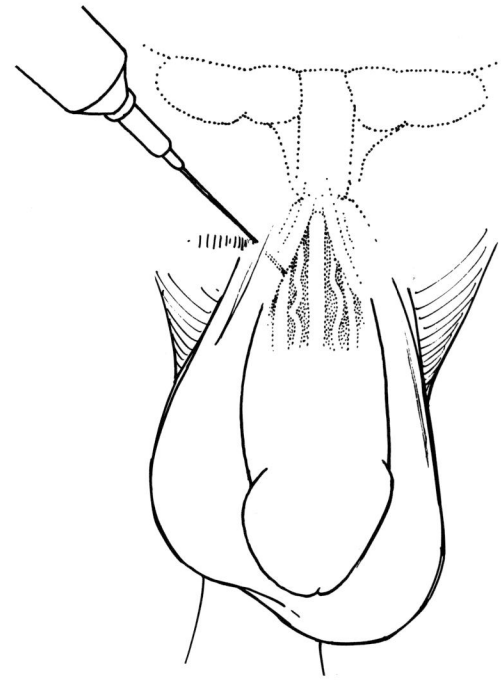

Ilioinguinal, Iliohypogastric, and Genitofemoral Nerve Blocks for Orchiopexy and Hernia Repair

71 *Anatomic relationships*: The iliohypogastric nerve from T-12 and L-1 exits through the transversalis muscle just medial to the anterior superior iliac spine and runs between the transversalis muscle and the internal oblique muscle 2 to 3 cm medial to the spine. The ilioinguinal nerve from L-1 arises slightly below and runs parallel to the iliohypogastric nerve and continues between the internal and external oblique muscles. The genitofemoral nerve from L-1 and L-2 runs over the surface of the psoas major muscle to divide just above the inguinal ligament into the genital and femoral branches. The genital branch enters the inguinal canal behind the cord.

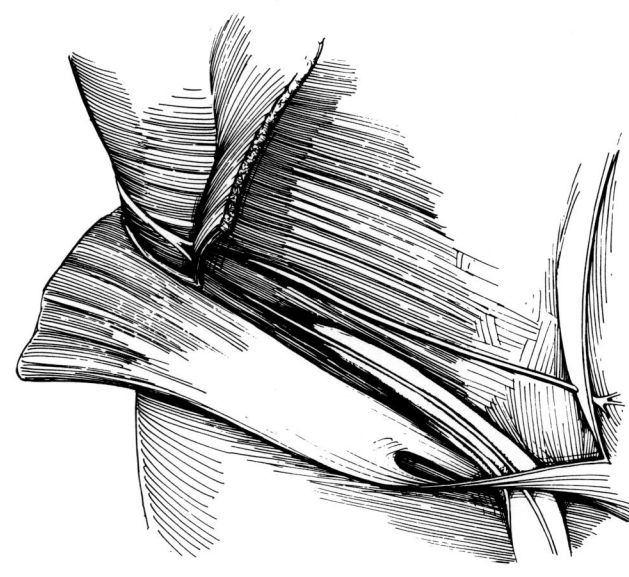

72 *Procedure*: Palpate the anterior superior iliac spine, and mark a point 2.5 to 3 cm medial and 2 to 3 cm caudal to it. Insert a 22-gauge needle to touch the inner surface of the iliac bone and inject 5 to 7 ml of bupivacaine solution as the needle is withdrawn. Repeat the procedure more medially, injecting 5 to 7 ml of solution just beneath the fascia of the three muscle layers. For block of the genitofemoral nerve, palpate the pubic tubercle, and inject 5 to 7 ml of the anesthetic solution in the muscle layers laterally, cranially, and medially. Supplement the nerve block with subcutaneous injections fanned out to the inguinal fold laterally and the midline medially.

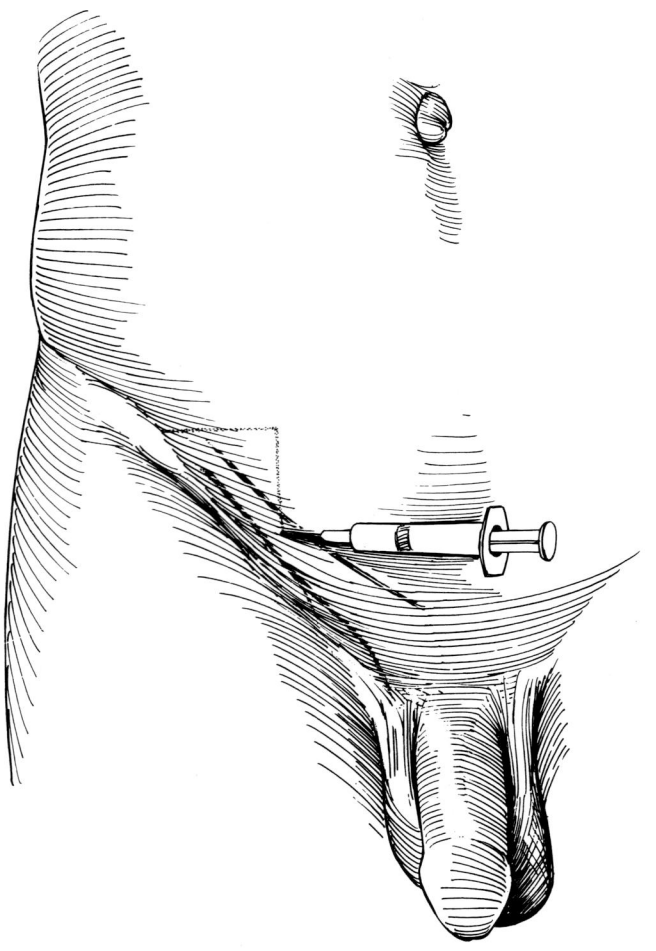

Pudendal Nerve Block

73 *Anatomic relationships*: The pudendal nerve arises from S-2, S-3, and S-4, runs laterally and dorsally to the ischial spine and sacrospinous ligament, and divides into the perineal nerve and the inferior rectal nerve. Plan to block the nerve as it passes the ischial spine.

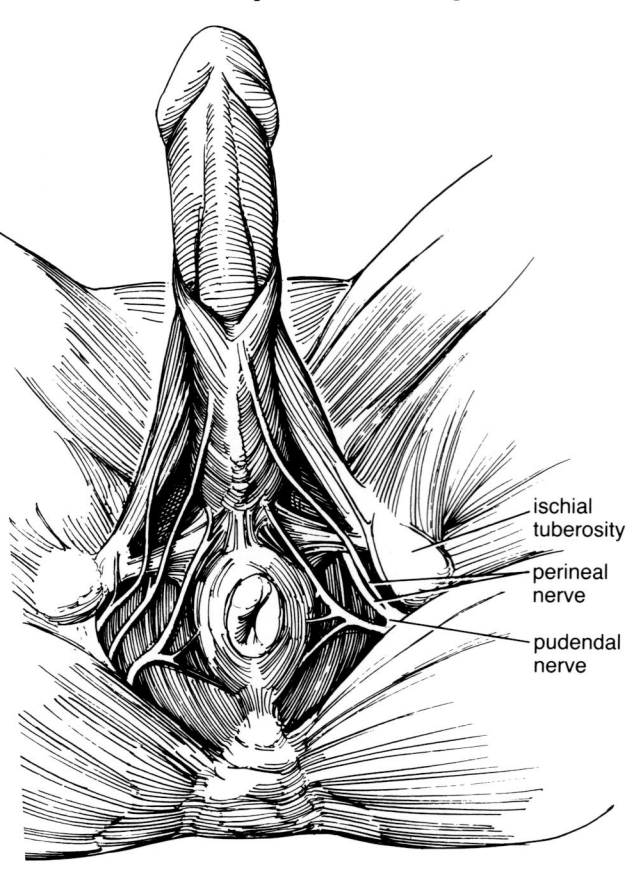

ischial tuberosity

perineal nerve

pudendal nerve

74 *Procedure*: With the child in the lithotomy position, insert the index finger in the rectum and palpate the ischial spine. Make a skin wheal 2 to 3 cm posteromedially to the ischial tuberosity. Insert a 12- to 15-cm, 20-

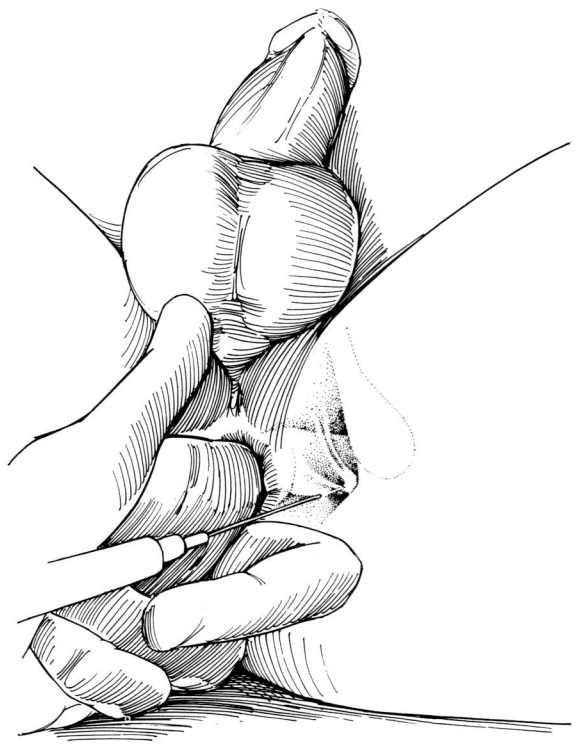

gauge needle on a 10-ml syringe in a posterior and lateral direction to pop the needle through the sacrospinous ligament. Use the index finger as a guide to determine that the needle comes in contact with the bony prominence of the ischial tuberosity. Aspirate and inject 5 to 10 ml of local anesthetic laterally and under the tuberosity to anesthetize the inferior pudendal nerve. Move the needle to the me-

dial side of the tuberosity and inject another 10 ml after aspiration. Then advance the needle 2 to 3 cm into the ischiorectal fossa and inject 10 ml. Finally, guide the needle dorsolaterally to the ischial spine and pop the needle through the sacrospinous ligament there. Aspirate for blood and inject 5 or 10 ml of the agent. Repeat the procedure on the other side.

Trans-sacral Block

75 *Anatomic relationships*: A layer of highly vascular fatty tissue lies between the two layers of bone. This continuation of the lumbar epidural space contains the posterior primary divisions of the sacral nerve, which exit through the posterior foramina to supply the buttocks and the anterior primary divisions, which exit through the ventral foramina to innervate the perineum and part of the leg.

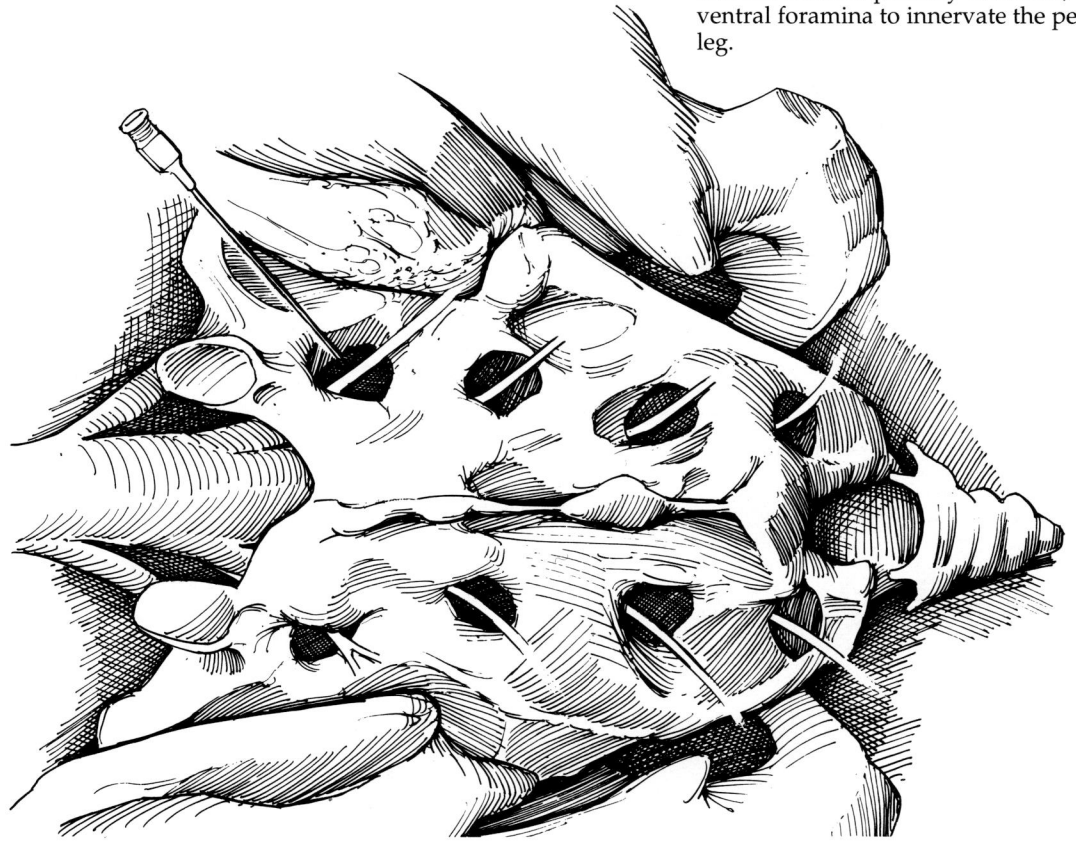

76 *Procedure*: Place the sedated child prone with a pillow under the hips. Palpate and mark both posterior superior iliac spines. Mark a point 1.5 cm medial and 1.5 cm cephalad to the posterior superior iliac spine to locate the first sacral foramen. Draw a line from this point to the lateral surface of the sacral cornua. Mark points 2 cm apart below the first foramen for the other three foramina.

Inject the agent subcutaneously to raise wheals. Insert a 12-cm, 22-gauge spinal needle containing a stilet perpendicular to the surface to contact the rim of the selected foramen. Move the rubber marker on the needle to a point 1.5 cm from the skin surface. Withdraw the needle slightly and angle it 45 degrees caudally and 45 degrees medially to insert it into the foramen up to the marker, for a depth of 1.5 cm. Inject 1.5 to 2 ml of anesthetic agent. For total caudal anesthesia, inject 15 to 25 ml. Hazards include producing a subarachnoid block and injecting the agent intravascularly in the large venous plexus.

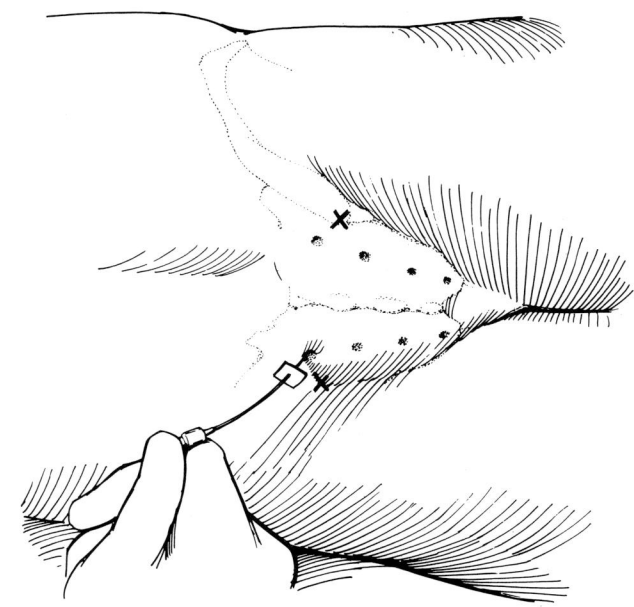

REPAIR OF VASCULAR INJURIES

Control the bleeding with digital pressure. Immediately increase the exposure; obtain blood; provide a second IV line and suction set; and obtain appropriate instruments, sutures, and assistance.

Venous Injuries

Laceration of the Vena Cava

77 Have your assistant compress the vessel digitally at the site of injury. Free the vena cava from the aorta, and have the flow blocked above and below with sponge sticks.

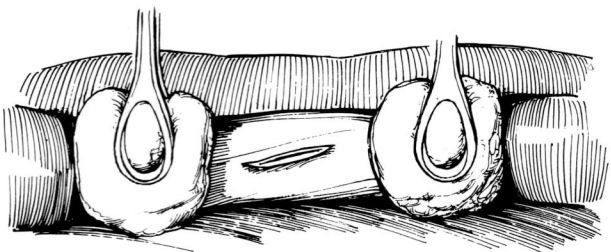

78 Grasp the edges of the laceration with several fine Allis clamps. This will allow dissection for better exposure. Run a 6-0 vascular suture down the laceration, as the clamps are removed successively. If this fails, keep pressure on the bleeding point and free the circumference of the vena cava on either side. Ligate the end of the laceration with a 2-0 silk tie, then oversew with the same suture.

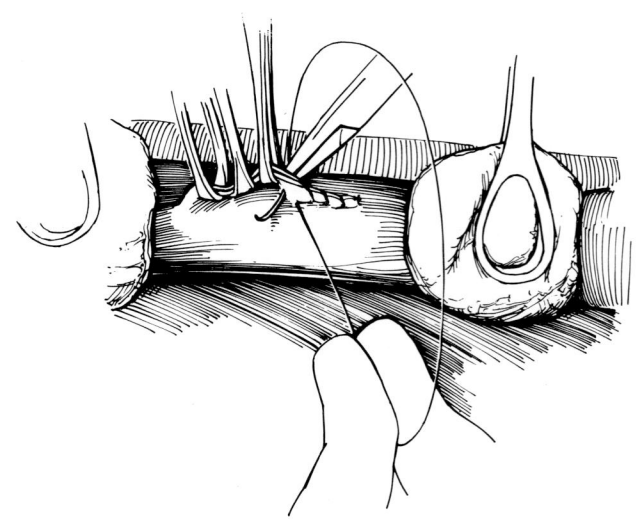

Pelvic Venous Plexus

79 Immediately pack the area of injury with moist sponges. Avoid blind clamping. Attach shoulder braces and place the child in the steep Trendelenburg position to empty the pelvic veins. Orient yourself to the anatomic distribution of the pelvic veins before attempting repair. Slowly remove the pack. Clamp and tie the bleeding vein or compress it distal to the tear with a sponge stick, and suture it with a 5-0 arterial monofilament suture (Prolene). Blind suture ligation can result in an arteriovenous fistula. If exposure is still not adequate, expose the ipsilateral internal iliac artery and clamp it with a vascular clamp at its origin from the common iliac artery. You may have to clamp both internal iliac arteries. Now remove the pack and control the vessel. If control still is not obtained, permanently ligate the internal iliac arteries and place a pack to be removed 48 hours postoperatively.

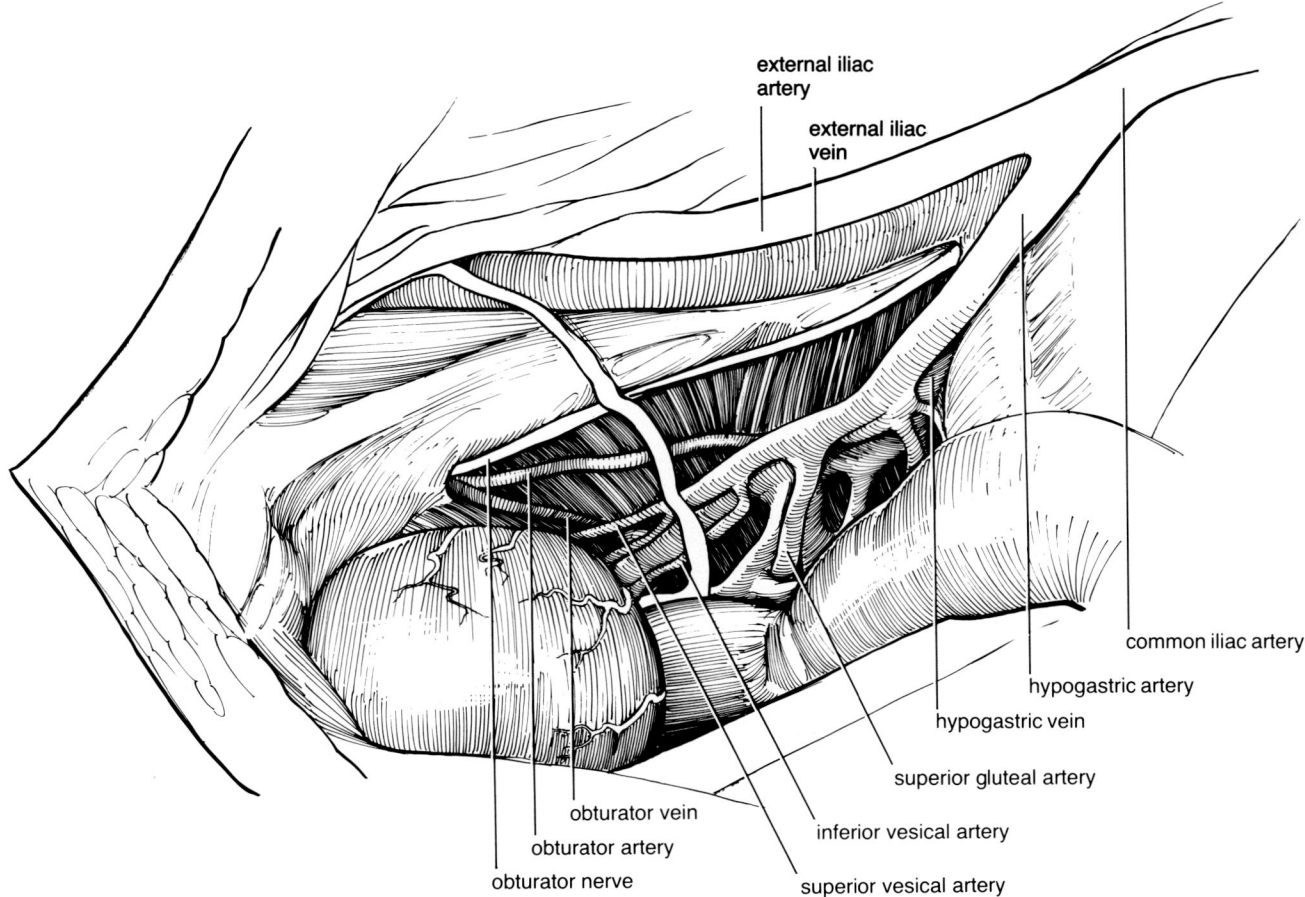

external iliac artery

external iliac vein

common iliac artery

hypogastric artery

hypogastric vein

superior gluteal artery

inferior vesical artery

superior vesical artery

obturator vein

obturator artery

obturator nerve

Common and External Iliac Veins

Note. Collaterals are numerous and can dilate in a few days after acute occlusion of a major vein.

Maintain direct pressure over the site. Visualization is facilitated by the more superficial location of these veins, compared with the hypogastric and pelvic veins, so that Trendelenburg tilt and proximal occlusion of the common iliac artery usually are not needed. Obtain proximal and distal control with sponge sticks and vascular clamps.

80 Repair the vein after longitudinal or transverse laceration or complete division if tension and venous constriction can be avoided. Carefully suture the edges of the defect with a 5-0 or 6-0 monofilament suture. Place a continuous over-and-over stitch; take small bites (1 to 2 mm deep and 1 mm apart). Inspect the vein for constriction.

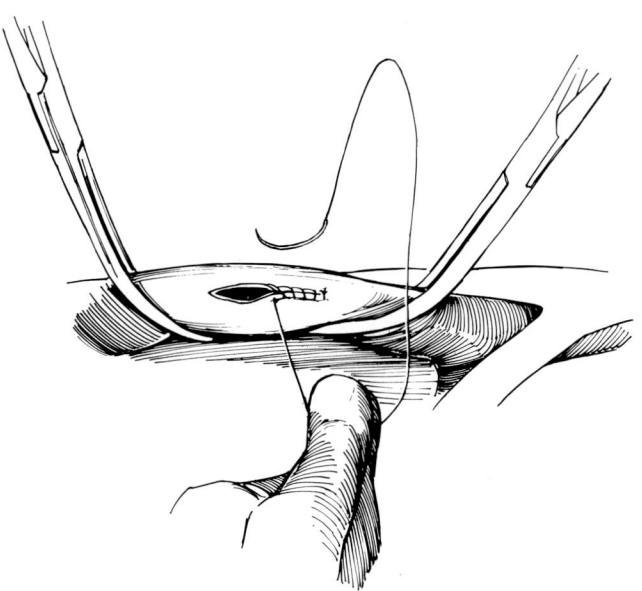

81 **A,** When the caliber of the vein has been significantly reduced, substitute a venous patch graft.
Expose the saphenous vein in the opposite leg. Resect a
suitable length; open it longitudinally and excise the
valves. Trim one end of it to fit the defect; manipulate the
patch by the edges to be trimmed to avoid intimal trauma
and later platelet deposition and thrombosis. Suture the
trimmed end to an end of the defect with a double-armed
5-0 or 6-0 monofilament mattress suture. **B,** Fasten the
midportions of the patch to the corresponding part of the
laceration with monofilament sutures. Trim the distal end
and coapt it with a second double-armed mattress suture.
Complete the anastomosis by running the two mattress
sutures, starting at each end and tying them to each other
in the middle on each side. Release the vascular clamps
one at a time.

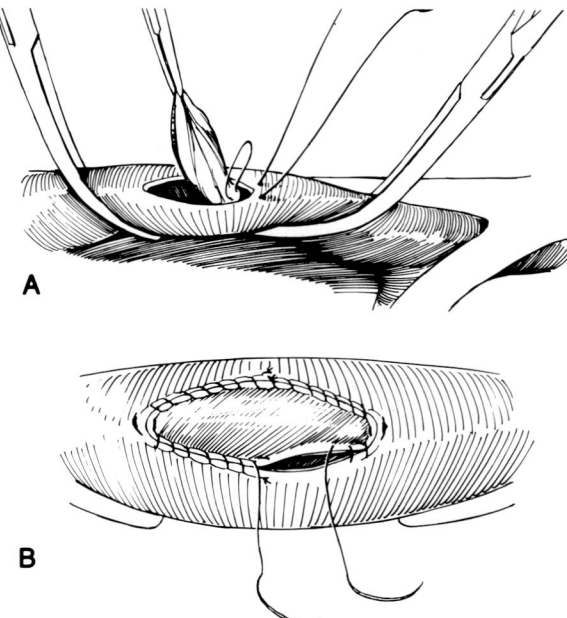

82 **A,** For repair after transection of a vein, trim the
ragged edges obliquely; do not spatulate them.
Mobilize the vein proximally and distally so that it will
come together without tension. If tension is inevitable, resort to ligation unless the pelvic collaterals have been disrupted and gangrene is inevitable. In this case, place a
vein graft. **B,** Place two double-armed 5-0 monofilament
sutures. **C,** Run one down each side.

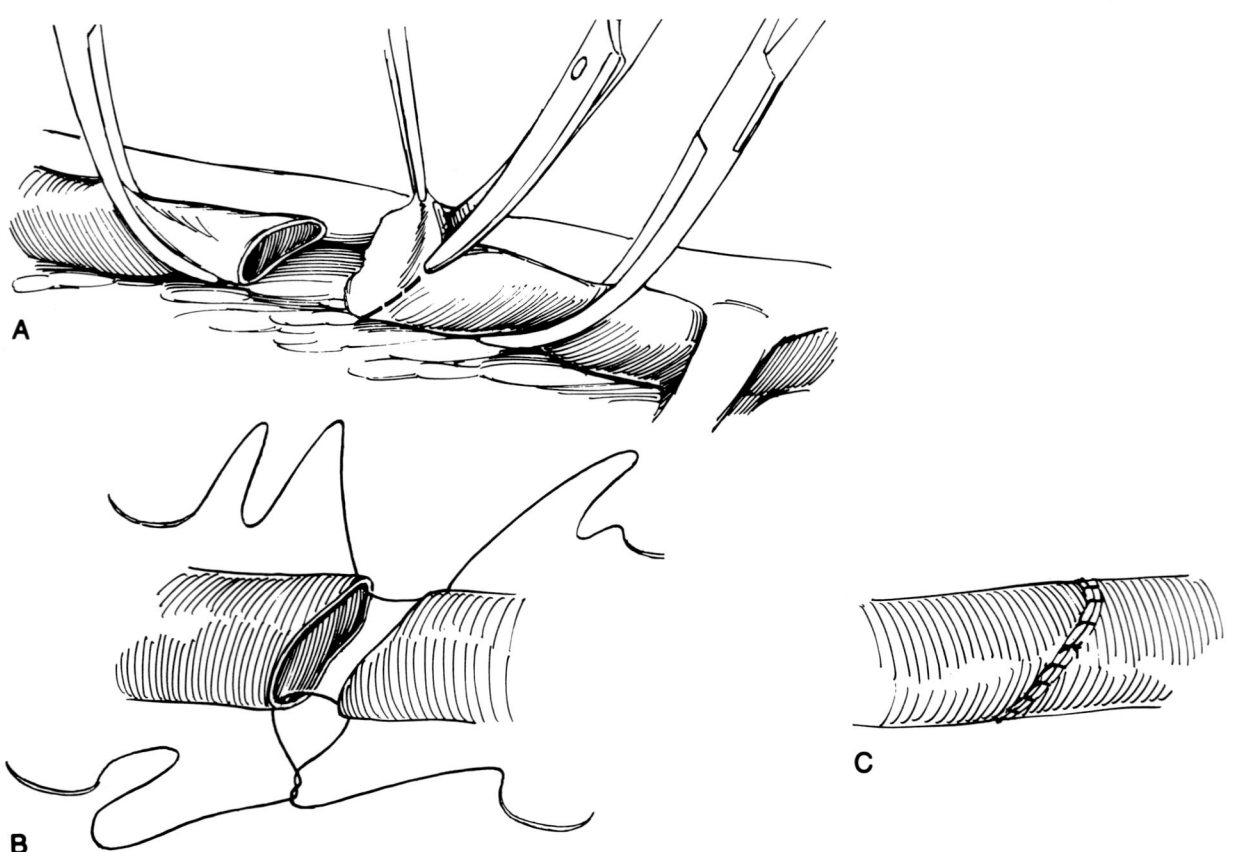

83 **A,** If near-total venous occlusion of the iliac vein is present, as after disruption of pelvic collaterals, with the possibility that the limb may be lost, a saphenous tube graft may be attempted, although subsequent thrombosis is quite likely. Obtain a vein graft 6 or 7 cm long from the opposite saphenous vein, one large enough to allow for contraction of the vein and to allow it to be used doubled. Mark the proximal end with a suture to indicate the direction of the valves. Trim the saphenous vein to a length twice that of the defect. Open the vein longitudinally with Potts scissors, and cut it in half transversely. **B,** Suture one side of each half together with a running 5-0 monofilament suture. **C,** Place the combined segments over a catheter of the same size as the iliac vein to be replaced, maintaining the correct orientation. Trim the other side and suture the graft around the catheter. Cut the catheter next to the graft, and gently slide the graft free. **D,** Suture the graft in place as for an end-to-end anastomosis.

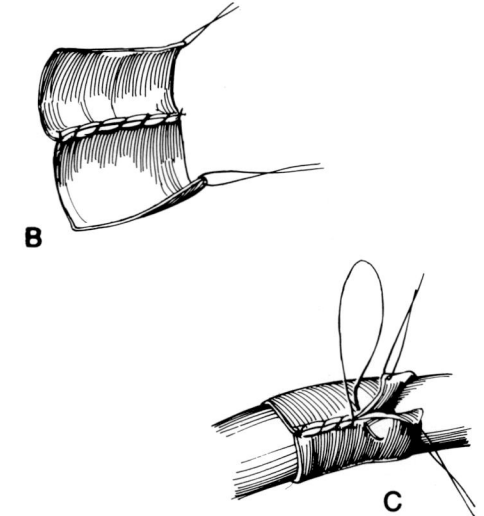

B

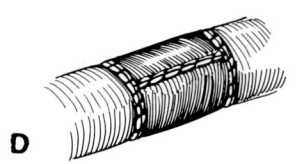

C

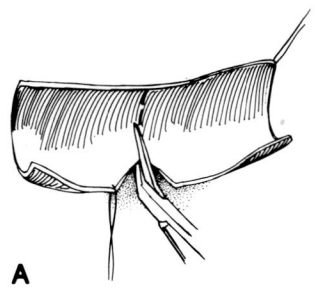

A

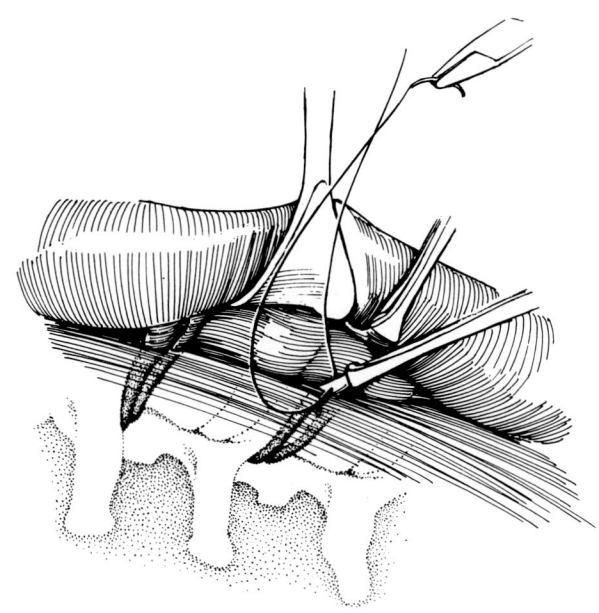

D

Lumbar Veins

84 As you slowly remove the pack, gently grasp each end of the lumbar vein with an Allis clamp. Suture ligate them with 6-0 monofilament sutures. Pack the site for a longer period until the bleeding stops if the cut end retracts into the intervertebral space. Then expose it and sew over the end of the vein.

Arterial Injuries

Aortic Laceration

85 Control proximal flow by quickly preparing two sponge sticks to hold a tightly folded (4 × 8) sponge between. Have the assistant apply firm pressure with the loop of gauze without entering the field. Control backbleeding yourself with digital pressure.

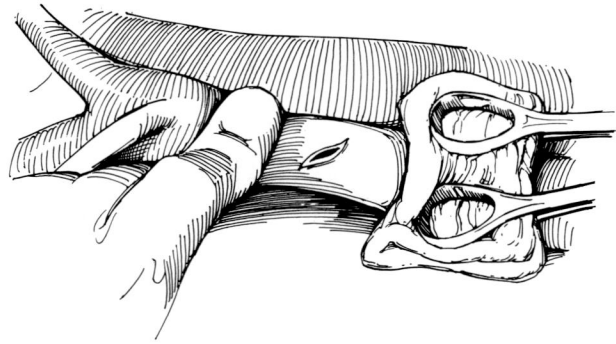

Laceration of the Branches of the Internal Iliac Artery

86 Temporarily occlude the abdominal aorta just above its bifurcation with one hand to reduce the bleeding. Clamp and ligate the cut artery. This can be done without risk of ischemia. Alternatively, maintain pressure on the bleeding point with a stick sponge while you free up the artery proximally and distally for several centimeters. Apply an arterial clamp proximally only tight enough to stop blood flow; be wary of dislodging a friable arterial plaque. Divide and ligate the vessel. When diffuse pelvic bleeding is present, consider ligation of the internal iliac artery.

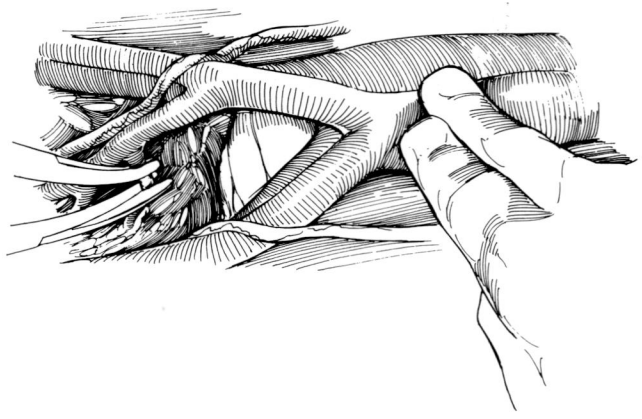

External Iliac Artery Laceration

87 **A,** Maintain compression over the defect with a sponge stick or fingers. Free the vessel proximally and distally. Apply vascular clamps, minimally closed. Place a running, over-and-over 4-0 or 5-0 monofilament suture. **B,** If the laceration is tangential or irregular, divide, trim, and reanastomose the artery. Up to 1 cm can be lost without consequent tension. Check the anastomosis for a strong pulse and absence of a thrill. Otherwise, redo the anastomosis. One can insert an arterial graft, although this is seldom necessary in the iliac arteries.

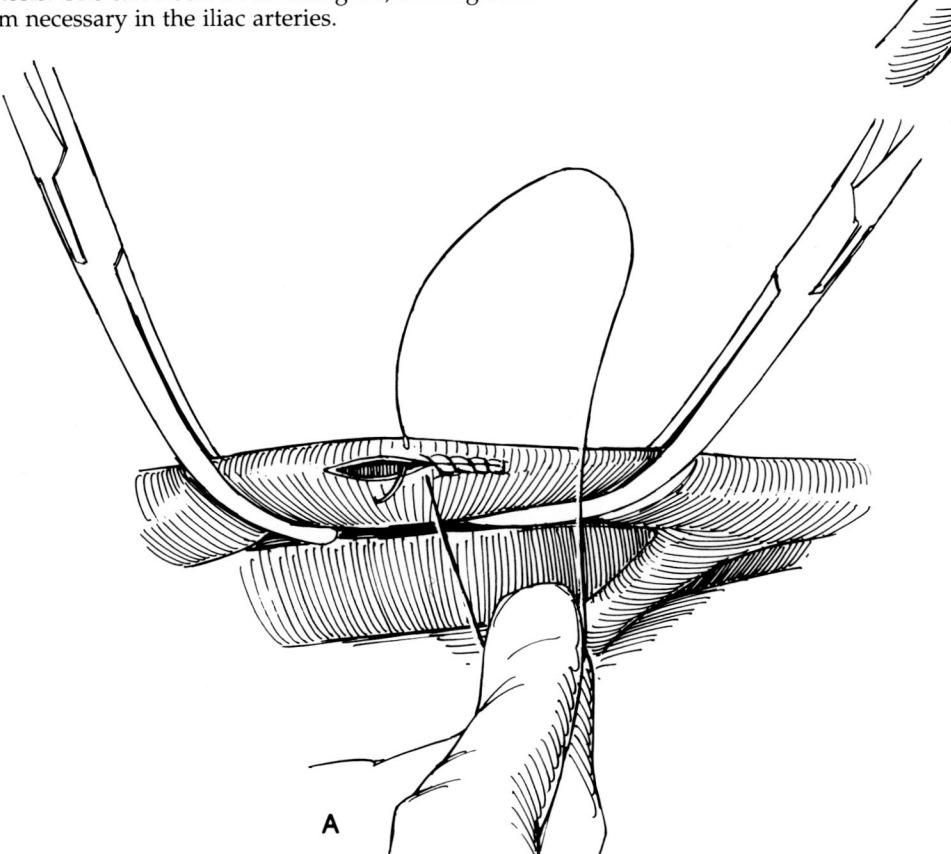

Loss of Control of a Renal Artery

88 **A,** With loss of control of the *left* renal artery during flank nephrectomy, especially during donor nephrectomy when a long segment of artery is removed, compress the pedicle area. Expose the aorta just below the diaphragm and compress it. Identify, clamp, and suture ligate the stump of the artery. **B,** Before clamping the *right* renal artery, dissect the vena cava away from the aorta above and below so that the aorta may be clamped in an emergency. If aortic clamping has not been done, control the stump with sponge stick or digital pressure while the aorta is freed from over the vena cava. Clamp and suture ligate the stump.

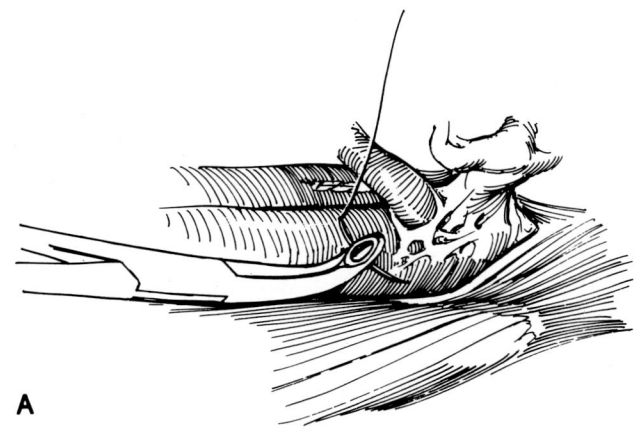

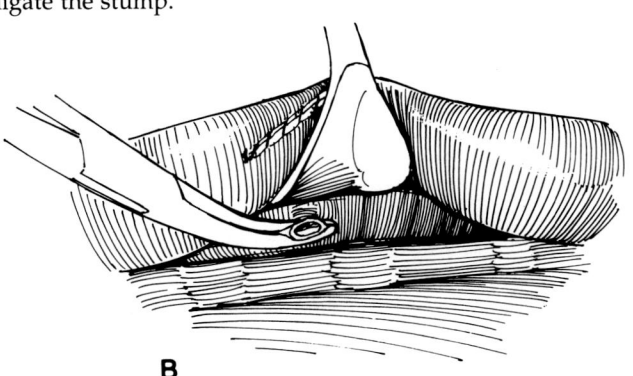

Necessary Arterial Resection

Remove the segment of a major vessel involved in the disease process after controlling blood flow proximally and distally. A vascular surgeon should then be called for assistance.

89 A, If the wound is not infected, select a knitted Dacron graft of a size similar to that of the artery, place it in a sample of the patient's blood, and allow clot-ting. Aspirate the intraluminal clot before use. Anastomose the less-accessible end first with a 4-0 monofilament continuous suture. Stretch the graft to flatten the crimps and trim it to length. **B**, Begin the second anastomosis on the back side, and run it up both lateral walls with a double-armed suture. Before the last sutures are placed and tied, release the proximal clamp to flush the graft. Complete the anastomosis and release the distal clamp, followed by the proximal one.

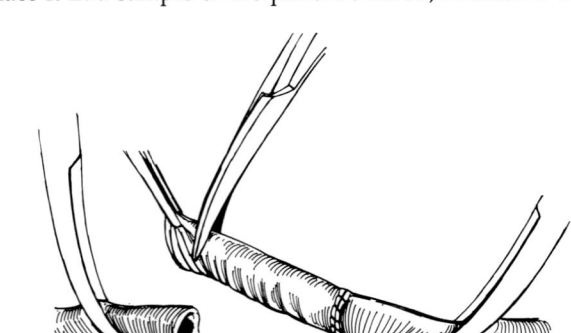

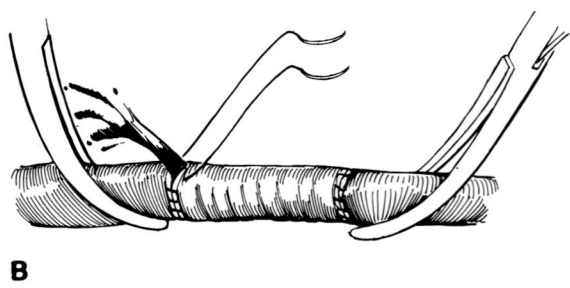

CLOSURE OF BOWEL LACERATION

Small Bowel Closure

90 A and **B**, For a transverse tear, place Lembert sutures of 4-0 silk at the mesenteric and antimesenteric ends of the laceration.

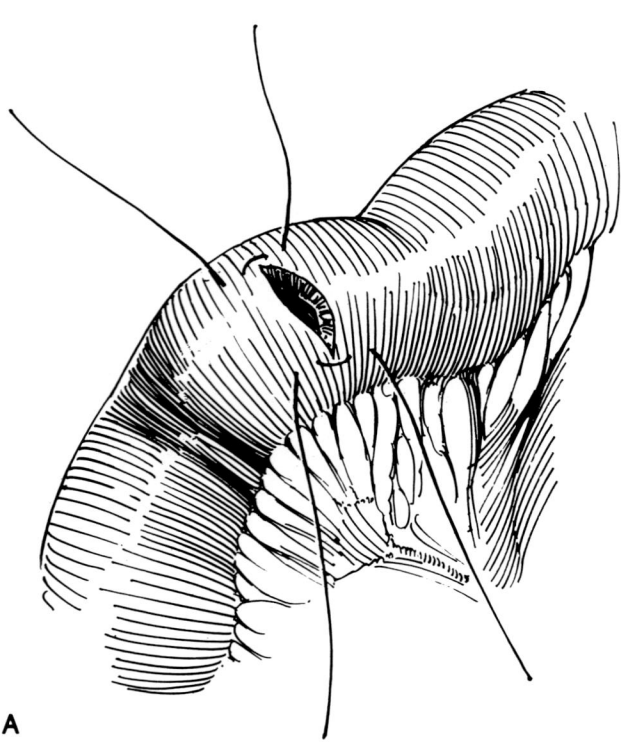

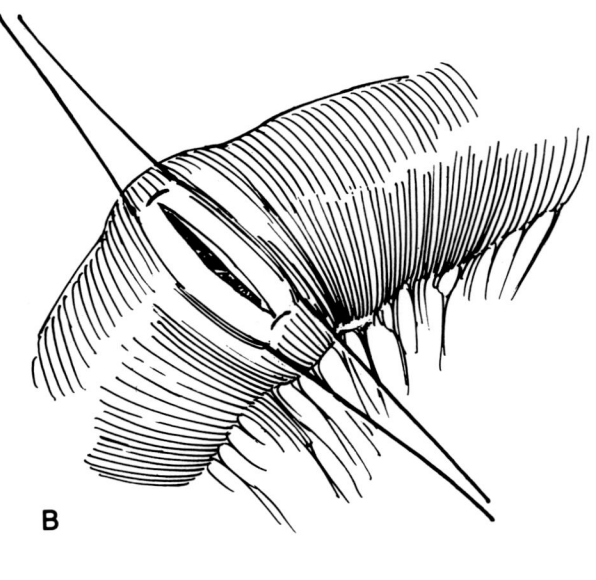

91 **A** and **B,** Convert a short linear laceration (one less than 3 cm in length) into a transverse one to avoid narrowing the lumen. Tag the sutures and have your assistant put gentle traction on them.

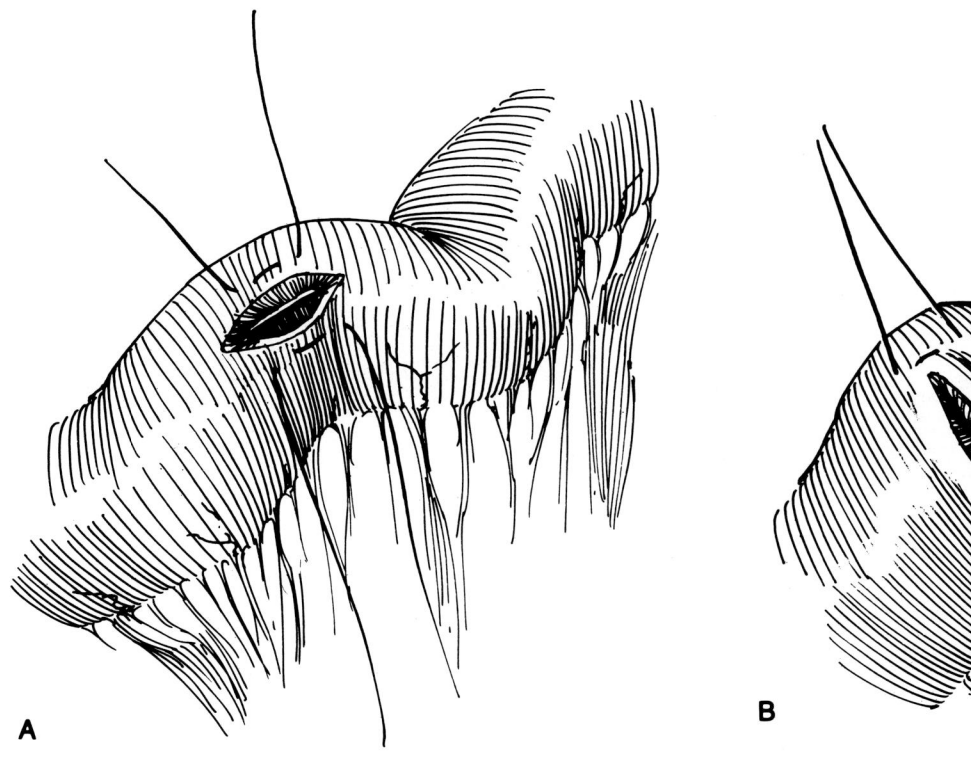

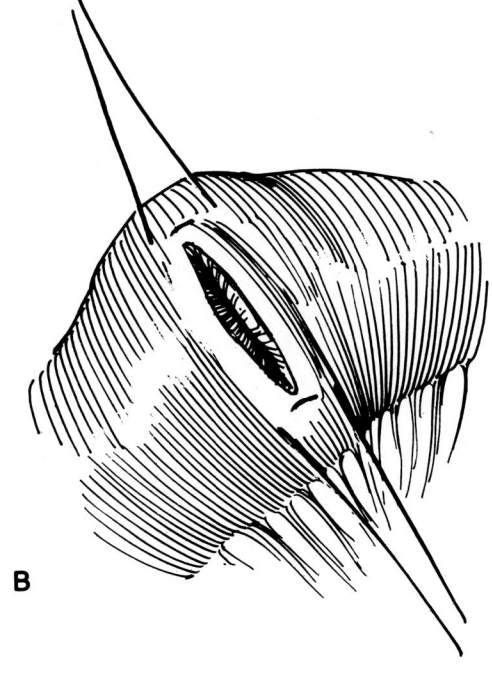

A

B

92 Place additional Lembert sutures, first at the midpoint, then midway between those already placed, dividing each remaining gap in half with bites of 3 to 4 mm through the serosal-muscularis-serosal layers on each side. The sutures should penetrate the tough submucosa but not enter the intestinal lumen. Next, place sutures 4 mm apart to close the remainder of the defect.

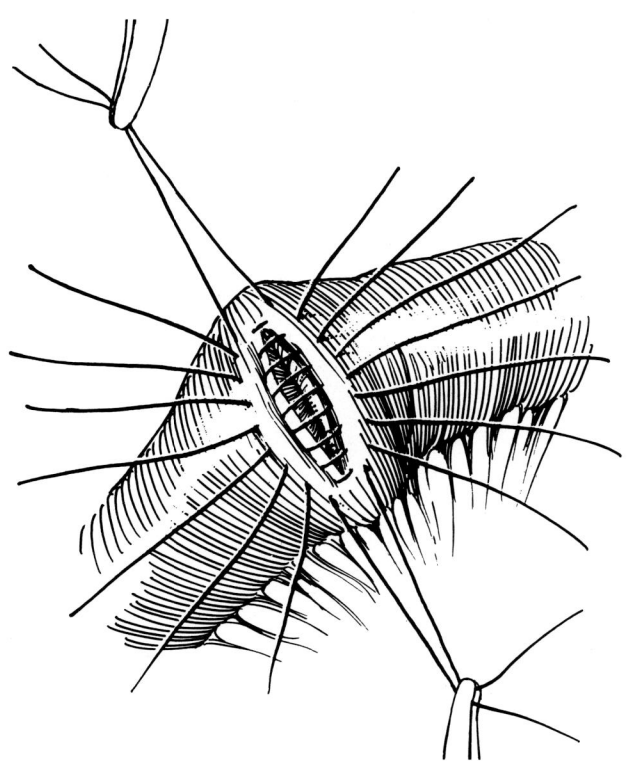

93 Have your assistant depress the edges under the sutures as you tie them.

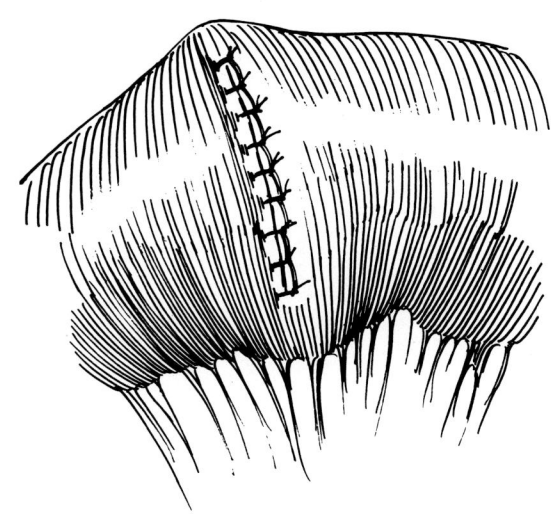

For lacerations longer than 3 cm, close them longitudinally. Very long lacerations require resection and end-to-end anastomosis.

Large Bowel Closure

94 Occlude the bowel above and below the lesion with intestinal clamps (not with tapes, which could harm the vessels) passed through the mesentery. Trim the edges of the defect. Place a row of vertical mattress 4-0 synthetic absorbable sutures.

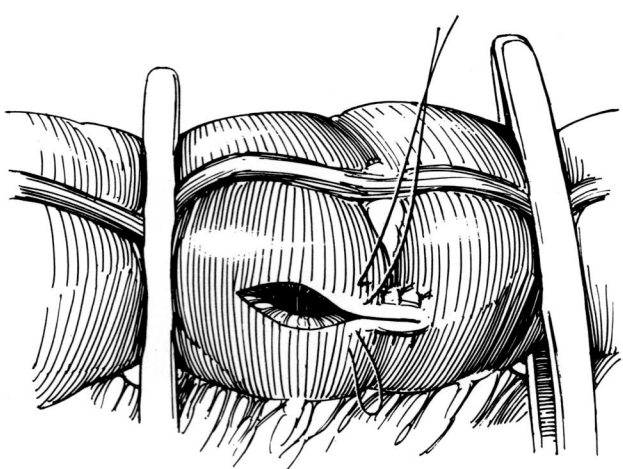

95 Place a second row, using Lembert sutures to invert the bowel over the first row.

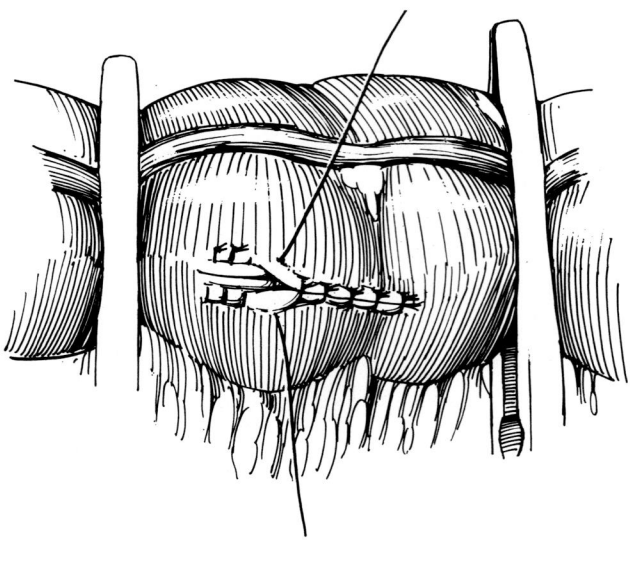

SECTION 3
Kidney

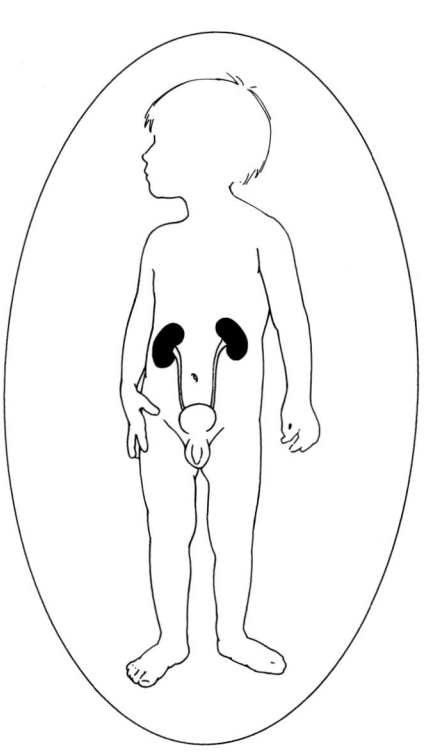

PART I

SURGICAL APPROACHES

CHAPTER 7

Selection of Incision

The kidney may be approached anteriorly, laterally, or posteriorly.

An *anterior transperitoneal route* is an excellent approach for major procedures on the kidney, ureter, and adrenal in infants and young children with protuberant abdomen, providing maximum exposure. This wide access is gained from an *anterior subcostal incision* (for localized lesions) or better from an *anterior transverse (chevron) incision* (ideal for excision of bilateral Wilms' tumors and for neuroblastoma and pheochromocytoma) or a *midline (vertical) incision* (useful for gastric augmentation procedures). The costal margin in children is high, so it does not limit a direct approach to the kidneys as much as in an adult. An anterior incision provides an opportunity to evaluate other intra-abdominal organs and gives superior access to the renal vessels and better control of the great vessels should they be injured. The disadvantages are the limited access that is obtained in obese older children and the risk of generating intestinal adhesions.

An *anterolateral extraperitoneal approach* through an *anterior subcostal incision* provides greater exposure in infants than it does in adults because of the wide costal flare and the more relaxed abdominal musculature. In debilitated children, a firm closure is ensured, because stress is distributed among the three fascial layers of the anterior abdominal wall. This approach induces fewer problems with ventilation than the standard flank incision, reduces postoperative pain, and allows earlier mobilization. The *pediatric extended anterior incision* benefits from its exten-

sion onto the anterior abdominal wall. It is a valuable incision for the removal of Wilms' tumor.

A *subcostal extraperitoneal lateral approach* through a *subcostal, transcostal,* or *supracostal incision* has the advantage of reaching the kidney, where it lies closest to the surface and is especially valuable in obese adolescents. If necessary for wider exposure for extensive surgery on the kidney, a lateral incision can be extended into a *thoracoabdominal incision* or converted into a *dorsal rib flap.* The disadvantages of these lateral incisions are the need to divide large muscles, the risk of injuring nerves, the need to make a relatively large incision, and the fact that the vascular pedicle lies on the opposite side of the kidney from the one exposed. In spite of these limitations, a lateral incision may be safer in neonates, even for bilateral pyeloplasties that require two flank incisions, to avoid the intestinal adhesions with resultant intestinal obstruction that are associated with a transabdominal-transperitoneal approach.

The *lumbar approach* is ideal for more limited reconstructive operations in children. A *dorsal lumbotomy* avoids division of muscles and nerves and heals quickly with minimal pain. Although the exposure is limited, it provides the most direct approach to the ureteropelvic junction, and because it avoids crossing muscles and nerves, it is followed by minimal postoperative discomfort and a quicker recovery. In adolescents, it is suitable for renal biopsy and at least for simple pyelolithotomy. The skin incision is placed obliquely to follow Langer's lines, easily accomplished in the child.

CHAPTER 8

Anterior Subcostal Incision

EXTRAPERITONEAL APPROACH

1 *Position*: Place the child in the supine oblique position with the buttocks flat and the shoulders turned up 30 to 40 degrees. For infants, place a folded towel under the sacroiliac joint; for adolescents, flex the table in addition to placing a sandbag. *Incision*: Start the incision in the midline anteriorly, one third of the distance from the xiphoid to the umbilicus. End the incision on the left at the tip of the 11th rib near the anterior axillary line. Curve it to avoid the costal margin.

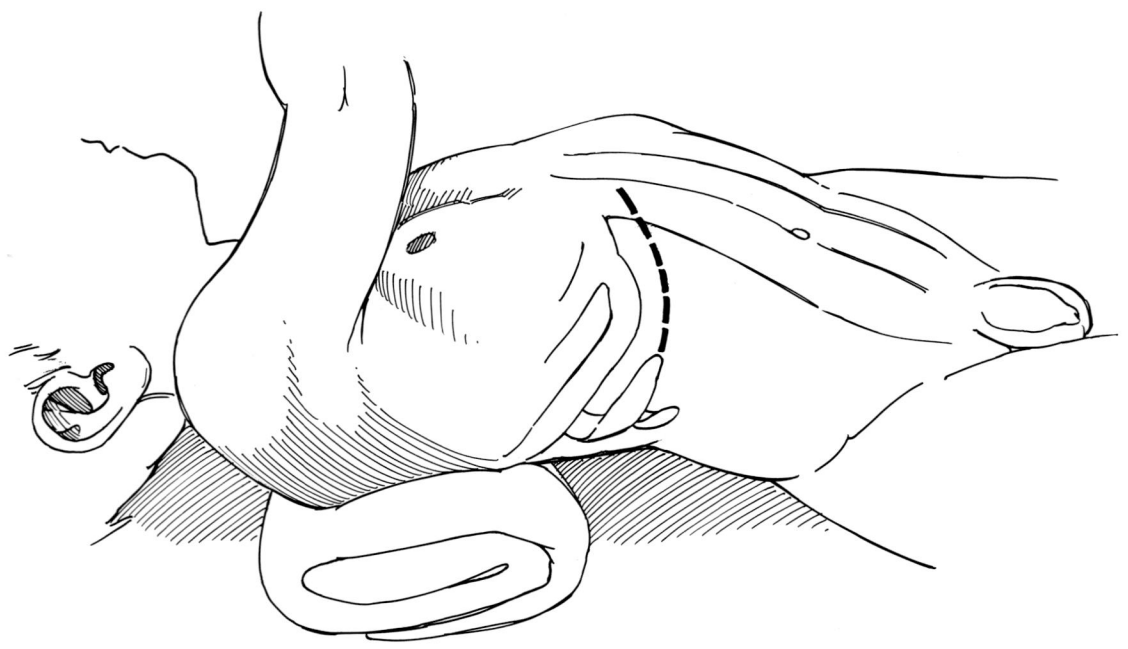

2 Divide the left side of the anterior rectus sheath and the external oblique muscles in the line of the incision for a short distance. If the rectus muscle must be divided, clamp, divide, and ligate the superior epigastric artery behind it.

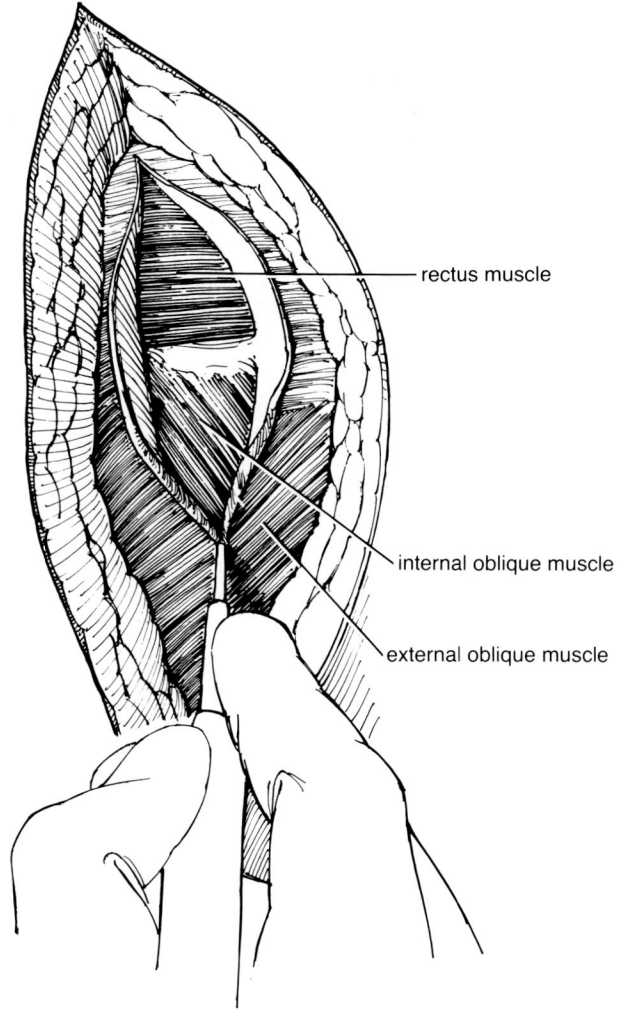

rectus muscle

internal oblique muscle

external oblique muscle

3 Divide or bluntly split the internal oblique and digitally separate the fibers of the transversus abdominis, starting as far posteriorly as possible where the peritoneum is less adherent. Incise the transversalis fascia and also its condensation at the lateral margin of the rectus muscle as the peritoneum is bluntly stripped down from the transversalis fascia covering the inferior portion of the anterior abdominal wall. Free the peritoneum superiorly as well.

For more exposure, divide some of the contralateral rectus sheath. Further exposure can be gained by extending the incision posteriorly as a flank incision or by cutting across both rectus muscles to open the peritoneum as a chevron incision (page 81).

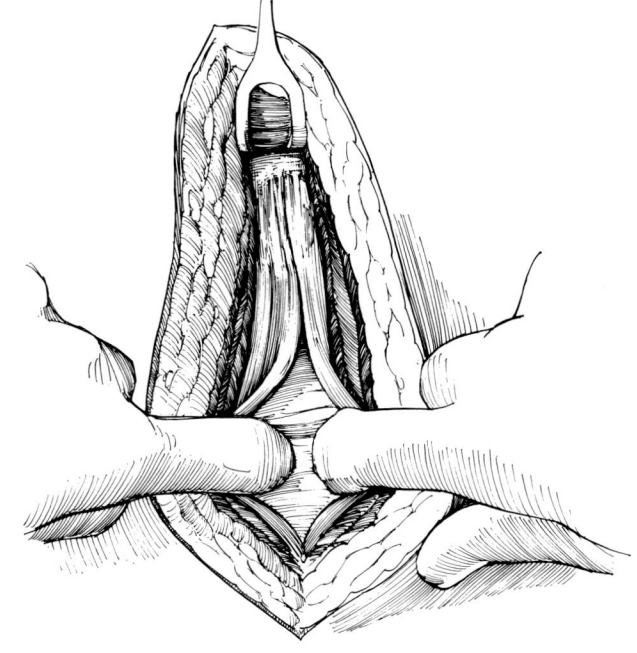

4 Use one hand to sweep far posteriorly to the lateral edge of the psoas muscle in the extraperitoneal space, then bluntly strip the peritoneum from the overlying muscle layer. The peritoneum is quite adherent here; use a peanut dissector of a sponge stick to avoid tearing it. Some sharp dissection with the scissors may be required. Make a transverse incision through the transversalis fascia as it passes behind the posterior rectus sheath and a sagittal incision through it as it descends into the pelvis.

Free the peritoneum from the transversalis fascia for a distance of at least a few centimeters above and below the wound so that it may be mobilized anteriorly to expose the posterior lamella of Gerota's fascia.

The limitations in exposure with the anterior incision are not primarily of muscular origin but originate with the transversalis fascia enveloping the peritoneum. Thus, the broadest exposure can be gained by incising this layer in two directions: (1) a transverse incision through its condensation as the posterior rectus sheath and (2) a sagittal incision through the fascia as it descends into the pelvis beneath the lower musculature, the peritoneum having been separated from it medially.

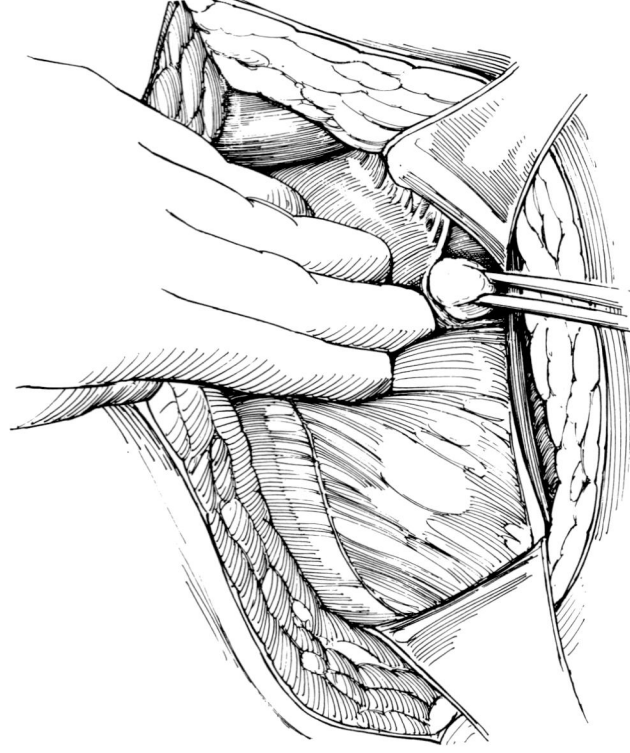

5 Enter Gerota's fascia over the lateral aspect of the kidney; reflect the fascia anteriorly.

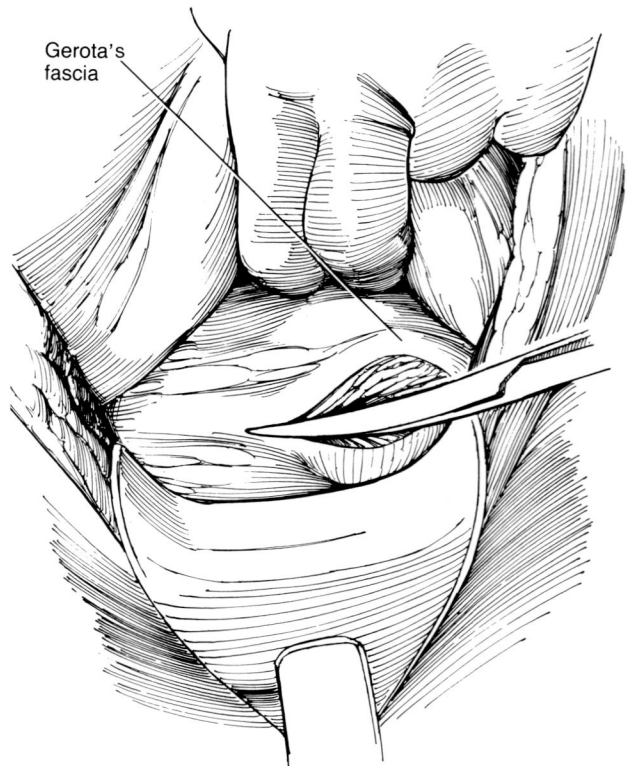

Gerota's fascia

6 **A** and **B,** Carry the peritoneum anteriorly with Gerota's fascia. Dissect the perirenal fat from the kidney so that the posterior portion remains behind the kidney to isolate it from the posterior body wall. Expose the posterior and anterior surfaces of the kidney. Close the wound in layers after providing for a Penrose drain.

Intraoperative problems may arise with this incision if the upper pole is large or adherent, but initial control of the pedicle reduces the risks. Bleeding from an accessory vessel may require extension of the incision across the midline. Pressure of the retractor on the 10th and 11th intercostal nerves may produce temporary hypesthesia postoperatively.

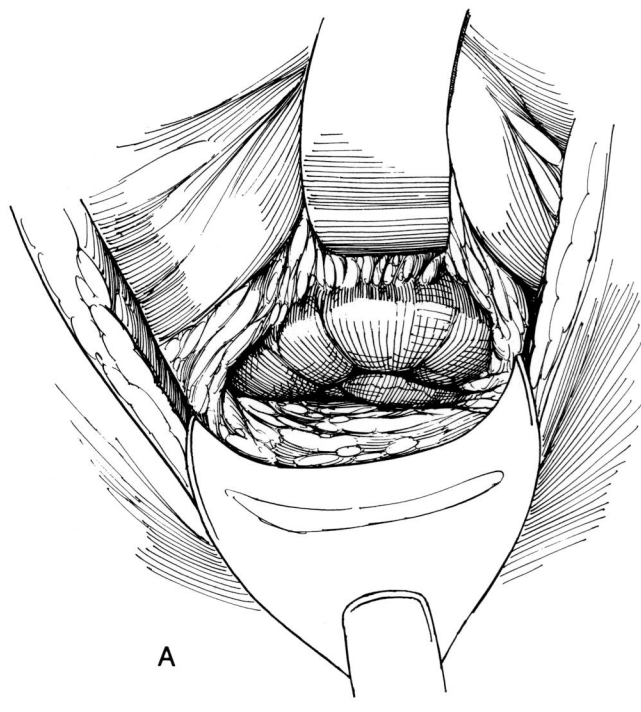

A

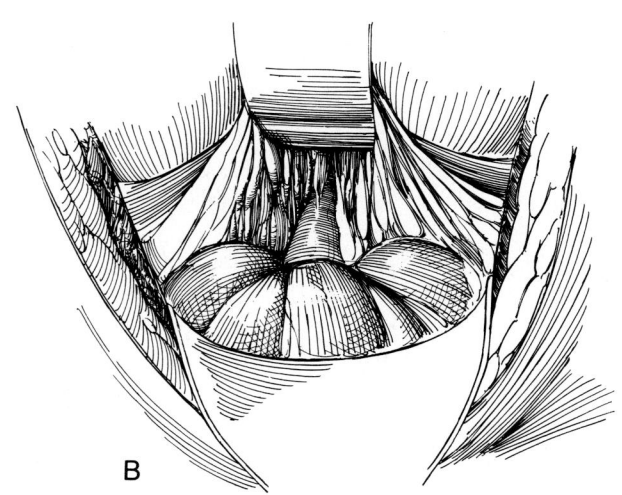

B

TRANSPERITONEAL APPROACH

7 Bluntly separate the fibers of the internal oblique and transversus muscle as previously described, and expose the outer surface of the peritoneum. Divide the peritoneum in the line of the incision.

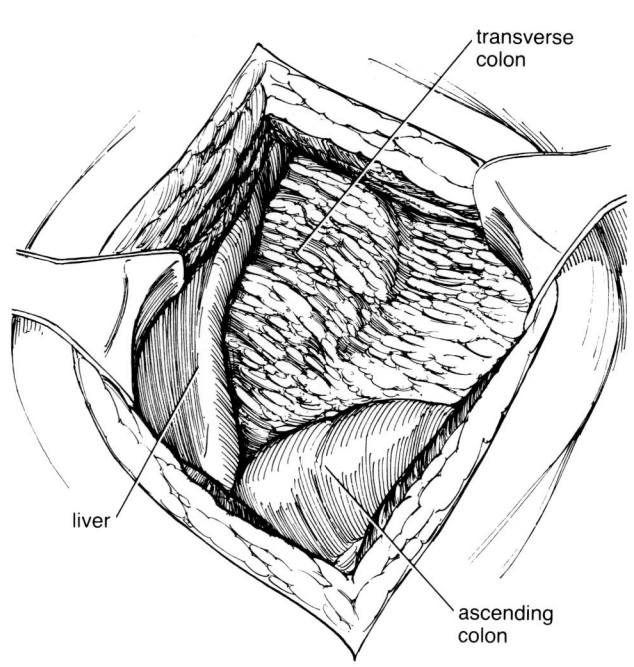

transverse colon

liver

ascending colon

8 **A,** *Right kidney:* The Kocher maneuver allows direct approach to the *right* renal hilum. Make an incision in the posterior peritoneum lateral to the second portion of the duodenum, and expose the anterior surface of the vena cava, posterior to the portal vein and anterior to the renal vein. **B,** Identify the right gonadal vein emptying anterolaterally into the vena cava, any accessory polar veins, and the large adrenal vein that enters posterolaterally 4 to 6 cm cephalad of the renal vein.

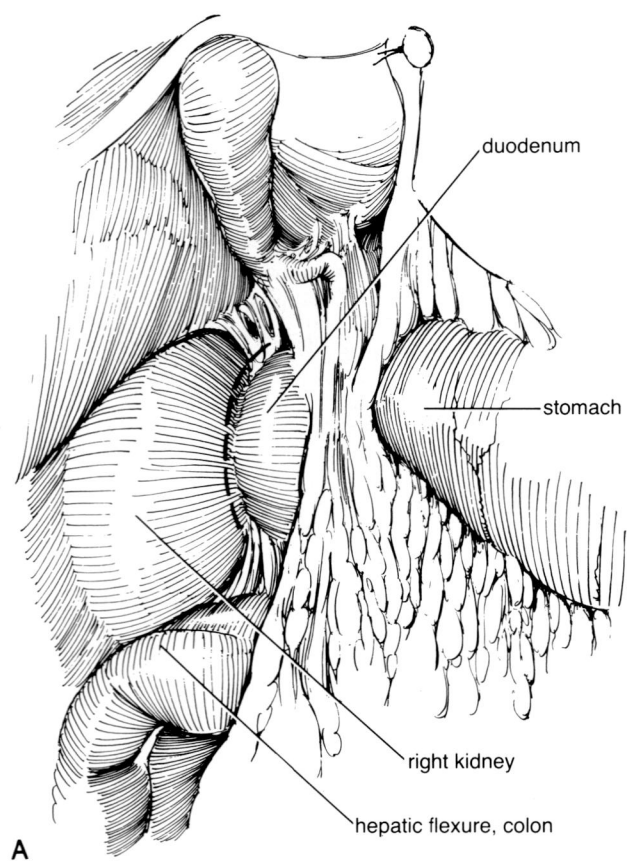

duodenum

stomach

right kidney

hepatic flexure, colon

A

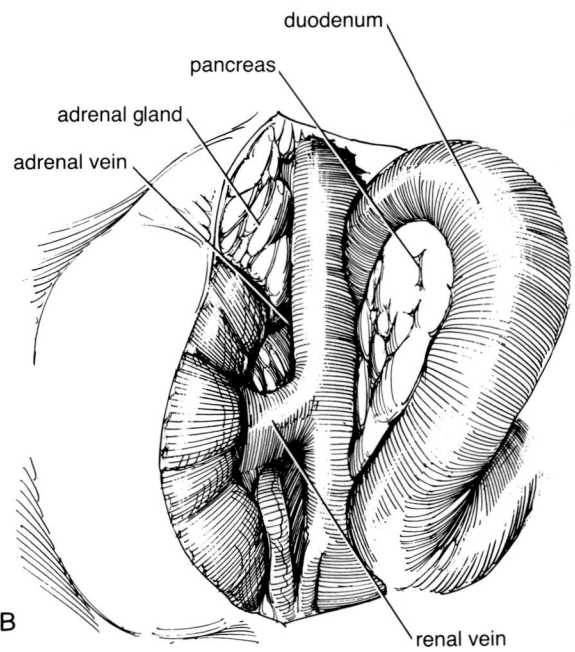

duodenum

pancreas

adrenal gland

adrenal vein

renal vein

B

9 **A,** *Left kidney:* For approach to the *left* renal hilum, make a vertical incision in the posterior peritoneum just caudad to the ligament of Treitz beside the fourth portion of the duodenum, and expose the anterior surface of the aorta. **B,** Identify the left renal vein as it crosses the aorta and the anterior-lying left gonadal artery, as well as the inferior mesenteric vein and the superior mesenteric artery.

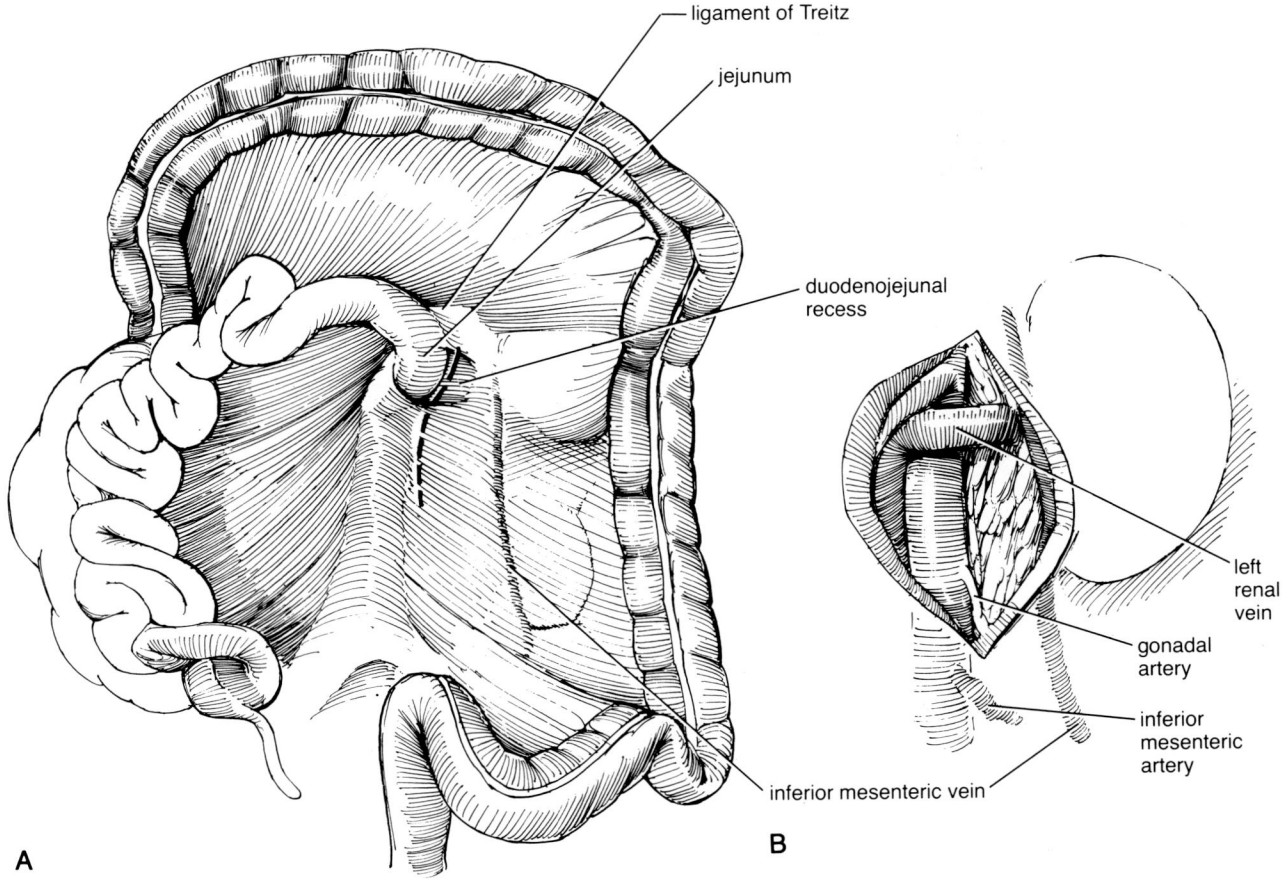

ligament of Treitz

jejunum

duodenojejunal recess

inferior mesenteric vein

left renal vein

gonadal artery

inferior mesenteric artery

A

B

10 **A,** The adrenal may be approached through the lesser sac as an alternative. **B,** Divide the gastrocolic portion of the omentum to enter the sac anterior to the pancreas and behind the stomach. Retract the colon inferiorly, incise the retroperitoneum just below the pancreas, and continue by dividing the splenocolic and renocolic ligaments to expose the left renal hilum.

Before closure, insert a drain if it is needed and bring it out extraperitoneally through a stab wound. It is not essential that the peritoneum be reattached behind the colon. Place a running synthetic absorbable suture to join the edges of the peritoneum and posterior rectus sheath. Approximate the transversalis and internal oblique muscles with interrupted synthetic absorbable sutures. Close the external oblique fascia and anterior rectus sheath similarly. Complete the closure of the subcutaneous layer and the skin.

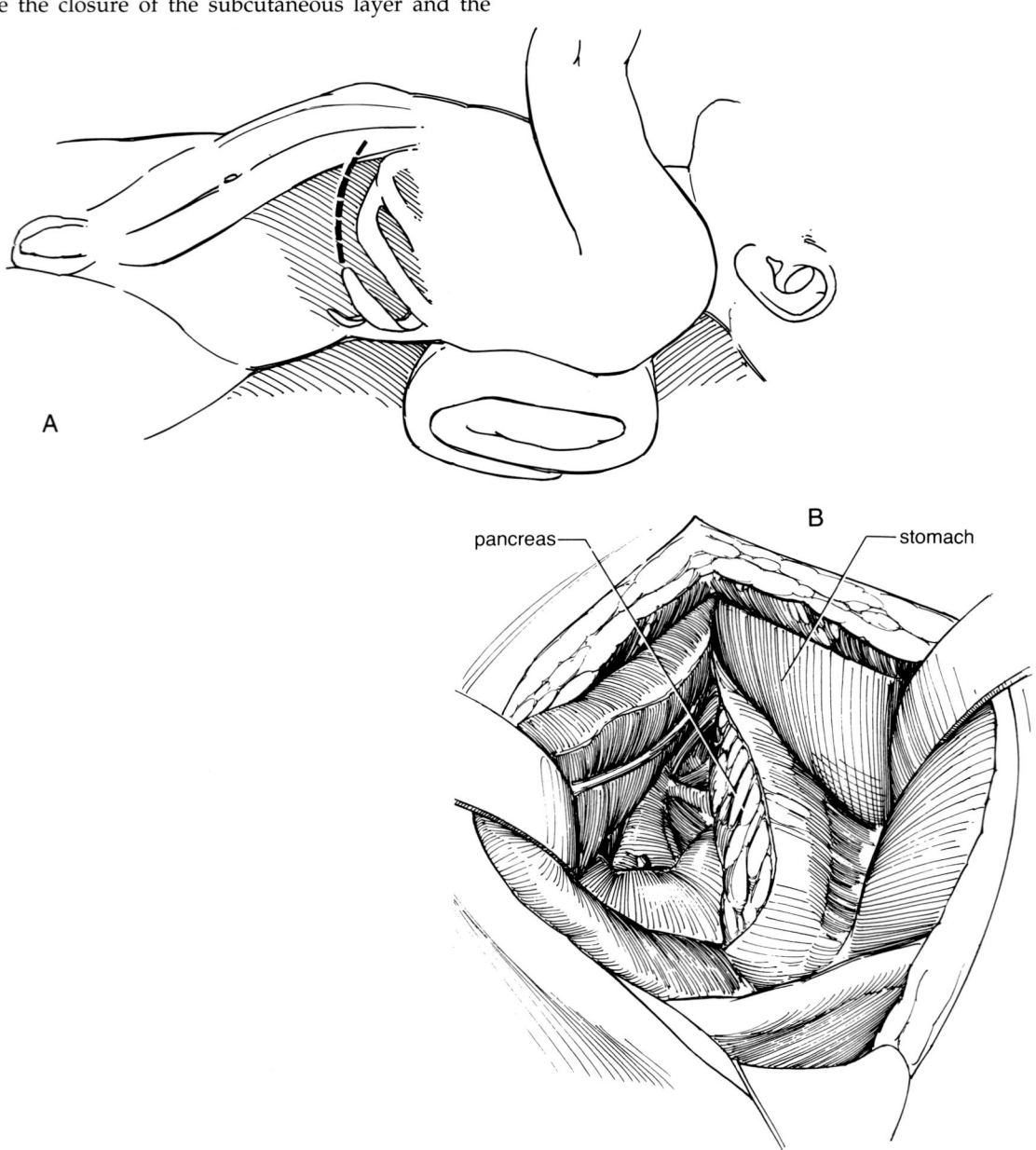

Commentary by H. Norman Noe

This incision by design allows a transperitoneal approach with the specific advantage of allowing early access to renal pedicle and retroperitoneal nodes. In a child, a transverse incision allows adequate exposure and, if necessary, can be extended if access to the contralateral kidney or other intra-abdominal organs is required. Care particularly should be taken on the left side to avoid injury to the pancreas or superior mesenteric artery when attempting to dissect the mesentery medially to gain access to the renal pedicle. If extension of this incision is required posteriorly and pleural entry is encountered, simple evacuation of the pleural cavity with a small catheter and suturing of the pleura usually are adequate, as is management without the necessity of formal placement of a chest tube.

CHAPTER 9

Pediatric Extended Anterior Incision

An extended anterior incision provides excellent exposure for excision of Wilms' tumor and also is valuable for bilateral simultaneous pyeloplasty.

1 *Position*: Place the child in a 30-degree oblique position with the lumbar spine over the break in the table. Flex the table to accentuate the renal area. Placing a rolled towel under the child's back or raising the kidney rest may improve the position.

Make a long transverse incision above the umbilicus, ending at the tip of the 12th rib on the involved side. For large tumors, make the incision higher so that it will extend through the 11th or 10th intercostal space, or consider a thoracoabdominal approach.

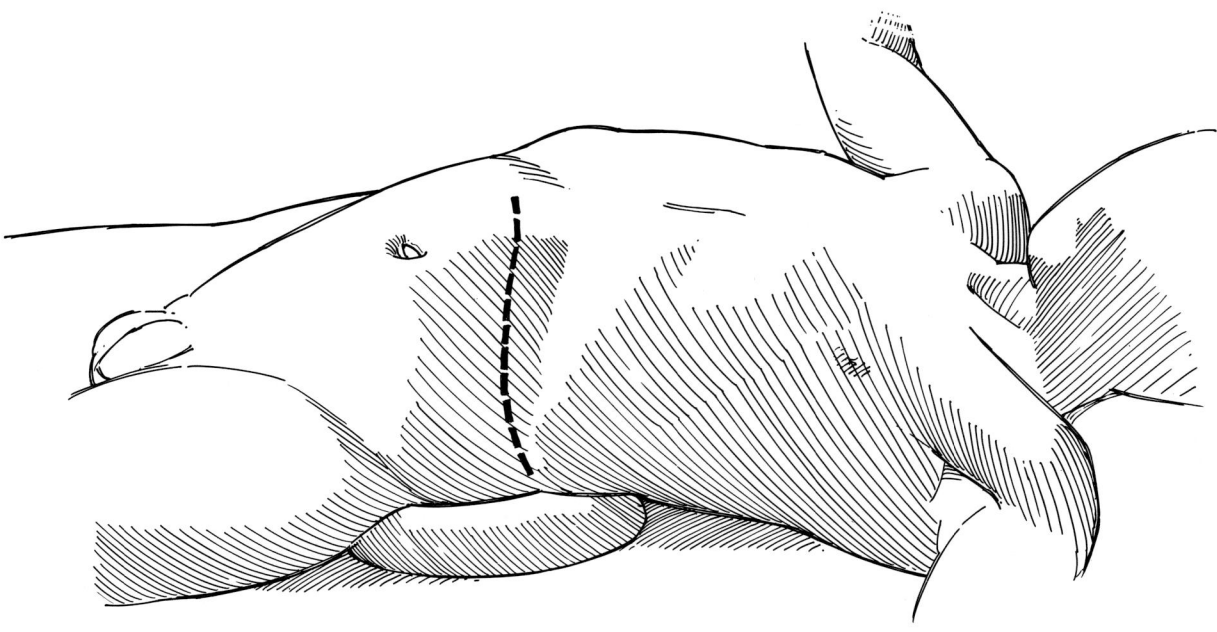

2 Divide the anterior rectus sheath and both rectus abdominis muscles. Divide and ligate the superior epigastric vessels. After opening the posterior sheath, insert two fingers under the body wall and divide all layers with the cutting current as far back as the tip of the 12th rib and extending forward beyond the linea semicircularis of the rectus sheath. Open the peritoneum and carefully contain the bowel with packs. Divide the falciform ligament above.

Assess operability by palpating and visualizing the para-aortic nodes, liver, and spleen and by looking for any direct tumor invasion into adjacent structures.

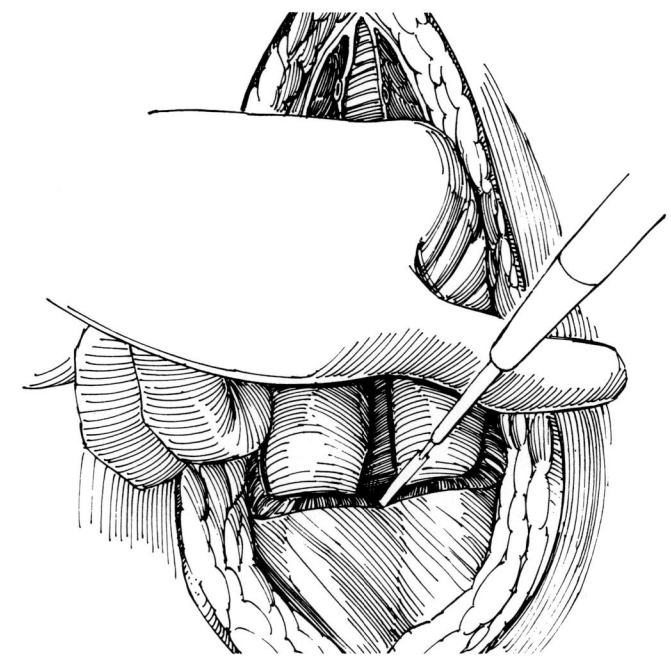

3 To gain access to the aorta through an incision in the retroperitoneum, displace the small bowel toward the opposite side and have your assistant hold the descending colon medially. Incise along the white line of Toldt to free the colon, then divide its attachments to the spleen on the left (or to the liver and gallbladder on the right). Gingerly dissect the colonic mesentery from the surface of Gerota's fascia over the tumor, taking care to preserve the colonic blood supply within it. For tumors on the right side, a Kocher maneuver will permit dissection of the duodenum and pancreas from the anterior aspect of the kidney.

Identify the aorta and vena cava. The inferior vena cava may be compressed and displaced by a tumor on the right side, and in its collapsed state it is easily divided and removed with the specimen. In addition, because with large tumors the vessels may be displaced and distorted, make positive identification of the artery and vein to the *opposite* kidney. If in doubt, place vascular tapes around the respective vessels.

It is good practice before closing to open Gerota's fascia on the opposite side and expose the kidney to look for tumor involvement.

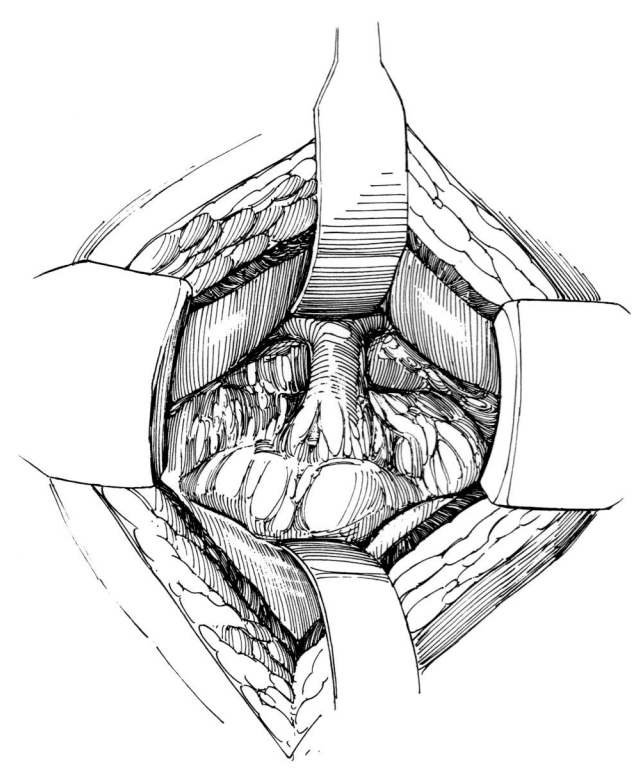

Commentary by H. Norman Noe

This incision by design allows a transperitoneal approach with the specific advantage of allowing early access to renal pedicle and retroperitoneal nodes. In a child, a transverse incision allows adequate exposure and, if necessary, can be extended if access to the contralateral kidney or other intra-abdominal organs is required. Care particularly should be taken on the left side to avoid injury to the pancreas or superior mesenteric artery when attempting to dissect the mesentery medially to gain access to the renal pedicle. If extension of this incision is required posteriorly and pleural entry is encountered, simple evacuation of the pleural cavity with a small catheter and suturing of the pleura usually are adequate, as is management without the necessity of formal placement of a chest tube.

CHAPTER 10

Anterior Transverse (Chevron) Incision

The anterior transverse (chevron) incision is used for bilateral upper retroperitoneal exposure by extension of an anterior subcostal incision across the midline.

The incision gives generous simultaneous access to both sides of the retroperitoneum. It is best to remove a large renal or adrenal mass on the left side, because there is more exposure when dividing the splenocolic ligament so as to avoid injury to the spleen. Avulsion of the right adrenal vein from the vena cava is avoided by the improved access to the upper retroperitoneum. The exposure allows the caudate lobe of the liver to be lifted from the cava to allow safe division of the small hepatic veins. The incision is most valuable when access to both sides of the retroperitoneum is required for left renal neoplasms invading the cava, for bilateral renal or adrenal tumors, or for large residual abdominal masses remaining after chemotherapy for metastatic testis tumor.

The incision may be converted to a thoracoabdominal approach by extending either limb upward below the 11th rib and dividing the diaphragm to expose intrathoracic extension of neoplasms. Or, by splitting the sternum at the apex, a wide V incision is formed that allows pursuit of renal cancer with caval involvement that extends to the suprahepatic level.

1 *Position*: Place the child in a supine position, hyperextended over a folded towel. *Incision*: From the tip of the 11th rib, incise the skin toward the midline below the costal margin to just below the xiphoid process. Continue down the opposite side to the tip of that 11th rib. If you are uncertain about operability or the need for such an extensive incision, make only half of it first.

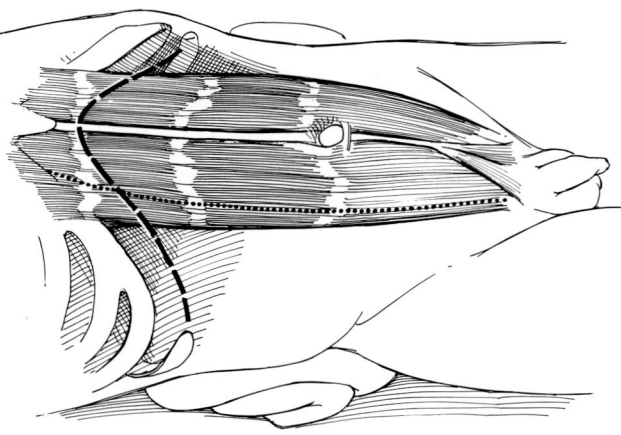

2 After incising the subcutaneous tissue, divide both sides of the anterior rectus sheath. Insinuate a finger under the rectus muscle and divide it with the cutting current. Ligate the superior epigastric artery as it is encountered.

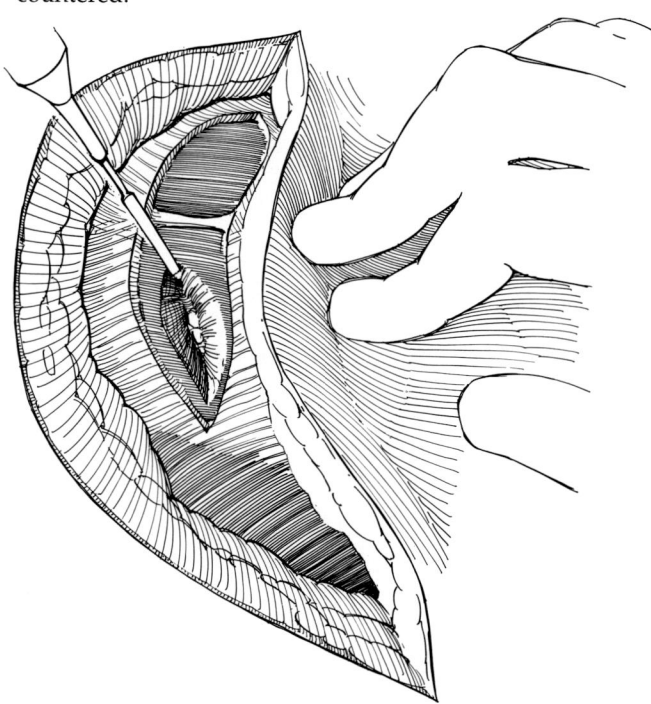

3 Divide the external and internal oblique investing fascia and muscles and split the fibers of the transversus abdominis. Incise the transversalis fascia and enter the peritoneal cavity just lateral to the posterior rectus sheath.

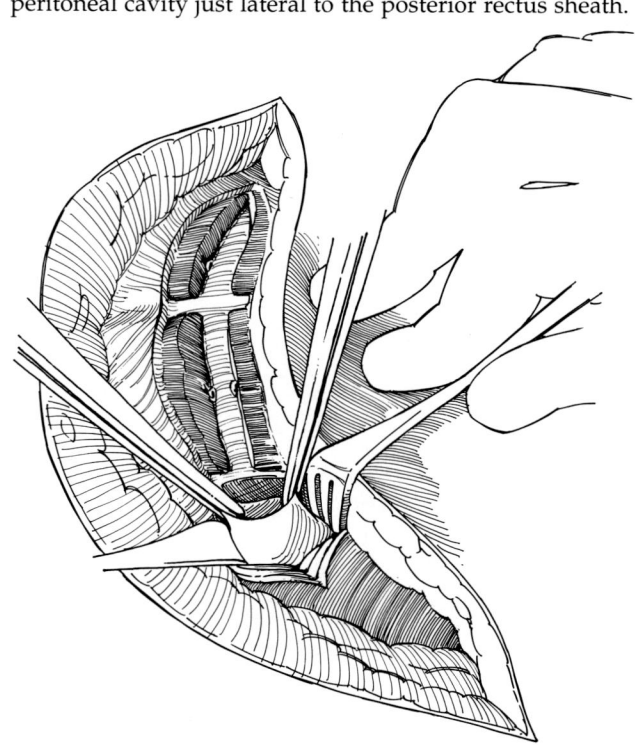

4 Complete the incision with cutting current or scissors against one or two fingers inside the abdomen. Divide the round ligament of the liver between clamps and ligate each end.

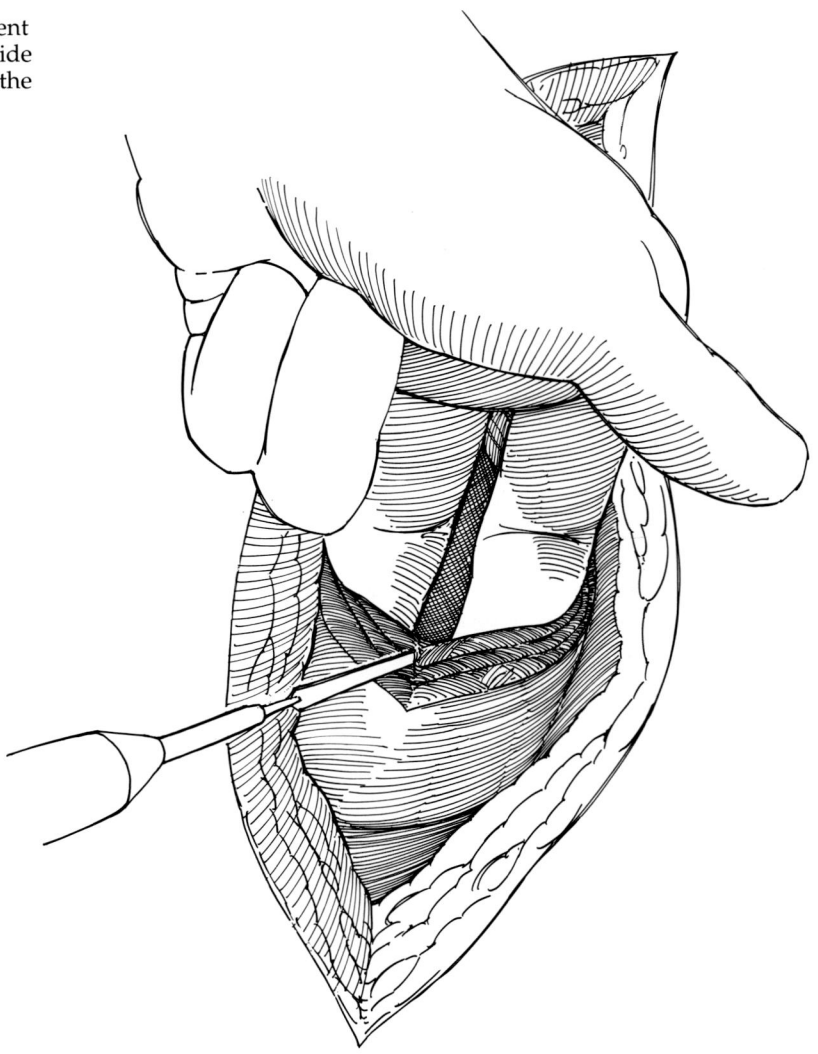

5 *Closure*: Remove the towel from under the back and straighten the table if flexed. Reapproximate the round ligament of the liver. Place three heavy sutures through the skin and linea alba at the apex of the incision to secure the linea alba in the midline; tie them when the rest of the closure is completed. Close the peritoneum, transversalis fascia, posterior rectus sheath, and linea alba in one layer with a running suture. Approximate the internal and external oblique muscles and the anterior rectus sheath with interrupted stitches of the same material. Alternatively, all fascial and muscular layers may be quickly closed employing a Prolene running suture. Close the subcutaneous tissue and skin and tie the three midline retention sutures over bolsters.

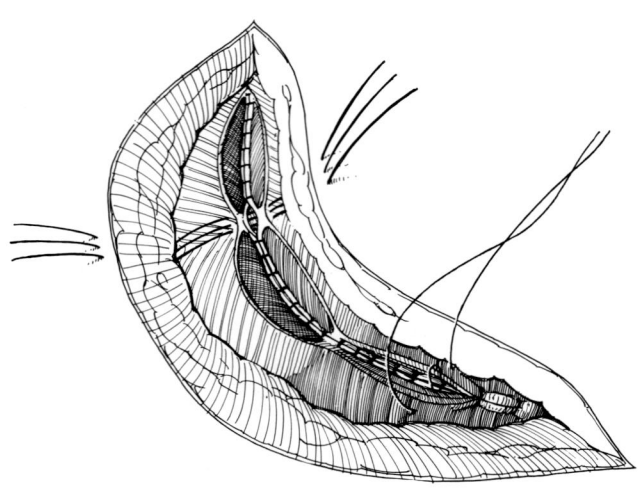

Commentary by H. Norman Noe

This incision allows wide exposure of both kidneys, the renal pedicles, and the great vessels. It should be used when large bulky tumor masses are present or if extensive retroperitoneal and intra-abdominal dissection will be needed. The transverse incision actually provides superior exposure to a vertical incision in a child and should be utilized, particularly if bilateral renal disease is suspected. Although many advocate a wide transverse approach for simultaneous pyeloplasty, it has been our philosophy to remain extraperitoneal where at all possible if a simple benign retroperitoneal disease process requires surgery. Thus, for bilateral pyeloplasty, it would seem preferable to perform each procedure through an anterior extraperitoneal subcostal incision as opposed to a single incision involving a transperitoneal approach, which would introduce the potential for intra-abdominal injury as well as prolonged postoperative ileus.

CHAPTER 11

Midline Transperitoneal Incision

1 *Position:* Place the patient supine with a rolled towel under the side of the lesion. *Incision:* Make an incision in the midline from the xiphoid to just below the umbilicus. For greater exposure, end the incision at the symphysis.

2 Divide the subcutaneous tissue with the cutting current and identify the fine decussations of the fused aponeuroses of the muscles of the anterior abdominal wall forming the linea alba. The rectus sheath here is covered with a delicate investment that may be opened to be certain of the position of the midline.

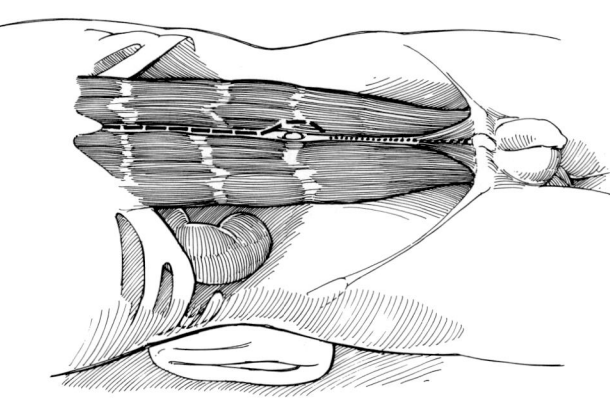

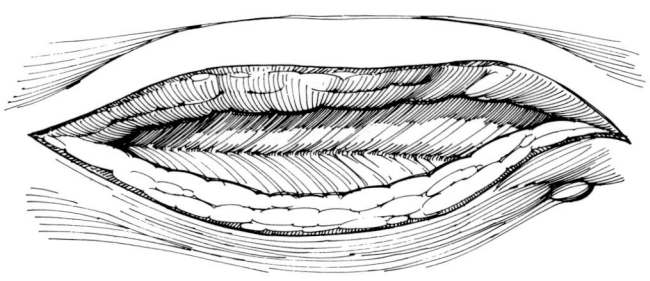

3 **A** and **B,** Incise through the linea alba into the very loose properitoneal fat covering the peritoneum. Successively elevate the areolar tissue and fat with two forceps to tent the peritoneum and incise the properitoneal tissue carefully between, taking care with each grasp not to include any bowel. **C,** After three or four such maneuvers, the peritoneum itself will be tented up. As the peritoneum is penetrated with the knife, air will enter and the bowel will fall away.

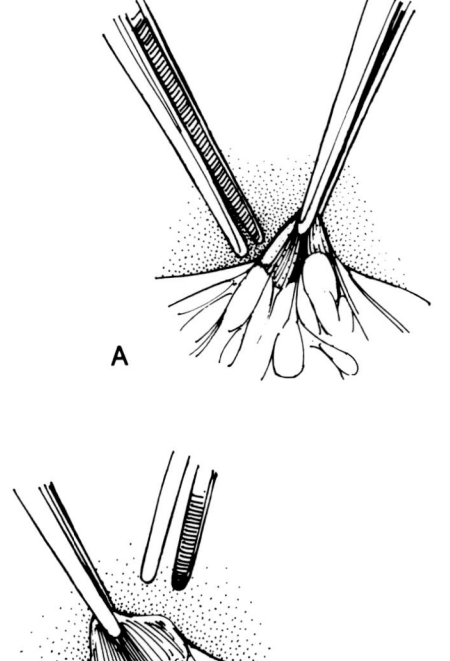

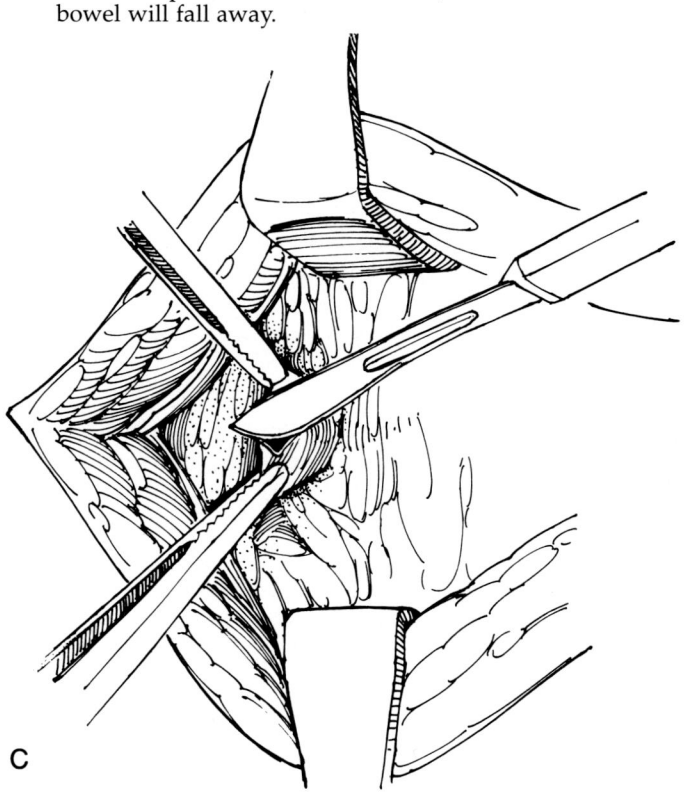

4 Hold each edge of the peritoneum in a curved clamp and open it in both directions with curved scissors while protecting the abdominal contents with a finger of the left hand. Divide and ligate the ligamentum teres.

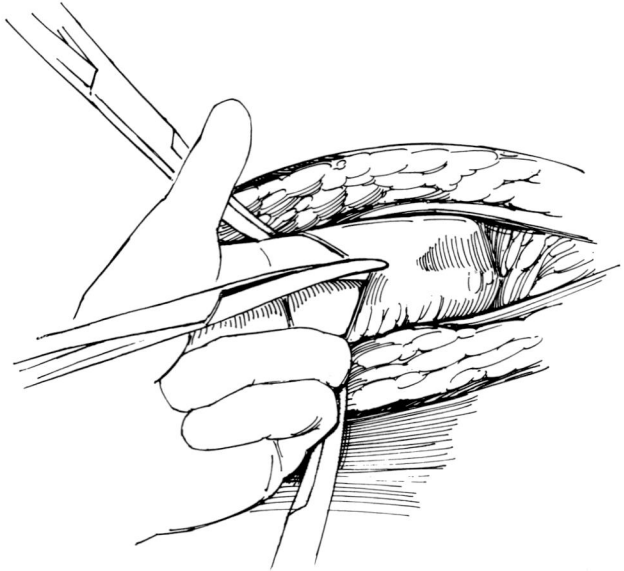

Closure: Tie a length of monofilament (Prolene, Novofil, or nylon) suture with six or seven knots at the xiphoid end. Run the suture continuously to the other end of the wound, catching only the fascia and ignoring the peritoneum. Tie the end securely. For greater safety, use three such sutures, each closing one third of the wound. Alternatively, close the peritoneum with a running absorbable suture, then close the fascia with sutures of interrupted synthetic absorbable sutures, either as simple sutures or figure-eight sutures. These are spaced in infants at distances equivalent to the standard rule for adults of 1 cm apart and 1 cm deep.

Because wound disruption requires special attention in adolescents (as it does in adults) place figure-eight interrupted Prolene stitches, incorporating all layers including the peritoneum, where the peritoneum may be grasped. These sutures must be tied square with multiple knots to prevent slipping, and the knots must be placed so that later they will not protrude under the skin. Approximate the subcutaneous tissue with fine sutures of synthetic absorbable material and close the skin with a fine absorbable subcuticular suture, with fine skin clips or removable sutures placed as end-on mattress stitches to elevate the skin edges.

Abdominal dehiscence may be a complication of any major abdominal operation, heralded by serosanguineous (pink) discharge from the wound that is an indication that intestines are lying subcutaneously. Hold the wound with tape or, if bowel is apparent, cover it with a sterile towel. Place a nasogastric tube and start intravenous fluids. In the operating room, with anesthesia, rinse each intestinal loop with saline solution and replace it in the abdominal cavity. Wash the omentum and cover the replaced bowel with it. Place through-and-through sutures of braided nylon, and thread a length of red rubber catheter on each before tying. Start antibiotics.

Commentary by Harry M. Spence (1962 and 1993)

Having long been a devotee of transperitoneal nephrectomy for Wilms' tumor in children and hypernephroma in adults, I feel reasonably qualified to express some thoughts on the indications and technique for transperitoneal renal surgery. I am prompted to make these remarks in view of the somewhat overly enthusiastic current trend that all operations on the kidney be done by this approach. Please regard my remarks as personal opinions and not ex cathedra.

First and foremost, there is no better approach for a Wilms' tumor or hypernephroma, large or small. The advantages are that the renal pedicle can be ligated and cut early, obviating to some extent manipulative metastases and cutting down on bleeding from the fragile distended veins, usually found with kidney tumors. Operability (ie, movability) can be determined early, as well as the presence or absence of metastasis. The entire mass with its fatty capsule intact can be removed *in toto*. Thus, this appeals to me as a good cancer operation.

I formerly used the Hugh Cabot T- or L-incision, combining a vertical midline and a transverse component from the midline incision to the flank. This gives unexcelled exposure, but the lateral portion is time consuming, both to make and to close. After watching the aortic graft experts, I have come to prefer the midline incision from ensiform to pubis. To be really adequate it *must* extend from ensiform to pubis. Closure with interrupted cotton or wire gives a sound wound. Neither the simple transverse nor the subcostal incision has given me the type of exposure I like. Furthermore, they are both more tedious to close.

Apart from tumors, I restrict the transperitoneal approach to the horseshoe kidney and the ectopic kidney. In both of these conditions, it facilitates handling the blood supply, which so often is anomalous. In the case of horseshoe kidney, it permits one to section the isthmus, do any necessary revision of the ureteropelvic junction, and anchor each lower pole outward at one operation.

Beyond these three specific indications for the transperitoneal approach, I believe the conventional flank route gives superior exposure for nephrectomy, pyelolithotomy, nephrolithotomy, nephrostomy, upper and lower pole resection and pyeloplasty, as well as decortication of large cysts. Of course, one must have adequate exposure so that the necessary manipulation can be done under vision and not by feeling blindly. These requirements in turn demand proper position on the table, good light, and a relaxed patient.

Update 1993. From the armchair of retirement, I make the following observations:

1. Regarding indications, I failed to mention that in traumatic injuries to the kidney (with or without accompanying damage to the abdominal viscera), the obvious choice is the midline transperitoneal approach.
2. The "modified chevron" for removal of renal tumors is enjoying an enthusiastic vogue at our institution (University of Texas, Southwestern). The "modified" translates into more than a simple subcostal, yet less than the "full" chevron incision originally described by Richard Chute. From my armchair, I see no advantage over the standard midline technique illustrated here.
3. The type of closure described by Hinman seems preferable to my use of cotton, as was advocated formerly.

CHAPTER 12

Paramedian Incision

Whether the paramedian incision is stronger than one made in the midline is questionable because the true midline incision may be closed in one layer with heavy sutures. The rectus-retracting incision illustrated keeps the rectus abdominis muscle intact, but it does disturb the blood supply where it enters at the tendinous intersections. An alternative is to split the rectus and retract the halves.

1 *Position*: Supine. *Incision*: From the xiphoid to below the umbilicus (for nephrectomy) or to the symphysis pubis (for renovascular operations). Place the incision 3 cm from the midline.

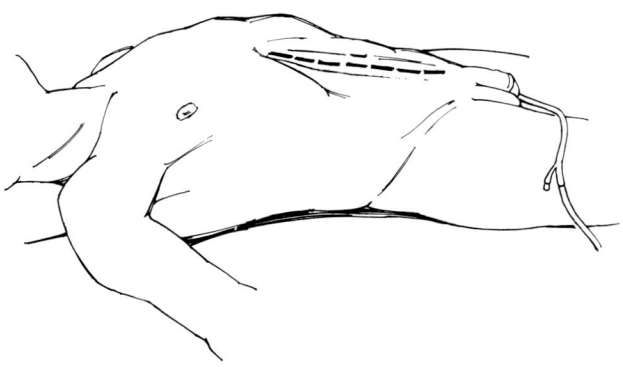

2 Incise the rectus sheath, also 3 cm to the right of the midline. Free the anterior surface of the rectus muscle from the sheath by retraction with clamps.

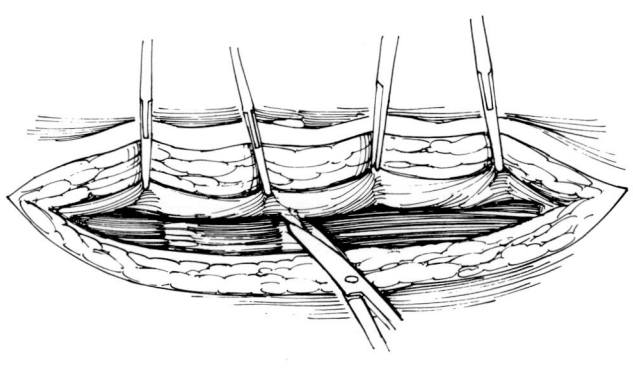

3 Insert U.S. Army retractors and free the medial and undersurfaces of the muscle, taking care to preserve the intrinsic blood vessels and nerves. Cut sharply at the tendinous insertions.

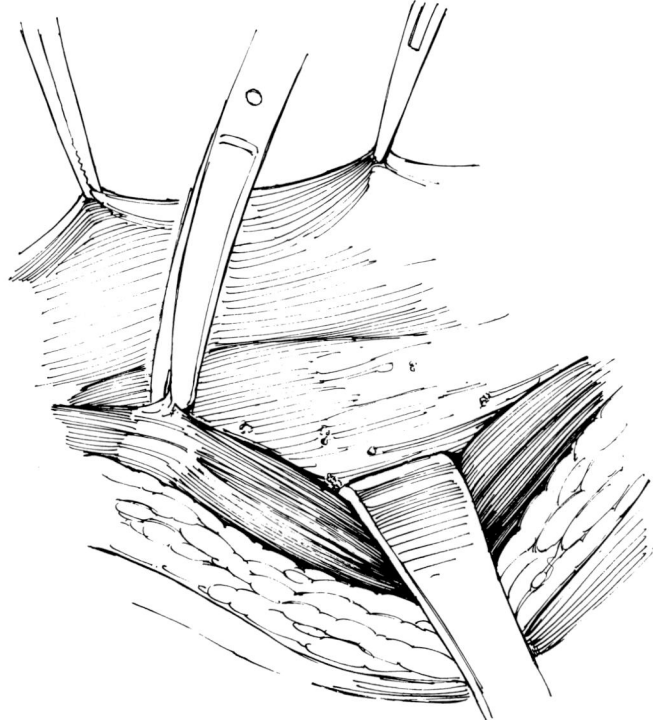

4 Divide the posterior rectus sheath, then open the peritoneum by carefully lifting it with two pairs of smooth forceps on either side and cutting into the tented area.

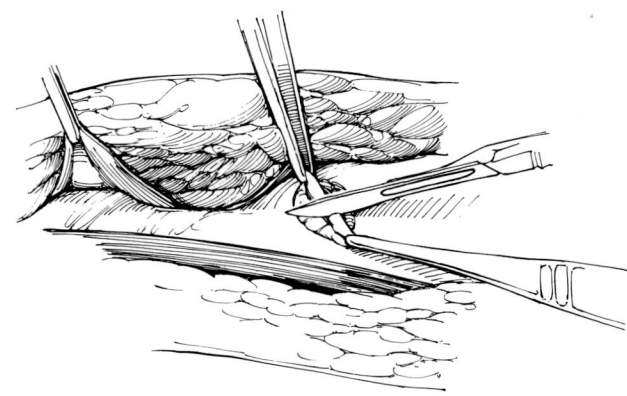

5 Insert two fingers and divide both structures to both ends of the incision. Proceed with the intra-abdominal operation.

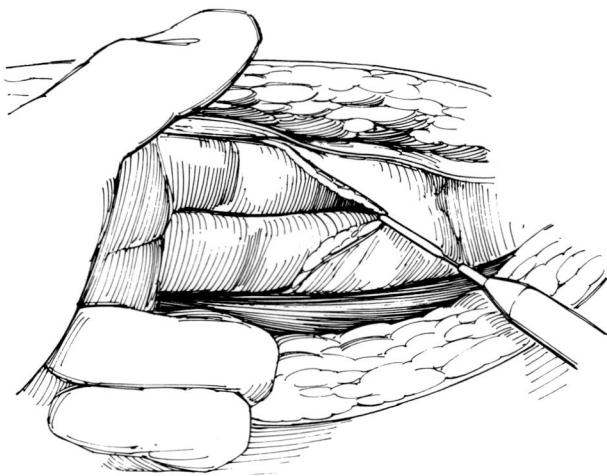

6 Close the peritoneum and posterior sheath in one layer with a running absorbable or nonabsorbable suture. Close the anterior sheath with interrupted sutures of the same material. Retention sutures occasionally may be needed.

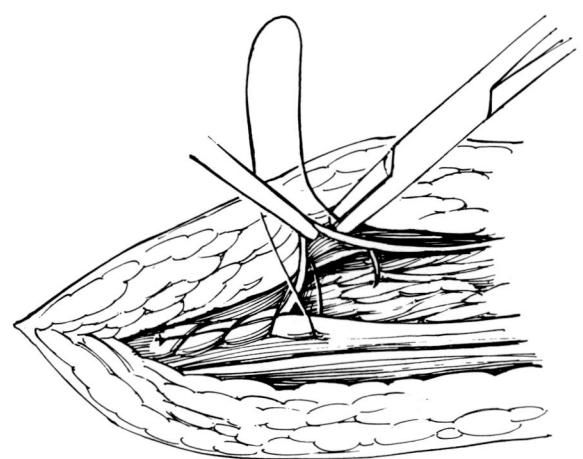

Comment

Access may be obtained to all four quadrants of the abdomen, allowing major vascular and posttrauma reconstruction. It may be used for bilateral lymphadenectomy and for major undiversion procedures. It is easy to open and close, but special precautions are needed to prevent dehiscence. It is, however, associated with a high incidence of postoperative bowel adhesions that result in obstruction.

CHAPTER 13

Subcostal Incision

A subcostal incision provides limited access and requires almost as much effort to make as a supracostal incision. It may be used for placement of a permanent nephrostomy, drainage of a perinephric abscess, and perhaps for removal of stones from the upper ureter, although the lumbotomy approach is better. Moreover, open procedures seldom are necessary with the availability of percutaneous methods. Other incisions are more suitable for access to the renal pedicle.

1 By drawing a horizontal line on the urogram from the lateral border of the rib cage, access can be evaluated, because only structures below that line will be adequately exposed.

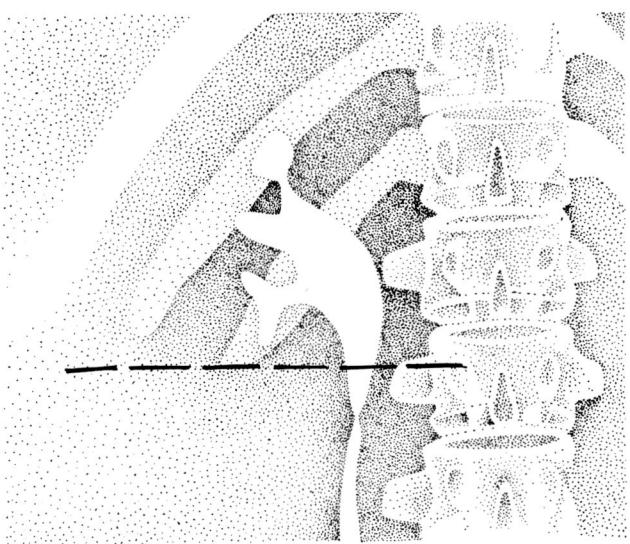

3 Incise the latissimus dorsi and serratus posterior inferior muscles, cutting back from their anterior free borders. Use the cutting current to minimize blood loss and trauma to the tissue secondary to application of multiple clamps and ligatures.

2 *Position*: Place the child in the flank position with a rolled towel under the 12th rib. In the adolescent for whom the kidney lift is used in conjunction with table flexion, watch for hypotension from poor venous return, mediastinal shift, and displacement of the liver.

Incision: Start the incision at the lateral border of the sacrospinalis muscle, 1 cm below the lower edge of the 12th rib. Follow the lower border of the rib anteriorly, curving the incision caudally as it crosses the anterior abdominal wall to avoid the subcostal nerve. End it near the lateral border of the rectus abdominis muscle. With a rudimentary 12th rib, place the incision well below the 11th rib.

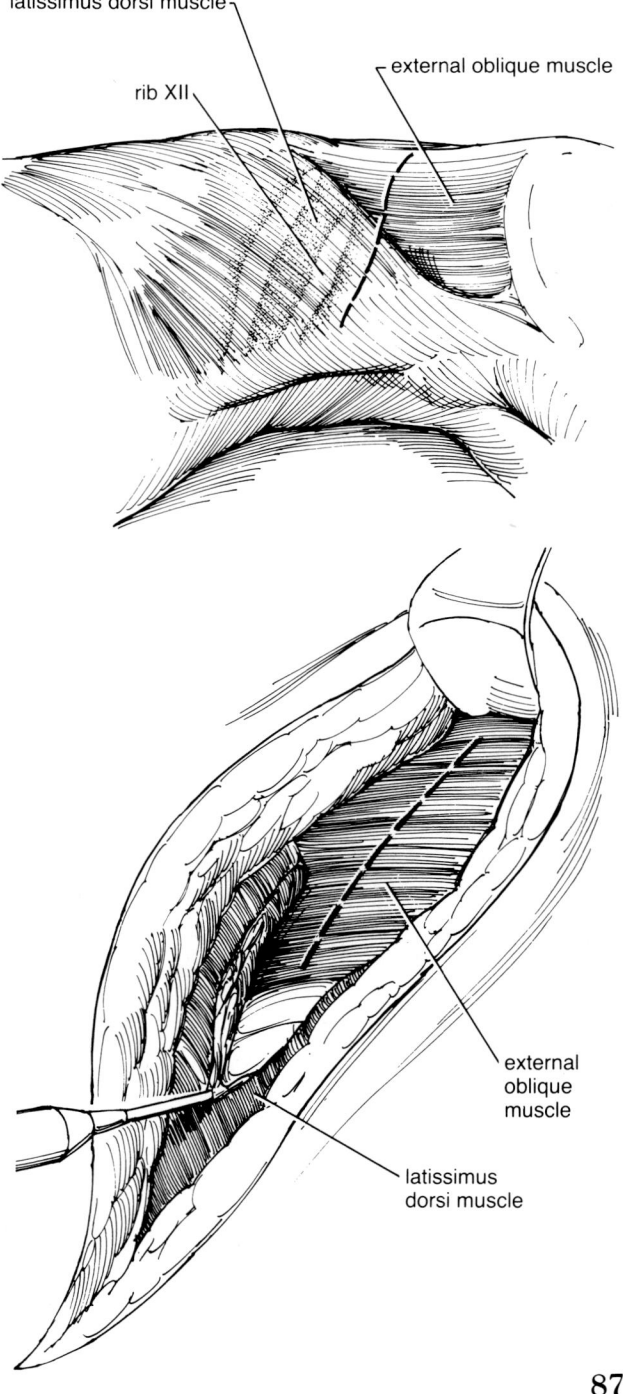

4 Incise the external and internal oblique muscles, starting at their posterior free border, and incise the serratus posterior inferior. Watch for the 12th intercostal neurovascular bundle that lies between the internal oblique and transversus abdominis muscles. It is necessary to free it and push it upward. Divide and ligate the small intercostal veins accompanying it.

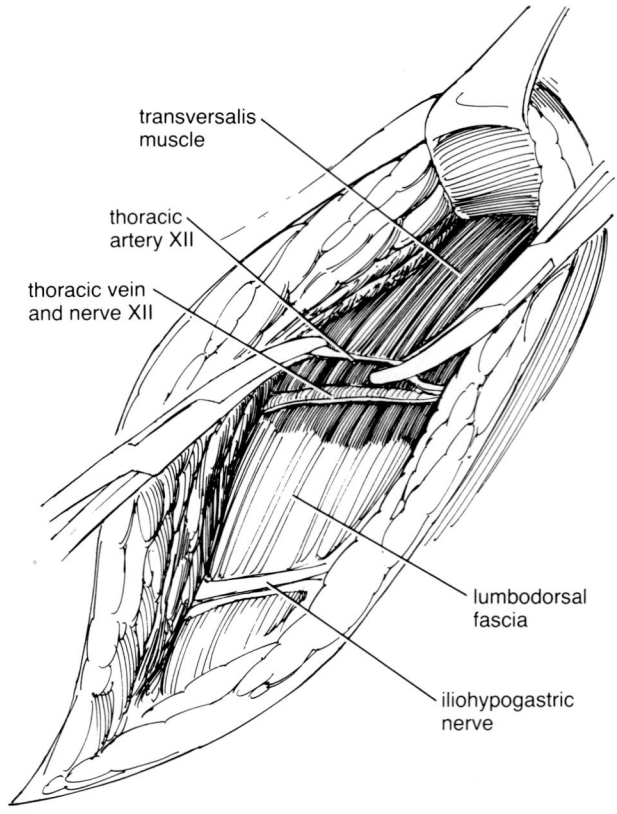

transversalis muscle

thoracic artery XII

thoracic vein and nerve XII

lumbodorsal fascia

iliohypogastric nerve

5 Identify the firm white lumbodorsal fascia and incise it in midincision. This allows insertion of two fingers to push the peritoneum forward before completing the incision through the muscle, thus avoiding cutting into the peritoneum. The fingers also aid hemostasis. Sharply cut the fascia to its junction with the anterior musculature. Incise and digitally split the transversus abdominis, thus exposing the peritoneum, which can be bluntly dissected and pushed anteriorly.

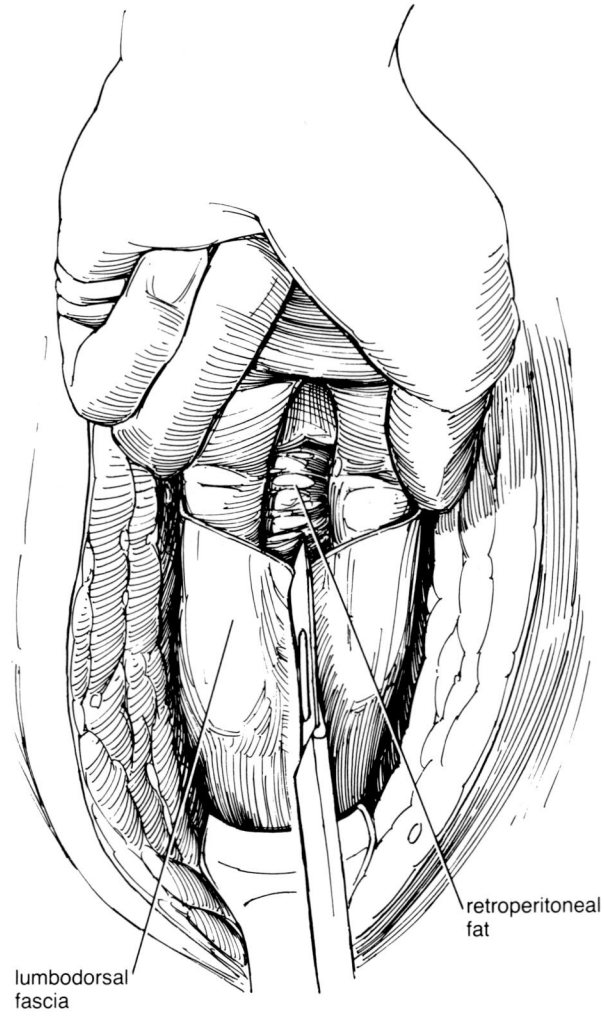

retroperitoneal fat

lumbodorsal fascia

6 Incise the posterior layer of the lumbodorsal fascia, working back from the anterior border of the sacrospinalis muscle, along with a few fibers of the serratus posterior inferior. Divide the sacrospinalis muscle with the cutting current so that the costotransverse ligament is exposed.

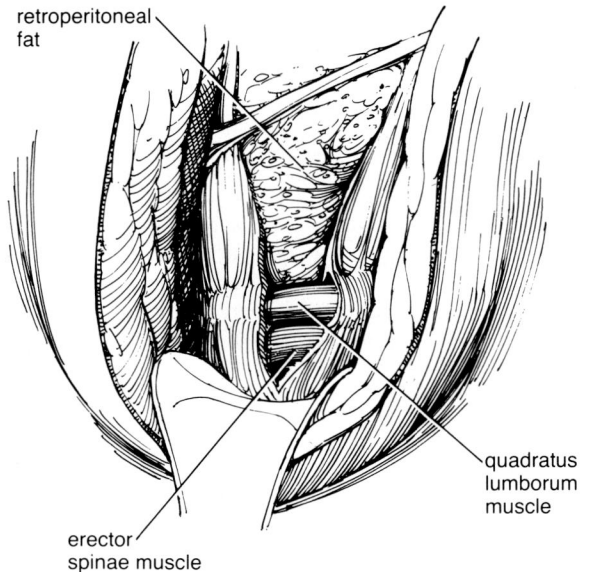

retroperitoneal fat

quadratus lumborum muscle

erector spinae muscle

7 While elevating the rib, cut the costotransverse ligament with partially opened Mayo scissors with the curved side down to avoid cutting the intercostal artery or entering the pleura, which lies beyond the tip of the transverse process. Free the subcostal nerve further and move it superiorly. Insert a self-retaining retractor and proceed with entry into Gerota's fascia.

Extension of the incision: If, after exposing the kidney, you have insufficient room and find that the kidney lesion is higher than was anticipated, make a costal extension to allow surgical control, as for a dorsal flap procedure (page 109). To do this, lift up the deep margin of the intercostal muscle at the angle of the rib. Elevate the serratus posterior inferior fibers attached to the lower edge of the 12th rib. Bluntly and sharply expose the periosteum of the rib. Incise the periosteum; scrape and strip it from the rib for a short distance. Resect 2 cm of the rib. Divide the diaphragm close to the body wall with Metzenbaum scissors. Swing the anterior rib segment over the upper rib and hold it up with a retractor.

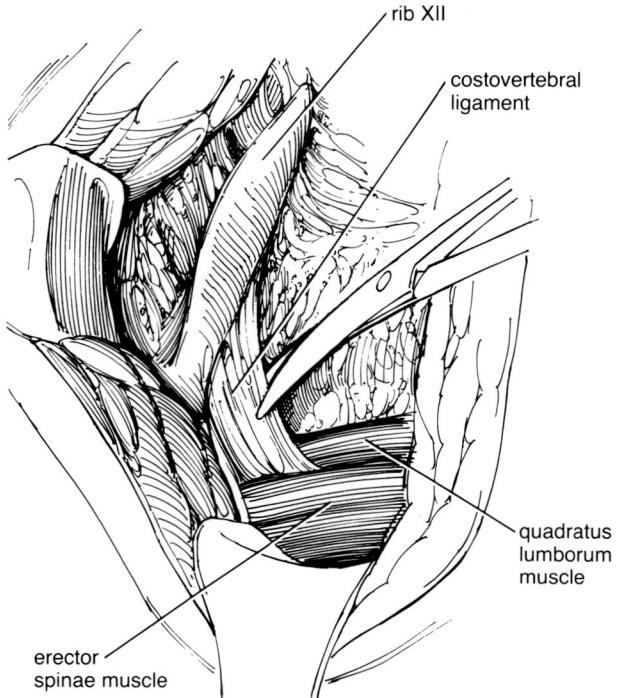

rib XII

costovertebral ligament

quadratus lumborum muscle

erector spinae muscle

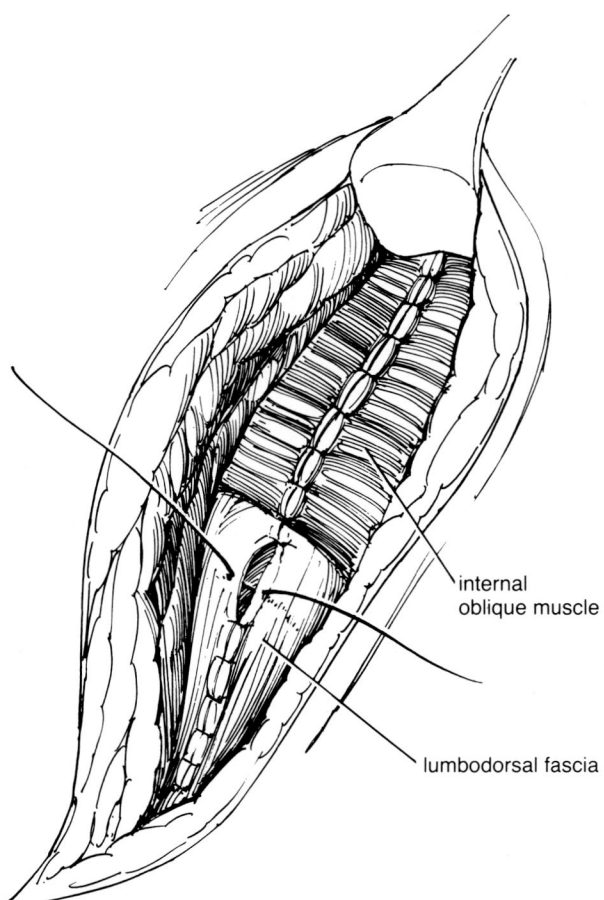

internal oblique muscle

lumbodorsal fascia

8 *Closure*: Lower the kidney rest and flatten the tabletop. Insert a Penrose drain to exit through a stab wound and an infant feeding tube to supply bupivacaine analgesia postoperatively. Start anteriorly to close the transversus abdominis and internal oblique muscles in one layer with interrupted sutures of 2-0 synthetic absorbable sutures. Alternatively, close the flimsy transversus muscle first. Work posteriorly and close the lumbodorsal fascia by approximating the aponeurotic portion of the transversus abdominis muscle and the posterior layer of the lumbodorsal fascia. Approximate the external oblique muscle, beginning anteriorly, and the serratus posterior inferior and latissimus dorsi muscles, beginning posteriorly, with interrupted 2-0 synthetic absorbable sutures. Close the skin.

To allow observation of the kidney bed for any oozing during closure, before lowering the kidney lift, insert figure-eight sutures through all layers and clamp the ends. Lower the lift and tie them in sequence.

CHAPTER 14

Transcostal Incision

Where functioning renal tissue is to be retained and drainage or infection anticipated, the lateral retroperitoneal incision may be appropriate. The choice of a subcostal, 12th rib, or supracostal 11th rib incision would depend on the position of the kidney, location of the lesion, previous surgical incisions in the flank, and experience of the surgeon. The transcostal incision approaches the upper retroperitoneum through the bed of the 12th rib. It may be used for simple or partial nephrectomy and for simple adrenalectomy in older children and adolescents, although a supracostal incision is easier to make and gives equal or better exposure.

Instruments

The special rib instruments used by thoracic surgeons are necessary: Snyder and Alexander periosteal elevators, Matson and Doyen rib strippers, guillotine rib cutter, rongeurs, and self-retaining retractor.

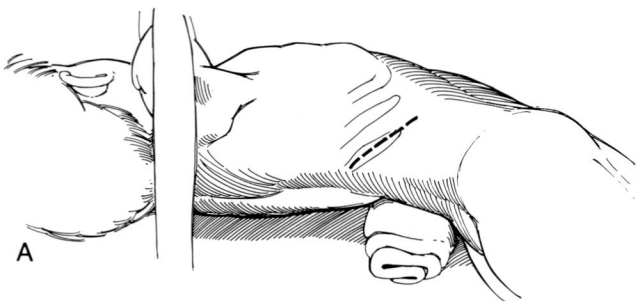

A

1 *Position:* Place the patient in the flank position over the break in the table and the kidney rest. Palpate the 12th and the 11th ribs and scratch the skin vertically in several places along the course of the 12th rib to guide the incision and to help align the skin at the time of closure. **A,** Incise the skin starting at the margin of the erector spinae muscles, running obliquely following the 12th rib and ending at the lateral border of the rectus abdominis. If the rib cannot be felt through a thick body wall, estimate its site and cut through enough of the subcutaneous tissue so that it can be palpated. **B,** Once the rib can be felt, divide the external oblique muscle and the latissimus dorsi muscle directly over its center line with the electrosurgical blade to expose its periosteal surface. Incise the periosteum sharply with a knife blade.

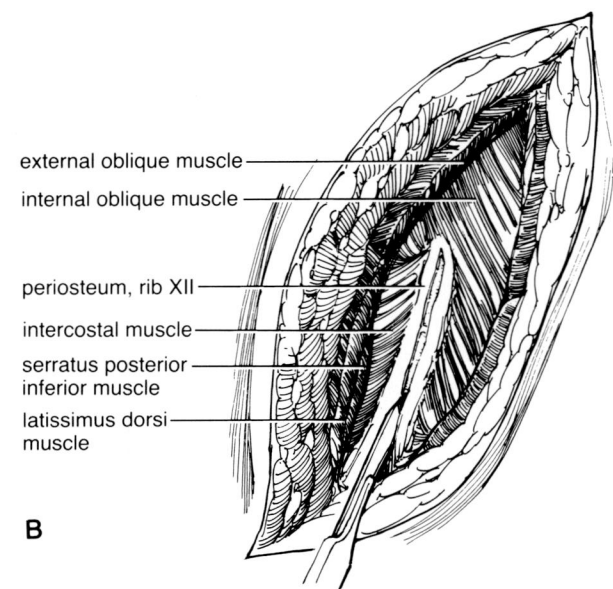

external oblique muscle

internal oblique muscle

periosteum, rib XII

intercostal muscle

serratus posterior inferior muscle

latissimus dorsi muscle

B

2 **A,** Scrape the periosteum from the rib with the chisel end of the Alexander periosteal elevator, beginning at the junction with the neck. Use small strokes to free it from the convex surface of the rib, and then free the upper and lower edges. A dry sponge also may be used to strip back muscle and periosteum. Finally, run the elevator along both edges at an angle to free the periosteum under them. **B,** The curved blades on the other end of the Alexander elevator are useful here to free the periosteum from the edges of the rib. **C,** Because of the angle of attachment of the intercostal muscles, the Matson rib stripper is pushed anteriorly on the upper edge of the rib and posteriorly on the lower.

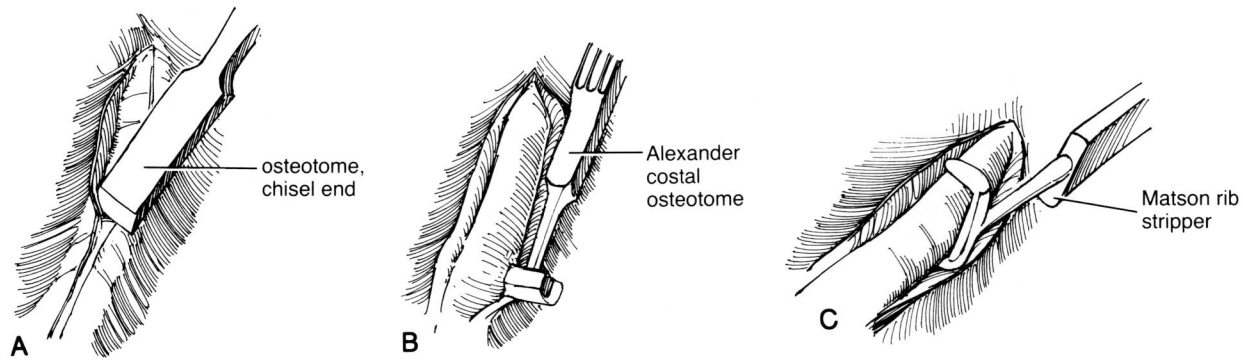

3 Insinuate the Doyen rib stripper under the rib inside the periosteum. Lift up on the shaft and pull back along the undersurface to the angle of the rib. Depress the handle and push forward to the tip of the rib, thus using each of the cutting edges effectively. Alternatively, but not as cleanly and easily done, the rib may be excised extra-periosteally. To do this, omit incising and freeing the periosteum, but proceed immediately to insertion of the Doyen rib stripper superficial to the transversalis fascia, forcibly separating the rib from the muscles and fascia inserting on it.

4 Grasp the rib with a Kocher clamp to steady it. Insert the rib cutter with the blade on the medial side and pull (or push) it well posteriorly to divide the rib as far back as possible. After division, use rongeurs to trim more of the rib if needed and to round the edges. Press bone wax into the cut end if it is bleeding (rare with the 12th rib). After lifting up the posterior end, cut the anterior fibrous attachment of the rib with Mayo scissors and remove it.

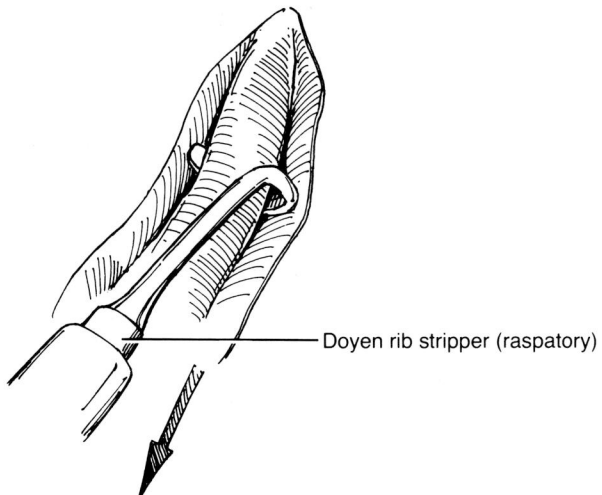

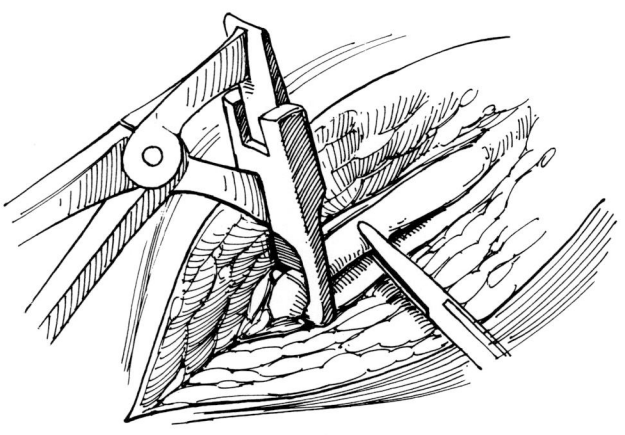

5 Incise the posterior layer of periosteum at the anterior end under the site of the rib tip to enter the retroperitoneal space. Insert a finger to depress the pleura and peritoneum, then extend the incision both ways with scissors. Spare the branches of the 12th intercostal neurovascular bundle by palpating them and letting them move caudally. Watch out for a vessel joining the 12th and 11th bundles anteriorly.

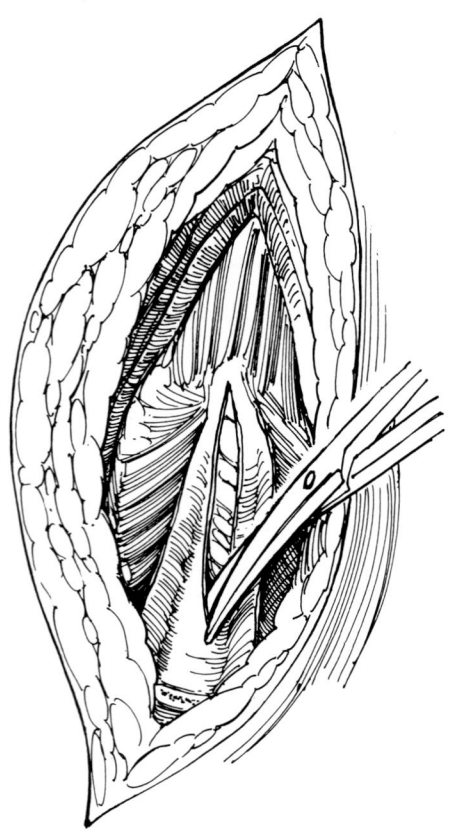

6 Divide the internal oblique muscle electrosurgically. Incise the thin fascia over the transversus abdominis and then digitally split the muscle to the anterior end of the wound.

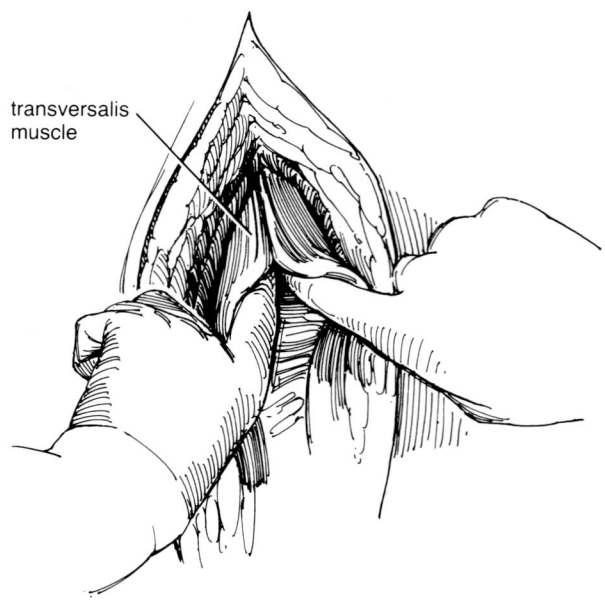

transversalis muscle

7 Identify the pleura posteriorly; have the anesthetist inflate the lung for easy visualization. (For the repair of pleural tears, see page 118.) Gently dissect the pleura from the endothoracic fascia beneath the 11th rib. At the same time, cut the attachments of the diaphragm against the body wall with Metzenbaum scissors. Separate the diaphragm from the retroperitoneal connective tissue to allow its displacement superiorly.

Free the peritoneum thoroughly by blunt dissection from the transversalis fascia on the undersurface of the abdominal wall not only medially but superiorly and inferiorly as well. This will facilitate placement of retractors and achieve optimal exposure.

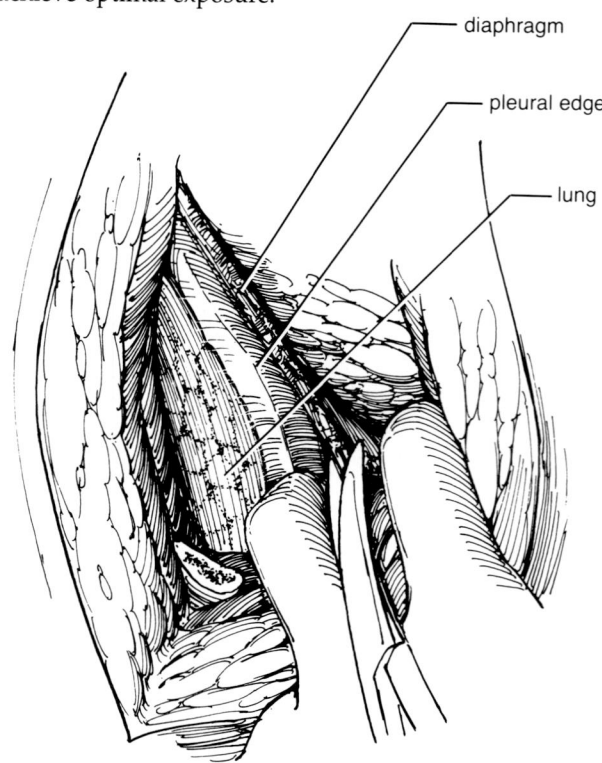

diaphragm

pleural edge

lung

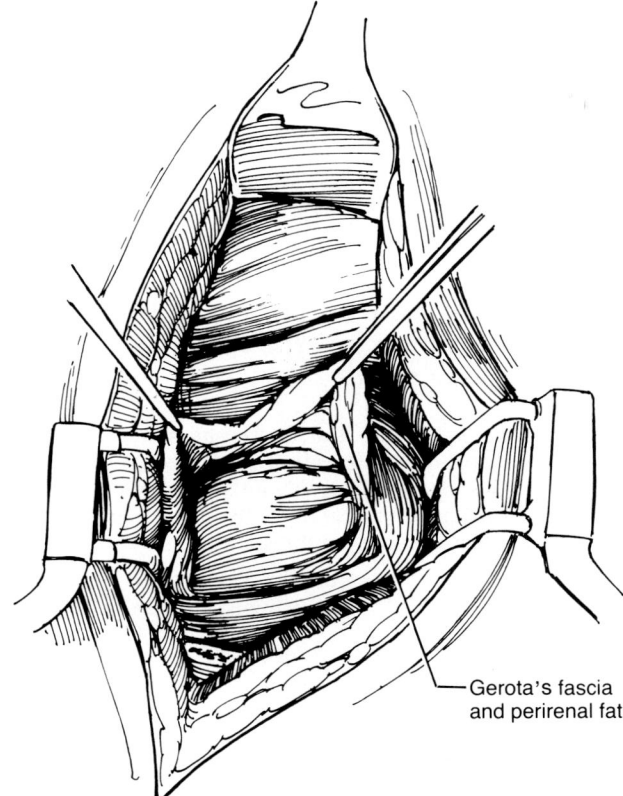

8 Insert a self-retaining retractor. Enter Gerota's fascia bluntly to displace part of the perirenal fat posteriorly and expose the kidney.

Gerota's fascia and perirenal fat

9 *Closure*: Insert a Penrose drain through a separate stab wound. Have the anesthetist lower the kidney rest and flatten the table. Pull the shoulder back if it has fallen forward. Note that rotation of hips and shoulders in opposite directions opens or closes flank incisions.

Approximate the anterior layer of the cut periosteum, beginning posteriorly at the superior margin, catching it superficially to avoid the intercostal bundle. Then, close the combined transversus and internal oblique muscles; begin anteriorly using interrupted synthetic absorbable sutures. Close the external oblique along with the posterior inferior serratus muscles and approximate the latissimus muscles with the same suture material. Do not cinch the sutures too tightly. Approximate the subcutaneous tissue obliquely so that the caudal part of the wound does not sag posteriorly. Close the skin following the scratches made initially. Suture the drain to the skin; do not place a safety pin through it in young children.

See Chapter 15 for Commentary.

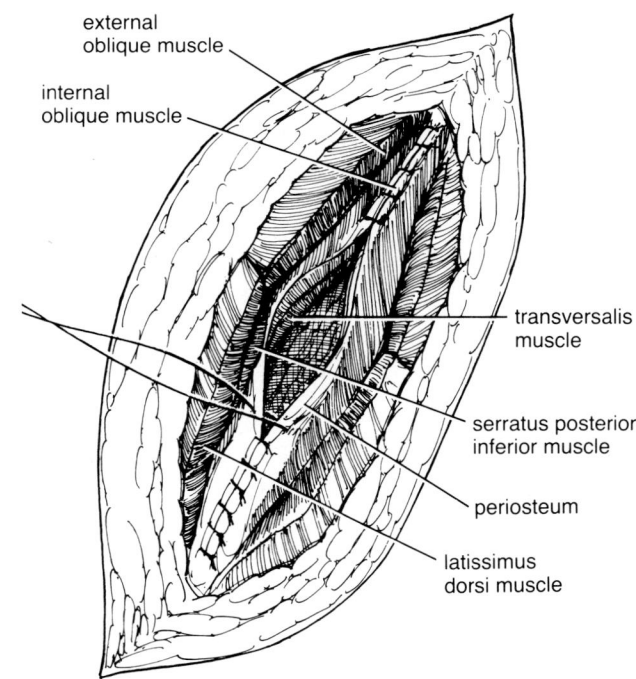

external oblique muscle

internal oblique muscle

transversalis muscle

serratus posterior inferior muscle

periosteum

latissimus dorsi muscle

CHAPTER 15

Supracostal Incision

An incision just above the 12th or 11th ribs is easier to make than a transcostal incision and gives equal or better exposure.

1 *Anatomic orientation*: The intercostal space provides wide exposure of the kidney and adrenal gland between the ribs by dividing the intercostal muscles and costovertebral ligament, followed by detachment of the lateral attachments of the diaphragm.

Review the kidney-ureter-bladder film to ascertain the length of the 11th and 12th ribs and decide above which one to incise for the appropriate exposure. If the 12th rib is long, a supracostal incision between it and the 11th rib gives excellent exposure; going above the 11th rib is reserved for patients with short or absent 12th ribs or for those requiring greater exposure, as for radical nephrectomy or adrenalectomy.

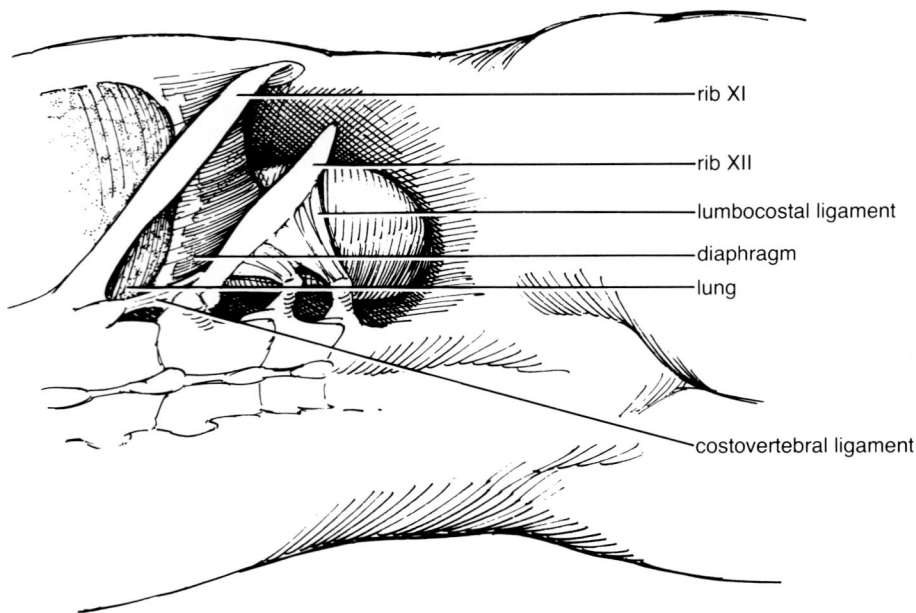

- rib XI
- rib XII
- lumbocostal ligament
- diaphragm
- lung
- costovertebral ligament

2 **A,** The muscle layers are shown as they are exposed and traversed in making the incision. **B,** The route of the incision is through the skin, dividing the latissimus dorsi and serratus posterior inferior and the external intercostal muscles. **C,** Cut the internal intercostal and enter the retrocostal space. Divide the attachment of the extrapleural fascia to the posterior surface of the rib; this leaves the intercostal nerve against the rib in its own compartment. **D,** Cut the extrapleural fascia and divide the diaphragm along the posterior body wall.

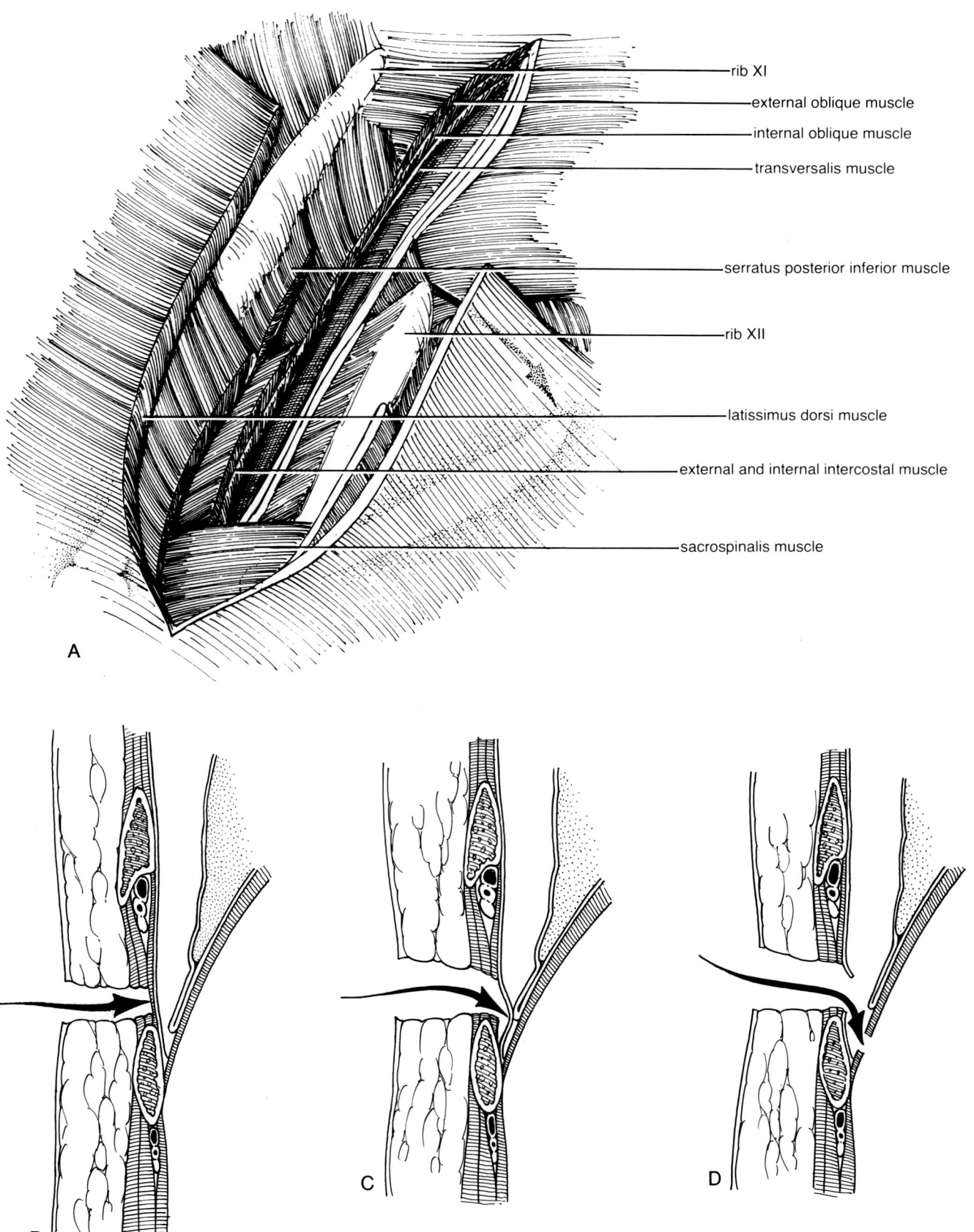

rib XI

external oblique muscle

internal oblique muscle

transversalis muscle

serratus posterior inferior muscle

rib XII

latissimus dorsi muscle

external and internal intercostal muscle

sacrospinalis muscle

A

B

C

D

3 *Position*: Use a flank position. If the incision is to be extended to or across the midline, place a folded towel under the chest to displace the child posteriorly at an angle of 30 degrees. *Incision*: Palpate the line of the chosen rib and mark the skin with vertical scratches to facilitate its alignment at the time of closure. Start the skin incision obliquely over the selected rib and extend it anteriorly to its tip. Posteriorly, carry the incision to the margin of the erector spinae muscle group, exposing the external oblique and latissimus dorsi.

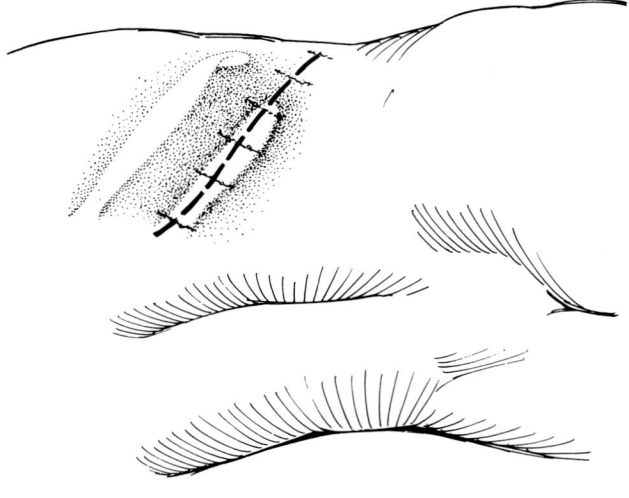

4 Cut directly down onto the rib through the overlying muscles with the cutting current. This divides the external and internal oblique muscles and the latissimus dorsi, as well as the serratus posterior inferior. Make the cut right down *to* the periosteum. Incise the layer of the abdominal wall where its layers coalesce just anterior to the tip of the rib.

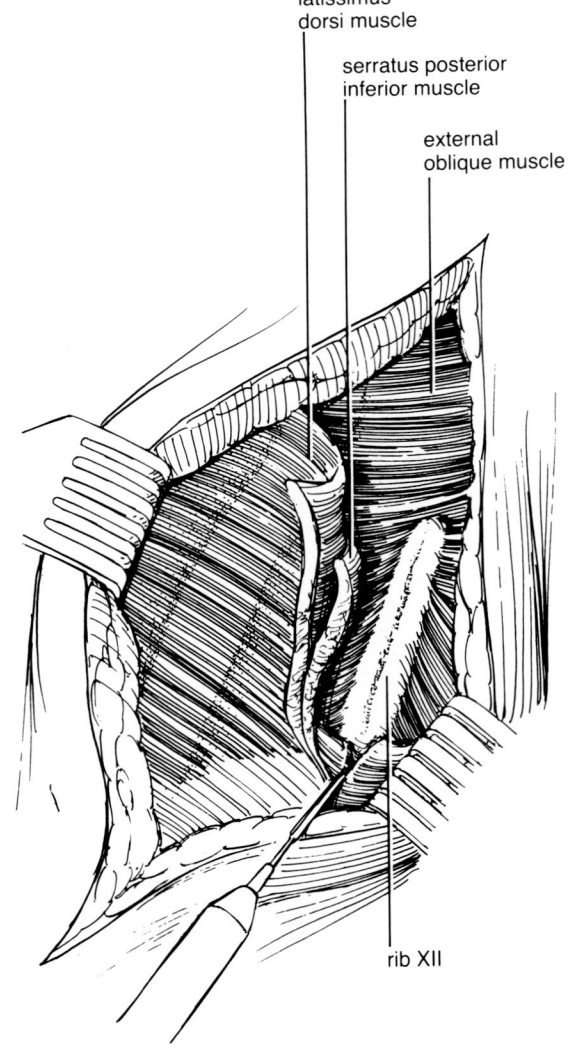

latissimus dorsi muscle

serratus posterior inferior muscle

external oblique muscle

rib XII

5 **A,** Reduce the setting for the cutting current. Divide the external intercostal muscle along the upper margin of the rib. Start at the tip of the rib, which is away from the pleura, dividing the muscles for an inch or so. **B,** Insinuate the index finger to displace the extrapleural fascia and the pleura and progressively divide the inner intercostal muscle against the fingertip, separating it from the rib throughout its length. This leaves the intercostal nerve against the rib.

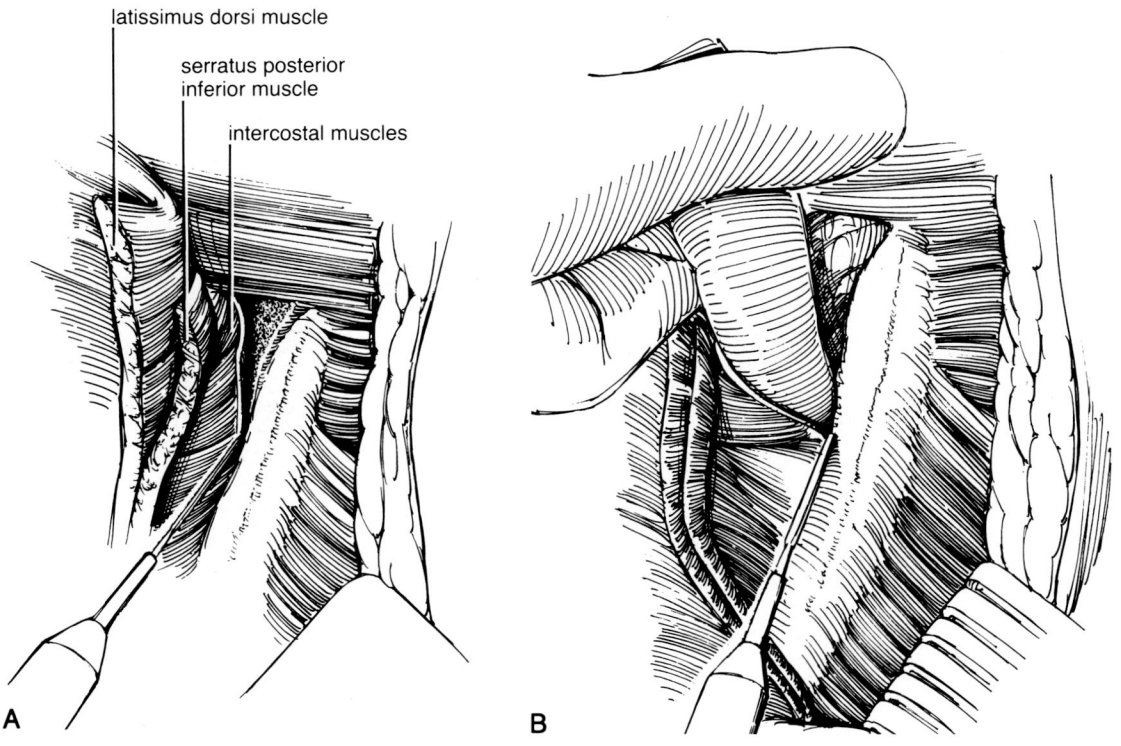

latissimus dorsi muscle

serratus posterior
inferior muscle

intercostal muscles

A

B

6 Using a finger, separate the thin extrapleural fascia from the undersurface of the rib. The extrapleural fascia splits into two layers to form a tunnel that contains the intercostal nerve (see Figure 2C). Carefully divide the external layer. As the posterior part of the wound is reached, the pleura can be pushed down by the index finger, away from the intercostal muscle and rib.

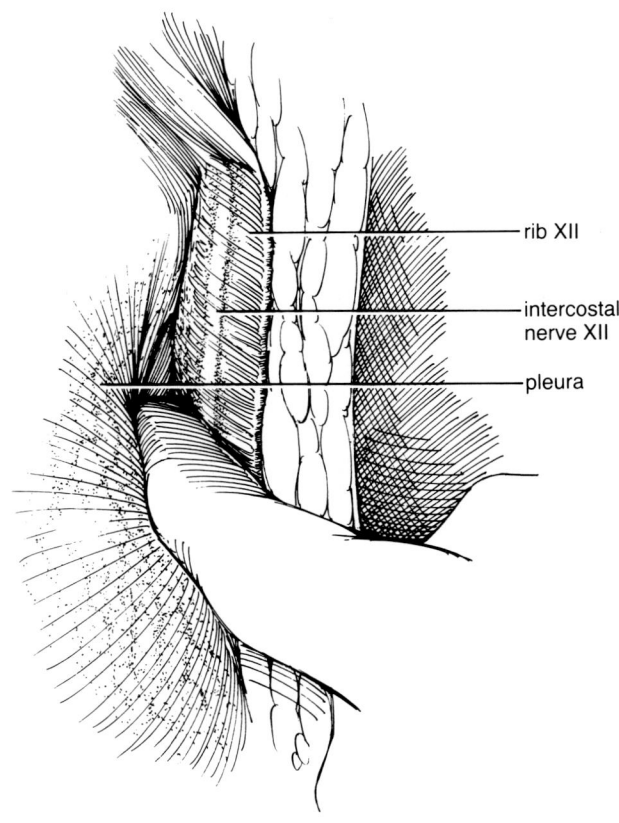

rib XII

intercostal
nerve XII

pleura

7 Run the pad of the left index finger dorsally along the top edge of the rib until it meets the sharp edge of the costovertebral ligament. Insert the slightly opened heavy curved scissors, curve down, over the rib and under the finger. Hug the top of the rib with the scissors to divide the ligament sharply and at the same time avoid the intercostal bundle that lies below the upper rib. The lower rib can now pivot on its costovertebral joint (both the 11th and 12th ribs have a single attachment to the vertebra) and be retracted inferiorly and held with a self-retaining retractor out of the way. To prevent the retractor from being levered out of the wound, support the handle with rolled towels stabilized with towel clips.

Complete the anterior part of the incision by dividing the external and internal oblique muscles and splitting the transversus abdominis sufficiently to allow the lower rib to be fully retracted downward until it lies alongside the lateral border of the quadratus lumborum muscle. To incise the anterior layers earlier would risk tearing the pleura before it had been freed from the 12th rib.

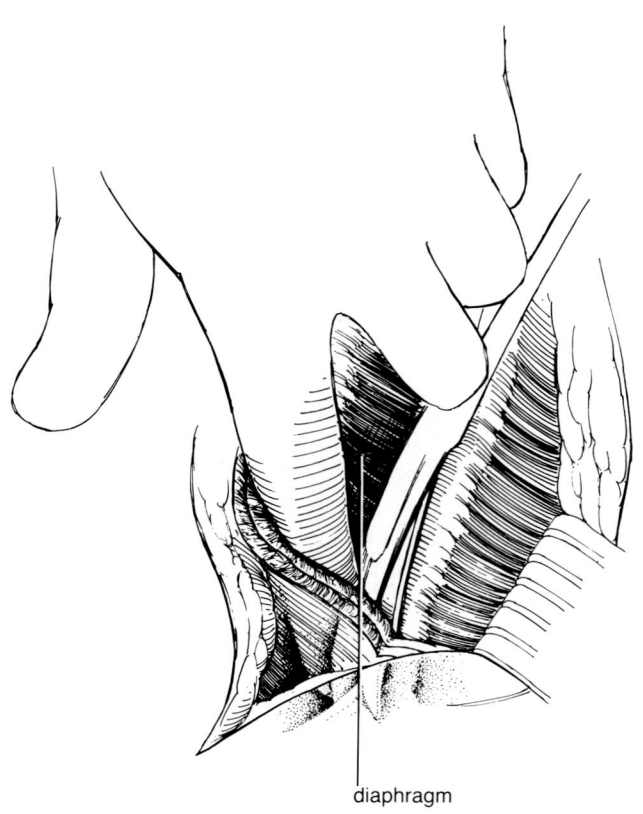

diaphragm

8 Push the diaphragm away from the undersurface of the rib and from the lateral arcuate ligament over the quadratus lumborum muscle.

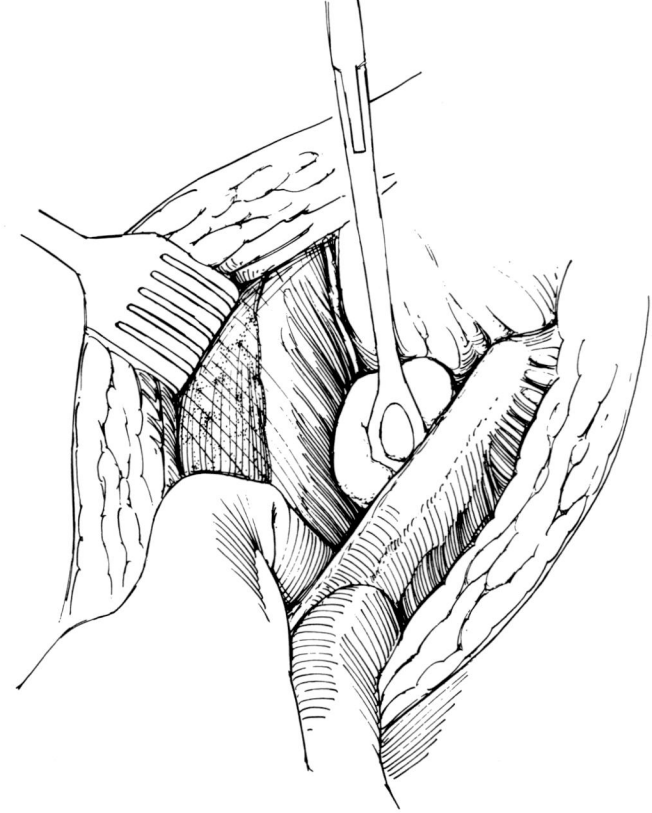

9 Divide the diaphragm close to its origin, using scissors. Coagulate those vessels encountered. Stay well away from the pleura, especially as the division is started anteriorly. As the diaphragm is freed, the pleura will now rise out of the way.

For exposure of the renal pedicle, peel the peritoneum from the transversalis fascia with a cherry sponge in one hand while depressing the peritoneum with a lap tape with the other. This should be done even if the incision is to be extended across the midline by dividing one or both rectus muscles, because it is difficult to retract the peritoneum from the body wall once it has been opened.

10 Place a retractor, open Gerota's fascia laterally, and expose the kidney through the perirenal fat.

The supracostal 11th incision differs from the supracostal 12th only in that the pleura extends lower and is more exposed to possible entry during its dissection from the inner aspect of the 12th rib, to which it is somewhat adherent, and during the division of the diaphragm at its origin.

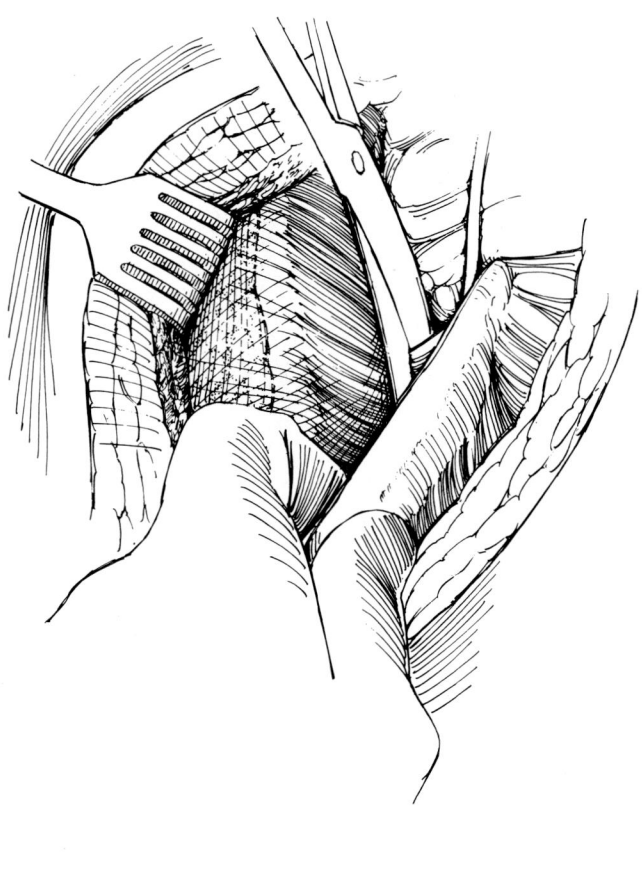

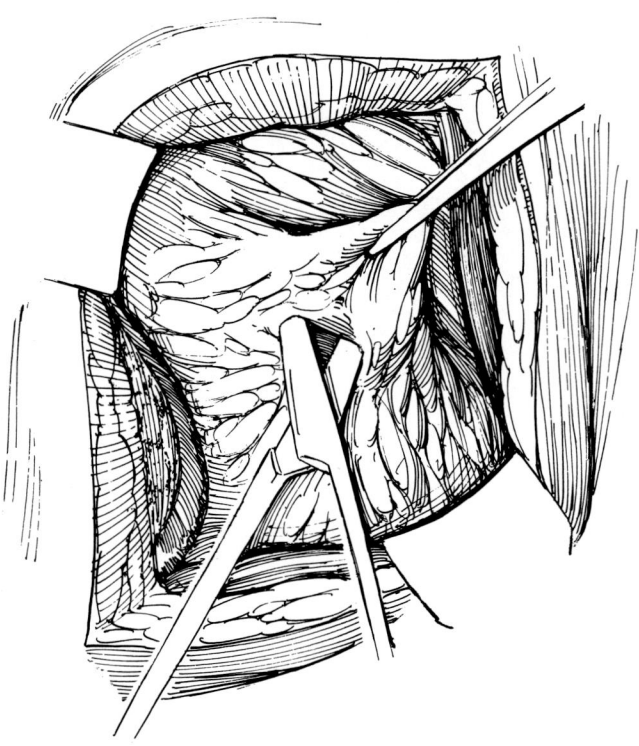

Closure: Begin closure by partially straightening the table to allow the edges of the wound to come together.

11 Place a figure-eight synthetic absorbable suture into the condensed tissue at the tip of the 12th rib and bring it through similar tissue below the eleventh rib and tie it. The rib pivots upward into its original position.

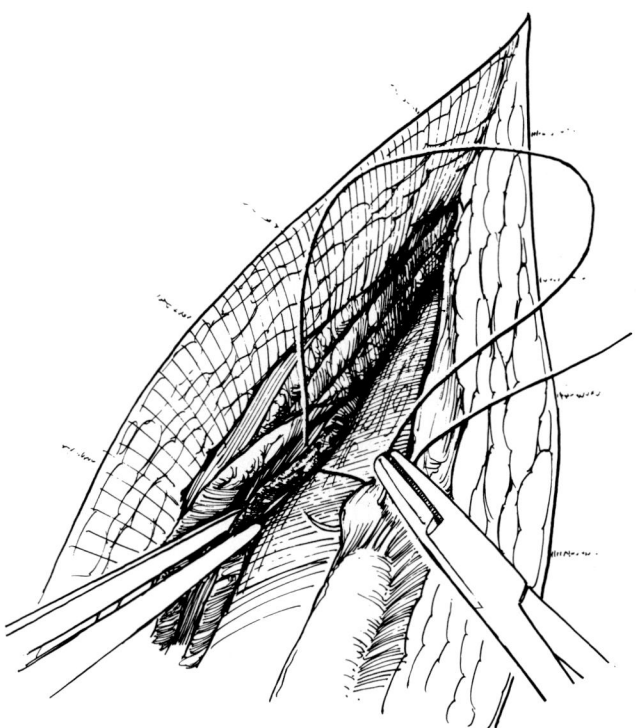

12 A and B, Starting posteriorly, pull the detached diaphragm and intercostal muscles out through the intercostal space and stitch them progressively to the edge of the muscles below the incision external to the inferior rib (serratus posterior inferior posteriorly and latissimus dorsi anteriorly) with interrupted sutures of synthetic absorbable sutures. Because this also closes the pleura if it has been inadvertently opened, the anesthetist must expand the lung before the final sutures are tied. Never encircle the lower rib with a closure suture—this risks damage to the intercostal vessels in the notch on its inferior surface.

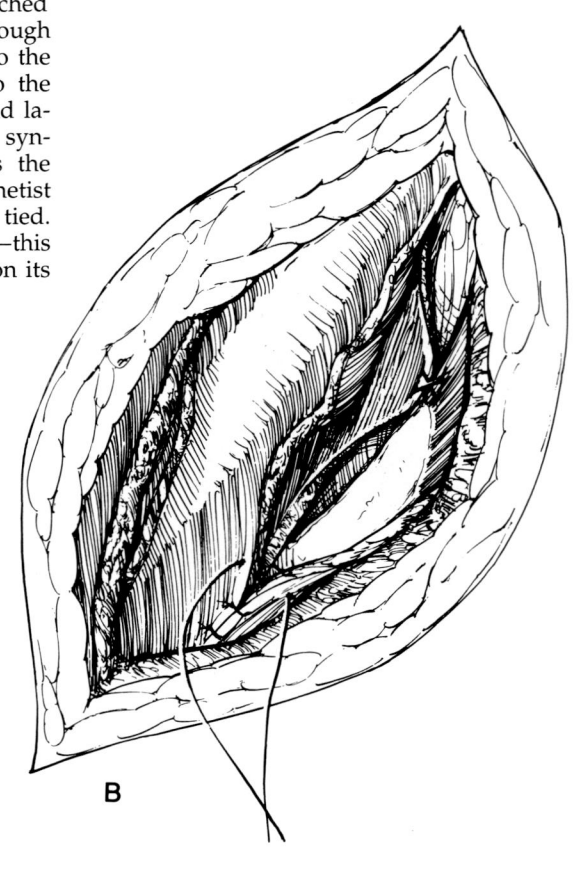

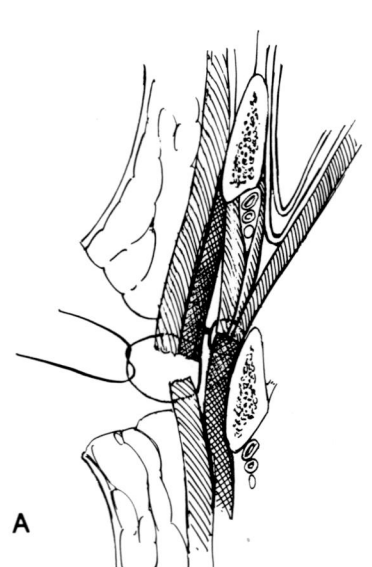

13 Stitch the upper margin of the incised latissimus dorsi to the external surface of the serratus, then to the lower margin of the latissimus dorsi. Place a Penrose drain through a stab wound below the 12th rib to allow the escape of trapped air and exudate and close the subcutaneous tissue and skin. If the pleura had been entered, leave a small catheter in the pleural space and put it under water as a seal.

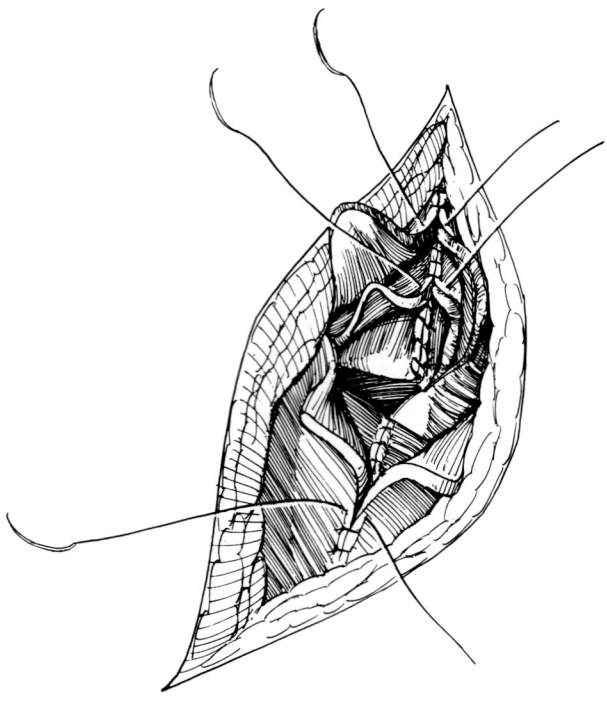

Commentary by A. E. MacNeily and William E. Kaplan

The surgeon's choice of incision for access to the pediatric kidney depends on many factors: the site of pathology (upper pole, lower pole, or ureteropelvic junction), the need for access to the more distal ureter (*eg*, nephroureterectomy), the presence of orthopedic abnormalities (*eg*, myelomeningocele), and the surgeon's own personal bias.

In general, we prefer to begin our approach off the tip of the 12th rib, proceeding anteriorly, as for the subcostal approach. If greater posterior exposure is required to the upper pole, the incision is extended posteriorly in a fashion analogous to that for the supracostal incision. Otherwise, greater posterior exposure is obtained by extending the incision subcostally. Rarely is the transcostal approach necessary in the pediatric population.

Special care must be observed to avoid incising the peritoneum, as it extends surprisingly far posteriorly in children. This is especially important on the right side, where the appendix can easily be mistaken for the tortuous ureter, often seen just distal to a congenital ureteropelvic junction obstruction!

Inadvertent peritoneotomy is closed at the time of its recognition with fine absorbable sutures.

A subcostal incision provides limited access with almost as much effort as a supracostal incision but may be used for placement of a permanent nephrostomy, drainage of a perinephric abscess, and perhaps for removal of stones from the upper ureter, although this is seldom necessary with the availability of percutaneous methods. Other incisions are more suitable for access to the renal pedicle.

Position: In the adolescent for whom the kidney lift is used in conjunction with table flexion, watch for hypotension from poor venous return, mediastinal shift, and displacement of the liver. Use the cutting current to minimize blood loss and trauma to the tissue secondary to application of multiple clamps and ligatures.

Extension of the incision: If, after exposing the kidney, you have insufficient room and find that the kidney lesion is higher than was anticipated, make a costal extension to allow surgical control, as for a dorsal flap procedure (page 109). To do this, lift up the deep margin of the intercostal muscle at the angle of the rib. Elevate the serratus posterior inferior fibers attached to the lower edge of the 12th rib. Bluntly and sharply expose the periosteum of the rib. Incise the periosteum; scrape and strip it from the rib for a short distance. Resect 2 cm of the rib. Divide the diaphragm close to the body wall with Metzenbaum scissors. Swing the anterior rib segment over the upper rib and hold it up with a retractor.

To allow observation of the kidney bed for any oozing during closure, before lowering the kidney lift, insert figure-eight sutures through all layers and clamp the ends. Lower the lift and tie the sutures in sequence.

CHAPTER 16
Thoracoabdominal Incision

For major surgery, provide overnight hydration with lactated Ringer's solution. To reduce blood loss, controlled sodium nitroprusside–induced hypotensive anesthesia can be used.

TRANSTHORACIC APPROACH

The transthoracic approach is applicable for radical nephrectomy (page 169), ileal ureter (page 255), and retroperitoneal tumors and node dissection (page 547).

If in doubt about operability, make the anterior segment first as the extrathoracic approach described in "Extrathoracic 11th Rib Approach" (page 104).

1 *Position*: With the patient near the ipsilateral (in this case, the right) side of the table, place the pelvis almost flat just below the break. Rotate the upper torso 40 degrees and support it with a rolled towel or sandbag. Place the upper arm across the chest onto a padded Mayo stand or suspend it on an anesthesia screen. Protect the left axilla with a pad. Hyperextend the table and hold the patient in position with wide strips of adhesive tape from shoulder to tabletop posteriorly only and from hip to tabletop both anteriorly and posteriorly. *Incision*: Identify the 10th rib and mark the overlying skin with needle scratches or marking pen ink. For large renal tumors, place the incision above the ninth rib. Incise the skin and subcutaneous tissue directly over the rib, extending the incision anteriorly across the rectus muscle high in the epigastrium and well above the umbilicus. Curve the incision inferiorly to avoid injury to the intercostal nerve and its branches as they emerge from under the rib lying above. It can be extended across the midline to the contralateral costochondral junction (short-dashed line); for retroperitoneal dissection, a midline or paramedian extension is useful (dotted line).

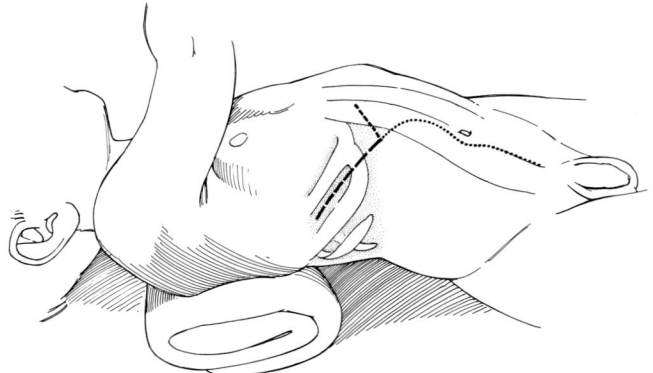

2 Incise the latissimus dorsi, posterior inferior serratus, and external oblique muscles with the cutting current, then divide the internal oblique muscle by cutting directly on the convex surface of the 10th rib. Carry the incision well posteriorly to allow division of the costovertebral ligament.

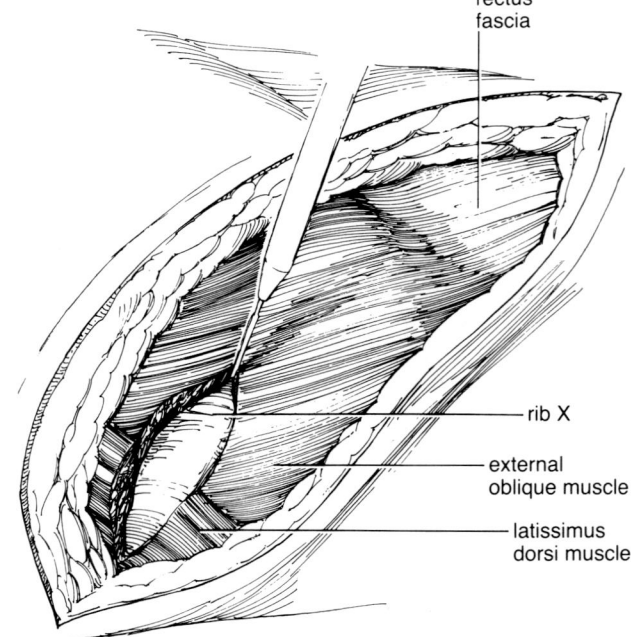

rectus fascia

rib X

external oblique muscle

latissimus dorsi muscle

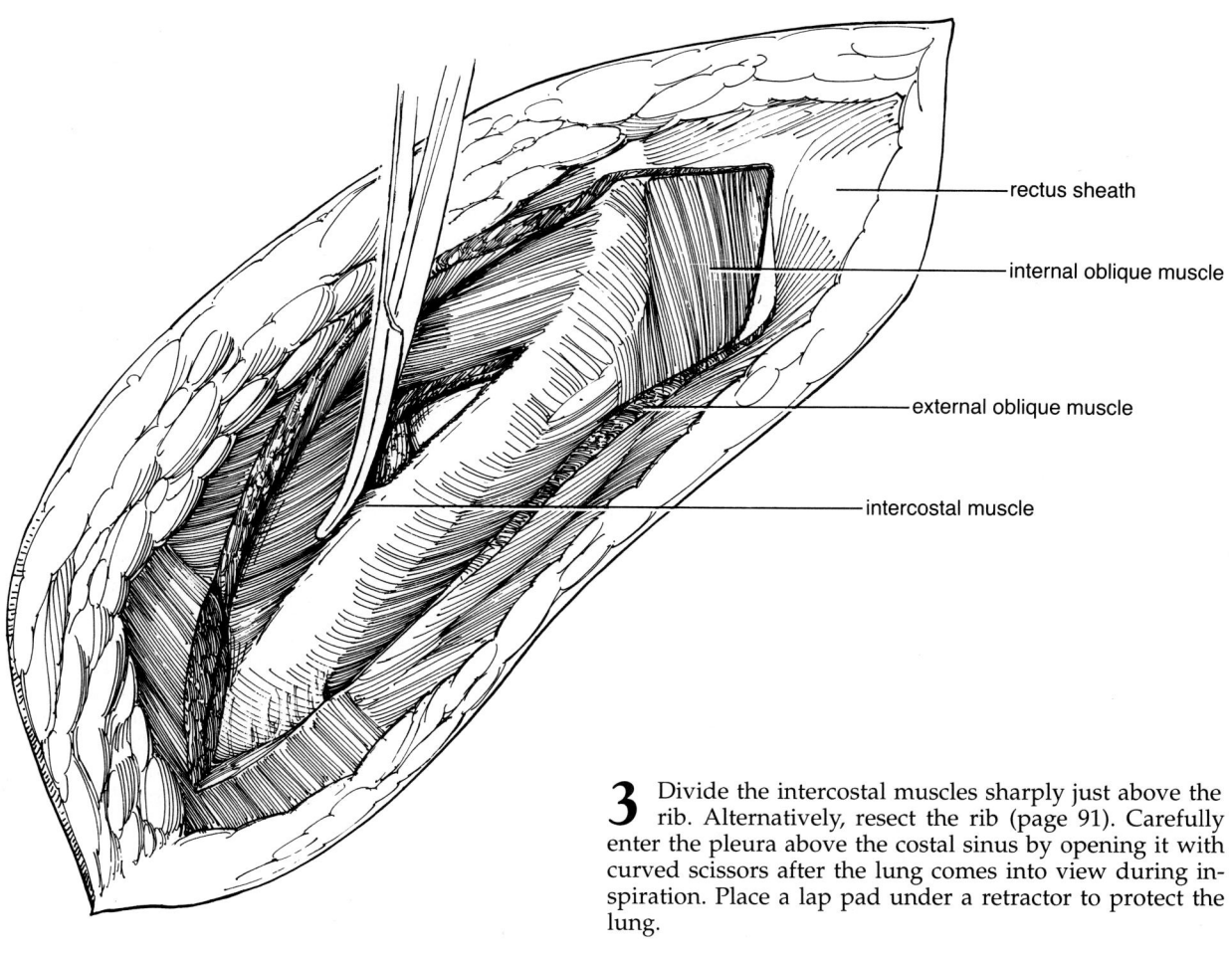

rectus sheath

internal oblique muscle

external oblique muscle

intercostal muscle

3 Divide the intercostal muscles sharply just above the rib. Alternatively, resect the rib (page 91). Carefully enter the pleura above the costal sinus by opening it with curved scissors after the lung comes into view during inspiration. Place a lap pad under a retractor to protect the lung.

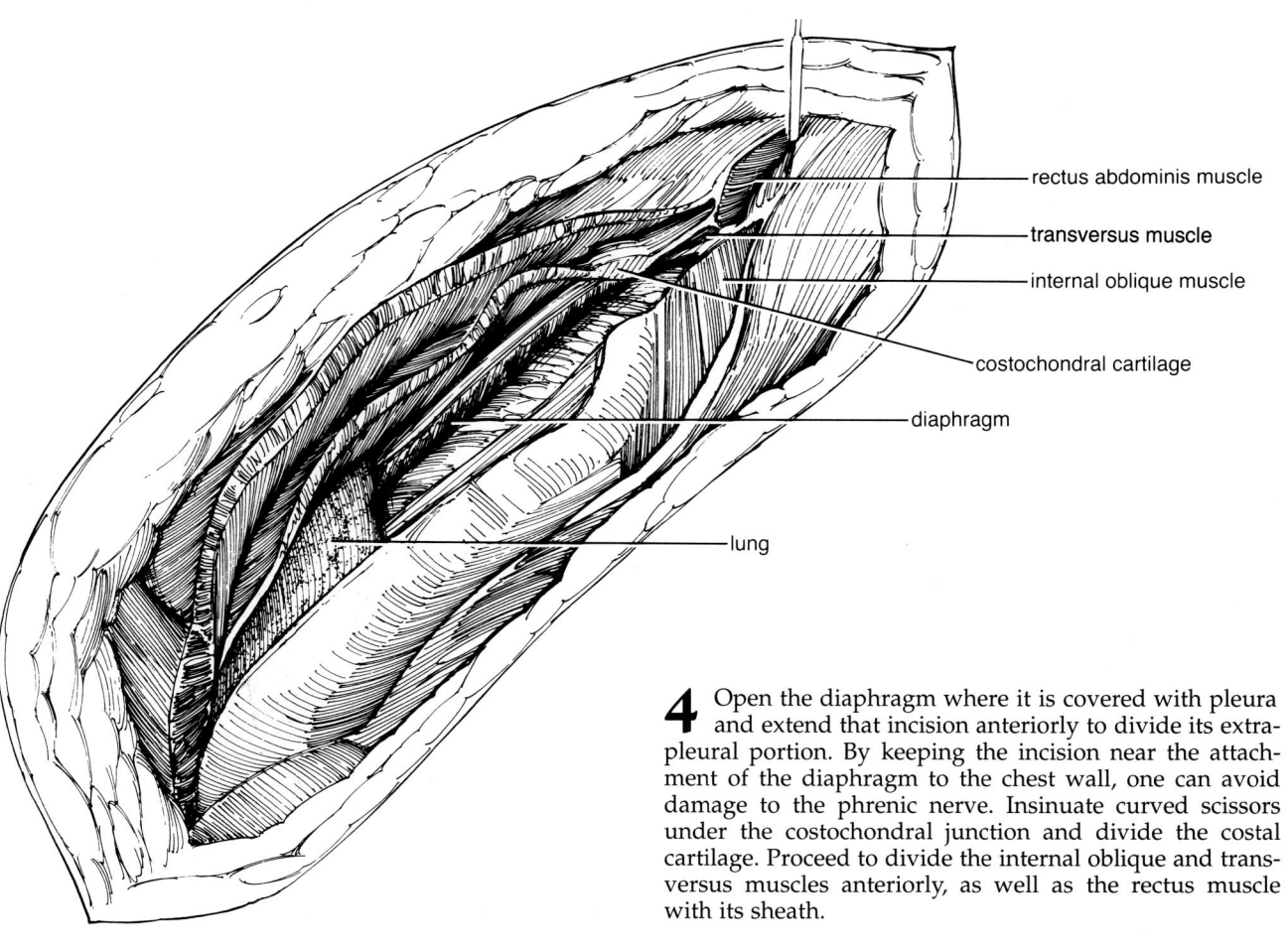

rectus abdominis muscle

transversus muscle

internal oblique muscle

costochondral cartilage

diaphragm

lung

4 Open the diaphragm where it is covered with pleura and extend that incision anteriorly to divide its extrapleural portion. By keeping the incision near the attachment of the diaphragm to the chest wall, one can avoid damage to the phrenic nerve. Insinuate curved scissors under the costochondral junction and divide the costal cartilage. Proceed to divide the internal oblique and transversus muscles anteriorly, as well as the rectus muscle with its sheath.

5 Open the peritoneum. Insert a retractor at the tip of the 10th rib, catching the ends of cartilage in its slots. Displace the liver on the right (and the spleen on the left) upward to expose the posterior peritoneum. Grasp the lateral edge of peritoneum near the diaphragm and dissect the avascular plane between Gerota's fascia and the peritoneum. Continue the dissection medially to identify the superior mesenteric artery, which in turn allows location of the right renal vein.

Proceed with radical nephrectomy or adrenalectomy. If more exposure is needed, continue the incision across the midline. For retroperitoneal node dissection, extend the incision inferiorly in the midline or as a paramedian inci-

sion. For adrenalectomy, provide two incisions in the diaphragm. Make the first one laterally between the lumbo-costal arch and the tendinous portion of the left leaflet. This will allow access to the adrenal area. Proceed with adrenalectomy. Before closure, place a second incision in the diaphragm more anteriorly, running parallel to the muscle fibers between the left leaflet and the site of attachment of the costal cartilages. Incise the peritoneum beneath and proceed with abdominal exploration and palpation of the other adrenal.

For even better exposure, make a single incision that extends medially from the lateral margin of the diaphragm.

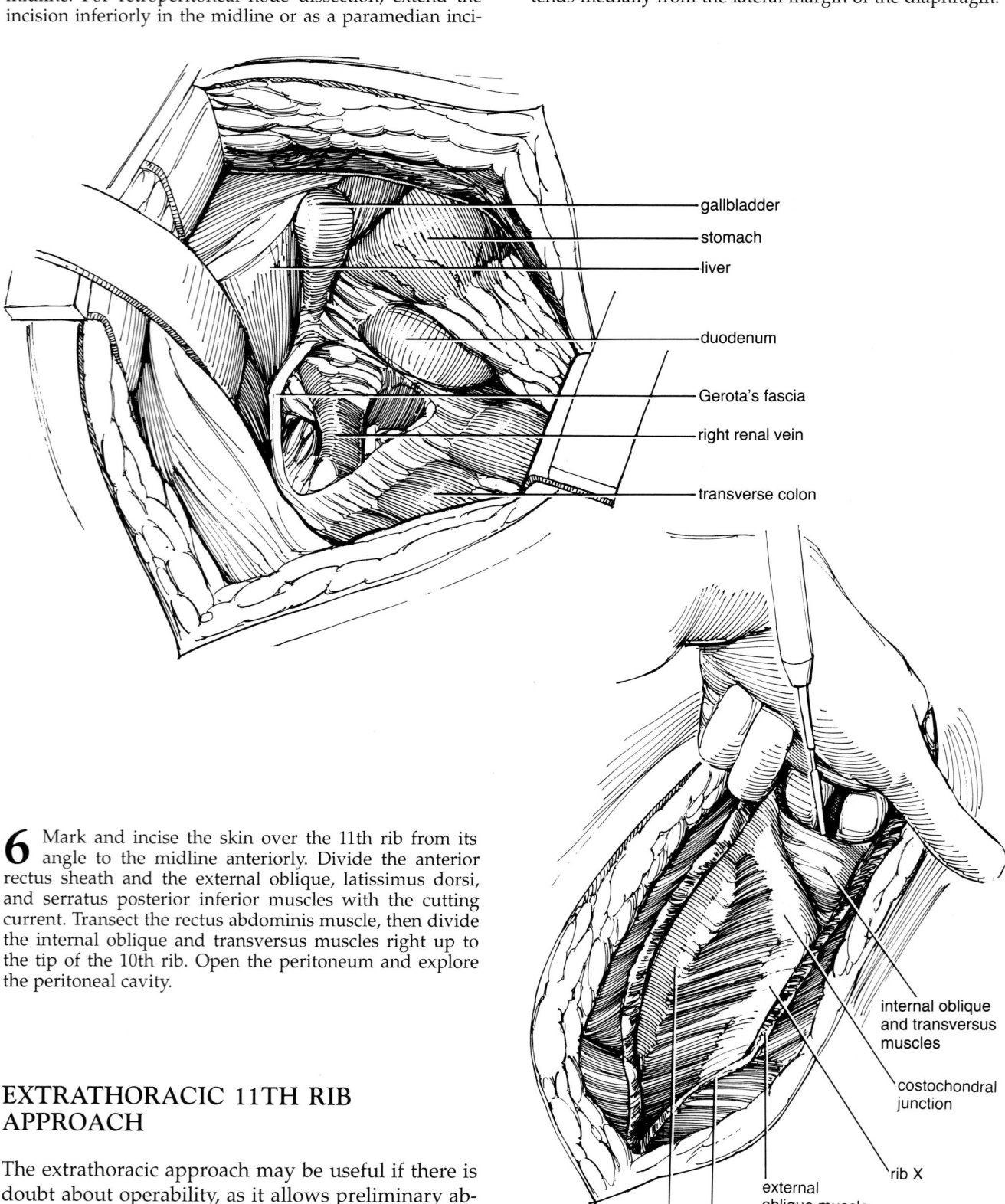

gallbladder

stomach

liver

duodenum

Gerota's fascia

right renal vein

transverse colon

internal oblique and transversus muscles

costochondral junction

rib X

external oblique muscle

latissimus dorsi muscle

rib IX

6 Mark and incise the skin over the 11th rib from its angle to the midline anteriorly. Divide the anterior rectus sheath and the external oblique, latissimus dorsi, and serratus posterior inferior muscles with the cutting current. Transect the rectus abdominis muscle, then divide the internal oblique and transversus muscles right up to the tip of the 10th rib. Open the peritoneum and explore the peritoneal cavity.

EXTRATHORACIC 11TH RIB APPROACH

The extrathoracic approach may be useful if there is doubt about operability, as it allows preliminary abdominal exploration. In some cases, the lesion is more accessible than expected and can be removed without entering the chest.

7 Protect the liver with the fingers of the left hand and divide the cartilaginous arch between the 9th and 10th ribs.

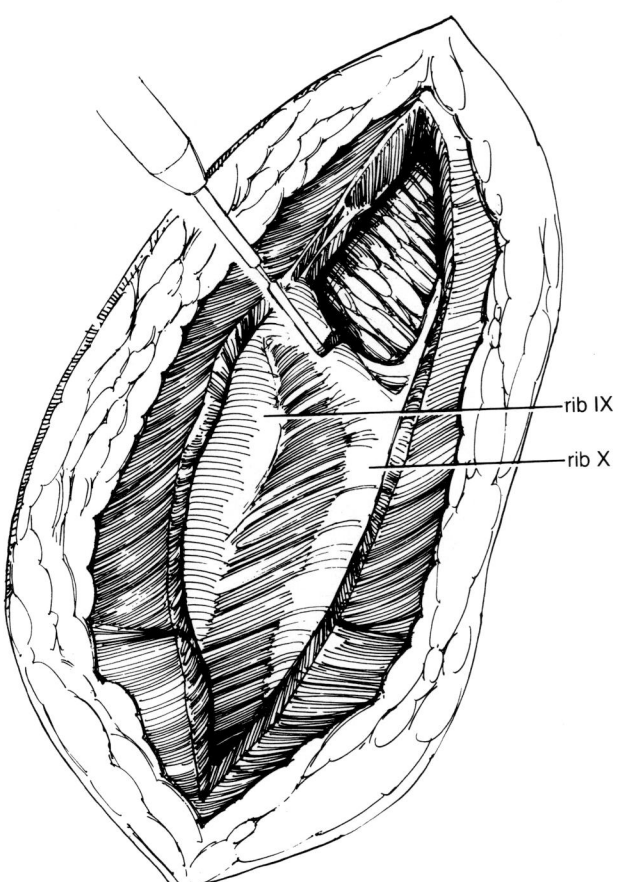

rib IX
rib X

8 Cautiously divide the intercostal muscles against the upper edge of the 10th rib with scissors or electrode, exposing the diaphragm first, then the pleura. Ask the anesthetist to expand the lung. Carefully dissect the pleura from the undersurface of the 10th rib and reflect it upward with the diaphragm. This maneuver is facilitated by dividing slips of the diaphragm first and then reflecting the pleura cephalad. Alternatively, enter the pleura as just described. Divide the costovertebral ligament and hinge the 10th rib downward.

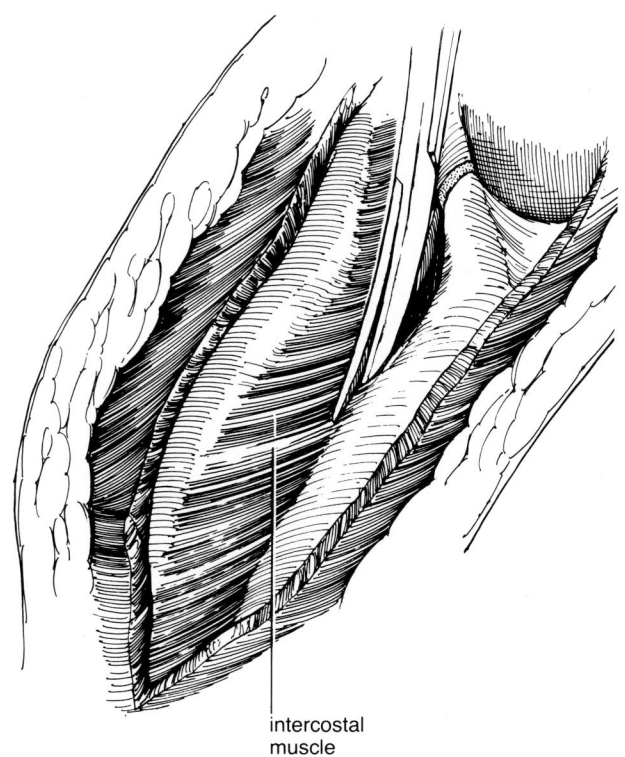

intercostal
muscle

9 Incise the diaphragm about 2 cm below the pleural reflection behind the rib. By staying near the insertion of the diaphragm into the chest wall, one can avoid damage to the phrenic nerve.

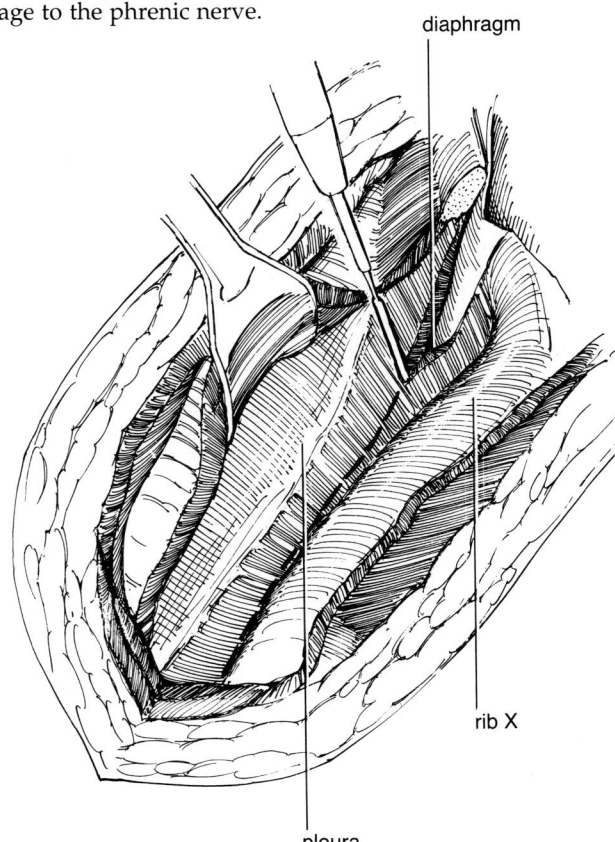

diaphragm

rib X

pleura

10 Tack the upper edge of the diaphragm to the serratus posterior inferior and latissimus dorsi muscles to protect the pleura. Open the peritoneum completely and divide the posterior rectus sheath. Insert a self-retaining retractor to separate the ribs and place an abdominal retractor as well. Proceed with radical nephrectomy or other procedure.

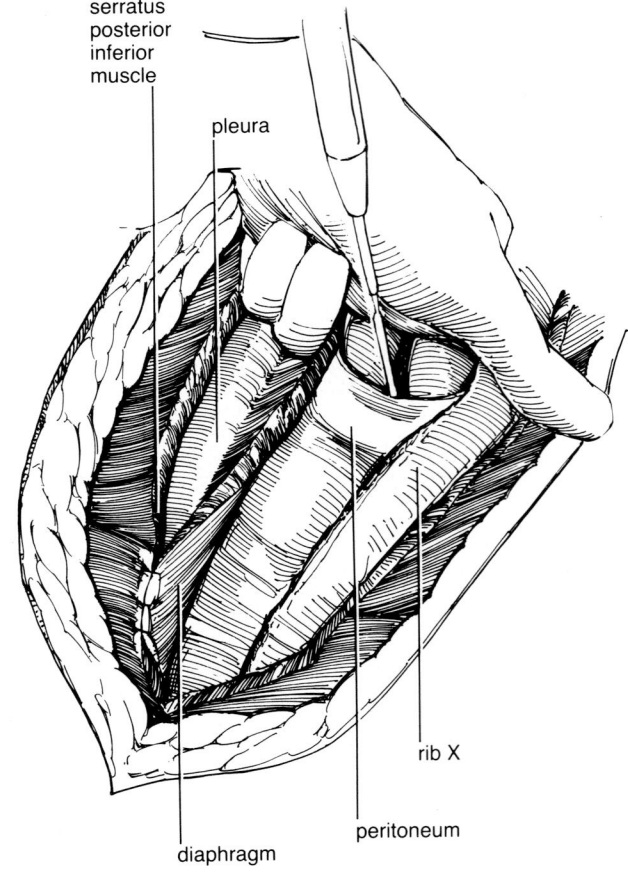

serratus
posterior
inferior
muscle

pleura

rib X

peritoneum

diaphragm

11 *Closure*: Close the posterior peritoneum with running 3-0 or 4-0 synthetic absorbable sutures. Place a retroperitoneal drain (optional) through a stab wound. Approximate the diaphragm with horizontal mattress sutures of 4-0 Maxon with the knots buried. Inject 5 ml of 0.75 percent bupivacaine into the area of the intercostal nerves percutaneously at the posterior end of the incision or place an epidural catheter into this area for postoperative infusion of local anesthetic agent. Protect the lung with a finger in the pleural space beneath and avoid entering the costal veins. Place a 3-0 monofilament nylon suture through the cut edges of the costal arch but do not tie it. Insert a 14 F Robinson catheter in the pleural cavity and close the pleura and intercostal muscles with a running fine synthetic absorbable suture. Alternatively, install a 20 F chest tube, bringing it out through a stab wound in the posterior axillary line, suturing it to the skin with heavy silk. Preplace several interrupted sutures near the costophrenic sinus. Tie the suture in the costal arch and then the sutures over the costophrenic sinus.

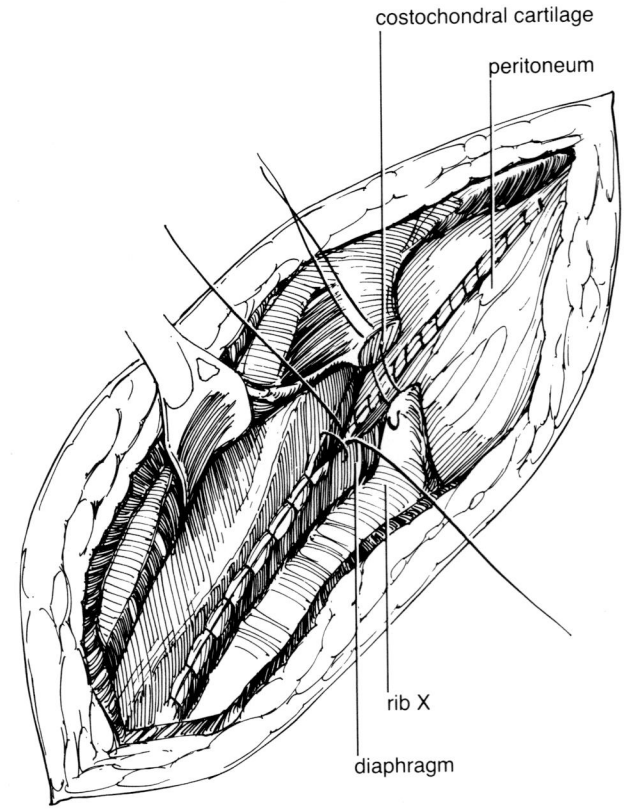

costochondral cartilage

peritoneum

rib X

diaphragm

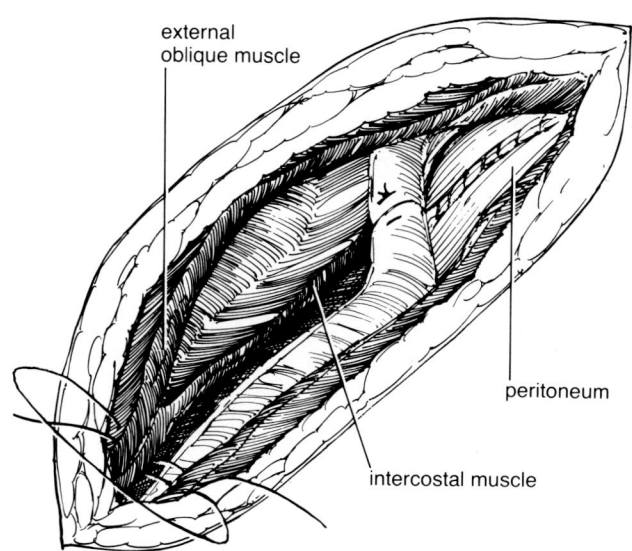

external oblique muscle

peritoneum

intercostal muscle

12 Close the thoracic part of the incision by first placing figure-eight 2-0 or 3-0 synthetic absorbable sutures through all the muscular layers of the chest wall; include the anterior pleural edge and the diaphragm in the last few sutures. Tie these sutures successively, beginning posteriorly. Suture the peritoneum with a running 4-0 absorbable suture; approximate the posterior and anterior rectus sheaths and the muscle layers with 2-0 or 3-0 synthetic absorbable sutures. Close the subcutaneous tissue and skin.

Commentary by Howard M. Snyder III

The thoracoabdominal approach is less frequently needed in children than in adults because of the increased flexibility of children's ribs that enables a subcostal incision that is extended across the midline to provide exposure for most renal procedures. The two situations in which the thoracoabdominal approach is most useful are adrenal surgery, as when one deals with an adrenal tumor, or when one is faced with a very large tumor of the kidney, most commonly Wilms' tumor. On the right side, the thoracoabdominal incision should be perhaps more frequently used for large renal tumors than on the left. A good way to judge whether a thoracoabdominal approach will be necessary is to look at the anteroposterior size of the tumor with respect to the space between the posterior abdominal wall and the undersurface of the ribs anteriorly. If there is very little room for the tumor to be moved, gaining adequate exposure of the upper portion of the kidney may be difficult without a thoracoabdominal incision. A last situation in which wide exposure of the kidney is essential and the thoracoabdominal approach may thus be useful is in kidney transplant donor nephrectomy, where wide exposure of the kidney and the vessels is essential to enable an atraumatic nephrectomy. Often for this, the extrapleural supra 11th rib incision works nicely.

CHAPTER 17
Dorsal Flap Incision
(NAGAMATSU)

Although rarely needed in children because of the flexibility of their ribs, the dorsal flap incision can obtain exposure well above the kidney and is an alternative to the thoracoabdominal incision (page 102) in adolescents. A subcostal or 12th rib incision can be extended with this technique if it proves inadequate. Instruments are the same as those used for the transcostal incision.

1 **A,** *Position and Incision*: Lateral, rotated 15 degrees anteriorly over the kidney rest with the table flexed. Support the upper arm. After the child has been taped in position, the table may be rotated anteriorly or posteriorly to facilitate making the lumbar or the dorsal incisions. **B,** Start the skin incision at the level of the ninth interspace, run it vertically down the edge of the sacrospinalis muscle, then curve it anteriorly along the upper edge of the 12th rib to meet the lateral rectus sheath at the level of the 10th interspace. If there is uncertainty about the extent of lesion, make only the abdominal portion of the incision to allow preliminary palpation and visualization.

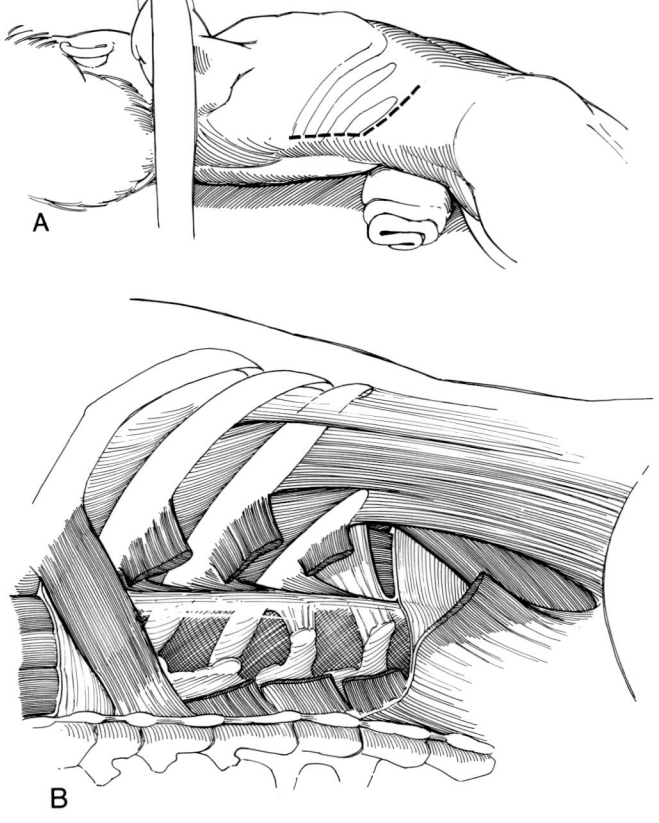

2 Divide the latissimus dorsi and the posterior inferior serratus muscles over the three lower ribs medial to their angles. Avoid the intercostal bundle. Divide the lumbocostal ligament and the tendinous slips of the sacrospinalis muscle before they insert into the two lower ribs. Mark each end of the lumbocostal ligament to aid in approximation at closure.

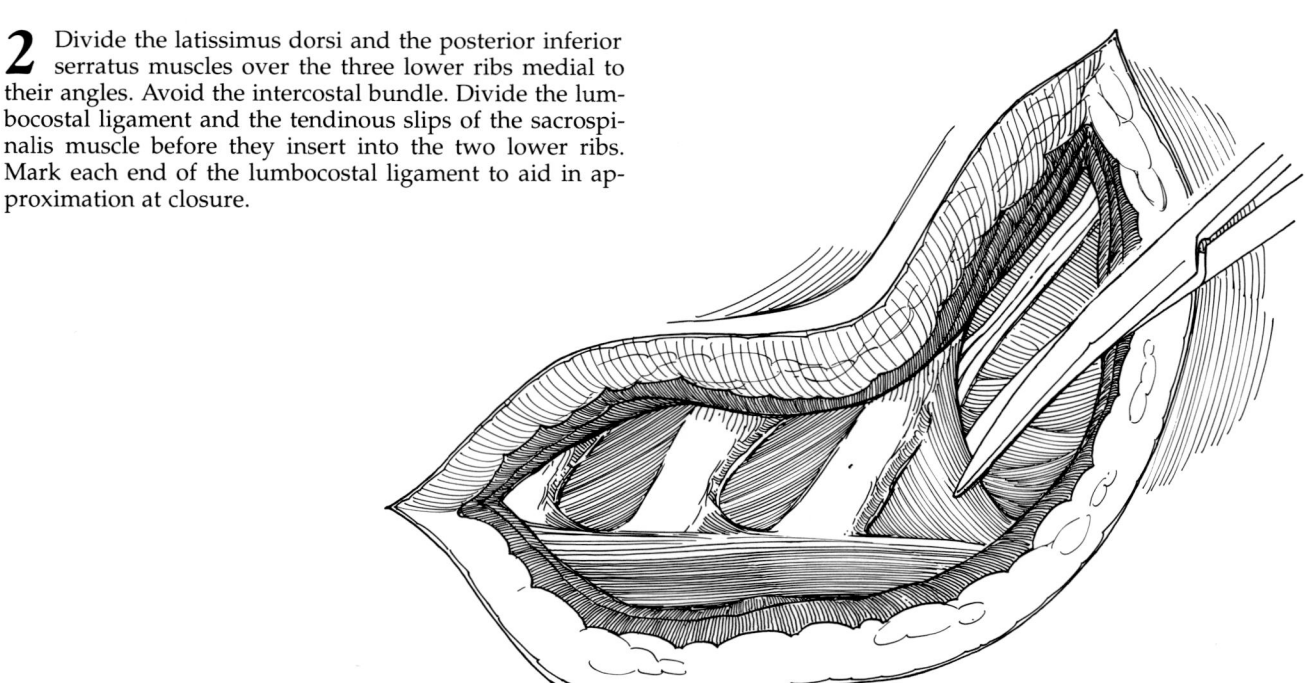

3 Open the periosteum and resect half-inch segments of the lower two ribs with the guillotine rib resector medial to the rib angle, after carefully freeing them from the pleura with the Davis periosteal elevator and the Doyen rib elevator, using the technique described elsewhere (Chapter 14). It is important that these segments be removed posterior to the nubby thickened angle of the rib both to provide a deep fulcrum for upward mobilization of the rib cage and to avoid pleural injury, because the pleura is reflected away from this area. Divide the lumbocostal ligament. It usually is not necessary to divide the lumbocostal arch of the diaphragm to free the pleura; let the diaphragm swing up with the lower rib cage. Do not isolate or dissect the 10th and 12th intercostal bundles.

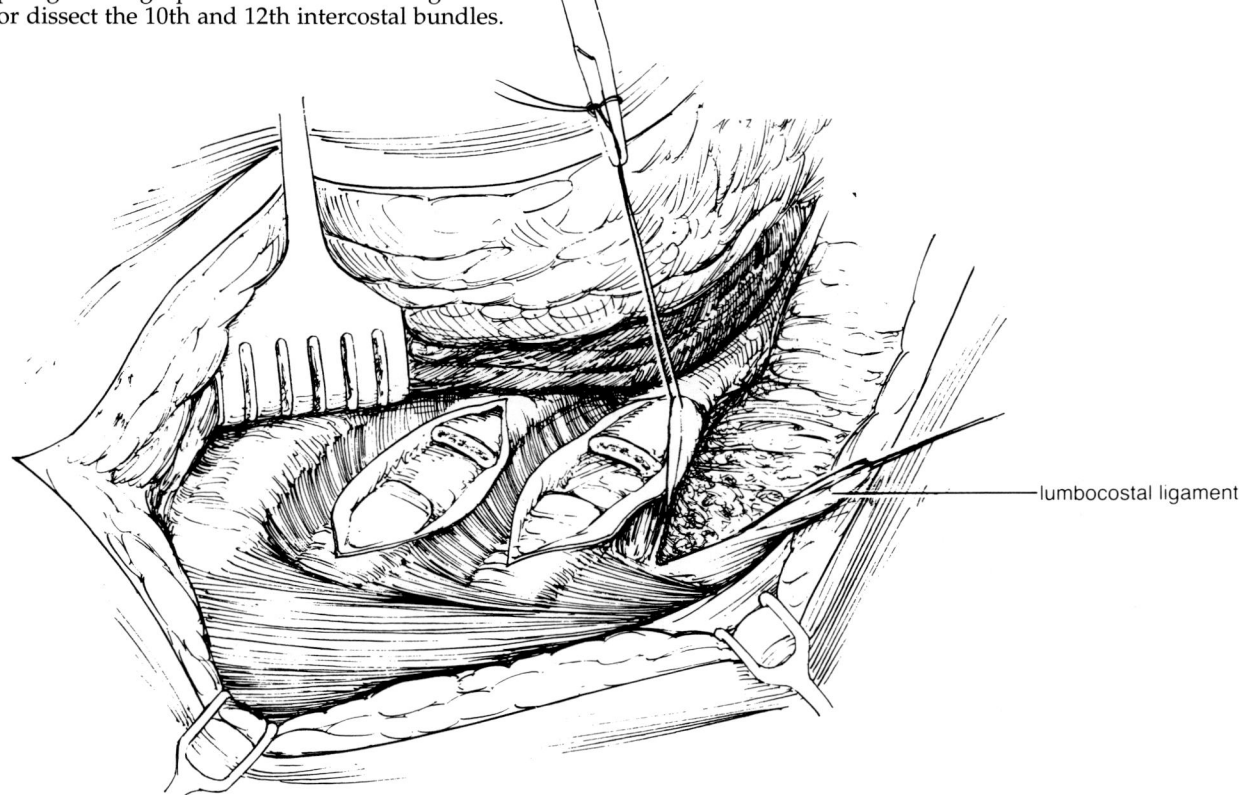

lumbocostal ligament

4 Complete the incision below the 12th rib anteriorly as for a subcostal incision (page 87), freeing the peritoneum from the undersurface of the transversus abdominis. Divide the lumbocostal fascia. Retract the lower part of the incision along with the iliohypogastric nerve. Proceed with the renal operation.

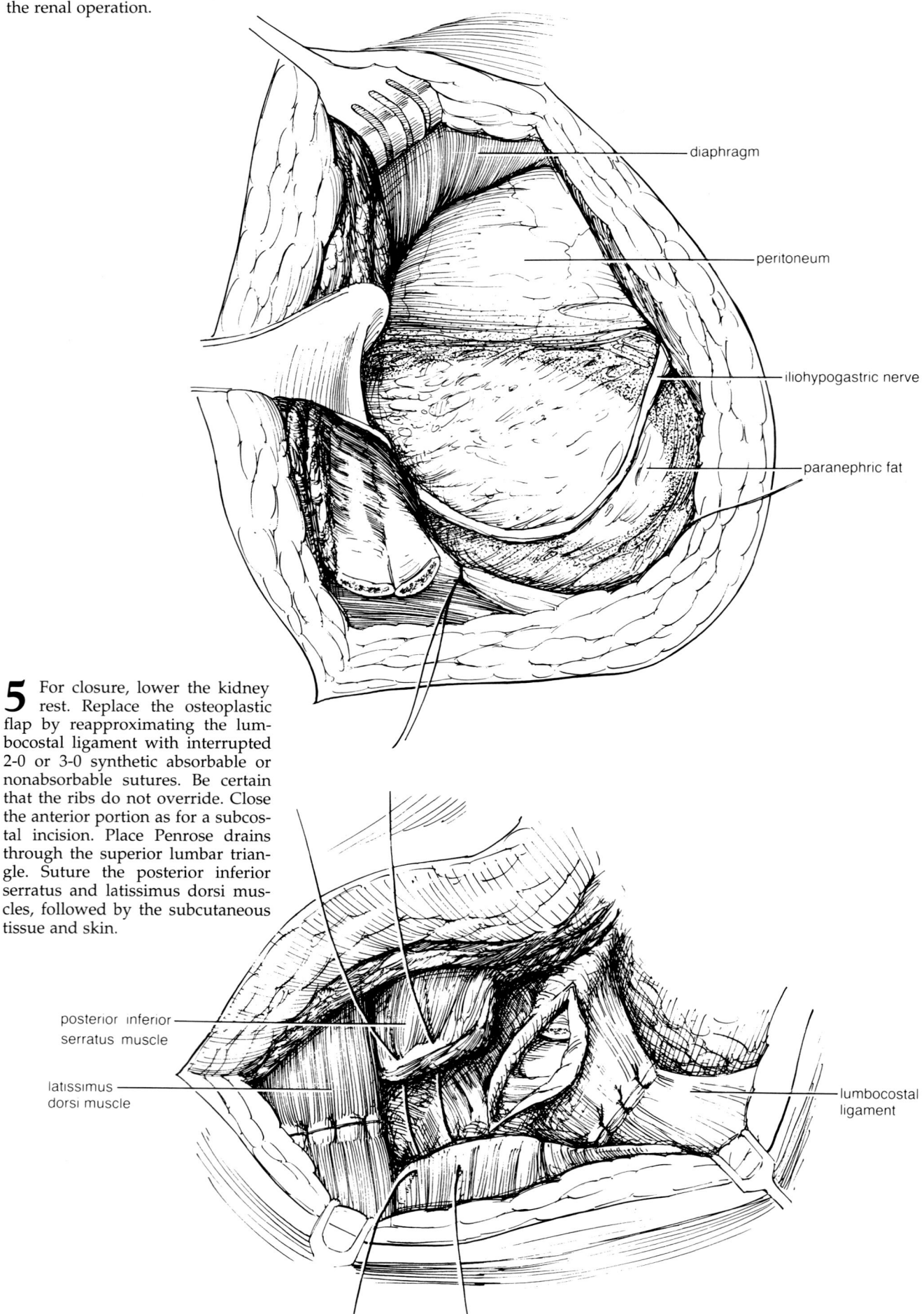

diaphragm

peritoneum

iliohypogastric nerve

paranephric fat

5 For closure, lower the kidney rest. Replace the osteoplastic flap by reapproximating the lumbocostal ligament with interrupted 2-0 or 3-0 synthetic absorbable or nonabsorbable sutures. Be certain that the ribs do not override. Close the anterior portion as for a subcostal incision. Place Penrose drains through the superior lumbar triangle. Suture the posterior inferior serratus and latissimus dorsi muscles, followed by the subcutaneous tissue and skin.

posterior inferior serratus muscle

latissimus dorsi muscle

lumbocostal ligament

Commentary by George R. Nagamatsu

Detailed sequential anatomic maneuvers were carried out on the warm cadaver during the development of this operation. This was followed by the initial operative cases fully detailed in the original descriptions. Clinical experience through the years has demonstrated the flexibility of this operation and simplified these steps, greatly reducing the operative time without compromising its aim of adequate exposure of the upper retroperitoneum in most cases without entering the pleural cavity. In the original communication, 44 cases were tabulated at the Bronx Veterans Administration Medical Center. The versatility of this exposure has been extended as a modification of the Young bilateral simultaneous lumbar exposure and as an optional extraperitoneal approach for bilateral retroperitoneal lymph node dissection in testis tumor in combination with a Cherney type of incision.

The key lumbocostal ligaments anchoring the lower two ribs are divided. Often, the fixed overhanging rib cage springs upward together with the attached pleura and the lateral crus of the diaphragm, demonstrating the attained mobility by this division. By the same token, accurate reapproximation of this ligament is the first step in the closure to follow. Prior to this division, therefore, both ends of the ligament are marked with sutures, thus ensuring correct realignment of the ribs without overriding. In the original description, division of the lateral crus of the diaphragm and, on occasion, the medial crus below the reflection of the pleura was depicted. However, this does not contribute to the procedure, and further manipulation in this area is contraindicated.

In proceeding with the abdominal limb as for a subcostal incision to meet the rectus sheath, it now will be possible in most cases of large renal tumors to assess their removability and early accessibility to the renal pedicle, often anteriorly. With the double advantage afforded by the now-unroofed costal overhang and the abdominal exposure, initial clamping of the renal artery under direct vision often is feasible. If it is necessary to open the peritoneum, especially in the right-sided cases, this may be done freely without compromising the final result. Allow the distended tense kidney to decompress its component of blood content, then clamp the renal vein. The now-limp imprisoned organ severed at the pedicle will allow radical removal with tender manipulation, minimizing cell bolus implants. Further toilet as indicated now can proceed visually in the wide-open field.

With increased familiarity of the technique and the avoidance of surgical manipulation after division of the lumbocostal ligaments as described, pleural injury is rare. Should it occur, notify the anesthetist, protect the area with a pad, and proceed with the operation. Attempts to suture the pleura at the time of injury are to be avoided. At the conclusion of the operation, close the rent around a small catheter buttressed with overlying muscle and fascia and remove the catheter at the last suture, with the lung expanded by the anesthetist. Small Penrose drains ordinarily are placed at the superior lumbar triangle. However, in cases of pleural injury, place these drains at the anterior portion of the incision. A chest film at the conclusion of the operation and the following morning is desirable. Postoperative management and ambulation do not differ in routine. With experience, the simplified bony mobilization requires only 5 to 10 minutes.

Several decades of long-term follow-up of patients managed with this type of incision have disclosed no restriction of lumbodorsal mobility. Cartilaginous or bony reunion at resected rib sites with normal realignment is found, owing to the key required reapproximation of the lumbocostal ligament.

CHAPTER 18

Dorsal Lumbotomy

UNILATERAL POSTERIOR LUMBOTOMY

Unilateral posterior lumbotomy provides less access to the kidney than flank approaches, but it has many uses in pediatric urologic surgery, including pyeloplasty, open renal biopsies, removal of small kidneys, simultaneous bilateral renal operations, large pelvic stones, and stones fixed in the upper or mid-ureter. It can be combined with coagulum and/or nephroscopy for free stones, although it is often difficult to nephroscope all calyces. It is unsuitable for malignant lesions or malpositioned kidneys. If the skin incision is made somewhat transversely, the disadvantage of a scar resulting from crossing Langer's lines is obviated without sacrifice of exposure.

1 *Instruments*: Provide Gil Vernet retractors and long curved retractors. For stone cases, include a flexible nephroscope and coagulum.

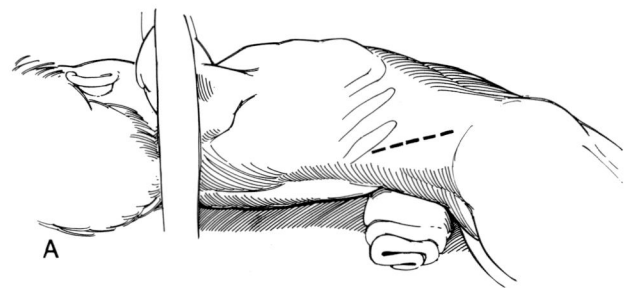

A

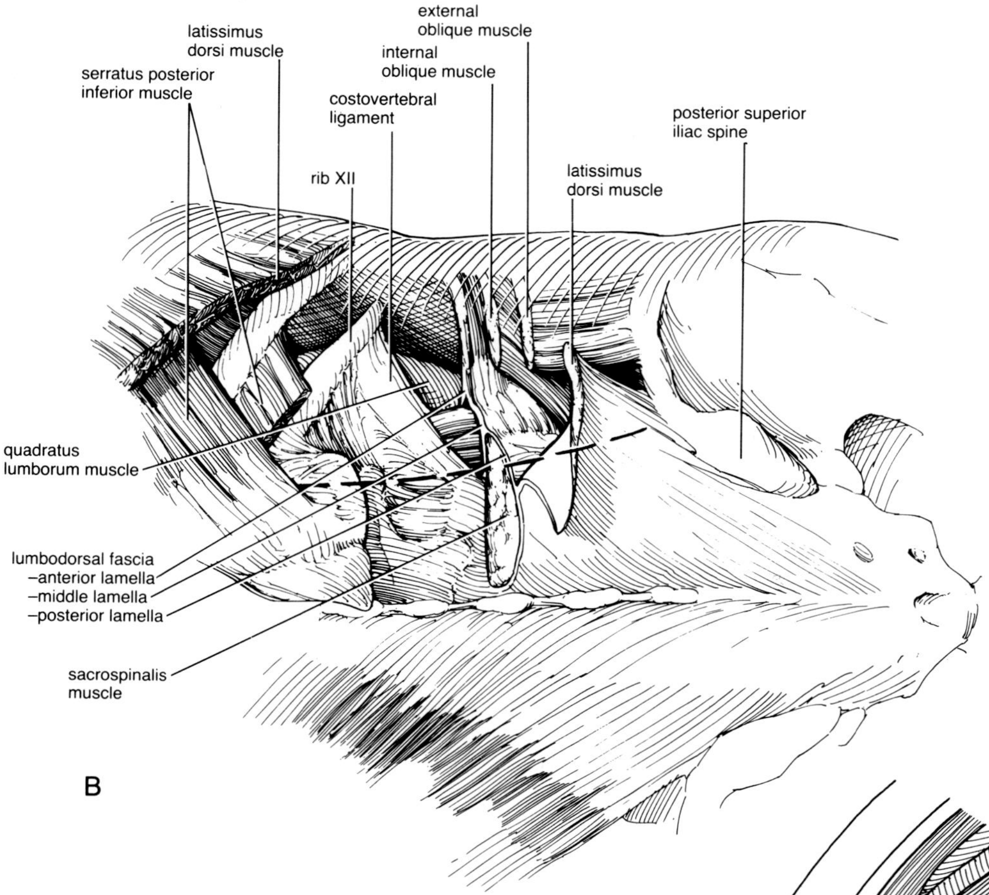

B

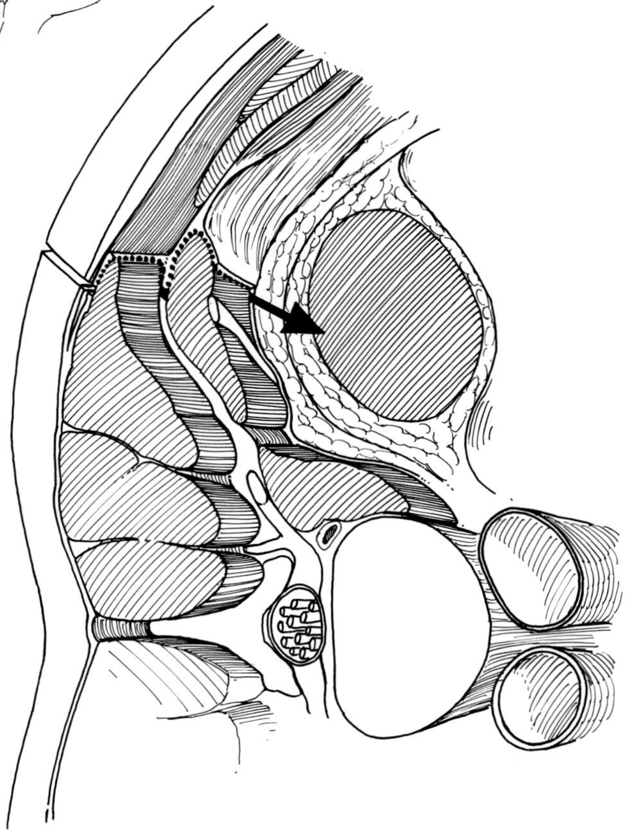

serratus posterior inferior muscle

latissimus dorsi muscle

costovertebral ligament

rib XII

internal oblique muscle

external oblique muscle

latissimus dorsi muscle

posterior superior iliac spine

quadratus lumborum muscle

lumbodorsal fascia
—anterior lamella
—middle lamella
—posterior lamella

sacrospinalis muscle

A, *Position*: After tracheal intubation, place the child in a modified lateral position, rotated forward 30 to 45 degrees. It is usually better not to flex the table, because this puts tension on the muscles of the back. For renal biopsy, the lateral position without flexion with the knees bent keeps the kidney from falling away from the surgeon and is less limiting on respiration. *Incision*: Make an oblique skin incision more or less along the skin lines (Langer's lines) that extend from the angle of the 12th rib, where the lateral border of the sacrospinalis muscle crosses the lower margin of the rib (approximately 5 to 6 cm from the spinal processes), down to the iliac crest at a point one third of the distance from the anterosuperior iliac spine to the spinal processes. **B,** and **C,** Approach is made anterior to the sacrospinalis and quadratus lumborum muscles via the lumbodorsal fascia.

C

2 After making the skin incision, free the subcutaneous tissue to make a vertical incision in the posterior projection of the latissimus dorsi and posterior inferior serratus muscles.

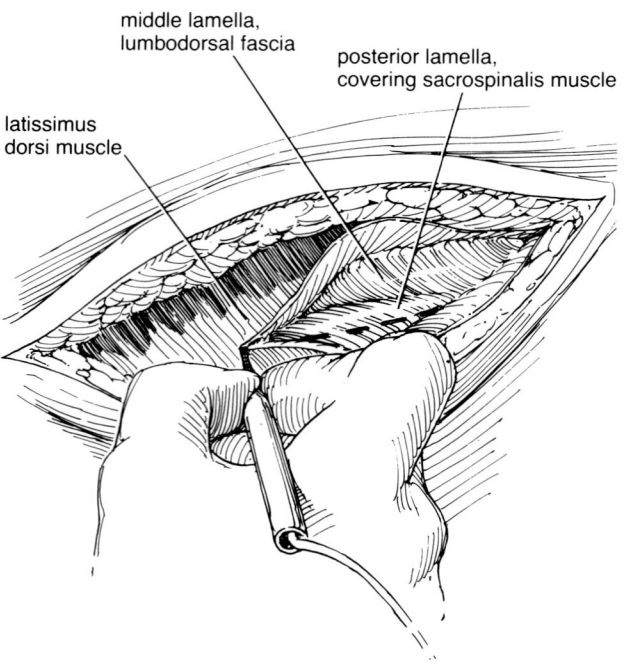

middle lamella, lumbodorsal fascia

posterior lamella, covering sacrospinalis muscle

latissimus dorsi muscle

3 Divide the posterior lamella of the lumbodorsal fascia vertically to expose the sacrospinalis muscle.

posterior lamella, lumbodorsal fascia

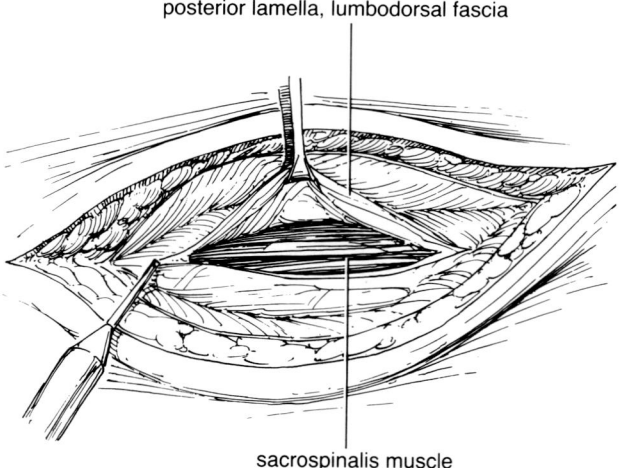

sacrospinalis muscle

4 Elevate the lateral edge of the cut lumbodorsal fascia with Allis forceps to allow medial retraction of the lateral edge of the sacrospinalis muscle.

quadratus lumborum muscle

middle lamella, lumbodorsal fascia

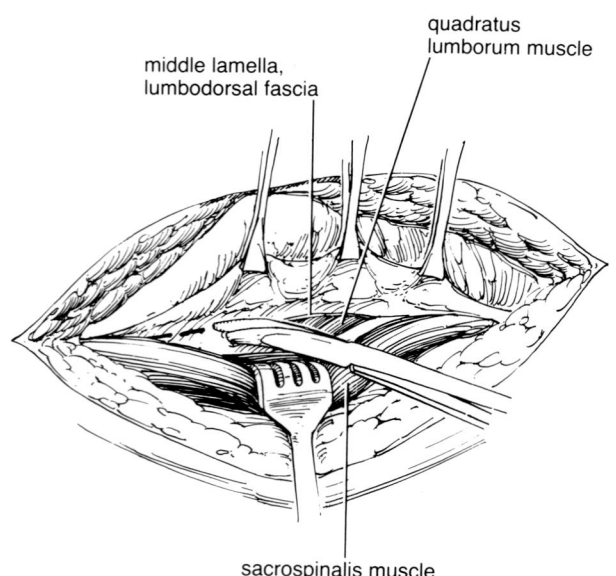

sacrospinalis muscle

5 Bluntly dissect the lateral margin of the sacrospinalis muscle to expose the subcostal vessels and the costovertebral ligament. Under vision, divide the ligament with scissors. Incise the exposed fused middle and anterior lamellae of the lumbar fascia approximately 1 cm under the edge of the quadratus lumborum muscle, down to the iliac crest. This fascia surrounds the quadratus lumborum muscle and is the origin of the internal oblique and transversus abdominis muscles. Watch out for the iliohypogastric nerve under the fascia during exposure and closure.

quadratus lumborum muscle

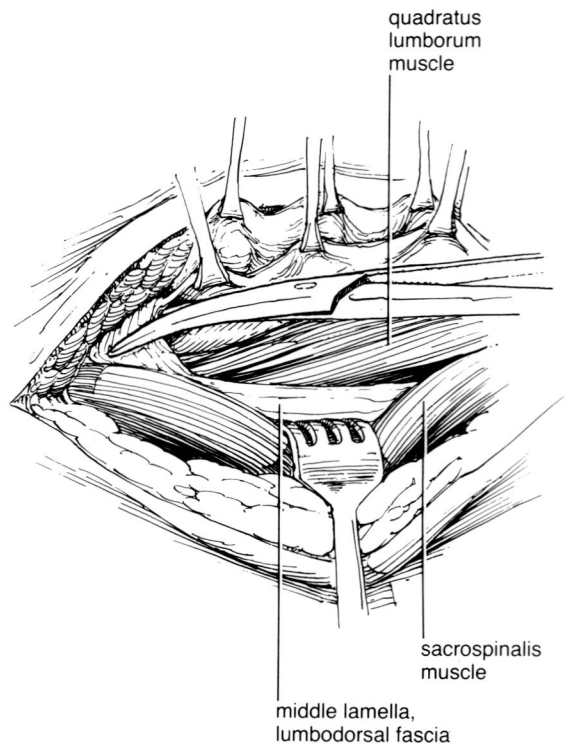

sacrospinalis muscle

middle lamella, lumbodorsal fascia

6 Retract the quadratus lumborum muscle dorsally, exposing the anterior lamella of the lumbodorsal fascia. Incise the anterior lamella of the lumbar fascia between the subcostal and iliohypogastric nerve, coursing obliquely across. Extend the incision in the lumbodorsal fascia cephalad to divide the costovertebral ligament and allow upward rotation of the 12th rib.

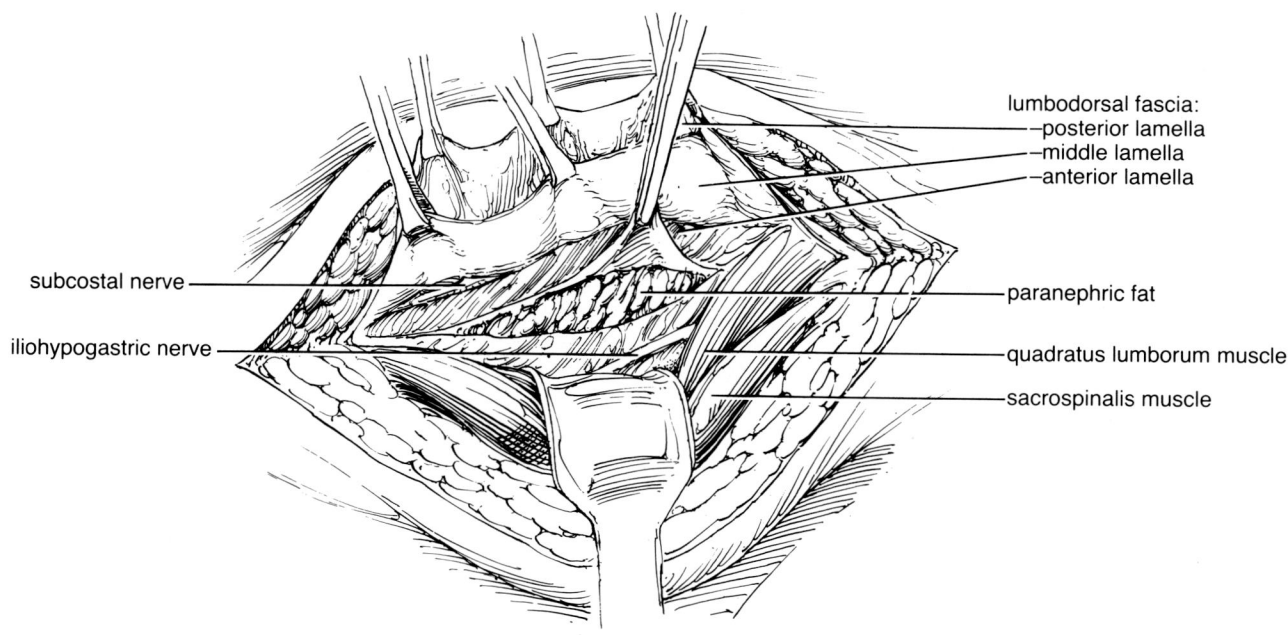

lumbodorsal fascia:
—posterior lamella
—middle lamella
—anterior lamella

subcostal nerve

iliohypogastric nerve

paranephric fat

quadratus lumborum muscle

sacrospinalis muscle

7 Pick up Gerota's fascia with two forceps at the cranial end of the wound and incise it. Extend the opening caudad with two fingers. If exposure is not adequate, especially if a radiograph is needed, resect 1-cm segments of the 11th and 12th ribs, taking care to stay out of the pleura.

Alternatively, extend the incision anteriorly as a T. Insert a laminectomy retractor.

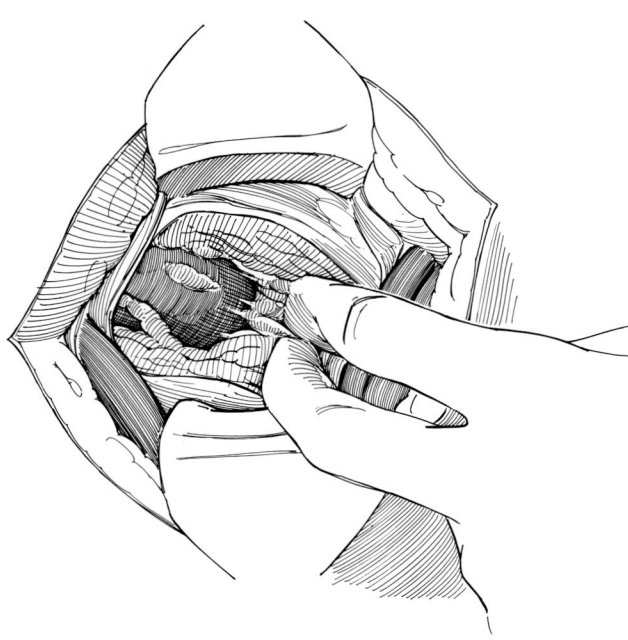

8 Pick up the ureter and begin renal dissection at the hilum.

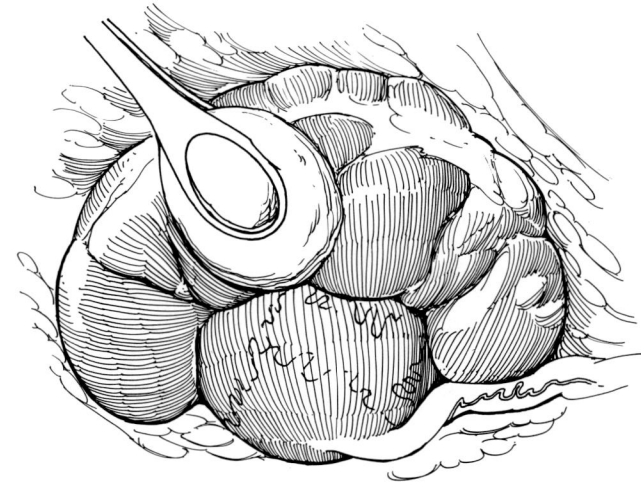

9 For pyelolithotomy, Gil Vernet retractors can be inserted to control the kidney position and assist in removal of the stone.

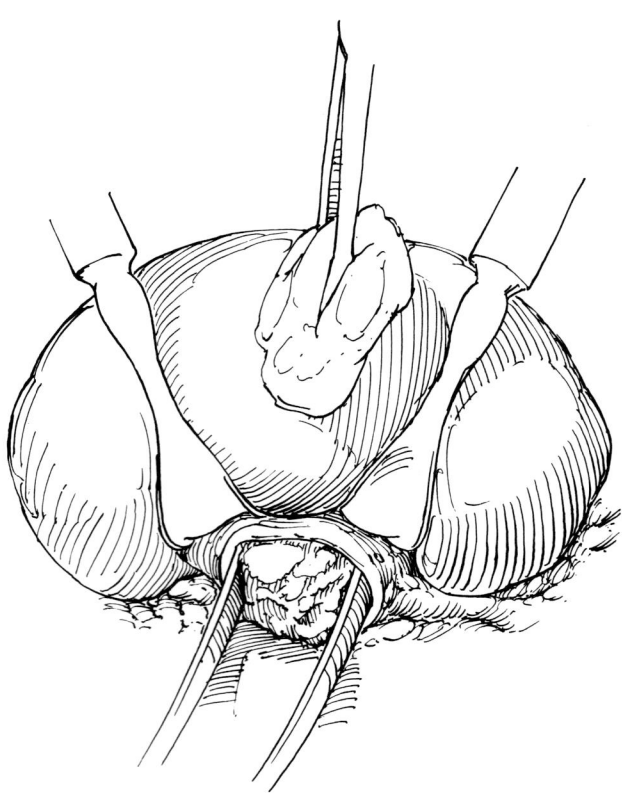

10 Insert a Penrose drain on completion of the procedure. Close the incision with six to eight 2-0 or 3-0 synthetic absorbable sutures in the two layers of the lumbodorsal fascia. Tie the second layer after the kidney rest has been lowered. If the latissimus dorsi and posterior inferior serratus muscles were divided, reunite them. Approximate the subcutaneous tissue and skin.

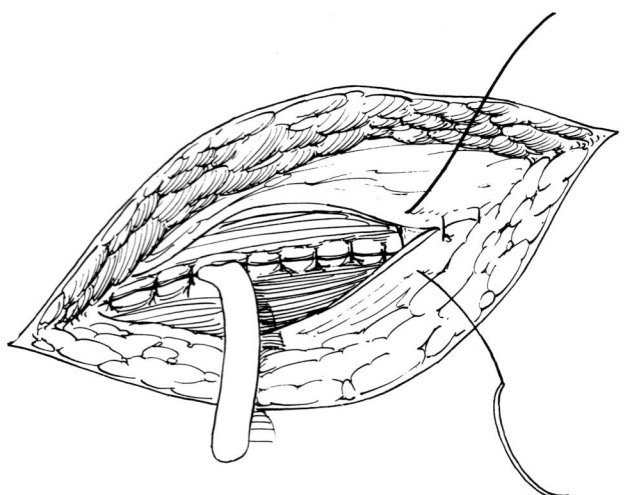

Extended Dorsal Lumbotomy

If the exposure is limited by the presence of the 12th rib above and the iliac crest below, mobilize the 12th rib by dividing the costovertebral ligament and resecting a 2-cm segment from it posterior to the angle. Incise the diaphragm up to the level of the 11th rib, keeping close to the 12th rib to avoid the pleura. The subcostal (12th) nerve and the iliohypogastric nerve now cross the incision and are freed; at least the latter must be preserved. Insert a self-retaining retractor and open Gerota's fascia vertically.

BILATERAL POSTERIOR LUMBOTOMY

An alternative to bilateral posterior lumbotomy is a posterior approach with rib resection (page 108). Bilateral posterior lumbotomy is used for simultaneous nephrectomy in transplant patients and for simultaneous adrenalectomy.

11 *Position*: Place the child prone with bolster support under shoulders and pelvis to avoid compression of chest and abdomen, and allow diaphragmatic breathing. Flex the table slightly. Provide a ring retractor with blades reversed.

Place one surgeon and one assistant on each side of the table to allow simultaneous exposure.

Incisions: Make oblique skin incisions (dashed lines) more or less along the skin lines, each of which extends from the angle of the 12th rib, where the lateral border of the sacrospinalis muscle crosses the lower margin of the rib (approximately 5 to 6 cm from the spinal processes), down to the iliac crest at a point one third of the distance from the anterosuperior iliac spine to the spinal processes. Proceed as for unilateral dorsal lumbotomy, placing the self-retaining retractor to compress the muscles medially.

For bilateral simultaneous exposure of the adrenal glands (Chapter 14), make two 12th-rib incisions (dotted lines).

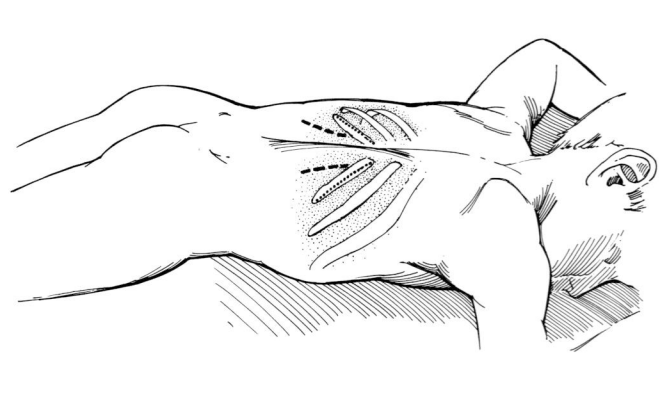

Commentary by Sakti Das

Dorsal lumbotomy is relatively easier in children than in adults, because the large longitudinal muscles in the anesthetized child can be retracted more effectively for wider access. The depth of the wound and thus the working distance of the target organs are shorter, often requiring only the insertion of Army-Navy retractors. Very young patients are positioned laterally and taped to the table with a towel roll beneath the contralateral flank.

During bilateral dorsal lumbotomy when the patient has been placed prone, one must carefully dissect along the anatomic plane and avoid entering the peritoneum, which gets pushed dorsally. I find that an assistant holding a deep Deaver retractor and adjusting retraction to my needs is more helpful than self-retaining retractors. For pyelolithotomy, it is wise to develop the renal sinus first so that Gil-Vernet retractors can be inserted to retract and stabilize the kidney from respiratory movements. An intraoperative flexible nephroscope should be available as an adjunct to coagulum for extraction of smaller free-lying renal calculi.

Closure of the tenuous middle lamella of lumbar fascia is not necessary and is fraught with the danger of catching the iliohypogastric nerve, which runs closely adjacent. The strong vertically disposed and overlapping sacrospinalis and quadratus lumborum, as well as the thick posterior lamella of the lumbar fascia, provide adequate strength to the closed wound.

The dorsal lumbotomy has not gained wide acceptance because of its relatively restricted exposure compared with the flank incision. However, because no significant muscles are divided in this transfascial approach, the postoperative morbidity is appreciably less and recovery is faster. Starting with open renal biopsies, one can use this approach for most open lithotomies from the kidney and upper ureter, as well as for simple nephrectomies. More recently, all of our pyeloplasties have been done through dorsal lumbotomy. In addition to the indications mentioned in the text, I have also done partial nephrectomy of ectopic upper moiety through the dorsal lumbotomy.

CHAPTER 19

Repair of Pleural Tear

If the pleura has been mobilized and possibly torn, have the anesthetist inflate the lung to identify the defect before closing the wound. Then have the lung deflated to draw the lung margin away from the site of the tear. Insert a small red Robinson catheter into the pleural space through the tear. Start a running 4-0 plain catgut suture; tie it beyond the anterior end of the pleural defect, continue around the catheter, and tie it beyond the end of the defect. Alternatively, include the diaphragm on one side and the intercostal muscles on the other (avoid the intercostal vessels and nerve). For small defects, have the anesthetist inflate the lung while you aspirate pleural air through the catheter with a large syringe, then tie the suture as the catheter is withdrawn.

If the defect is larger, leave the catheter in the pleura until the entire wound is closed, taking care not to position a Penrose drain near it. Place the end of the catheter underwater, and have the anesthetist fully inflate the lung. Remove the catheter when no more bubbles appear. Expose a portable chest film in the postanesthesia care unit. If there is any possibility that the lung itself has been perforated, guide the catheter from the wound and place it underwater in a sterile vacuum system (Pleur-Evac). A pleural tear that involves injury to both the underlying lung and the intercostal vessels in the chest wall usually results in hemopneumothorax. Here, insert a large right-angle tube with all the holes within the chest. The tube must be fastened to the chest wall with a silk suture that closes the skin firmly around the tube and also grasps the catheter so that it will not be inadvertently withdrawn. Add a seal of petrolatum gauze around the tube and connect it to continuous drainage using a three-bottle suction apparatus. Make a portable upright chest radiograph to make sure the lung is expanded and all fluid has been evacuated from the pleura. When no air has been aspirated for 8 hours, remove the tube.

CHAPTER 20

Splenorrhaphy and Splenectomy

SPLENORRHAPHY AFTER AN INTRAOPERATIVE INJURY

Intraoperative injury of the spleen usually is the result of capsular avulsion by forcible retraction of the spleen away from the retroperitoneal surface, where it is held by the splenomental fold that lies between the greater omentum and the medial aspect of the lower pole of the spleen. Splenectomy should be avoided, especially in children; splenorrhaphy and segmental splenectomy usually are reasonable alternatives.

First, cover the avulsed area with hemostatic gauze (Avitene), and firmly hold it with a dry lap pad. Avoid holding it with a retractor, which will usually make the tear worse or start a new one. Remove the pad and trim any excess gauze. Add more gauze if an area is still bleeding. If necessary, place a row of 3-0 or 4-0 synthetic absorbable mattress sutures over it. Bolsters of hemostatic gauze can be inserted under the longitudinal loops of the suture to decrease cutting into the capsule.

If the bleeding is brisk and time is needed for repair, open the lesser sac and compress the tail of the pancreas over the splenic vessels. Mobilize the spleen by incising the lienorenal ligament to be able to deliver the spleen and tail of the pancreas into the wound. The splenic vessels are then readily compressed, and the splenic wound itself can be tamponaded and repaired under direct vision. Proceed with splenorrhaphy using interlocking mattress sutures placed in the capsule 1 cm from the edge. For gross injury, stretch polyglycolic acid–knitted mesh over the spleen, and sew the edges of the mesh together to either encase the entire spleen or cover one pole as a cap (see "Repair of Renal Injuries," Chapter 26). Resort to splenectomy only if all conservative measures fail.

SPLENECTOMY

The vasculature to the spleen, being somewhat like that of the kidney, allows segmental splenectomy. Selective ligation is possible because the splenic artery, before it reaches the spleen, gives off a superior polar artery supplying the upper segment of the spleen. Near the hilus, it divides again into two branches to the middle and lower polar segments. By preliminary ligation of one of these vessels, a segment of the spleen may be removed along a rela-

tively avascular plane. For partial splenectomy, a Frazier neurosurgical suction tip helps in the identification and clipping of intrasplenic vessels. The argon-beam coagulator may be used for parenchymatous dissection, although blunt dissection with pressure hemostasis usually is adequate. The splenic vein pursues a tortuous course above the pancreas, allowing it to be ligated at one of its anterior bends. Accessory spleens may be encountered, usually with independent blood supplies, and should be preserved.

Start by gently retracting the greater omentum and transverse colon inferiorly with the right hand. With the left hand, reach over the top of the spleen, and rotate it anteriorly and medially to incise the attachments to the peritoneum, followed by those to the kidney, diaphragm, and colon.

Slide the left hand more laterally to hook the fingertips under the medial edge of the peritoneum that was just divided. Avoid traction injury to the splenic capsule or vessels. Incise the posterior parietal peritoneum superiorly and inferiorly to the pancreas and release the final attachments of the splenocolic and splenodiaphragmatic ligaments. Place one or two lap tapes into the bed to insure hemostasis and to keep the spleen from dropping back into the wound. Identify the gastrosplenic ligament and the short gastric vessels where the spleen abuts the stomach. Be sure to work high on the greater curvature of the stomach in a caudad to cephalad direction to expose and avoid tearing the most cephalad short gastric vessels. Doubly clamp the splenic vessels sequentially, divide them, and have your assistant tie them beneath the clamps. Be sure not to clamp or ligate any part of the stomach.

Lift the spleen with the left hand. Hold the tail of the pancreas out of the way with the left thumb and index finger during dissection of the vessels under direct vision and during clamping. Dissect the artery from the vein before it divides into its branches. Clamp and ligate the artery first; contraction of the spleen gives the patient a transfusion. Clamp each vessel with three clamps. If the pedicle is small, it may be clamped *in toto* but with some risk of an arteriovenous fistula.

Cut between the distal clamps. Tie beneath the first clamp with a 2-0 or 3-0 synthetic absorbable suture and remove the clamp. Repeat for the second clamp. Remove the packs from the bed. If any bleeders are seen, oversew them with 4-0 synthetic absorbable sutures. Drainage is not necessary.

POSTOPERATIVE PROBLEMS

Because of the risk of overwhelming infection, administer 14-valent pneumococcal polysaccharide vaccine and penicillin.

Commentary by Barry A. Kogan

I would give the following three admonitions, realizing that prevention is the best treatment: (1) use an incision that provides excellent exposure; (2) when doing a difficult left nephrectomy, take down the lienorenal and splenocolic ligaments first; and (3) place padded retractors carefully.

Avoid taking out the spleen of a child unless absolutely necessary. If splenectomy (or mobilization of the spleen to better repair an injury) is necessary, a Babcock clamp can be placed on the stomach and used to gently pull it into the wound, allowing better visualization of the short gastric vessels and the peritoneal attachments of the spleen. Tears of the short gastric vessels are troublesome and difficult to repair; hence, good exposure of these vessels is the key.

CHAPTER 21

Repair of Incisional Hernia

Factors involved in postoperative incisional hernias in children are debility, postoperative deficiency of protein and vitamin C, previous wound infection, postoperative sepsis, vertical incisions, failure to use nonabsorbable sutures or retention sutures when indicated, and excessive postoperative coughing. Realize that bulging of the flank after lateral incisions is more often caused by denervation weakness of the muscles than an actual hernia involving the peritoneum. For this reason, repair may be done because of cosmetic indications or local discomfort, because there is little risk of intestinal incarceration. Provide prophylactic antibiotics before and after the operation.

IMBRICATED REPAIR

1 *Position*: Lateral or oblique, depending on the site of the hernia. Place a nasogastric tube if the hernia involves the peritoneum. **A,** *Incision*: Make an elliptic incision and excise the scar. **B,** Extend the incision through the subcutaneous layer circumferentially, exposing normal fascia away from the defect first. Have your assistant elevate the wound edges with large rake retractors. Mobilize the flaps from the fascia, and define the area of the defect. Do not open the hernia sac prematurely. Meticulous hemostasis is important.

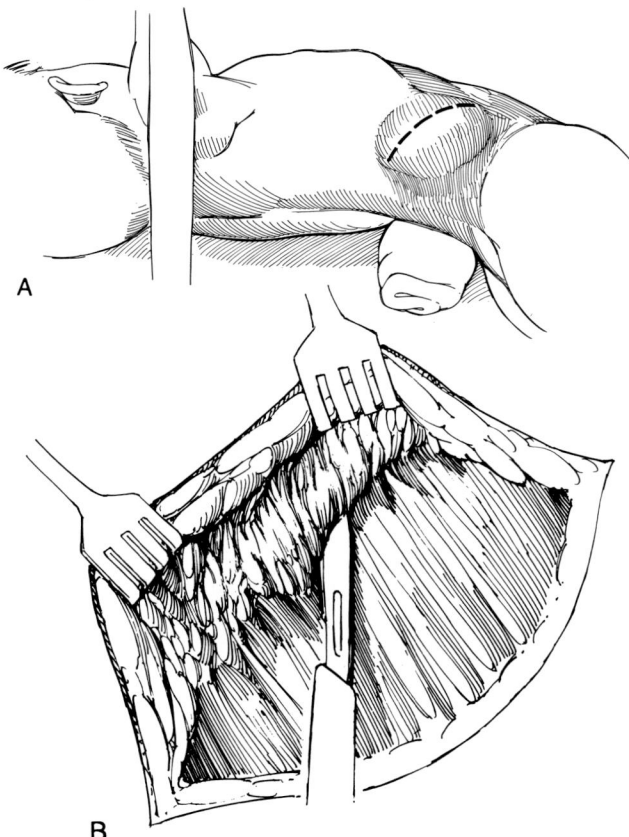

2 Deliberately open the sac, which is made up of attenuated fascia and peritoneum. If adherent, free the peritoneum from the intestinal contents. Trim the edges of the defect until sound fascia is reached.

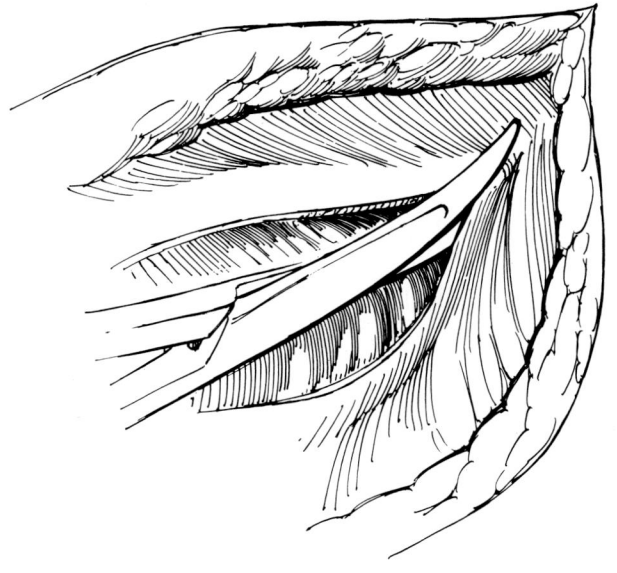

3 Imbricate the fascia in a side-over-side (vest-over-pants) technique with heavy synthetic absorbable sutures placed as interrupted mattress stitches. Do this by entering the upper fascia 2 or 3 cm from its edge and then passing through the lower fascia 1 cm from its edge. Exit from the lower flap 1 cm lateral to the stitch, then exit from the upper flap 1 cm lateral to the original site of entry. Clamp the ends of the suture. Repeat these stitches 1 cm apart for the length of the defect. Tie them sequentially, as your assistant keeps tension on the rest.

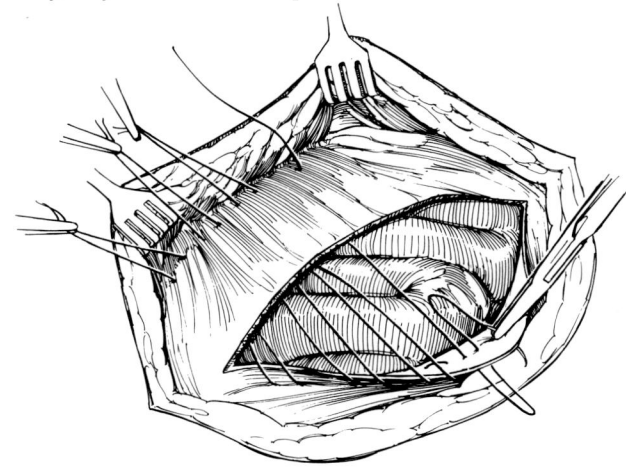

4 Run a heavy synthetic absorbable suture under the flap just below the first row of sutures. Take care not to go through the fascia and involve the underlying bowel in the stitch.

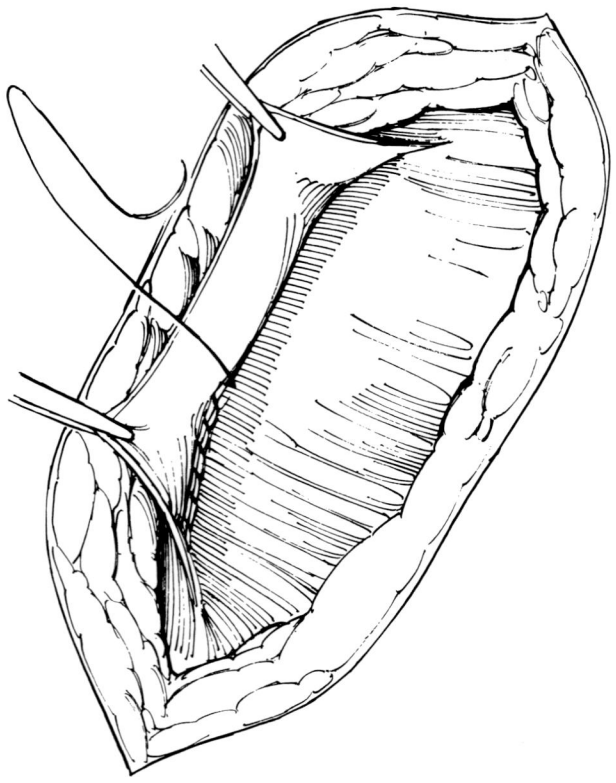

5 Place a row of interrupted figure-eight sutures of heavy synthetic absorbable material between the upper flap and the adjacent lower (posterior) flap. Insert two suction drains in the subcutaneous space, but do not place sutures there. Close the skin with subcuticular sutures. An abdominal binder may be used over the dressing. Nasogastric suction may not be necessary if all oral fluids are withheld until good propulsive peristalsis is heard.

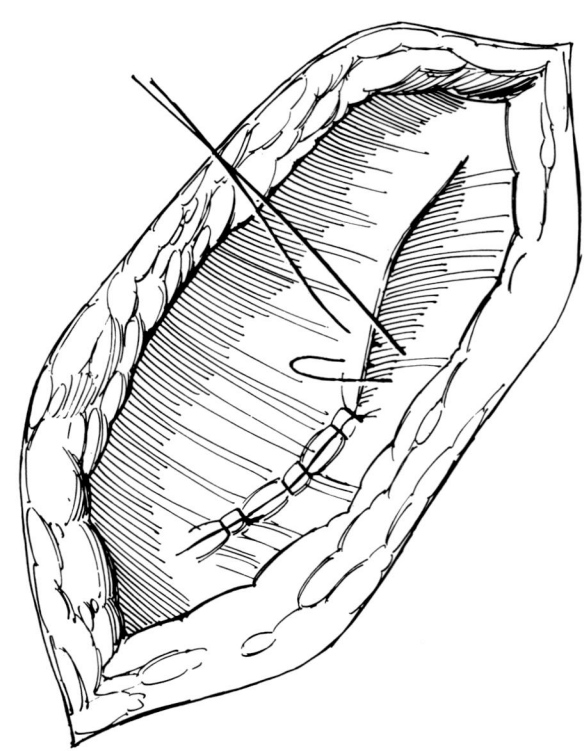

AUGMENTED REPAIR OF LARGE DEFECTS USING SYNTHETIC MATERIALS

Proceed as previously described, clearing the fascial surfaces of fat. Be certain of asepsis and hemostasis. Close the peritoneum separately with 3-0 or 4-0 synthetic absorbable sutures, if possible. Cut a large enough piece of polypropylene mesh to shape and to overlap the edges by 2 cm. Suture the mesh to the aponeurosis with interrupted 2-0 or 3-0 nonabsorbable sutures. If there is any question about asepsis or hemostasis, do not use polypropylene mesh. If the wound becomes infected, the mesh would have to be removed. However, tantalum mesh can be used safely if asepsis is in doubt. A stronger repair is obtained by placing the mesh under the fascial layer rather than on top. It should extend beyond the fascial edges by 3 to 4 cm. Close the subcutaneous tissues and skin over suction drains.

Alternatively, if you have been able to close the defect edge to edge with interrupted sutures, strengthen it by running a firmly placed monofilament nylon suture back and forth both vertically and horizontally to "darn" the defect. However, this last technique encourages closure with tension, which is associated with recurrence. If this technique is used at all, relaxing fascial incisions placed well lateral to the defect should be used.

POSTOPERATIVE PROBLEMS

Infection is the greatest concern and must be treated aggressively. *Recurrence* of the herniation is not as common as persistent bulging of the area.

PART II

KIDNEY RECONSTRUCTION

The indications for repair of the ureteropelvic junction (UPJ) for hydronephrosis and the ability to estimate the potential for recovery are currently controversial. Now that fetal ultrasonography is routine, more cases are detected that require a decision for management soon after birth.

Imaging techniques applied to renal trauma similarly offer the opportunity for early treatment but require judgment so that unnecessary procedures

can be avoided. Vascular surgeons developed procedures that experienced urologists with some special training are able to apply to the vessels supplying the kidney. The harvesting of kidneys for renal transplantation and the implantation itself are simple extensions of those techniques. The place of endopyelotomy in children has not yet been determined but, because of its simplicity, is being increasingly substituted for open repair.

CHAPTER 22

Pyeloureteroplasty

Clear the urinary tract of infection if possible. Ascertain the presence and degree of obstruction by radioisotope and pressure-flow studies. It seldom is necessary to obtain a ureterogram to visualize the ureter when a preoperative hydrated ultrasound study does not show a megaureter behind the bladder or dilation of the upper ureter below the UPJ.

In a neonate, perform ultrasonography to evaluate the extent of the renal pelvic dilation, but delay further evaluation for 4 weeks. Then obtain a voiding cystourethrogram and a renal scan. If obstruction is present, repairing the lesion within the following month is reasonable. Retrograde and antegrade studies seldom are needed. Pyeloplasty, rather than nephrectomy, almost always should be done in infants, regardless of the amount of renal damage, especially if the contralateral kidney does not show compensatory hypertrophy, because every nephron may be needed in later life, when single-nephron hyperperfusion supervenes. In bilateral cases, both sides may be corrected at the same session through anterior subcostal or posterior lumbotomy incisions. Use magnification, together with fine instruments and sutures.

DISMEMBERED PYELOPLASTY
(ANDERSON-HYNES)

Approach the pelvis through a dorsal lumbotomy incision in infants; in older children, use an anterior subcostal incision (as shown in Figure 1A), taking care to stay out of the peritoneal cavity.

1 **A,** *Position*: Supine with a rolled towel or sandbag under the flank. In older children, slightly flex the table to place some tension on the flank muscles. *Incision*: Incise the skin and subcutaneous layer from the tip of the 12th rib to within a fingerbreadth or two of the linea sem-ilunaris at a point two fingerbreadths above the umbilicus. Mobilize the colon. For bilateral cases, separate subcostal incisions are better than a single transperitoneal one (or use a lumbotomy approach). If this is a secondary opera-tion, make the new incision one rib higher, and work from normal tissue to that previously involved. **B,** Open Gero-ta's fascia laterally to preserve the dorsal layer with its contained perinephric fat to cover the repair later. Dissect sharply and bluntly while rotating the kidney clockwise on the right and counterclockwise on the left to expose the posterior aspect of the pelvis. Free as little as possible of the kidney itself, and leave some fat attached for traction and manipulation. Have your assistant hold the lower pole up and anteriorly with a sponge stick to expose the junc-tion posteriorly.

2 **A,** Carefully expose the ureter below the UPJ first, taking care not to interfere with the segmental blood supply to this area. Place a small Penrose drain or vessel loop around the ureter. For secondary operations, locate the normal part of the ureter distally and dissect up from normal to abnormal. Dissect as short a length of the ureter as possible and preserve its adventitial vessels. **B,** Palpate and look for aberrant lower-pole vessels, which are com-mon with this anomaly; they usually can be moved out of the way, because their division could result in segmental renal ischemia and systemic hypertension.

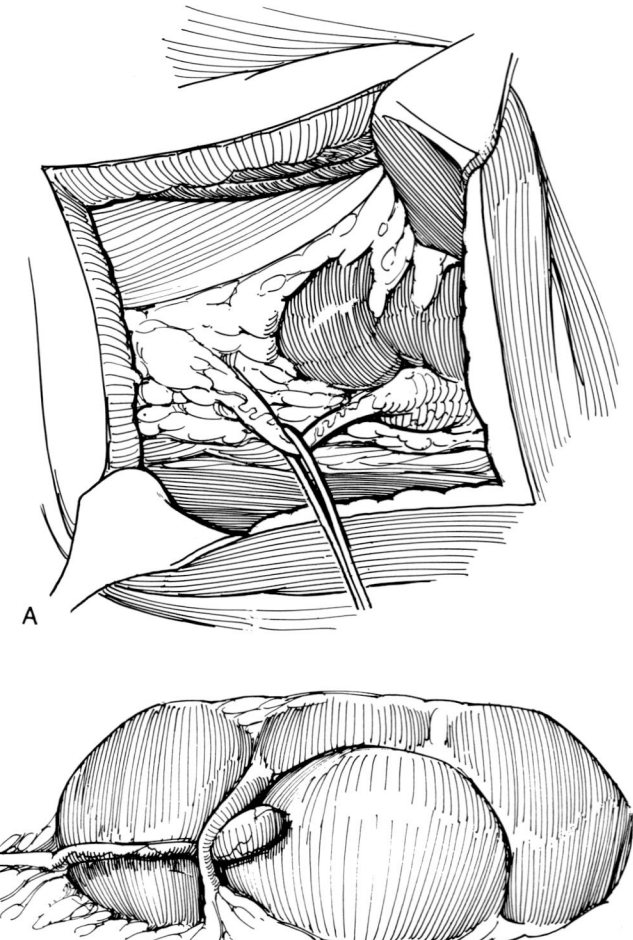

A

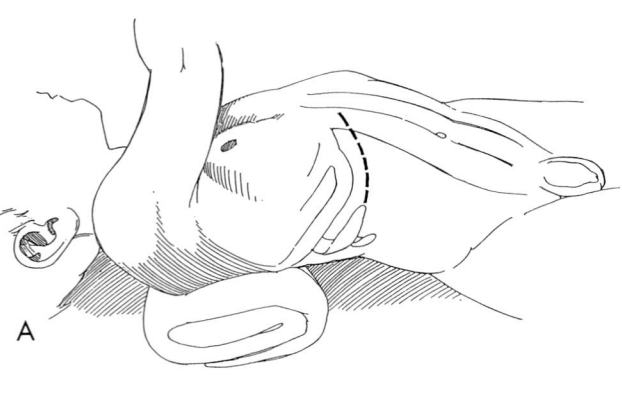

A

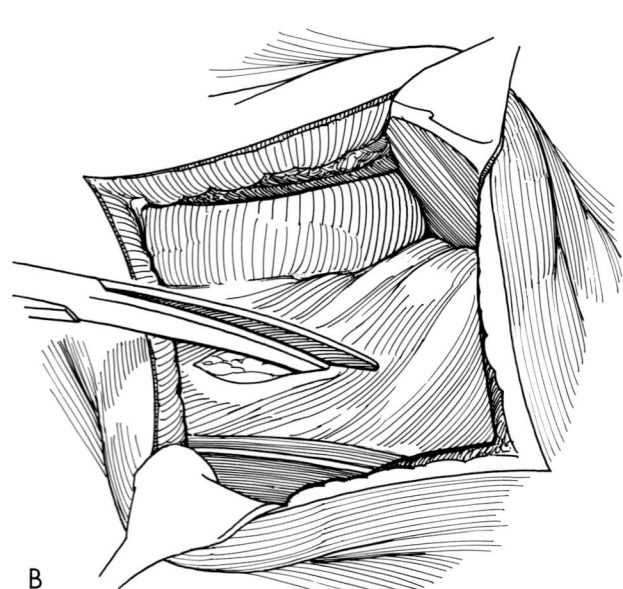

B

B

3 After exposure of the UPJ, make a decision about what type of operation to use. Obstructions usually are high-insertion anomalies at the UPJ, usually without stricture. They may lie just below the UPJ because of stricture or, rarely, may involve the upper ureter as a stricture or ureteral valve. It is necessary to ask whether the ureter is long enough to allow dismemberment and excision of the UPJ. A modified Anderson-Hynes pyeloplasty usually is suitable, although a Foley Y-plasty works well with high insertions of the ureter, and for a long dependent junction, the Culp or Scardino techniques may solve the problem of providing sufficient ureter for approximation.

Place a stay suture in the ureter at its junction with the pelvis; divide the ureter obliquely and spatulate it on its less-vascularized lateral surface for a distance equal to the length of the proposed V-shaped flap. This step often may be done more accurately after the pelvic flap is formed. Whether it is necessary to pass a 5-F infant feeding tube distally to check for narrowing of the upper ureter is not agreed on; it could instigate strictures.

(A modification of the Anderson-Hynes pyeloplasty divides the ureter transversely and spatulates it, excises the pelvis, and forms a V flap at the caudal rim. The V flap is inserted into the spatulated ureter to provide a tapered junction).

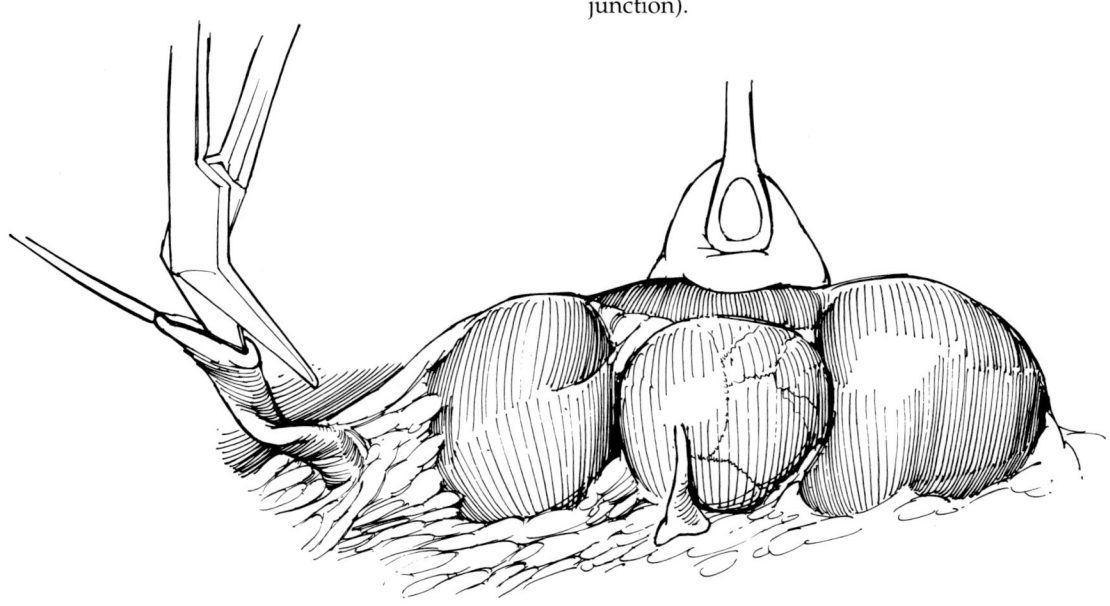

4 With the pelvis full, map out the proposed diamond-shaped incision with a skin-marking pen, angling the caudal triangle medially to form a V flap. An angled Satinsky clamp can be useful to identify and immobilize the site to be cut. The kidney can be brought up into the wound with vein or Gil-Vernet retractors or rotated with a sponge stick. Place stay sutures of 7-0 catgut at the angles of the diamond. Because considerable pyelectasis is the rule, include a portion of the pelvis; reduction pyeloplasty is part of the repair. *Caution*: Do not remove too much pelvis, especially in a bifid system, and keep well away from the calyceal necks, which can be surprisingly close to the edge; otherwise, closure will be difficult, and infundibular stenosis could result. Incise for a short distance along one of the planned lines with a #11 hooked blade.

5 Use Lahey or Potts scissors to complete the resection, cutting from inside one stay suture to inside the next. Remove the specimen.

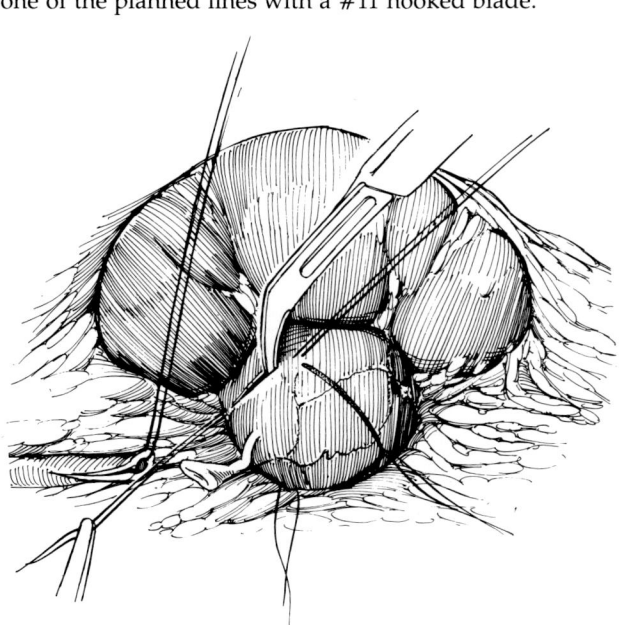

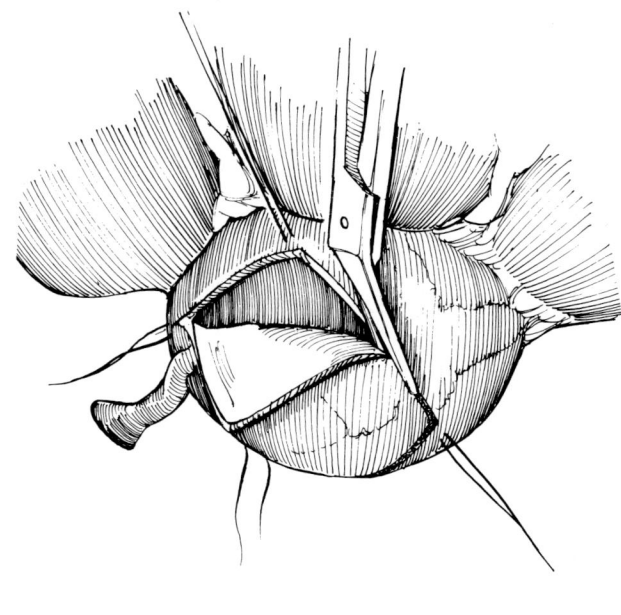

6 **A,** Insert an infant feeding tube of suitable size into the ureter to prevent catching the far wall in a suture. Using loupes, place one 5-0 or 6-0 (or 7-0 in neonates) synthetic absorbable suture adjacent to the apex of the V-shaped flap from outside in, then out through the apex of the ureteral slit. Place a second suture 2 mm away from the first. Tie both sutures with four square knots and cut the short ends. Use the ureteral stay suture for manipulation; do not use forceps. Alternatively, use a double-armed suture and run one end up the back wall from inside the lumen and the other up the front wall. **B,** Catch the mucosa minimally to include more muscularis and adventitia in the stitch.

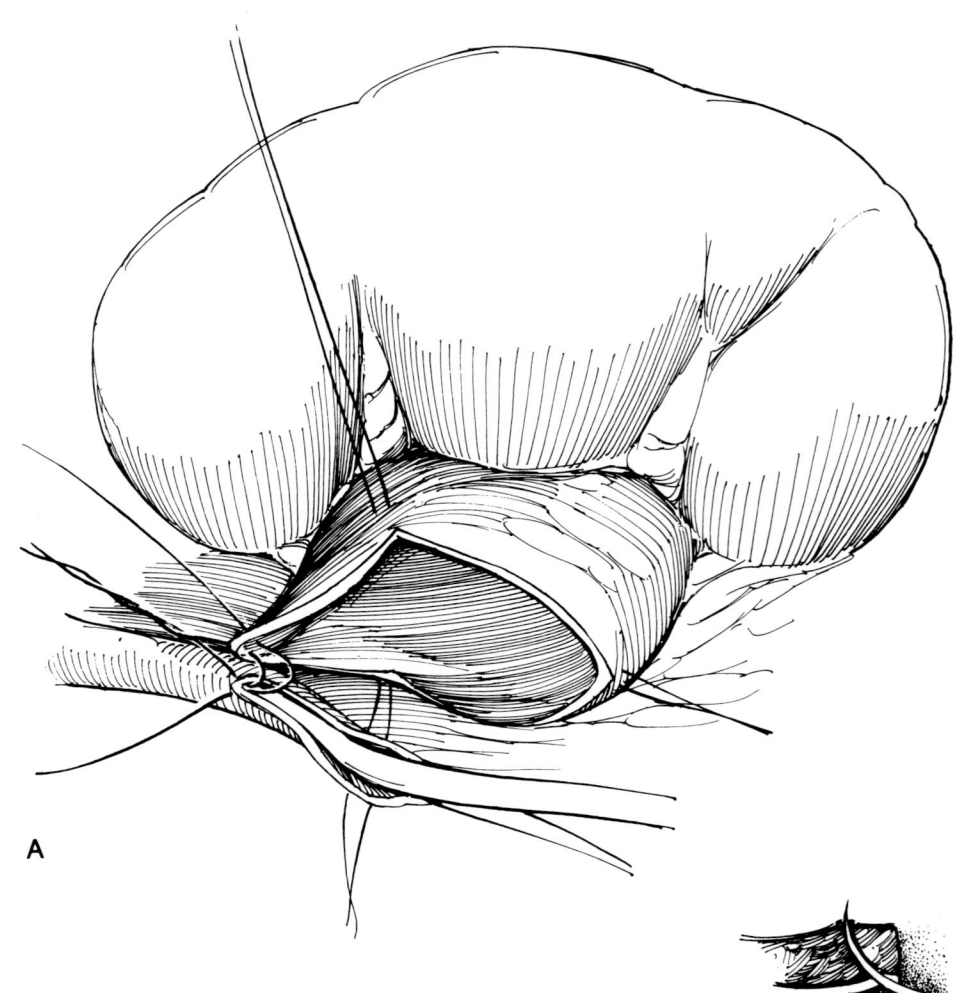

A

B

7 **A,** Continue the first suture to the tip of the ureter on the far side as a continuous stitch, locked at every four or five bites. Do the same for the second suture on the near side. Remove the feeding tube, and irrigate the pelvis and calyces free of clots. This is especially important with an anterior approach, because the clots tend to lie in the calyces. **B,** Tie the two sutures together, cut one, and continue with the other to close the pelvic defect.

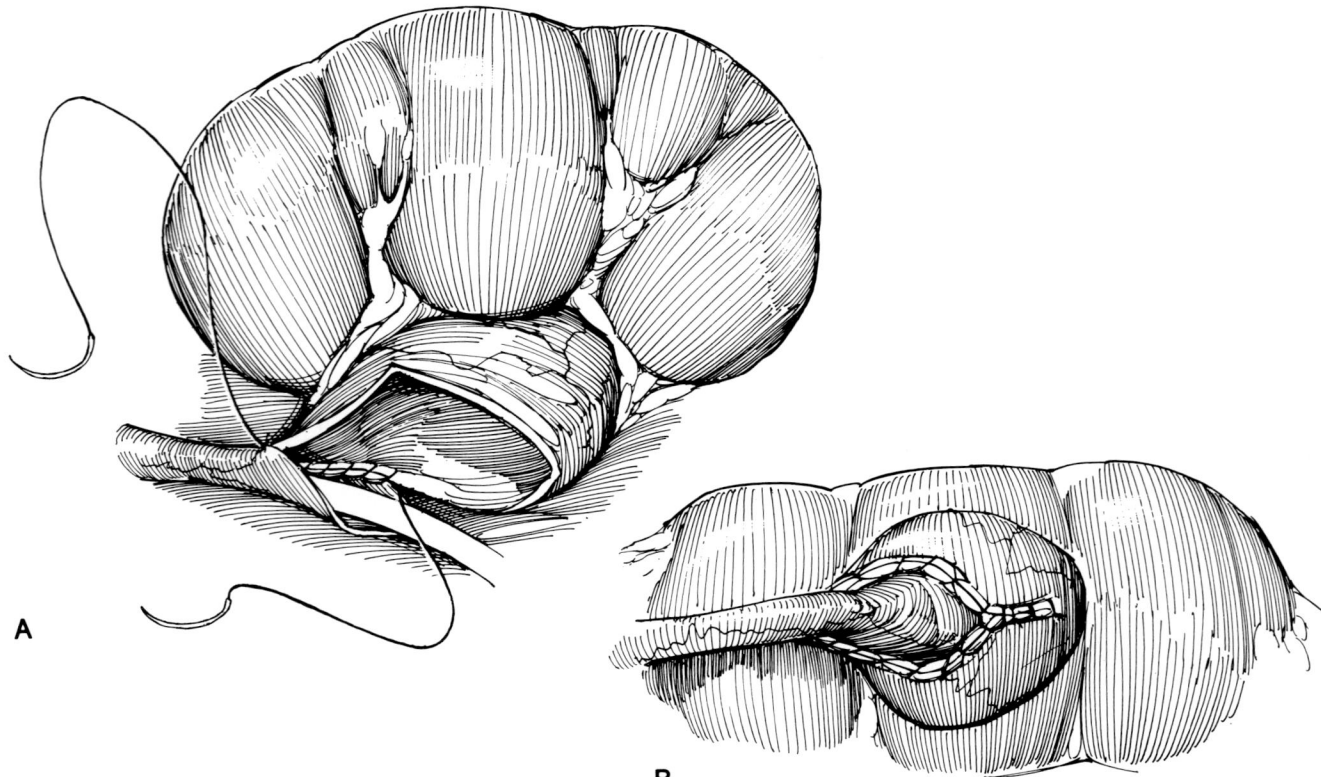

A

B

8 Alternatively, form a pursestring around the central defect by starting a third suture from the upper end.

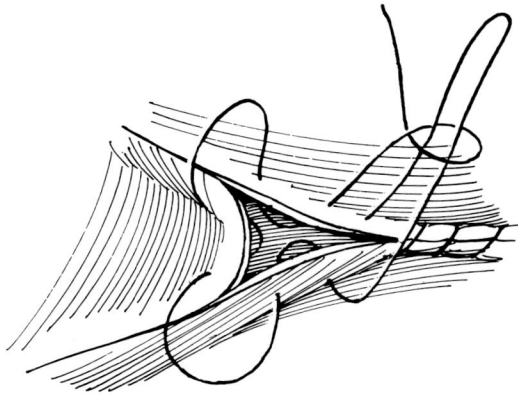

9 Inject saline with a fine needle through the pelvic wall to test for watertightness and for patency of the anastomosis. Add a suture or two, if needed, to close a leak. Use an omental wrap (page 272) if the tissues appear poorly vascularized or if the operation is the second one.

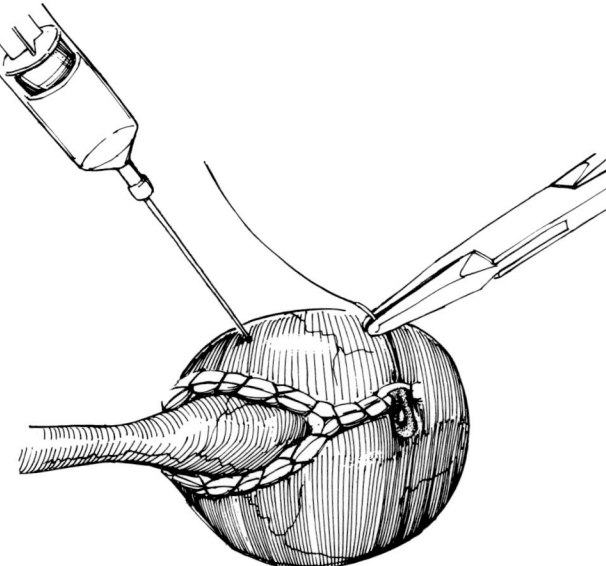

10 Insert a Penrose drain and fasten it near, but not touching, the anastomosis or the ureter below it by the long-suture technique. Alternatively, use a suction drain; accurate drainage is important. If the kidney has been mobilized, hold it up with a nephropexy stitch, which is needed more often with a flank approach. Tack the two edges of Gerota's fascia together around the kidney with fine plain catgut. Close the wound in layers, leading the drain laterally so that the child will not lie on it. If leakage occurs, an adhesive stomal bag may be applied, but it rarely should be necessary.

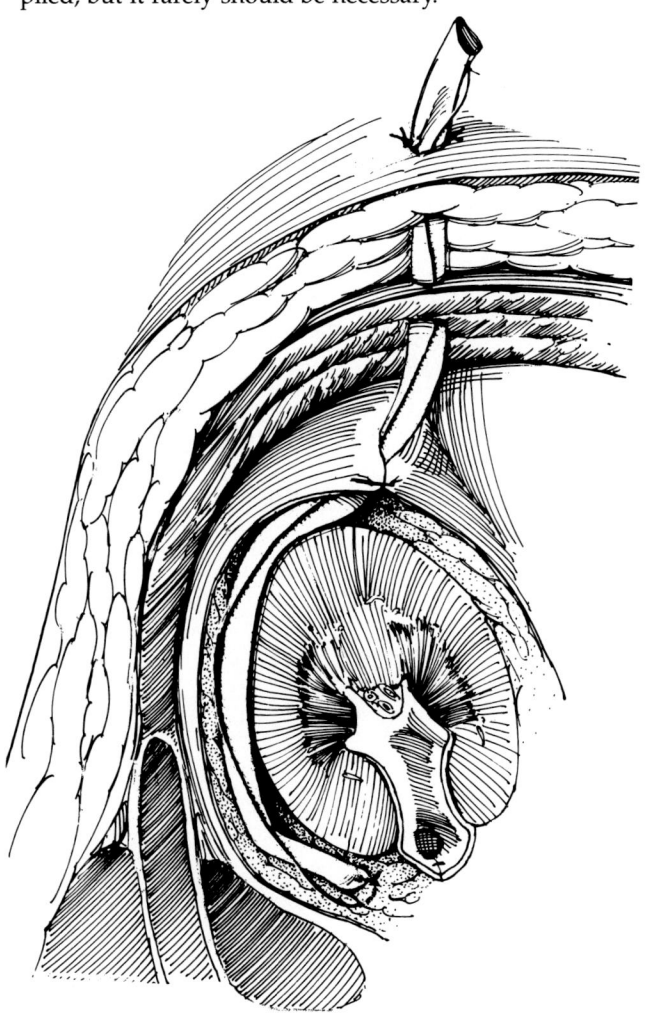

11 **A,** If the repair appears tenuous or the kidney is infected, insert a nephrostomy tube with (page 140) or without a double-J stent, a kidney internal splint/stent (KISS) catheter that stents and exits through the pelvic wall, or soft silicone tubing before closing the pelvis. The pros and cons of stenting are described on page 6. **B,** A Cummings tube, combining nephrostomy and stent, is an alternative; if such a stent is too long, it may enter the bladder and siphon off the bladder contents, which can be disturbing to the patient and the surgeon. In general, avoid placing a stent, although it may prevent kinking by a large floppy pelvis. A compromise may be to place a nephrostomy tube in an infant or to use both a tube and a double-J stent in any difficult repair.

Insert a balloon catheter to prevent backpressure on the repair, and remove it in 24 to 48 hours. Consider giving suppressive antibiotic therapy. Avoid irrigating a nephrostomy tube. Discharge an infant in 48 hours with the drain in place. Shorten the drain 2 days after drainage stops, and then remove it. If a stent has been placed, take it out in 10 to 12 days when a nephrostogram shows the anastomosis to be watertight, unless repair was difficult. Remove the nephrostomy tube if it drains readily when filled while held vertically or after a trial of intermittent clamping and checking for residual urine.

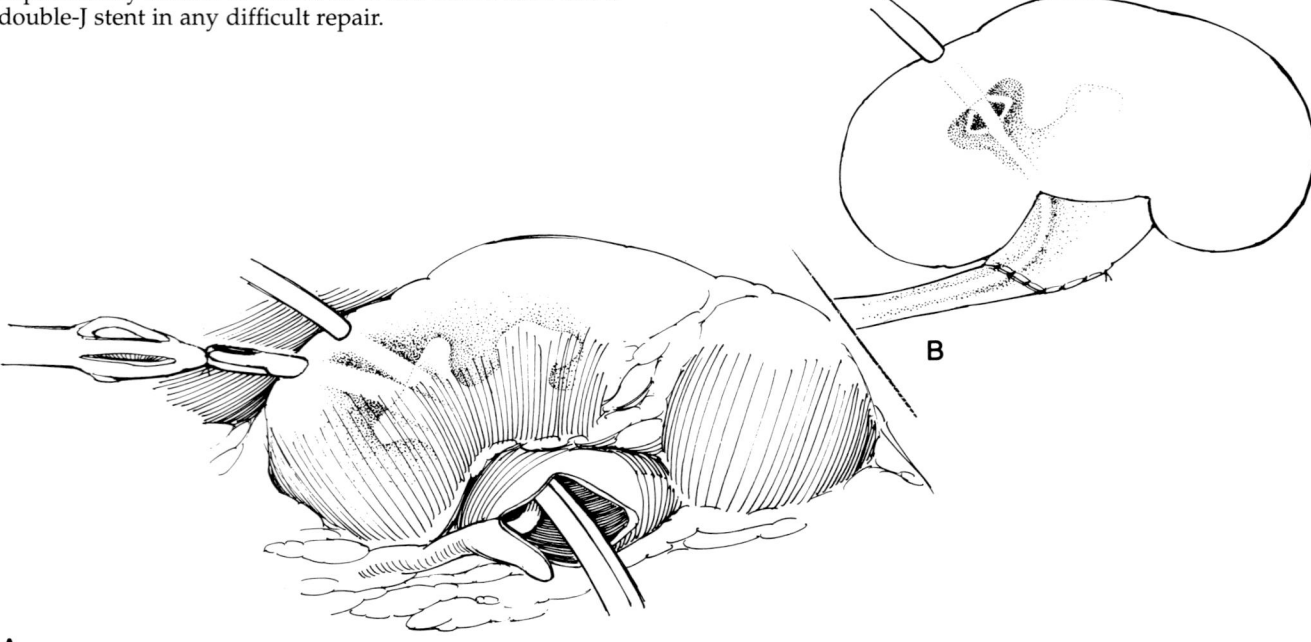

A

YV-PLASTY
(FOLEY)

The Foley Y-plasty is effective for a high insertion of the ureter. It preserves the small extrarenal pelvis in cases with intrarenal dilation.

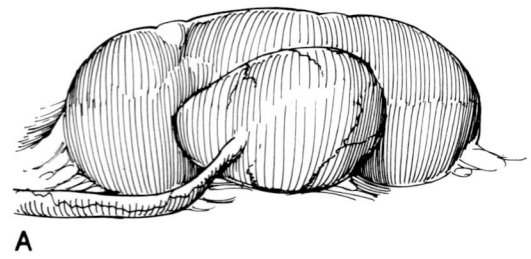

A

12 **A,** Free the ureter but preserve the adventitia. **B,** Draw the ureter cephalad with a Penrose drain. Mark a long Y-shaped incision between three stay sutures. Incise the pelvis between the stays with a #11 hooked blade, and open it with Potts scissors, forming a V with arms equal to the length of the ureteral incision. At this point, consider placing a nephrostomy tube, with or without a stent.

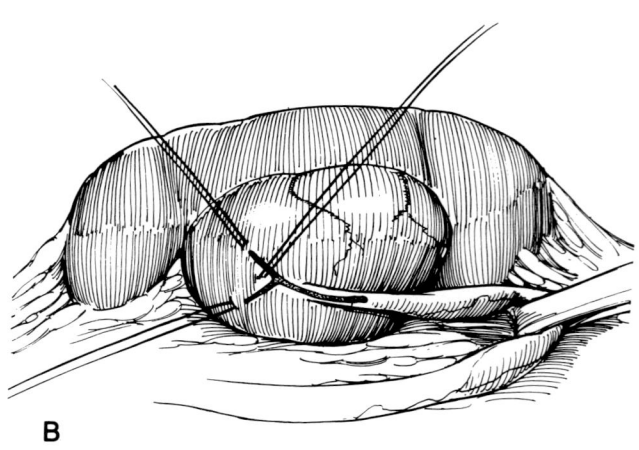

B

13 Suture the apex of the flap to the apex of the ureteral incision by placing a 7-0 synthetic absorbable suture in through the apex of the V and out through the apex of the ureteral incision, and tie it. Include a minimal amount of mucosa.

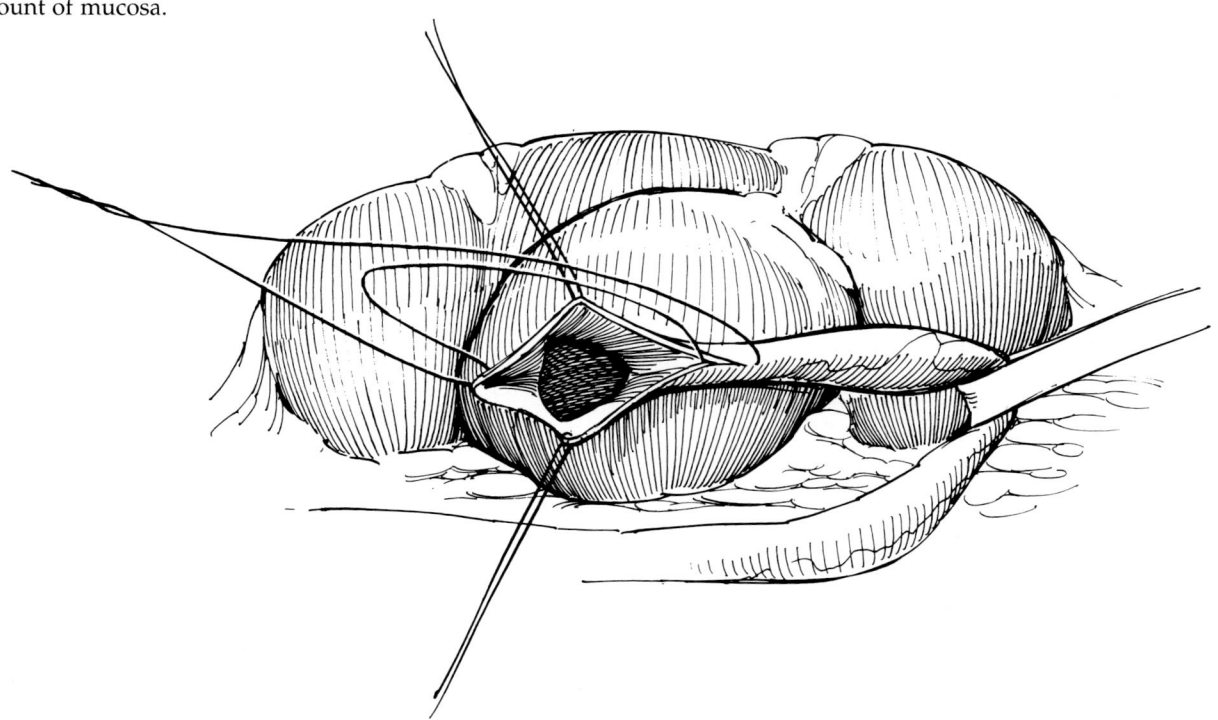

14 **A** and **B,** Place interrupted 4-0 synthetic absorbable sutures down both sides of the V to make a watertight anastomosis. Alternatively, two sutures may be run continuously, as in the dismembered technique. Pad the area with perirenal fat, and provide drainage accurately.

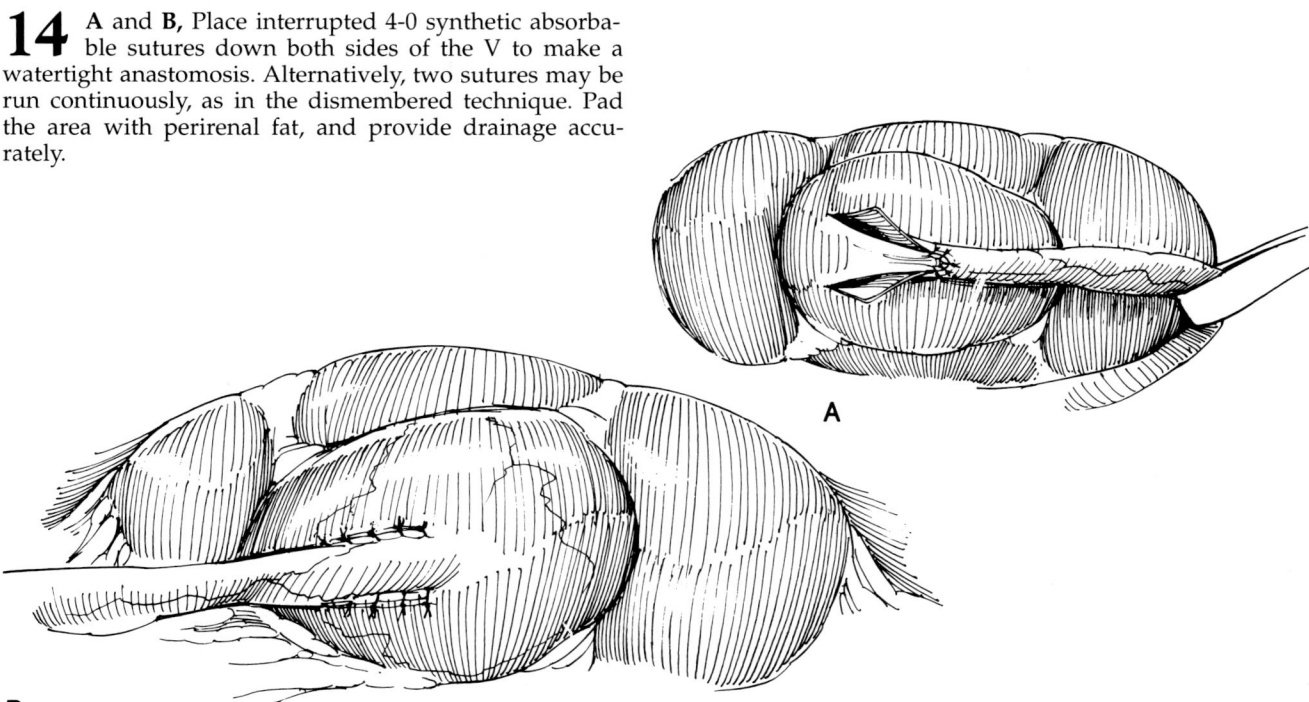

A

B

PELVIC FLAP PYELOPLASTY
(CULP OR SCARDINO)

Use the Culp procedure for low defects; select the Scardino variation for cases with higher insertion of the ureter. If much ureter has been lost, do a calycoureterostomy (page 253).

15 **A,** Mark a spiral (Culp) flap, running obliquely around the enlarged pelvis and extending the incision down the ureter for a distance equal to the length of the flap. The Scardino incision (not shown) runs vertically from the UPJ. **B,** Incise the flap, and hold it down with a stay suture. **C,** Approximate the posterior edge of the flap with the lateral ureteral edge with a running 5-0 or 6-0 synthetic absorbable suture. **D,** Close the anterior edge of the flap and pelvis with similar sutures. It helps to suture over a small infant feeding tube.

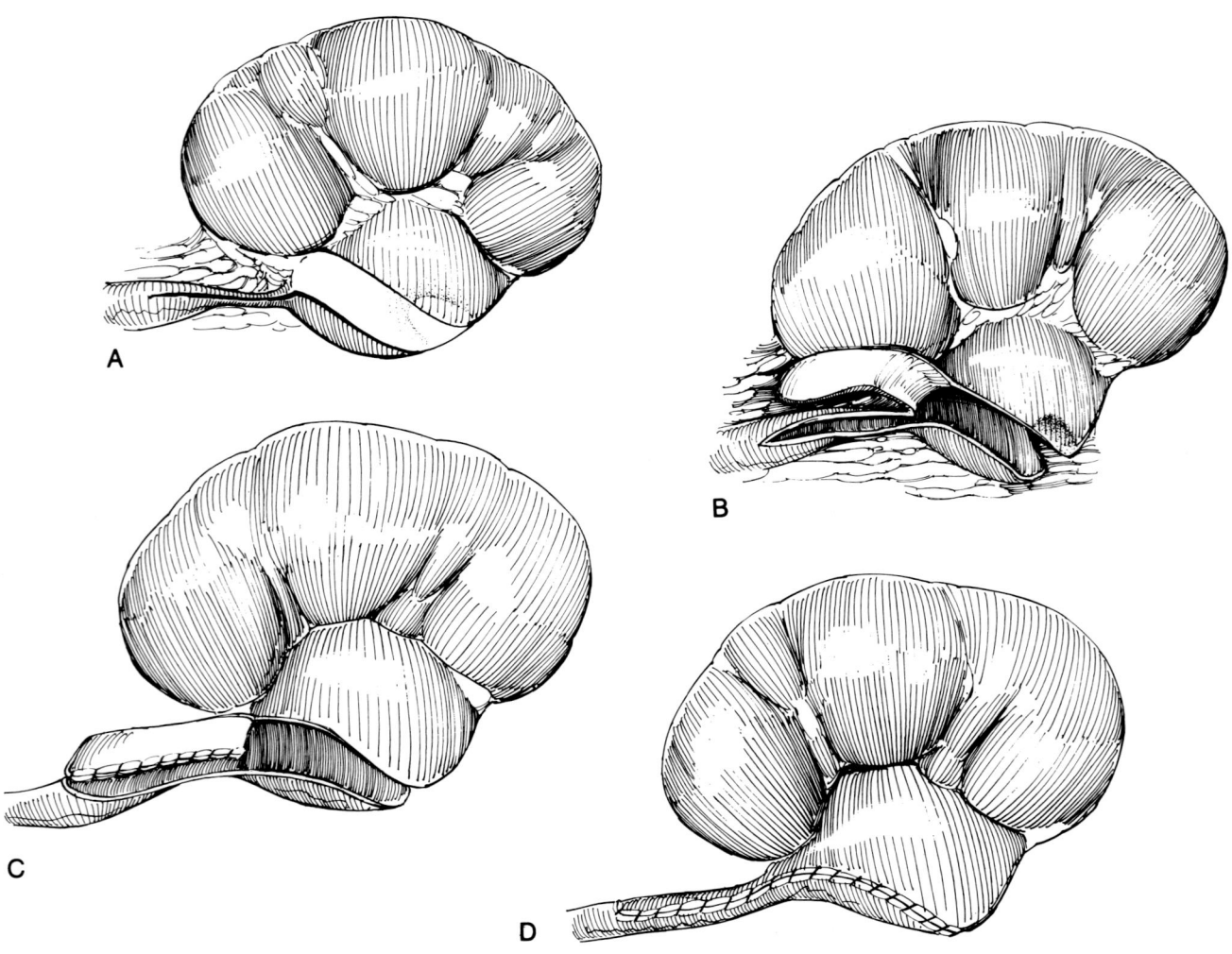

INTUBATED URETEROTOMY
(DAVIS)

Intubated ureterotomy is sometimes used for long, scarred defects near the UPJ that are not amenable to endoscopic incision.

16 With a #11 knife blade, incise the pelvis just above the UPJ between two stay sutures. Open the ureter, using the Potts scissors, until normal caliber is reached.

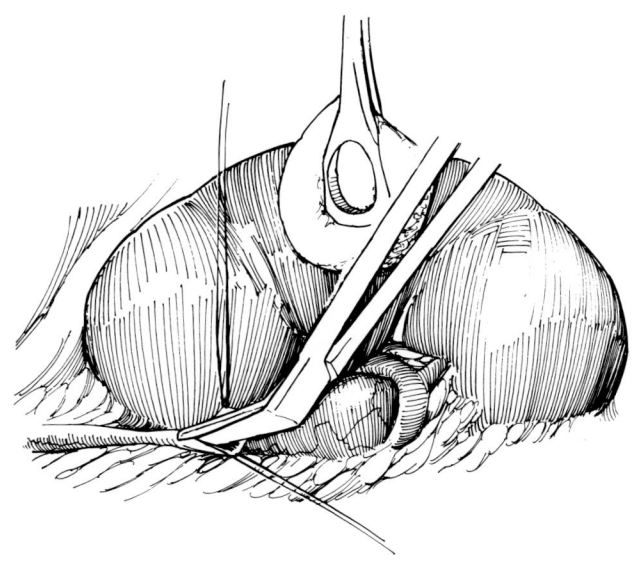

17 Insert an 8 F silicone stent and a nephrostomy tube. Tack the edges of the defect together loosely with 5-0 synthetic absorbable sutures.

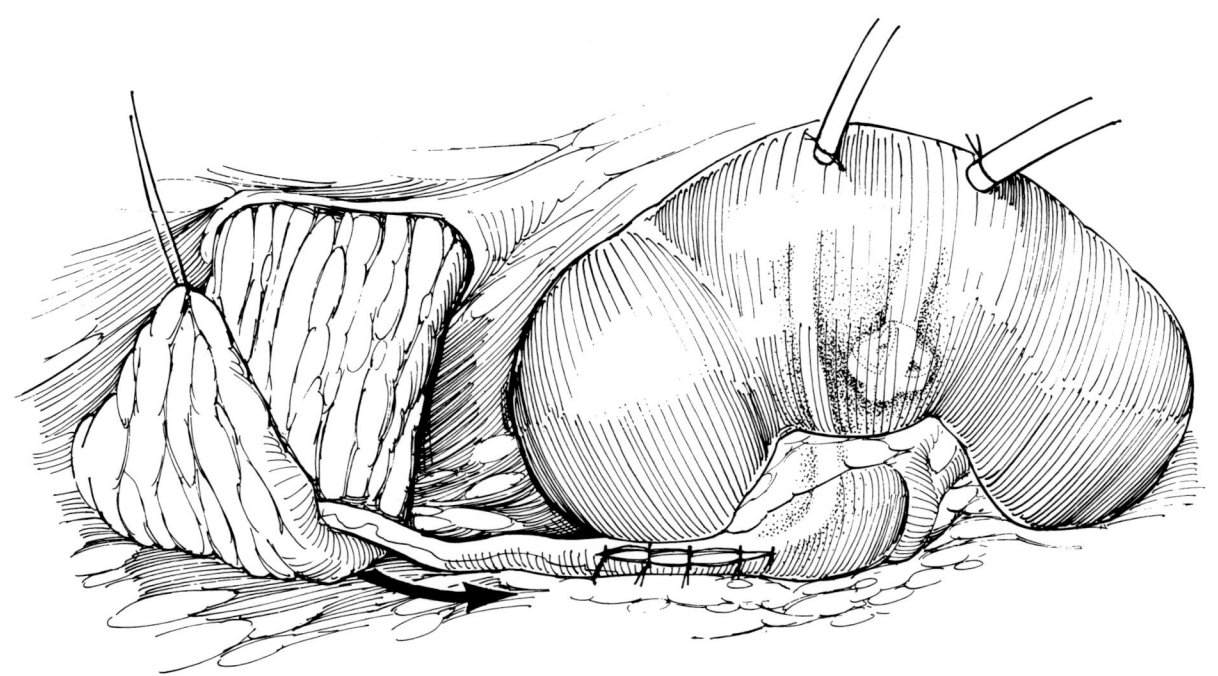

18 For a lower defect, incise it laterally over a small-caliber double-J stent. Place a few fine sutures to hold the ureter loosely against the stent, being careful not to constrict it.

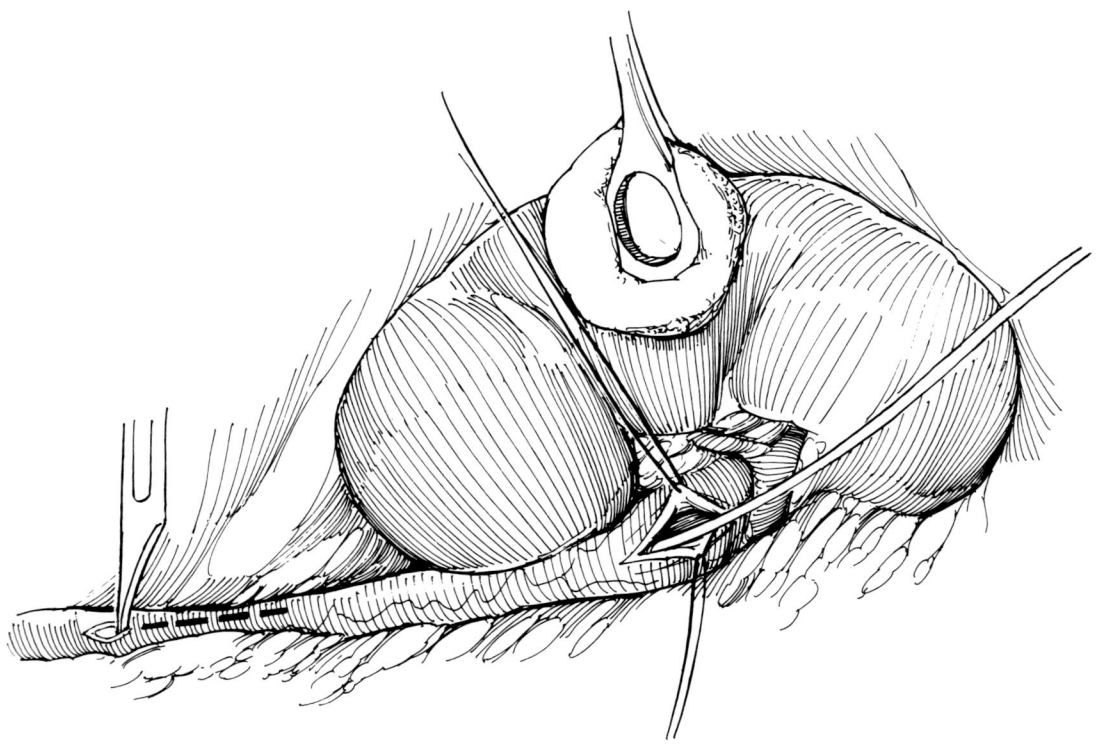

19 Close the pelvic defect after placing a nephrostomy tube. Tack retroperitoneal fat around the defect, or bring the omentum through the posterior peritoneum and wrap it about the ureter, a better alternative. Drain the area very accurately. Leave the stent in place at least 6 weeks, testing for sealing with nephrostograms before and after removing it.

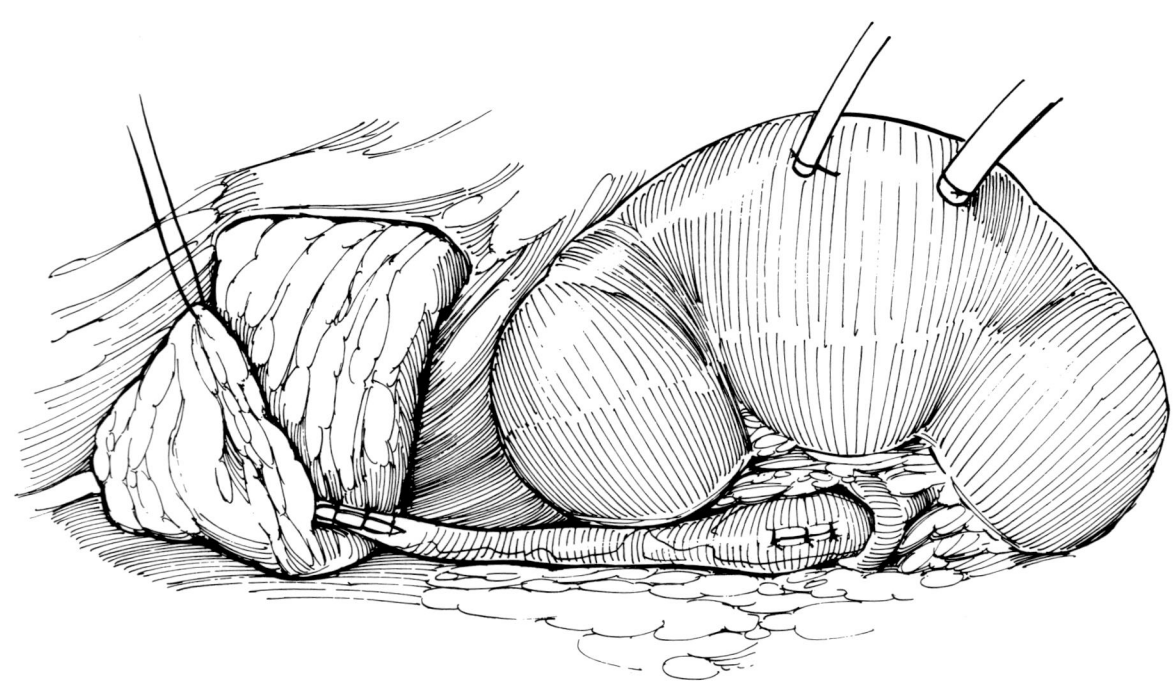

FOLLOW-UP

At 3 months, obtain a voiding cystogram and a renal scan. Repeat the scan in 6 months. Improvement in drainage is not to be expected after 6 months. Children will exhibit good growth of the parenchyma after repair ("catch-up" growth), but parallel improvement in the pyelogram should not be expected.

POSTOPERATIVE PROBLEMS

Bleeding can jeopardize the repair by the formation of clots that obstruct. Its source is usually the nephrostomy tract. If this cannot be tamponaded, immediate reexploration may be required. In general, avoid irrigation of the nephrostomy tube, because it introduces infection and can disrupt the suture line.

Acute pyelonephritis indicates infection behind obstruction. If a nephrostomy tube was not inserted at operation, place one percutaneously. *Urinary leakage* may occur within the first 24 hours because of an overfull bladder (an argument for leaving a balloon catheter in the bladder for the 1st day). Drainage lasting over a week should be investigated, because subsequent peripelvic and periureteral fibrosis will harm the anastomosis. First, be sure the drain is not in contact with the anastomosis or with the ureter below it. Shorten it and subsequently remove it. An intravenous urogram may identify the leak and detect obstruction. Leakage may be handled by percutaneous nephrostomy or by passage of a stent from either below or above. If a stent has not been used, insert a double-J stent from below, except in the small child, as soon as obstruction is suspected. A urinoma may form when a flank drain is removed too soon; passing a curved clamp down the drainage tract usually can relieve this problem. If the drain has fallen out, replace it with a cut-off small Robinson catheter, with extra holes passed through the fascia and transfixed to the skin. Before removing a stent, fill the system with contrast medium to test for leakage. Remove the drain only after being sure the ureter is intact.

Obstruction at the UPJ after the stent is removed can be managed by leaving the nephrostomy tube in place, placing a tube percutaneously until a nephrostogram shows an open tract, or passing a double-J stent from below. To detect silent obstruction, check the renal status by sonography at 4 to 6 weeks, by a diethylenetriamine penta-acetic acid scan at 3 months, and by an intravenous pyelogram at 6 months. For obstruction that persists, attempt intubation from below. If these measures fail, allow the area to heal, and proceed with formal percutaneous balloon dilation or retrograde or percutaneous incision of the stricture. Place an 8 to 10 F nephrostomy tube percutaneously for access and diversion. Obtain an antegrade ureterogram to visualize the defect under fluoroscopy. Negotiate the stricture with a guide wire, and dilate it with a balloon catheter, 5 to 8 F. Place a ureteral stent made from an infant feeding tube with extra side holes to allow drainage from the pelvis and bladder. For strictures, but not for fistulas, cap the stent when the antegrade drainage is satisfactory after resolution of the initial hematuria. Remove the stent in 4 to 6 weeks by exchanging it for a nephrostomy tube over a guide wire, then obtain an antegrade pyelogram to be sure the ureter is intact. Clamp the tube if it is intact; remove the tube in 2 or 3 days if the child does well. If the ureter appears narrow, perform a perfusion pressure test. A few cases will need formal reoperation; however, the explanation may lie not in ureteral disease but in the initial involvement of the pelvis in extensive fibrosis. Pathologic examination of the resected portion of the pelvis, instead of showing muscular hypertrophy, may show fibrosis that explains the poor function after a technically adequate repair. Other alternatives are transplanting the kidney to the true pelvis (page 244) and constructing an ileal ureter (page 255).

Other postoperative problems include granuloma formation around catgut sutures, wound infection, incisional hernia (page 121), and those problems associated with broken stents (page 40).

Commentary by Max Maizels

After the decision to perform pyeloplasty, I perform the following procedures, based on my experience and opinions.

Preoperatively, it is worthwhile to ensure that satisfactory imaging of the ureter has excluded a coexistent problem. Usually, it is enough to do an ultrasound study in a state of overhydration (either after oral administration of fluids in children who can comply, or immediately after a renal scan during which IV fluids and/or furosemide has been administered). The ultrasound study would detect ureteral dilation, either behind the bladder, as a megaureter, or below the UPJ, consistent with upper ureteral obstruction. Naturally, a satisfactory voiding cystourethrogram should have been performed to be sure that coexisting reflux is not a confounding issue. It is also worthwhile to consider the status of the contralateral kidney. Usually, the kidney is normal. Should it show compensatory hypertrophy, as detected on ultrasound by measurement of length and depth, it is unlikely that the hydronephrotic kidney is worth salvaging, and nephrectomy is the better option. This is unusual nowadays, because children present in infancy before pathologic processes have had years to progress. Should the clinical circumstances indicate that the obstruction is bilateral, consider repairing both sides simultaneously by posterior lumbotomy incisions. *At the time of surgery*, when the child is anesthetized, examine the abdomen by deep palpation to examine the kidneys. This provides information as to the mobility and location of the kidney and whether a tense renal pelvis will be encountered. When the site of obstruction is likely to be below the level of the ribs, the prone position is the satisfactory one. A Foley catheter is not necessary if external renal drainage is to be provided (see following paragraphs). The bladder can be emptied by the Credé maneuver after induction of anesthesia before surgery is started. It can be helpful in small infants, particularly chubby ones, to mark the site of the anticipated incision prior to surgery. This can be done conveniently with a needle scratch marking the upper and lower limits of the incision. One caveat involving optimizing the prone position for pyeloplasty is to be sure that the abdominal contents are capable of falling away and are not compressed by towels, rolls, or a heating pad underneath. An angled Satinsky clamp can be applied to the renal pelvis to identify and immobilize the site to be excised during the dismembering process. Once the kidney has been exposed, obstructions are usually found at one of three sites: at the UPJ (high-insertion anomaly with or without UPJ stricture and/or ureteral kink), just below the UPJ (as a stricture), or in the upper ureter (stricture or valve of the ureter). It is important to be confident that an actual pathologic segment can be identified. This can be pursued by instilling saline into the renal pelvis by a needle puncture and observing the response. Most commonly, a flaccid pelvis will become tense, and the lesion will be seen as a white, fibrotic nondistensible segment, perhaps only 3 or 4 cm long at or below the UPJ. The whiteness is related to inherent fibrosis.

Stenting has emotional advocates and opponents. This emotionalism probably stems from exceptionally good anecdotal experiences with stenting or exceptionally bad ones. It may very well revolve around the fact that stenting for pediatric patients has involved the use of catheters, which provided drainage via side holes. Naturally, the small-lumen catheters used in pediatric surgery may become blocked with inflammatory exudate or blood easily and obstruct the repair. Today, an alternative catheter, the KISS catheter, is available. The drainage lumen of this catheter is designed as a trough, rather than side holes, so its potential for obstruction is much less. The catheter may be used as a nephroureteral stent and may exit through the renal pelvis analogous to a catheter that stents the ureter after tapered reimplantation that exits from the bladder.

While *performing the anastomosis*, avoid multifilament suture material, which may drag adjacent areolar tissue through the suture tracts. A few days after surgery, the areolar tissue within the tract can become necrotic and lead to flank urine drainage. Monofilament synthetic sutures greatly obviate this undesirable sequela.

When beginning the anastomosis, it is helpful to first stabilize the repair by placing the first suture using a double-armed 7-0 monofilament absorbable suture placed as a mattress at the apex and tied with the knot outside the lumen. A running closure is performed along each wall of the spatulated ureter to the dismembered pelvis. It is helpful to first sew the wall farthest from the surgeon (from inside the lumen) and then sew the nearer wall. Just prior to closing of the pyelostomy, the pelvis can be irrigated through the indwelling stent to ensure that blood clots and tissue are not retained. It is most unusual to encounter a calculus. Most UPJ obstructions are associated with a markedly dilated renal pelvis, although, rarely, the dilation will be intrarenal. In that instance, a conventional dismembered pyeloplasty is not conducive to a good result; rather, the Foley YV-plasty preserves the available ureter and pelvis while it maximizes the ability for drainage.

An *indwelling ureteral stent* may be needed. A handy routine to follow is to permit the stent to offer closed external drainage for the day after surgery. On the 1st postoperative day, it is routine that there be minimal flank drainage, and the KISS catheter can be capped. This encourages internal antegrade drainage. Commonly, the flank drainage remains minimal over the course of the 1st postoperative day. The drain can be removed on the 2nd day, at which time the child can be discharged. The nephroureteral stent remains indwelling over the course of the next 5 to 7 days, at which time it is removed in the outpatient unit. As the catheter had been sutured to the pelvis only with 7-0 Dexon, it offers little resistance to removal after the skin sutures are cut. A Foley catheter is not used routinely to drain the bladder, because the KISS catheter drains the repaired kidney for the day after surgery.

After surgery, it is important to maintain good liaison with the pathologist for mutual examination of the specimen for changes in the pelvic wall, muscular hypertrophy, or fibrosis of the ureteropelvic complex that are enough to account for the obstruction. If these changes do not sufficiently account for the obstruction, one should be suspicious of the value of pyeloplasty for this case. Noting the extent of the fibrosis may permit prediction of the ability of the kidney pelvis to drain, because extensive fibrosis later may account for inefficient pelvic drainage, despite a technically successful result.

CHAPTER 23

Surgery of Horseshoe Kidneys

1 The vascular supply to horseshoe kidneys is quite variable, with the isthmus and lower poles frequently receiving blood from the common iliacs. The gonadal vessels pass over these lower renal vessels. The ureters lie nearer the midline than normal. Realize that the isthmus itself rarely is obstructive and that symphysiotomy seldom is indicated.

The approach to the horseshoe kidney depends on the objective of the operation. For correction of unilateral ureteropelvic junction (UPJ) obstruction or for nephrectomy, an anterior subcostal extraperitoneal incision provides good access (page 72). To operate on both pelves and divide the isthmus as well, a longer supraumbilical transverse incision, going transperitoneally and then reflecting the ascending and descending colon to reach the retroperitoneum, gives excellent exposure and is recommended for children. In adolescents, a long midline incision is required.

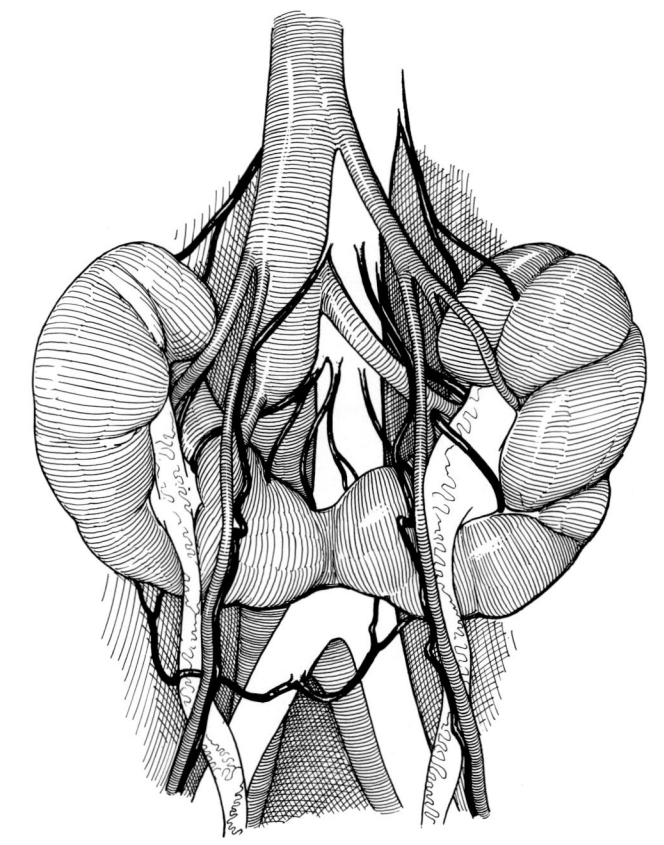

PYELOPLASTY

2 Approach the pelvis through an anterior subcostal incision. Mobilize the colon, and move Gerota's fascia and perirenal fat medially to provide cover for the repair later.

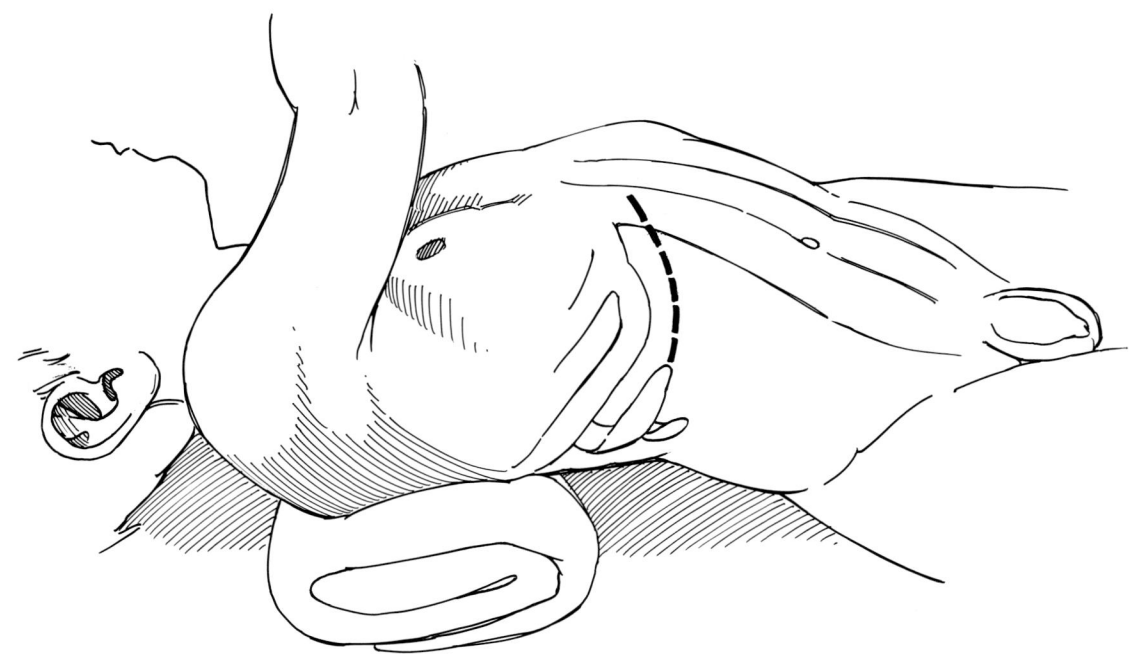

3 **A** and **B,** A modified Anderson-Hynes pyeloplasty usually is suitable (page 123). Place a stay suture in the ureter at the UPJ; divide and spatulate the ureter. Position the flap high on the pelvis so that when it is turned down, its apex will not reach the isthmus; contact could compromise the repair. Mark it with three stay sutures. **C** and **D,** Suture the ureter to the flap, starting at the apex of the flap and using two running 5-0 or 6-0 synthetic absorbable sutures with an occasional locked stitch. Install a Penrose drain fixed by the long-suture technique (page 6), and bring it out extraperitoneally. Replace Gerota's fascia and perirenal fat around the drain.

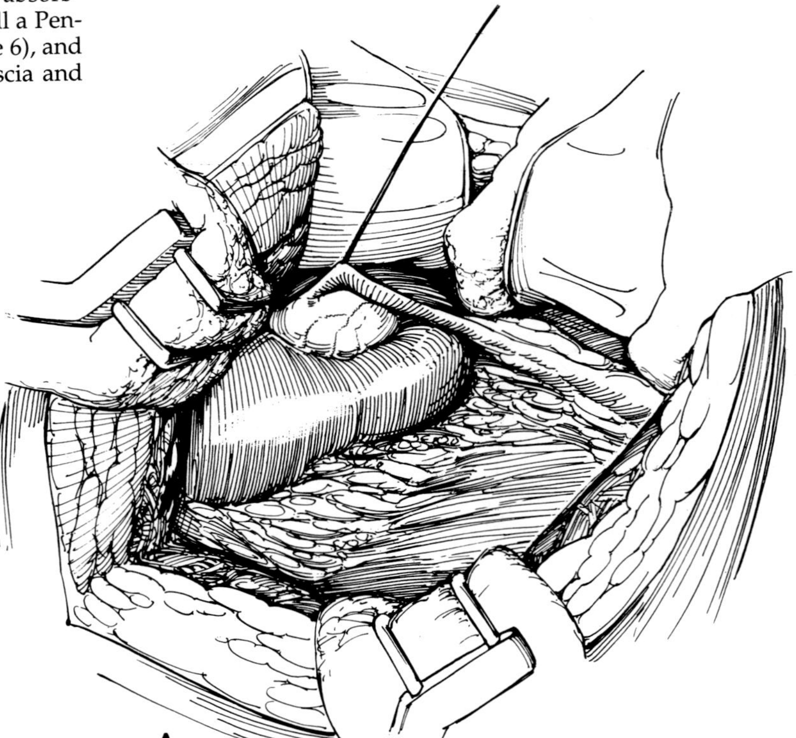

A

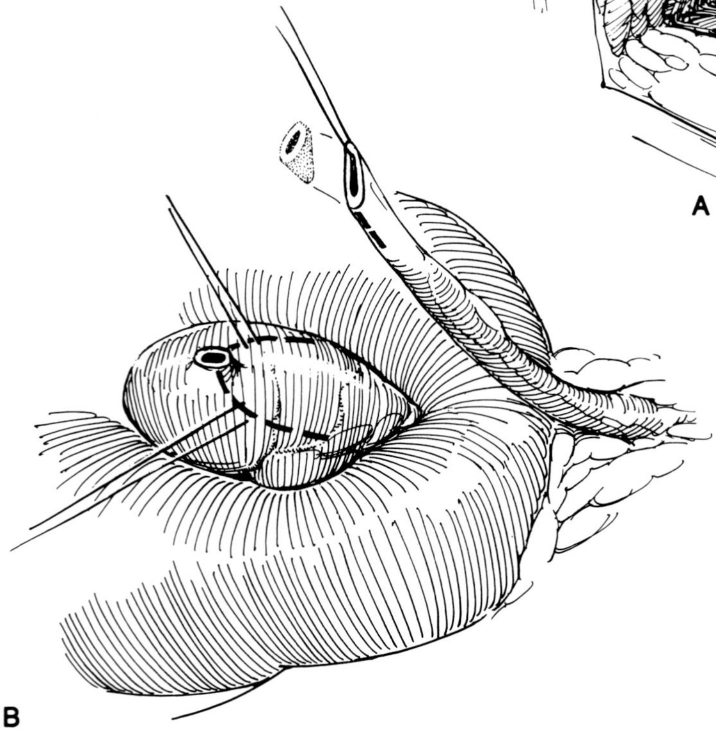

B

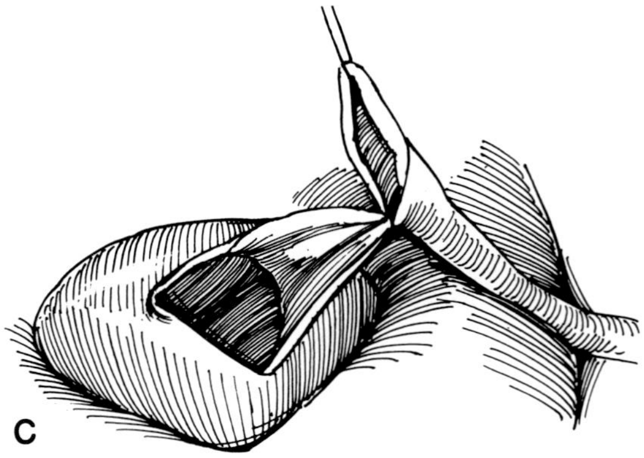

C

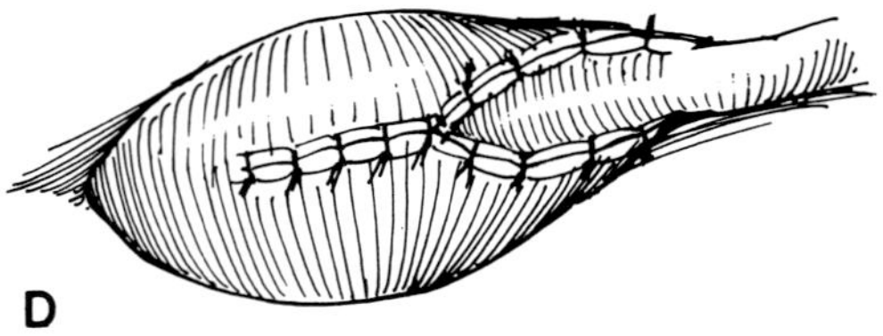

D

4 **A,** The Foley Y-plasty (page 128) can be used with high insertions. Hold the ureter cephalad with a Penrose drain. Incise the ureter vertically to its insertion into the pelvis. From this point, form a V with arms equal to the length of the ureteral incision. Consider placing a nephrostomy tube with or without a stent. **B,** Place a 4-0 synthetic absorbable suture in through the apex of the V and out through the apex of the ureteral incision and tie it. **C,** Place interrupted 4-0 synthetic absorbable sutures down both sides of the V to make a watertight anastomosis. Isolate the area with the perirenal fat, and provide drainage accurately. Use a similar incision and approach for pyelolithotomy in the horseshoe kidney.

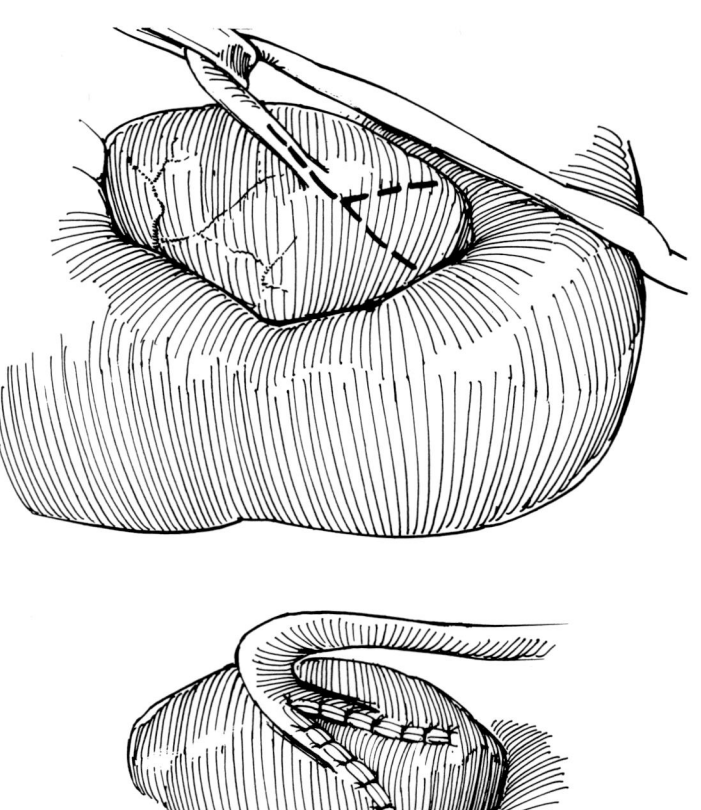

A

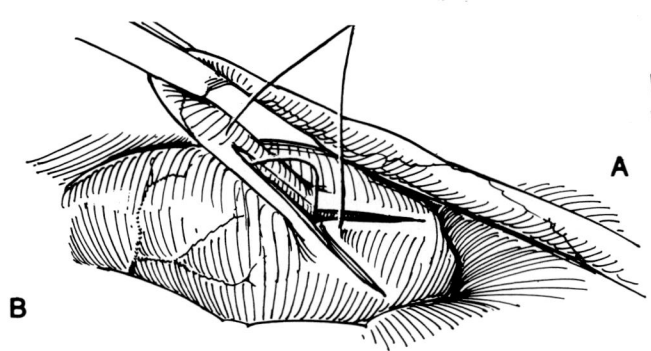

B

C

HEMINEPHRECTOMY

5 A and B, Obtain wide exposure through a transperitoneal incision—long transverse in children or long midline in adolescents. Incise the peritoneum over the aorta and vena cava to get exposure of the vascular pedicles, as for radical nephrectomy (page 169). Free up the upper pole and divide the ureter. Proceed to expose the remainder of the anomalous vascular supply, and individ-

ually clamp, ligate, and divide each artery and then each vein supplying the affected kidney. Divide the isthmus last by making a V-shaped incision that leaves a notch in the remaining portion of the isthmus to aid in closure. Because of vascular fixation, minimal rotation of the lower pole can be achieved.

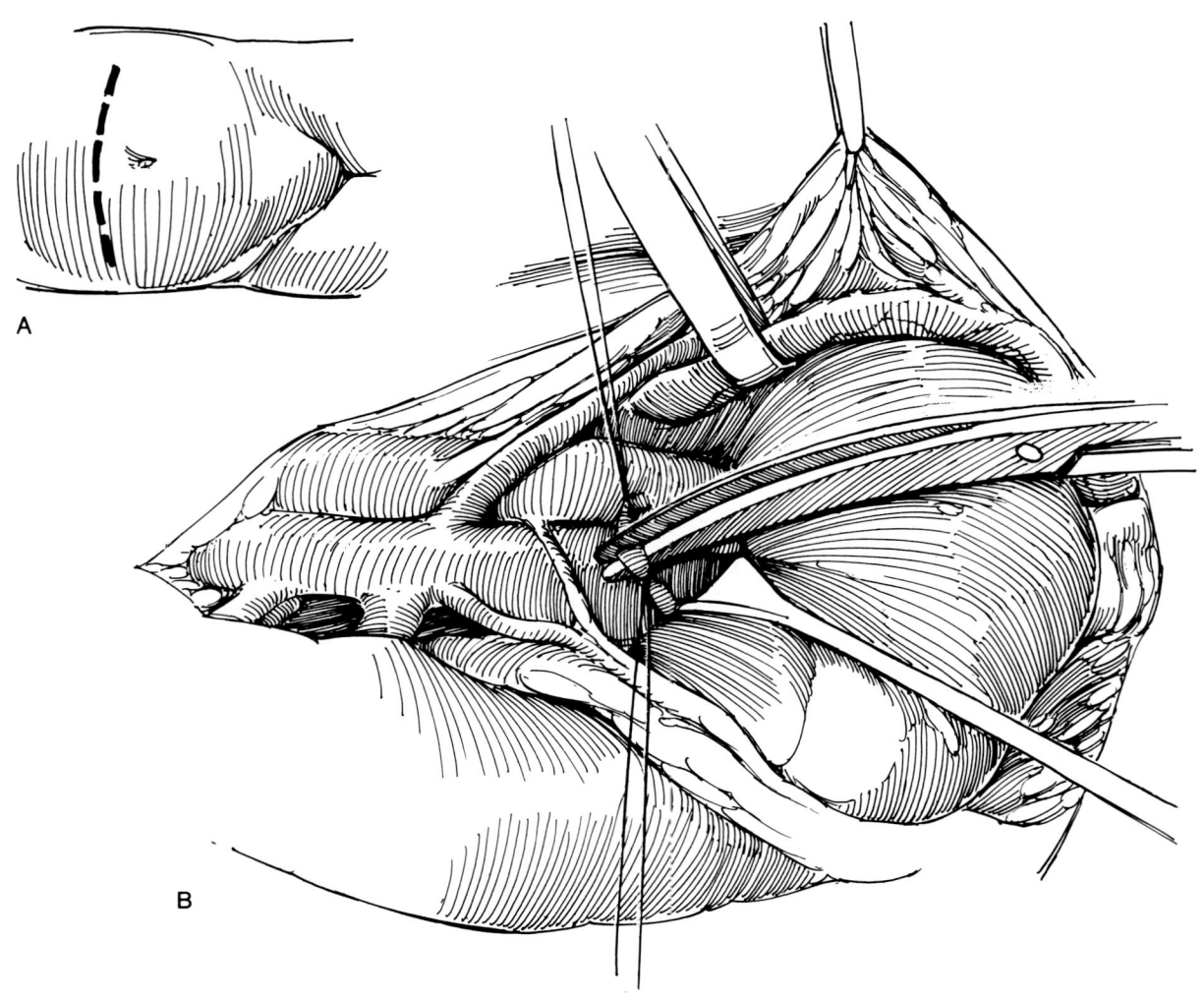

A

B

DIVISION OF THE ISTHMUS

Division of the isthmus rarely is indicated alone, because ureteral obstruction usually is caused by high insertion rather than impingement on the isthmus. Division does allow the kidneys to be rotated into a slightly more normal position for direct drainage from the pelves after pyeloplasty or for radiography after removal of a staghorn calculus.

Mobilize the ascending colon and cecum along the white line, and move it across the great vessels. Enter Gerota's fascia laterally; take care to preserve it to cover the repair. Expose the isthmus by blunt dissection, and dissect the vessels entering it from the aorta and vena cava. In some cases, vessels may come from the iliacs.

6 Identify the center of the isthmus by observing lobulation, by palpating the thinnest portion, and by inspecting the radiographs to avoid entering a calyx. Place a padded bulldog clamp on any vessel that supplies the isthmus, and observe for ischemia. Lift the isthmus and loop the posterior vessels. Ligate and cut only those vessels that prevent division of the isthmus; spare every vessel possible. If the isthmus is thin, place a Satinsky clamp on either side, divide between, and close the exposed ends with running sutures. For a thick isthmus, incise and peel back the capsule. Divide the parenchyma bluntly with the back of the knife. Avoid entering a calyx. If a calyx is transected, close it meticulously. Resect any devascularized tissue. Place figure-eight 4-0 synthetic absorbable sutures to transfix the arcuate vessels. Digital compression is useful to reduce blood loss during suturing.

7 Close as much of the capsule as possible, using running or interrupted 4-0 synthetic absorbable sutures. Mattress sutures with hemostatic gauze bolsters incorporating capsule and parenchyma may be used if necessary. When lateral rotation of the lower pole is necessary, division of one or more arteries to the area of the isthmus may make it possible. Resect any resultant ischemic tissue. Lift the lower pole of each kidney, and place a mattress 3-0 synthetic absorbable suture over fat bolsters. Pass the suture superiorly and laterally into the psoas muscle. Have your assistant push the kidney cephalad with a sponge stick, holding the stump away from the ureter while you tie the suture.

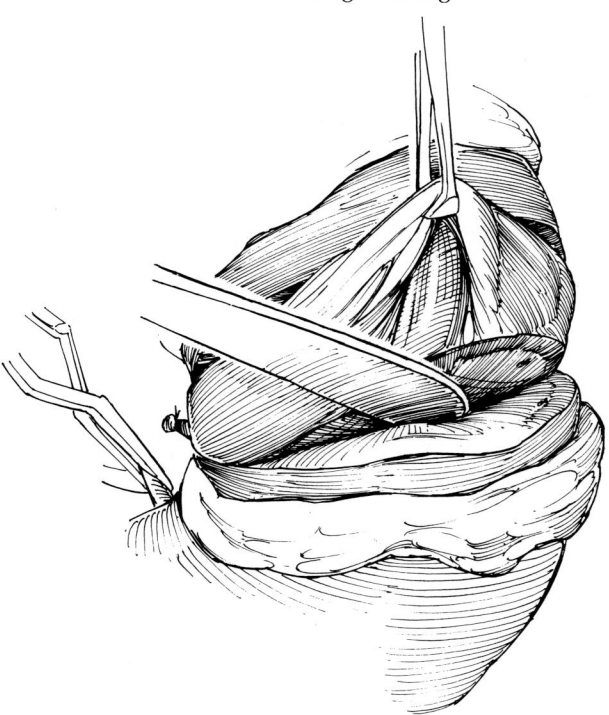

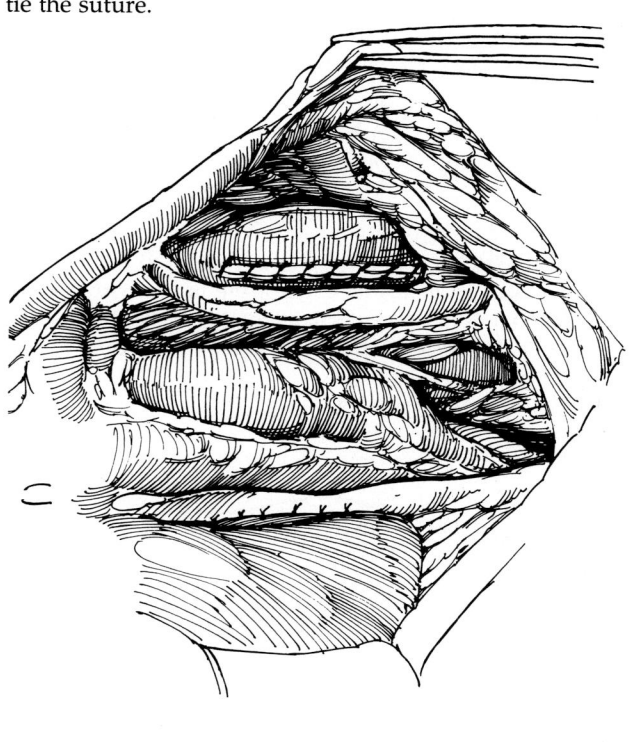

Commentary by Panos P. Kelalis

Symphysiotomy seldom is necessary and certainly should not be a part and parcel of procedures dealing with the reconstruction of the UPJ in horseshoe kidneys. At times, symphysiotomy may become necessary for drainage, in association with nephropexy. In such cases, and whenever a concern is raised that the isthmus may be inhibiting drainage and when significant hydronephrosis is noted (with thinning of the renal parenchyma), an attractive alternative is ureterocalycostomy.

Ureterocalycostomy (page 253) is easy to perform, achieves excellent drainage, and makes division of the isthmus unnecessary. In fact, in the presence of significant hydronephrosis, ureterocalycostomy is the procedure of choice to bypass obstruction at the UPJ. In children with horseshoe kidneys, the incidence of vesicoureteral reflux is high. A voiding cystourethrogram always should be done to exclude reflex-producing secondary UPJ obstruction.

Commentary by David Innes Williams

I would advise great caution in operating on hydronephrosis in horseshoe kidney without confirming genuine obstruction. Also, a cautious approach to nephrolithotomy is advisable, with consideration of noninvasive measures first. Before undertaking nephrectomy for nephroblastoma, chemotherapy is mandatory; these nephrectomies, in my experience, have been extremely difficult.

CHAPTER 24

Nephrostomy

Percutaneous nephrostomy often is the better temporary alternative to open placement of a nephrostomy, although the quality of drainage is inferior. Ureterostomy *in situ* is a simple, quick procedure compared with nephrostomy, and the catheter emerges in a more comfortable position for the child.

1 **A,** *Position:* Flank position with the table flexed. *Incision:* Make a subcostal incision (page 87). **B,** Expose the renal pelvis. Hold the edge of the hilum with vein or Gil Vernet retractors. Alternatively, for large pelves, approach the pelvis from its anterior surface.

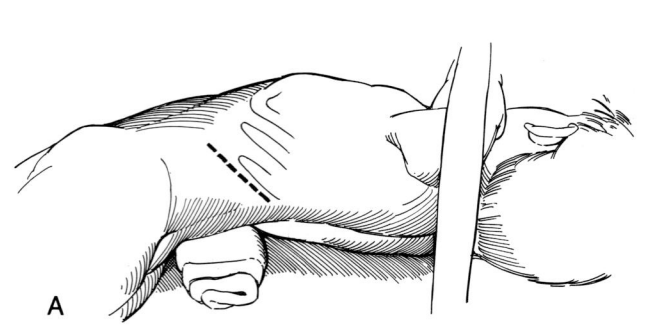

A

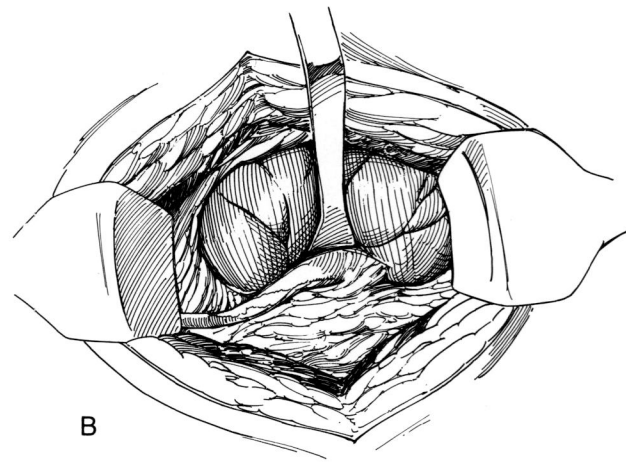

B

140

2 **A,** Place two 5-0 synthetic absorbable sutures in the pelvis well away from the ureteropelvic junction, and make a 1- to 2-cm incision parallel to the border of the hilum with a hooked knife blade. Prepare a small Malecot catheter by transfixing the tip with a #1 silk suture. (A whistle-tip, plastic Foley catheter has the advantage that it may be replaced by merely passing a guide wire through it down the ureter.) Insert a long curved clamp or, in adolescents, a Randall stone forceps with a suitable curvature, and pass the tip into a lower calyx. Press it firmly into the parenchyma while palpating for the tip. Cut the capsule in

a radial direction over the clamp to allow it to exit. Open the clamp slightly to dilate the tract. Grasp the suture on the catheter in the clamp. **B,** Ask the assistant to steady the kidney. Stretch the tip of the catheter by pulling the clamp with one hand and the catheter with the other or by inserting a curved clamp from outside between the wings to reduce their diameter. Gradually move both hands in concert to draw the catheter through the tract and out of the pelvis. Because the pelvis often is thinned, little force is needed. Cut the suture, then draw the catheter back until it fits in or near the lower calyx.

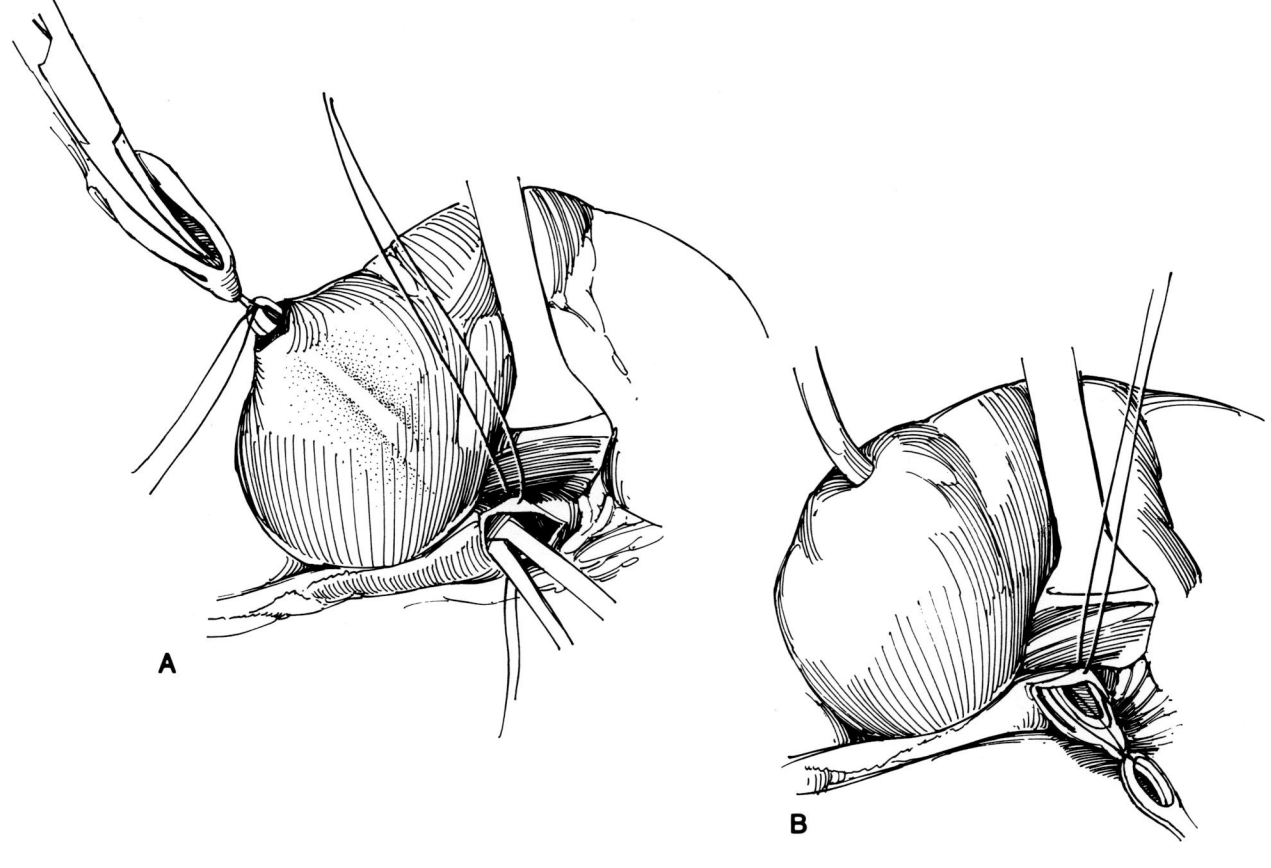

3 Suture the catheter to the capsule with a figure-eight 4-0 synthetic absorbable suture over fat bolsters. Bring the tube out through a separate stab wound in the flank placed well anteriorly so that the child will not lie on it. Fix it to the skin with a silk suture. Close the pyelotomy incision with a running 5-0 synthetic absorbable suture. Place a Penrose drain, and replace the perirenal fat and Gerota's fascia.

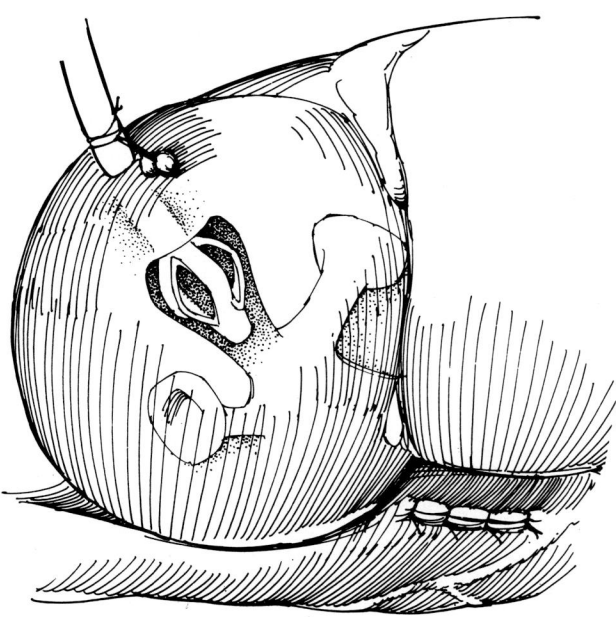

ALTERNATIVE TECHNIQUE

4 Prepare a Malecot catheter by cutting the distal end obliquely and making a vertical slit in it to create an eye. After inserting the clamp through the parenchyma, grasp a length of moistened umbilical tape and draw the end out through the pelvis. Pass a mosquito clamp through the eye of the catheter, bring the tape through, and tie it. Draw the tape and catheter out through the cortex, and position the catheter as described. Take care not to saw the parenchyma.

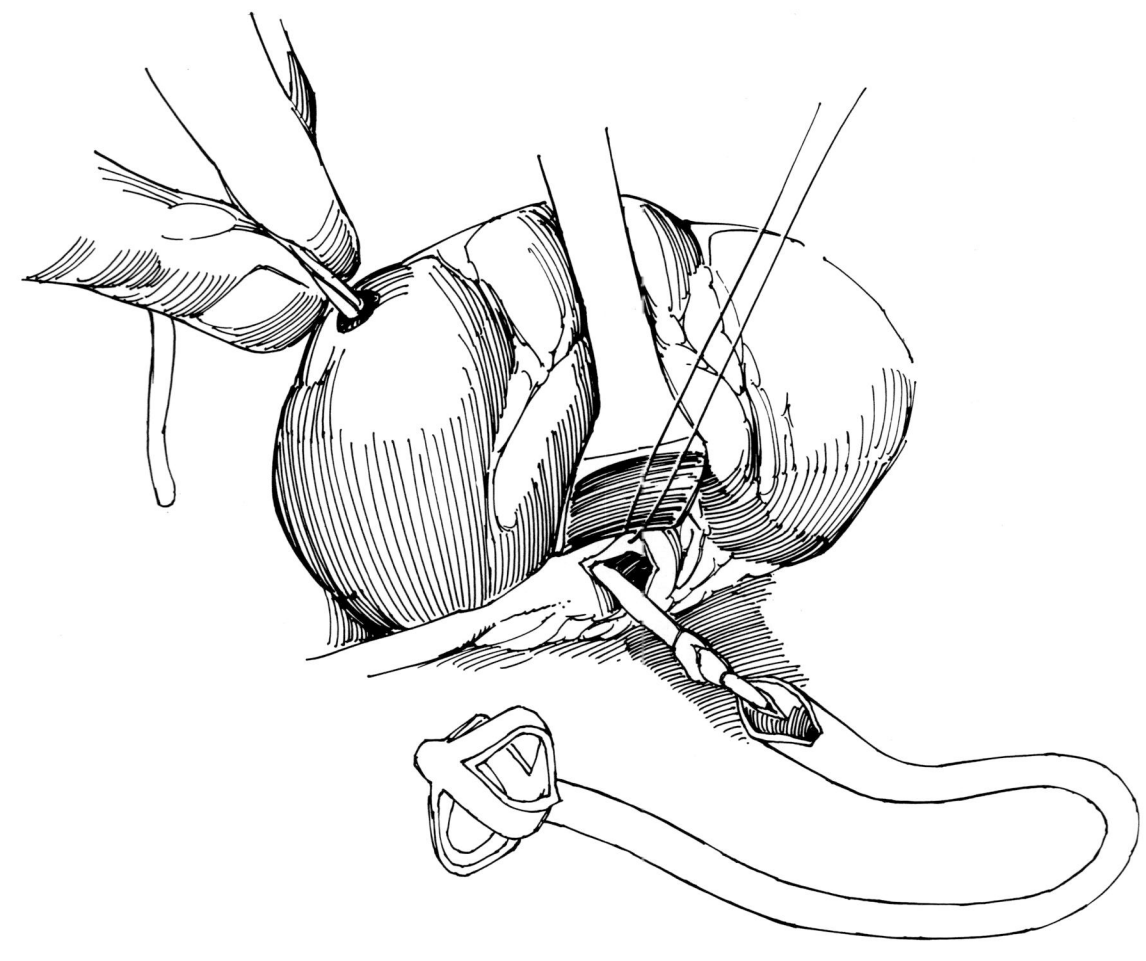

Commentary by Robert Kay

Although percutaneous nephrostomy has replaced the need for open nephrostomy in acute obstruction, sepsis, or other emergent situations, there still is a role for the open placement of a tube in the kidney. In most cases, this is done simultaneously with a reconstructive procedure such as pyeloplasty or ureterocalicostomy. It is important that the procedure is understood so that it is a part of the surgeon's armamentarium.

The only difference that I add to Dr. Hinman's well-described procedure is that I use a pediatric right-angle clamp. The tips are small and can be insinuated through the cortex to the capsule. Opening the clamp slightly dilates the tract so that the Malecot catheter can be grasped directly without the need for the suture. I fix the catheter only to the skin, not the kidney.

There are three problems that can occur in the placement of a nephrostomy tube. First, bleeding may be seen. In almost all cases it will stop spontaneously, but not without producing some anxiety. By placing traction on the catheter into the calyx, bleeding will stop in most cases. Second, too large a tract allows dislodgment of the catheter from the kidney. If this looks like it might occur, a pursestring may be placed in the capsule around the catheter to hold it in place. Finally, the catheter can be so placed that it blocks the UPJ, creating obstruction in the postoperative period. It is important that the end of the tube be placed in the calyx or near the infundibulum and be allowed to block the dependent portion of the newly created UPJ.

URETEROSTOMY *IN SITU*

For temporary diversion, expose the upper ureter retroperitoneally. Make a short ureterotomy, and insert an infant feeding tube into the renal pelvis. Fix it in place with a suture in the ureteral wall. Make a stab wound in the anterior axillary line, draw the tube out, and stitch it to the skin with a heavy silk suture.

END URETEROSTOMY

If both ureters are dilated, after bringing the less-dilated ureter across the midline, either bring them both through the body wall side by side or form an end-to-side anastomosis of the smaller to the larger one, which is brought to the skin in the lower quadrant (preferable to a midline subumbilical stoma). Form a stoma by everting the ureter to form a nipple (page 213).

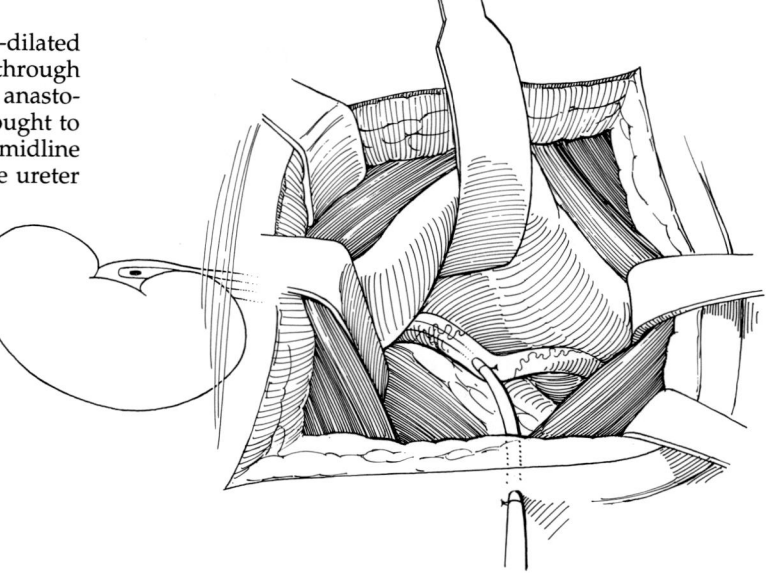

POSTOPERATIVE PROBLEMS

In cases of *excessive hematuria,* clamp the tube and allow a clot to form; this might disrupt the repair. *Inadvertent removal of the tube* is due to inadequate suturing and taping to the skin. These fastenings must be checked daily and replaced immediately if loose. After a week or two, the tube probably can be replaced with a small silicone balloon catheter on a stilet. Insert it to the same depth indicated by the color change on the catheter that was removed. Inflate the balloon with 3 ml of water and check its position with a gravity nephrostogram.

Obstruction to drainage requires gentle irrigation. First, give an intravenous push of mannitol to be certain dehydration is not the cause. If this fails to induce drainage, make a gravity nephrostogram to be sure the end of the tube is in the right position. If it is displaced, reposition it percutaneously. *Continued drainage* after removal of the tube suggests distal obstruction, which must be looked for radiographically and treated with retrograde intubation. *Stones* may form in patients with chronically alkaline urine. Use a silicone tube, and change it every 6 weeks.

Commentary by Robert Kay

In situ ureterostomy is a rare procedure today. I have seen it only once in my career; it was in a patient with a transureteroureterostomy, in whom the tube crossing the anastomosis created an obstruction to the ipsilateral kidney. It is an important technique to know, however, so that in unusual situations, the surgeon can feel comfortable in using it.

CHAPTER 25

Open Renal Biopsy

Open biopsy is preferable to needle biopsy in children, who frequently are uncooperative, and in adolescents (1) with solitary or small contracted kidneys and very poor renal function, (2) who are very obese, or (3) have some bleeding tendency.

Avoid biopsies in patients with severe hypertension and uncorrected coagulopathies. Use general anesthesia.

1 **A,** *Incision*: Approach the kidney through a dorsal lumbotomy incision (page 18). An alternative is the subcostal incision (page 13). **B,** Incise Gerota's fascia over the lower pole of the kidney, and mobilize the perirenal fat caudad to expose the renal capsule. Insert a narrow Deaver retractor between the kidney and the fat to draw the kidney down. Insert two fine stay sutures on either side of the proposed incision. Insert a third suture in the parenchyma, and make a deep elliptic incision into the

cortex around it. Lift the specimen out on the suture and place it on saline-moistened, coated gauze (not in formalin). At the same time, make a needle biopsy of the deeper cortex. Close the capsule by tying each of the stay sutures to itself and then to each other. If bleeding is appreciable, carefully rotate a taper-cut needle swaged with 5-0 or 4-0 chromic catgut through the renal cortex to cross at the depth of the incision as a horizontal mattress suture. Tie it carefully over pieces of fat with two-handed square knots to avoid tearing the suture from the tissue. Place a second suture if necessary for hemostasis. Then obtain a needle-biopsy specimen under direct vision to obtain material from the deep cortical and juxtamedullary levels. If the site bleeds, close it with a figure-eight suture. Approximate Gerota's fascia, then the muscles, fascia, and skin in layers. Close the skin with synthetic absorbable subcuticular sutures. If skin clips are used in immunosuppressed children, leave them for 10 or 12 days. Divide the biopsy tissue directly on the gauze, and fix the three portions in formalin, in 2 percent glutaraldehyde, and by quick freezing, respectively.

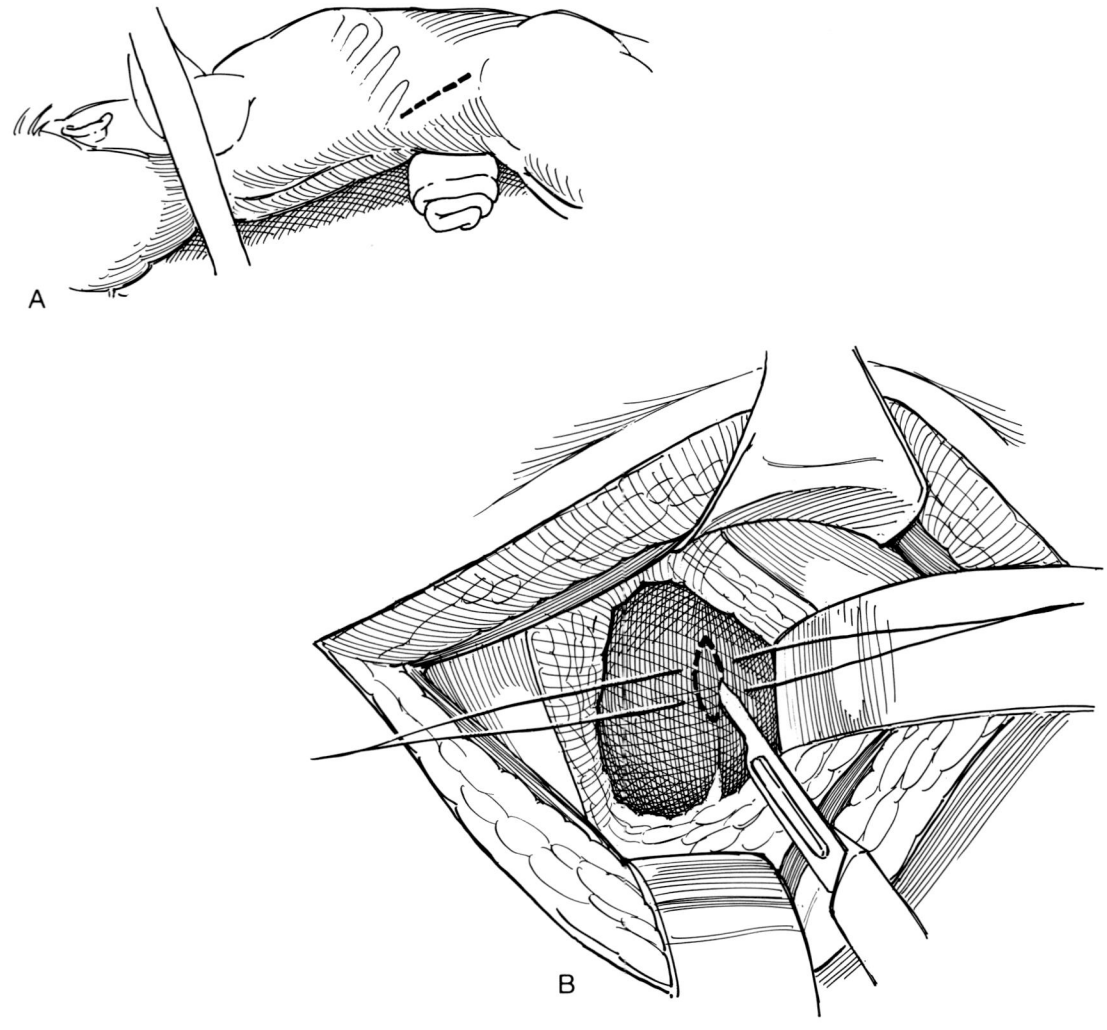

POSTOPERATIVE PROBLEMS

Bleeding occurs, especially in hypertensive children or those with minor coagulation problems. *Gross hematuria* usually will stop after 24 hours of bed rest. A *retroperitoneal hematoma* may form. *Wound infection* is uncommon.

Commentary by Robert Kay

Open renal biopsies continue to be required, despite increasing proficiency by pediatric nephrologists with percutaneous approaches. The dorsal lumbotomy approach is quite useful because of the low morbidity. However, in exceptionally muscular or obese children, the subcostal incision may be more appropriate. As opposed to the use of fat, as proposed in the text, we prefer a synthetic thrombogenic material such as oxidized cellulose (Oxycel). In most cases, the incision can be very small, and with the muscle-splitting approach, postoperative pain and complications are minimal. The two biggest problems the surgeon may encounter are bleeding and biopsy of the wrong organ. Bleeding can be controlled by sutures and thrombogenic material. There have been cases in which biopsies of the liver, on the right side, and the spleen, on the left side, have been performed when the surgeon has been misoriented. It is important to realize that the complication can occur, if rarely, in order to avoid it.

Commentary by Stephen R. Shapiro

I favor a small anterior subcostal incision for open renal biopsy, especially when there is a possibility of bleeding (*ie*, patient with bleeding tendency), because this allows better control. I have not used a suture in the parenchyma, and I have not found an open needle biopsy to be necessary; instead, I use a #11 blade to obtain a deep wedge of renal tissue that can be gently coaxed out without crushing it. Although this may cause some minor bleeding, the latter can be well controlled with the chromic catgut sutures described in the text. It is important to use chromic catgut sutures on the kidney, rather than polyglycolic acid or similar sutures, because chromic catgut is less likely to cut through the renal tissue. In an extreme case, the Argon beam coagulator can be used for fine control of bleeding within the renal parenchyma.

CHAPTER 26

Repair of Renal Injuries

EXPLORATION, EXPOSURE, AND REPAIR

Obtain urine for microscopic analysis, either by having the child void or by catheterization; in either case, collect the urine after the first 30 ml has passed. More than five red blood cells per high-power field is significant to detect injury, although vascular avulsion may be missed when the kidney becomes functionless, and no red blood cells will be found in the urine. Make an intravenous urogram (IVU) to stage

the injury by inserting a large-bore IV catheter and rapidly injecting up to 2 mg/kg of contrast material. A nephrotomogram can be made with the same injection. If the results of these studies are normal, observe the child. If the results are somewhat abnormal, obtain a computed tomographic (CT) scan, and decide whether observation, aortography, or operation is appropriate. When markedly abnormal or major renal bleeding is occurring, proceed to operation.

1 *Incision*: Make a midline transperitoneal incision (page 83). First, explore the abdomen for associated injury. Repair injuries to the liver, spleen, and bowel first, unless renal bleeding is so rapid that blood cannot be replaced. In the meantime, apply laparotomy sponges to the kidney area to aid in control of renal bleeding. Lift the small bowel and place it on the chest in a plastic bag. Identify the aorta if possible. If the aorta is covered by hematoma and cannot be palpated, identify the inferior mesenteric vein, and incise the posterior parietal peritoneum medial to it over the site of the aorta for 10 cm from the ligament of Treitz. Dissect through the medial portion of the hematoma to expose the aorta, watching out for the inferior mesenteric artery. Avoid disturbing the perirenal hematoma by not dissecting laterally near the kidney.

2 Dissect along the aorta superiorly to reach the next landmark, the left renal vein where it crosses anteriorly. Place a vessel loop around it, and retract the vein superiorly to expose first the left renal artery and then the right one. Beware of the left posterior lumbar vein that comes off the renal vein. Place vessel loops around the renal artery of the injured side to make it ready for placement of a vascular clamp, but unless bleeding is heavy, do not apply the clamp at this time.

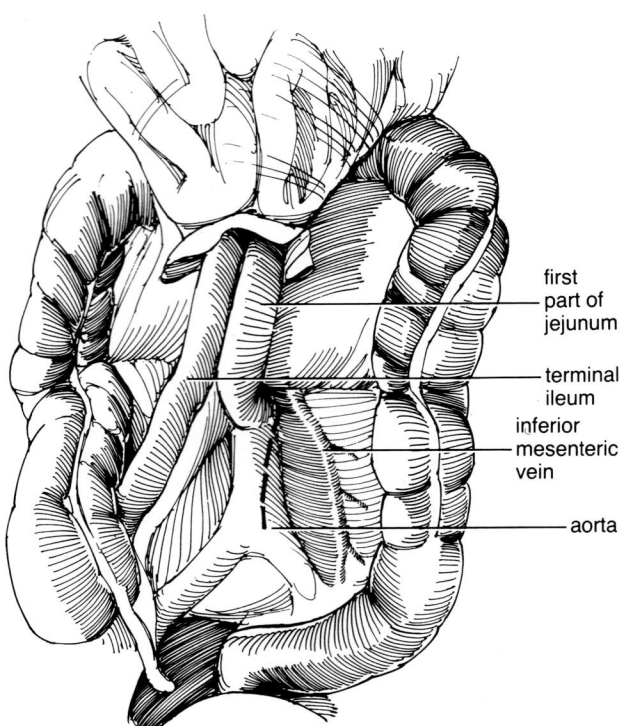

first part of jejunum

terminal ileum

inferior mesenteric vein

aorta

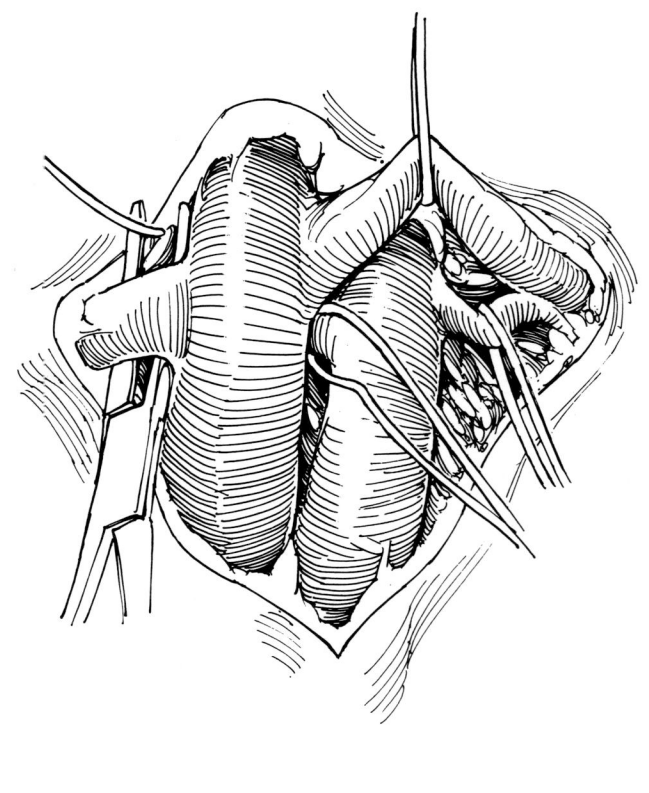

3 For left renal injury (as shown), incise the parietal peritoneum lateral to the descending colon, and reflect the colon medially to expose the hematoma inside Gerota's fascia. Dissect directly into the hematoma through the fascia and the perirenal fat to reach the kidney. Free all aspects of the kidney to be able to examine it carefully. If the bleeding warrants, clamp the artery with a vascular clamp before proceeding with definitive repair of the renal defect(s). However, in most cases, compression with the fingers is sufficient.

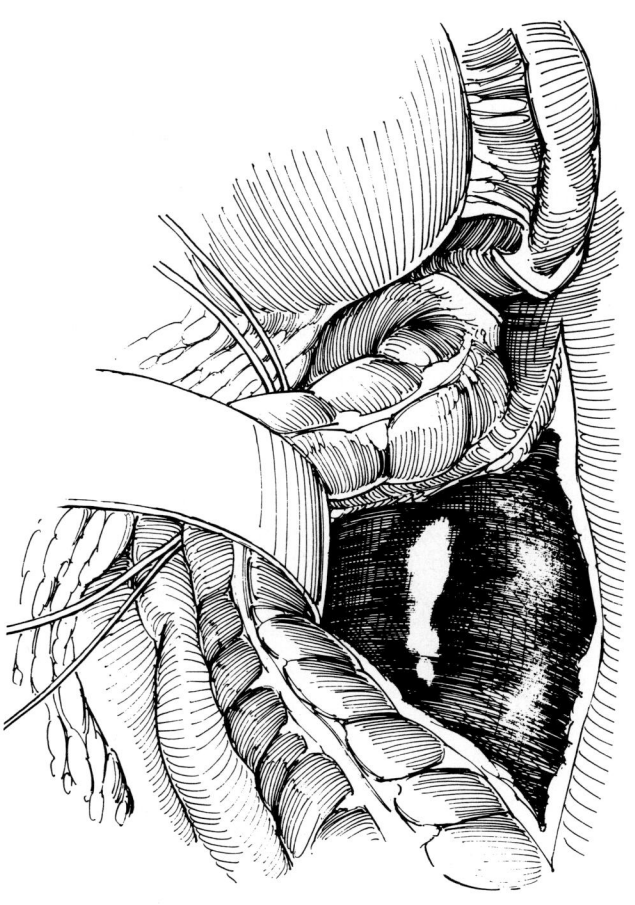

4 Remove the intrarenal hematoma residing in a laceration, and ligate the contributing intrarenal arteries and veins. Resect any necrotic tissue, and secure hemostasis by placing fine figure-eight 4-0 chromic catgut sutures on the interlobar, arcuate, or interlobular vessels; catgut sutures slide through tissue better than do woven nonabsorbable ones. Ligate a segmental artery if it supplies blood to less than 15 percent of the kidney; if the resulting infarction is greater than that, remove that portion of the kidney. If there is a major injury of the upper or lower pole, elect partial nephrectomy (page 161). If you think reconstruction will take more than 30 minutes, cool the kidney with slush (see page 162). Injured segmental veins can be ligated without worry of renal infarction because of intrarenal collateral circulation.

5 Make a watertight closure of any open calyces or infundibula with running 4-0 chromic catgut sutures. Be certain that there is no leakage by pinching the upper ureter closed while injecting a small amount of dilute methylene blue directly into the renal pelvis. Close any residual openings. Apply patches of gelatin sponge or microfibrillar collagen to persistently oozing areas.

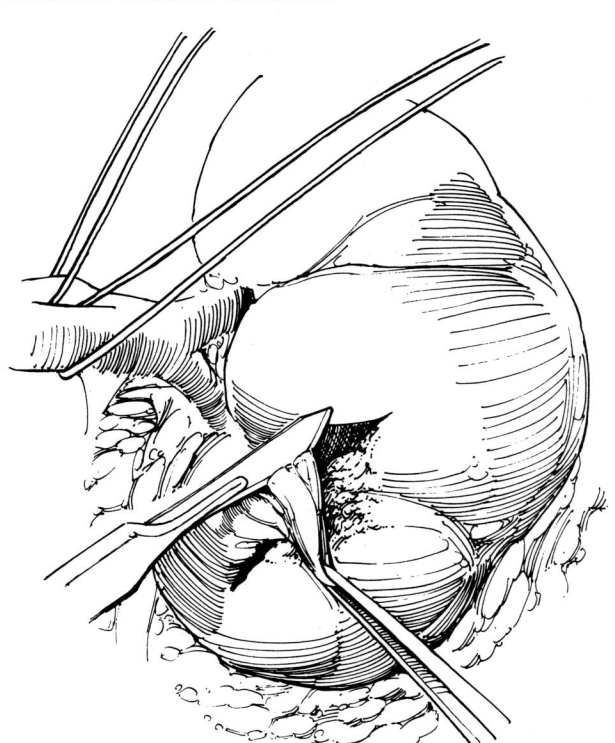

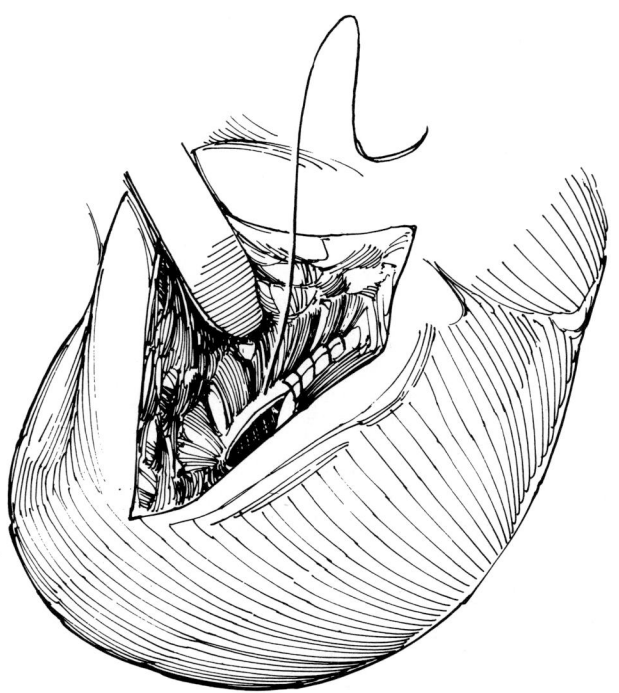

6 **A,** Cover the defect with any available capsule, and hold it in place with mattress sutures over fat bolsters.

B, Alternatively, apply a long bolster of gelatin sponge held with mattress sutures in the capsule. The capsule often is destroyed; in that case, use a pedicle flap of omentum (page 272) brought through a window in the mesocolon and tacked in place with interrupted 4-0 chromic catgut sutures. Because the calyces usually have been opened and there is risk of urinary leakage, insert a closed-system (Jackson-Pratt) drain that exits retroperitoneally from the flank through a stab wound; closed drainage is preferred to Penrose drainage, because it decreases the chance of infecting the retroperitoneal hematoma.

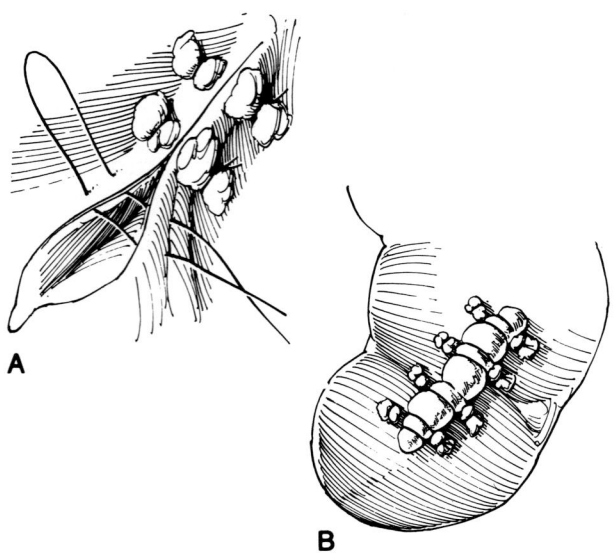

7 For renal artery thrombosis, remove that segment of the artery, and replace the defect with vascular graft obtained from the saphenous vein or hypogastric artery. Close lacerations of the main renal vein with fine vascular sutures, but ligate a lacerated venous branch and depend on internal collateral circulation. With deceleration injury to the renal artery, the defect usually is at the origin of the artery from the aorta, leaving the artery suitable for autotransplantation.

Continue gastric suction for 3 or 4 days, then ambulate the patient. Follow the blood pressure and hematocrit data closely and provide IV fluids to achieve a high urine output.

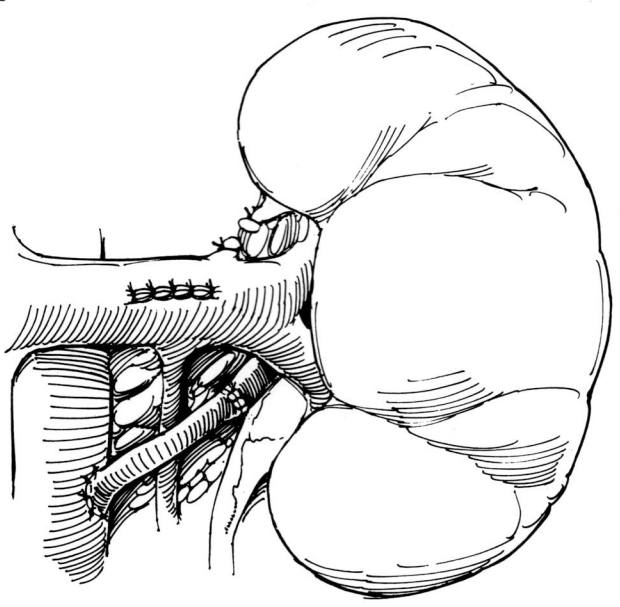

POSTOPERATIVE PROBLEMS

Watch for *delayed bleeding, infection* with abscess formation, continued open or closed *urinary leakage, arteriovenous fistula,* and, later, *hypertension.* Obtain a follow-up IVU 3 months after injury.

Commentary by Jack W. McAninch

In the pediatric age group, renal injuries occur most commonly from blunt trauma. The presence of five red blood cells or more per high-power field in the urine is indicative, and imaging studies should be done (IVU and/or CT) to stage the injury. The major indication for exploration is renal bleeding, but large segments (more than 15 percent) of nonviable tissue associated with a parenchymal laceration and urinary extravasation constitute relative indications. If the renal vessels on the injured side are isolated before exploration of the kidney, they can then be clamped should heavy bleeding be encountered when Gerota's fascia is entered. Total renal exposure is important, because multiple injuries may be present.

It is important to place vessel loops on the renal vasculature before exploring the hematoma and kidney. Complete renal exposure is necessary, because more than one injury may exist. Clamping of the renal artery usually is not necessary. Bleeding often can be controlled with finger compression. All clot and nonviable tissue should be removed and hemostasis obtained, as recommended in the text. The use of microfibrin collagen hemostatic sponge is helpful when small amounts of bloody oozing persist on the repaired surface.

Aggressive débridement of nonviable tissue should be done by sharp dissection. Bleeding vessels are individually suture ligated, and the collecting system is closed watertight. The fracture margins can be approximated by closing the capsule over bolsters. When capsule has been destroyed, omentum or a free graft of peritoneum can be used to cover the defect. Omentum is my choice because of its viability and support of wound healing.

When the collecting system has been opened, a drain should be placed only until one is certain that urine is not draining and then should be removed (48 hours). This will help avoid infecting the retroperitoneum and the hematoma.

Injuries to the main renal artery seldom can be repaired with adequate return of renal function, in approximately 20 percent; in many such cases, multiple associated injuries make renal arterial reconstruction—a time-consuming process—unfeasible. In most cases, renal vein injury can be repaired. Segmental artery injury without parenchymal laceration should be ligated; the infarcted tissue will be reabsorbed, and hypertension seldom occurs.

A watertight closure of the collecting system is important. A simple method to check the closure is to occlude the upper ureter by finger compression and inject 5 ml of dilute methylene blue into the renal pelvis. Any small openings are easily noted and closed; follow with coverage of the defect (*eg,* omentum) to provide added security. Closed-system (Jackson-Pratt) drains are preferred to decrease the potential for infecting the retroperitoneal hematoma. These reconstructions should take less than 1 hour in most instances. It is important to move through the process expeditiously; otherwise, the trauma surgeon becomes impatient as the child's temperature drops along with the blood volume.

CHAPTER 27

Renal Transplantation

In most children, preoperative voiding cystourethrography provides adequate information on bladder dynamics. In those children with voiding dysfunction or prior urinary diversion, formal urodynamic studies and cystourethroscopy are necessary. Cycling the defunctionalized bladder for a week or two through a suprapubic trocar catheter will allow assessment of its potential. Do any necessary bladder augmentation at least 3 months before transplantation, then check to make sure the storage and evacuation system works. It is important to determine if the bladder has adequate capacity, empties without residual urine, and has a functional continence mechanism. In children with prior urinary diversion, intermittent catheterization may be necessary in cases with adequate capacity but incomplete emptying.

Because an adult kidney usually is used for renal transplantation in small children weighing 20 kg or less, use a transperitoneal approach, and position it behind (lateral to) the cecum. Older children who require transplantation into a conduit also need a transperitoneal approach. Otherwise, the retroperitoneal approach has fewer technical problems and avoids leakage of peritoneal dialysate. Choose the site for the vascular anastomoses so that the arterial supply and venous drainage will be adequate. In a small child, anastomosis to the vena cava and the aorta or common iliac artery is necessary. Ureteral implantation may be difficult because of multiple previous procedures. If all else is impossible, make a direct ureteral (or even pelvic) anastomosis into the bladder, or anastomose the renal pelvis or ureter to the native ureter.

Dialyze the child the day before operation, if possible, to ensure metabolic and electrolyte balance.

Make a midline incision from the xiphoid to the symphysis pubis. Reflect the right colon medially by incising the lateral posterior parietal peritoneum, and develop the retroperitoneal space down to the lateral aspect of the bladder. Remove the right kidney if necessary.

Free the vena cava from the level of the right renal vein to its bifurcation; sometimes it is necessary to mobilize both proximal iliac veins. Identify, doubly ligate, and divide the lumbar veins in the area of the proposed renal vein anastomosis. Mobilize the aorta distally from just below the renal arteries to, and including, both common iliac arteries. Initiate blood transfusion to compensate for the relatively large volume of blood that will be required to fill the adult kidney.

Perform an end-to-side anastomosis of the shortened renal vein to the vena cava superiorly, using 5-0 or 6-0 cardiovascular sutures, as in an adult.

Isolate a segment of aorta by placing two pediatric vascular clamps inferiorly on the common iliac arteries and one superiorly on the aorta. Perform end-to-side anastomosis of the spatulated renal artery to the lower aorta with running or interrupted 5-0 or 6-0 cardiovascular sutures. Remove the superior clamp on the inferior vena cava first and then all three inferior clamps. Finally, release the superior aortic clamp very slowly and keep it in place in case reclamping is necessary.

TRANSVESICAL URETERAL IMPLANTATION

For a description of the extravesical (Barry) technique designed for transplantations, see page 211. An alternative to ureteroneocystostomy is anastomosis of the recipient ureter to the donor pelvis when the donor ureter is short or circulation is compromised.

Open the partially filled bladder anteriorly. Select a site on the floor of the bladder as near and as lateral to the ureteral orifice as possible and make a short transverse incision through the mucosa. Make a second transverse incision proximally, and dissect a tunnel between them with curved scissors. The length of the tunnel will be proportionate to the size of the child, with a maximum of 2.5 cm in adolescents. Draw an 8 F Robinson catheter through the tunnel retrogradely.

Pass a right-angle clamp obliquely through the bladder wall from outside just above the upper end of the tunnel. The tract must provide a smooth oblique exit for the ureter, which after transplantation will have a more anterior course than the normal ureter. Stretch the hiatus large enough so that it cannot obstruct the ureter. Draw the catheter through the hiatus with a clamp below the spermatic cord in males, and fasten it to the tip of the ureter with a 2-0 suture. Pull the ureter gently into the bladder, leaving it a little redundant outside the bladder.

Trim and spatulate the end of the ureter, leaving 1 cm protruding. Anchor the apex with a 5-0 synthetic absorbable suture to the trigonal muscle and mucosa. Place several mucosal sutures on either side and at the apex. Test for absence of constriction with an infant feeding tube. Close the mucosa over the hiatus. A stent is not needed.

Close the cystotomy in one layer with a running full-thickness 3-0 or 4-0 synthetic absorbable suture. Just catch the edge of the mucosa, and take a good bite of the muscularis and adventitia. Carry the stitches beyond the ends of the incision to avoid leakage. Close the peritoneal incision lateral and inferior to the right colon to extraperitonealize the ureter and graft. To prevent lymphoceles, some surgeons make a 12- to 15-cm incision in the peritoneum below and medial to the kidney and pull a tongue of omentum through it and drape it over the graft. Flood the wound with a solution of bacitracin and neomycin and aspirate it. Obtain perfect hemostasis; these patients may bleed from azotemic coagulopathy as a spastic vessel opens. You may or may not want to insert a retroperitoneal suction drain. Close the abdomen appropriately. Place a balloon catheter through the urethra into the bladder.

BLADDER AUGMENTATION WITH RENAL TRANSPLANTATION

For a patient with a small contracted bladder and end-stage renal failure, perform ileocystoplasty (page 440) prior to transplantation, and colocystoplasty (page 444), cecocystoplasty (page 452), or ileocecocystoplasty (page 463) as a first stage. Left nephrectomy can be done at the same time.

At the second stage, mobilize the right colon, and remove the right kidney. Transplant the donor kidney into the right iliac fossa, and tunnel its ureter retroperitoneally to exit near the augmented bladder. Anastomotic alternatives include ureteroureterostomy and implantation into the bladder or into an ileal nipple, if that has been formed.

POSTOPERATIVE PROBLEMS

Hyperacute rejection is heralded by swelling and discoloration of the kidney soon after it is revascularized. It must be differentiated from renal vein obstruction or thrombosis. Take a biopsy specimen to confirm the diagnosis of hyperacute rejection. If the results are positive, it may be advisable to remove the kidney; if doubtful, leave the kidney in place and hope for reversal.

Try not to confuse the signs and symptoms of *rejection* with those of *urologic complications*. Use ultrasonography and renal scintigraphy to differentiate among acute tubular necrosis, rejection, and urinary obstruction. One can resort to intravenous pyelography, cystography, and even retrograde or antegrade pyelography. Percutaneous nephrostomy is diagnostic for total or partial obstruction and, moreover, is therapeutic.

Renal rupture is an unusual complication secondary to acute rejection and requires emergency nephrectomy.

Urinary infection with or without pyelonephritis may occur, especially if reflux persists. *Urinary leakage* may occur at the ureterovesical anastomosis or from the bladder closure; it may result from necrosis of the distal ureter.

Ureteral obstruction, when seen in the 1st week or so, usually is caused by edema, but hematoma, lymphocele, or technical error may be the cause. Later, periureteral fibrosis or contraction of the ureter from partial ischemia can cause obstruction. In any case, the diagnosis of obstruction must be made at once; the alternative is sepsis and loss of the graft. Treatment is by percutaneous diversion or by transurethral insertion of a silicone stent. Some cases may respond to percutaneous transluminal ureteroplasty. If these measures are inapplicable or if they fail, reoperate and reimplant the ureter or resort to pyeloureterostomy, ureteroureterostomy, crossed ureteropyelostomy, or even calycocystostomy combined with a psoas hitch.

Ureterocutaneous fistulas, identified by nuclear scanning and ultrasonography, are the result of devascularization during harvesting and implantation, especially from live donors. Rejection may play a role. Intervene at once on development of a fistula to avoid wound and systemic infection or even a fatal outcome. Insert a nephrostomy tube percutaneously or place a stent endoscopically. If these measures fail to stop the leak, do a ureterovesical or pyelovesical anastomosis with a Boari flap or a psoas hitch; alternatively, consider an anastomosis of the ureter or pelvis to one or another residual terminal ureter. A nephrostomy tube or silicone stents may be needed in complicated situations. Fistulas can occur from a calyx if a renal pole is devascularized. Partial nephrectomy or an omental patch is a good treatment.

Vesicocutaneous fistulas are not common when the bladder has been opened through normal wall and closed carefully. When a cystostomy has been found to be necessary in an infant because of the small urethra, it may not close spontaneously. Delay treatment of fistulas by using prolonged urethral drainage, suction drainage, and antibiotics, but do not be afraid of surgical excision and closure of the tract.

Lymphoceles, although often confused with extravasation, appear several weeks after surgery rather than at once. Look for reduced renal function, local swelling, genital edema, ipsilateral iliofemoral venous thrombosis, and increased blood pressure and weight. Aspiration with the aid of ultrasonography will identify lymph, which has lower levels of creatinine and potassium than does urine. If a lymphocele recurs, marsupialize it into the peritoneal cavity.

Renal artery stenosis comes from a defective anastomosis, chronic rejection, or kinking or torsion due to excessive length. In children, the inadequate size of the recipient vessels may be the cause. It will occur both early and late. Look for hypertension; although this may be due to rejection or renal disease, do an angiogram, especially if you find a diastolic bruit or a decrease in renal function. Use selective renin determinations to be sure the kidney is the cause of the hypertension, and locate the lesion with anteroposterior and oblique views on digital subtraction imaging. Delay treatment if renal function is stable and hypertension can be controlled medically. In any case, try transluminal angioplasty before proceeding with a difficult surgical procedure, which carries a real chance for loss of the graft.

Arterial thrombosis usually comes either from tearing of the intima when the kidney is secured or during perfusion; however, rejection and poor anastomotic technique may be factors, as well as hypercoagulability, arteriosclerotic disease in the recipient artery, or embolus. Treatment is usually prompt nephrectomy.

Venous thrombosis is secondary to errors such as kinking of the graft when the kidney is put in place. It is hard to distinguish the signs of swelling of the graft, oliguria, and proteinuria from those of rejection. Perform renal venography when suspicion is aroused, and reexplore immediately to do a thrombectomy.

Acute tubular necrosis is a complication in the immediate postoperative period. Follow the patient with nuclear scans to check on blood flow and evidence of rejection and with sonograms to rule out obstruction and extravasation.

Watch for *vascular problems,* such as hemorrhage (reoperate immediately); occlusion secondary to intimal injury and, rarely, renal vein thrombosis; impotence from interference with blood flow in the pelvis; wound complications (look for pelvic abscesses and fluid collections by sonography and computed tomographic scans); urinary complications, such as leakage at the ureteroneocystostomy from ischemia, detected by sonography and requiring formation of a ureteropyelostomy reinforced with omentum; and rejection of the graft, which calls for immunosuppression.

Nephrectomy after transplantation can be difficult because of the rejection reaction and the adherence of the kidney to the recipient artery and vein. The operation is best done by the original transplant surgeon, who can most effectively clear these vessels. Allograft nephrectomy more than 1 or 2 weeks after transplantation usually should be done subcapsularly because of perinephric fibrosis.

It may be advisable to remove the kidneys before transplantation for poorly controlled renin-mediated hypertension, persistent urinary tract infection, renal stones, prior urinary diversion, or severe reflux. Use bilateral posterior incisions (page 116) because of their low morbidity and mortality. Polycystic kidneys may require removal in two stages through the flanks. Bilateral nephroureterectomy is recommended for a patient with existing urinary diversion. Native nephrectomy usually is performed weeks before transplantation.

Commentary by John M. Barry

The transplantation of adult kidneys into small children is technically challenging; however, the results are better than when kidneys from very young donors are used because of technical difficulties, including thrombosis, urinary fistula, and ureteral obstruction.

A skilled pediatric nephrologist is indispensable in the preoperative preparation and postoperative management of these small patients, especially when a living related donor is unavailable for preemptive transplantation. The skillful use of chronic peritoneal dialysis and dietary supplementation by a small indwelling feeding tube presents the pediatric renal transplant surgeon with a well-prepared patient in positive nitrogen balance.

Adequate intraoperative fluid administration is important. A central venous pressure (CVP) greater than 10 cm H_2O and a systolic blood pressure (BP) greater than 100 mm Hg before the vascular clamps are removed will allow adequate perfusion of the transplanted kidney. The anesthesiology team must still be prepared to rapidly infuse another 250 to 300 ml of intravenous fluid as soon as the kidney is revascularized because of the loss of blood volume into the adult kidney transplant. Close monitoring of the CVP and aggressive replacement of urine output are important in the early postoperative period. Some centers prefer to use 5 percent albumin infusions because of third-space fluid losses or the development of postdialysis ascites. At times, inotropic infusion is necessary to maintain adequate systolic BP when the CVP is already in the target range of 8 to 10 cm H_2O.

Although the quality of life of pediatric kidney transplant recipients is not ideal, it is superior to that achieved with chronic dialysis. Growth retardation and delay in puberty are but two of the problems faced by small children who receive kidney transplants. The best growth following renal transplantation is observed in patients who are no older than 5 years of age at the time of engraftment.

PERCUTANEOUS PLACEMENT OF HEMODIALYSIS CATHETER

Vascular Access by Radial Artery–Cephalic Vein Shunt

Provide a cutdown tray, electrocautery, two winged Ramirez shunt tubes, vessel tips (two small, two medium, and two large), a straight connector, neomycin-bacitracin irrigating solution, 100 ml heparinized saline, a 10-ml syringe with plain tip, and 1 percent lidocaine.

1 Use the nondominant arm, if possible; prep and drape it. Apply a tourniquet and mark the courses of the distal cephalic vein and radial artery in the forearm. Mark a transverse incision four fingerbreadths above the wrist in an adolescent—closer in a child—to keep the shunt clear of the wrist. Infiltrate the area with local anesthesia, and incise the skin. Do not place the shunt higher than necessary in case it must be replaced later. Use electrocoagulation for hemostasis.

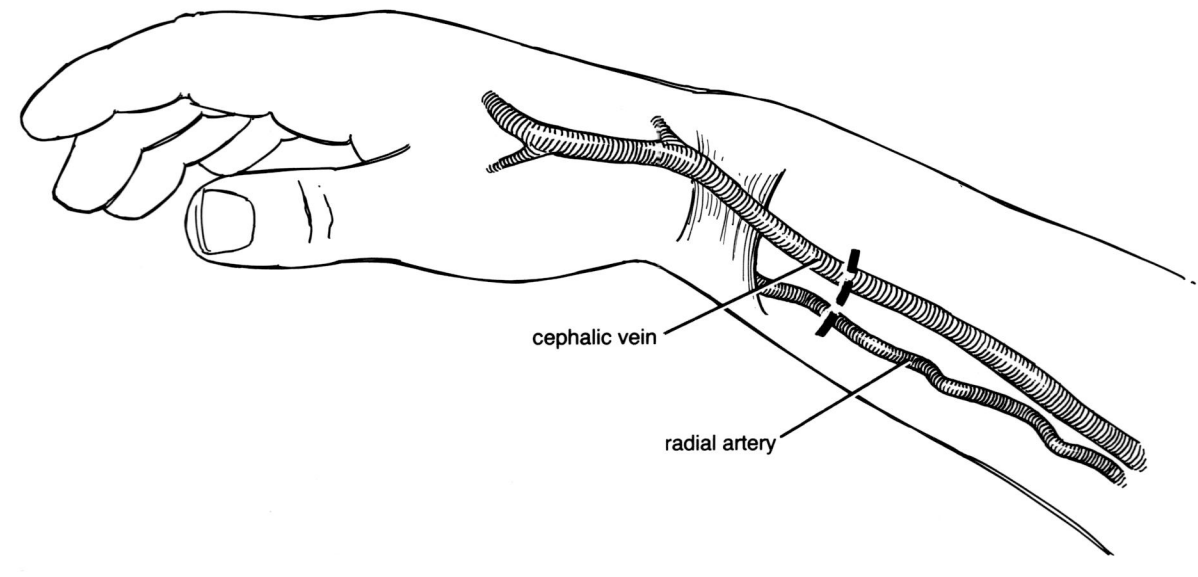

cephalic vein

radial artery

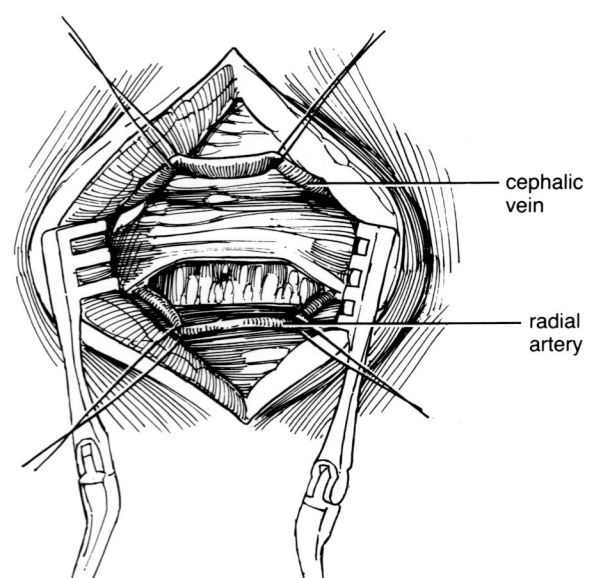

cephalic vein

radial artery

2 Isolate 1.5 to 2 cm of the cephalic vein using a mosquito clamp, and pass two 2-0 silk sutures around it. Palpate the radial artery through the antebrachial fascia, and incise the fascia longitudinally for 1.5 to 2 cm to expose the artery. Ligate any muscular branches with fine silk. Isolate a segment of the artery, and pass two ligatures of 2-0 silk around it.

3 Select the appropriately sized vessel tip for both vein and artery, and insert each into its trimmed winged shunt until the etched areas are within the tubing. Tie them in place with a 2-0 silk ligature, using three knots, then cut one end of the ligature. Fill the tubing with heparinized saline, and clamp the other end. Skill is needed to have the loop run easily through the incision in the skin and to prevent the cannulas from being kinked where they enter the vein or artery.

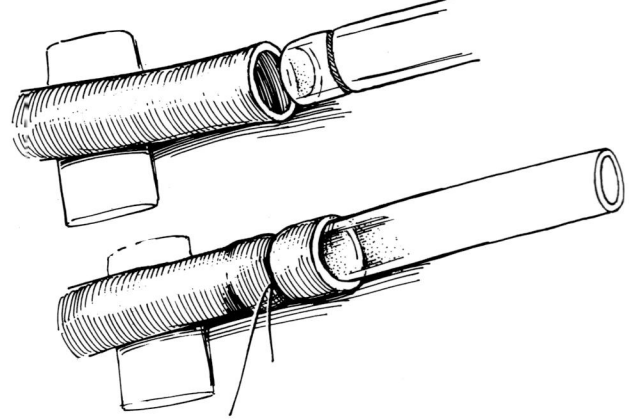

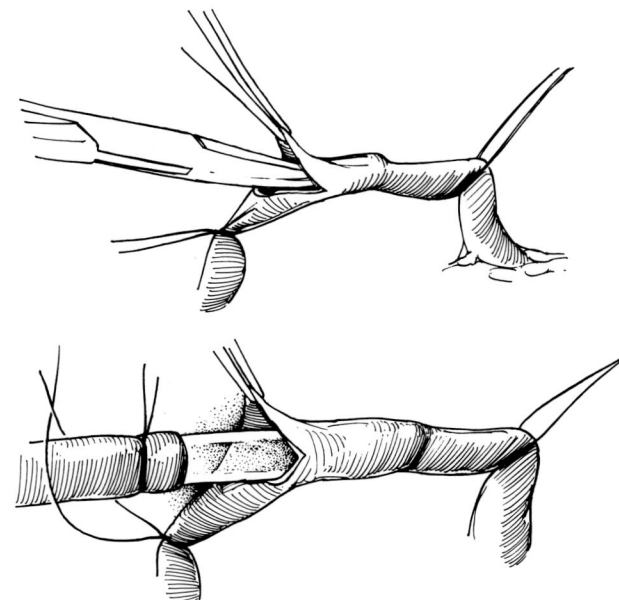

4 Return to the exposed cephalic vein and tie the distal ligature, leaving the ends long. Pass a #11 blade obliquely, halfway through the vein, keeping the cutting edge up. Lift the edge, dilate the lumen gently with a curved mosquito clamp, and insert the vessel tip.

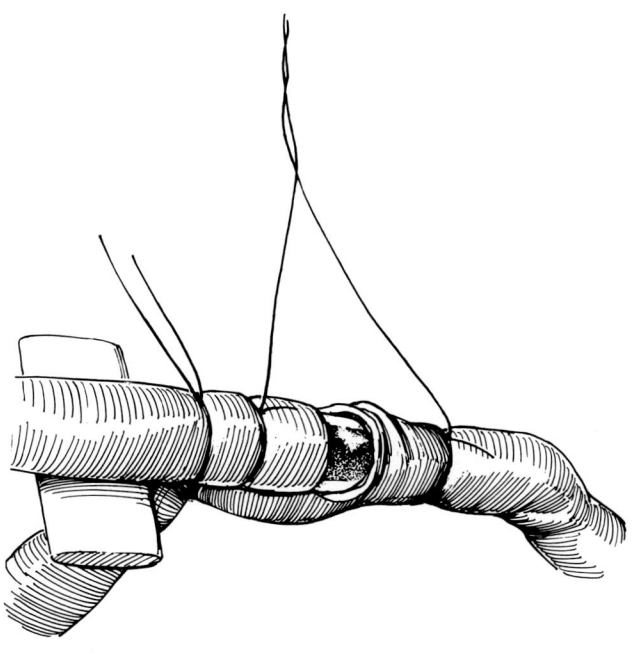

5 Tie the proximal ligature around the vein and vessel tip, and cut one end. Tie the other end to the remaining end of the ligature, holding the tip in the tubing. Pass the ends of the distal ligature around the shunt tubing, tie them, and cut the ends. Make a subcutaneous tunnel distal to the incision to seat the wings of the shunt. Irrigate the tubing with heparinized saline and reclamp it. For the radial artery, tie the distal ligature and leave it long. Put traction on the proximal ligature for hemostasis, and cut the artery as was done for the vein. Dilate the artery gently, and insert the vessel tip with attached shunt. Tie the ligatures as described for the vein.

6 Pass the shunt tubing from both artery and vein through stab wounds in the skin. Relax the traction ligature on the artery and let the tubing fill. Place the shunt connector to join the two assemblies, and fix it with shunt tape. Close the wound in two layers, using a running 4-0 synthetic absorbable suture for the skin. Alternatively, other wrist veins and the ulnar artery can be used.

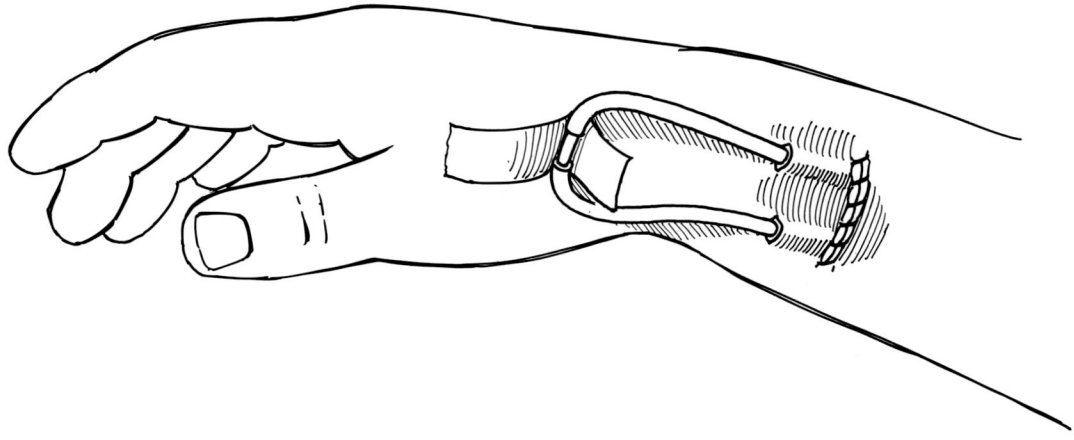

POSTOPERATIVE PROBLEMS

Clotting of the shunt in the early postoperative period is corrected by prepping the field and then separating the tubing at the connector. Pass a #3 Fogarty embolectomy catheter into the venous side, partially inflate it, and draw it out. Irrigate the tubing with heparinized saline on a plain-tipped syringe. Repeat the procedure on the arterial side, and reconnect the tubing. Mild anticoagulation will help, but recurrent thrombosis necessitates moving the shunt to other vessels.

Commentary by John M. Barry

Artery-vein shunts are rarely indicated in children. When hemodialysis is needed, place double-lumen catheters in the internal jugular, subclavian, or femoral vein. In children with adequate vessels in their extremities who require long-term dialysis, create arteriovenous fistulas with native vessels or with a subcutaneous synthetic graft.

PART III

KIDNEY EXCISION

CHAPTER 28

Simple Nephrectomy

For *retroperitoneal masses*, obtain a sonogram and an intravenous urogram. If the mass is renal and cystic, do a radioisotope scan. Nonfunction of the mass indicates multicystic kidney or advanced ureteropelvic junction (UPJ) obstruction. If functional, do a voiding cystourethrogram. Reflux identifies megaureter and duplication. Absence of reflux can mean UPJ or ureterovesical junction obstruction, duplication, or ureterocele. If the renal mass is solid by sonography, a computed tomographic (CT) scan is needed to detect Wilms' tumor, neuroblastoma, or mesoblastic nephroma.

Subject an adrenal mass detected by sonography to CT scan to differentiate solid neuroblastomas from cystic adrenal hemorrhage. The CT scan also will help identify retroperitoneal lymphomas and sarcomas. For Wilms' tumor, if CT scan and sonography show a unilateral tumor, proceed with nephrectomy. If nephrectomy is not possible, perform a biopsy preparatory to chemotherapy and delayed nephrectomy. If tumors are bilateral, perform a unilateral total and a contralateral partial nephrectomy or a bilateral partial nephrectomy; if that is not possible, obtain a biopsy preparatory to chemotherapy. In a solitary or fused kidney, do a partial nephrectomy or a biopsy if partial nephrectomy is not possible. For pyonephrosis, consider percutaneous drainage for 3 months before removing the kidney.

For renal carcinoma (rare in children) radical excision of the kidney with nodal dissection for malignancy appears not to add to the rate of cure. However, removal of tumor from the vena cava is beneficial.

Extracorporeal techniques have proved to be of value in few cases. In the past few years, partial nephrectomy has gained advocates who apply it not only to tumors in solitary kidneys but also to small tumors that are being diagnosed through widespread use of sonographic and scanning procedures.

SELECTION OF INCISION

For infants and children, the anterior subcostal incision usually provides the best exposure. For adolescents, a lateral approach (particularly the 12th rib supracostal incision) is most commonly used. However, the flexion that is required decreases vital capacity and venous return to the heart, and thus it may not be tolerated by obese patients. A further disadvantage is that the kidney is approached before the vessels can be secured. Flank wounds are more prone to subsequent muscular weakness from stretching the intercostal nerves. The advantages are (1) simplicity of the dissection through the flank and (2) the absence of organs or vessels in the retroperitoneum. The pleura and peritoneum are readily repaired, if entered. If the exposure proves to be limited, it can be increased by segmental resection of the overlying ribs (page 108). Good visualization of the kidney is obtained, making inspection and repair easy. Even the pelvis is well exposed when the kidney is rotated anteriorly. Closure in layers with dependent drainage makes for a secure wound.

The classic subcostal flank incision is better if reoperation is a possibility, although it has the disadvantage of often proving to be too low (page 87). The alternatives are resecting the 12th rib (page 90) or, better, going just above it through a supracostal incision (page 94). Entering above the 11th rib is not much more difficult and gives appreciably better exposure. Of course, the more extensive thoracoabdominal (page 102) and dorsal flap (page 108) incisions provide still better access to the renal area for large tumors.

An anterior approach, whether transverse (page 81), subcostal (page 87), or midline (page 83), provides superior exposure to the vascular pedicle of the kidney for renal trauma and neoplasm. Anterior approaches are somewhat more difficult than those through the flank and risk both injury to the viscera and later formation of intestinal adhesions. The upper pole is remote, and the renal pelvis lies under the renal pedicle. The peritoneal cavity may become contaminated if the urine is infected. Wound separation is more common than in flank incisions. A posterior approach through a dorsal lumbotomy is quicker and carries less morbidity but provides more limited exposure (page 112).

ANTERIOR SUBCOSTAL APPROACH

Give intravenous crystalloid fluids preoperatively. Have blood available in case of a vascular accident. Provide endotracheal anesthesia and adequate relaxation.

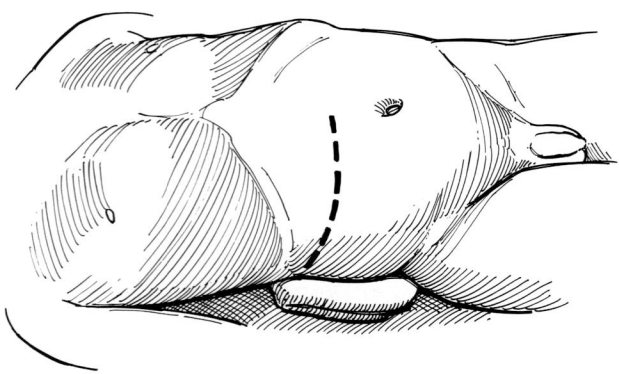

1 *Position*: Place the child on the operating table in a semioblique position, with a folded towel under the flank. *Incision*: Perform an anterior subcostal incision, as described on page 87.

2 Bluntly push Gerota's fascia medially off the psoas muscle, carrying the peritoneal reflection with it. Install a self-retaining retractor.

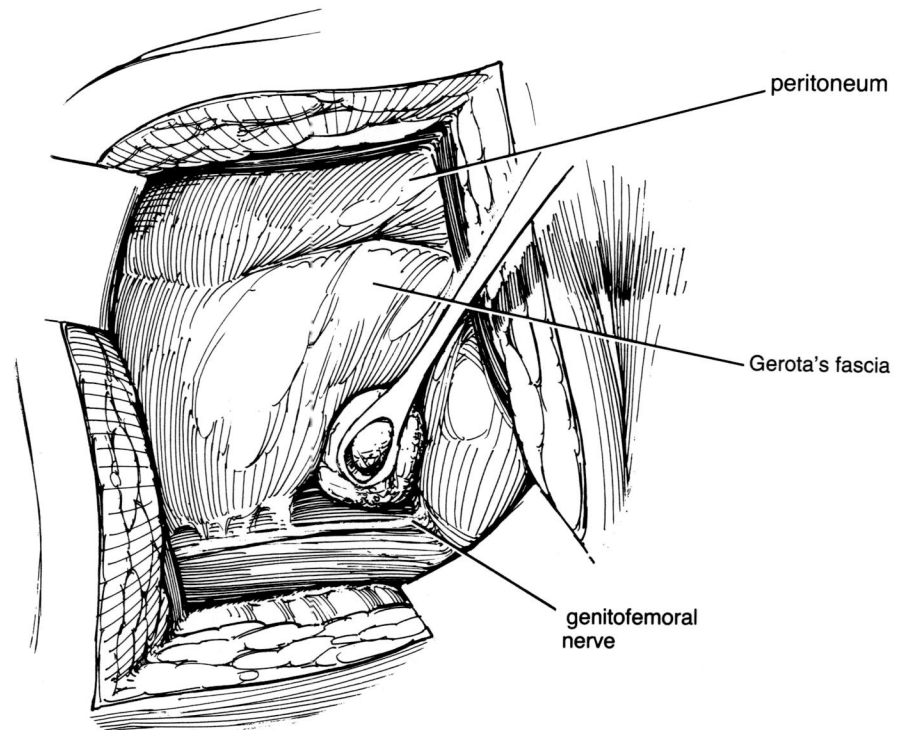

peritoneum

Gerota's fascia

genitofemoral nerve

3 Insert a Kelly clamp through Gerota's fascia into the pale, lemon yellow–colored perirenal fat. Open Gerota's fascia longitudinally with the scissors through the length of the incision. Fingers also may be used to separate the thin fascia.

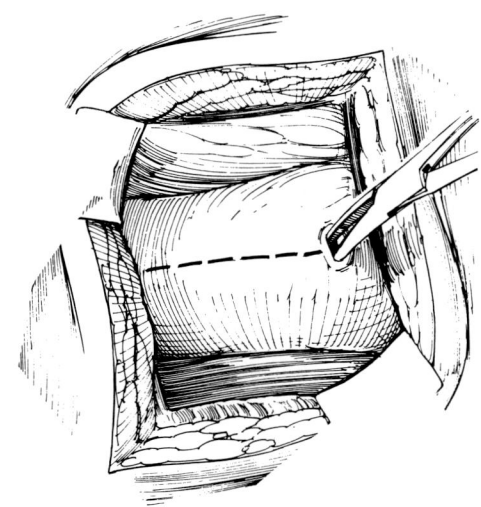

4 Bluntly and sharply dissect the perirenal fat from the lower pole of the kidney. Do the easy parts first, gradually working toward the more adherent areas. Take care ventrally where the peritoneum may be adherent. Open the peritoneum if adherent bowel is suspected. Gerota's fascia should be held medially in two curved clamps by the assistant. Watch for aberrant blood vessels, especially near the poles. An area resistant to dissection may well contain a vessel. Aspirate the contents of a large hydronephrosis to aid in exposure. Dissect sharply under vision near the pedicle. Fulgurate the emissary veins and do not dissect under the capsule. Identify the ureter on the peritoneal side of the wound. Free it with a right-angle clamp, and encircle it with a Penrose drain to allow it to be freed further. Be aware that the gonadal vein is readily torn.

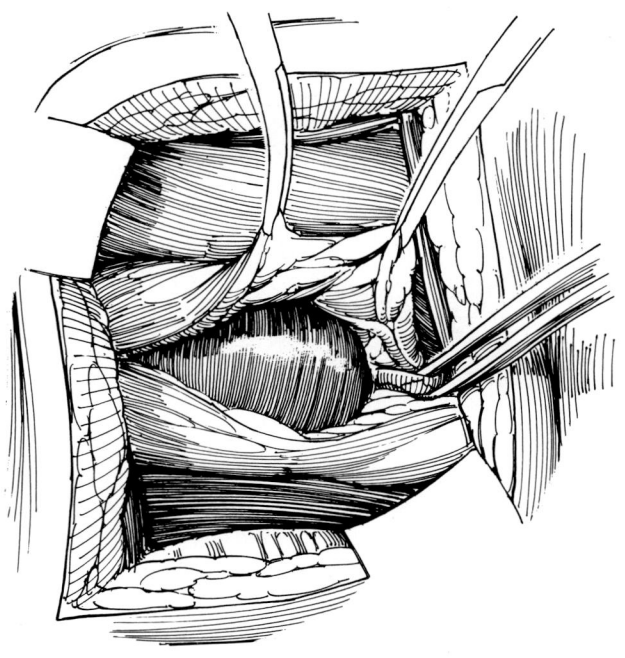

5 Doubly clamp and cut the ureter. Ligate both ends with absorbable suture material, leaving the proximal suture long enough for traction and identification. Dissect proximally along the ureter to free the pelvis.

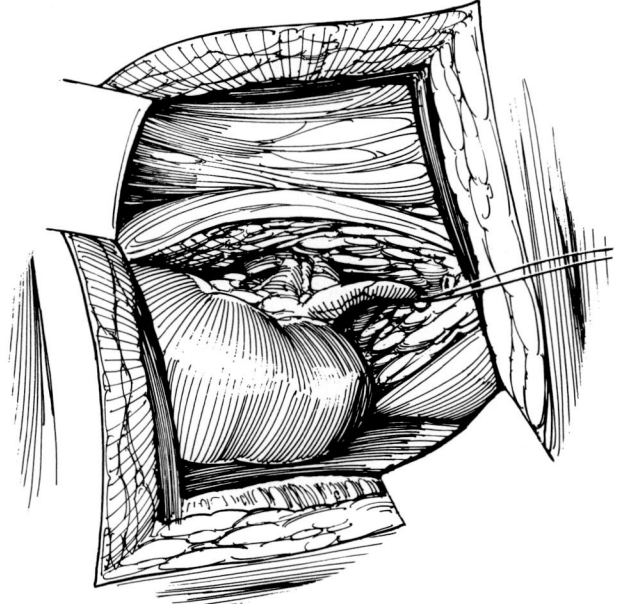

SECURING THE PEDICLE

Complete the dissection of the tissue anterior to the pedicle, trimming it approximately 1 cm away from the hilum. Identify the renal vein anteriorly, dissect it for a short distance, and encircle it with a vascular loop. If dealing with a neoplasm, remove obvious lymph nodes for staging (for radical nephrectomy, see Chapter 33). Start near the hilum, using sharp and blunt dissection to move the perihilar tissue medially to identify and dissect the artery.

6 A, One method of ligation is to doubly clamp the artery and divide it between clamps; do the same for the vein and remove the specimen.

B and C, Tie the artery with a 1-0 synthetic absorbable suture, reinforced with a second 1-0 synthetic absorbable suture as a stick tie. Ligate the vein with a 1-0 synthetic absorbable suture.

7 A preferable method of pedicle ligation, rather than to clamp the vessels, is to pass a right-angle clamp under the artery and draw two ligatures successively around it. Then, doubly ligate the artery. Do the same for the vein. If the right renal vein is short, use two Satinsky clamps on the vena cava and oversew the cuff after removing one clamp.

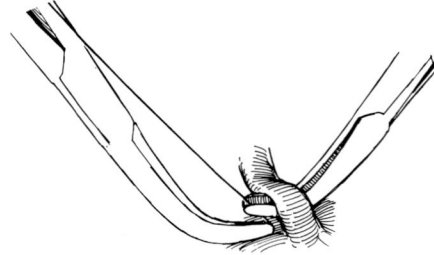

LOSS OF CONTROL OF THE PEDICLE

Remain calm. Palpate the source of the spurting blood to be able to compress the vessel digitally for 10 minutes. Alternatively, compress the artery and vein with a stick sponge. Take time to obtain a second suction line, more blood, and some 5-0 vascular sutures and vascular clamps. Tell the anesthetist of the situation. First, replace the blood loss. Do not clamp blindly, but get exposure, compress the aorta above the renal artery, and clamp the artery with a vascular clamp or try to visualize one end of the hole and put a suture in it. Tie the suture and hold it up as you put a stitch in the part that your assistant exposes next. Run the vascular suture up the defect and down again, as your assistant slowly rolls the packs away and you apply suction.

Alternatively, hold a finger over the hole and grasp the vessel with the tip of a Kocher clamp. Pulling up on it stops the bleeding so the vessel can be suture-ligated. For the vena cava, Allis clamps are adequate.

On a rare occasion, it may be advisable to close the wound around a clamp. In this case, return the patient to surgery for its removal, and be prepared to manage any further bleeding.

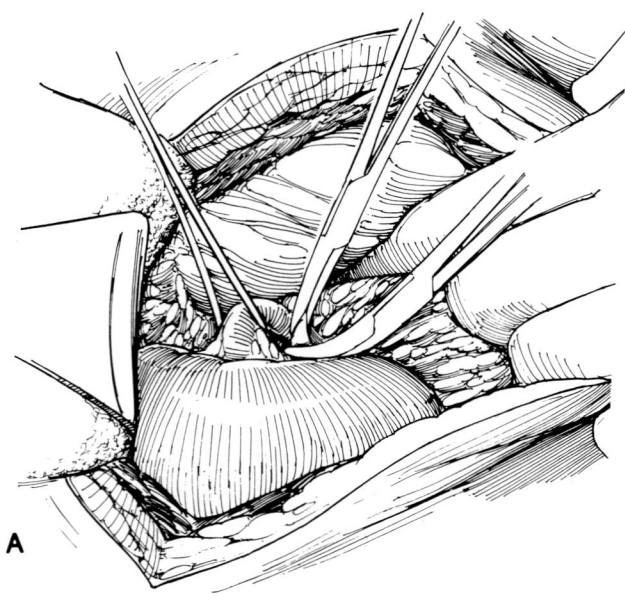

A

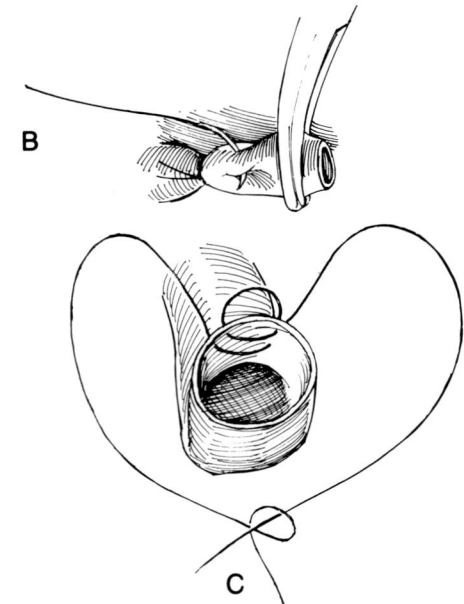

B

C

CLOSURE

Fill the wound with saline solution and look for bubbles, because the pleura might have been breached. If the pleura does require closure, proceed as described on page 83, and expose an upright chest film in the postanesthesia care unit. Beware of tension pneumothorax from either a torn pleural adhesion or an actual laceration of the lung. When the pleura is intact, insert a Penrose drain to be left for 24 hours to let the air and serum out of the wound and allow observation for bleeding. Inject 0.25 to 0.5 percent bupivacaine into the appropriate intercostal nerve, or insert a small feeding tube adjacent to the wound to allow subsequent bupivacaine administration. Close the wound with 3-0 or 4-0 synthetic absorbable sutures. If this is a secondary operation, insert the sutures in the muscle first, then tie them successively.

ANTERIOR TRANSPERITONEAL APPROACH

Divide the parietal peritoneum lateral to the descending or ascending colon. Enter the plane between the peritoneum and Gerota's fascia, and bluntly separate these structures until the aorta or vena cava is approached. For nonmalignant conditions, enter Gerota's fascia over the medial border of the kidney and expose the vein and artery. On the left side, secure the renal artery with a heavy silk ligature by retracting the vein caudad; on the right, secure it between the vena cava and aorta. Then the vein may be clamped, ligated, and divided. Place a second tie on the artery, divide it, and oversew the end with 4-0 arterial suture. The kidney can be easily removed inside Gerota's fascia. Drain the area through the flank by a stab wound.

SECONDARY NEPHRECTOMY

Have adequate blood available. Prepare the bowel. This is especially important in a child when the bowel may need to be resected.

Choose a new site for the incision, if possible, and be sure to give yourself enough exposure. The kidney will be adherent to the body wall; therefore, it is very easy to cut right into the kidney without realizing it. Open the peritoneum anteriorly to safeguard the duodenum and colon. One can even work transperitoneally.

Palpate the renal artery first, and approach it through the layers of tough fibrofatty tissue. Once you can get a right-angle clamp under the renal artery, draw a suture through and ligate it. The vein, if short, may require a Satinsky clamp, oversewn on the vena cava. Now free the upper pole, keeping close to the capsule to avoid the adrenal gland (also see "Subcapsular Nephrectomy," page 160).

POSTOPERATIVE PROBLEMS

Hemorrhage can arise from the renal artery, aorta, or vena cava. A vessel in spasm may be overlooked during closure. *Ileus* can be a problem secondary to retroperitoneal dissection about the celiac axis. Even after a flank approach, the patient should not resume oral intake until peristalsis returns.

Commentary by Charlotte Massad

Simple nephrectomy frequently is used for removal of small renal units (as in cases of multicystic dysplasia or reflux atrophy); therefore, small anterior subcostal, flank, or posterior incisions generally suffice. Serial aspiration of presenting cysts can facilitate the removal of even large cystic kidneys through a small incision. I generally do not obstruct the ureter early in the dissection of a functioning kidney, because the resulting dilation can interfere with the hilar dissection; rather, the ureter is isolated with vessel loop and followed proximally to the vessels without division until the arterial supply is interrupted. In infants, it is possible to perform a near total ureterectomy from an anterior subcostal incision, whereas older children generally require two incisions. I generally do not drain the retroperitoneum in the uncomplicated nephrectomy, because postoperative bleeding seldom is a problem.

Regional anesthesia is effective for postoperative pain relief for kidney surgery. In infants, high-volume caudal epidural bupivacaine (Marcaine) (with or without epinephrine or morphine) can be used, and in older children, lumbar epidural bupivacaine (either continuous or "one-shot") is safe and effective for regional analgesia. Of course, the bladder should be drained as long as these blocks are in effect, and if narcotics are used, respiratory monitoring is necessary.

Commentary by Fray F. Marshall

Simple nephrectomy usually is not performed for malignancies, including Wilms' tumor, for which the perinephric tissue with Gerota's fascia needs to be removed. Rupture of a tumor also is less likely if this is done. With improved radiographic techniques, especially CT, the necessity for exploration of the contralateral kidney may be less mandatory. In older children with larger tumors or large hydronephrotic kidneys, a flank approach can be considered. Most of the time, this lateral approach will not create significant respiratory embarrassment, even in obese patients. Subcostal incisions are sometimes low but allow transabdominal exposure, which sometimes is needed. We have not had to close a wound around a clamp, and we do not generally place drains following a nephrectomy.

Subcapsular Nephrectomy

Removal of the kidney inside the capsule seldom is needed in children in whom tissue planes are more readily dissectible. Should it be necessary, approach the kidney at a level different from the previous surgery (flank if previously anterior; 12th rib if previously subcostal). Be careful because the kidney capsule may lie just below the transversalis fascia so that the parenchyma will be entered easily owing to the lack of pararenal or perirenal fat remaining in this area. Before concluding that subcapsular nephrectomy is necessary, try separating the perirenal fat from the capsule with blunt dissection in the usual way. Only if this proves impossible, proceed subcapsularly. Incise the scarred perirenal tissue and the capsule from the lateral border medially to the hilum, and grasp the edge with a Mayo clamp. Insert a finger beneath this layer, and bluntly peel the capsule from the parenchyma, working anteriorly until the hilum is reached.

Draw back on the kidney while retracting the capsule medially. Palpate the renal artery; it is usually small. Incise the turned-back capsule directly in line with it.

Dissect the renal artery first, if possible, although it lies behind the vein. Triply ligate the artery in continuity and divide it. Treat the renal vein similarly. If separation of the vessels is not possible, place two pedicle clamps and divide between them. Rotate the kidney cephalad and place a Penrose drain around the ureter below the scar tissue. Divide and ligate it. Continue the dissection along the ureter to reach and free the renal pelvis. Remove as much perirenal tissue as feasible with the specimen. Close with adequate drainage, to be continued longer than that for an uncomplicated case.

Commentary by Fray F. Marshall

Subcapsular nephrectomy sometimes is performed for nephrectomy after renal transplantation, but it is not considered for any malignancy. If there has been significant infection or previous exploration, the easiest path of dissection may be subcapsular, although this approach is needed infrequently.

CHAPTER 30

Partial Nephrectomy

Consider partial nephrectomy for children with bilateral tumors or a tumor in a solitary kidney. The operation may be necessary in the presence of chronic renal failure. Partial nephrectomy provides functional renal reserve at the cost of a technically more difficult operation with a greater chance of local recurrence and more manipulation of the tumor.

Removal of the lower pole for stone disease in a thin-walled lower calyceal stump is a reasonable objective of partial nephrectomy. Calycopyelostomy with anastomosis of the opened lower pole calyx to the incised renal pelvis is an alternative.

For a complicated case, obtain a renal arteriogram. A computed tomographic (CT) scan will precisely delineate the extent of the tumor. This information will help not only plan the line of excision but detect major arterial disease.

Have the child well hydrated before occluding the arterial blood supply. If the problem might become complex, prepare iced slush for renal cooling. With a solitary kidney, if it will be severely stressed by ischemia, vascular access may be arranged preoperatively for postoperative dialysis (page 151).

Extracorporeal surgery for partial nephrectomy is an alternative for large tumors to avoid spillage and incomplete resection but rarely is necessary, and it carries a higher risk. After removing the kidney *in toto*, cool it and flush the main artery with iced Ringer's lactate solution until clear. Remove the tumor, avoiding injury to the major vessels and ureter. Take special care not to interfere with the vessels supplying the ureter and renal pelvis. Perfusion via artery or vein helps identify vascular branches. After closing the collecting system and parenchyma, transplant the kidney into the iliac fossa.

Bilateral tumors require preliminary node dissection with frozen-section biopsy examination before proceeding. Perform radical nephrectomy on the most-involved side and a partial nephrectomy on the other kidney. Preserve at least one of the adrenal glands. A better alternative may be to proceed in two stages, preserving renal tissue on one side at the first operation, giving chemotherapy, and then preserving as much as feasible on the other side at a later operation. It is even possible to take a third look. Note that with asynchronous bilateral tumors, one of them probably represents a metastasis.

Make preparations for cooling, even though warm ischemia time seldom exceeds 30 minutes. Start intravenous (IV) mannitol administration (see "Radical Nephrectomy").

1 **A**, *Position*: Lateral, over a kidney bolster. *Incision*: A supracostal incision is best for adolescents, but a pediatric extended anterior incision is suitable for children. If autotransplantation is a possibility, use an anterior approach (Chapter 9).

With the flank approach, open Gerota's fascia in the lateral plane, and free the entire kidney. Leave the perirenal fat around the tumor undisturbed.

B, Dissect the vascular pedicle sufficiently to allow use of vascular clamps. Place a vascular tape around the artery. Dissect the vessels entering the hilum, especially those leading to the involved portion of the kidney.

Palpate for hilar nodes (left para-aortic for left-sided tumors; right paracaval for the right) if the operation is for carcinoma, and send suspicious nodes for frozen-section examination.

Inspect the kidney to determine the practicality and the site of heminephrectomy. To determine the line of demarcation, place a bulldog clamp temporarily on the identified artery and observe for blanching. IV indigo carmine dye may give a line for resection. Place a vascular tape around any accessory vessels. Ligate and divide polar vessels that directly supply the segment to be removed. The plane of excision must follow the radial direction of the renal segments.

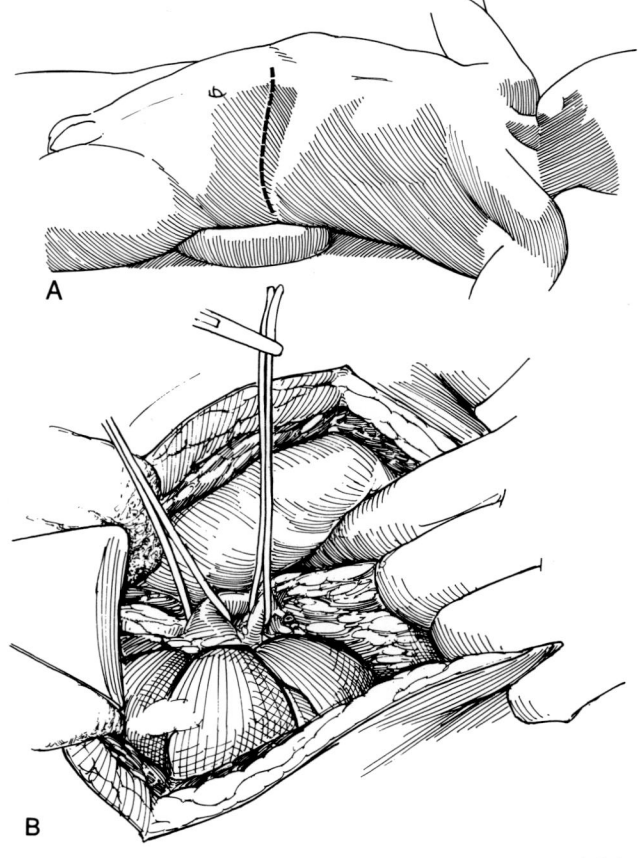

A

B

POLAR PARTIAL NEPHRECTOMY

2 Apply a padded rubber dam, clamp the artery in a padded clamp, and cool the kidney, unless ischemia time is estimated to be less than 30 minutes. Ask the anesthetist to inject furosemide or give 20-percent mannitol IV. Incise the capsule 1 to 2 cm distal to the site of the proposed resection, unless this is over tumor, in which case, move the incision proximally. Reflect the capsule from the normal parenchyma with the back of the knife.

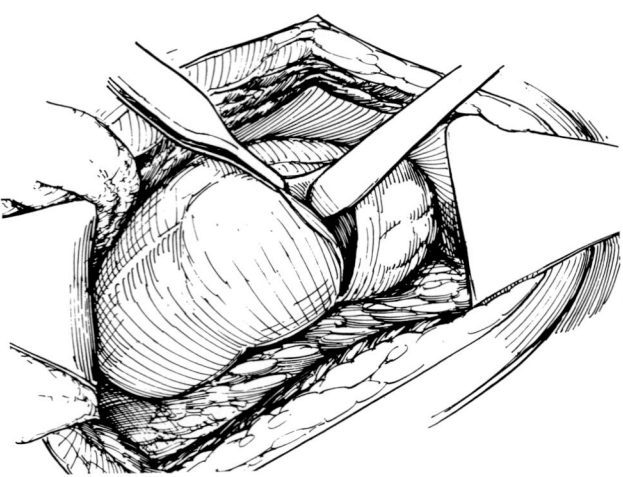

4 Bluntly incise the parenchyma, using the knife handle, leaving 1 cm of normal tissue on the side of the tumor. Follow the normal plane (neither guillotine nor wedge) between the renal lobules. Progressive slices may be removed if the disease process extends more proximally, unless dealing with carcinoma, in which case it must be treated by nephrectomy.

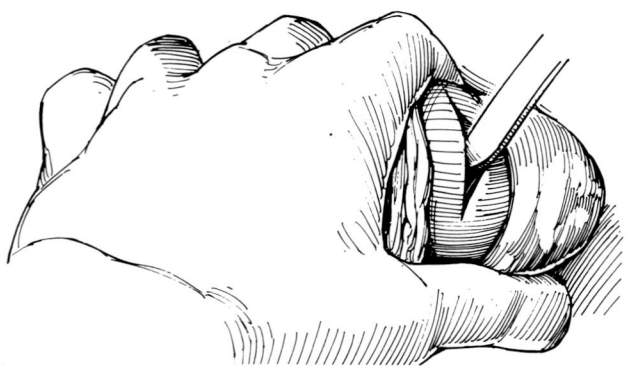

3 Place a rubber-shod bulldog clamp on the artery. In some cases, finger compression of the parenchyma may substitute for vascular clamping. It is not necessary or desirable to clamp the renal vein if the main renal artery is occluded.

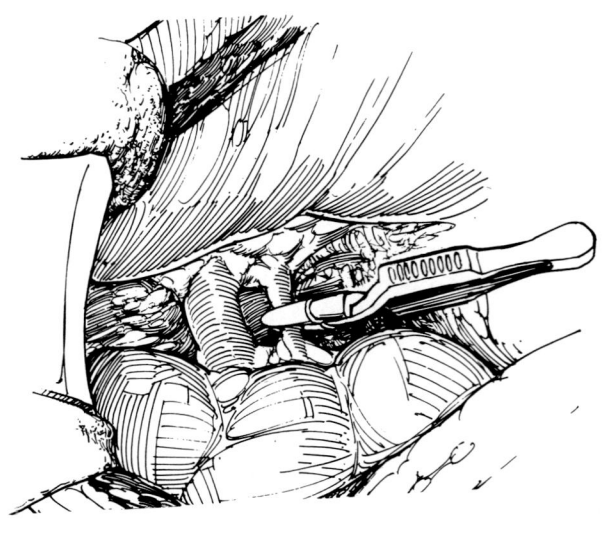

5 Use the thumbnail, if desired.

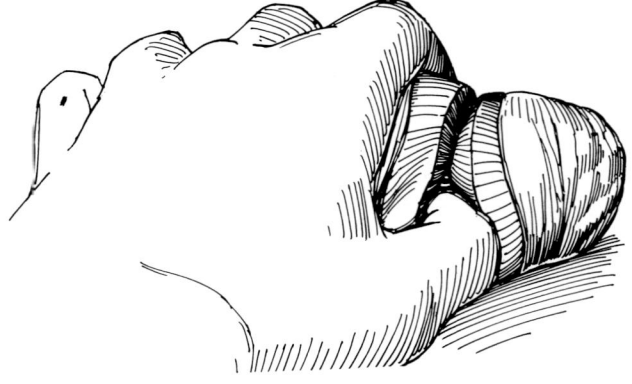

6 Sharply divide the arcuate vessels with Lahey scissors and suture-ligate them with figure-eight, 4-0 or 5-0 chromic catgut sutures. Cut each calyceal infundibulum with knife or scissors. Excise them as distally as possible in stone cases.

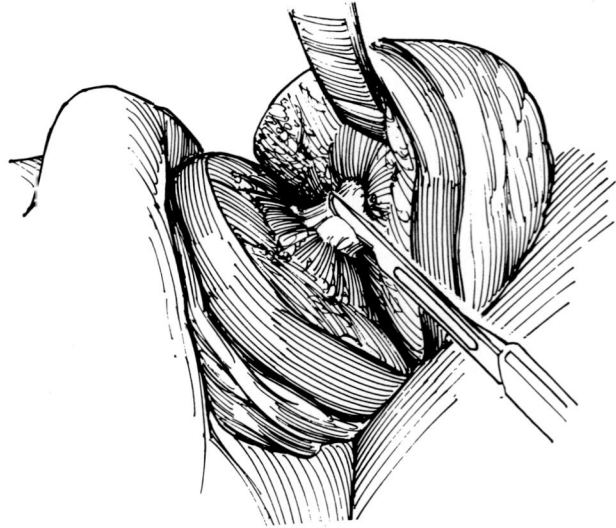

7 Suture-ligate all remaining arcuate vessels, paying special attention to the large venous collectors near the hilum. Work rapidly but accurately. Electrocoagulation cannot be used because of the electrolytes in the urine, although argon-beam laser coagulation, if available, may be effective. Ligate the interlobar vessels with sutures that include the adjacent infundibulum. Release the bulldog clamp momentarily to allow identification and ligation of remaining open vessels. Place a self-retaining ureteral stent, if desired. Close the infundibulum with a 4-0 or 5-0 continuous synthetic absorbable suture to make the suture line watertight. If the operation is for a tumor, send specimens of appropriate margins for frozen-section examination.

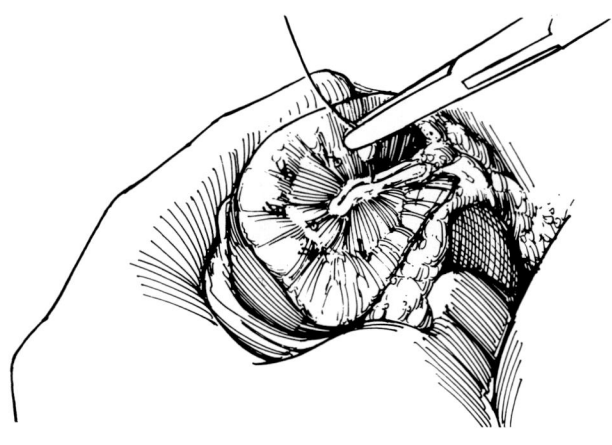

8 If possible, close the kidney on itself (it will be limp because the artery is clamped), or close the capsule alone, using 3-0 or 4-0 chromic catgut mattress sutures; enclose fat pads obtained from the properitoneal fat in the loops. A free peritoneal graft can substitute for an inadequate capsule, or pull the omentum through the retroperitoneum and apply it as a wrap. Absorbable collagen may be applied for hemostasis. Release the bulldog clamp, and compress the kidney at the suture line for several minutes to ensure hemostasis. If this does not stop the bleeding, an arterial branch was not controlled and the kidney must be cooled after arterial clamping and reopened. If urinary output decreases after release of the clamp, give furosemide IV. Perform a nephropexy to keep the lower pole away from the ureteropelvic junction and ureter.

Suture a Penrose drain adjacent to the repair by the long-suture technique (page 127), or, less desirable, place a closed suction drain to exit through a stab wound. Close Gerota's fascia to cushion the repair inside perirenal fat. Complete the wound closure. Drain for at least 7 days. If leakage does occur, perform a retrograde ureterogram and place a J stent.

Within the 1st postoperative month, obtain a sonogram and CT study of the kidney as a baseline, and follow with sonograms every 3 months for the first 2 years.

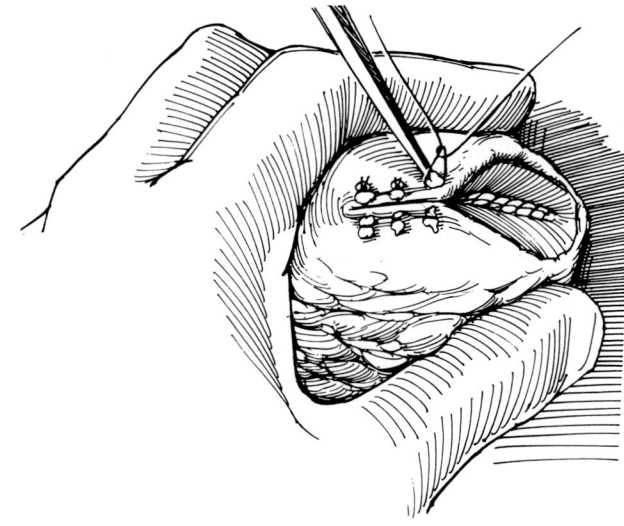

WEDGE RESECTION FOR PERIPHERAL TUMORS

9 Incise the capsule 2 cm away from the tumor margin. Consider clamping the renal artery if the resection will be extensive.

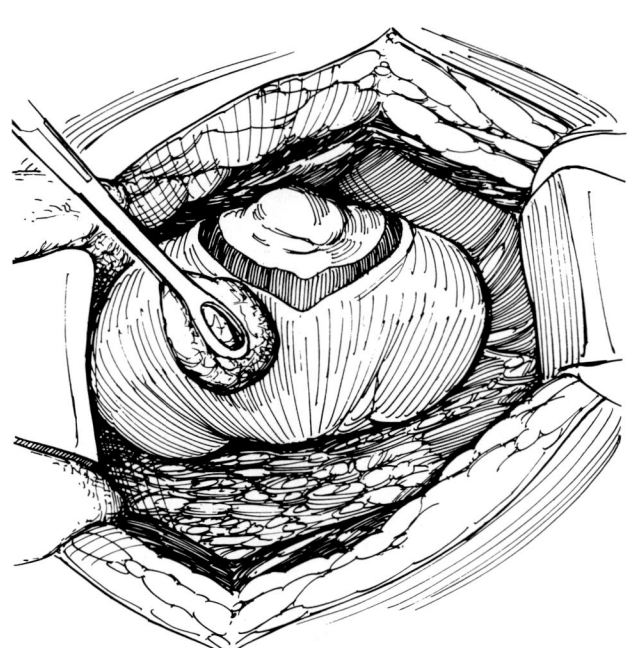

10 Remove a wedge by following the nephrons to include normal parenchyma beyond the tumor. Secure hemostasis by suture ligation, as previously described.

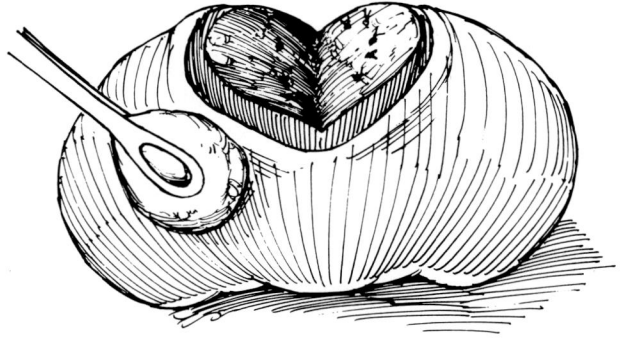

11 Before closing the collecting system, insert an internal stent. **A,** Close the defect with mattress sutures and fat bolsters to the capsule.

B, If the defect is large, fill it with retroperitoneal or omental fat.

C, Suture the two poles together or apply hemostatic gauze or a free peritoneal graft.

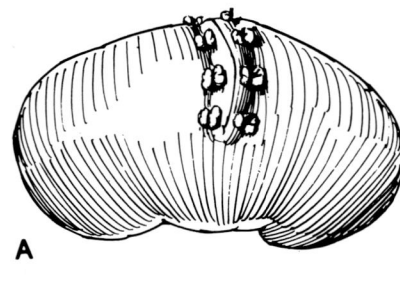

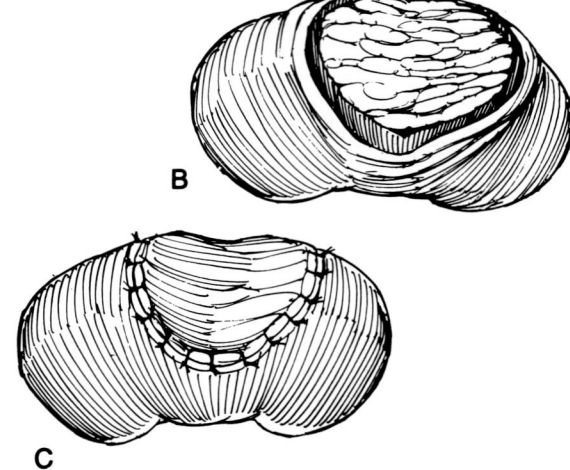

ENUCLEATION

Enucleation is done for a very small tumor and is the only possibility for a patient with multiple tumors in a solitary kidney. However, malignant cells may extend into the pseudocapsule and lead to local recurrence. Rather than simply enucleating, remove a layer of normal parenchyma, if it can be done without entering a major vessel or calyx. Vascular control is not needed.

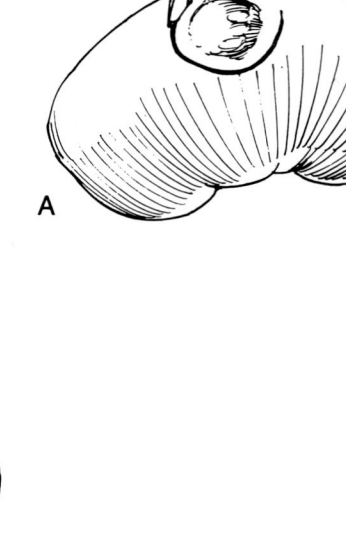

12 **A** and **B,** Incise the capsule around the tumor. Bluntly enucleate the tumor by following the plane outside the compressed pseudocapsule of fibrous renal tissue, which is relatively avascular. The calyces are not entered. Fulgurate the false capsule, preferably with an argon-beam laser, and pack it with oxidized cellulose or omentum, as necessary, to control oozing. Close the capsule as in other techniques.

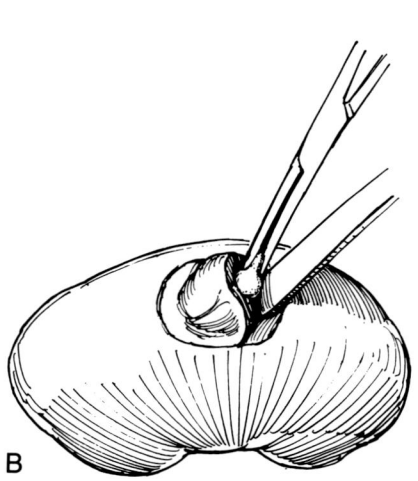

POSTOPERATIVE PROBLEMS

If leakage occurs, look for *distal obstruction. Urinomas* and *fistulas* are uncommon but occur with wedge resections that are closed with large mattress sutures. A resection following the plane of the lobules followed by closure of the calyx with a watertight suture is best. Placement of a ureteral catheter rarely is necessary.

Wound infections can occur and often follow operations done in the presence of infected stones. *Renal artery thrombosis* and *damage to the intima* are rare

traction complications. *Secondary nephrectomy* is reported in fewer than 3 percent of cases. A brief period of *renal insufficiency* may follow partial nephrectomy in a solitary kidney, and gradually decreasing renal function may occur later in children with reduced renal parenchyma as a result of hyperfusion.

Commentary by Fray F. Marshall

Partial nephrectomy often is considered when a child has a ureteral duplication and dysplastic upper pole segment. Resection along the collecting system often is helpful in this circumstance, after radiologic investigation has been made of the entire duplicated system.

In partial nephrectomy for tumors, extracorporeal surgery rarely is necessary. It is associated with a somewhat higher risk, especially with a solitary kidney. If operations are required on both kidneys, sometimes these procedures are better staged than performed at the same time. Sequential operations reduce the likelihood of postoperative dialysis.

In terms of technique, the renal artery and vein can be occluded together, because, particularly on the right side, venous bleeding can be significant. To help delineate segments of the kidney, the renal artery never is injected directly, because that arterial segment can be injured. If delineation of various segments of the kidney is necessary, a bulldog clamp can be placed on one branch of the renal artery, and systemic methylene blue can be given IV. To facilitate hemostasis, we have employed the argon-beam coagulator in some instances. It is very important to delineate the collecting system, including injecting it with dilute methylene blue. We have not used double-J stents in our partial nephrectomy patients. Rather than a Penrose drain, we have used closed urinary drainage. We have not recommended enucleation except in the rare circumstances of small multiple tumors or with von Hippel-Lindau disease.

Commentary by Barry A. Kogan

Partial nephrectomy is an important procedure in pediatric urology. I use it primarily in cases of bilateral Wilms' tumors. I believe a CT or magnetic resonance imaging scan is essential to help preoperative planning but almost never find a need for renal arteriography. Although I agree that ischemia time rarely exceeds 30 minutes, I do pay particular attention to careful isolation of the vessels, cooling of the kidney during ischemia, and administration of mannitol and/or furosemide several minutes prior to clamping. Because most of my cases are for bilateral Wilms' tumors, I generally would perform these via a transabdominal approach, although a flank incision in selected cases is easier and less morbid.

From a technical standpoint, after removing the tumor and ligating the larger vessels, I generally lay a piece of thrombin-soaked Gelfoam in the bed prior to closing the kidney and capsule over the top. In peripheral lesions, it often is possible to avoid clamping the artery, and the illustrations demonstrate nicely that vascular control in these cases can be obtained by pressure on the kidney from the assistant's hand. I have not had occasion to place a ureteral catheter in these cases, but if the resection were extensive enough, it might be appropriate.

CHAPTER 31
Pediatric Heminephrectomy

Pediatric heminephrectomy is an operation for the diseased upper pole in duplicated systems.

1 *Position:* Place the infant supine with the involved side slightly elevated. *Incision:* Make an anterior subcostal extraperitoneal incision (page 79). Open Gerota's fascia posteriorly, and mobilize the usually scanty fat anteriorly to free the entire kidney. Rotate it anteriorly and expose the upper-pole ureter, pelvis, and renal pedicle from behind. The line of demarcation usually is obvious on inspection and palpation.

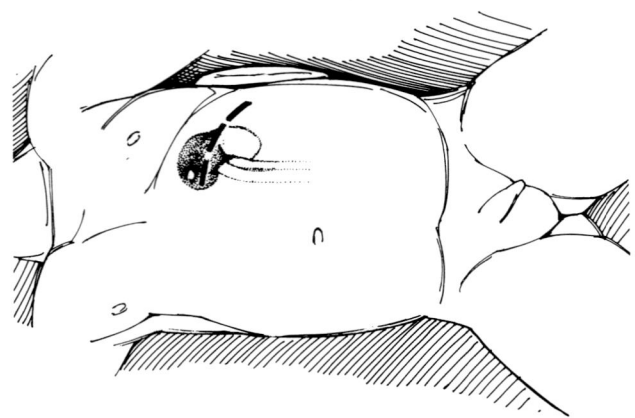

2 Identify both ureters and trace the larger one to the upper pole. Free this ureter from its bed as distally as is feasible, at the same time avoiding interference with the blood supply of the other ureter. Divide it but do not ligate the distal stump (especially if it is infected) unless it has refluxed. Place a traction suture or clamp on the proximal end and pass it under the upper-pole vessels, taking great care not to avulse small branches to the upper pole. Lifting the ureter helps identify the vessels before division while completing the proximal dissection into the hilum. Locate and dissect out the blood supply to the upper segment. If a vessel is not clearly separate from those going to the rest of the kidney, pass a 4-0 synthetic absorbable suture around it, occlude it with traction, and note the area of blanching. If you see that it is a part of the upper pole that becomes ischemic, tie the suture and divide the vessel. It seldom is necessary to occlude the main blood supply; if it is, give intravenous mannitol before applying the clamp.

Note the deep groove between upper and lower moieties and the difference in thickness and color of the parenchyma. Feel for the pulsation of the arteries to the lower pole. Incise the renal capsule circumferentially 2 cm distal to the now-obvious line of demarcation, and peel it back with a knife handle.

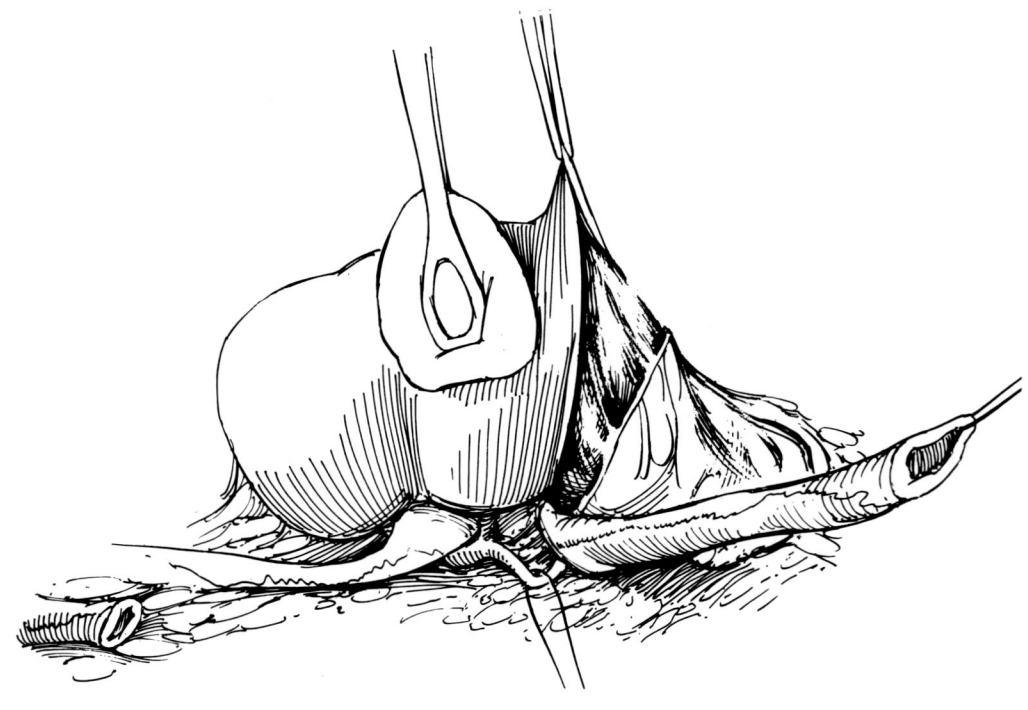

3 Transect the renal parenchyma with a knife blade or cutting current, knife handle, or scissors along the plane of demarcation, which will be found to be concave. Sharp dissection is needed because of the fibrous character of the parenchyma. Insert the index finger into the upper-pole renal pelvis; this helps identify the plane between the upper and lower pole. If in doubt, err on the side of leaving some upper-pole tissue behind. The residual upper-pole tissue and portions of calyces may be trimmed later. As the separation proceeds, place a figure-eight 4-0 synthetic absorbable transfixion suture on any major vessel, especially on those associated with the calyx and pelvis. Remove the calyceal lining if it is not contained in the specimen. Avoid opening into the upper calyx of the lower segment; if done, close the calyx with a running 4-0 synthetic absorbable suture.

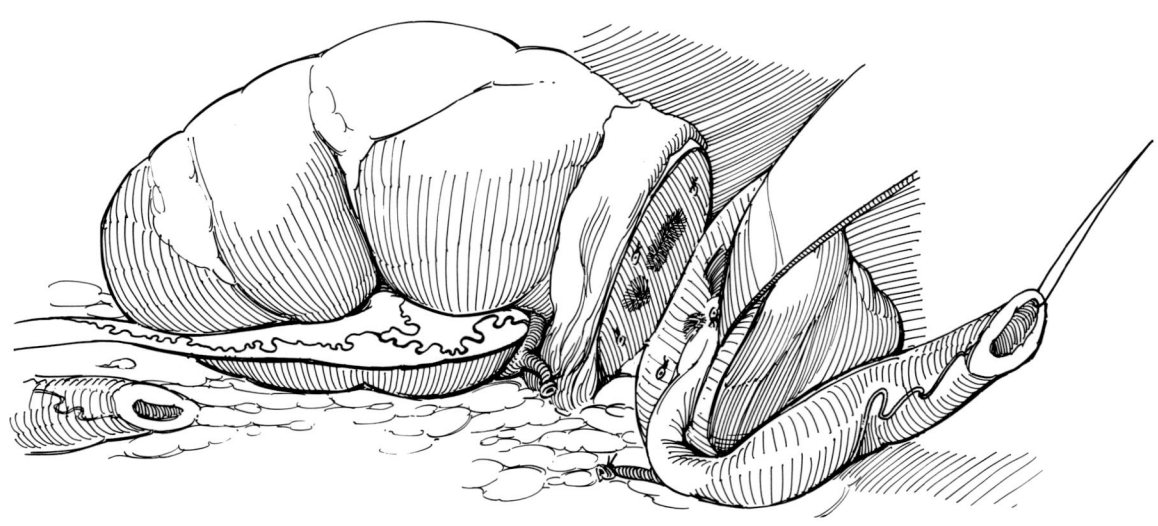

4 Close the capsule over the exposed parenchyma with a running 4-0 synthetic absorbable suture. Place a mattress 3-0 synthetic absorbable suture over fat bolsters in the capsule of the posteroinferior surface of the kidney to suture the mobile residual kidney to the posterior body wall as a nephropexy to maintain the renal axis and prevent torsion of the vasculature of the remaining segment and kinking of the relatively redundant lower-pole ureter. Tack a Penrose drain adjacent to the area of transection by the long-suture technique (page 6), reapproximate the perirenal fat and Gerota's fascia, and close the wound in layers.

For the rare case requiring lower-pole heminephrectomy, the procedure is similar, except that extreme care must be taken to preserve the vascular supply to the upper pole, which usually is a branch from the main vessel to the lower pole.

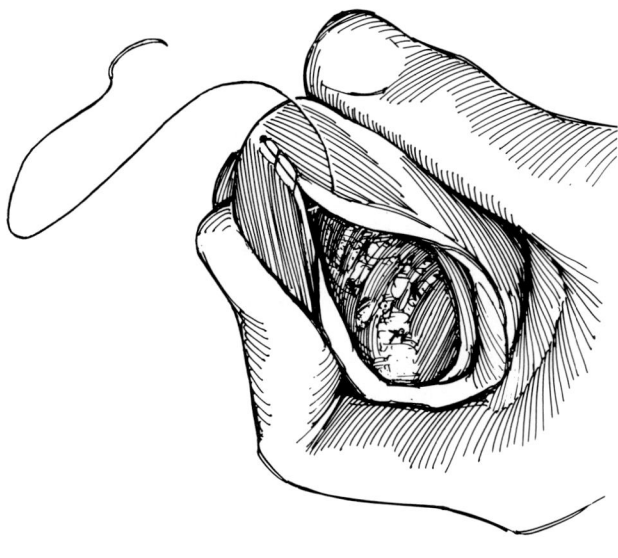

Commentary by Terry W. Hensle

In general, heminephrectomy in the pediatric patient is done for problems associated with duplication anomalies such as ectopic ureterocele and, less often, ectopic ureter. Often, the ureter associated with the upper pole is very large, and the upper pole itself is very small and frequently dysplastic.

It is of utmost importance for the surgeons to have adequate exposure of the upper pole to perform this procedure safely. It cannot be obtained adequately by putting downward traction on the ectopic ureter. Complete dissection and mobilization of the upper pole avoid disrupting small feeding branches to the upper pole, which can be avulsed by the traction method of exposing upper-pole lesions.

Great care also must be taken when transposing the transected upper-pole ureter upward. Frequently, there are small feeding vessels associated with the main blood supply to the upper-pole segment. These can easily be disrupted or avulsed simply by pulling the upper-pole ureter beneath the upper-pole blood supply on a traction suture. The upper portion of an abnormal ureter should be cleaned carefully to make sure that all of the small branches have been either ligated or electrocoagulated prior to transposing the ureter.

If the surgeon takes care with good exposure initially and adequately deals with collateral blood supply, the operation goes along rapidly and without excess tissue trauma or blood loss.

CHAPTER 32

Nephroureterectomy With Node Dissection

THORACOABDOMINAL APPROACH

Obtain an intravenous urogram to visualize a filling defect; obtain a computed tomographic scan to rule out a nonopaque stone. Tissue for cytologic examination can be obtained from voided urine or, better, from a brush biopsy specimen.

For renal pelvic carcinoma, nephroureterectomy is indicated. In doubtful cases, ureteropyeloscopy can visualize the tumor. If doubt remains, inspect the pelvis or calyx by open or percutaneous methods and do a biopsy. In a solitary kidney, resect and fulgurate the tumor endoscopically. For an upper- or midureteral lesion, excise and reanastomose the ureter. For a lower-ureteral lesion, resect the ureter and reimplant it in the bladder after taking a frozen section from the cut end. If the tumor is of a high grade, do a nephroureterectomy.

The purpose of nephroureterectomy is removal of the kidney, ureter, and bladder cuff in continuity, including the regional lymph nodes. The operation can be done through one or two incisions. If the ureter contains the tumor, reverse the order of the operation, and approach the ureter first.

POSTOPERATIVE PROBLEMS

Pneumothorax can occur if the chest tube fails to function. *Urinary drainage* through the bladder incision is rare.

Commentary by Thomas S. Parrott

Nephroureterectomy for a tumor rarely is indicated in the pediatric population. Transitional-cell carcinoma (TCC) of the renal pelvis or ureter is infrequently encountered in infants and children. There are only five reported cases of TCC arising from the renal pelvis in children through 1975. Rarely, Wilms' tumor patients will have ureteral metastases, in which case partial ureterectomy should be performed *en bloc* with the renal specimen. Whether it is better to remove a cuff of bladder in such circumstances, as for transitional-cell tumors, has not been proved. When large, bulky transitional-cell tumors are encountered in the older child, the thoracoabdominal approach with node dissection, as outlined in this chapter, should prove quite satisfactory. Because most transitional-cell tumors are not massive, the need for routinely opening the chest in children, with its increased morbidity, is suspect. The subcostal transabdominal approach, used routinely in Wilms' tumor cases, should prove best in most cases. The issue of whether to remove interaortocaval nodes in addition to those nodes overlying and lateral to the ipsilateral great vessel is controversial when dealing with children. With longer life expectancy, the issue of ejaculatory impotence, which can accompany complete node dissection, becomes important. In the absence of a clear mandate for total retroperitoneal node removal, the modified approach, as recommended by many for testis tumor, would seem prudent.

I totally agree that the two-incision approach is preferred in infants and children. The bladder incision can be made in a low transverse fashion, as for ureteral reimplant surgery. Subcutaneous flaps are developed, and the midline is entered vertically. The operator stands on the patient's opposite side from the tumor, mobilizes the peritoneum medially, then divides the round ligament (in females) or mobilizes the spermatic cord (in males). The next landmark is the obliterated hypogastric artery (lateral umbilical ligament), which is divided as it crosses over the ureter. Ureteral mobilization is thus enhanced by identifying and dividing this structure. Usually, the dissection from above is encountered at this point, and the tumor specimen is brought down into the lower exposure. The bladder may then be opened as described.

One cannot stress enough the importance of dividing renal hilar tissue between clips or ligatures. Never try to cauterize this lymphatic tissue, because lymphatic leakage is apt to occur, and chylous ascites may complicate the postoperative course. The use of Penrose drains for the kidney incision is optional; however, it usually is best to drain a bladder incision through a separate stab.

CHAPTER 33

Radical Nephrectomy

CHOICE OF INCISION

The single most useful incision in children is the pediatric extended incision. Although it takes longer to make than a flank incision, it does provide better exposure and has the advantage that the chest is not entered. It is not necessarily the most suitable incision for a very large tumor in older children (especially if the lesion is at the upper pole, in which case a thoracoabdominal incision is needed). An anterior transperitoneal approach does allow early control of the arterial blood supply and, consequently, the least blood loss, but a vertical incision has certain disadvantages compared with a transverse one: it is 30 times weaker, it requires placement of stay sutures in a debilitated patient, it is more prone to allow splenic injury, it fosters adhesions, and it provides poorer renal exposure. If tumors are bilateral, it is advisable to operate on the second side at another time.

RIGHT TRANSVERSE APPROACH

1 **A,** *Position:* Right semioblique. *Incision:* Extended pediatric anterior incision (page 79). The surgeon stands on the right. Open the peritoneum fully. Insert a Balfour or ring retractor while packing the liver and gallbladder superiorly. Palpate the abdominal viscera and nodes. Shifting the liver medially is made easier by incising the lateral ligaments. Pack the liver superiorly, but avoid injury to the underside.

B, Retract the ascending colon medially. Pick up the parietal peritoneum, and incise it over the kidney near the colon. Extend this incision from the aortic bifurcation to above the renal pedicle. With large tumors, the peritoneum covering the kidney often is infiltrated by the tumor. Consequently, incision becomes difficult. It may be advisable to begin the incision at the caudal end of the tumor, where the layers are intact. If the tumor has grown in the direction of the colon, detachment may be difficult. Avoid injury to the mesocolon.

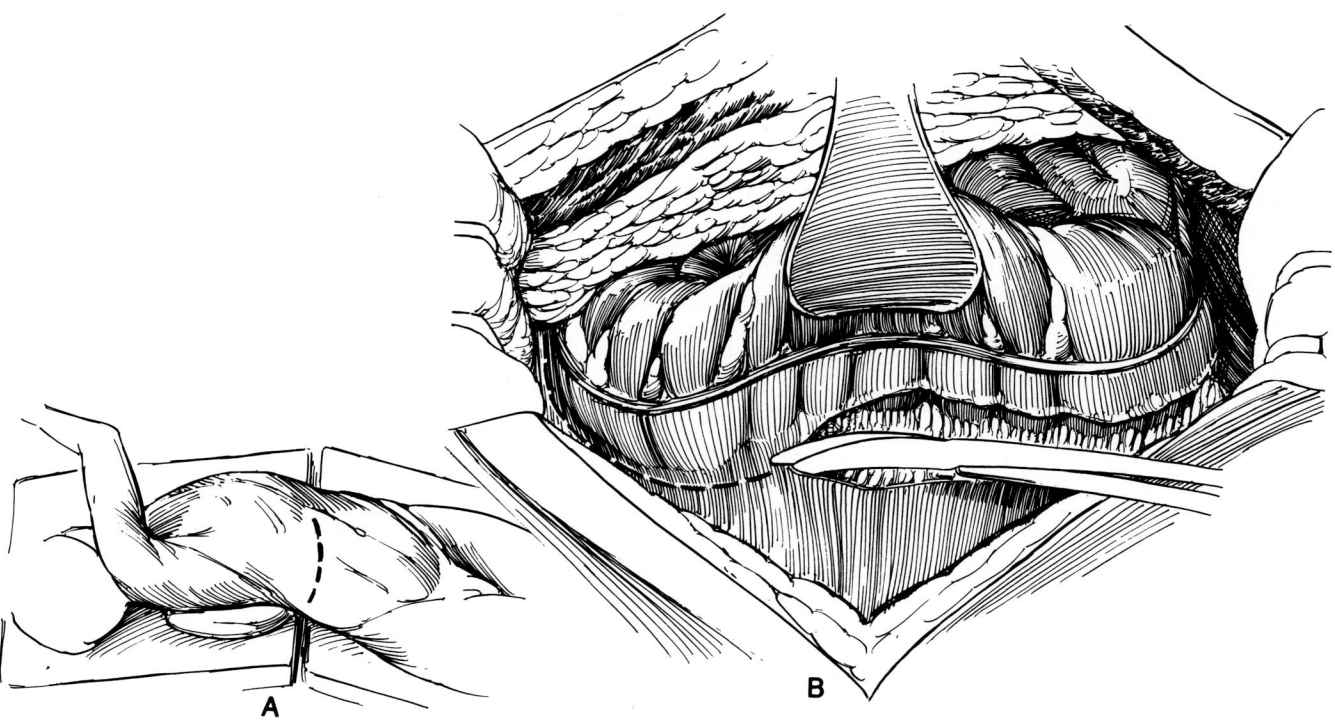

A

B

2 Mobilize the hepatic flexure of the colon and kocherize the duodenum by blunt dissection. The second part of the duodenum may be closely connected to the tumor. Detach it as follows: (1) carefully divide the connecting fibers by sharp dissection, and only then begin blunt dissection. Here there is danger of injury to the duodenum with necrosis and perforation as a consequence; (2) in this region, do not coagulate—at the most, use only bipolar coagulation; (3) if the duodenum is lacerated, repair it in three layers around a tube brought out through a stab wound; (4) if the duodenal injury produces an expanding intramural hematoma, clamp and ligate the bleeding vessel, then close the serosa; (5) hold the bowel medially with retractors over moist laparotomy tapes; (6) place laparotomy tapes over the inferior edge of the wound and hold them with a retractor blade; (7) beware of injury to the liver from inadequately padded retractors—repair it with interrupted horizontal mattress sutures; (8) it is very important to occasionally moisten the bowel and to watch it for compromised circulation.

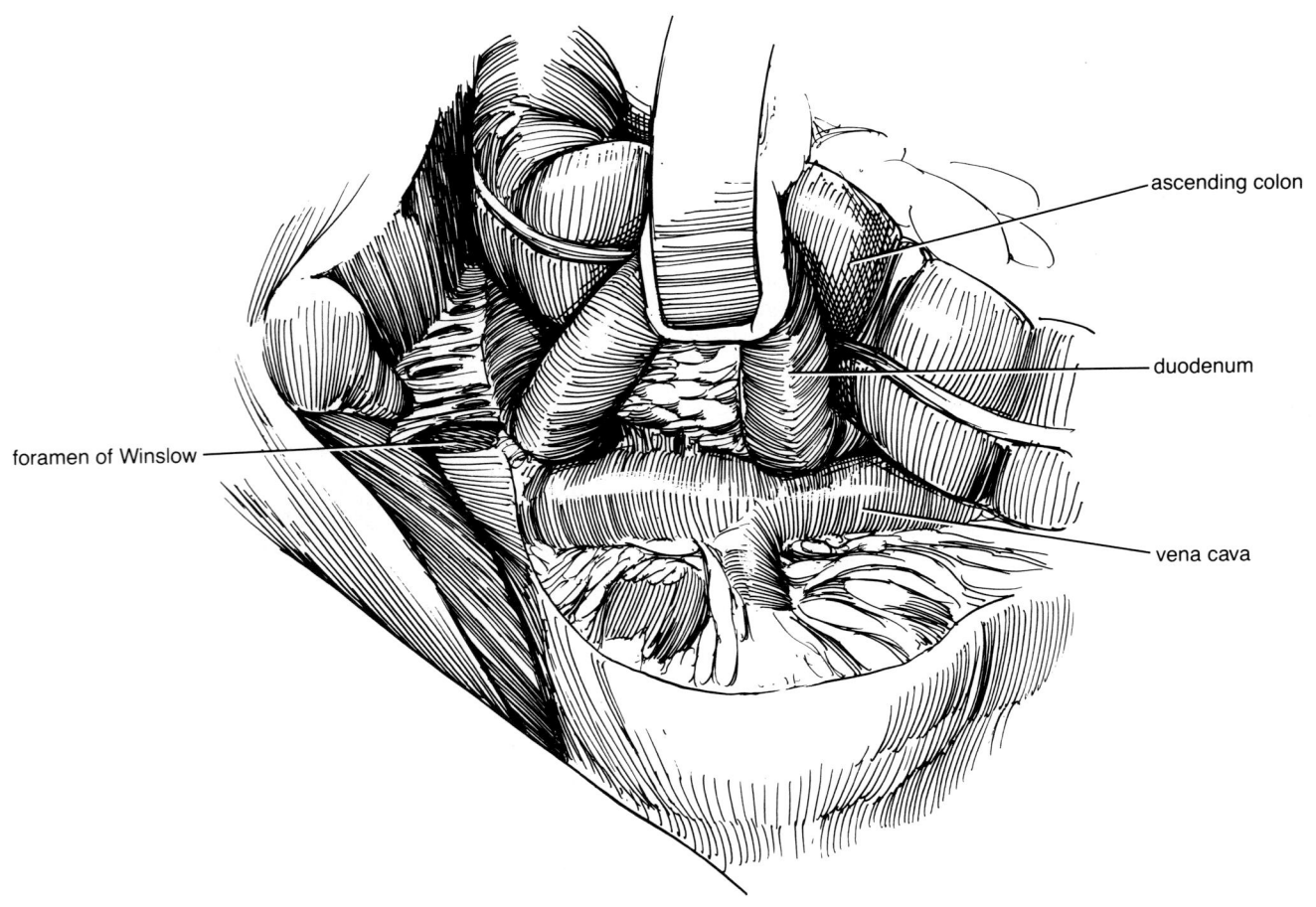

ascending colon

duodenum

foramen of Winslow

vena cava

3 **A,** Dissect on the left side of the vena cava, and free the left renal vein. Keep close to the anterior surface of the aorta to avoid the lumbar veins. Palpate, then expose the right renal artery by elevating the left renal vein and gently retracting the vena cava toward you. For large tumors that overlap the vena cava, it is easier to begin the dissection of the cava in the caudal region, below the lower pole of the kidney, then slowly work up, while applying clips on the aortic side of the vena cava.

B, Pass a right-angle clamp beneath the right renal artery, grasp a ligature, pull it through, and tie it close to the aorta. Place a second suture and tie it. Clamp and divide the artery, and ligate the distal end. A suture tie may be placed on the proximal stump. A better method may be to put one tie on the artery and proceed to divide the vein before completing ligature of the artery. **C,** Dissect the right renal vein. If the vein is large, the dorsal dissection of the renal vein with a right-angle clamp can be tricky. Beware of injury to the vein from too-aggressive drilling on the hidden dorsal side. Carefully dissect it by spreading

the clamp. Palpate the vein gently for any firmness, suggesting a tumor thrombus. (For management of a thrombus, see page 180.) Watch for the entrance of the main adrenal vein into the vena cava. If it is avulsed, grasp the stump with an Allis clamp, and close it with a running 5-0 vascular suture. Alternatively, place one Satinsky clamp, then place a larger one beneath it; remove the top one, and oversew the stump. If the adrenal is injured, oversew the edge.

Watch for lumbar veins that come into the renal vein or vena cava at this level. When they are encountered, pass a ligature on a right-angle clamp, and tie the large renal vein. With any large tumor infiltrating in the region of the hilum, it is advisable to apply a Satinsky clamp to the vena cava and to oversew the cut venous stump secondarily. Dissect the vein distally, then clamp, divide, and ligate it. Leave the distal suture on the renal vein sufficiently long to be used later by the pathologist for purposes of identification.

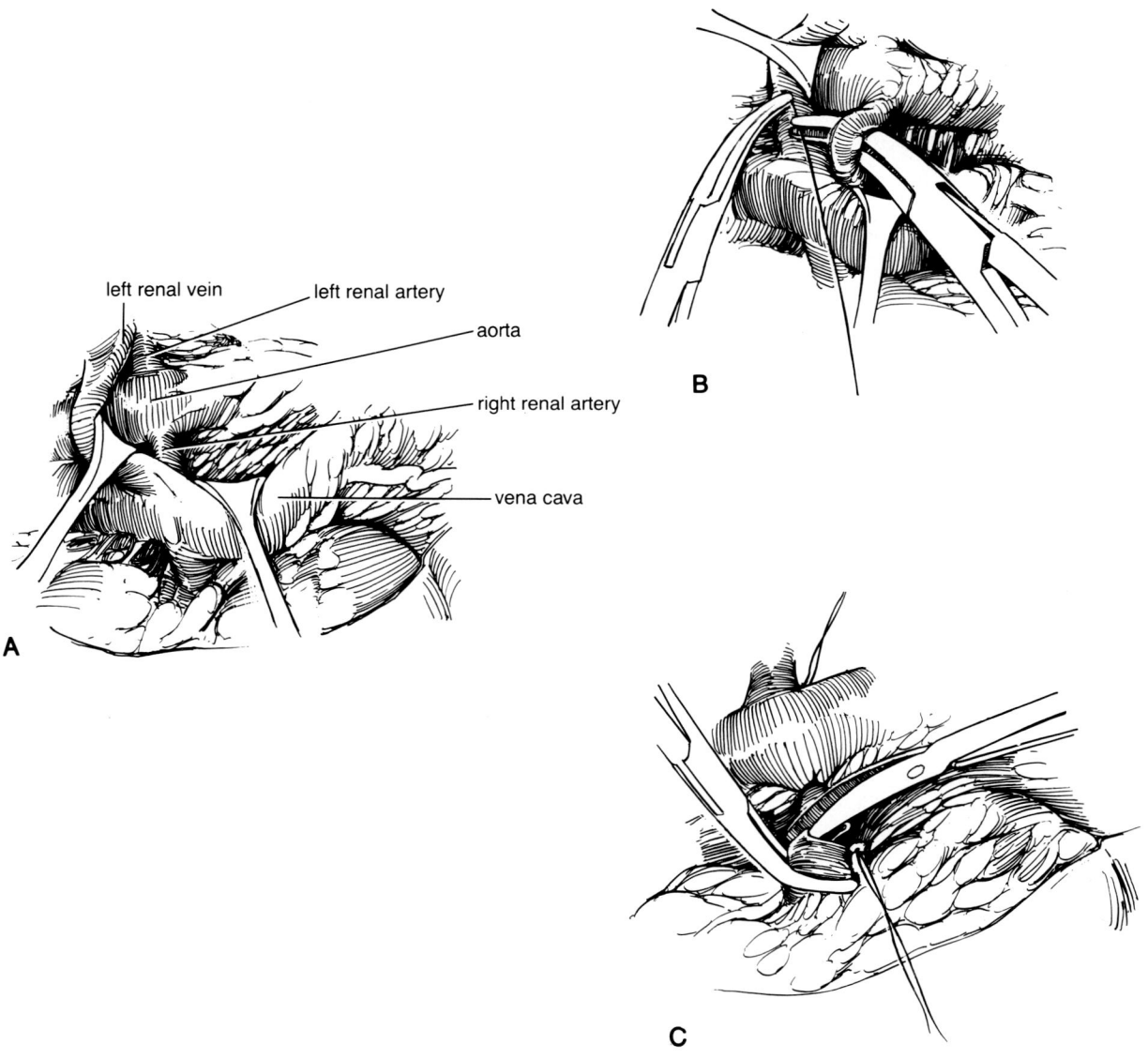

left renal vein left renal artery

aorta

right renal artery

vena cava

A

B

C

4 Clear the anterior surface of the vena cava, and ligate the gonadal vein. Free the lymphatic tissue from the vena cava, moving in a lateral direction toward the right. Clip all lymphatic vessels.

Mobilize the ureter and gonadal vein bluntly to the level of the bifurcation of the aorta. Lift them into the wound; clamp and ligate them with 1-0 silk ligatures, leaving the proximal suture long enough for identification later. If ureterectomy is to be done for transitional cell neoplasms, free the distal end as low as is feasible; divide and tag it for recovery from below. Pick up the lateral edge of the peritoneum below the tumor, and incise it vertically up to the liver, then medially to just above the adrenal gland.

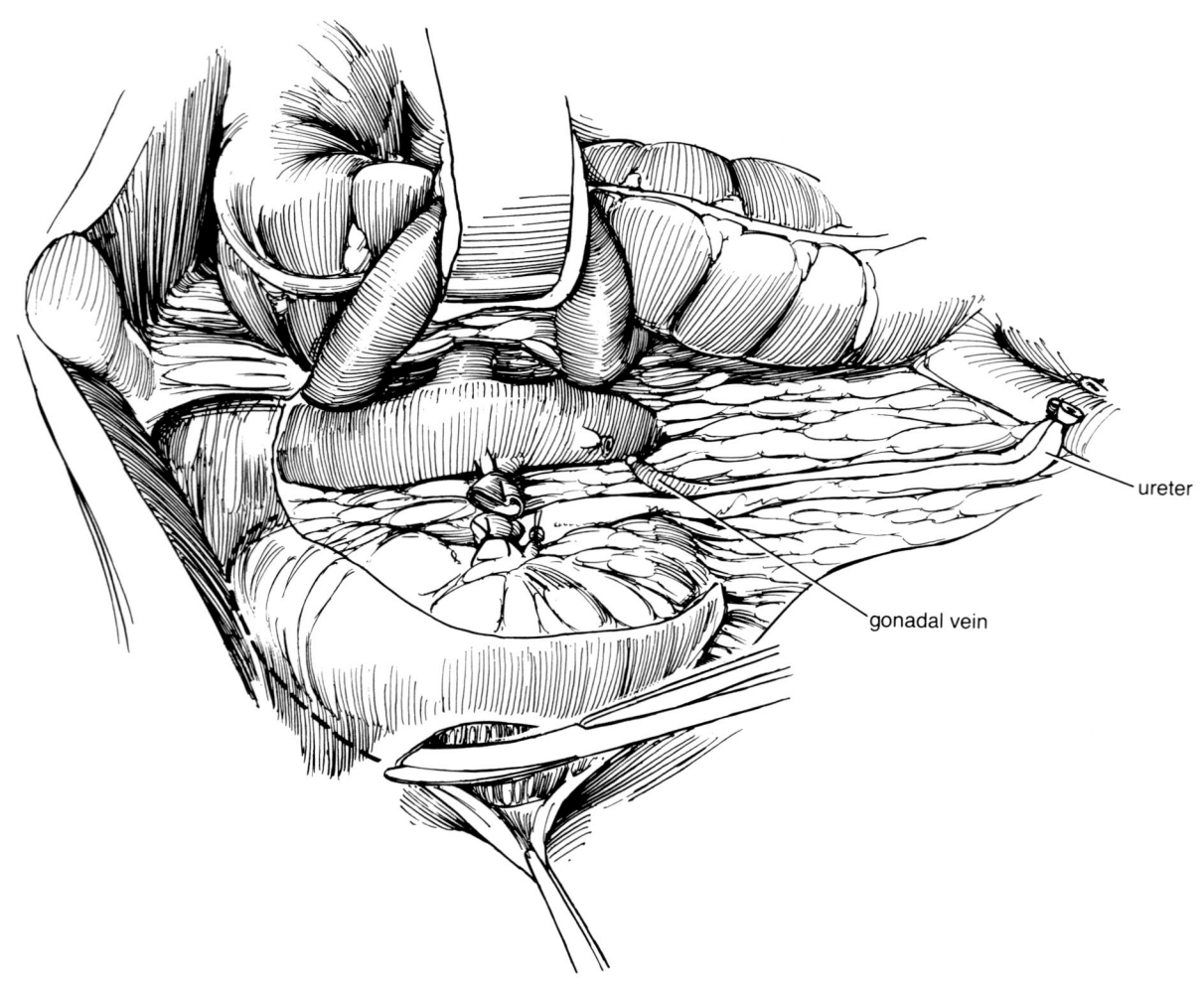

ureter

gonadal vein

5 Lift the lower pole of the kidney with the left hand, and mobilize Gerota's fascia that encloses the kidney from the posterior body wall. Clip small vessels as they are encountered, and doubly clamp and ligate large collateral veins. Alternatively, clip these veins with large clips.

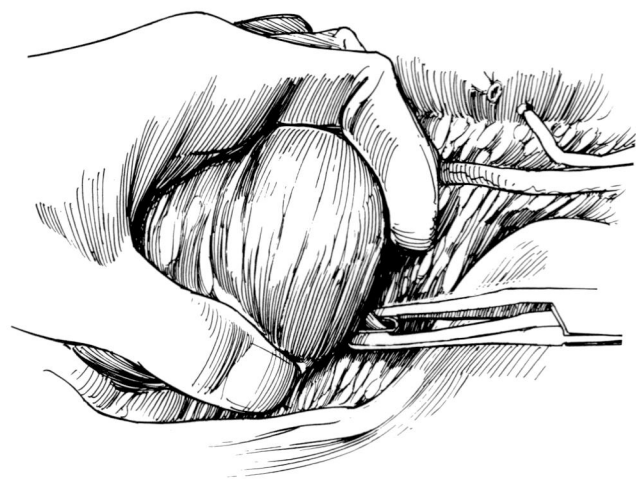

6 Pull down on the upper pole of the kidney to expose the adrenal gland, as the connective tissue and vascular and peritoneal attachments are progressively divided. Dissection is easier if one proceeds laterally along the posterior body wall toward the crus of the diaphragm. The cranial connections to the adrenal gland must be divided carefully step-by-step between clips. Clip the small vessels and especially the lymphatics. If the tumor is restricted to the lower pole, adrenalectomy is not necessary, but it is necessary with all tumors of the upper part of the kidney.

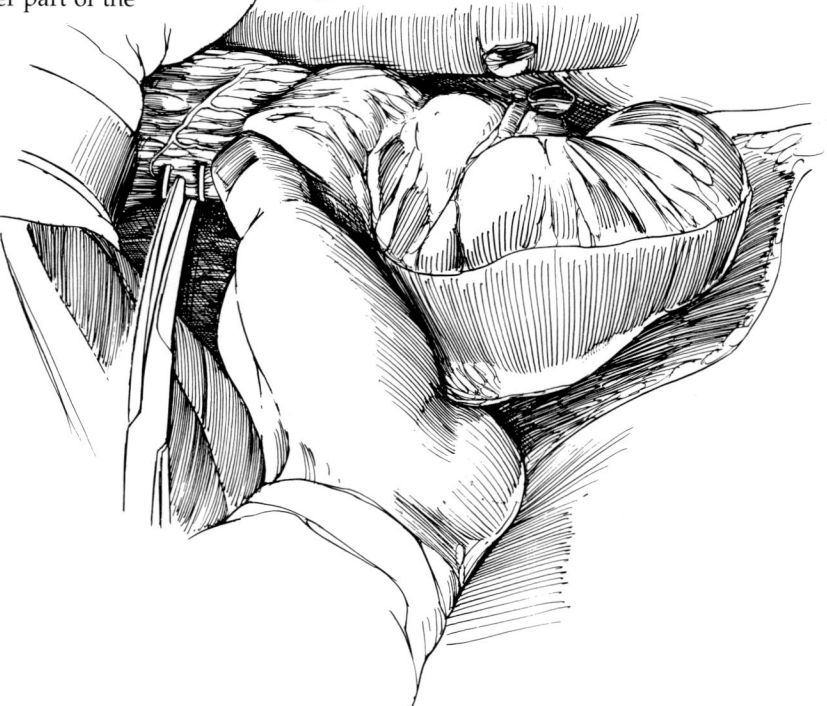

7 Displace the kidney caudally and laterally to visualize the vena cava and expose the right adrenal vein, which is divided between ligatures. Avoid the small veins bridging between the liver and vena cava, but clip and divide the lymphatics and small adrenal arteries. Unresectable tumors are those with medial extension to the aorta, vena cava, superior mesenteric vessels, and celiac axis. It is of little use to excise part of the tumor; complete removal provides the patient's only chance for cure.

Remove the tumor mass. It may be sensible to oversew the stumps of the renal artery and vein with 5-0 arterial silk. Close the defects in the mesocolon to prevent internal hernias. Check blood pressure; if below normal, anticipate possible bleeding from small vessels now in spasm.

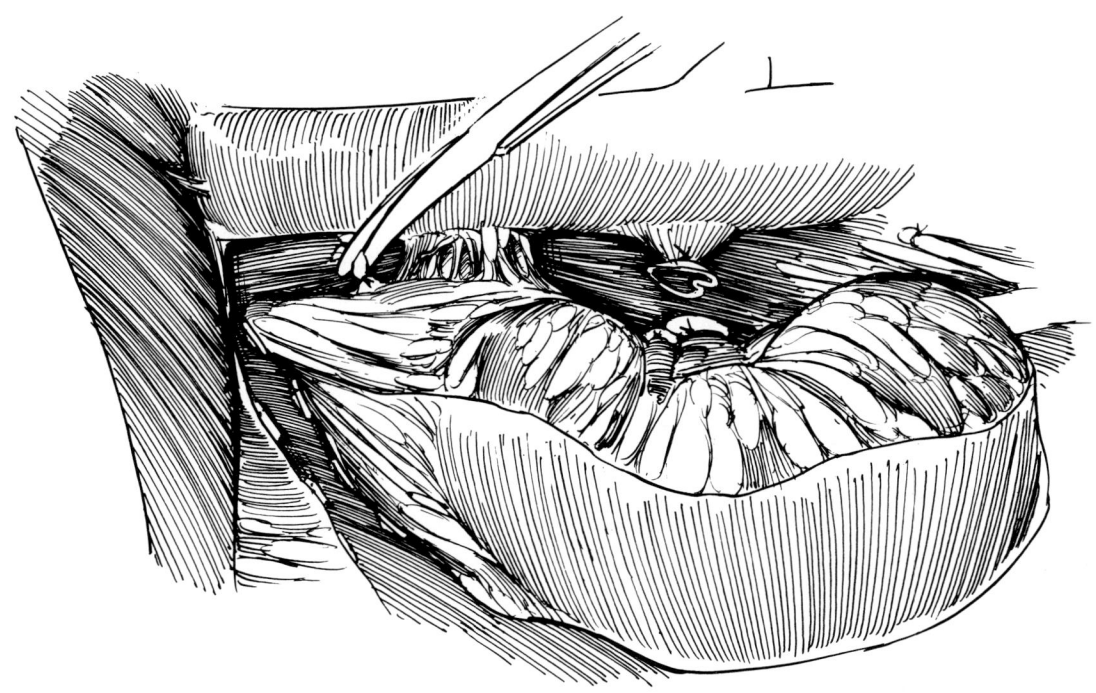

REGIONAL LYMPHADENECTOMY FOR RIGHT RENAL TUMORS

Generally, it is considered worthwhile to perform limited regional removal of hilar, paracaval, and para-aortic lymph nodes, with resection of the corresponding interaortocaval nodes. The lymphadenectomy should extend as far as the suprarenal vein above and to the level of the inferior mesenteric artery below.

8 **A,** Draw the vena cava toward you, and lift the left renal vein caudad. Clear the lymphatic tissue from the aorta, and pass it under the stump of the right renal vein. Clip all lymphatic vessels.

B, Continue along the aorta to its bifurcation. The lumbar arteries and veins may or may not need division.

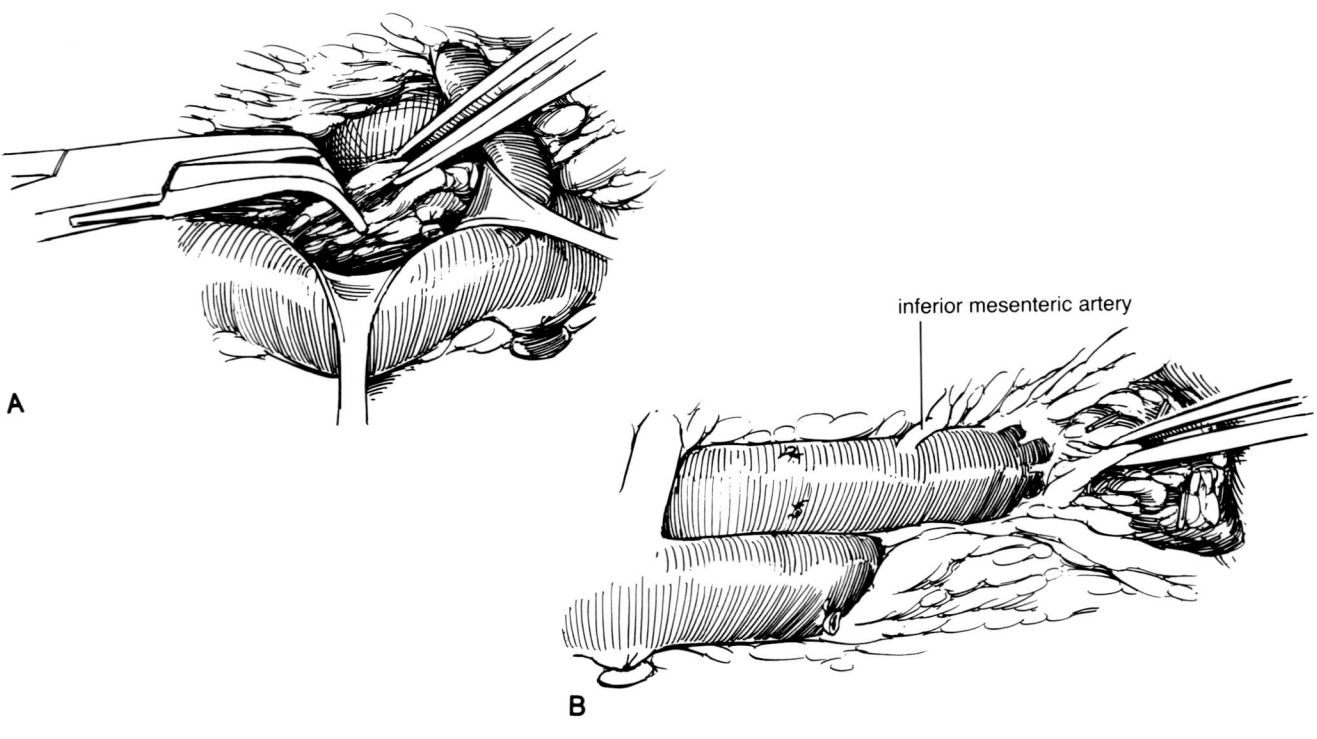

inferior mesenteric artery

9 **A,** Retract the vena cava to the left, and dissect the tissue from behind the vena cava and from the right side of the aorta.

B, Proceed down to the level of the aortic bifurcation.

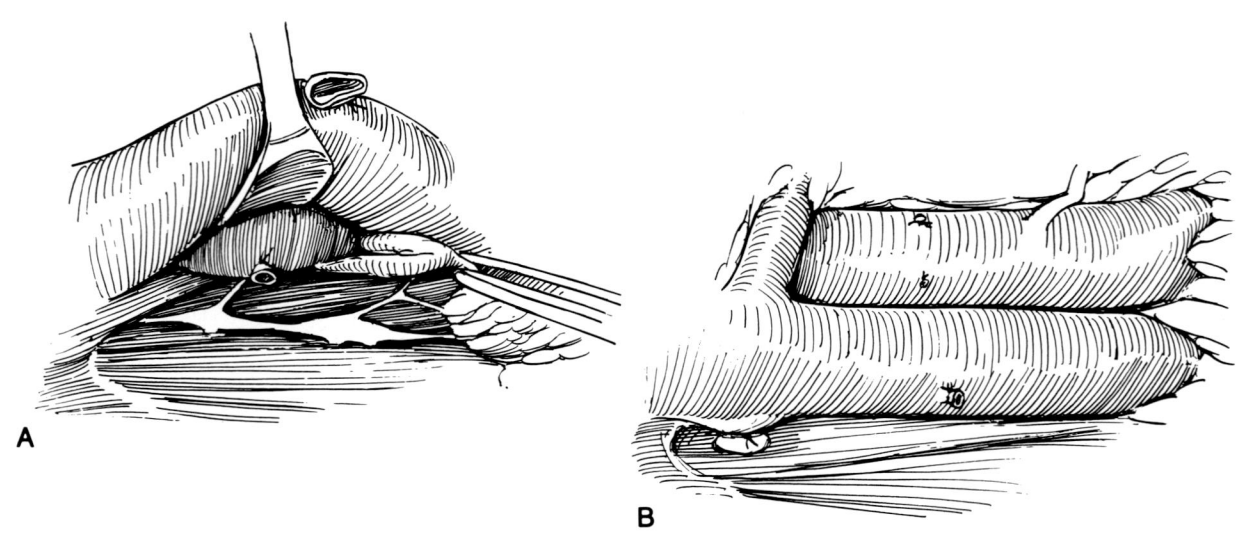

LEFT LATERAL APPROACH

This incision may be preferable in adolescents and obese older children, but for very large tumors, the thoracoabdominal approach is best (page 108).

10 A, *Incision:* Make an 11th-rib supracostal incision, extending anteriorly (page 94). An anterior transverse incision also may be used (page 81). Open the peritoneum.

B, Pack the spleen, pancreas, and stomach upward and to the right side, which may not be easy in obese patients. Place the self-retaining retractor and cover the intestine with a moist pack. Beware of injuring the spleen with a retractor, and be sure to inspect it before closing the abdomen.

Pick up and incise the posterior peritoneum lateral to the descending colon from the bifurcation of the aorta to a point above the adrenal gland. Divide the lienorenal ligaments to mobilize the pancreas and spleen upward and to the right. The pedicle of the left kidney can be exposed by freeing the greater omentum from the transverse colon and splenic flexure and by retracting it and the stomach, spleen, and pancreas upward, while moving the large intestine downward. Watch for infiltration and invasion of the mesocolon, the colon itself, and the tail of the pancreas. Preoperative studies often give little evidence for the involvement of these structures.

If the pancreas is injured, obtain a consultation from a general surgeon. Close a simple laceration with synthetic absorbable mattress sutures, and drain the retroperitoneum with a sump drain. If the pancreatic duct also is injured, resect the tail of the pancreas, ligate the duct, close the capsule, and drain freely.

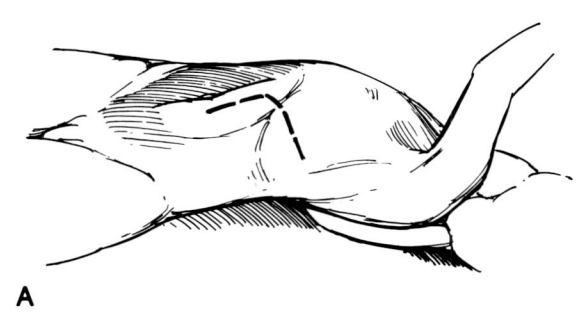

A

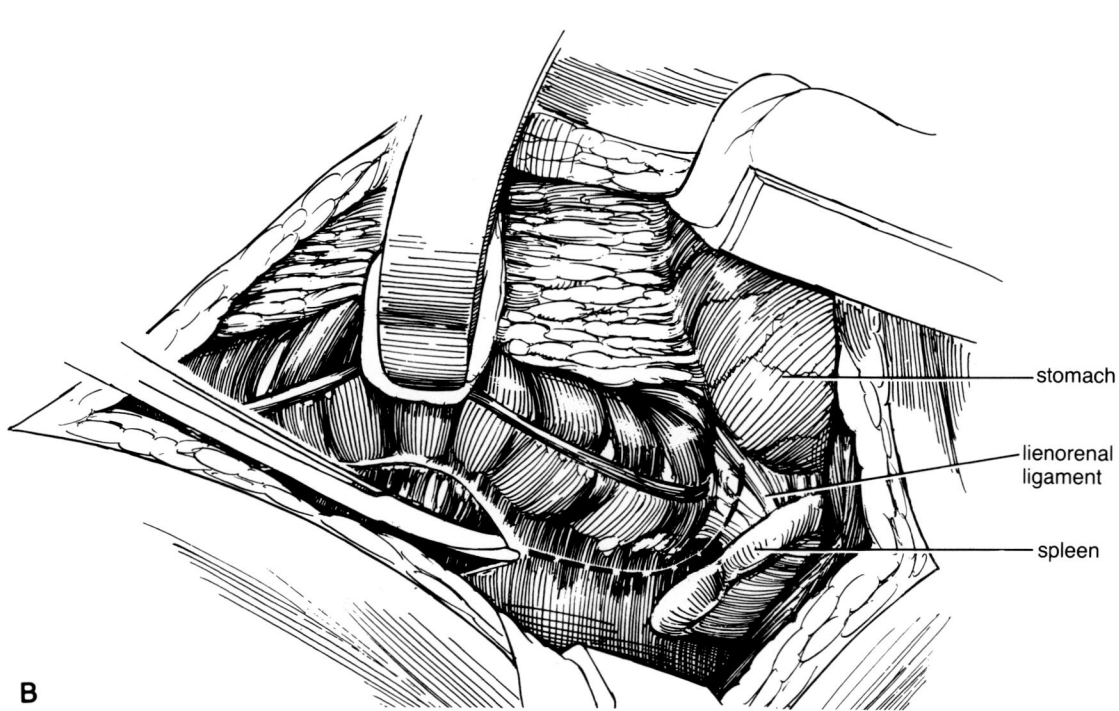

stomach

lienorenal ligament

spleen

B

11 Dissect medially to expose the aorta. If the tumor is large with medial extension or if the patient is obese, it may be difficult to uncover the aorta. Begin the dissection caudad to the renal hilum. Locate the renal vein where it crosses the aorta. For large tumors with involved lymph nodes, the dissection of the renal artery can be difficult because of its dorsolateral junction with the aorta. Remove the connective tissue and lymphatics to expose the left renal artery by downward traction on the left renal vein. In many cases, the mesocolon has attached itself to the anterior surface of the tumor, making this dissection difficult. In addition, look for connections between the tail of the pancreas and the tumor and for the splenic vessels, with a cranially situated tumor. Place a ligature around the renal artery close to its origin and tie it. Generally and theoretically, it is better to ligate the artery first. On approaching the pedicle from the front, however, it sometimes is easier to ligate and divide the vein first, after which the artery is easily exposed and quickly clamped and ligated.

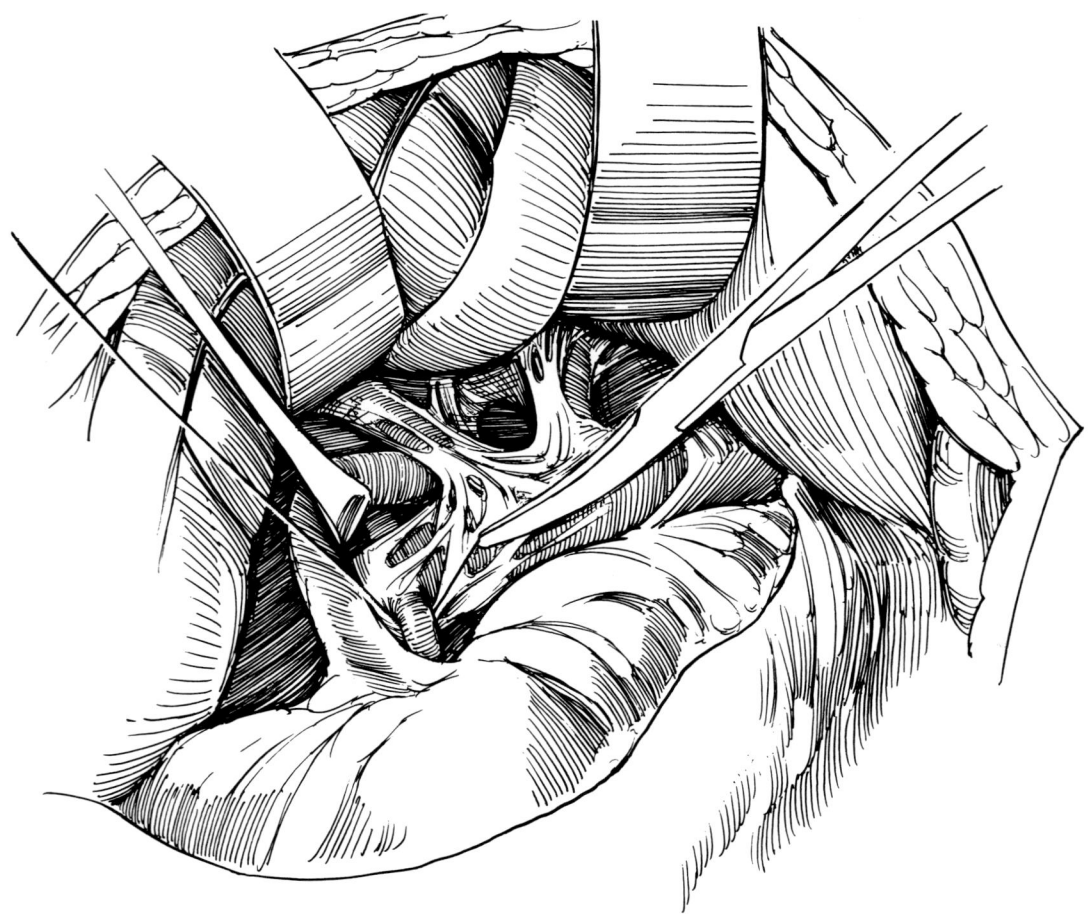

12 Dissect the left renal vein as it crosses over the aorta. Palpate it carefully for contained thrombus. Doubly clamp, divide, and ligate it. Dissect it laterally to locate and divide the lumbar vein. You need not expose the adrenal or gonadal veins; they will be included in the *en bloc* dissection. Complete the dissection of the left renal artery, and clamp it distally. Divide and ligate the left renal artery both proximally and distally.

Free the ureter and the gonadal veins as low as is feasible, and divide them between clamps. Ligate the tissue distally and proximally with a ligature. Leave the sutures long on the side of the specimen. If ureterectomy is planned, as for transitional-cell carcinoma, dissect the ureter distally as far as it is accessible.

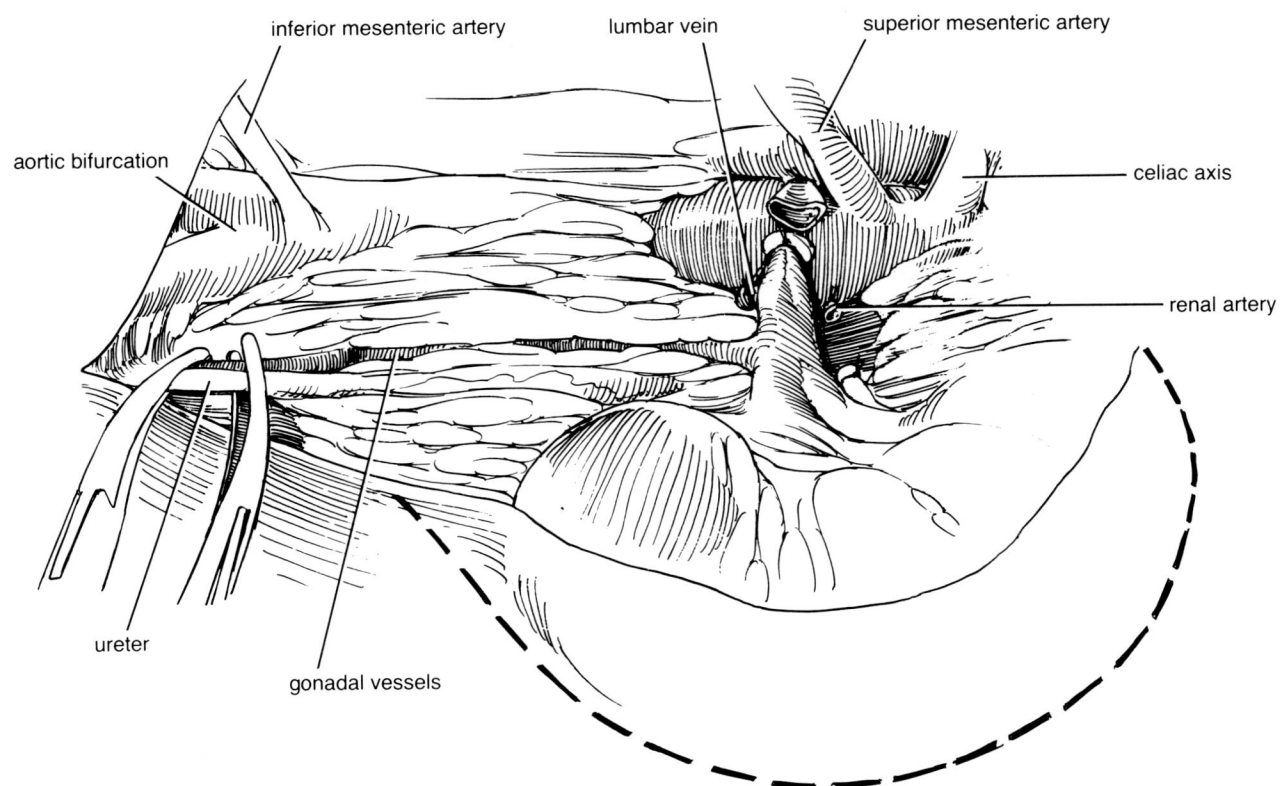

inferior mesenteric artery

lumbar vein

superior mesenteric artery

aortic bifurcation

celiac axis

renal artery

ureter

gonadal vessels

13 Divide the peritoneum laterally over the lateral border of the kidney. Free the posterior and lateral surfaces of the specimen by blunt and sharp dissection outside Gerota's fascia. Work from the caudal end of the dissection up to the medial border while dividing any additional vessels so that the lower pole of the kidney can be completely freed. Clip each vessel as it is encountered; use large clips on large collateral veins.

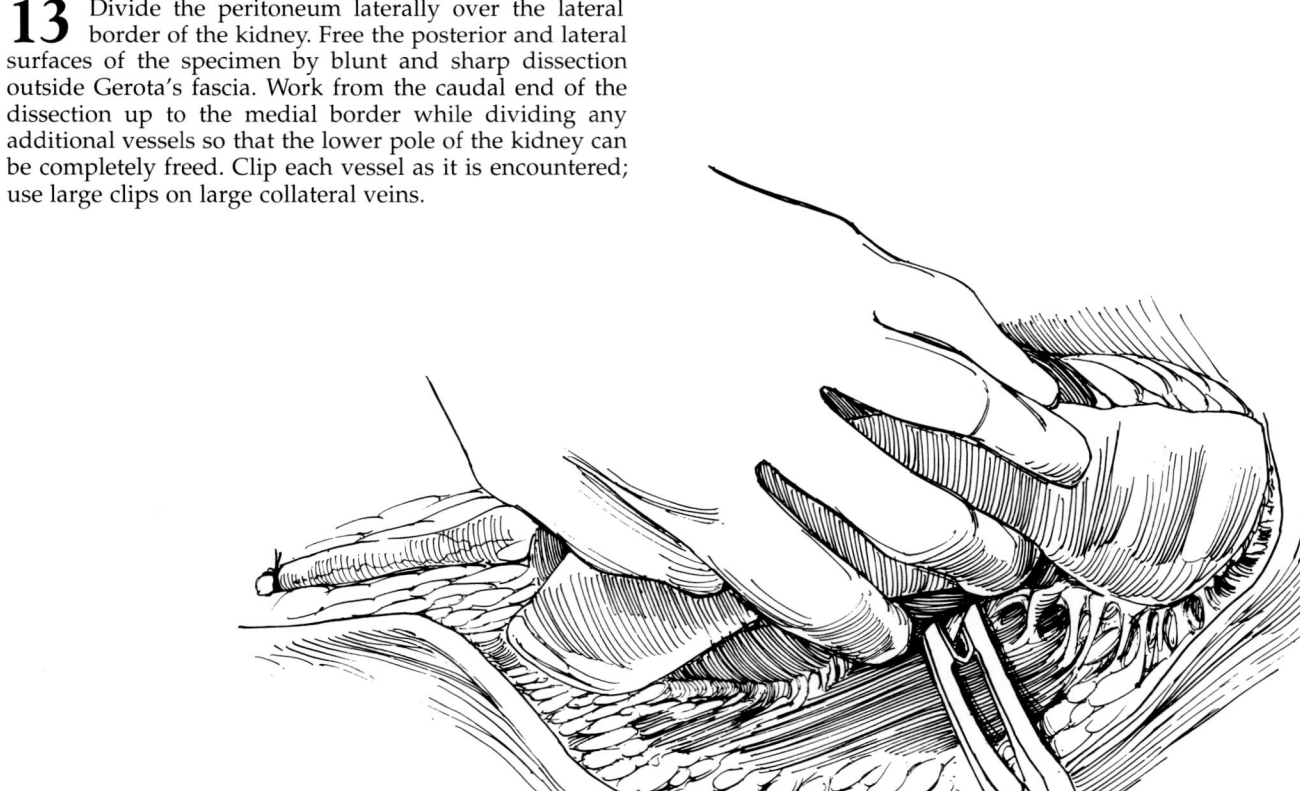

14 Complete the step-by-step dissection on the cranial and medial borders by pressing the kidney downward and laterally, to work along the crus of the diaphragm and expose the remaining small vessels and the adrenal artery. Remove the specimen.

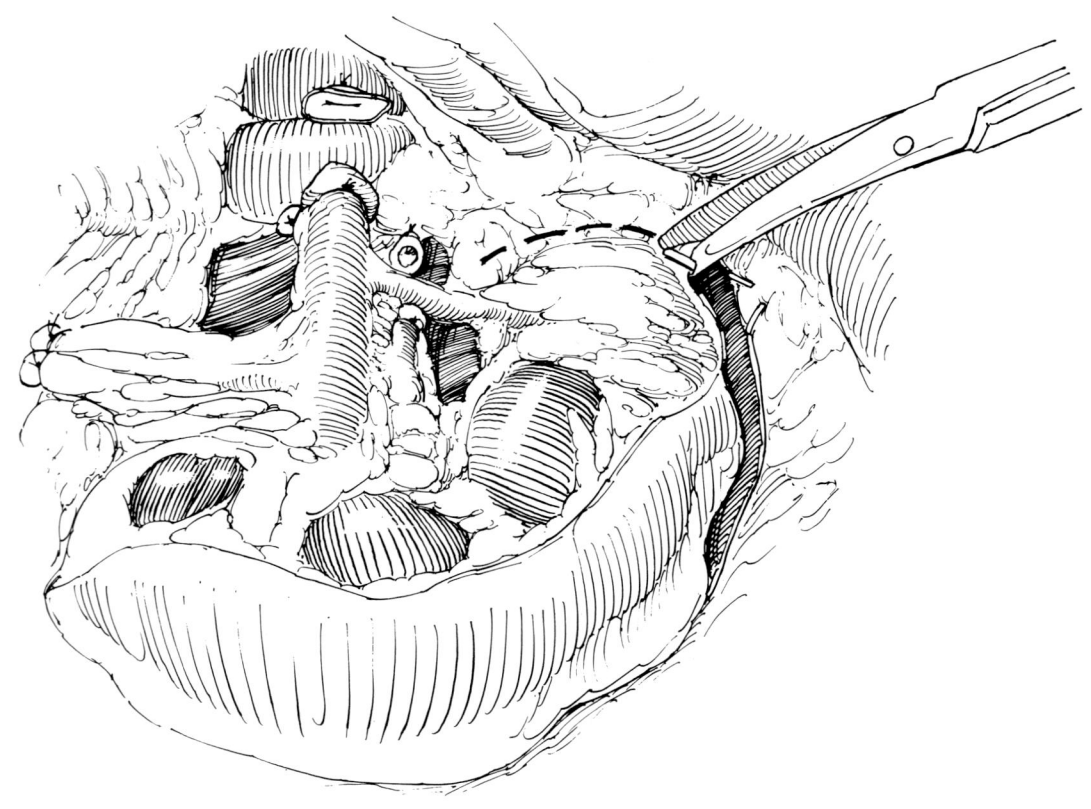

REGIONAL LYMPHADENECTOMY FOR LEFT RENAL TUMORS

15 Retract the vena cava to the right to dissect the lymphatic tissue from the anterior and lateral surfaces of the aorta. Clip or ligate all the lymphatics at the upper margins.

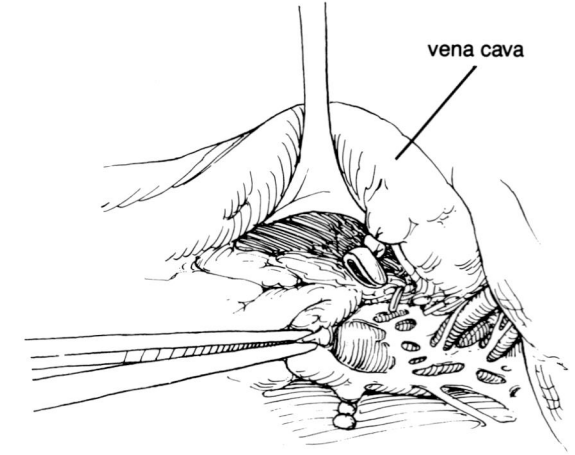

vena cava

16 Dissect down along the aorta, preserving the superior mesenteric artery (SMA), as well as the celiac ganglia and splanchnic nerves, which lie on the aorta at its origin. Continue down between the vena cava and aorta and along the lateral surface of the aorta to the inferior mesenteric artery. Lumbar vessels need not be taken. Remove the specimen after appropriately marking it with silk ties for orientation. Check the spleen for injury (page 119). Close the wound in layers around a Penrose drain.

Bilateral tumors require preliminary node dissection with frozen section biopsy examination before proceeding. Perform radical nephrectomy on the most involved side and a partial nephrectomy on the other kidney, as previously described. Preserve at least one of the adrenal glands. Alternatively, proceed in two stages, preserving tissue on one side at the first operation, then on the other later. Note that with asynchronous bilateral tumors, one of them probably represents a metastasis.

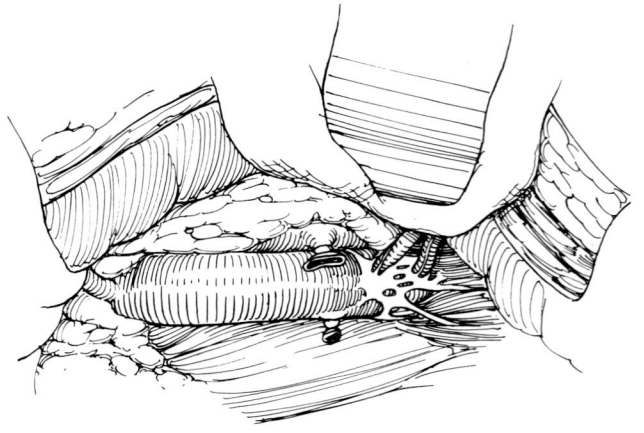

POSTOPERATIVE PROBLEMS

For a *collapsed lung* that fails to expand, arrange for bronchoscopy. A *tension pneumothorax* can occur if the lung is inadvertently cut or if an old adhesion separates with a tear. In an emergency, push a needle into the second intercostal space, then insert a pleural drain attached to a water seal (page 118). *Pleural effusions* should be aspirated. *Bleeding* from the wound usually comes from a loose vessel in the muscle layers. Pressure on the area often will arrest it.

Pancreatic injury may not be recognized intraoperatively. After operation, an elevation of serum amylase levels, an alkaline drainage from the wound, or a retroperitoneal collection of fluid is highly suggestive. Analyze the fluid for amylase and obtain a computed tomographic (CT) scan to identify the pocket, then drain it. Expect spontaneous closure of the fistula, but hyperalimentation will be required during that time. The *spleen* may be injured if the splenocolic and lienophrenic attachments are not divided to allow the spleen to be swung up out of the way.

Vascular injuries should be minimal if adequate exposure is obtained through a large incision with mobilization of the bowel. On the right side, the adrenal vein is vulnerable to injury where it enters the deep side of the vena cava. If your assistant will lift up the right lobe of the liver and retract the vena cava while you are dissecting carefully, laceration or avulsion will be avoided. The SMA or the celiac vessels are at risk when large tumors create distortion. If one of these vessels is transected, reanastomosis with a borrowed arterial segment may be necessary.

Pulmonary complications of atelectasis and lobar collapse can be prevented by proper inflation and suctioning. The diaphragm can be injured during retrocrural dissection of nodes lying above the renal hilum, as the crus is divided and resutured. The diaphragm also is traversed in the thoracoabdominal approach and, to prevent later herniation, requires reapproximation with interrupted sutures, with a running fine suture on the pleural surface.

Commentary by Thomas S. Parrott

Radical nephrectomy is a very important operation. Anyone dealing with renal malignancies in children should be thoroughly familiar with the concepts outlined in this chapter. Almost all renal tumors in children, especially the most common nephroblastoma, can be satisfactorily approached through a subcostal transperitoneal incision.

Rarely it is preferable to open the chest, because even large upper-pole renal tumors usually can be safely removed with the less-morbid abdominal approach. If more exposure is required when employing the traditional incision, the subcostal incision can be extended to a T shape, carrying the arm of the T into the thorax. However, this should rarely be necessary.

Currently, controversy exists on whether the opposite kidney should be completely mobilized and its anterior and posterior surfaces carefully inspected for tumor. Recent evidence suggests that a normal CT scan is adequate for determining that the opposite kidney is normal, and mobilization should therefore be unnecessary. Whether contralateral mobilization and inspection is undertaken is a surgical choice; however, the need for accurate information is absolutely essential. The surgeon's responsibility is to assess tumor spread accurately to allow for proper staging and precise treatment. This is particularly important in Stage 5 (bilateral) disease, because in recent years, the objective of surgery in bilateral Wilms' tumor cases has changed from ablation to preservation of as much renal tissue as possible.

Preliminary ligation of the renal pedicle is desirable but may not be technically possible when large anterior-projecting tumors are encountered. Under such circumstances, the tumor may be mobilized initially and the vessels divided only after the tumor has been satisfactorily encircled, allowing the operator to grasp the pedicle between the thumb and forefinger. At such times, I often find it helpful to stand on the opposite side of the tumor, allowing for adequate retraction of the abdominal wall away from the tumor. On rare occasions, the extent of tumor may be so great as to make the attempt at its total removal hazardous to the immediate survival of the patient. This is especially true with lesions involving the root of the mesentery at the take-off of the SMA, when the duodenum is significantly involved, or when the head of the pancreas is clearly infiltrated. In such circumstances it may be prudent to take adequate biopsies, including sampling of regional nodes, and to mark the extent of the tumor with clips prior to closure. Chemotherapy and radiation may reduce the size of the tumor, making second-look procedures technically easier and far less hazardous.

Metastasis to regional lymph nodes occurs in approximately one third of cases, and it is now clearly evident from the National Wilms' Tumor Study (NWTS) that lymph node involvement affects prognosis. Accurate staging requires knowing whether lymph nodes are involved or not; however, there is no good evidence that total lymph node removal influences survival in Wilms' tumor cases. Excision of hilar nodes and selective sampling of paracaval and interaortocaval nodes are essential.

The interested reader should commit to memory the anatomic relationships shown in Figure 12. Realizing the proximity of the SMA take-off to the left renal vein is essential in avoiding damage to the former structure when tumor surrounds the left renal pedicle. Other surgical pitfalls to be avoided when performing nephrectomy on the left side include damage to the pancreas and spleen. Careful retraction and division of the splenorenal ligament should prevent the latter.

CHAPTER 34

Vena Caval Thrombectomy

Insert an intra-arterial and a Swan-Ganz catheter to be prepared for large blood losses. Determine the extent of the thrombus by a coronal cut on magnetic resonance imaging (MRI). Use contrast venacavography for a patient with suspected cardiac involvement or for a patient in whom the extent of the thrombus is unclear on MRI.

Classify the case into one of three groups: Group 1, infradiaphragmatic infrahepatic extension; Group 2, supradiaphragmatic intrapericardial or suprahepatic extension; and Group 3, supradiaphragmatic intracardiac extension. Consider collaboration with a vascular surgeon. Intraoperative ultrasonography may help define the status.

Commentary by Andrew C. Novick

One of the unique features of renal, adrenal, and certain retroperitoneal malignancies is their frequent pattern of growth intraluminally into the venous circulation. In extreme cases, this growth may extend into the inferior vena cava with cephalad migration as far as the right atrium. The absence of metastases in some children with direct vena caval involvement from a malignancy remains intriguing. In most cases, an aggressive treatment approach is warranted if the tumor is localized and complete surgical removal can be accomplished.

Accurate preoperative information regarding the presence and complete extent of an inferior vena caval (IVC) tumor thrombus is essential to determine the appropriate operative approach. Computed tomographic scanning and ultrasound will detect gross renal vein and IVC involvement but are unreliable in delineating the cephalad extent of a thrombus. Inferior vena cavography has been the most accurate diagnostic study for assessment of IVC thrombi; however, a single antegrade study may be insufficient with complete caval occlusion; in such cases, a second retrograde injection of the IVC is needed to define the distal limits of the thrombus. Recent data indicate that MRI is an accurate noninvasive method for delineating the full extent of IVC thrombi, and this is now the preferred caval imaging modality at most centers. Inferior vena cavography is reserved for patients in whom MRI findings are equivocal or when MRI is contraindicated.

Renal arteriography remains an important preoperative study in patients with renal malignancy and an IVC thrombus. Large caval thrombi often demonstrate hyper-

vascularity with distinct arterial supply from the renal artery. When this finding is observed on arteriography, we perform renal arterial embolization 2 to 3 days before surgery. We have observed several cases of definite shrinkage in the size of a caval thrombus following such embolization, which has facilitated its intraoperative removal.

In performing surgical removal of an IVC thrombus, it is essential to obtain control of the cava above the thrombus to prevent intraoperative embolization of a tumor fragment. Temporary occlusion of the infrahepatic IVC can be done safely, but occlusion of the suprahepatic IVC often causes a profound decrease in venous return with hypotension; additional disadvantages of the latter maneuver when removing a caval thrombus include backbleeding from hepatic and lumbar veins and occasional swelling of the liver from venous congestion, which interferes with exposure. Use of an intraoperative caval-atrial venous shunt is another available technique for use in this setting.

Cardiopulmonary bypass (CPB) with deep hypothermic circulatory arrest (DHCA) offers several advantages for removal of a supradiaphragmatic vena caval thrombus. Because formal isolation and control of the distal IVC are not necessary, extensive retrohepatic or intrapericardial caval dissection is avoided. There is no need for occlusion of the porta hepatis, ligation of multiple lumbar veins, or aortic cross-clamping to prevent hemorrhage. CPB with DHCA allows direct visual inspection of the entire vena caval lumen in a completely bloodless field. An atriotomy can be performed easily, which facilitates removal of not only atrial thrombus but also friable or adherent pieces of thrombus in the intrahepatic IVC. The risk of sudden, massive intraoperative hemorrhage or distal tumor thrombus embolization is lessened. Finally, DHCA allows up to 60 minutes of safe ischemia in a bloodless field for the performance of vena caval thrombectomy or resection and appropriate caval reconstruction. The maximum period of safe ischemia with occlusion of the suprahepatic IVC and porta hepatis is no more than 30 minutes.

We have found that CPB with DHCA is a safe and effective approach. There have been no ischemic or neurologic complications and no cases of perioperative tumor embolization. The most common postoperative complication has been hemorrhage requiring surgical reexploration, which has occurred in 8 per cent of patients. CPB is associated with temporary platelet dysfunction, and this effect may be augmented with superimposed DHCA. This problem generally is managed with platelets, fresh-frozen plasma, desmopressin acetate, aminocaproic acid, or a combination of these. Recent data also suggest that high-dose aprotinin has a dramatic ability to normalize coagulation after CPB and to reduce transfusion requirements.

CHAPTER 35

Excision of Wilms' Tumor and Neuroblastoma

EXCISION OF WILMS' TUMOR

Carefully stage the tumor preoperatively. Use abdominal ultrasonography to evaluate the involved kidney and also to assess the contralateral one. Ultrasonography may detect vena caval involvement. Computed tomographic (CT) scan indicates the extent of renal involvement and assesses the stage of the tumor. It is particularly useful in determining response to chemotherapy and assessing operability. Should the vena cava not show or appear to be involved on ultrasonography, order a venacavogram. Angiography is reserved for bilateral cases or those in horseshoe kidneys. Include a CT scan of the chest to detect small metastatic lesions.

Establish reliable vascular access for fluid and blood replacement in the neck or upper extremities, not in the legs where intraoperative interference with the vena cava may block inflow. If intestinal involvement is suspected, use an oral bowel flush preoperatively. For a tumor in a horseshoe kidney, plan to remove the isthmus as well as that half of the kidney.

1 *Position:* Tilt the involved side at an angle of 30 degrees, elevated on a rolled towel. Place intravenous lines in the upper extremities. *Incision:* Use a generous pediatric extended anterior incision (page 79) one or two fingerbreadths above the umbilicus. A flank approach is not suitable, because it makes staging by access to the lymph nodes and contralateral kidney impossible. An extension into a thoracoabdominal incision through the bed of the 9th or 10th rib is reserved for very large upper-pole lesions, especially with ipsilateral pulmonary metastases. A self-retaining ring retractor can be placed after the falciform ligament has been divided. Assess the extent of the tumor, then cover it with a moist laparotomy pad. Inspect the liver for metastases, and look for nodal and vena caval involvement to determine if primary excision is possible. If the operation is obviously going to be extremely difficult, back out and intervene with chemotherapy, radiation therapy, or both. If the pseudocapsule has been broached, mark the edges with titanium clips for following the tumor later and applying radiation. Avoid spilling tumor into the peritoneal cavity, and if spillage seems imminent due to necrosis of the tumor, pack the area with laparotomy tapes as one would do to block pus.

Reflect the colon and the peritoneum over the contralateral kidney, free the kidney from Gerota's fascia, and inspect both anterior and posterior surfaces. Perform a biopsy on any suspicious lesions, because bilateral Wilms' tumor must be managed differently from a unilateral tumor.

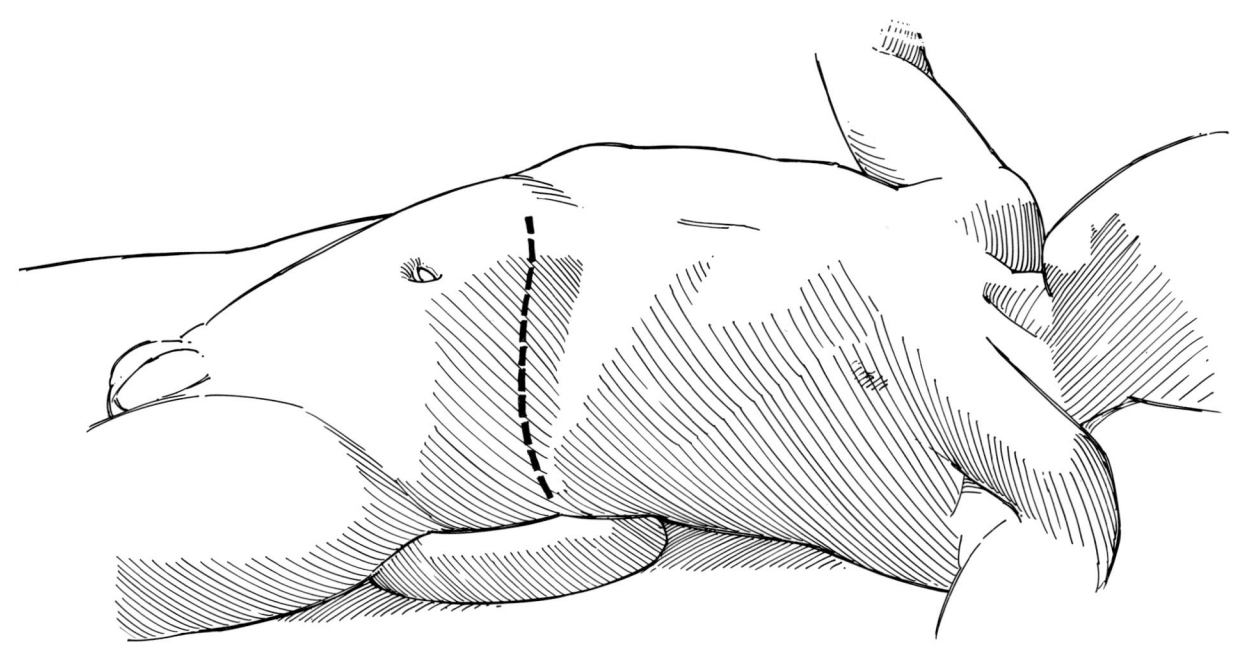

2 Displace the small bowel medially. A bowel bag may be helpful. Retract the colon laterally. Incise the parietal peritoneum vertically over the aorta along the root of the mesentery. Divide the ligament of Treitz, allowing the duodenum to be mobilized upward and to the right. An alternative approach is to incise the white line and mobilize the colon medially.

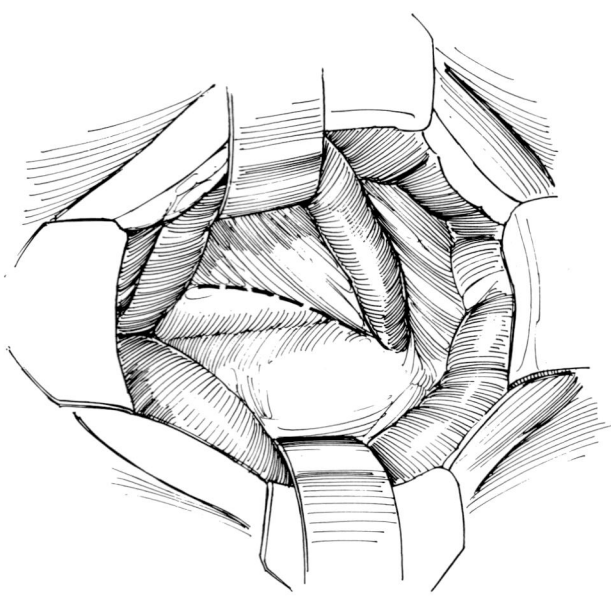

4 A and B, Palpate the vena cava for extension; if a thrombus is present, proceed as described in Chapter 34. Place a small Satinsky clamp on the vena cava just proximal to the insertion of the left renal vein. Ligate the vein distally and divide it proximally. Run a continuous 5-0 or 6-0 vascular suture over the stump, and remove the clamp.

Continue dissection para-aortically on the left as well as between the aorta and vena cava down to the bifurcation, avoiding the inferior mesenteric artery. Expose and control the lumbar vessels. Elevate the spleen and pancreas. Dissect cephalad to ligate the small adrenal arteries, and remove the nodal tissue. This tissue is sparse in children; *en bloc* dissection should not be attempted.

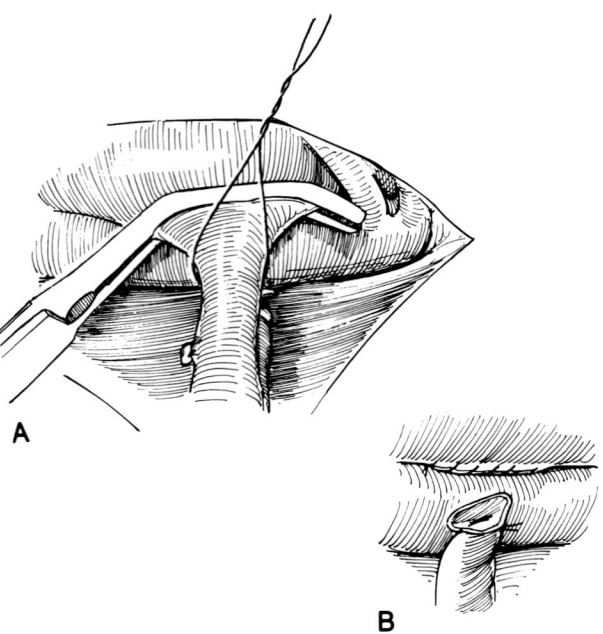

A

B

LEFT-SIDED TUMOR

3 Dissect the anterior surface of the vena cava to the level of the superior mesenteric artery (SMA), which must be identified, and to the origin of the left renal pedicle. Begin to selectively sample the lymphatics over the vena cava and to dissect over the left renal vein. Complete resection of all nodal tissue is not necessary. Dissect the left adrenal vein starting where it crosses the aorta and then the left gonadal vein. Tie each of them in continuity and divide them.

Take care not to injure the renal vein—it is attenuated over the tumor; the opposite renal vein may be confused with it. Retract the left renal vein downward with a vascular loop, and dissect the nodal tissue about the renal artery. Palpate the vein for tumor extension. Thrombi usually are not invasive and are readily extractable, but as many as 1 in 10 enters the vena cava and deserves preoperative imaging. Ligate the renal artery proximally, then doubly clamp and divide it. Ligate each end under the clamp. The tumor will now be softer and less likely to rupture.

It may be necessary to mobilize a segment of the inferior vena cava to rotate the tumor and venous drainage away from the renal artery so that it may be ligated. To do this requires identification and cautious ligation of the lumbar veins. Sometimes it is not feasible to reach the renal artery with the vein in place, in which case divide and ligate the vein first, although this causes severe congestion of the kidney.

Now turn attention to the friable parasitic veins. Dissect enough to ligate them to avoid blood loss and the chance of tumor spillage.

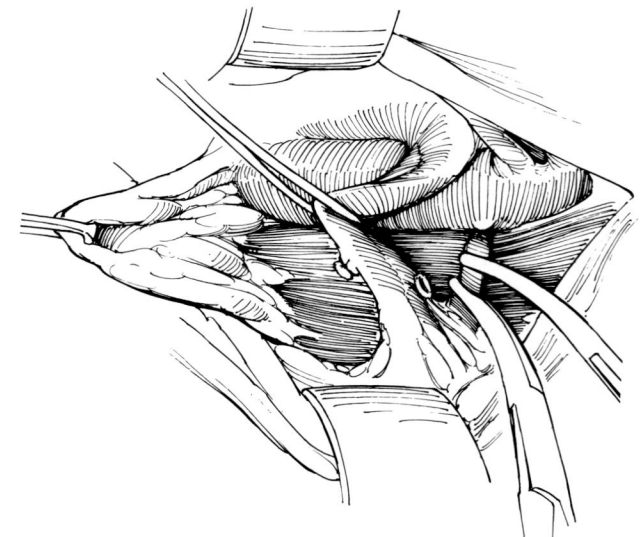

5 Hold the descending colon medially, and incise the parietal peritoneum laterally along the white line. Bluntly separate the mesocolon from Gerota's fascia. Hold the spleen and tail of the pancreas out of the way with padded retractors. Be careful to avoid spillage of tumor while removing the tumor with Gerota's fascia and the enclosed pararenal fat. Bluntly work a hand over the top of the mass, and mobilize Gerota's fascia and the kidney. Include the adrenal gland with upper-pole tumors. An engorged accessory vein may run from the upper pole to the vena cava. Extension into the liver may occur on the right side, which usually can be resected inside a pseudocapsule after mobilization of the liver. It may be necessary to resect part of the diaphragm if involved. Divide the ureter well below the kidney, and remove the specimen. Complete extirpation may require resection of a segment of spleen, stomach, or colon, the tail of the pancreas, or portions of the diaphragm or psoas muscle, but do not be heroic. Avoid splenectomy because of the risk of pneumococcal sepsis. Tag the nonresected portion with titanium clips to aid in postoperative radiation and for a second-look operation. Irrigate the wound with normal saline, and obtain complete hemostasis. Insert a Penrose drain retroperitoneally to exit through a stab wound in the flank. Replace the colon to cover the dead space from the tumor, tack the retroperitoneum together anteriorly, and close the wound in layers.

Whether lymph node dissection should be done has not been decided, but a sampling should be done for staging.

Should the tumor not be resectable, place at its margins titanium (a material that does not interfere with the CT beam) clips to follow the tumor during chemotherapy and radiation treatment.

RIGHT-SIDED TUMOR

6 **A** and **B,** Expose the retroperitoneum as described in Steps 1 and 2. Separate the hepatic flexure of the colon and the right and transverse colon from the duodenum, liver, and gallbladder. After retracting the duodenum medially and exposing the great vessels, selectively resect the nodal tissue over the vena cava and below the renal vein. Draw the cava to the right, and retract the left renal vein cephalad with a vascular tape. Clear the right renal artery, ligate it in continuity, doubly clamp it, divide it, and ligate both ends. Ligate the right renal vein close to the vena cava, doubly clamp it, divide it, and ligate both ends; use suture ligation of the proximal end, because the vein is short. Continue the nodal sampling caudally, removing some right paracaval tissue while dividing and ligating the gonadal vessels.

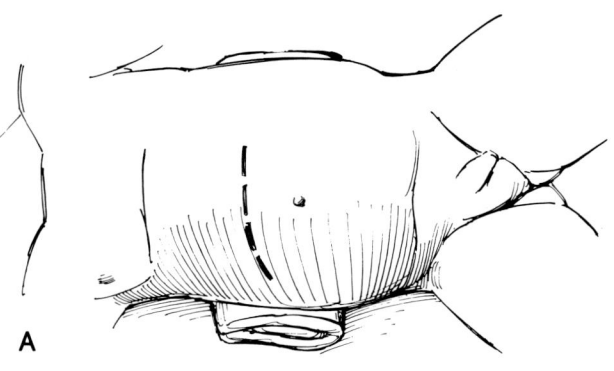

A

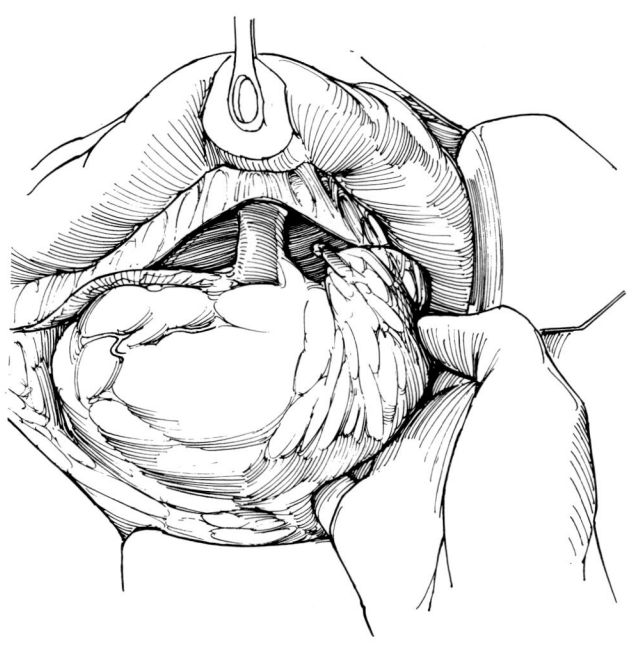

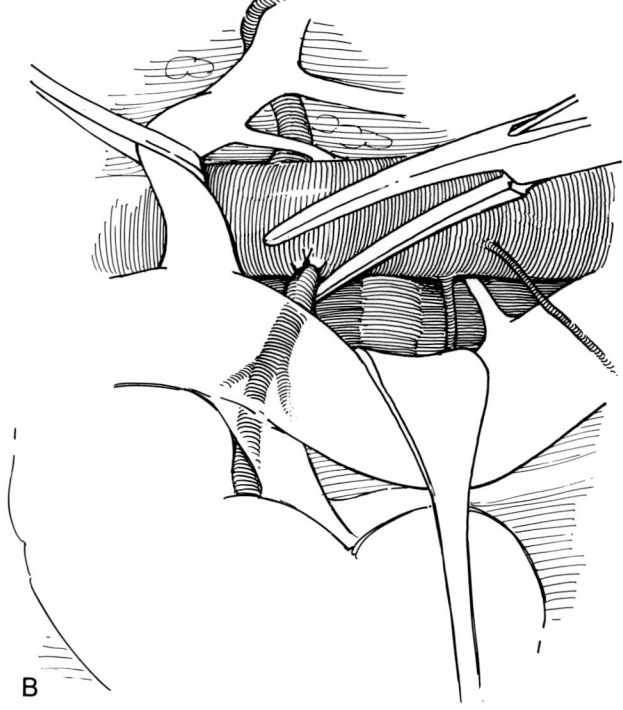

B

7 Incise the parietal peritoneum lateral to the ascending colon, separate the mesentery from Gerota's fascia, and move the duodenum medially over the vena cava.

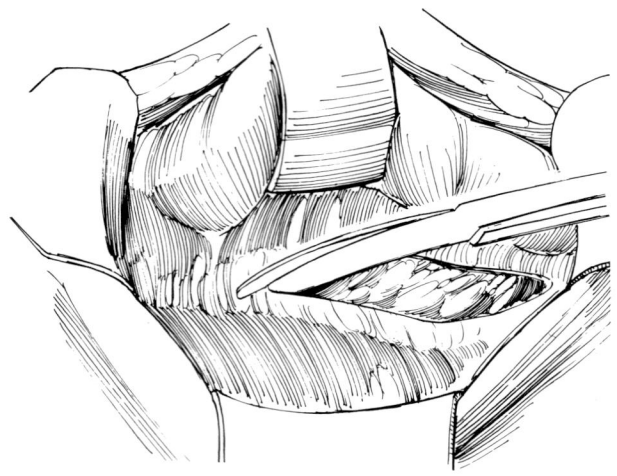

8 Dissect and divide the adrenal vein. Draw the renal artery from beneath the vena cava. Now place a hand over the top of the mass, and strip Gerota's fascia from the body wall, to include the adrenal gland if the tumor is in the upper pole. Care is needed because the right adrenal vein is short and situated partially behind the vena cava (page 196). The pseudocapsule of a large tumor may be adherent to the undersurface of the liver but may be dissected free. If the liver is involved with tumor, a wedge must be removed *en bloc* with the specimen (rarely is hepatic lobectomy required). Divide the ureter as low as is feasible, and remove the specimen. Ligate the ureteral stump with an absorbable suture. Close the wound with drainage, as previously described.

Should hepatic lobectomy be necessary, free the coronary and triangular ligaments, and successively dissect the porta hepatis and the right hepatic artery, hepatic duct, and right branch of the portal vein. If the segmental hepatic structures are identified with the help of an ultrasonic probe and an ultrasonic dissector, less liver need be removed.

The remainder of the operation proceeds as described for the left side.

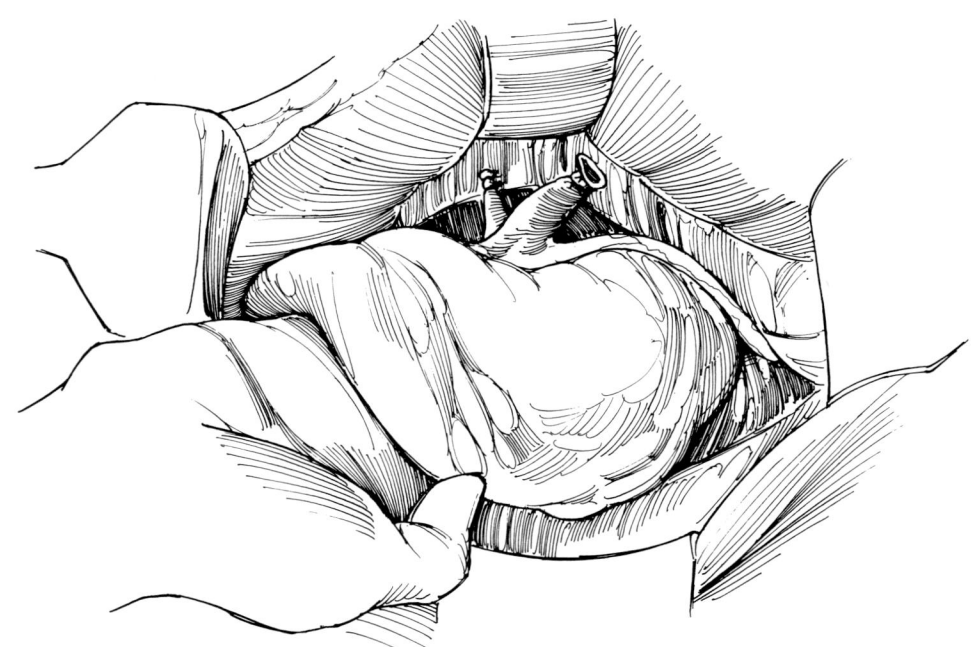

Postoperatively, stage the tumor as follows: *Stage I,* completely removed with kidney; *Stage II,* completely removed but partly outside kidney; *Stage III,* residual local tumor; *Stage IV,* hematogenous metastases; and *Stage V,* bilateral. Determine favorable or unfavorable histology, and proceed with chemotherapy and radiation therapy.

BILATERAL TUMORS

For small *bilateral Wilms' tumors* at the poles, perform partial nephrectomies. For one large and one small tumor, perform a radical nephrectomy on the most involved side and a partial nephrectomy on the other kidney. Preserve at least one of the adrenal glands. Alternatively, proceed in two stages, preserving renal tissue on one side at the first operation, then on the other side later. If both kidneys are extensively involved, take a biopsy specimen from both of them and obtain representative lymph nodes from each side. Give chemotherapy postoperatively and return for a second look, intending to conserve as much renal tissue as possible in a case with favorable histology. Substitute radiation therapy after intensive chemotherapy in a case with unfavorable histology; later, take a second look. At that point, it is reasonable if the tumor cannot be resected to give further therapy and make a third attempt at removal. Bilateral nephrectomy with renal transplantation is the last resort, because immunosuppression fosters return of the neoplasm.

For *involvement of the vena cava*, a condition that may be detected during preoperative B-mode ultrasonography, proceed as described on page 180.

Lung metastases require both chemotherapy and radiation. Arrange for removal of persistent lesions by wedge resection or lobectomy.

POSTOPERATIVE PROBLEMS

Vascular injury can occur during the procedure. The celiac axis, the contralateral renal artery, the SMA, and the aorta below the renal origin could be ligated inadvertently if the aorta, vena cava, and contralateral renal vessels are not visualized. Ligation of the inferior mesenteric artery is not harmful in a child, especially if done close to the aorta to preserve the marginal artery. The left renal vein should not be divided during a right-sided operation in a child. If it is cut inadvertently, anastomose it to the vena cava while providing diuresis.

Air embolism or tumor embolism can occur during vena caval manipulations. *Bowel ischemia* and necrosis result from interference with the mesenteric blood supply, especially after radiation therapy. *Pancreatic fistulas* occur if the resected end of the tail is not carefully oversewn with a running nonabsorbable suture. *Splenic injury* is secondary to retraction (page 119). *Chylous ascites* can arise if the cisterna chyli is torn but usually will respond to several paracenteses. *Atelectasis* or pneumothorax may occur if the diaphragm was involved or if wedge resection of the lung was performed.

Commentary by Martin A. Koyle

Although surgery still maintains an important place in the therapy for the patient with Wilms' tumor, improvement in survival over the past two decades of children with this tumor primarily has been a result of advances in chemotherapy. Today, there is controversy as to whether chemotherapy should be used primarily to downsize large tumors, tumors of high stage, and tumors with inferior vena cava extension with the hope of making subsequent nephrectomy easier or even allowing a partial renal-conserving approach.

Prior to surgery, it is imperative to use the excellent radiologic armamentarium that we have available. In the child with an abdominal mass, ultrasound is performed first to confirm renal origin, to determine whether the mass is solid or cystic, and to ensure patency of the inferior vena cava in the case of solid tumor. CT scan has become the modality of choice to image Wilms' tumor, the contralateral kidney, and the liver. Its primary fault is its inability to assess the lymph nodes and the venous system accurately. In those cases where tumor vascular extension is suggested by ultrasound, we then proceed with magnetic resonance imaging examination of the venous system. Seldom today need we proceed with an invasive study such as a venogram; however, in rare instances, this may be necessary. At surgery, a lifeline for chemotherapy and vascular access is placed first unless the diagnosis is in doubt. Place a nasogastric tube and Foley catheter prior to final positioning of the patient. In a patient with a unilateral lesion, we prefer elevating the affected side 25 to 30 degrees using padding. With small tumors, we will then proceed with a unilateral subcostal incision (Kocher), which can be extended across the midline as a chevron if necessary. The latter, of course, is our primary approach for larger tumors or those for which venous control is necessary. When control of the suprahepatic inferior vena cava is necessary, the incision is extended as an inverted Y using a midline sternotomy.

Rather than place a self-retaining retractor, I generally have used a heavy suture (# 1 Prolene) placed through the posterior rectus in the inferior margin of the wound. Traction is applied on the suture, and it is clipped to the drape, thus separating the incision nicely. I then use moist laparotomy sponges to pack the bowel out of the way, preferably within the abdomen itself, because exteriorized bowel can become dusky and edematous. With large tumors, however, this may not be possible, in which case it is important to inspect the exteriorized small intestine from time to time and even replace it into the abdomen if it does become engorged and congested.

Generally, unless the lesion is extremely large (despite our success using preoperative CT staging for bilateral disease) the contralateral normal kidney is explored first to rule out bilateral disease. If bilateral disease is encountered, biopsy specimens are taken from both sides rather than performing nephrectomy. The nodes also are biopsied, allowing accurate staging of the lesion. In proceeding with nephrectomy, it cannot be overemphasized how important it is to identify the anatomic structures properly. We have seen the inadvertent complication of complete vena cava excision as well as unsuspected superior mesenteric artery ligation during nephrectomy, and both were unrecognized during the postoperative period before referral to our center. I prefer to identify the ureter first and work cephalad along the great vessels, identifying the inferior mesenteric artery as the first major distal aortic branch. All lymphatic tissue is mobilized toward the affected kidney and ultimately is removed *en bloc* with the specimen. Moving cephalad, once the renal vein is located, it is dissected free. On the left side, the gonadal and adrenal vein tributaries, as well as any lumbars that may drain into the left renal vein, are ligated and divided. The artery is then identified, doubly ligated proximally and singly distally, and divided. If the tumor does not shrink and the vein does not become less engorged, one should suspect an additional renal artery, which may be present in as many as 20 percent of cases. After gaining arterial control, the vein can be ligated and transected in a fashion similar to the artery. I have used simple ligatures—not suture ligatures—on these vessels. Few data support the concept of traditional radical nephrectomy rather than simple nephrectomy for Wilms' tumor, but it is preferable to take all regional nodes with the specimen and remove the kidney within Gerota's fascia. Unless it is a superior-pole tumor, I do not routinely take the adrenal gland on the affected side. It is important, even after achieving good vascular control, to avoid damaging the friable parasitic veins that may run along the surface of the capsule of the kidney. One also must be very gentle in mobilizing the mass to avoid rupture of these tumors, which can be large and necrotic.

With respect to partial nephrectomy, an angiogram generally is not necessary preoperatively. The patient should be well hydrated prior to surgery. With large lesions, especially if clamping of the renal artery is anticipated, a central venous pressure line should be placed, and an arterial line considered. During surgery, the main renal artery is identified and mobilized to the first branch, which usually is the posterior segmental artery. In most cases, clamping of the renal artery will not be necessary; however, the surgeon should be prepared to do so. Thus, ice slush should be available at a moment's notice. Mannitol is given before the artery is clamped, and furosemide is administered after the clamp subsequently is released.

Cautery is useful to circumscribe the lesions with a rim of contiguous normal tissue and to fulgurate the base of the excised mass. The argon coagulator also is useful for large lesions to achieve excellent hemostasis. I pack the raw areas with Surgicel gauze and spray topical thrombin over it, because in most cases, the defect or raw edge cannot be readily approximated and compressed. In the rare situation when the surgeon must consider removal of an adjacent structure, it is best instead to take a biopsy specimen of the mass and come back for a second look in an attempt to resect the lesion after chemotherapy. In redo cases, I often have found it useful to mechanically prep the bowel in case there is a surgical misadventure. Unlike with neuroblastoma, for which there is no effective multimodal therapy, I feel strongly that there is no need to perform heroic surgery for Wilms' tumor, because such surgery could lead to significant morbidity or jeopardize the patient's life, unless all medical therapies have been exhausted.

One wonders whether in the future, with continued improvement in radiologic staging, patients eventually will undergo primary laparoscopy to assess the contralateral kidney, lymph nodes, and liver and then undergo either biopsy and pretreatment or a nephrectomy via a retroperitoneal approach to minimize morbidity.

EXCISION OF NEUROBLASTOMA

Excretory urography usually shows downward and lateral displacement of the kidney without intrarenal distortion by a tumor with stippled calcifications (in approximately 60 per cent of cases). CT scans define the tumor and aid in determining when to operate. Radionuclide scans detect skeletal metastasis, assisted by bone marrow aspiration.

The operation is performed as described for Wilms' tumor except that it is more difficult because of tumor adherence to neighboring organs. The aim should be to remove all of the tumor but, in fact, the tumor may involve structures such as the celiac axis and the portal system. It is not worthwhile to remove adjacent organs. Severe hemorrhage is possible, so debulking may be the safer procedure. Mark the margins with titanium clips, and resort to chemotherapy, radiation therapy, or a combination. Return in 3 months for a second look.

Commentary by H. Norman Noe

There is no instance in pediatric urology in which proper surgical planning and precise technical execution are more important than in the excision of neuroblastoma. Of primary importance are gaining early control and ligation of the vascular pedicle to the tumorous kidney. Incision of the parietal peritoneum directly over the great vessels usually provides proper access for early ligation of the artery and thus avoidance of forced collateral venous drainage and a potential embolic phenomenon in the process of dissection. There are times, however, with very bulky tumors when this simple approach will not suffice. In these cases, incision of the peritoneum lateral to the colon can allow separation of the colonic mesentery anteriorly from Gerota's fascia, leaving the fascia intact and giving access to the inferior and medial portions of the hilum.

On occasion, mobilization of a substantial segment of the inferior vena cava with careful identification and ligation of the lumbar vessels is necessary to rotate the tumor and venous drainage away from the renal artery to allow proper ligation. Forceful retraction of the renal vein on the affected side, which still can occlude venous return and force collateral venous drainage, should be avoided. For larger tumors, it also is important that the SMA is identified early in the course of dissection to avoid injury to that important structure. Once vascular control at the pedicle has been achieved, it still is important to avoid damaging the thin, friable parasitic veins, which, in some tumors, can be quite numerous and prominent. Proper treatment and ligation of these parasitic vessels can minimize blood loss and the chance of tumor spillage.

Gentle dissection once the vascular pedicle has been clamped usually allows removal of the tumor with Gerota's fascia and its enclosed fat to be accomplished without rupture of the tumor. Although it is unlikely that it will be necessary to resect adjacent structures because of tumor invasion, one still must be prepared and have planned for just such a contingency.

CHAPTER 36

Calyceal Diverticulectomy

If stones are present, extracorporeal shock-wave lithotripsy may be used first with the hope that the fragments will pass. Consider a percutaneous approach directly into the diverticulum, then dilate the calyceal neck. A large nephrostomy tube may be left through the diverticulum for 2 weeks, anticipating obliteration of the cavity. Open excision is an alternative.

1 After exposure of the appropriate area of the kidney, check the location of the diverticulum by palpation or, if deep, by aspiration with an 18-gauge needle. Use intraoperative ultrasonography for small fluid-filled diverticula and those containing stones.

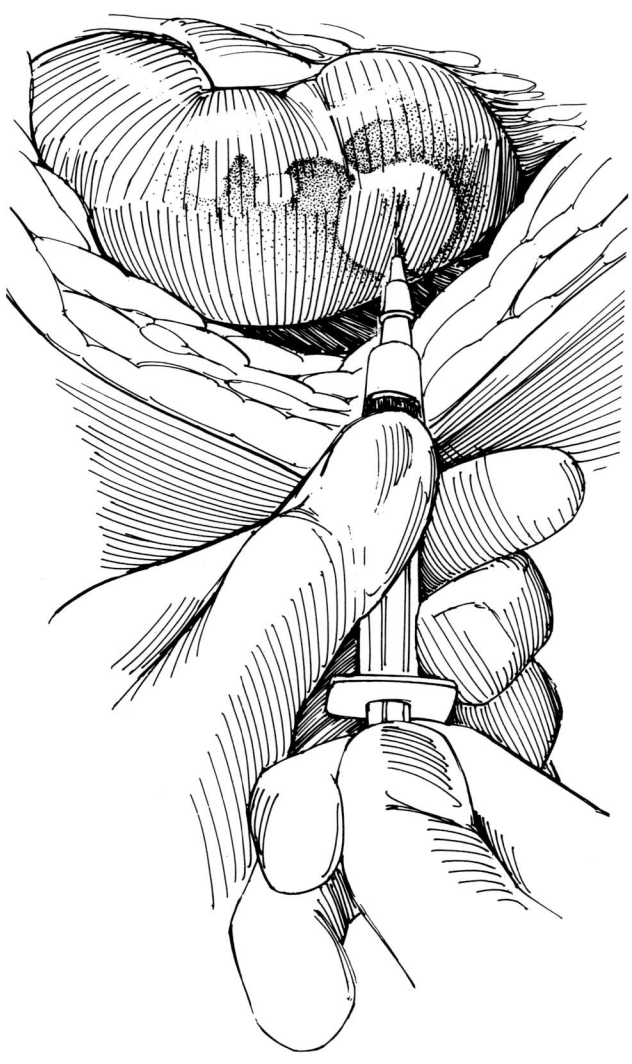

2 **A,** Incise through the parenchyma into the diverticulum, and trim excess cortex and capsule. Marsupialize the edges of the diverticulum with interrupted 3-0 synthetic absorbable sutures. A wedge excision may be needed. The transitional epithelial lining seldom needs to be removed.

B, If necessary, inject dilute methylene blue into the renal pelvis to identify the narrow neck of the diverticulum. Incise the neck circumferentially, and invert the wall with 3-0 synthetic absorbable sutures. Pack the cavity with perirenal fat, and place a Penrose drain to the area. Consider partial nephrectomy for deeper, larger, or polar diverticula.

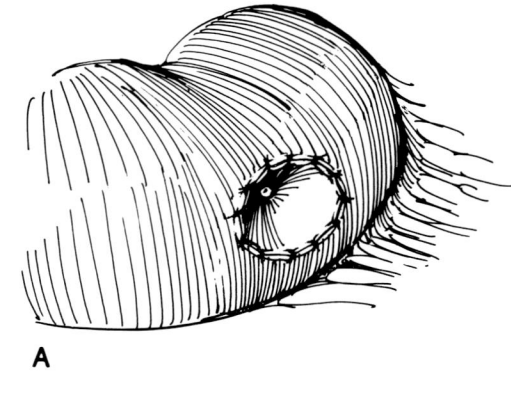

A

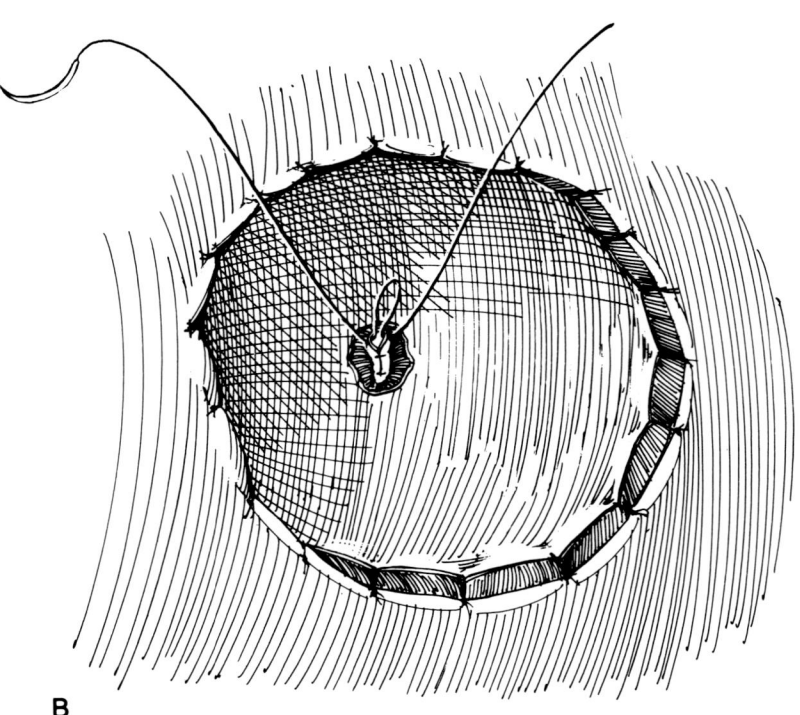

B

POSTOPERATIVE PROBLEMS

Prolonged urinary drainage indicates incomplete closure of the diverticular neck. Other problems are similar to those after a partial nephrectomy.

Commentary by Joseph D. M. de Vries

Clinical diverticula, which originate from a minor calyx and are lined by transitional epithelium, can vary from the size of a pea to that of a ping-pong ball, with an incidence of 3 per 1000 in both children and adults. Sometimes the differentiation with a solitary cyst can be extremely difficult. One must remember that the latter seldom occurs in childhood; the presence of a cystic Wilms' tumor must be excluded in these cases.

Unfortunately, size seldom correlates with clinical symptoms; even the smallest ones can provoke severe colicky pains when involved with infection or stone formation.

Always think to exclude tuberculosis of the kidney!

If we are dealing with a clinically important solitary lesion, we always try first to solve the problem by a percutaneous route. For adults, we puncture the kidney directly on the stone, but in children, we prefer an open procedure through a posterior lumbotomy as the least traumatic approach, because no muscles need be cut. If the overlying parenchyma is still substantial, we use the Cavitron ultrasonic aspirator instrument to remove it without any blood loss. The marsupialization is performed with only three or four stitches, and after the neck of the diverticulum is inverted, we use collagen tissue spray to firmly fix perirenal fat at the bottom and the edges of the diverticulum instantly. In this way, postoperative leakage of urine should not occur.

The increasing experience with endoscopic-laparoscopic procedures today makes their use for this purpose feasible. We now remove (small) kidneys and adrenal tumors by this route, making it possible to discharge the patient after 1 day of hospitalization; so far, however, we have no personal experience with this procedure treating calyceal diverticula. If one has no experience with the percutaneous operative procedure and an open operation is contraindicated, an alternative method is simply to puncture the cyst, leave a pigtail stent, and perform chemolysis of the stone, using mostly an acid irrigation fluid, such as Renacidin, depending on the component of the stone mass.

If during the operation no passageway to the pyelocalyceal system can be found, we suspect a "simple" cyst, because the epithelial lining is capable of excreting fluid. If we are unable to remove this epithelium completely, we must put in an omental flap to prevent new diverticulum formation.

SECTION 4
Adrenal Gland

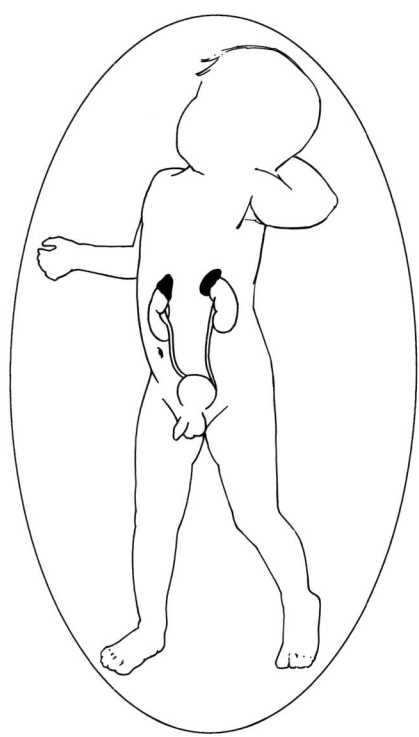

CHAPTER 37

Preparation and Approaches to Adrenal Surgery

PHEOCHROMOCYTOMA

Measure plasma catecholamines, such as epinephrine (adrenal source), norepinephrine (extra-adrenal source), metanephrine, and normetanephrine. An oral clonidine-suppression test may be useful in doubtful cases. Localize the tumor. In children (in whom 10 per cent of tumors are bilateral; 10 per cent, multiple; and 10 per cent, extra-adrenal) tumor localization is done by computed tomographic (CT) scan, magnetic resonance imaging using both T_1 and T_2 images (pheochromocytomas light up on T_1; adenomas are hypodense compared with metastatic lesions), radionuclide studies with metaiodobenzyl guanidine (^{131}MIBG) scan, positron emission tomographic scan, or rarely, venous sampling.

Preparation. A day or two ahead of time, provide the child with whole blood equivalent to 2 units in an adult, regardless of blood-volume studies. Avoid stimulatory diagnostic procedures. Preoperative and intraoperative adrenergic blockade with prazosin or phenoxybenzamine or a catecholamine-synthesis inhibitor such as α-methyltyrosine, while preventing hypertensive crises, does make the detection of small extra-adrenal tumors more difficult by blunting the sudden rise in blood pressure during exploration, which may be the only indication of their presence. For dysrhythmia during the operation, use intravenous (IV) lidocaine or propranolol. To be safe, have two experienced anesthesiologists at the table and adequate monitoring equipment.

Place one IV catheter to monitor central venous pressure. Insert a second IV catheter for fluid administration. To the connector next to the vein, attach the tubing from the bottle containing the drug for control of excess blood pressure. Keep the connection close to the vein to avoid dead space and resultant delay in getting the drug into the circulation. Monitor intra-arterial pressure with a cannula in the radial or brachial artery. Maintain electrocardiogram tracings continuously. Induce anesthesia with thiopental sodium. For an anesthetic agent, avoid halothane and tubocurarine chloride; methoxyflurane is preferred, along with succinylcholine and nitrous oxide. Use sodium nitroprusside or phentolamine to reverse hypertensive crises that occur with intubation or manipulation of the tumor. In any case, stabilize the patient before beginning the operation. A hypotensive episode during surgery requires the vigorous administration of whole blood and plasma volume expanders to fill the vascular spaces consequent to removal of α-adrenergic stimuli. Sympathomimetic amines can be used as backup. Vasoconstrictors, however, have the risk of precipitating renal shutdown and cerebral ischemia. For hypotension after removal of the tumor, expand the blood volume with fluids and whole blood.

Incision. An anterior transabdominal incision through a high modified chevron-shaped incision (page 81) is the approach of choice for pheochromocytoma because of the bilaterality of this condition and the high incidence of extra-adrenal sites—especially in children, in whom these tumors are often bilateral and multiple (20 to 30 per cent). However, newer imaging techniques for localization of pheochromocytoma make a lateral approach tempting, because it results in far fewer complications. A good rule is to avoid a lateral approach in children whom you suspect to have extra-adrenal pheochromocytomas. An anterior approach also is preferred in infants for excision of neuroblastoma, which often is infiltrating and thus not confined to the adrenal. For the same reason, approaching anteriorly through a modified chevron incision is suitable for tumors greater than 10 cm in diameter in patients of any age. Also, if a child must undergo reoperation for adrenal disease, the exposure will be much better through the peritoneum than through the flank. However, the disadvantages of an anterior incision are several: the exposure takes longer to obtain, and the approach to the adrenal is not as direct. Furthermore, the adrenals usually are found to lie surprisingly deep and high. Postoperatively, ileus is common, and intestinal adhesions may become a problem.

In any case, a radical adrenalectomy is required to remove adjacent neural crest tissue.

Postoperative Support. Continue monitoring the blood pressure, because acute hypotension is still a risk, especially if the child is moved. Correct it with fluids. Check the blood glucose level to detect hypoglycemia before it can become fatal. Follow up with metanephrine and vanillylmandelic acid levels every 6 months for 3 years and yearly for another 4 years. Recurrent (residual) tumors, with recurrence of symptoms, are not infrequently found in the opposite adrenal but are small and easily excised.

OTHER ADRENAL TUMORS

Preparation for surgery and the surgical approach to an adrenal lesion other than pheochromocytoma and neuroblastoma depend on the type and function of the lesion. Localization has become so exact that exploration using bilateral exposure rarely is necessary. Endocrine support and supplementation are critical to a successful outcome.

To prevent adrenal insufficiency during and after such a stressful procedure, prepare any child or adolescent scheduled for adrenal excision with steroids by giving cortisone acetate in appropriate doses orally for 2 days preoperatively. Supplement this with an IV dose both immediately before and immediately after surgery. Subsequent therapy depends on the amount of adrenal tissue left after surgery.

CUSHING'S SYNDROME

The cause of Cushing's syndrome may be excess adrenocorticotropic hormone (ACTH) production by the pituitary gland in 70 per cent of cases; a primary tumor of the adrenal cortex in 20 to 25 per cent; or extra-adrenal tumors, such as oat-cell carcinomas of the lung or tumors of the thymus, in 5 to 10 per cent.

Rule out pituitary tumor. Measure serum cortisol levels. Perform a dexamethasone-suppression test. If the cortisol level is depressed, the diagnosis is bilateral hyperplasia. An autonomous tumor is present if no depression occurs. Measure ACTH levels to detect ectopic production of the hormone.

For adrenal-dependent Cushing's syndrome, localize the tumor before exploration with radionuclide studies (65 per cent accuracy) or CT scan (80 per cent accuracy). Venous sampling can be very accurate. For pituitary-dependent Cushing's syndrome, consider pharmacologic agents directed at the pituitary (bromocriptine) or the adrenal (mitotane), pituitary irradiation, trans-sphenoidal hypophysectomy, or bilateral adrenalectomy. Realize that adenomas, cysts, cortical carcinomas, and myelolipomas may be difficult to differentiate. For perioperative endocrine control with Cushing's syndrome, give cortisone acetate in a dose equivalent to 100 to 200 mg intramuscularly (IM) in the adult the evening before and the morning of surgery. Immediately after the operation, give another 100 mg IM.

Start water-soluble cortisol IV at a rate of up to 10 mg/h. Give cortisone acetate IM every 8 hours on days 1 and 2 and every 12 hours on days 3 and 4. Start a maintenance dose orally twice a day along with fludrocortisone daily for a month.

CHAPTER 38

Surgical Approaches to the Adrenals

POSTERIOR APPROACH

The posterior approach is ideal for small, well-localized benign adrenal tumors, providing adequate access with the lowest morbidity. However, do not use it for pheochromocytoma in children, for large adrenal tumors with their parasitic blood supply, or for malignant tumors with the potential for intra-abdominal extension. For these cases, use the wider field obtained by an anterior approach.

ANTERIOR APPROACH

Choose an anterior transabdominal approach through a modified chevron incision (page 81) for pheochromocytomas that may be bilateral or at sites distant from the adrenal. For well-localized pheochromocytomas or for large masses, especially in obese children, use the thoracoabdominal incision (page 102); it is safer and avoids traction on the tumor.

Approach to the Left Adrenal for Pheochromocytoma

Localize the tumor with magnetic resonance imaging (MRI) and perhaps also with metaiodobenzyl guanidine (^{131}MIGB) scan. In children, multiple tumors are not rare.

1 **A,** *Position:* Place the child supine. *Incision:* Make a pediatric extended anterior incision (shown) or a chevron incision (page 81). **B,** Rather than reflecting the splenic flexure, approach the adrenals through the lesser sac. Mobilize the colon medially by incising the splenocolic ligament. For more exposure, ligate the inferior mesenteric vein and divide the ligament of Treitz. Dissect the pancreas from the surface of the adrenal gland. Incise the retroperitoneum just below the lower border of the pancreas and open Gerota's fascia.

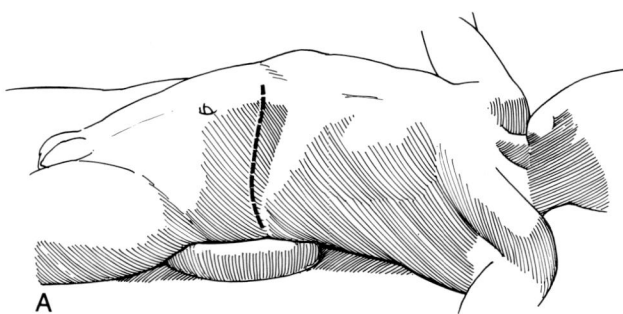

A

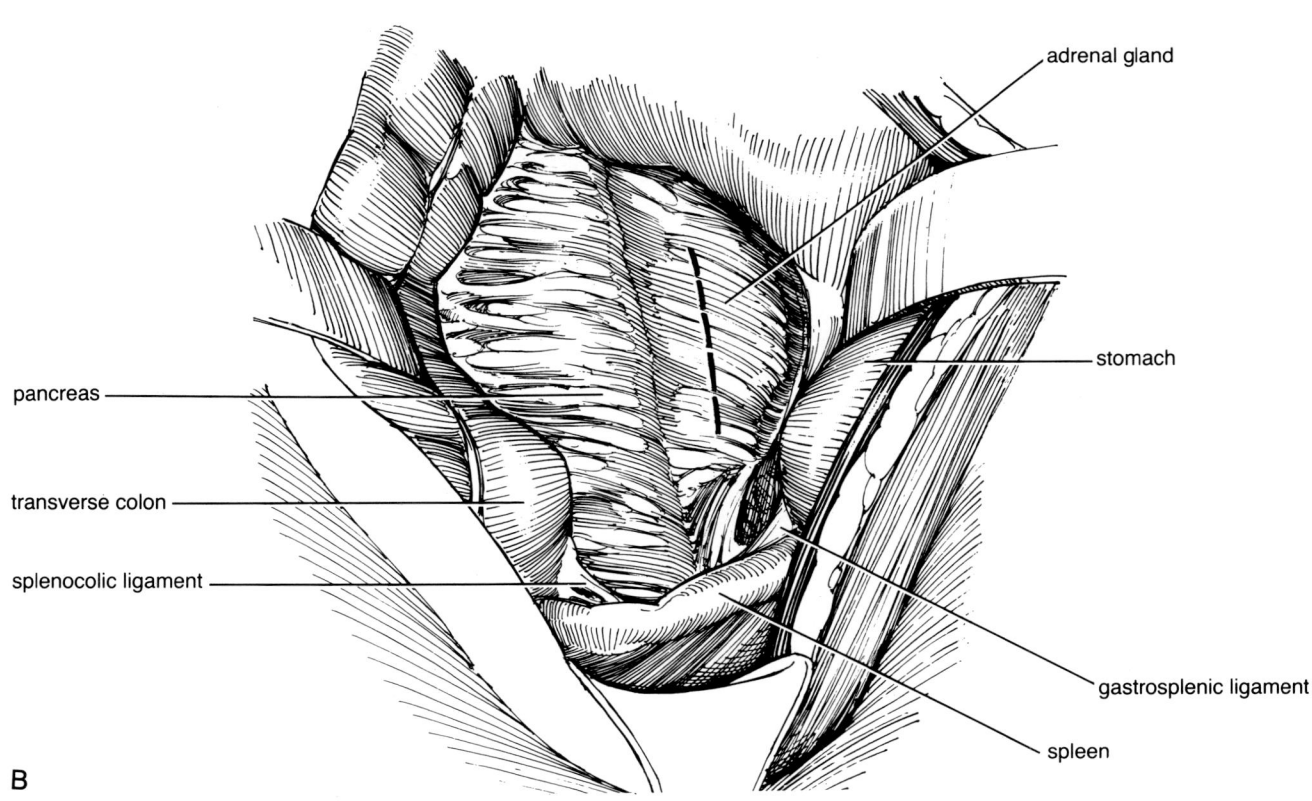

adrenal gland

stomach

pancreas

transverse colon

splenocolic ligament

gastrosplenic ligament

spleen

B

2 Place retractors; use a large ring retractor. Realize that pheochromocytomas, especially large ones, are soft and friable, and some are malignant, so any break in the capsule can cause recurrence. **A,** Carefully free the gland from its bed inferiorly. **B,** Dissect it laterally to the superior margin of the left renal vein and locate the adrenal vein, which may empty into the inferior phrenic vein or even directly into the vena cava.

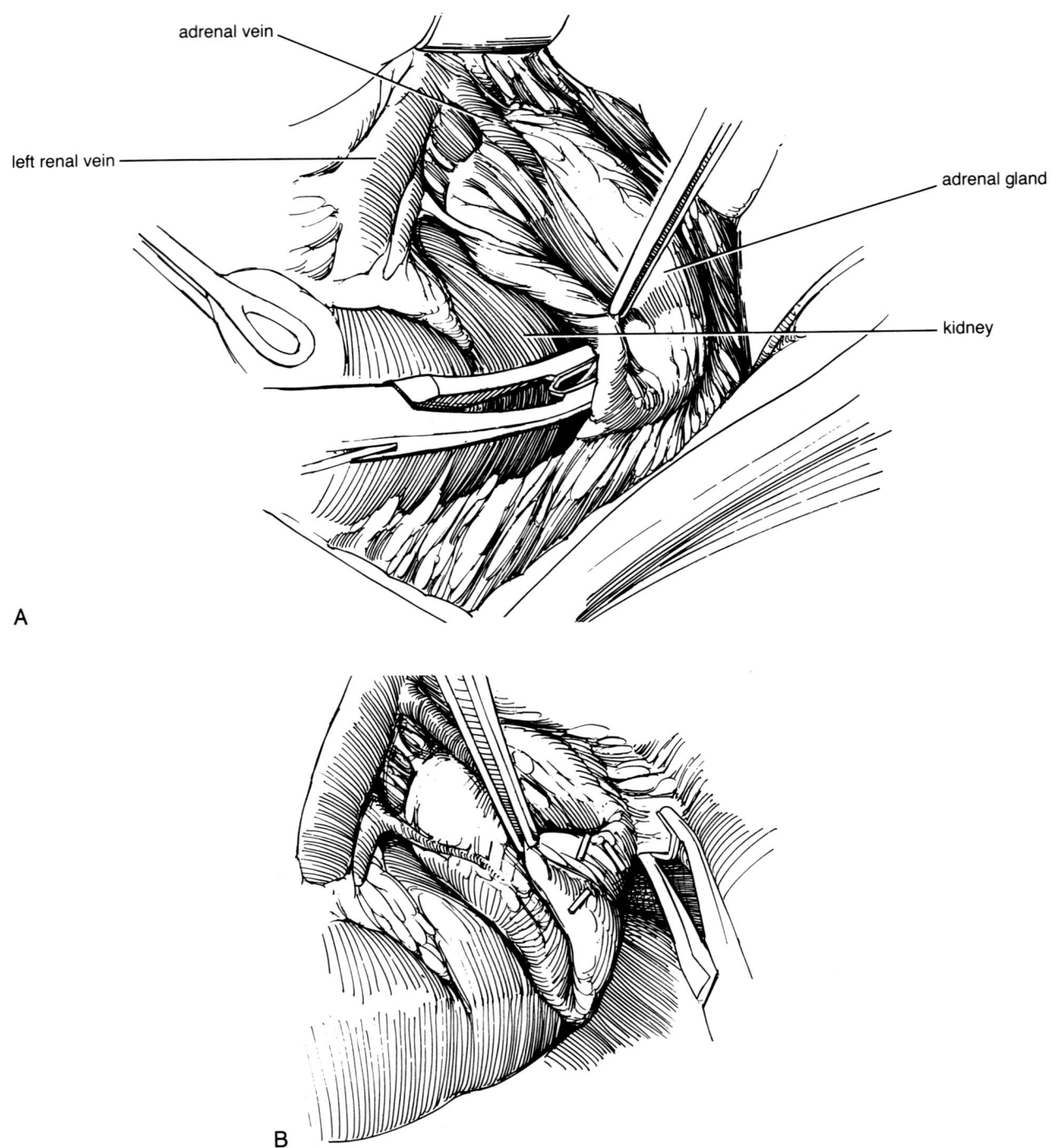

3 Dissect out the vein and notify the anesthesiologist. Pass a 2–0 silk ligature and be ready to ligate the vein proximally. If the patient is stable, avoid venous congestion, which increases friability, by delaying venous ligation until the arterial inflow is controlled. Otherwise, clamp and divide the vein and ligate it beneath the clamp. Leave the distal ligature long for traction.

For either left or right pheochromocytomas, if malignancy is suspected, as evidenced by fixation or by invasion of local tissues, proceed with regional lymphadenectomy. Look for other tumors in the para-aortic region by opening the posterior peritoneum over the aorta and palpating the renal pedicle on both sides and the groove between the aorta and vena cava to a point below the bifurcation. Close the retroperitoneal incision. Reapproximate the gastrocolic ligament, and close the abdominal wound.

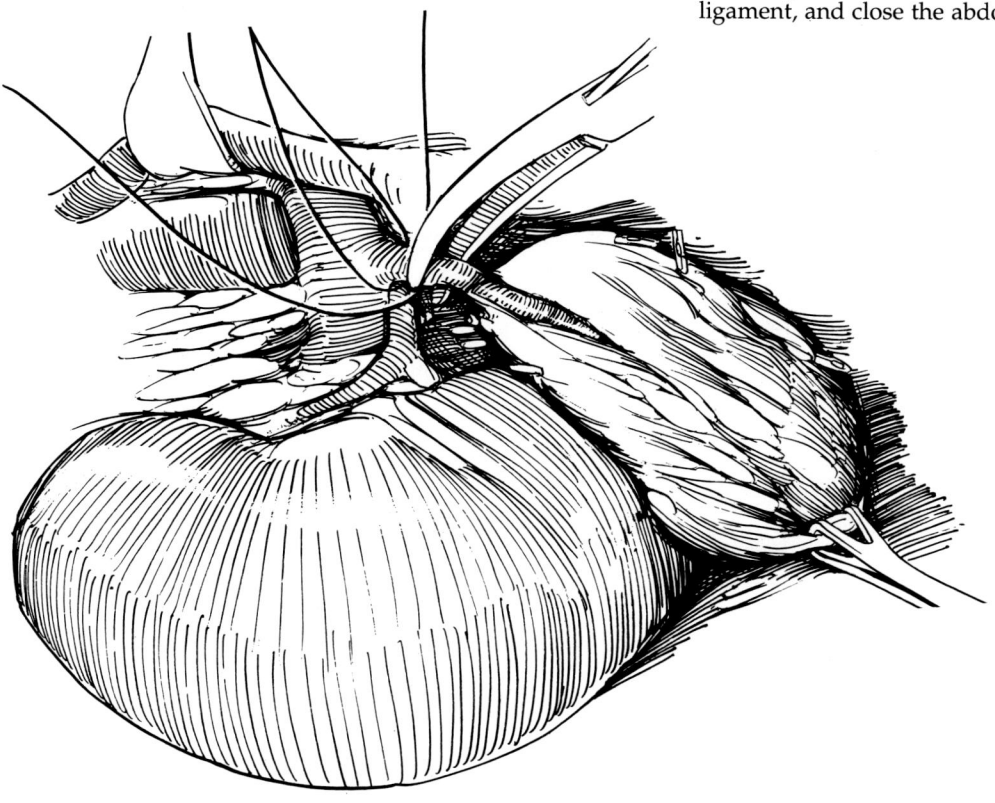

Approach to the Right Adrenal for Pheochromocytoma

4 **A,** The exposure here will not be as wide as on the left side. Make an extended pediatric anterior incision or a chevron incision (page 79, 81). A thoracoabdominal incision is an alternative (page 102). **B,** Retract the liver and perform a wide Kocher maneuver to mobilize the duodenum. Free the hepatic flexure of the colon, using clips as needed, to expose the right colic artery. Continue to incise the parietal peritoneum to the level of the cecum.

duodenum

right kidney

adrenal gland

B

A

5 Pull the kidney down and dissect the right adrenal laterally, as described for the left adrenal.

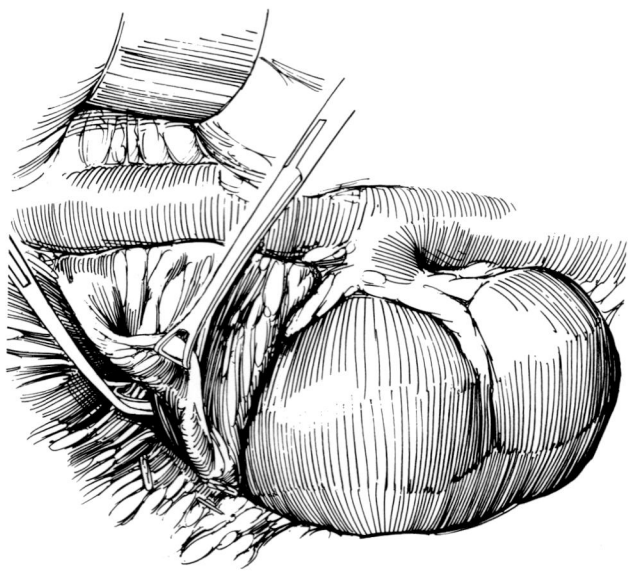

6 Clip the branch from the phrenic artery.

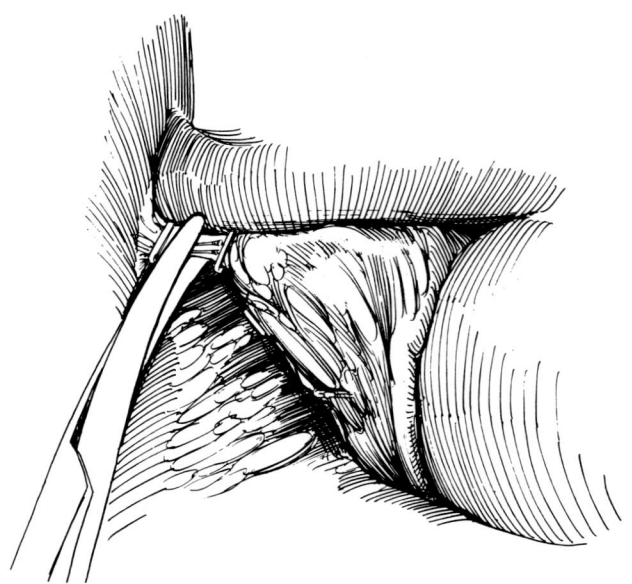

7 Expose the adrenal vein entering the vena cava by dissecting from above downward. Take great care not to injure the thin-walled vein or tear the vena cava. Gently retract the vena cava with a long vein retractor. Notify the anesthesiologist, place a 2-0 silk suture around the vein, and ligate it near the vena cava. If the vein is short and wide, insinuate a Satinsky clamp onto the cava and use that for control instead of using a ligature alone. Tie or place a hemoclip distally. Individually clip the small arteries from the aorta; do not try to tie them. Remove the specimen. Close the retroperitoneum and the wound.

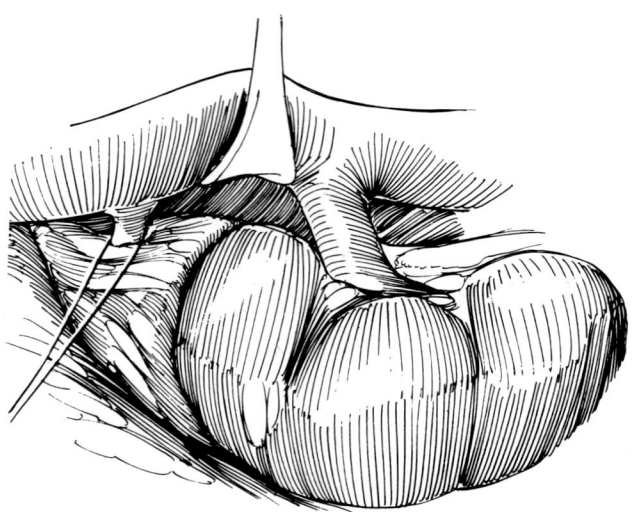

SIMULTANEOUS BILATERAL EXPOSURE

8 With the child prone and a pillow under the abdomen (not shown), either make a bilateral lumbotomy incision or resect the 12th rib bilaterally.

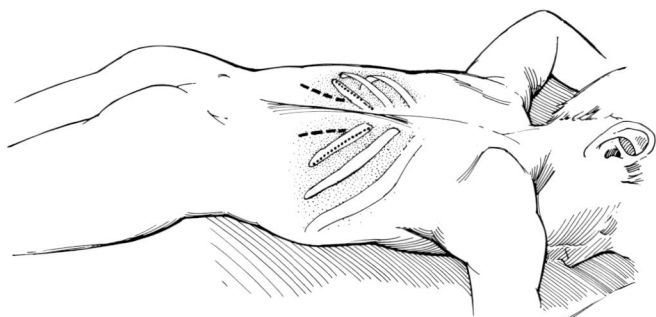

Postoperative Problems

Adrenal insufficiency and *hypotension* are related to the preoperative diagnosis and the amount of adrenal tissue remaining. Appropriately monitored therapy (Chapter 37) will replace the deficits. *Other complications* are similar to those after nephrectomy (page 159). Pneumothorax and pancreatic and splenic injury are not uncommon, nor are wound infections, retroperitoneal hemorrhage and hematomas, and thrombophlebitis. More particular to adrenalectomy are injuries to the portal vein, to the vena cava at the entrance of the adrenal vein, and to the hepatic vein—all of which are managed intraoperatively. Subdiaphragmatic abscess can be an additional complication.

Commentary by E. Darracott Vaughan Jr.

I generally use a flank or lateral approach in patients with adrenal adenomas (either incidental or causing Cushing's syndrome), smaller adrenal carcinomas, and well-localized pheochromocytomas. An anterior approach is limited to patients with multiple pheochromocytomas or bilateral adrenal lesions. Children are in the high-risk group for multiple pheochromocytomas; however, [131]MIBG scanning and MRI are extremely accurate in identifying multiple tumors, and if these tests show only a solitary lesion, I would use a flank approach, particularly on the right side where it is more difficult to isolate the adrenal vein from an anterior approach.

My standard rule in adrenal surgery is to leave the adrenal attached to the kidney and begin by dividing the most-posterior lateral attachments and then the superior attachments. This allows the operator to bring the adrenal gland down into a more accessible area. One exception is in patients with pheochromocytomas, in whom the initial dissection, particularly on the left, should be aimed at early control of the adrenal vein.

More recently, if a patient with the pheochromocytoma has very high levels of catecholamines or any evidence of cardiomyopathy, we would use not only phenoxybenzamine but also α-methyl-p-tyrosine to reduce catecholamine production.

Ureter

A repertoire of procedures is needed when the ureter must be resected or reinserted. Reimplantation into the bladder is most direct but not always possible. Mobilization of a wing of the bladder and anastomosis to the other ureter are alternatives. If such procedures are not applicable, fall back on mobilization of the kidney, autotransplantation, or ureteral substitution with bowel.

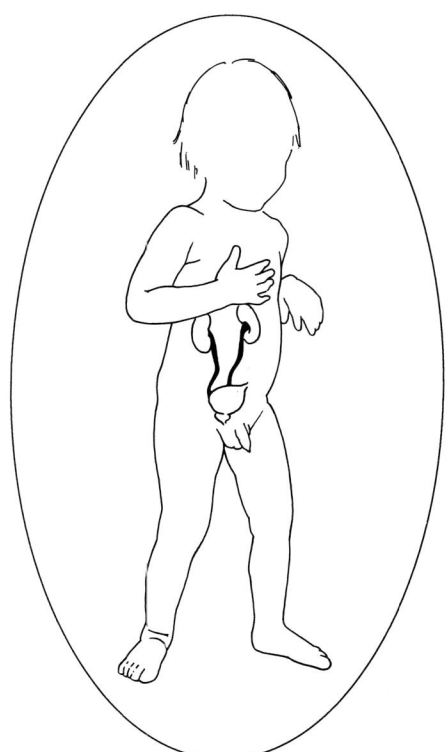

CHAPTER 39

Ureteroneocystostomy

Indications for antireflux surgery include breakthrough infection on suppressive antibiotics, severe reflux with previous episodes of pyelonephritis, and an anatomic abnormality of the orifice. Girls in whom reflux persists after puberty also may need operation.

For *vesicoureteral reflux,* obtain a dimethylsuccinic acid scan to assess for renal scarring and a voiding cystourethrogram. Ultrasonography can be useful as a screening procedure. Suggested protocols include the following: for *primary reflux* in single system, grade the reflux (it may not be necessary to observe the orifice cystoscopically, because its position correlates so well with grade of reflux); treat Grades 1 through 4 conservatively unless infection persists or parenchymal loss or scarring supervenes. For Grade 5, reimplant, or in duplex systems, perform pyelopyelostomy (page 230) or ureteroureterostomy (page 227). For *secondary reflux,* assess vesical urodynamic status for evidence of neurogenic or non-neurogenic bladder dysfunction; correct it with drugs and training before considering surgical treatment of the reflux, because implantation into such bladders often is unsuccessful. Every attempt should be made to obtain normal detrusor dynamics before operation.

Selection of Technique. For most cases in infants and children, the transvesical technique is used for small trigones or large ureters. The transvesical Politano-Leadbetter, distal tunnel advancement (Glenn-Anderson), or cross-trigonal (Cohen) technique is suitable for most cases, because simple advancement techniques may be done rapidly with minimal dissection. They are preferred for bilateral cases, because they do not interfere with perivesical nerves. The extravesical (Lich-Gregoir) or external tunnel (Barry) technique also is useful not only for unilateral "virginal" cases but also for more complicated ones. For megaureter, the ureteral tapering (Hendren) or folding techniques are used. For thick-walled bladders, the ureter can be dissected extravesically, repaired, and pulled through the original hiatus, to be advanced subepithelially, as in the Cohen technique.

Each technique has advantages and disadvantages; blind extravesical passage of the ureter as in the Politano-Leadbetter technique carries the risk of obstructing the ureter by kinking. The Glenn-Anderson advancement technique avoids this problem and is a good choice for the laterally placed ectopic ureteral orifice, although persistent reflux may be more common than with other techniques. The Cohen technique is easily performed but does have the limitation of making future catheterization difficult, even with flexible cystoscopes. The extravesical techniques are useful, especially with large ureters.

For *ureteral stenosis and injuries,* ureteroureterostomy in the lower ureter usually is technically difficult and not infrequently fails.

Suggested protocols are as follows: if the obstruction is low, do a ureteroneocystostomy with or without a psoas hitch (page 41); if higher, make a bladder flap (page 42A); if merely crushed, stent the ureter. Remember that a fibrotic or contracted bladder may be unsuitable for implantation or flap procedures. Consider performing ureteroureterostomy (page 227), using the appendix or transplanting the kidney (page 244) to bridge the gap. As a last resort, perform a ureteroileostomy (page 371) or even a cutaneous ureterostomy (page 360) or nephrectomy. In any case, avoid excessive ureteral mobilization and tension on the anastomosis. A nonrefluxing anastomosis may not be essential in an adult, making the anastomosis technically easier.

For bilateral megaureters, especially at reoperation, consider making a long reimplantation with a psoas hitch for one ureter and performing ureteroureterostomy for the other.

TRANSVESICAL TECHNIQUE
(POLITANO-LEADBETTER)

1 *Position:* Place the child supine in a frog-legged position, and insert a small silicone catheter into the bladder through the urethra. *Incision:* Make a small transverse lower abdominal incision (page 267) for primary operations; for secondary operations, a vertical abdominal incision may occasionally be required. Place a ring retractor. Incise the bladder vertically, then enlarge the opening with the two index fingers. A figure-eight suture may be placed where the incision approaches the retropubic space to prevent further tearing.

2 Place four stay sutures about the margin of the cystostomy, and drape them over the retractor for exposure (not shown), or place lateral retractor blades inside the bladder. Insert a moist pack in the bladder dome to be held with a Deaver retractor. Avoid rubbing the bladder wall, which can cause edema. Insert a 5 F infant feeding tube in the ureter and suture it to the orifice with a purse-string 4-0 synthetic absorbable suture.

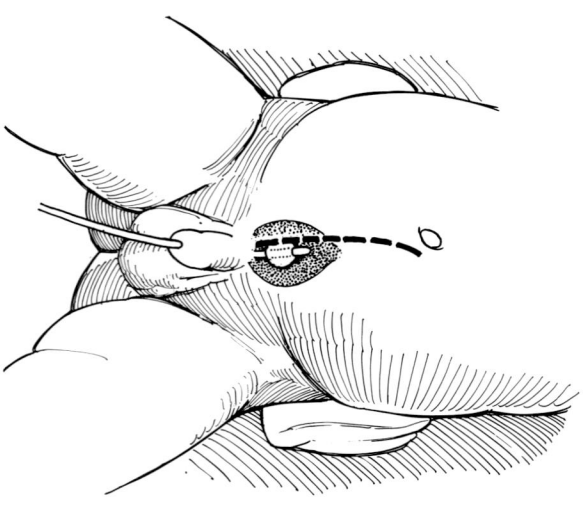

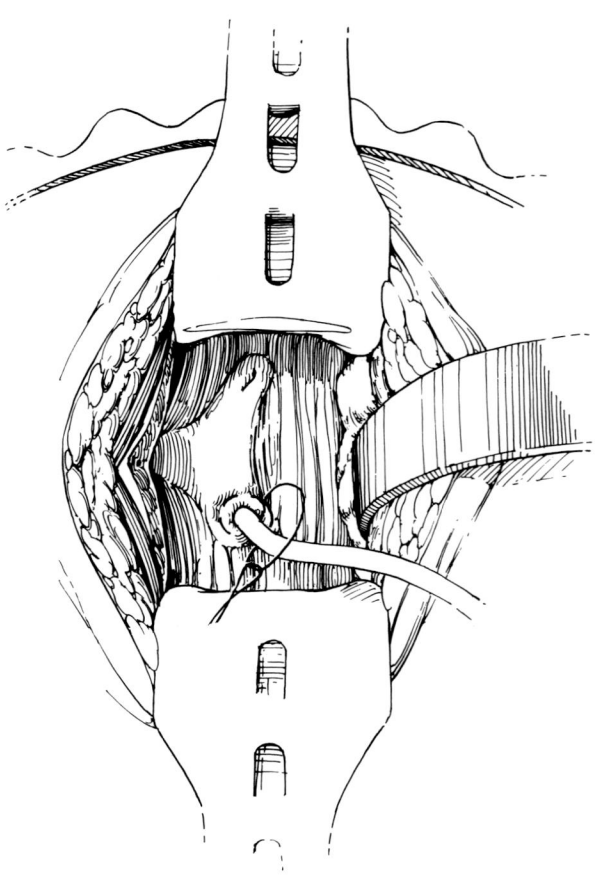

3 Gently lift the tube to draw the ureteral orifice into the bladder. Cut through the epithelium around the orifice with a hooked blade.

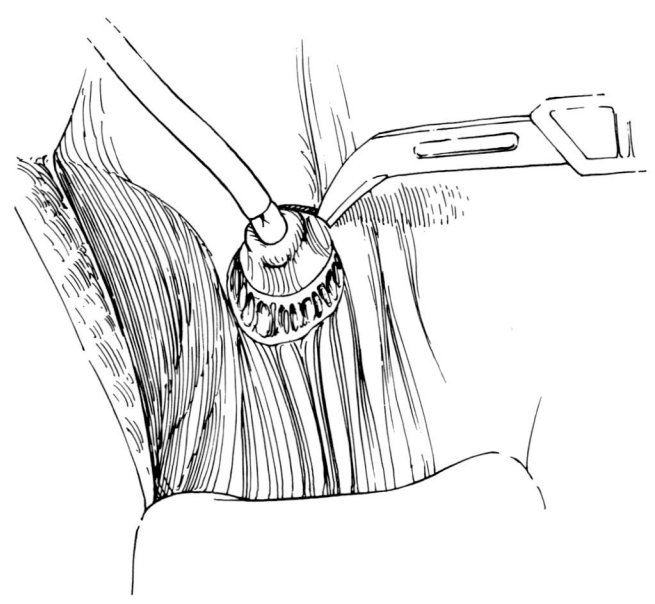

4 **A,** With tenotomy scissors held at right angles to the ureter, sharply divide the superficial trigonal muscles, which are clearly seen medially and inferiorly as the ureter is withdrawn. **B,** Develop a plane inferiorly next to the ureteral adventitia, and free the ureter of all attachments to Waldeyer's sheath bluntly and sharply, keeping away from its adventitial blood supply. Mobilize enough ureter by pushing the adherent peritoneum away with a peanut dissector to ensure tension-free respositioning. Preserve the ureteral adventitia, because stripping it results in ure-

teral ischemia and necrosis. Avoid kinking, twisting, or J-hooking the ureter. **C,** Insert traction sutures through the bladder wall medially and laterally to open the hiatus, and elevate the hiatus with a narrow Deaver retractor. Do not use forceps. Bluntly dissect between the ureter and bladder wall under vision with a large right-angle clamp or a Küttner dissector to free the peritoneal attachments. Avoid devascularization or perforation of the ureter. Be sure the clamp does not pass through peritoneum or bowel.

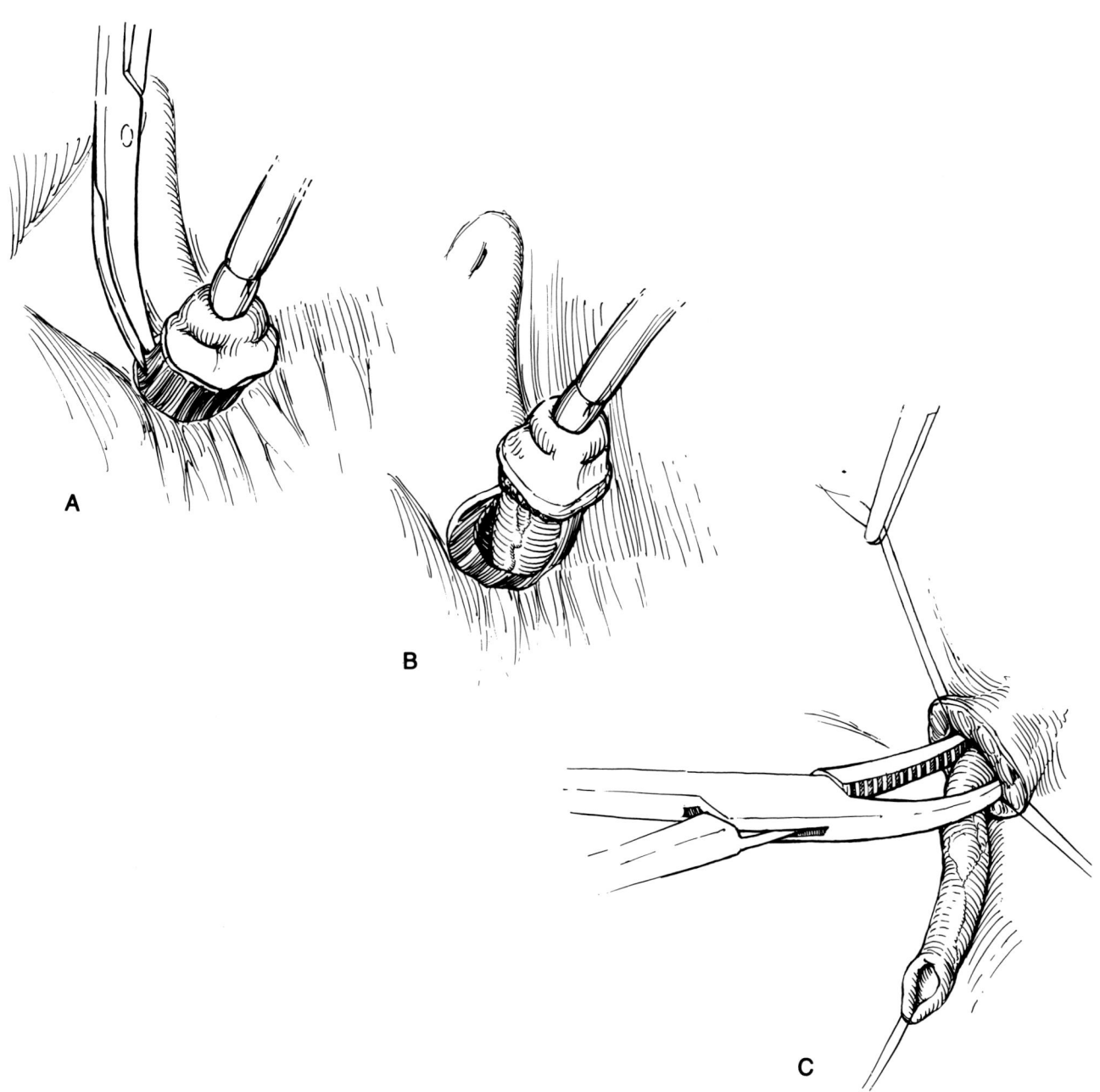

5 **A** and **B,** Insert a long Mixter clamp into the hiatus, and dissect along the outer surface of the bladder wall. Elevate the tip against the wall at a point 2.5 cm cephalad and slightly medial to the hiatus. A 3:1 or even 5:1 ratio of tunnel length to ureteral diameter is needed. Avoid placing the new hiatus any more lateral than the original one and be sure it is large enough. Incise onto the clamp. **C,** Catch the ureteral traction suture, and also the stent if it has not been removed, in a right-angle clamp, and draw it up through the tunnel and out the new hiatus. Pull the ureter into the bladder through the retrovesical tunnel, checking to be certain it is not kinked. Close the bladder wall behind the original hiatus with interrupted 3-0 or 4-0 synthetic absorbable sutures. If a longer tunnel is needed, incise the hiatus cephalolaterally and close the bladder wall below the ureter.

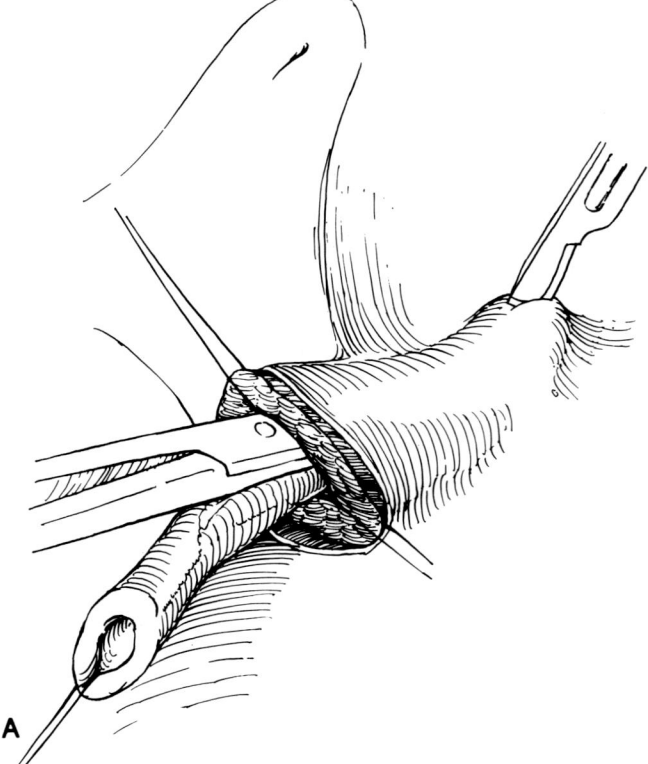

A

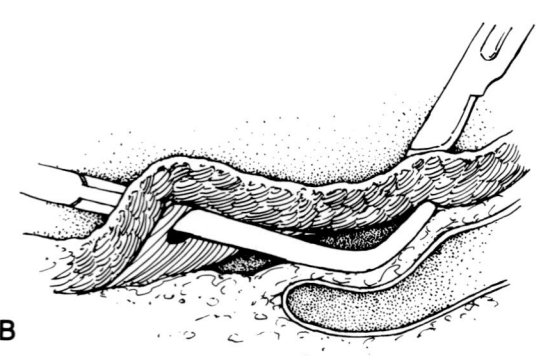

B

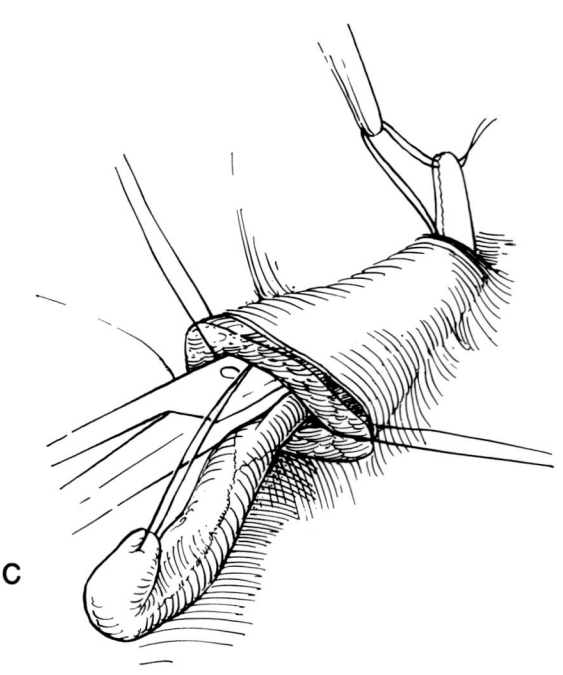

C

6 **A,** Dissect a subepithelial tunnel from the new hiatus to the old hiatus by cutting and spreading with small curved scissors. It may be easier in some cases to dissect from the other direction. If the roof is torn, merely tack it back after implanting the ureter. It is even possible to incise the intervening epithelium and dissect it back as two flaps to be subsequently approximated over the ureter. In any case, check the size of the tunnel by inserting a mosquito clamp. **B,** Pass a clamp, holding the stay suture down through the tunnel, grasp it with another clamp, and draw the ureter through. Again check the caliber of the tunnel and hiatus. The tunnel should lie within the square outlined on the trigone depicted in the inset.

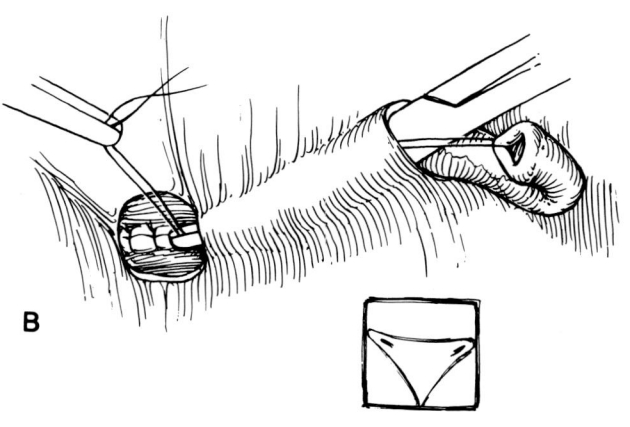

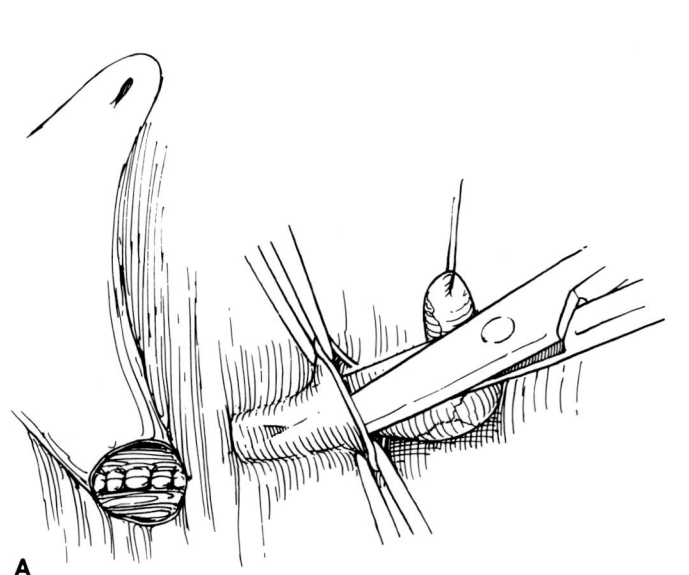

7 **A,** Trim the old meatus from the ureter, and, if needed, spatulate the end on the medial aspect. Anchor the tip with two sutures placed deeply into the trigonal muscle and through the vesical epithelium. **B,** Complete the anastomosis with carefully placed 4-0 or 5-0 synthetic absorbable sutures for an epithelium-to-epithelium coaptation. Close the upper epithelium incision vertically with the same suture material. Pass a 3.5 or 5 F infant feeding tube to be sure no ureteral kinks are present. Stent the ureter with this tube if desired. The stent will align the ureter and prevent possibly obstructive kinks or adhesions. Suture it with a 4-0 plain catgut suture to the opposite side of the bladder near the neck and bring it out through a stab wound.

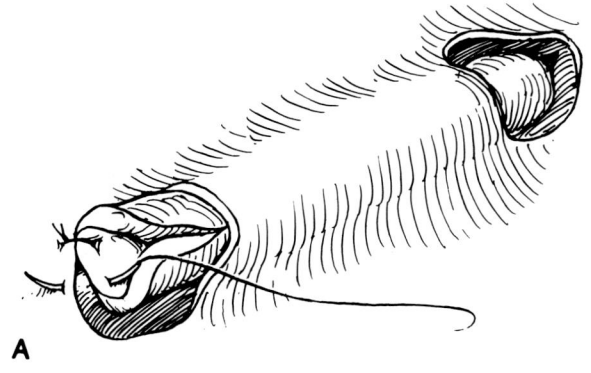

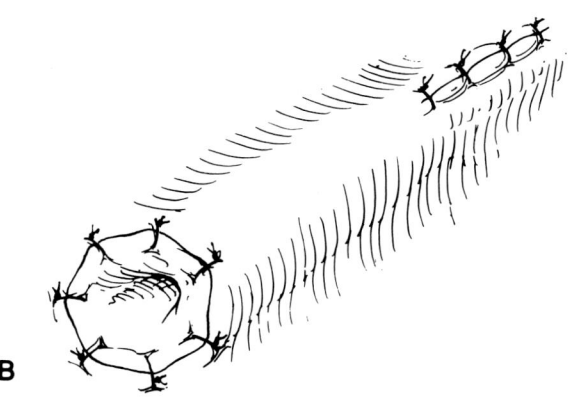

8 **A,** For additional length, tunnel distally. **B** and **C,** Draw the ureter through to the new hiatus and suture it there. Close the two epithelial defects longitudinally. **D,** Alternatively, advance the meatus by incising rather than tunneling the more distal epithelium and closing it over the ureter.

To drain the bladder in boys, insert a 14 or 16 F Malecot catheter. A small transurethral silicone balloon catheter also can be used effectively. Bring the catheter through a stab wound in the bladder and out just above the abdominal incision. In girls, the ureteral stents can be brought out easily through the urethra alongside a small balloon catheter. In many cases, it is easier to insert an 8 to 12 F red rubber catheter in the urethra, put a 2-0 silk stitch through its tip, and bring both ends of the suture through the bladder and abdominal walls so it may be tied over a gauze roll.

Close the bladder in layers with a running 4-0 subepithelial plain catgut suture, then with interrupted 3-0 chromic catgut or synthetic absorbable sutures to the muscle. Place a small Penrose drain in the space of Retzius and bring it out through a stab wound below the incision. Reapproximate the rectus muscles and fascia with 3-0 or 4-0 synthetic absorbable sutures. Close the subcutaneous tissue with fine plain catgut sutures and the skin with a subcuticular 4-0 or 5-0 synthetic absorbable sutures.

After operation, continue with prophylactic antibiotics. Obtain an intravenous urogram or sonogram at 6 weeks and a voiding cystourethrogram at 12 weeks. Monitor the urine by culture. If reflux is cured, stop the suppressive antibiotics, but continue checking the urine for infection. At 1 and 3 years postoperatively, obtain a renal ultrasound study to assess renal growth and rule out hydronephrosis.

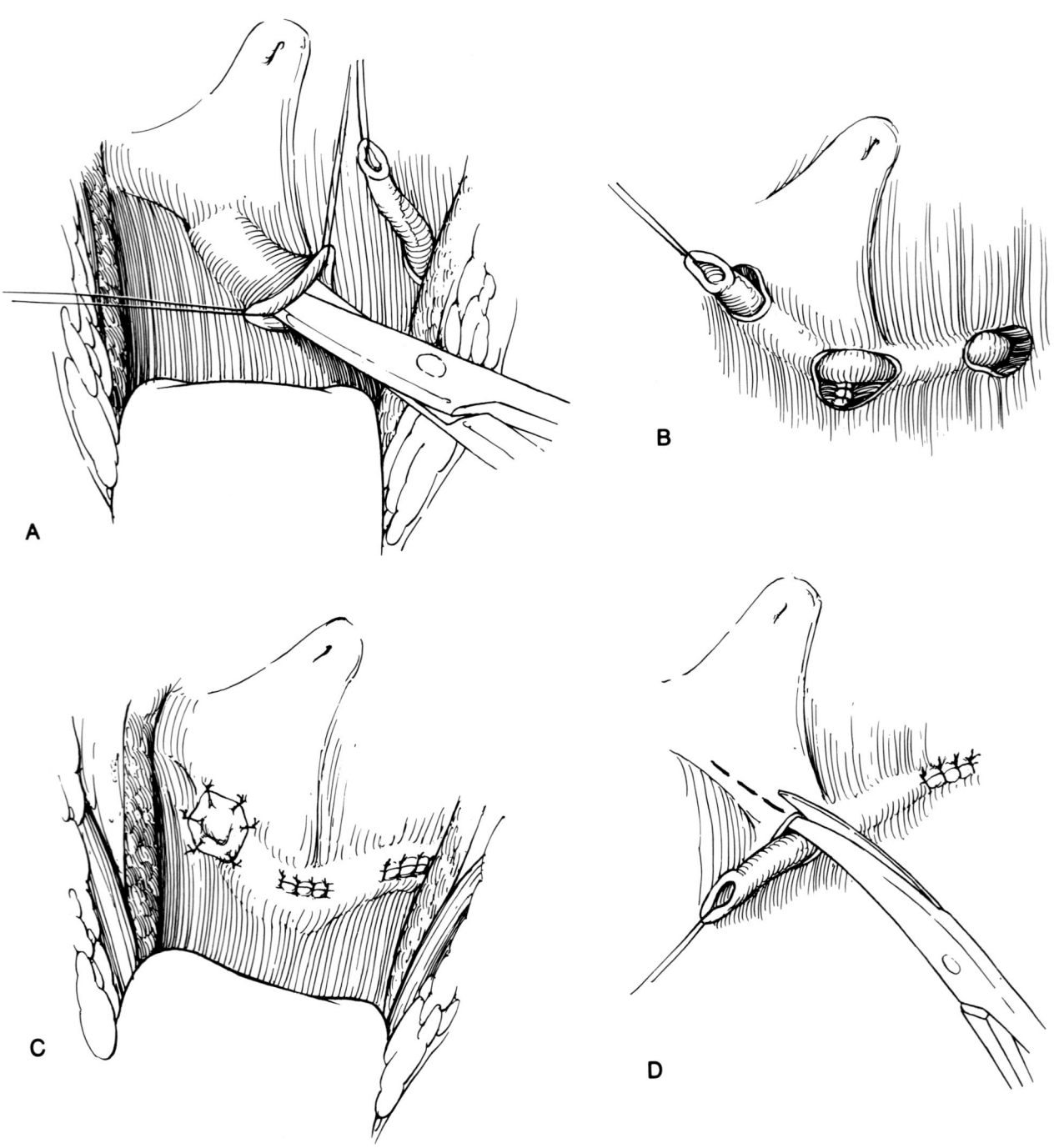

DISTAL TUNNEL REIMPLANTATION
(GLENN-ANDERSON)

This technique is done under direct vision without blind extravesical dissection. It fixes the ureteral orifice well down on the trigone, providing for maximal closure and prevention of reflux and an orifice that is catheterized readily.

9 **A,** Free the ureter as described. Create a subepithelial tunnel distally to form a new hiatus. **B,** Incise the entire thickness of the vesical wall above the original hiatus. Do not deviate laterally. **C,** Close the defect behind the ureter with interrupted 4-0 synthetic absorbable sutures. **D,** Draw the ureter through the tunnel with a right-angle clamp. Trim, fix, and anastomose it to the vesical epithelium. Close the original epithelial defect.

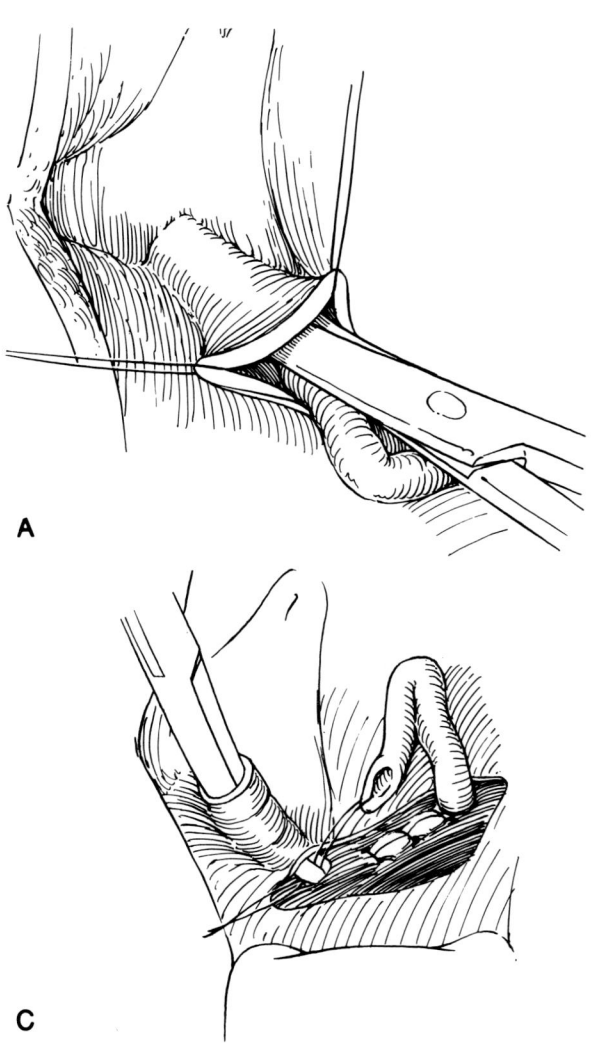

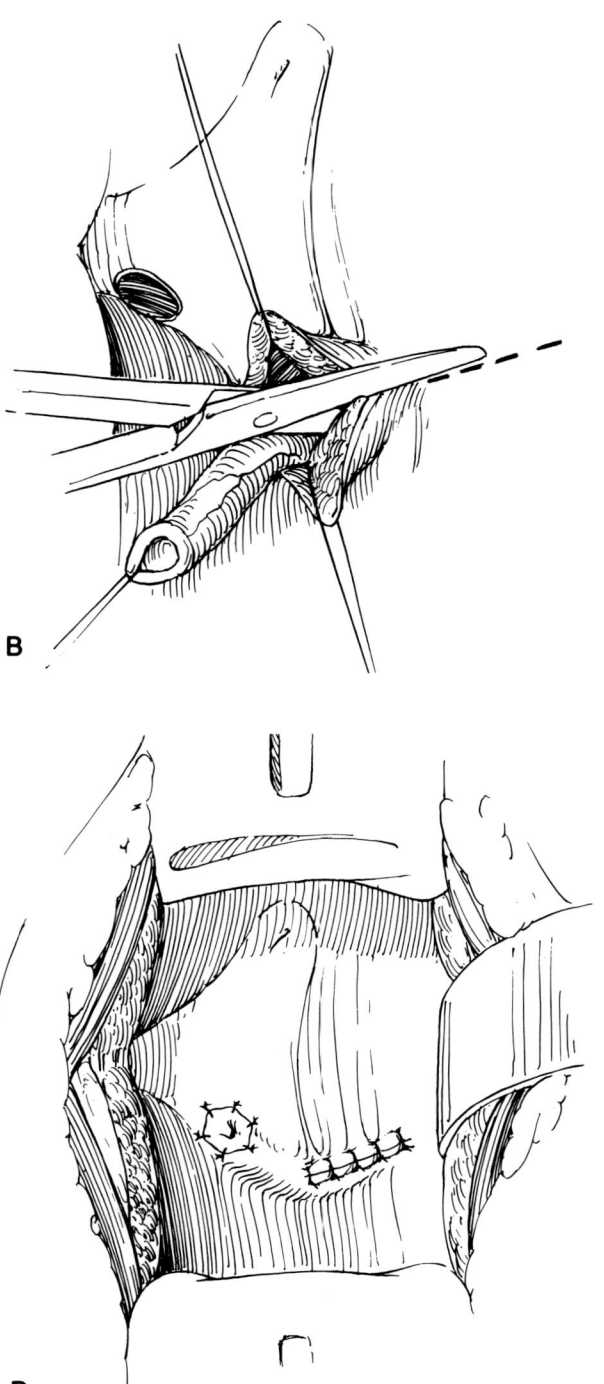

TRANSTRIGONAL TECHNIQUE
(COHEN)

Free the ureter as described previously. Assess the size of the hiatus; if it is too large, narrow it with two or three fine synthetic absorbable sutures. Be sure the ureter is freely mobile. If more exposure is needed, incise the superolateral margin of the hiatus with the cutting current, and lift the edge with small vein retractors. This maneuver also will allow a higher and, consequently, longer tunnel.

10 **A,** Incise the epithelium vertically just above and slightly lateral to the opposite ureteral orifice, depending on the size of the trigone. Pull up on that edge of the bladder with Allis clamps to tent the bladder wall. Insert Lahey scissors, and gently open and close them to advance across to a point approximately 1 cm above the opposite orifice. Of course, much depends on the size of the ureter and the trigone. When crossing the midline with the scissors, be careful not to let the tips go too deeply into the muscle. Take special care not to let the scissor tips curve too much anteriorly and go through the epithelium. When the orifices are pulled laterally and the intratrigonal area is stretched, this area becomes flatter. Remove the tube from the ureter. Insert a curved clamp, and draw the ureter through the tunnel by its traction suture until it lies free of tension. **B,** Trim the end, spatulate it if small, and anchor it with a 4-0 chromic catgut suture through all layers of ureter and bladder. Approximate the epithelium with 5-0 synthetic absorbable sutures, and close the original hiatus with the same material. Check the course of the ureter with an infant feeding tube.

11 **A,** For bilateral reimplantation, make a separate tunnel for the second ureter from the hiatus of the first ureter. Alternatively, bring this ureter through the original tunnel. **B,** Bring the second ureter to that epithelial opening and suture it in place. Insert a 3.5 or 5 F infant feeding tube to be sure the ureter has a smoothly curving course. One may tack the tube laterally to the epithelium with a 3-0 plain catgut suture and leave it as a stent. In boys, it may be advisable to place a Malecot catheter for 48 hours. It should exit from a stab wound. In girls, a Robinson catheter will suffice, held by a silk suture through the bladder dome and skin. Insert a Penrose drain, and close the bladder and wound in layers. Leave the stent in place for 48 hours.

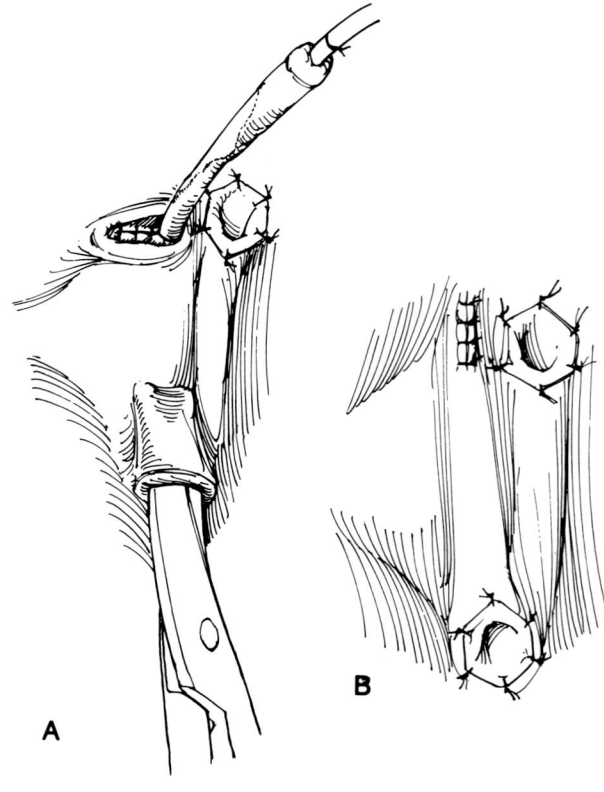

A

B

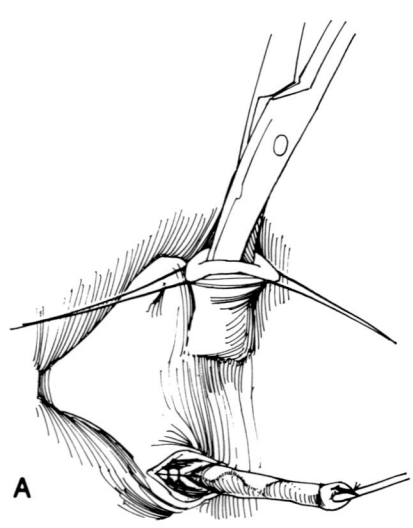

A

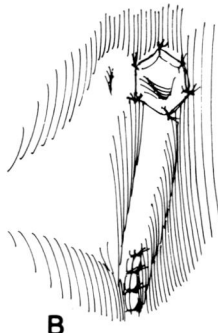

B

SHEATH APPROXIMATION TECHNIQUE
(GIL VERNET)

Make a transverse incision between the two laterally placed orifices to expose the underlying trigone. Catch the periureteral sheath at the inferior margin of each ureter with a single nonabsorbable mattress suture. Tie the suture to draw the ureters together in the midline.

EXTRAVESICAL TECHNIQUE
(LICH-GREGOIR)

Place an indwelling balloon catheter and fill the bladder to one-third capacity to aid in the dissection.

12 **A,** *Incision:* Make a lower midline incision (page 263) or better, a lower transverse (Pfannenstiel) incision (page 267). Superficially incise the fascia over the bladder, and draw it cephalad with a finger on either side of it to expose the obliterated hypogastric arteries. **B,** Insert a ring retractor. Dissect the obliterated hypogastric artery on one side to its crossing of the ureter. Undermine the artery with a right-angle clamp, tie it in continuity, and divide it. Avoid dissecting toward the origin of the artery and thus entering the venous plexus there. Expose the ureter and encircle it with a Penrose drain or surgical loop. Ligate the several perforating vessels behind the ureter, but dissect laterally to preserve as much of the adventitial vasculature as possible. Dissect toward the bladder, ligating certain uterine vessels as necessary.

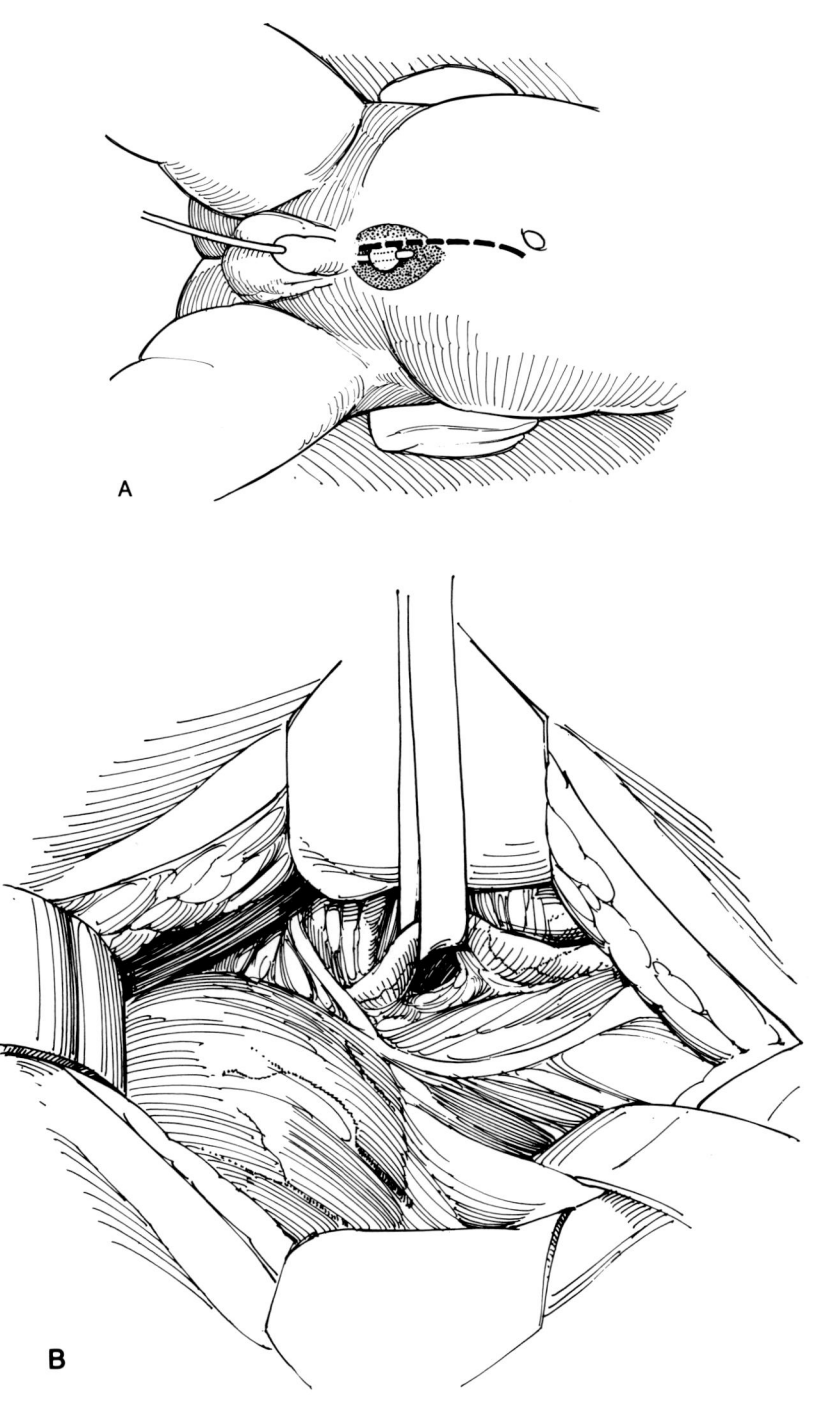

A

B

13 Lift the ureter in the Penrose drain sling. Separate the intramural portion of the ureter from the detrusor muscle circumferentially, using a Schnidt clamp to reach the vesical subepithelium.

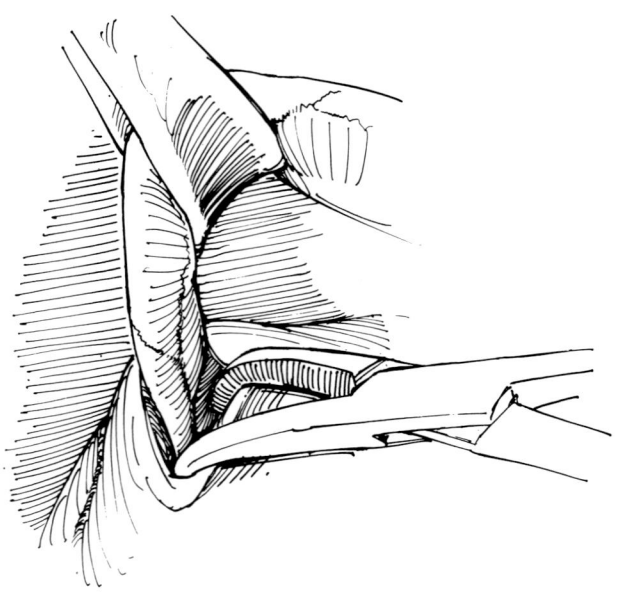

14 **A,** Divide the detrusor muscle down to the subepithelium with a #15 blade, cutting in a vertical direction for 2.5 to 3 cm from the ureter. Because this cut is made with the bladder rotated, the direction it should take may not be immediately apparent. Let the bladder drop back momentarily and follow the natural course of the ureter. **B,** Undermine the bladder muscle against the subepithelium to provide lateral flaps to cover the ureter. Make a Y-shaped incision proximally to release the flaps longitudinally. **C,** Close the muscle loosely over the ureter with 3-0 synthetic absorbable sutures. Avoid constriction of the ureter at the point of exit. Allow the bladder to fall back, insert a Penrose drain, and close the wound in layers.

The original Gregoir technique does not require mobilization of the intramural ureter. After exposing the junction of the ureter to the bladder, make a vertical incision on the posterior bladder wall just above the ureterovesical implantation, over a length of from 3 to 5 cm, according to the size of the child. Divide the detrusor muscle to the subepithelium, and undermine it slightly. Place the ureter into the groove in contact with the bladder epithelium, and close the muscle over the ureter with interrupted 4-0 chromic catgut or synthetic absorbable sutures. Start the suture exactly at the level of the ureterovesical junction. Place a second layer with a continuous suture in the adventitia of the bladder. Avoid constriction of the ureter at the point of exit.

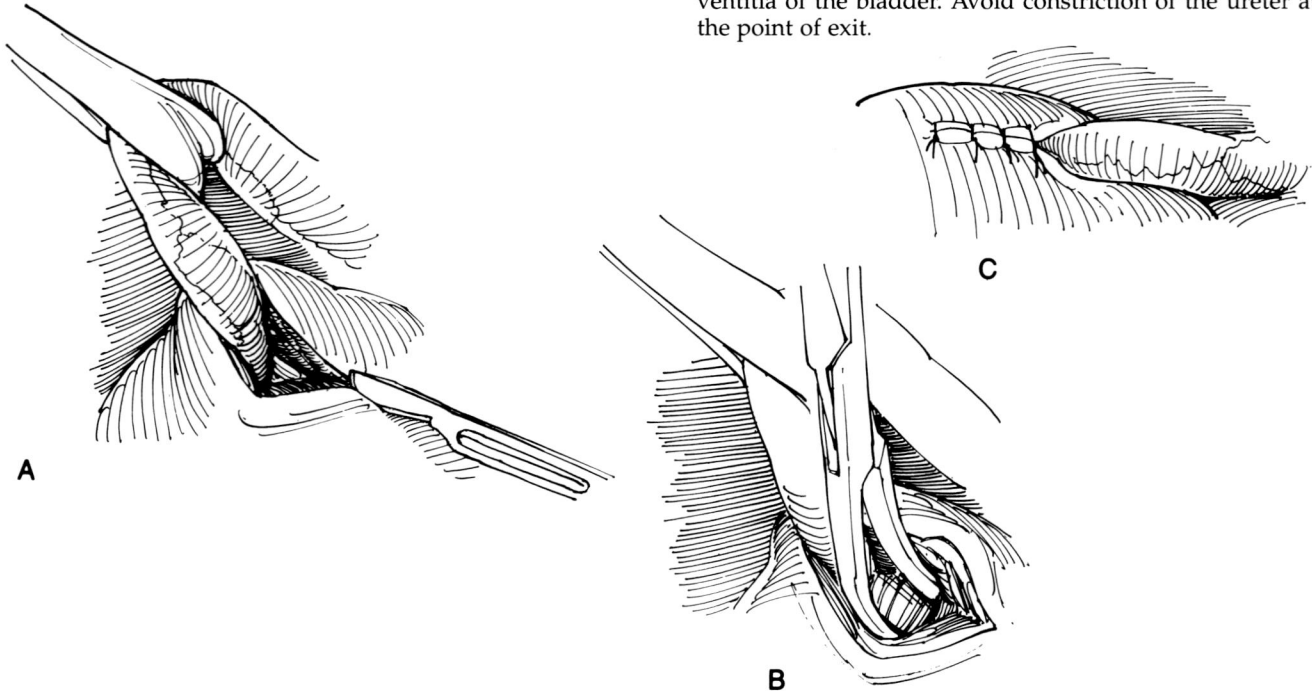

INTRA-EXTRAVESICAL TECHNIQUE
(PAQUIN)
(NOT ILLUSTRATED)

The intra-extravesical technique is useful for both children and adolescents.

Mobilize the ureter extravesically, as previously described. In adolescents, divide the superior vesical pedicle for access. Open the bladder, and make an epithelial incision medial to the original hiatus. Create a subepithelial tunnel beginning outside the bladder, and draw the ureter through it with a catheter passed in retrograde fashion. Alternatively in adults, consider a psoas hitch with direct subepithelial implantation (page 236).

EXTERNAL TUNNEL METHOD
(BARRY)

The external tunnel method is especially suitable for kidney transplantation.

Fill the bladder fairly full, and clamp the urethral catheter that is connected to closed sterile drainage. Place a stay suture in the bladder wall, and roll the bladder medially.

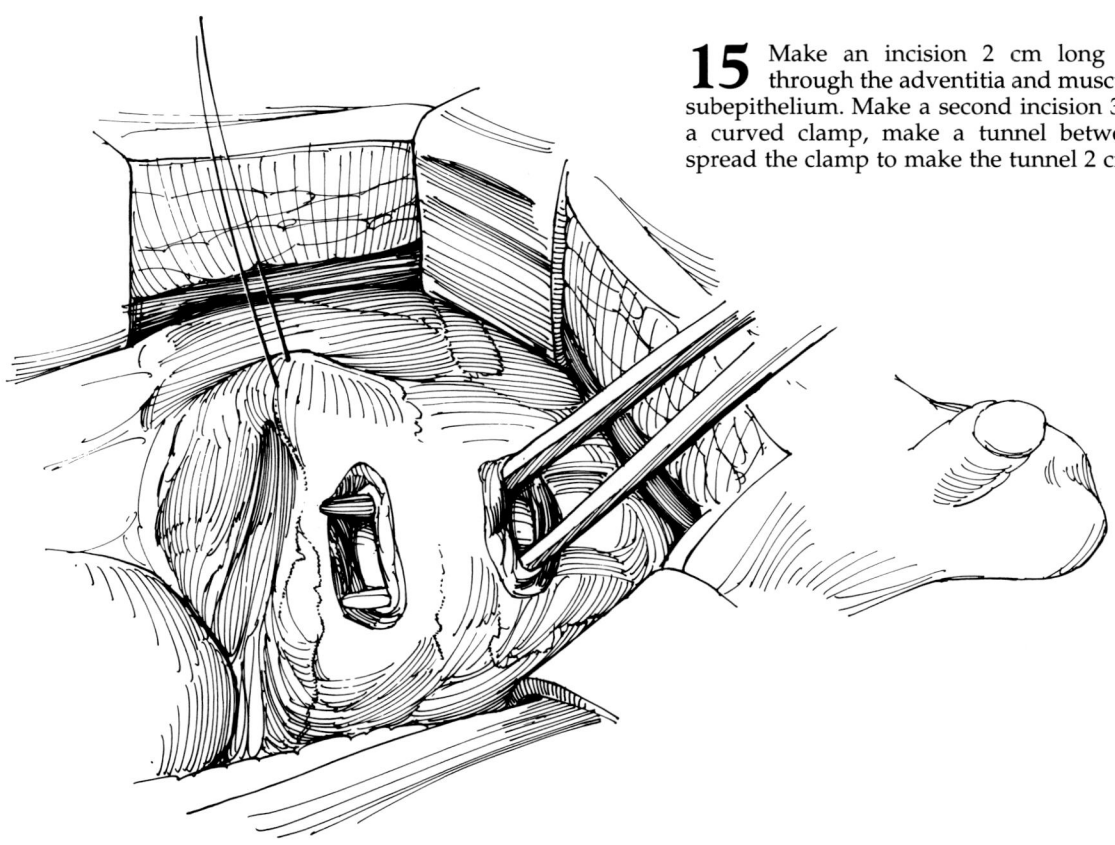

15 Make an incision 2 cm long with the scalpel through the adventitia and muscularis down to the subepithelium. Make a second incision 3 cm distant. With a curved clamp, make a tunnel between the incisions; spread the clamp to make the tunnel 2 cm wide.

16 Grasp the epithelium through the distal incision with vascular forceps. Have the circulating nurse release the urethral clamp and drain the bladder. If a small tear is made inappropriately in the epithelium, lift it with fine forceps and ligate it with a fine synthetic absorbable suture. Close larger tears with a running suture. Excise a button of epithelium.

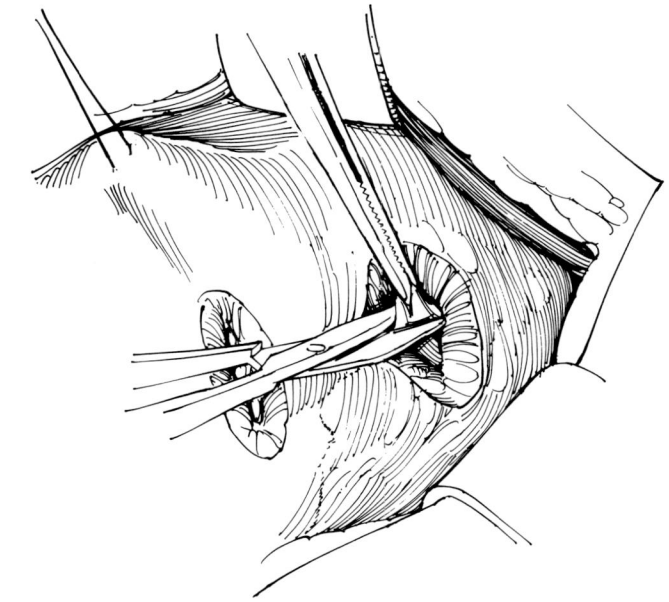

17 **A** and **B,** Draw the ureter through the tunnel, and suture it to the opening with three 4-0 synthetic absorbable sutures. Place a fourth suture through the full thickness of the tip of the ureter, cut the suture long, thread each end on a curved needle, pass it into the lumen and out through the bladder wall,2 cm distal to the epithelial opening, and tie the two ends together. Close the distal bladder opening with 4-0 synthetic absorbable sutures to all layers but the epithelium. Stents and drains are not needed. Leave the balloon catheter in place for 5 days.

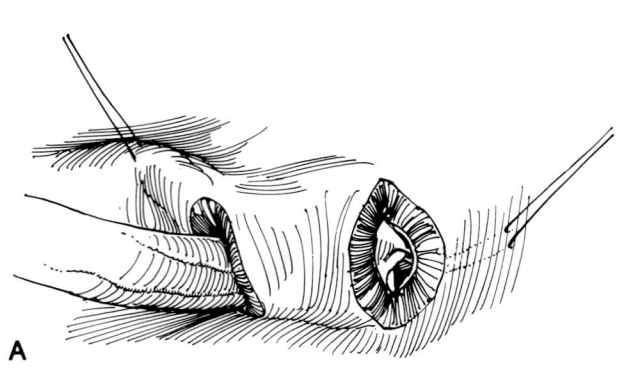

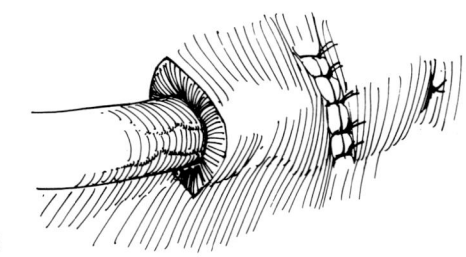

DETRUSORRHAPHY (HODGSON-ZAONTZ)

18 Insert a small balloon catheter attached by a Y-tube to a bag of sterile water and a drainage tube so that the bladder volume may be regulated during detrusorrhaphy.

Through a Pfannenstiel incision, rotate the bladder to expose the ureter extravesically. Place a vessel loop around it to use for traction to allow dissection to its junction with the bladder. Preserve as much of the periureteral vasculature as possible, but free the terminal ureter of its perivesical and muscular attachments. Distend the bladder moderately. Make limited incisions through the detrusor, one proximal and one distal to the attachment of the ureter (take care not to denervate the detrusor). Starting laterally, elevate the muscle from the epithelium, including the fibers from Waldeyer's sheath to form detrusor flaps. Expose the surrounding bladder subepithelium in a 5-cm arc about the orifice, taking care not to perforate it. (If the bladder epithelium is breached, empty the bladder and close the defect with a fine figure-eight suture before proceeding). Place traction sutures in the detrusor edges for aid in the dissection. The degree of pouching of the epithelium may be regulated by filling and emptying the bladder.

Use 3-0 or 4-0 synthetic absorbable suture (not catgut, which would be absorbed too quickly). Place the suture first through the muscle of the bladder wall at the lower edge of the opening from outside in to exit at the edge of the epithelial-muscularis dissection, then pass it through the ureteral muscle at the former ureterovesical junction at the 5 o'clock position. Finally, pass it distally to exit inside-out near the point of entry. This is a vertical mattress suture that forms a VEST-type stitch). Place a second suture in the same way at the 7 o'clock position of the ureter.

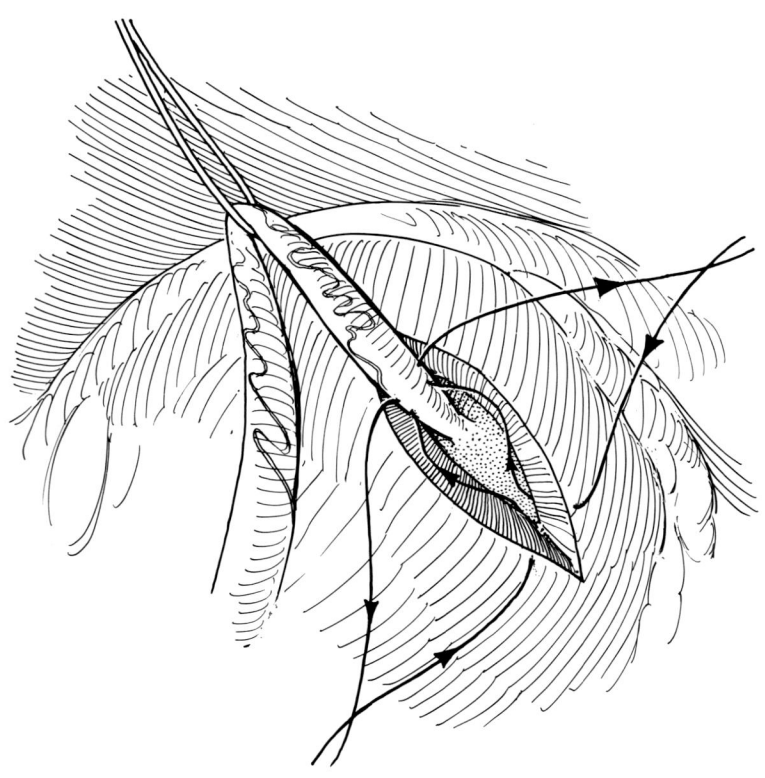

19 A and B, Tie the sutures to telescope the ureter into the bladder to form a long subepithelial tunnel. For duplex ureters, place an extra suture between them. Close the hiatus loosely with running or interrupted 4-0 synthetic absorbable sutures to back up the tunnel. Neither a stent nor a drain is needed. Leave the balloon catheter in place overnight to cope with the effects of atropinization; remove it the next day. Check for incomplete emptying, especially in bilateral cases, and be prepared to start clean intermittent catheterization.

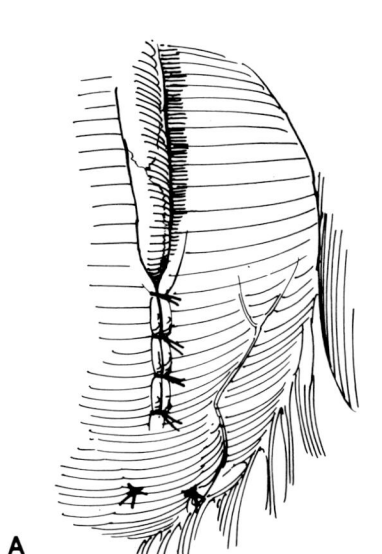
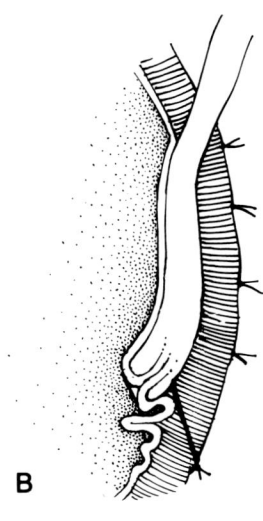

A

B

SPATULATED NIPPLE TECHNIQUE

The spatulated nipple technique is a method for direct anastomosis that is preferrable to the older fishmouth method. It may be used as a last resort if the ureter cannot be extended without tension.

20 A, Pass the ureter directly through the bladder wall near the hiatus, and incise the lateral border for a distance of 2 to 2.5 cm. B, Turn the ureteral wall back on itself and tack it in place with 4-0 chromic catgut or synthetic absorbable sutures. Anastomose the collar to the bladder epithelium.

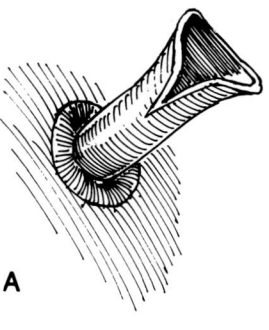
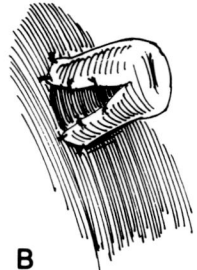

A

B

LAPAROSCOPIC URETERAL IMPLANTATION
(LICH-GREGOIR ADAPTATION)

Create a pneumoperitoneum and insert two 11-mm trocars, one in the left midclavicular line 5 cm above the umbilicus for the camera, and one in the midline below it for various instruments. Also insert two 5-mm trocars in the left and right midclavicular line at the level of the anterosuperior iliac spine for the dissecting instruments. Identify the obliterated hypogastric artery. Open the peritoneum over the iliac vessels, and identify the ureter.

21 A and B, Grasp the ureter with Babcock-type forceps to put tension on the periureteral tissue for blunt dissection of the terminal 2 or 3 cm. Incise into the muscle layer of the bladder wall electrosurgically for a distance of 3 cm proximal to the ureterovesical junction. Complete the trough by cutting with scissors and bluntly dissecting to expose the subepithelium.

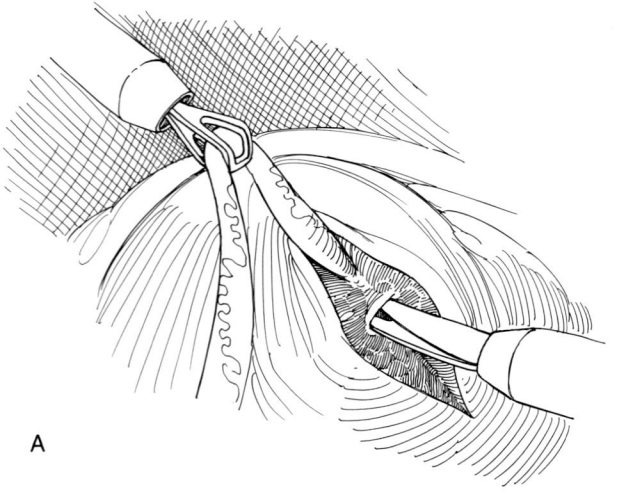

A

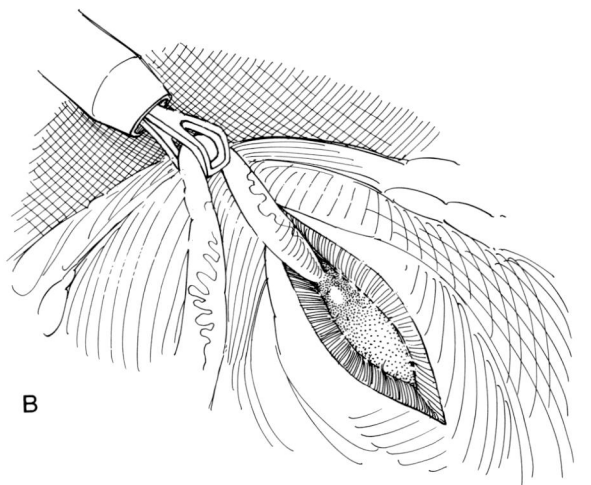

B

22 A, Place the ureter in the trough, and approximate the edges over the ureter distally with a pair of grasping instruments. Place a staple with the hernia stapler through the edges at the distal end to contain the ureter. B, Staple the rest of the incision together.

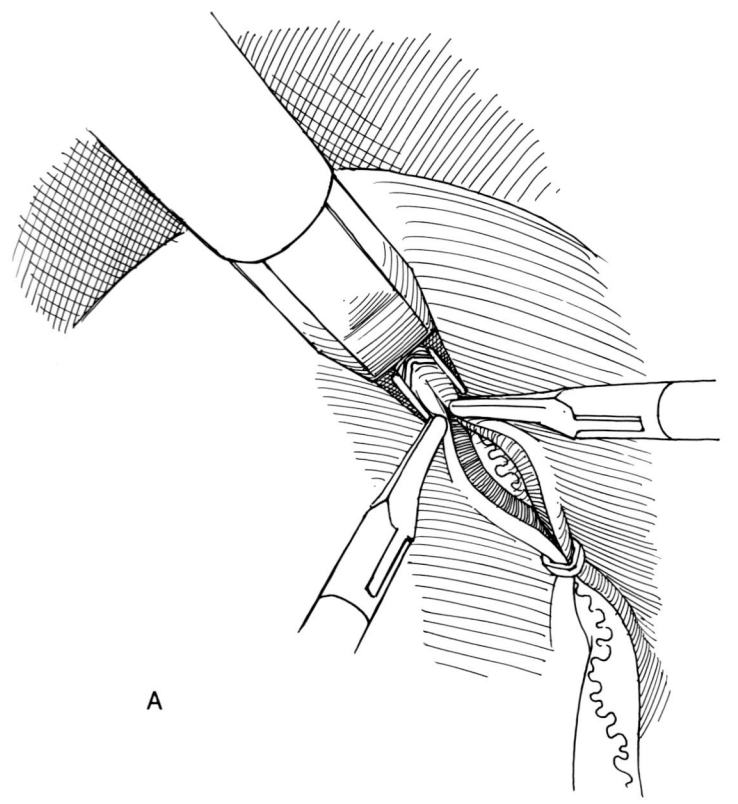

A

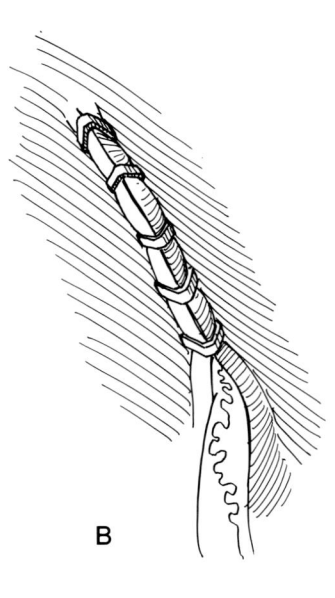

B

VENTRICULOURETERAL SHUNT

23 Divide the ureter 3 cm above the bladder. Anastomose the ureter to the bladder by an extravesical technique. Insert the shunt tube to a point 1 cm short of the ureteral orifice, and fix both tube and ureter to the external bladder wall. Perform a psoas hitch (page 236). Instead of reimplantation, one also may perform a transureteroureterostomy (page 246).

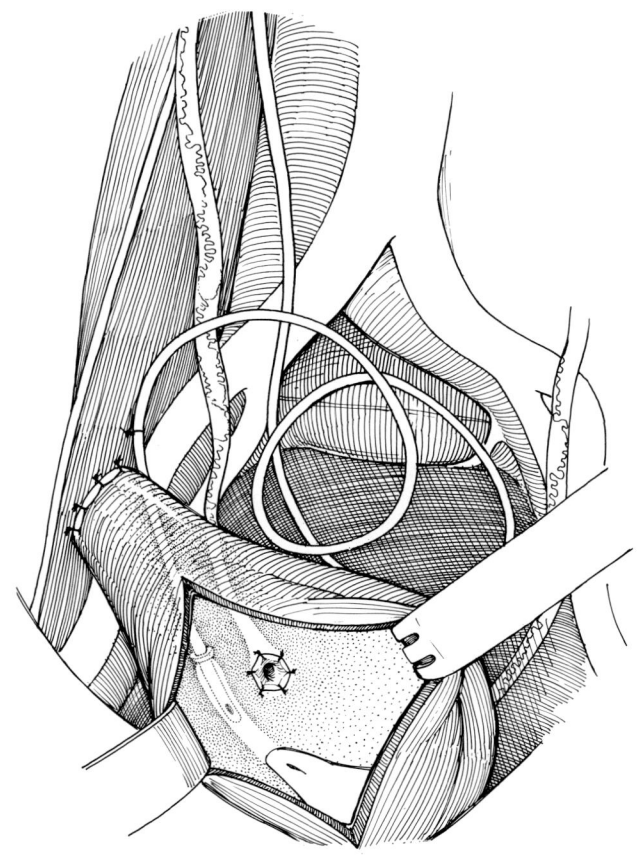

POSTOPERATIVE PROBLEMS

Previously unrecognized *bladder dysfunction* is the most common cause of problems with ureteral reimplantation. Dissection perivesically itself can cause bladder dysfunction. The *non-neurogenic neurogenic bladder syndrome,* if not recognized preoperatively, can lead to failure to correct the reflux or to secondary obstruction at the new orifice.

Persistent ipsilateral reflux usually is of low grade and will resolve spontaneously. The same is true of reflux occurring postoperatively on the other side, although both ureters usually are implanted whenever the other side shows any evidence of abnormality. Persistent reflux usually is due to technical failure, such as insufficient ureteral mobilization, too short a tunnel, or inappropriate placement of the orifice, or to ureterovesical fistulization; reoperation is necessary. Look for vesical dysfunction before reimplanting. *Ureteral obstruction* is due to angulation or obstruction at the hiatus, which may occur after removal of the stent, causing flank pain, nausea, vomiting, ileus, and even sepsis. Rarely will percutaneous nephrostomy be required. Obstruction that occurs soon after operation as a result of edema or contraction of the thickened bladder wall during spasm is especially troublesome in infants younger than 3 months of age and in those with dilated ureters preoperatively. In such patients, stenting should be routine. *Sepsis* means obstruction and must be handled by its release.

Late Obstruction. Ureteral obstruction is of concern if it persists longer than a few weeks and may require endoscopic manipulation or reoperation. If it occurs when the bladder is full, it is the result of extravesical ureteral angulation and a laterally placed hiatus. Too large a hiatus may allow compression of the ureter by a paraureteral diverticulum. An ischemic ureter due to too much dissection may contract and obstruct. In any case of continued hydronephrosis, look first for persistent bladder dysfunction, as well as residual valves and high urine output. The unrecognized dysfunctional bladder is the most common cause of failure of ureteroneocystostomy. Bladder augmentation may be required.

Extravasation, especially after tailoring, indicates early obstruction from edema, angulation, or constriction at the hiatus unless the catheter has been kinked. Prolonged stenting is indicated. *Gross hematuria* is not unusual. Clots indicate inadequate operative hemostasis, but they rarely require transurethral fulguration or reexploration. *Anuria* should respond to furosemide (Lasix) and adequate fluid support. Check the ureteral catheters for patency. If stents are not used, get an intravenous urogram and, perhaps, place catheters retrogradely or install a nephrostomy tube percutaneously.

Fever may occur postoperatively if the urinary tract had not been cleared of infection. Antibiotic administration continued for 4 to 6 weeks reduces the chance of chronic infection. Later recurrent infections are limited to the lower tract and usually are related to bladder dysfunction.

Life-long surveillance is needed after implantation. Start with a voiding cystourethrogram at 1 year and then yearly ultrasonographic studies for the first 5 years. Further study is needed if infection occurs.

REOPERATION

Look first for bladder dysfunction. If it is on a functional basis, it must be corrected by retraining before reoperation is attempted. For neurogenic dysfunction, it may be that augmentation cystoplasty is needed.

Approach a persistently refluxing ureter transvesically. Circumscribe the meatus, and open the entire subepithelial tunnel to allow removal of the intact ureter. Mobilize the ureter above the hiatus to get more than enough length. Reimplant with the Politano-Leadbetter technique.

For an obstructed ureter, if the obstruction is limited to the meatus, an endoscopic method such as passage of a stent, balloon dilation, or a limited intravesical procedure is adequate. For a more extensive obstructive lesion, approach the ureter extravesically to obtain an unoperated portion for reimplantation, ignoring the original intravesical portion. Should that leave the ureter too short, proceed with a psoas hitch. Resort to transureteral ureterostomy if the ureter is still too short. If both ureters are involved, one solution is to insert one ureter into the bladder with a psoas hitch and the other into the implanted ureter.

Commentary by Mark Zaontz

The Politano-Leadbetter transvesical reimplantation is a time-honored standard with high success rates if the technical aspects of this operation are strictly adhered to. Careful mobilization of the ureter is paramount to avoiding devascularization and subsequent ureteral ischemia, which can lead to complications including ureteral stricture and possible urinary leakage if ureteral necrosis occurs. One must avoid any tension on the ureter when advancing it to a new location. The most distal segment of the ureter should be freshened up and trimmed to ensure that good vascularity exists. Care should be taken to look extravesically as well as intravesically to ensure no kinking or twisting of the ureter has occurred. Likewise, the ureter should be brought through the most-immobile portion of the bladder posteriorly, with a hiatus that is not closed tightly, to avoid J-hooking and/or ureteral stenosis.

One tip that I have found useful to aid in freeing up the ureter and also with subepithelial tunnel dissection is the use of 1 percent lidocaine (Xylocaine) with a 1:100,000 epinephrine solution injected periureterally at the orifice and along the proposed subepithelial tunnel using a 26-

gauge needle. This decreases bleeding and provides ease of dissection in a readily defined plane.

As already described, the intravesical subepithelial tunnel is typically created by blunt or sharp undermining of the bladder epithelium in a superomedial or superolateral direction. An alternative method includes elevation of the epithelial leaflets created by sharp dissection. I use scissors that have a 135-degree angle. The blades of the scissors are tapered to a fine blunt tip, giving them the advantage and characteristics of both the right-angle Mixter clamp and the standard tenotomy scissors. The modified scissors provides ease in creating an appropriate subepithelial tunnel and minimizes the degree of epithelial trauma.

Once reimplantation is completed, it is important to be able to pass a 5 F feeding tube up to the level of the renal pelvis without impedance. This ensures that the course of the ureter is unobstructed. I generally leave a ureteral stent in at least one ureter if the procedure is bilateral to avoid the potential complication of anuria from postoperative edema.

The Glenn-Anderson ureteral advancement technique essentially lengthens the subepithelial tunnel by relocating the ureteral hiatus cephalad and advancing the ureteral orifice inferomedially. Mobilization of the ureter is the same as described for the Politano-Leadbetter procedure. Again, it is important not to close the detrusor hiatus too tightly to avoid ureteral kinking and obstruction. Generally, after closure of the detrusor hiatus, if a right-angle clamp can be insinuated between the superior margin of the hiatus and the ureter, then adequate closure has been obtained. A dilated ureter would be a contraindication for this technique unless adequate tunnel length can be obtained.

The Cohen transtrigonal technique has the advantage of advancing the ureter across the trigone in a natural continuation of the ureteral course. In this regard, the original ureteral hiatus is unchanged. These two factors explain the low risk of obstruction from this operation. A significant drawback of this otherwise highly successful technique is the difficulty of ureteral access at the bladder level postoperatively because of the new cross-trigonal position of the reimplanted ureters.

For any of the described intravesical techniques where ureteral stents are used, I prefer the 8 F Dow Corning cystocatheter, which I fenestrate prior to insertion. This setup has a nice trocar system to allow easy insertion through the skin and into the bladder through separate stab wounds. There is a hookup that allows the catheter to be connected to a leg bag for easy management postoperatively. As an alternative to this, the kidney internal splint/stent (KISS) catheter can be used with equal efficacy. This catheter comes in various French sizes. The portion of stent that resides in the ureter and bladder has a longitudinally open segment that makes potential clotting or obstruction of the catheter virtually impossible during the indwelling time.

The extravesical techniques are all similar in nature, with modifications as described. The main difference between the technique described by Lich-Gregoir and that of Hodgson is that the latter performs the extravesical technique with ureteral advancement. In Chicago, we termed this technique "detrusorrhaphy." An important tip in doing detrusorrhaphy involves ensuring that the detrusor incision, which usually is initiated with electrocautery, is made in the same direction that the ureter is heading to avoid unnecessary angulation of the ureter. Traction on the ureter after it has been dissected down to the epithelial junction helps define the path the ureter should be taking. The initial detrusor incision is usually more lateral than one would expect.

Prior to beginning any of the extravesical techniques, it is important to place an indwelling balloon catheter and to fill the bladder roughly one third to one half of its calculated volume with sterile saline. The catheter is hooked up to a drainage bag and is clamped until the ureteral repair is completed. This allows for easier dissection of the detrusor muscle off of the underlying epithelium. Stay sutures of chromic catgut should be used liberally to retract the margins of the detrusor muscle to allow for easier dissection. Tenotomy scissors and moistened Küttner dissectors are used to mobilize the detrusor muscle off of the epithelium. Should an inadvertent rent in the epithelium occur, this readily can be closed with 6-0 chromic catgut in a figure-eight fashion. If the ureteral hiatus is particularly close to the bladder neck, the majority of the detrusor dissection should occur in a cephalad direction, as opposed to distally toward the bladder neck. The critical portion of this procedure involves the advancement of the ureter onto the trigone toward the bladder neck with a pair of VEST-type sutures of 4-0 chromic catgut or polyglycolic acid. The sutures must engage the ureter in its seromuscular plane at the 5 and 7 o'clock positions, respectively, at the ureteroepithelial junction. The detrusor defect is closed with a running 4-0 polyglycolic acid suture. A second layer of interrupted Lembert sutures may be used to reinforce the initial closure. Care is taken to avoid making the exiting ureter too snug at the hiatus. No ureteral stents or drains are necessary, because there have been no reports of ureteral obstruction or urine leaks after detrusorrhaphy. The urethral catheter is left overnight and removed the following morning. The advantages of this operation include its high success rate, low morbidity, little or no hematuria, few bladder spasms, and absence of wound drains or ureteral stents. Additionally, hospital stay is usually only 1 or 2 days. Caution is advised in considering this operation for bilateral reflux. There have been numerous instances of prolonged urinary retention and the need for intermittent catheterization on a temporary basis. This has been thought to be caused by partial bladder denervation by the extravesical technique. Refluxing and obstructive megaureters can be corrected using the detrusorrhaphy technique as described, with the exception of disconnecting the ureter at the ureteroepithelial junction for tapering. The ureter is then intubated with either the KISS catheter or the Dow Corning cystocatheter. The stent is brought out through a separate stab wound in the bladder after passing it through the original epithelial rent. The tapered ureter is then reanastomosed to the epithelium with 5-0 chromic catgut in interrupted fashion. The advancement technique is the same as that described.

CHAPTER 40

Ureteroneocystostomy With Tailoring

Megaureters may be refluxing or obstructive and can result from either primary or secondary causes. An intravenous urogram shows a dilated ureter with a distal funnel shape. A voiding cystourethrogram in obstructed megaureter shows no reflux or outlet obstruction; it reveals reflux in refluxing megaureter. Isotope scan assesses renal function and drainage. Added furosemide can help differentiate hydronephrosis with or without obstruction. Perfusion pressure studies can be helpful in equivocal cases. If the narrowed distal segment causes functionally significant obstruction, excise, taper, and reimplant it.

If bilateral megaureter repair and reimplantation is required into a bladder with a small or reduced capacity, reimplantation of the better ureter combined with transureteroureterostomy may be advisable (page 246), especially because the extensive dissection required may result in voiding difficulties.

1 Identify the type of megaureter. **A,** Obstructive megaureter. **B,** Refluxing megaureter. **C,** Paraureteral diverticulum with megaureter, a condition usually associated with massive reflux. With obstructive megaureter, the hypertrophied helically oriented muscular coats become circular at the site of obstruction, proximal to the longitudinal bundles of the intramural segment.

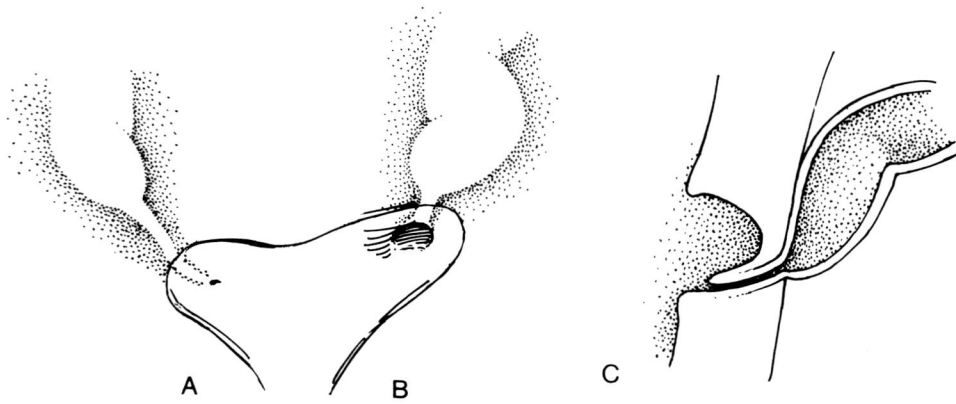

2 **A,** *Incision:* Lower transverse, unless there is great tortuosity so that the upper ureter also needs narrowing. **B,** Insert a ring retractor and open the bladder, holding its edges with stay sutures. Insert a catheter into the ureter, and suture it to the trigonal muscle. Dissect as much ureter as possible intravesically, as described for the ureteroneocystostomy (page 203).

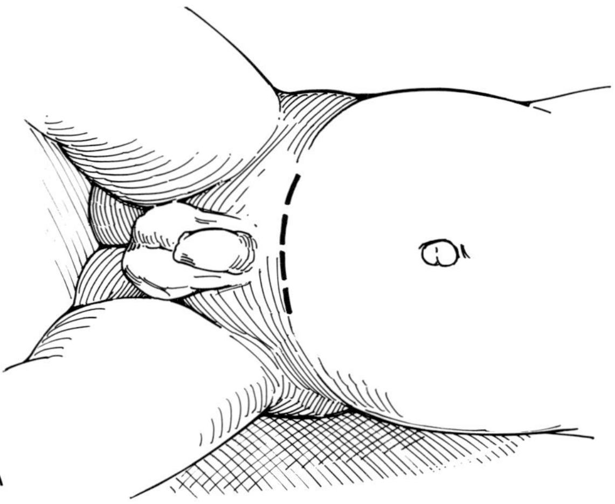

A

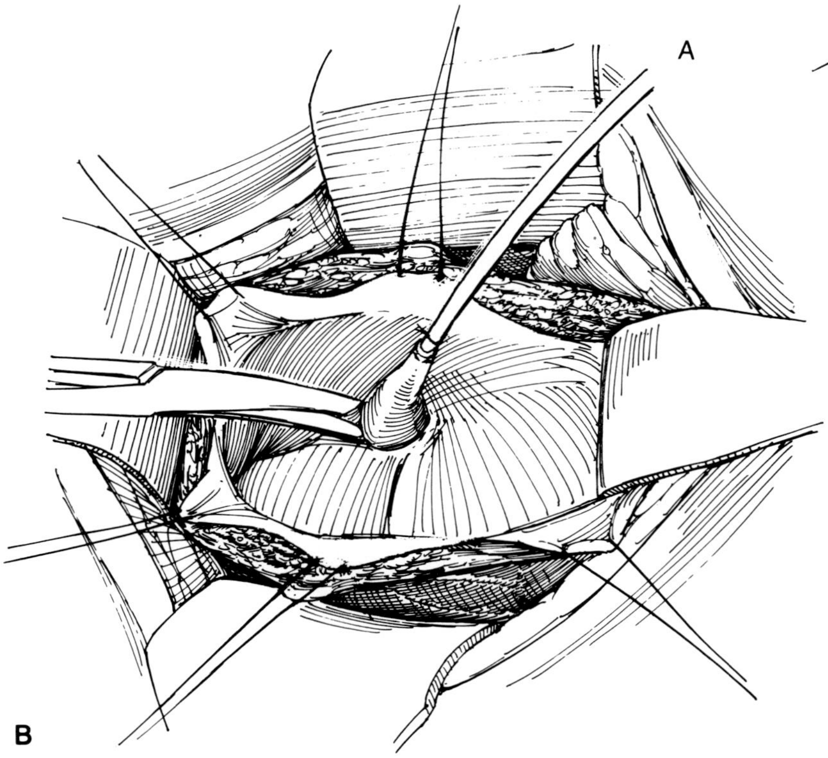

B

3 For very dilated, tortuous ureters, go extravesically to obtain a straight length of ureter free of kinks.

From outside the bladder, dissect along the hypogastric vein until the ligament of the obliterated hypogastric artery is reached. This route will cause the least damage to the vesical nerve supply. Divide the obliterated artery, exposing the ureter without any further sharp dissection, because the peritoneum swings off it. Pull the ureter out of the bladder, and rotate it into the paravesical field. Reclamp the catheter for traction. Cautiously free the ureter from the adjacent peritoneum, saving all the periureteral tissue by sweeping the peritoneal attachments toward the ureter, thus skeletonizing the peritoneum, not the ureter. This mobilization seldom needs to extend higher than the common iliac vessels, unless the ureter is very tortuous and so must be considerably shortened, such as with prune-belly syndrome.

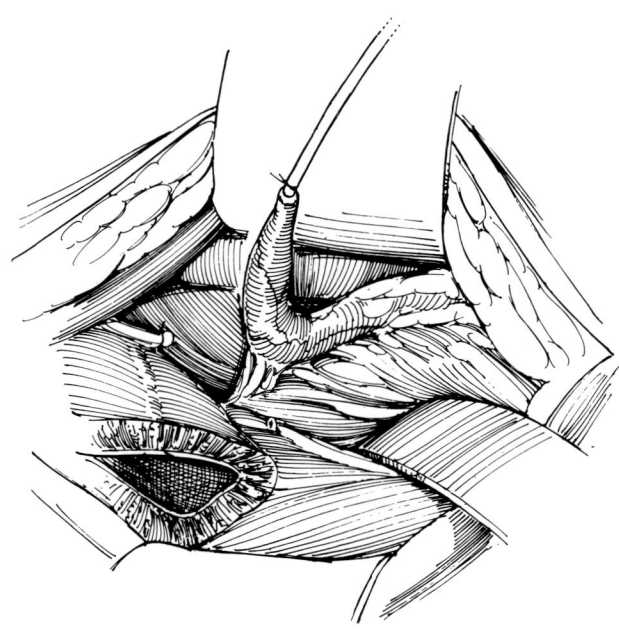

4 Dissect beneath the periureteral sheath on the lateral aspect of the ureter to allow insertion of scissors, then open the sheath (also on the lateral aspect) to expose the segment of ureter to be narrowed. Turn the sheath back, preserving the contained collateral vessels.

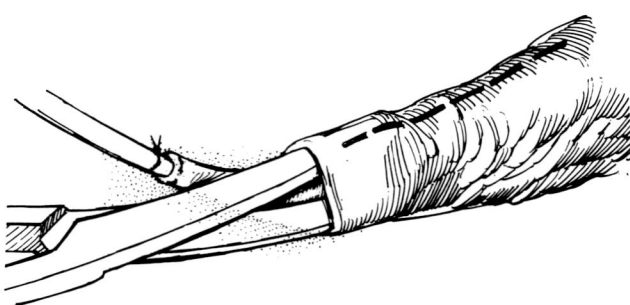

5 **A,** Incise the *lateral* aspect of the adventitia for a distance slightly longer than the length of the proposed tunnel, approximately 10 cm. Preserve the periureteral tissue with its vessels. Dissect the adventitia back from approximately half the circumference of the ureter. Distend the ureter with saline, and mark the portion to be excised with a marking pen. Usually, make the strip for excision approximately one third of the ureteral circumference, because some of the remaining wall will be used up in closure. Excise the longitudinal strip of ureteral wall freehand with scissors. Excising too much jeopardizes the blood supply and predisposes the ureter to stenosis. Leave the terminal segment as a handle. **B,** Close the proximal two thirds to form a tapered portion of the ureter with a running locking everting stitch of 5-0 synthetic absorbable suture. Complete closure of the distal third with interrupted sutures of the same material, because the length needed is uncertain at this stage. Take care not to constrict the lumen. Check the suture line with saline injection.

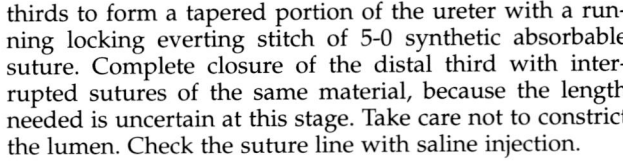

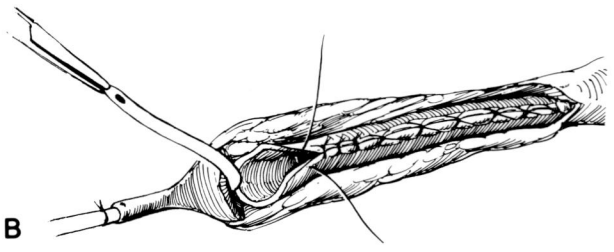

B

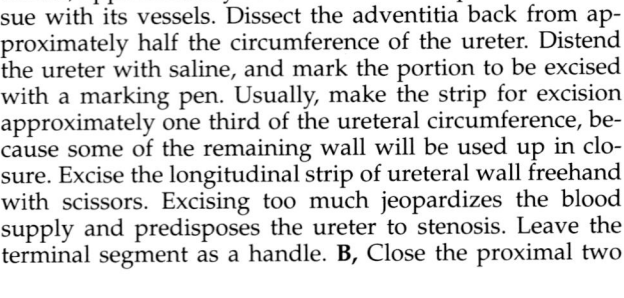

A

6 Close the preserved flaps of periureteral tissue that were previously around the ureter, using a loose running 4-0 or 5-0 synthetic absorbable suture.

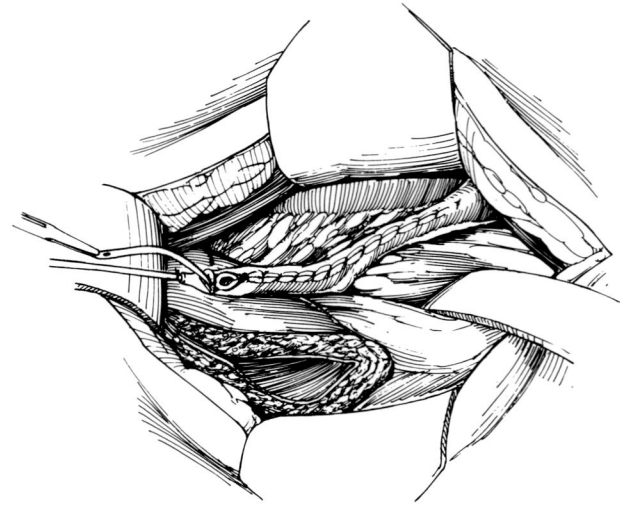

7 Return intravesically and close the original hiatus with several 4-0 synthetic absorbable sutures. One method of creating an intravesical tunnel is to incise the mucosa on the back wall of the bladder with a knife 1 to 2 cm distally and 3 to 4 cm proximally to prepare a long bed in which to lay the tapered ureter. Fold back the vesical mucosal flaps. Make a new hiatus through the muscle from inside the bladder at the proximal end of the incision, making sure that it is large enough. It is vital that the new hiatus be in the back wall of the bladder; if it is misplaced on the side wall, bladder filling will angulate and obstruct the ureter. Alternatively, a tunnel can be created by dissecting submucosally, as in a standard reimplantation.

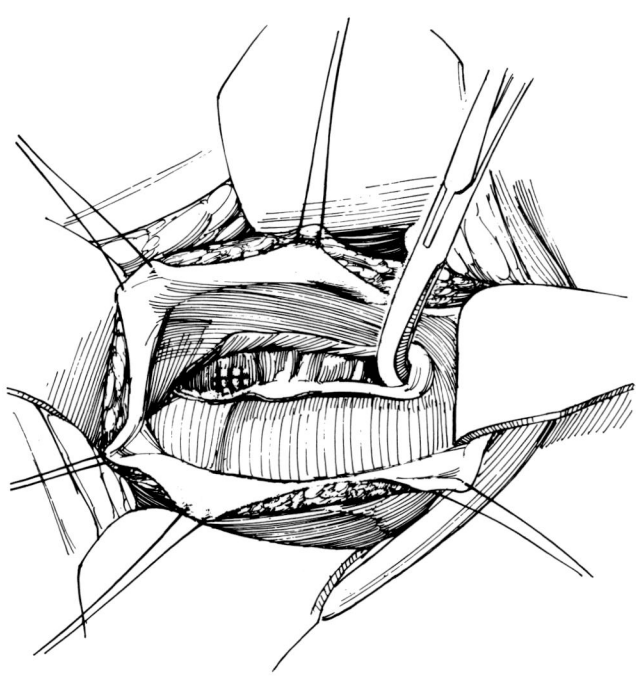

8 Draw the ureter through the new hiatus. The taper will end only a few centimeters above it, approximately at the level of the common iliac vessels. Be sure the suture line lies posterolaterally when the ureter is placed in its bed; this will reduce the incidence of fistula.

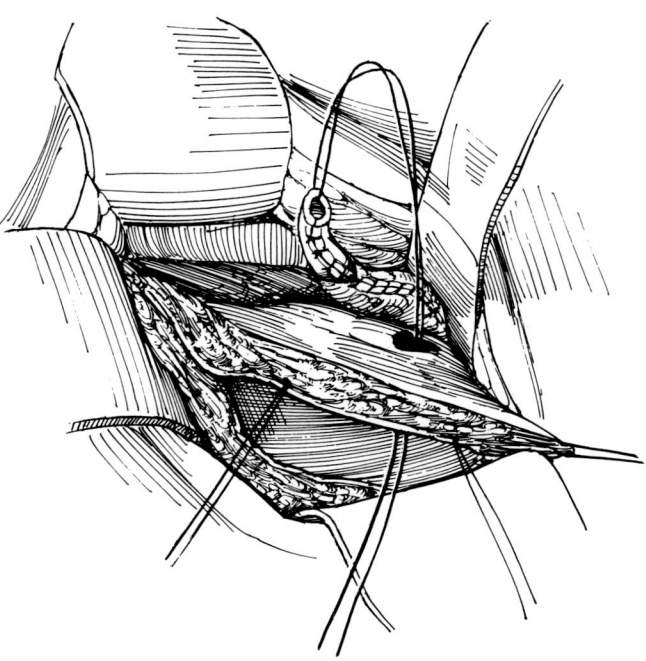

9 **A,** Cut the end of the ureter to an appropriate length, long enough to reach the site of the original hiatus. Place two stitches of 4-0 or 5-0 synthetic absorbable sutures in the bladder wall at the end of the tunnel to include muscle and mucosa and thus anchor the ureter in place, sutured side down. **B,** Complete a mucosa-to-mucosa anastomosis of the tip and, if using the open tunnel technique, close the mucosal flaps with interrupted fine stitches of 5-0 synthetic absorbable suture. The ureter also can be implanted by the cross-trigonal technique (see page 208).

Insert a fenestrated 5 F plastic catheter to the renal pelvis, and lead both it and a drain out through stab wounds. Leave the stent in place for 10 days. Drain the bladder in boys with a Malecot suprapubic catheter or urethral balloon catheter (a urethral catheter is suitable for girls), and remove the catheter a day after withdrawal of the stent.

In cases in which the bladder is small relative to the size of the ureter, and especially in reoperative cases, perform a psoas hitch (page 236). Close the bladder in two layers and provide a Penrose drain to the area. Leave a balloon catheter in the bladder until the stents are removed.

It is important that the tunnel be long enough (five times the diameter of the revised ureter), that the new bed be along the posterior wall of the bladder and that the hiatus not be situated laterally, that the tapering not be higher than the level of the iliac vessels, that the new suture line lie posterolaterally, and that the ureter not be angulated as the psoas hitch is made. With duplex systems, mobilize the ureters with their common sheath, while preserving as much adventitia as possible. If the ureters end in a common stem, excise the obstructive segment, taper both ureters along their lateral aspects, as described previously, and reimplant the two ureters together. If only one ureter is grossly dilated, excise its wall to tailor it and reimplant the two ureters. The infolding technique could be used but may result in a bulky mass for implantation. Alternatives include ureteroureterostomy with implantation of a single tapered ureter.

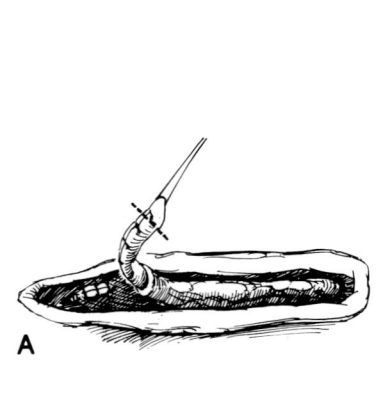

A

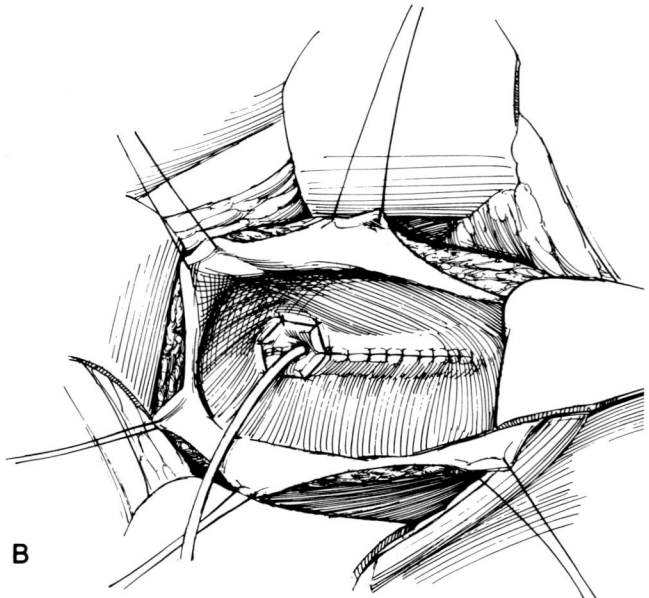

B

ALTERNATIVE IMPLANTATION TECHNIQUE

(HODGSON-ZAONTZ)

An extravesical implantation by a modification of the Lich-Gregoir technique (Figures 39–12 to 39–14) may be faster than a combined intravesical and/or extravesical method and as effective. It is not practical for an extremely dilated ureter or for bilateral cases. Dissect the detrusor from the bladder mucosa before detaching the ureter to make a space for the inversion (Figures 18 and 19 in Chapter 39). Tailor the ureter, excise the distal end, and reanastomose it to the bladder mucosa over a stent that is brought out above the incision. Insert two vertical mattress sutures, and draw the ureter beneath the mucosa.

Close the hiatus. Drain the bladder through the urethra or suprapubically.

ALTERNATIVE TAILORING TECHNIQUES

Ureteral Folding
(Kalicinski)

The ureteral-folding technique leaves intact the somewhat-helical ureteral blood supply that may be transected during tailoring and reduces interference with ureteral blood supply. However, it makes a bulky mass of ureter to be implanted. Excision is probably better for wide ureters and those in infants; folding works well for narrower ureters.

10 A, After dissection extravesically, pull the ureter into the bladder. Place a 10 F infant feeding tube in the ureter and with the fingers around the tube, pinch the walls to displace the tube medially. Run a 3-0 synthetic absorbable suture down the ureter on the lateral side, away from the catheter. Tie it several centimeters from the end, and continue the suturing with interrupted mattress sutures. B, Fold the free margin around the stented portion, and fasten it with multiple interrupted 4-0 synthetic absorbable sutures. Proceed with implantation by a standard technique. Stent the ureter for 4 or 5 days. C, Alternately, fold the lateral margins of the deflated ureter inward, and hold them with imbricating sutures.

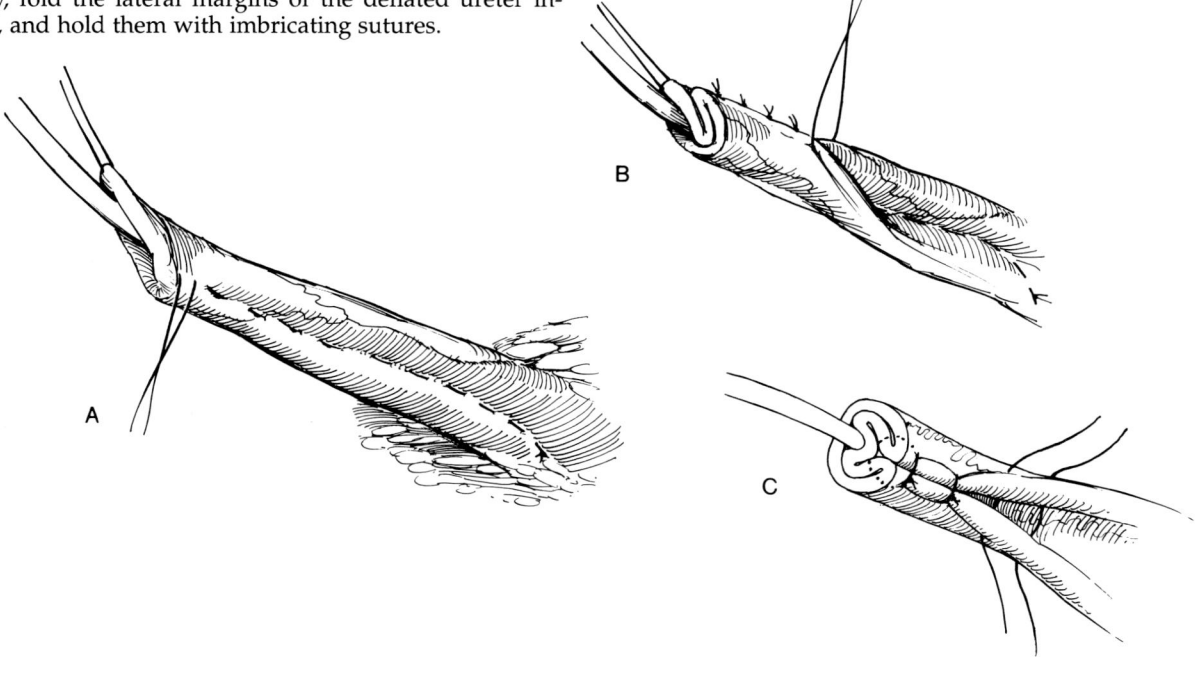

Ureteral Wall Excision
(Hodgson)

11 A, Pull the ureter into the bladder through the hiatus. Run a horizontal mattress stitch of 3-0 synthetic absorbable suture lateral to the stent, placing interrupted sutures distally. Cut the resulting free lumen longitudinally. B, Trim the edges to excise redundant ureteral wall. C, Run a second row of 3-0 synthetic absorbable sutures to approximate the edges. Proceed with implantation. Consider a psoas hitch for better support of the tunnel.

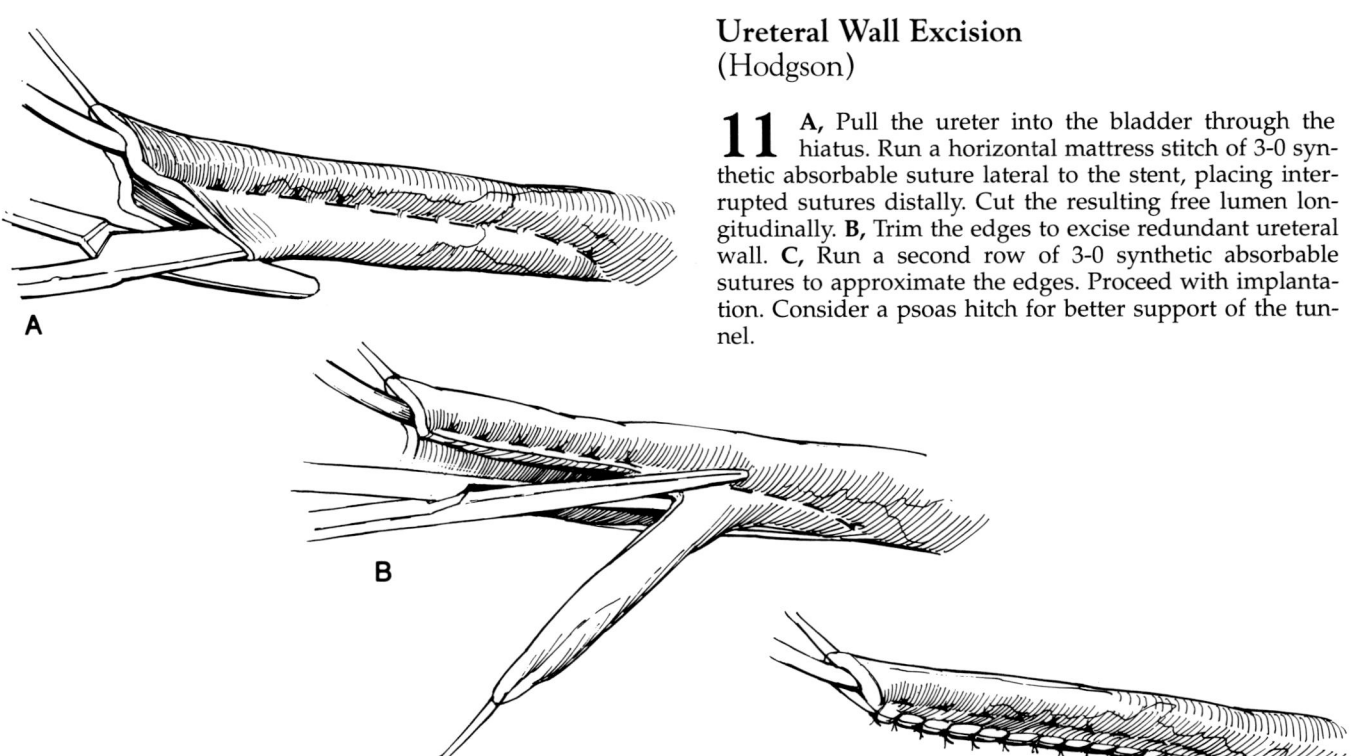

POSTOPERATIVE PROBLEMS

Bladder spasms are common. Use epidural continuous infusion of bupivacaine to greatly reduce the problem. Oral diazepam and oxybutynin also are useful.

Complications after tailoring procedures are more common than after simple ureteroneocystostomy but of a similar nature. *Obstruction* results from angulation or from ureteral stricture. *Reflux* is secondary to providing too short a tunnel. Get an intravenous urogram or ultrasound scan at 4 to 6 weeks postoperatively to assess obstruction and a radionuclide cystogram to check for persistent reflux. Do not hurry to reoperate, because it may take as long as 2 years for high-grade reflux to resolve after implantation. In addition, these patients often have decreased renal function with high urine output, placing an added load on the ureterovesical transport mechanism. Provide adjunctive measures postoperatively, such as intermittent catheterization if the bladder empties poorly; anticholinergic medication if there is poor compliance; and bladder augmentation if the bladder is small, scarred, and noncompliant. Careful follow-up for at least 5 years to detect silent malfunction is mandatory.

Commentary by James Mandell

The current controversy in pediatric urology is centered not on how but on when and if one should repair megaureter caused by ureterovesical obstruction. In newborns, the upper-tract dilation is likely to improve with time. If surgery is decided on, the various techniques provide an armamentarium of approaches that can be tailored for the situation at hand. With extremely dilated, tortuous ureters, the best approach is the standard intravesical and extravesical dissection with excisional tapering and closure in two layers. If the bladder is small or there is scarring from previous surgery, a psoas hitch may be useful. The use of transureteroureterostomy and intestinal augmentation for bladder salvage cases can be handy. With lesser degrees of dilatation and a normal bladder size and compliance, the intravesical approach with the classical tapering or the newer nonexcisional tailoring techniques (I prefer the Ehrlich modification) do well. The most common complication in such cases is postoperative reflux, and long tunnels are necessary. I like the crossed-trigonal tunnels for this setting.

Commentary by W. Hardy Hendren

Megaureter is not a diagnosis but a descriptive term for a ureter that is wide and sometimes very tortuous. Megaureters can be obstructive or refluxing. In cases of primary obstructive megaureter, the ureteral orifice looks normal endoscopically. There is a terminal segment 1 to 3 cm long that contains excess fibrous tissue and lacks muscle. Biopsy of the dilated ureter above that segment shows muscle hypertrophy. The kidney in cases of obstructive megaureter often is better preserved than in cases of refluxing megaureter. In cases of megaureter secondary to massive reflux, the ureteral orifice usually is dilated and often laterally placed. In some cases, there is a paraureteral diverticulum just above the orifice. Frequently, the kidney is

badly damaged in a case with massive reflux from a combination of backpressure from the bladder during voiding and infection. A few megaureters can have paradoxically both obstruction and reflux when the ureter ends ectopically in the bladder neck or urethra. In the resting state the ureter is obstructed, but during micturition it can show reflux.

Not all wide ureters need to be corrected surgically. For example, in boys, endoscopic ablation of urethral valves can reduce intravesical pressures, allowing secondary megaureter to then improve spontaneously. Similarly, megaureters in association with myelodysplasia can resolve when the bladder is emptied by intermittent catheterization.

When a large ureter must be corrected surgically, dissecting the ureter free from the bladder and shortening, tapering, and reimplanting it to provide normal drainage without reflux are involved. The tunnel length should be approximately five times the diameter of the ureter to be reimplanted, just as in ordinary ureteral reimplantation. Thus, tapering the terminal ureter makes it feasible to reimplant a dilated ureter and achieve a satisfactory ratio of tunnel length to ureter diameter. Ureteral peristalsis cannot be effective when the ureter is dilated, because the walls do not coapt. Tapering the lower ureter to improve peristaltic efficiency allows the ureter to empty actively. This effect results in improvement in dilatation of the upper tract.

When the ureter is not tortuous, the operative approach can be through a transverse lower abdominal incision. This approach affords adequate exposure of the lower pelvis, as would be customary for a usual ureteral reimplantation. However, when there is great ureteral tortuosity, as is often present in prune-belly syndrome, dissection higher into the gutters may be necessary to shorten excessive length of the ureter. In such cases, it is better to use a vertical transabdominal approach to provide greater operative exposure. The Denis Browne ring retractor is useful in this case. By sewing a catheter into its orifice, the ureter is mobilized intravesically. The ureter is freed using that approach, as long as it proceeds easily. Then, exposure is shifted paravesically to continue its mobilization upward. To locate the ureter with minimal paravesical dissection, which can cause nerve damage to the bladder, one dissects along the hypogastric vein to the obliterated umbilical artery-ligament. It is divided. This allows retracting the peritoneum cephalad. The ureter lies immediately beneath the ligament. Mobilizing the ureter and bringing it upward into the paravesical field are facilitated by dissecting along the anterior wall of the ureter from below, penetrating the paravesical tissue at the level of the ligament, and then pulling the ureter through to that point. When dividing the attachments of the ureter during its mobilization, it is important that they be divided as far from the ureter as is feasible. This retains as much as possible of the attached periureteral tissue for collateral blood supply. Unless the ureter is extremely elongated and tortuous, we generally mobilize it only as far as the point where it crosses the common iliac vessels.

Tapering the ureter is performed on its lateral aspect, because the main collateral blood supply is along its medial wall. Furthermore, when the suture line for tapering is closed, it should be placed posteriorly next to the detrusor muscle when the ureter is reimplanted into the bladder. This reduces the likelihood of a fistula forming into the bladder. We formerly employed special ureteral clamps, but in recent years we generally have not used them. The ureter is distended via the catheter used in its mobilization. A ligature around the tip of the ureter retains the saline within it. The periureteral sheath is opened by dissecting carefully between the sheath and the wall of the ureter on its posterolateral aspect. The sheath is incised and laid back approximately half the circumference of the ureter to expose the segment to be removed; this area is identified with a skin-marking pencil. Using sharp, straight scissors, the strip of ureter is removed; it must not be too wide. Trimming the ureter excessively will result in its being made too narrow, which will jeopardize its blood supply. Some added width will be taken up in the closure, which is done with a running, locking suture to avoid reefing the closure. The ureter is filled again with saline to make certain that it is watertight. The periureteral tissue is then closed over the ureteral suture line.

It is important that the new hiatus through which the ureter will be brought be in the back wall of the bladder. It is a common error to bring the ureter through the side wall, which will cause it to be angulated when the bladder fills. After closing the original ureteral hiatus, a bed is prepared for the ureter. This bed starts at the new hiatus, which is more cranial and more medial than the original hiatus. The bed extends downward to just above the bladder neck. Instead of making a submucosal tunnel, which often is used in ordinary ureteral reimplantation surgery, it is easier to lay back mucosal flaps before implanting the ureter. The ureter is brought through the new hiatus, taking care that there is no angulation or tension. It is laid in the bed prepared for it, with the ureteral suture line posteriorly against the bladder muscle. The ureter is trimmed to appropriate length. The two most distal sutures are placed in bladder mucosa and muscle to the 6 o'clock position of the ureter; this anchors it firmly. Remaining sutures close the mucosa of the bladder to the open end of the ureter and mucosa-to-mucosa closure covers the ureter. A small plastic drainage catheter is passed up the ureter to the kidney for 8 to 10 days while the repair heals. Contrast medium is injected before removing the catheter to make certain that there is no extravasation. After bilateral megaureter repair, catheters are removed on successive days—not simultaneously. Lower megaureter repair, when done as described, should have a complication rate almost as favorable as that for reimplantation of nondilated ureters, ie, less than 5 percent.

In some highly abnormal bladders (such as in boys with urethral valves or prune-belly syndrome or in patients with multiple previous operations), it may be impossible to get two good ureteral reimplants into the bladder. In many such instances, we have found it best to reimplant the better ureter, together with psoas hitch fixation of the bladder and transureteroureterostomy of the contralateral ureter.

In the majority of cases, successful repair of the lower ureter will result in straightening of tortuousity of the upper ureter and gradual reduction in its caliber. There are, however, some cases in which the upper ureter needs to be repaired. This is technically easier than repair of the lower ureter. The kinked ureteropelvic junction is straightened between the upper ureter, after it is shortened, and the renal pelvis. This may be all that is required. If the upper ureter also is quite dilated, it can be trimmed in the same fashion as the lower ureter. A temporary nephrostomy is placed when the upper tract is dilated. Contrast medium is injected through the nephrostomy tube a week later to be certain that there is free passage to the bladder and no extravasation. The tube is removed.

Kalicinski has described an infolding technique to narrow the functional lumen of the lower ureter, as illustrated. This technique was developed to lessen the risk of devascularizing the ureter while trimming it. This infolding also has been successfully used by other surgeons. It should be stated, however, that the likelihood of devascularizing the ureter by trimming should be minimal, if it is performed in the manner we have described. In more than 350 megaureter repairs in the past 28 years, ureteral fibrosis from devascularization rarely was a problem. Somehow it seems more appealing to place a trimmed ureter into a tunnel, rather than one with excessive bulk. Infolding the dilated ureter in experimental animals has been shown to result in spontaneous disappearance of the infolded segment in some cases, presumably from its devascularization from being infolded. Thus, it may be that both methods achieve a similar end after healing is completed. Like many problems in surgery, there often is more than one way to obtain the desired end result!

CHAPTER 41

Operations for Ureteral Duplication

Start with ultrasonography, followed by intravenous urography if sufficient functioning parenchyma remains. If function is minimal, a delayed renal scan may demonstrate a poorly secreting upper-pole system. Even with nonfunction, the decrease in number of calyces and the lateral and downward displacement of the lower-pole segment strongly suggest duplication. A delayed film may show contrast medium in the upper-pole segment when the ectopic orifice lies within the sphincter, and voiding cystography may show reflux in these cases. Clear urine continuing to leak after the bladder is filled with indigo carmine indicates an orifice distal to the internal sphincter. To locate it, cystourethroscopy and vaginoscopy are helpful.

Approach the operation knowing the degree of damage to the involved segment and whether reflux in the lower segment is present. Removal of the damaged upper pole with subtotal excision of the ureter usually is needed (page 166). However, with some function in the upper pole, reimplantation, ureteroureterostomy, and ureteropyelostomy are alternatives, depending on the length of the duplicated ureter.

URETERONEOCYSTOSTOMY FOR DUPLICATED URETERS

1 **A,** *Incision:* Use a lower transverse incision (page 267).
B, After opening the bladder, place a 5 F infant feeding tube into each ureter, and suture them in place with a 4-0 synthetic absorbable pursestring suture. With traction on both catheters, incise the mucosa around both orifices with a hooked knife, then develop a periureteral plane inside the sheath with Lahey scissors; free up the ureters well outside the bladder. Do not attempt to separate the ureters.

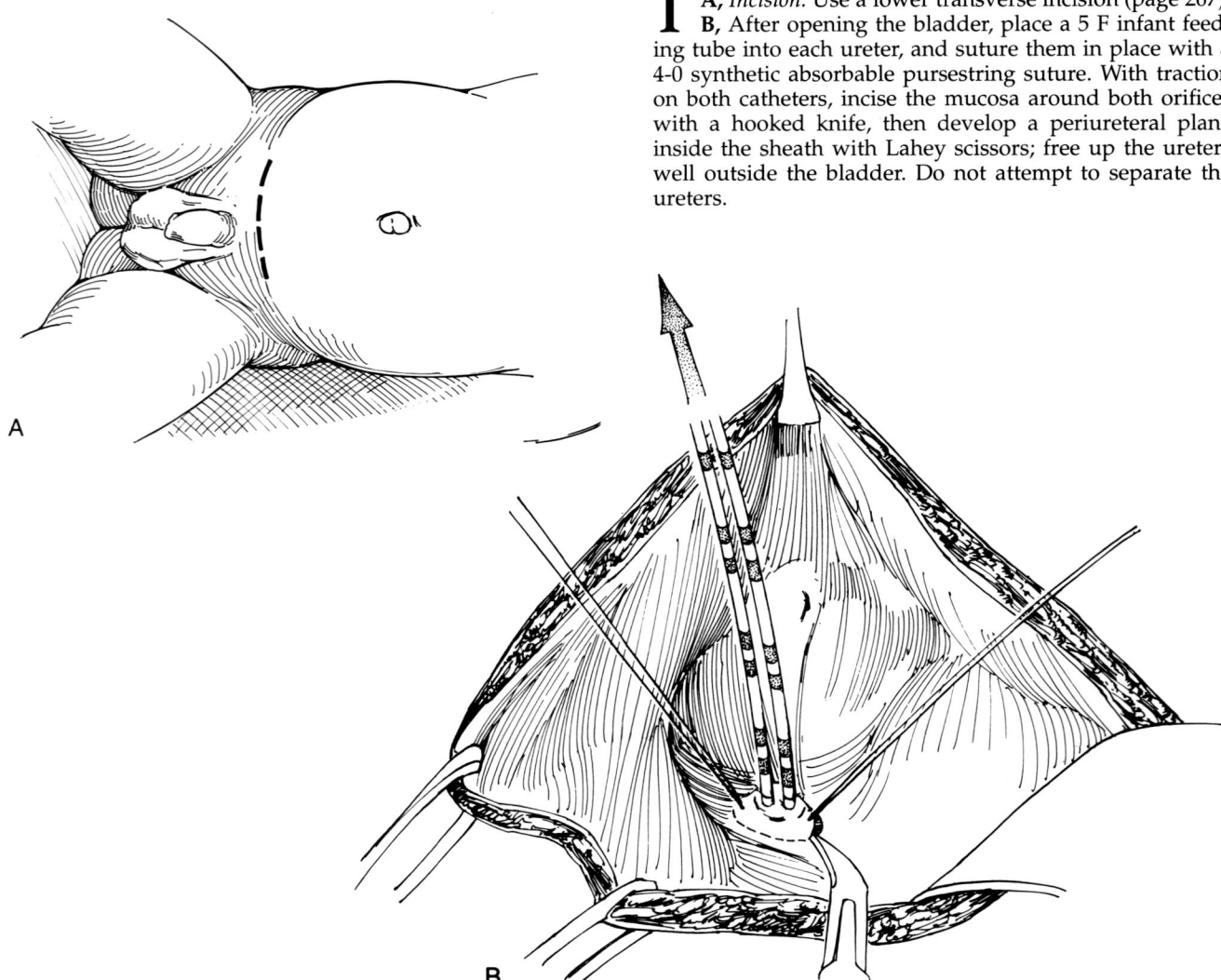

A

B

2 **A,** Usually trim and discard the distal end of the ureters. If the duplication is incomplete, trim the terminal segment of the ureter to expose two lumina. **B,** Suture both to the vesical mucosa, as described for ureteroneocystostomy (page 201) by the Politano-Leadbetter, Glenn-Anderson, or Cohen technique, suturing the luminal edges to each other and to the vesical mucosa. The ureters now may lie side by side, or the lower segment may be located closer to the vesical neck.

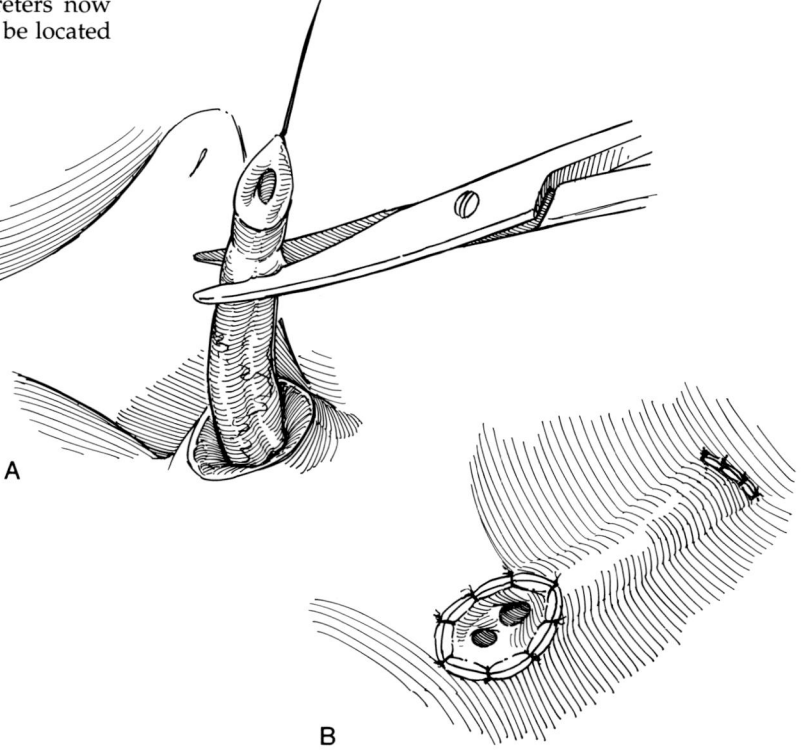

TRANSURETEROURETEROSTOMY FOR DUPLICATED URETERS

Anastomosis of the diseased ureter to the normal mate is used for ureteral dilatation and reflux of one part of a duplicated system. If the age and sex of the child permits, with the aid of a cystoscope, place a 5 F infant feeding tube in the recipient ureter transurethrally.

3 Through a lower transverse incision, expose the terminal portion of the double ureters extraperitoneally nearly to the bladder. Separate the ureters where they are readily accessible above their common sheath by sharp and blunt dissection, preserving the adventitia, and loop each of them with a small Penrose drain.

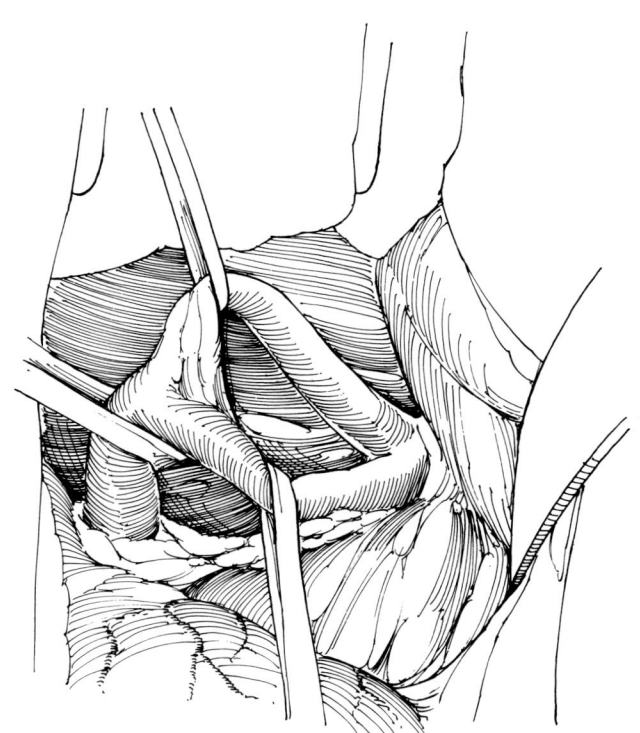

4 After placing a stay suture in the refluxing donor ureter, clamp and divide it obliquely below the suture. Ligate the stump as low as possible with a 3-0 synthetic absorbable suture.

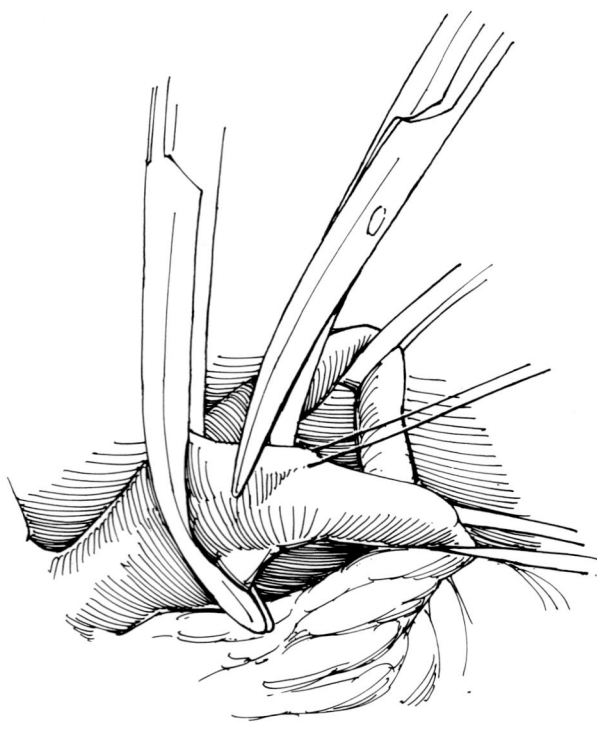

5 Place two stay sutures in the recipient ureter 1 to 2 cm apart, depending on its size, and incise between them with a hooked blade.

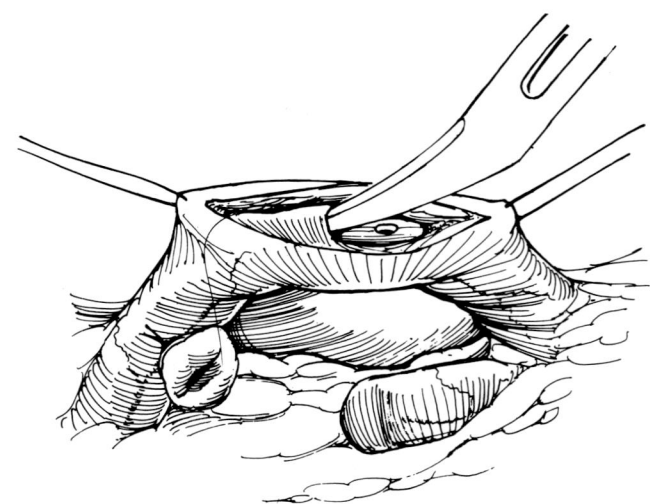

6 **A,** Withdraw the catheter from the recipient ureter, and pass it up the donor ureter. Insert a 4-0 or 5-0 synthetic absorbable suture through each end of the ureterotomy, then through the tip and through the base of the donor ureter. **B,** Tie them, then run each suture down the respective side with an occasional lock stitch. Tie each to the origin of the other. Drain accurately with a Penrose drain (page 127).

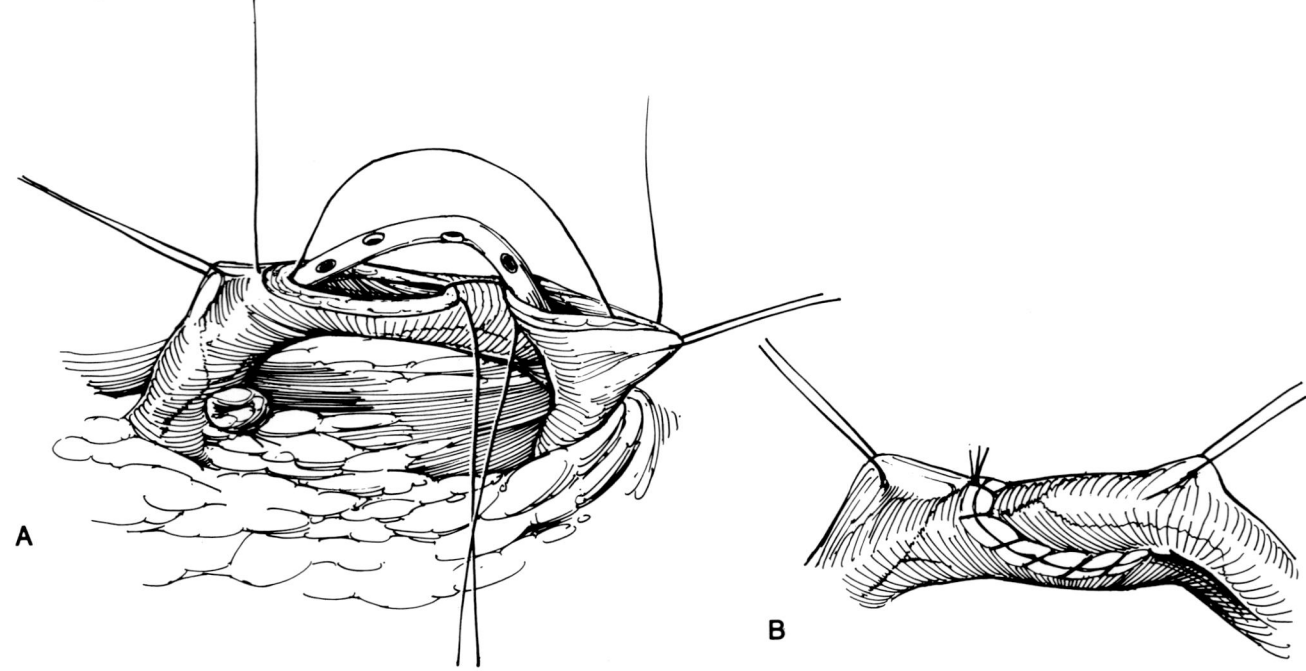

A

B

URETEROPYELOSTOMY

Anastomosing the upper portion of the diseased duplicated ureter to the ipsilateral renal pelvis eliminates ureteroureteral reflux but requires a recipient ureter of adequate caliber. Make an anterior subcostal extraperitoneal incision (page 87).

7 Expose both ureters near the renal pelvis and separate them on Penrose drains. Continue the dissection to expose the lower-pole pelvis.

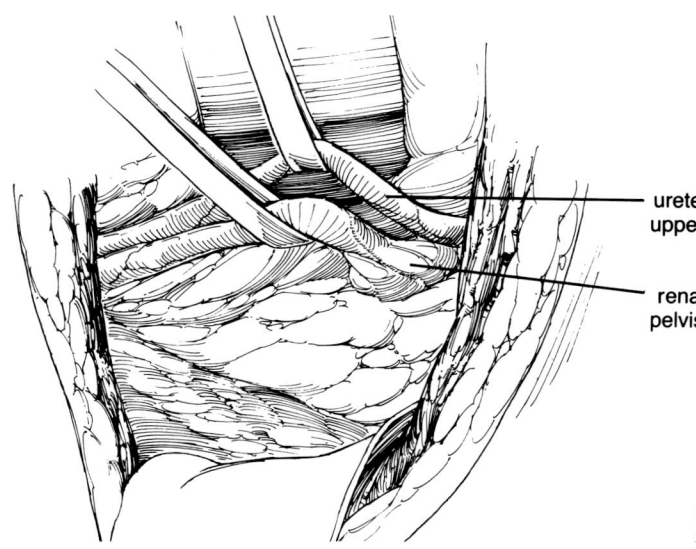

ureter to
upper pole

renal
pelvis

8 Place two stay sutures in the ureter to the upper pole 2 to 3 cm apart opposite the lower-pole pelvis, and incise between them with a hooked knife. Place two stay sutures in the lower-pole pelvis, and similarly incise between them.

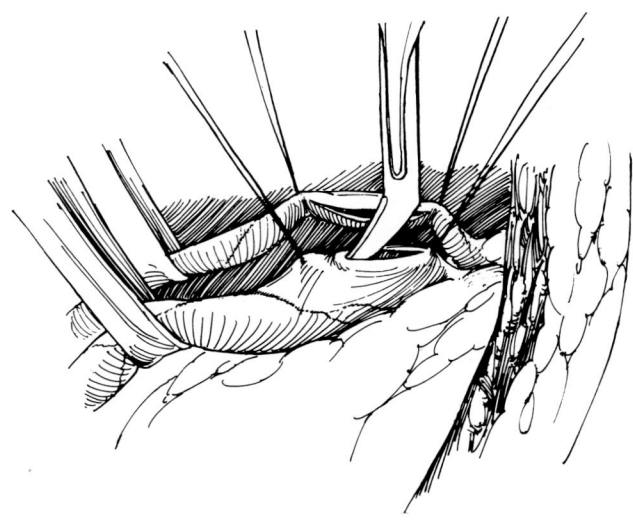

9 A, Place one 4-0 or 5-0 synthetic absorbable suture through each end of both incisions and tie them. Place a double-J stent or infant feeding tube if you are concerned about the anastomosis. B, Continue suturing down the far side with one suture and up the near side with the other, occasionally locking them. Tie each suture to the origin of the other suture. Drain the bladder with a urethral catheter for 2 or 3 days after operation.

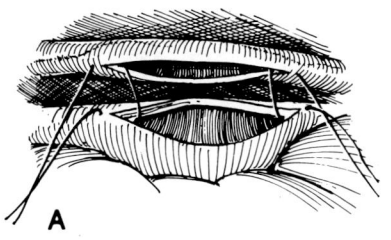

A

B

10 A similar procedure is possible between two dilated pelves as follows: **A** and **B,** by division and anastomosis; **C** and **D,** by making a U-shaped incision and connecting the limbs.

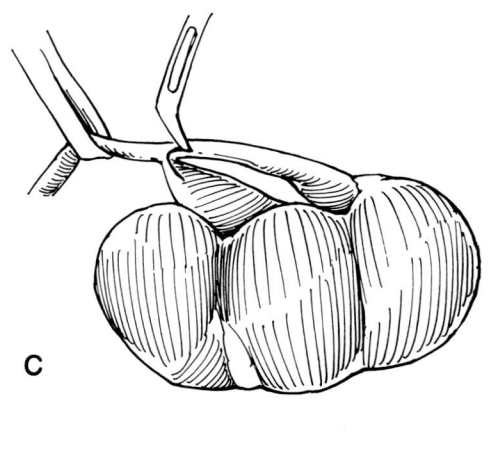

C

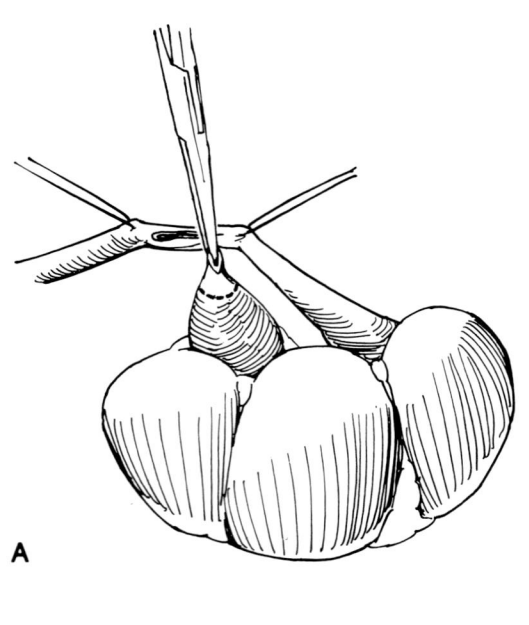

A

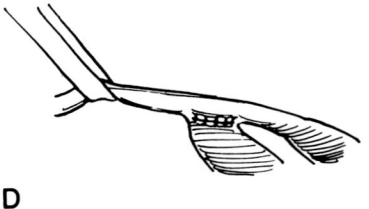

D

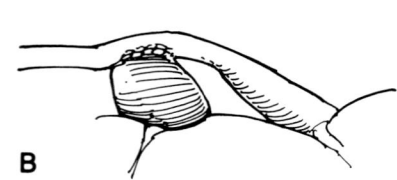

B

PARTIAL URETERECTOMY

11 It is not necessary to resect the entire ureter of a nonfunctional duplicated system. Leave the terminal portion in place, because it has a common wall and blood supply with its mate. After dissecting the extra ureter to within 1 or 2 in above the bladder, divide it and incise it with scissors down its anterior wall to near the bladder wall. Close the short stump with 4-0 synthetic absorbable sutures, or merely trim the edges. Drain the area for a few days.

Should reflux with infection persist in the residual ureteral stump, it must be excised. The transvesical approach shown on page 679 for excision of a utricular cyst can gain access to the stump, an approach less formidable than a dissection from above.

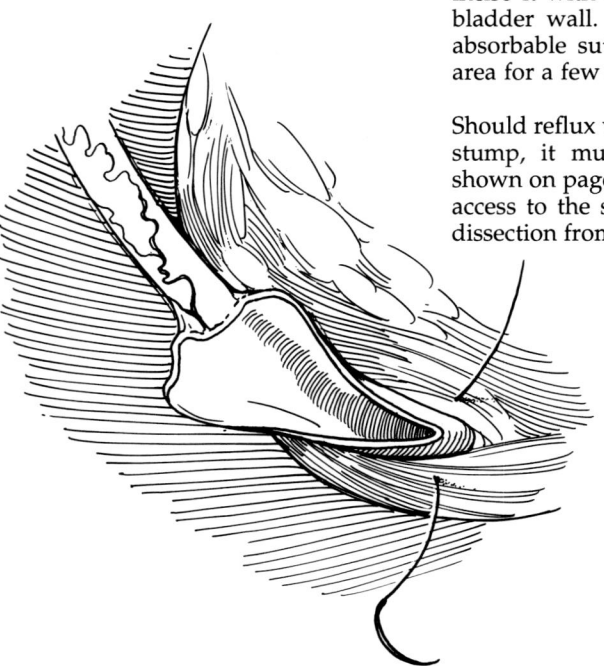

POSTOPERATIVE PROBLEMS

Complications are similar to those after ureteroneocystostomy (page 215) and include extravasation, gross hematuria, ureteral obstruction and anuria, persistent reflux, and sepsis.

Commentary by Claude C. Schulman

The question of how complete excision of the ectopic ureter should be frequently is raised during heminephrectomy in ureteral duplication. If no reflux is present in the ectopic ureter and the terminal portion is not too dilated, it may be preferable not to undertake total excision, because this is likely to jeopardize the delicate neighboring structures—particularly the ipsilateral ureter and the urinary sphincter. Simple removal of the lumbar ureter during heminephrectomy should be sufficient.

However, if reflux is present in the ectopic dilated ureter, which usually is the case when it opens in the bladder neck or urethra, complete excision might be necessary. Complete extravesical mobilization is carried downward to the bladder adventitia. For complete removal, the ectopic ureter is approached through a transvesical incision and pulled through the bladder. The ectopic ureter is dissected by freeing it from the trigonal mucosa down to its opening. After the ectopic ureter is removed, the trigone is reconstructed.

CHAPTER 42

Repair of Ureterocele

An intravenous urogram will demonstrate most of the characteristics of an ectopic ureterocele, such as obstruction of the upper segment and the typical off-center bladder deformity of variable size, but this study may not be necessary, because ultrasonography usually is adequate to delineate the relationships of the ureterocele and assess the degree of ureteral dilatation. Supplement ultrasonography with a voiding cystourethrogram to assess the bladder and to detect reflux into the ipsilateral ureter that leads to the lower pole and into the contralateral ureter that then must be concomitantly reimplanted. However, it is not the presence of reflux at the time of diagnosis, especially in newborns, that should dictate the approach. Indeed, a significant number of refluxing ipsilateral or contralateral cases disappear spontaneously in the newborn period when simple decompression by endoscopic puncture has been performed, so that upper-pole nephrectomy is often avoided. A voiding cystourethrogram made with dilute contrast medium may not only demonstrate the ureterocele but also provide information on the size, urethral extension, and support behind the ureterocele, and an oblique voiding film may give important information. Finally, function of the two renal moieties is assessed by radionuclide scan to deter-

mine if heminephrectomy is the more practical course. Cystoscopy at low pressure is done as part of the operation.

When the child is ill, percutaneously decompress the upper tract, drain the lower tract by catheter, or do both. Consider initial transurethral incision of the ureterocele not only as a temporizing measure but also for cure, because three quarters of selected cases, especially if not ectopic, will not require further treatment. If incision proves inadequate in ill infants as shown by ultrasonography and persistence of symptoms, turn to percutaneous renal drainage. Pyelostomy or ureterostomy may have to be considered.

For a ureterocele with little or no upper-pole function, do immediate endoscopic incision to relieve symptoms, then upper pole nephrectomy with drainage of the distal segment. If the upper pole functions, perform ipsilateral ureteropyelostomy (page 229) or ureteroureterostomy (page 227), and reimplant the orthotopic ureter if necessary because of reflux. If the function is good, proceed with excision of the ureterocele and reimplantation of both ureters together (page 226).

INTRAVESICAL REPAIR

If function of the upper-pole segments warrants their salvage, excise the ureterocele and reimplant both ureters together. Clear infection with appropriate antibiotics.

1 **A,** *Position:* supine. Before draping, visualize the ureterocele endoscopically while avoiding distention of the bladder, which may cause the ureterocele to flatten or prolapse extravesically, making assessment difficult. *Incision:* Use a transverse lower abdominal incision (page 267). Alternatively, make an oblique lower-quadrant muscle-splitting incision (page 270). **B,** Open the bladder with a Y-incision, apex caudad. Intubate the orifice of the ureterocele with an infant feeding tube. Identify the orifice to the lower pole and intubate it also. Place five traction sutures around the ureterocele to surround the orifice, and gather them together in one clamp. Insert infant feeding tubes in all three ureters and hold them in place with fine sutures (sutures not shown for clarity) With a hooked blade or needle electrode, incise the epithelium and subepithelium at the border of the ureterocele. Include the orifice to the lower pole.

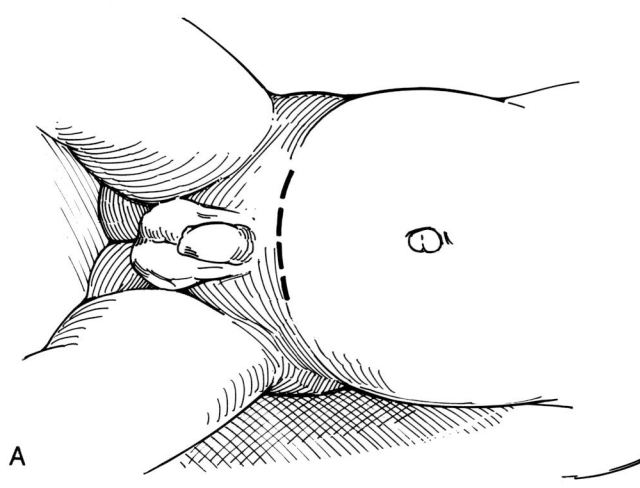

A

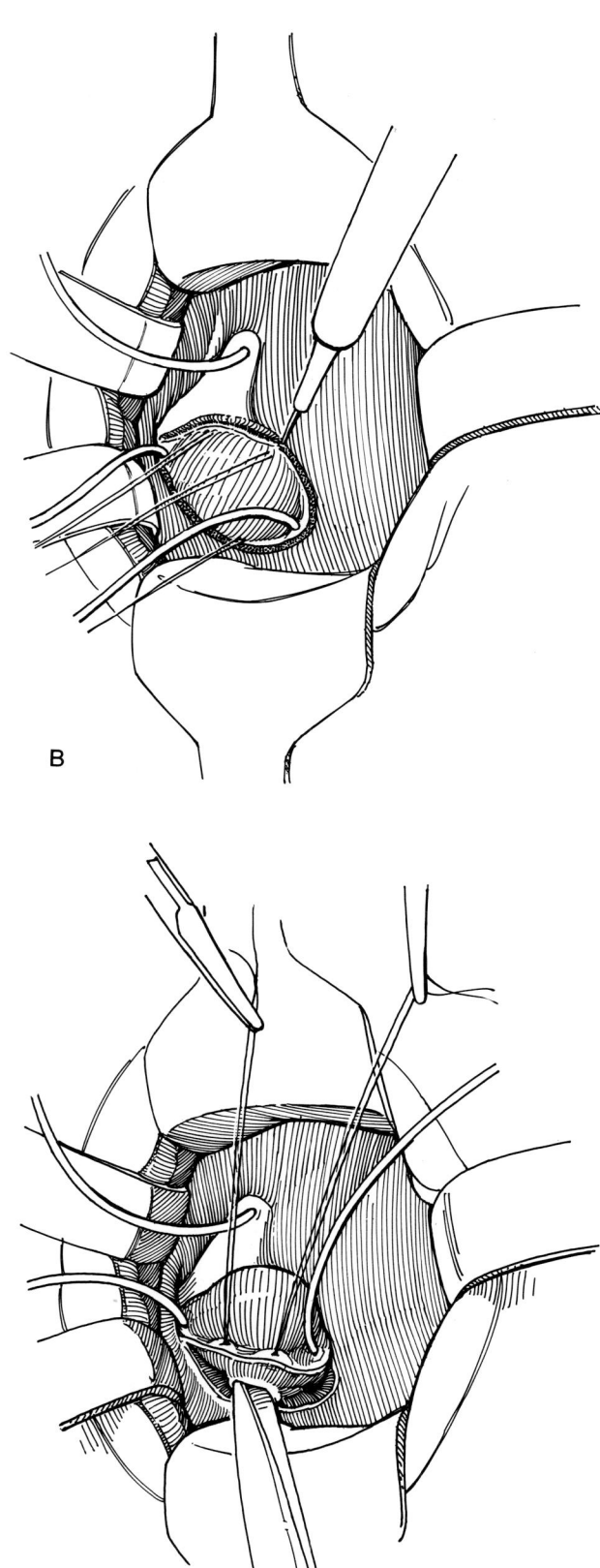

B

2 Elevate the lateral border with stay sutures, and separate the subepithelium from the underlying muscle of the bladder with fine scissors.

3 Dissect the combined ureteral complex through the ureteral hiatus, as for ureteroneocystostomy (pages 204–206). If the ureterocele extends into the urethra, the dissection requires great patience, because the wall of the ureterocele may blend with that of the trigone. If more exposure is needed, incise the anterior bladder wall to the level of the bladder neck, but not beyond. Proximally, continue the dissection of both ureters through the ureteral hiatus. Extravesical dissection usually is not necessary. Close the defect in the detrusor distal to the hiatus with 5-0 synthetic absorbable sutures.

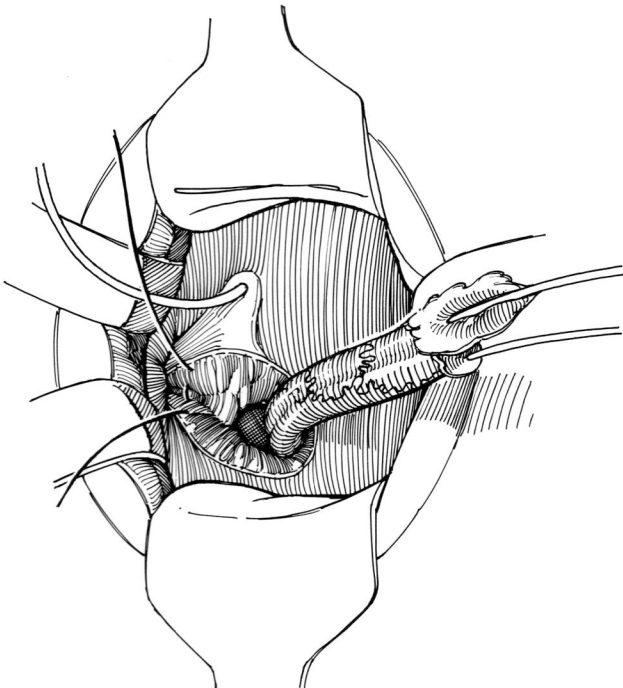

4 Close the vesical epithelium and subepithelium over the trigone. If the ureterocele is large, the weakened detrusor must be reinforced with transverse sutures. Remove the tubes from the double ureters. Place a stay suture through the epithelium-subepithelium above the contralateral orifice. Elevate the epithelial edge, and insinuate scissors beneath it to create a transverse tunnel that exits at the stay suture.

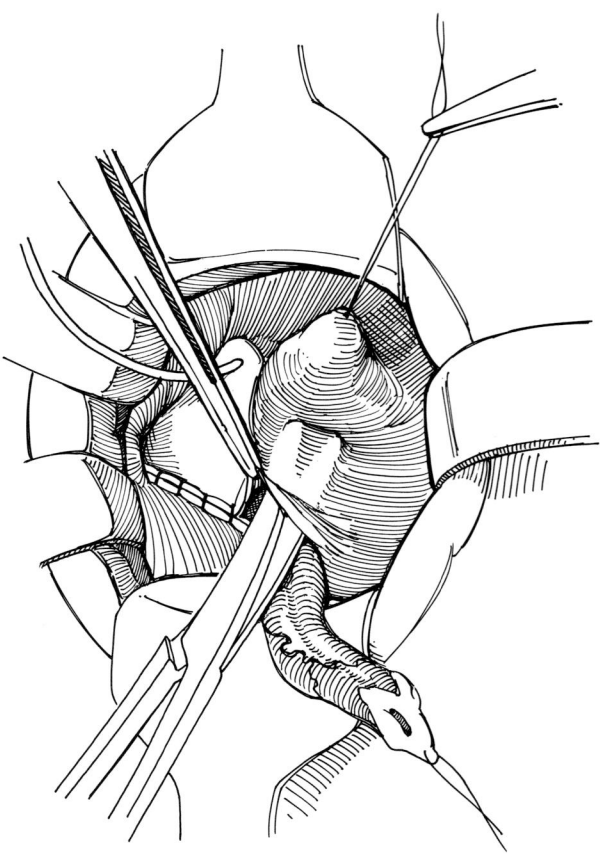

5 Pass a clamp from right to left through the tunnel to draw the combined ureters through on their stay suture, avoiding rotation and angulation. Suture the margins of the ureteral complex to the vesical wall with 5-0 synthetic absorbable sutures and complete the closure over the original hiatus. Intubation of the ureters is not necessary.

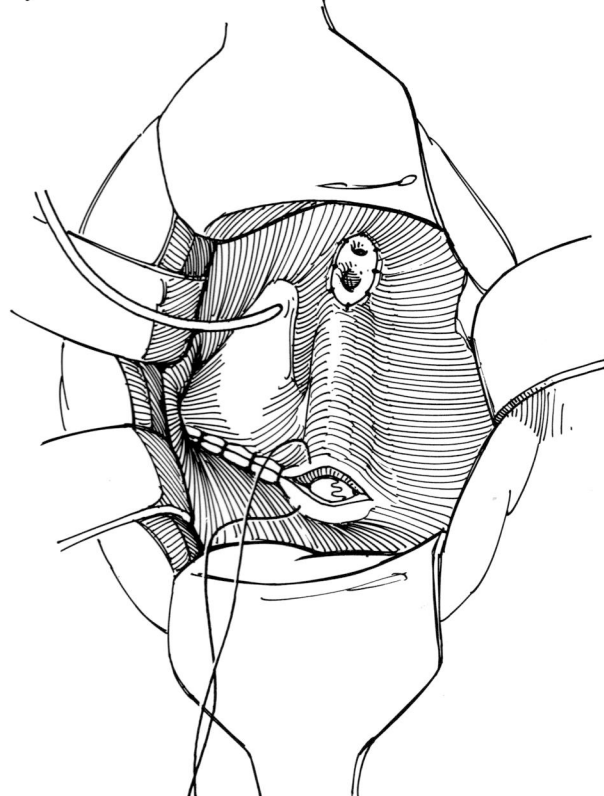

A *residual ureteral stump* after heminephrectomy is removed by following the steps just illustrated, except that the end of the accessory ureter is partially dissected from the ipsilateral ureter (page 230), preserving the joint blood supply, and the single ureter is implanted cross-trigonally.

POSTOPERATIVE PROBLEMS

Complications are similar to those after ureteroneocystostomy (page 215). *Infection* in a closed segment of ureter can lead to sepsis. *Incontinence* results from extensive suburethral dissection.

Commentary by Claude C. Schulman

Management of a large infant-type extravesical ureterocele depends on the child's age and clinical condition, presence of renal failure or sepsis, presence of associated lesions of the lower pole and contralateral kidney or bilateral ureteroceles, and expertise of the surgeon. No general agreement exists on the optimal treatment for an ectopic ureterocele. Of importance to the surgeon is the extravesical extension of the ureterocele, which causes bladder outlet obstruction, and the strength or weakness of the underlying detrusor muscle backing, which might appear as an extensive defect after excision of the ureterocele.

With few exceptions, a conservative approach cannot be justified, because dysplastic lesions or severe damage to the upper-pole parenchyma are associated with the ureterocele, and such procedures as ureteropyelostomy only should be considered in a solitary kidney or when both kidneys are damaged. Thus, in most patients, heminephrectomy is the procedure of choice. It is accomplished easily through a retroperitoneal flank incision, with resection of the proximal portion of the involved ureter.

The controversial question is whether excision of a ureterocele is necessary after upper-pole nephrectomy. Complete excision with extensive reconstruction of the floor of the bladder and reimplantation of the ipsilateral and sometimes contralateral ureter is advocated as the standard procedure by several pediatric urologists. This approach is considered when the ureterocele is large, when detrusor backing is weak, when ipsilateral and even contralateral reflux is present, and when the ureterocele extends down into the urethra. Complete dissection of the ureterocele may be difficult, particularly at the lower end, where it may adhere closely to the bladder neck and urethra. In these patients, a combination of intravesical and extravesical approaches is useful for complete downward dissection of the ureterocele with mobilization of the entire bladder. During dissection of the ureterocele, care should be taken not to injure the external sphincter area. When the ureterocele is unroofed, it is important to remove the entire wall of the ballooning portion, particularly near the bladder neck and in the posterior urethra, to avoid having a retained lip of incised ureterocele acting as a valvular fold and causing obstructive problems. After the ureterocele has been excised completely, the urethra and trigone should be reconstructed with reimplantation of the lower-pole ureter, and sometimes the contralateral lower-pole ureter, following the Politano-Leadbetter technique or the Cohen crossed-advancement procedure.

An essentially extravesical dissection has been advocated to avoid potential damage to the urethra or vagina. Individual skill and experience remain essential for the choice of approach.

In the last decade, an increasing number of authors have advocated a more conservative approach, consisting of heminephrectomy with removal of the upper-pole ureter to the level of iliac vessels, if excision of the ureterocele is not considered mandatory. Complete decompression of the ureterocele, as well as disappearance of mild to moderate reflux in the ipsilateral lower-pole ureter, can be anticipated in a significant number of cases. This approach avoids the risk and potential complications of extensive surgical reconstruction at the bladder level, because the bladder is never entered. The procedure is completed entirely through a single retroperitoneal flank incision. The ureteric stump is left open and drained so that urine remaining in the ureterocele and distal ureter empties in a retrograde fashion when the child voids and intravesical pressure rises.

If reflux was noted in the obstructed system or if the ureterocele was incised causing reflux, the distal stump is ligated. This more-conservative approach gives satisfactory results in approximately two thirds of cases. If the ureterocele fails to collapse and remains obstructive or if reflux persists in the lower-pole ureter, however, it is likely to result in recurrent infection, bladder outlet obstruction, bladder diverticulum, or reflux, all of which necessitate an additional operation through a suprapubic incision in a second stage some time later in one third of cases. This expectant approach also allows total reconstruction at a separate time—usually in easier and safer conditions—in naturally selected cases that really need it.

With the advent of prenatal ultrasonography, an increasing number of uropathies are discovered before clinical manifestations. In neonates and young infants, there also is a place for cystoscopic incision of asymptomatic ureteroceles discovered by ultrasonography. A small, careful horizontal incision is made at the base of the ureterocele, which does not seem to lead to reflux. This allows good drainage of the obstructed but otherwise salvageable kidney with a single or duplex system.

CHAPTER 43

Psoas Hitch Procedure

The psoas hitch procedure is useful in children in conjunction with urinary tract reconstruction after previous diversion when used with transureteroureterostomy and primary reimplantation, and for cases of persistent reflux or obstruction after ureteroneocystostomy or loss of the distal ureter. Estimate the capacity of the bladder to be sure it is sufficiently large and compliant. Provide antibiotic coverage.

1 **A,** *Position:* Supine, with children in the frog-legged position (adolescents are liable to anteromedial thigh pain with paresthesia in this position). Examine the bladder cystoscopically. Place a balloon catheter transurethrally and half fill the bladder. *Incision:* either a lower transverse (page 267) or a long lower midline (page 263) is suitable, in part depending on the position of previous incisions. The transverse incision may need to be extended on the involved side.

B, Mobilize the peritoneum medially. Free the vas deferens in boys; the round ligament may be divided in girls. Circumcise the peritoneal reflection on the dome of the bladder, and close the peritoneal defect with a running plain chromic catgut suture. Take care when freeing the peritoneum over the dome that the bladder wall is not overly thinned; saline instillation in the subperitoneal connective tissue will help this dissection. Follow the obliterated hypogastic artery down to the superior vesical pedicle. Divide the pedicle, ligating the vascular stump with a 2-0 synthetic absorbable suture. Dissect and excise the diseased segment of the ureter. Place a fine traction suture in the free end, and ligate the stump with a 2-0 synthetic absorbable suture. *Note:* it may be necessary to divide the superior vesical pedicle on the opposite side.

Alternatively, especially in secondary cases, open the peritoneum and mobilize the ureter extravesically while preserving its blood supply.

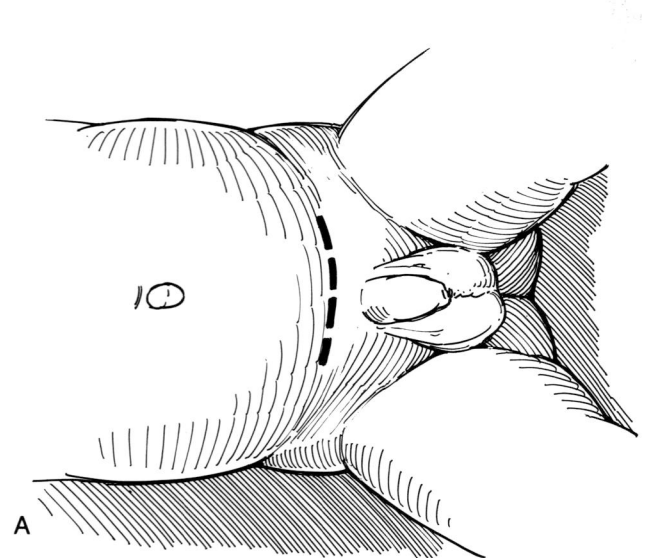

A

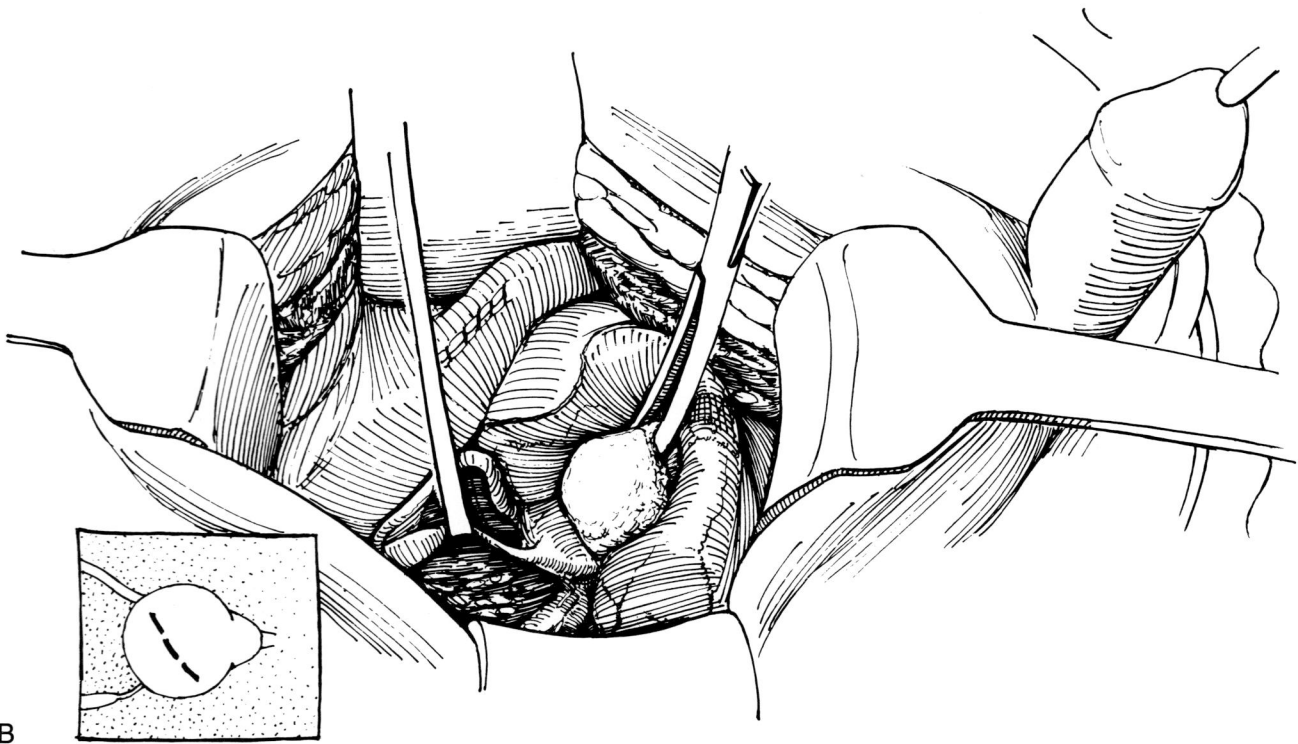

B

2 Place stay sutures just above the midpoint of the anterior bladder wall, and open the bladder near its equator semiobliquely between them with the cutting current. This incision should cut across the middle of the anterior wall at the level of its maximum diameter and should extend a little more than halfway around it. When it is closed vertically, the anterior wall of the bladder will be elongated somewhat more than half of the maximum circumference of the bladder. The apex of the bladder then can be lifted above the iliac vessels as high as with the Boari bladder flap.

3 **A,** Insert two fingers into the fundus of the bladder, and elevate it to meet the ureteral stump, thus converting the transverse incision into a vertical one.

B, Incise the margins of the elongated incision laterally, if necessary, to obtain additional length.

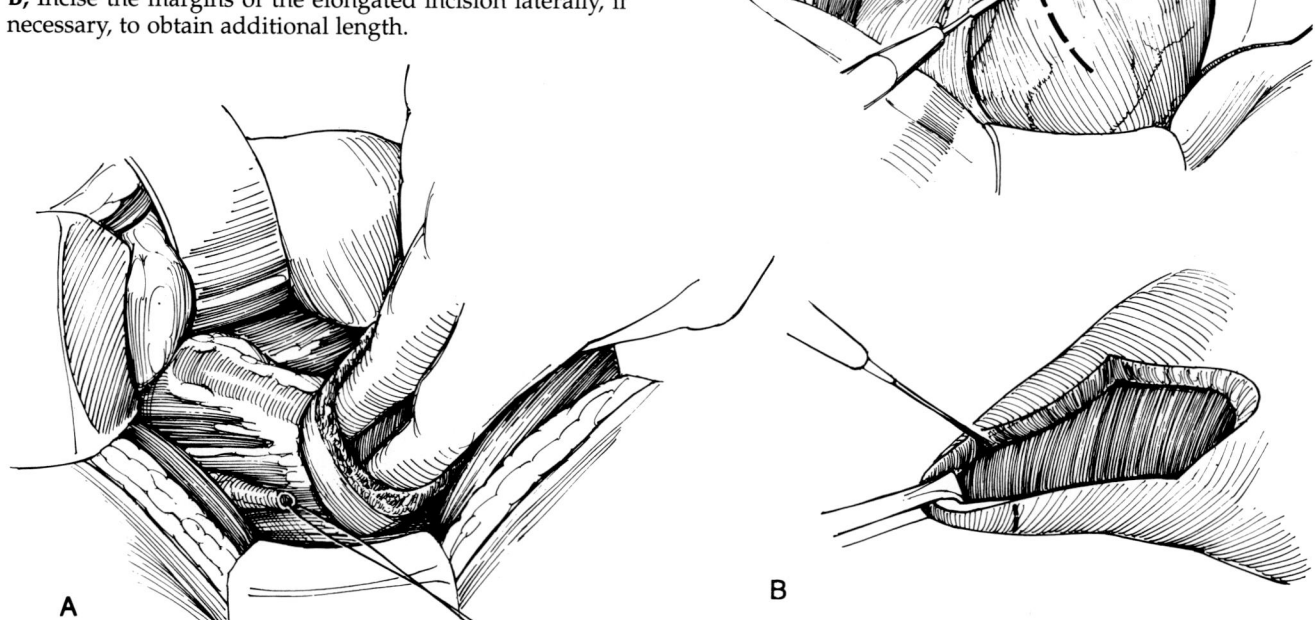

A

B

4 If the bladder still will not reach the end of the ureter with a 3-cm overlap for the anastomosis (in the adolescent), go to the contralateral side and dissect the peritoneum and connective tissue from the pelvic wall and from the lateral wall of the bladder to and, if necessary, including the superior vesical pedicle, which is clamped and ligated with a 2-0 synthetic absorbable suture.

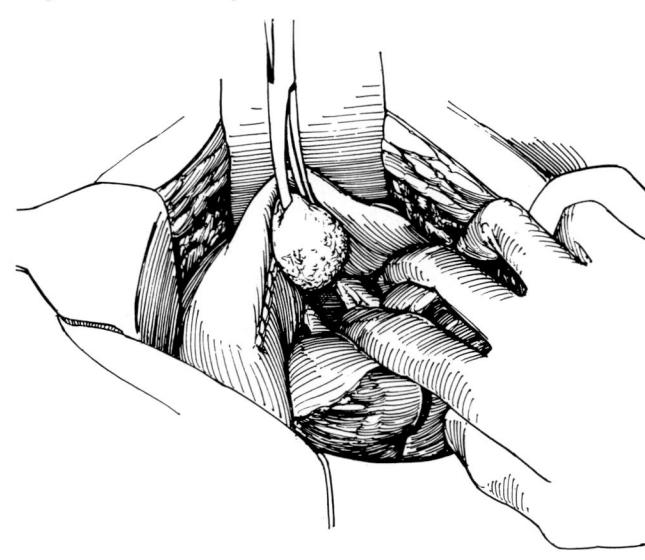

5 Insert two fingers into the bladder, and hold it without tension against the tendinous portion of the psoas minor muscle to determine where the ureter will enter. Place two heavy traction sutures from the bladder wall to the tendon for stabilization during ureteral implantation.

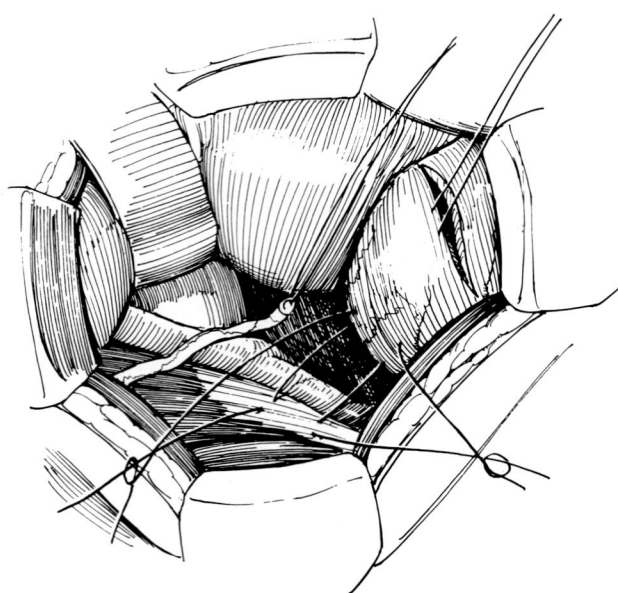

6 Perform a ureteroneocystostomy, as described in Chapter 39 on page 201. From within the bladder, incise the urothelium transversely at the proposed site of the meatus. Tunnel distally under the urothelium for 3 cm with Lahey scissors. Invert the scissors, and pass the tips obliquely through the bladder wall. Push the connector end of an 8 F infant feeding tube over the scissor blades, and draw the tube into the bladder. Tie the ureteral traction suture to the other end of the catheter, and draw the ureter into the bladder. Trim the end of the ureter obliquely, and hold it with a stay suture.

An alternative method to create the hiatus is to insert a peanut dissector into the bladder against the wall where the new hiatus will be created. With the cutting current, incise the wall against the dissector. Pass a clamp thought the defect, and draw the ureter in to check its position. Withdraw the ureter and create a suburothelial tunnel.

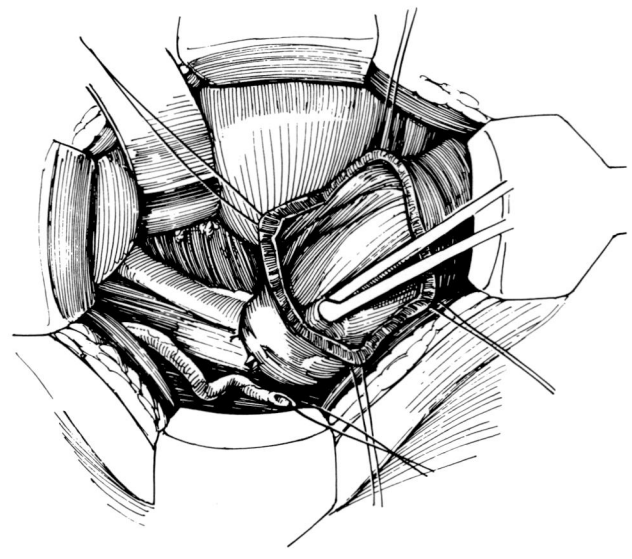

7 Place one 4-0 synthetic absorbable suture deeply into the bladder wall, then through the tip of the ureter. Complete the anastomosis with four or five interrupted sutures to include the vesical urothelium and half the thickness of the ureteral wall. If the bladder cannot be elevated high enough, resort to a direct (refluxing) anastomosis. Insert an 8 F infant feeding tube to the renal pelvis as a stent, and bring the end of the stent through the bladder and body walls in a stab wound. Alternatively insert a double-J stent. Suture the tube to the skin with #1 silk. Tack the ureteral adventitia to the bladder wall at the exit site with three or four interrupted 4-0 sutures.

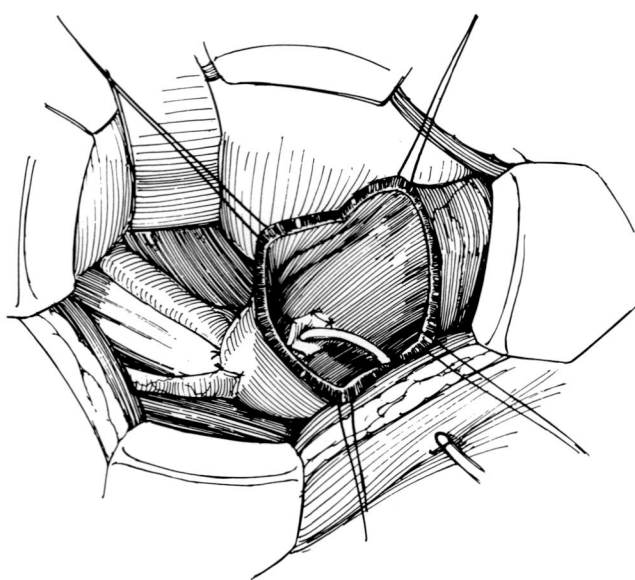

8 Hold the bladder wall against the psoas tendon 2 cm above the ureteral exit site by elevating it with two fingers within. Place five or six 1-0 or 2-0 synthetic absorbable sutures to fasten the bladder to the psoas minor tendon, if present, and to the psoas muscle above and lateral to the iliac vessels. If the tendon is not developed, take deep bites in the muscle itself to anchor to prevent distraction of the ureteric reimplantation by detrusor contraction. Take care not to include the genitofemoral nerve trunk. Tie the sutures loosely so as not to devitalize the bladder wall. Insert a suitable Malecot or balloon catheter into the bladder through a stab wound, especially if there is concern about healing. Check the closure of the peritoneum over the dome of the bladder if it had been opened. Close the bladder opening with a layer of running 3-0 plain catgut suture in the submucosa and with an interrupted layer of 2-0 synthetic absorbable suture in the muscularis and adventitia. Place a Penrose drain in the adjacent retrovesical area, and close the wound in layers. Remove the drains 2 or 3 days after drainage stops. Remove the stent in 1 week, and obtain a cystogram. If that shows no extravasation, remove the suprapubic tube.

Greater length might be obtained by substituting a vertical Z-plasty for the semioblique equatorial incision.

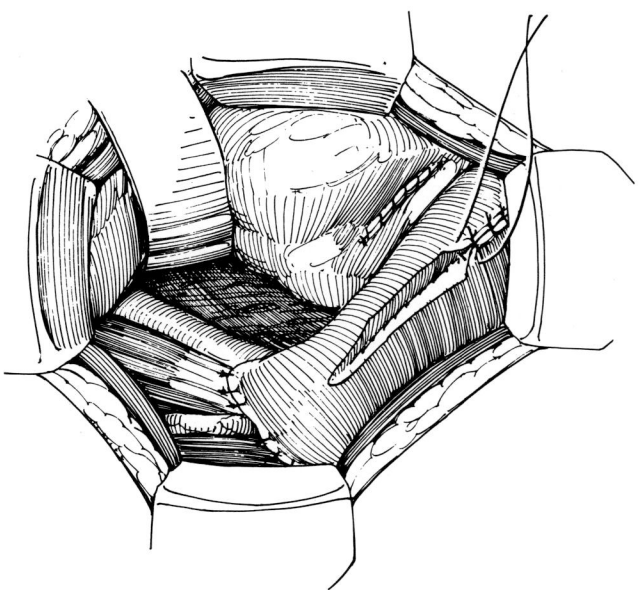

POSTOPERATIVE PROBLEMS

Prolonged urinary drainage is an indication for a retrograde cystogram to ascertain if the leak is at the ureterovesical anastomosis, in which case insertion of a double-J stent and a urethral catheter may allow the fistula to heal. *Obstruction* may be the result of restrictive construction of the tunnel and ureteral orifice or of ureteral angulation during fixation of the bladder extension. Endoscopic catheterization with insertion of a stent may correct the problem.

Commentary by Kevin A. Burbige

The vesical psoas hitch is a valuable technique, useful in compensating for significant amounts of lost ureteral length or for accomplishing a long submucosal tunnel during ureteral reimplantation by immobilizing the ipsilateral posterior bladder wall.

I have found the psoas hitch procedure useful in performing total urinary tract reconstruction where short ureters are common, especially after prior urinary diversion. It also is helpful in revising a failed ureteral reimplant when an adequate submucosal tunnel has failed to cure the reflux. I also have used it often in conjunction with a transureteroureterostomy when implanting a dilated ureter into a valve bladder where an extra-long tunnel is required.

My technique differs somewhat from that illustrated. If scarring from previous surgery is present, it often is easier to open the peritoneum and mobilize the cecum or sigmoid medially to expose the psoas. I perform the hitch prior to ureteral reimplantation by placing figure-eight sutures from the posterior wall of the bladder to psoas, starting inferiorly and working upward. I believe "walking" the hitch up the psoas gives added security. When a long tunnel reimplant is required, the superiormost anterior bladder wall just above the hitch can be split to facilitate the submucosal dissection and avoid "working under the eaves."

The surgeon must be careful to avoid tension when performing the hitch, or the bladder will pull away with filling postoperatively. Likewise, as Dr. Hinman points out, one must avoid mistaking the genitofemoral or ilioinguinal trunk for the psoas tendon and must protect the vas deferens in boys and the fallopian tube in girls. Cannulation or compression of either structure is to be avoided.

Complications inherent to any form of ureteral reimplantation (obstruction, urinary leakage) should be considered if the postoperative course is not smooth.

CHAPTER 44
Bladder Flap Repair
(BOARI)

A psoas hitch procedure is preferable to a bladder flap repair (page 236). Only rarely is the bladder so small that a hitch is not sufficient. Other alternatives are ureteroureterostomy (page 246), renal displacement, or renal autotransplantation (page 244). A relative contraindication to bladder flap repair is severe neurogenic bladder disease.

For bilateral injury, consider ureteroureterostomy with a psoas hitch, bladder flap, or a combination of the two. The appendix can be used to bridge a gap. Rarely is ileal substitution needed.

1 **A,** *Position:* Supine. Insert a balloon catheter, draped to be accessible during the operation. *Incision:* May be predetermined by the scars from the previous operations, which were the cause of the destruction of the distal ureter. Either a midline (page 263) or a transverse lower abdominal incision (page 267) is suitable.

B, Mobilize the peritoneum medially, along with the vas deferens or round ligament, to expose the normal ureter above the defect, usually best identified at or above the level of the bifurcation of the common iliac artery. Encircle it with a Penrose drain, and dissect it toward the bladder as far as is practical.

With an extremely scarred ureter, to avoid dissection in the retroperitoneum with the accompanying high risk of injury to the iliac vein while mobilizing the peritoneum laterally, a generally less desirable option can be used. Approach the ureter transperitoneally through a midline incision. Reflect the cecum or sigmoid colon medially to open the posterior peritoneum along the lateral gutter, and dissect the ureter distally over the iliac vessels as far as the bladder.

To prepare the bladder flap, dissect the peritoneum from the posterior lateral surfaces of the bladder. Infiltrate the subperitoneal tissue with saline to help with this dissection. Isolate and divide the urachal remnant.

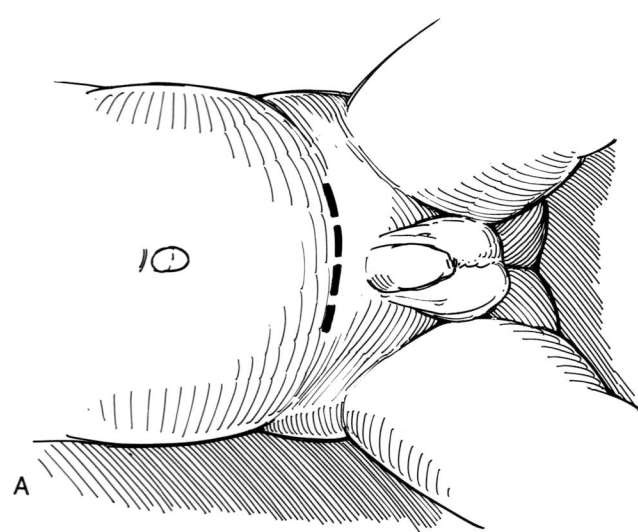

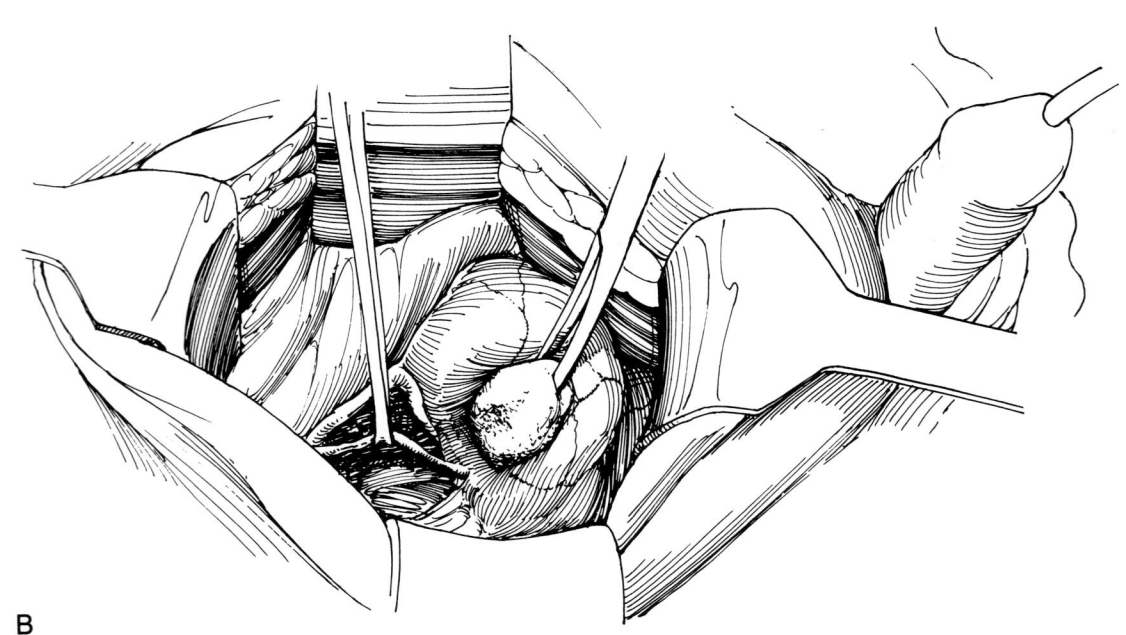

2 Excise the diseased portion of the ureter if practicable, and place a fine stay suture in the proximal normal end for traction. Ligate the distal end. Fully mobilize the bladder, including division of the both the superior and inferior vesical arteries on the opposite side. Try pulling the unopened bladder into a tube onto the psoas muscle. At this point, it may be seen that a psoas hitch is all that is needed. If not, proceed with making a bladder flap. Fill the bladder, and measure the length of flap needed on an umbilical tape, extending from the posterior wall of the bladder to the proximal cut end of the ureter. Mark the outline with a marking pen.

Place two stay sutures in the fixed portion of the bladder at the proposed base of the flap. In the adolescent, they must be placed at least 4 cm apart to provide a broad base. The longer the flap, the wider the base must be. Avoid scarred regions of the bladder. Place two more stay sutures at the distance measured by the umbilical tape to mark the distal end of the flap. Site the flap transversely, or, if greater length is required, make an oblique or S-shaped flap. Usually, 3 cm on a distended bladder is enough. Make the width of the flap at its distal end three times the diameter of the ureter to avoid constriction after tubulation. Now, outline the flap superficially with the weak coagulating current, which also can serve to fulgurate surface vessels. Recheck the dimensions of the flap. With the cutting current, cut through the bladder wall across the distal end of the flap inside the stay sutures. Place two stay sutures in the corners of the proposed flap, and cut the rest of it with the cutting current. Fulgurate bleeders as they are encountered (or ligate them with fine plain catgut ligatures). Inspect for vascularity, and trim ischemic areas accordingly. Insert a 5 F infant feeding tube in the contralateral ureter.

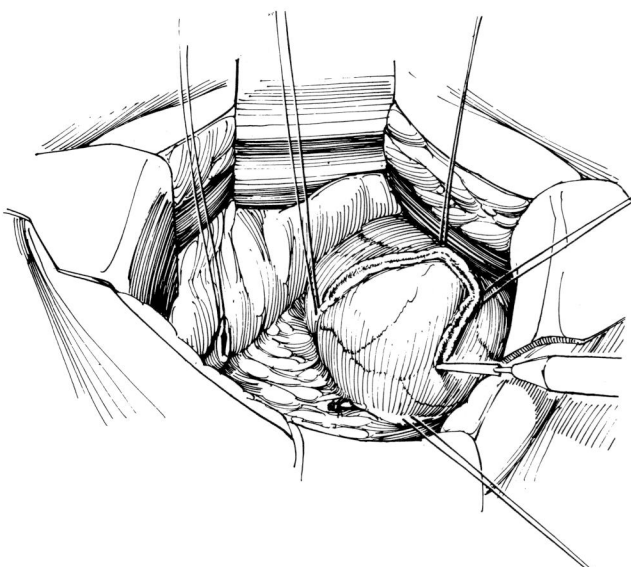

3 The flap should overlap the ureter by at least 3 cm to allow for a proper tunnel. If not, mobilize the ureter but leave its adventitia undisturbed, because it now derives all its blood supply from the renal pedicle. Omission of the tunnel by directly anastomosing the ureter to the bladder wall may be necessary in some cases. If the ureter is still too short, free the kidney inside Gerota's fascia, and move it down to gain 4 or 5 cm in ureteral length. Avoid tension at all costs.

Dissect a subepithelial tunnel with Lahey scissors for a distance of 3 cm, then bring the tip of the scissors through the epithelium. Injection of saline subepithelially helps formation of the tunnel. Install the broad end of an 8 F infant feeding tube (with the cap removed) on the tip of the scissors, and draw the tube up through the tunnel.

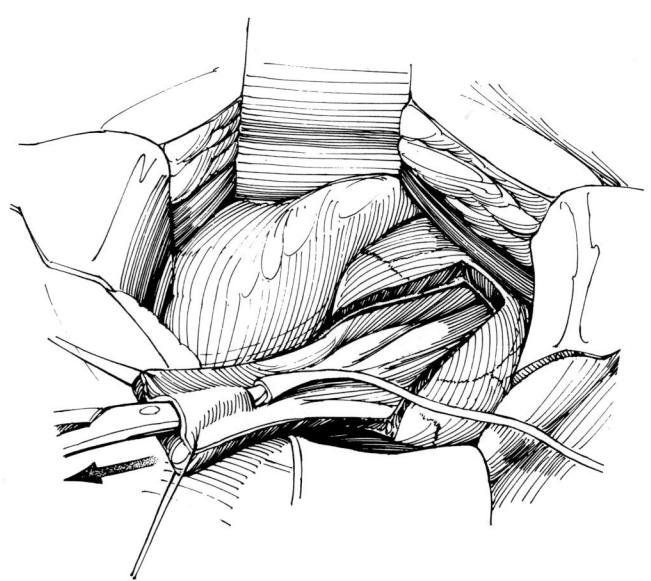

4 Attach the ureteral stay suture to the tube, and draw the ureter down through the tunnel. Spatulate the ureter after trimming it obliquely.

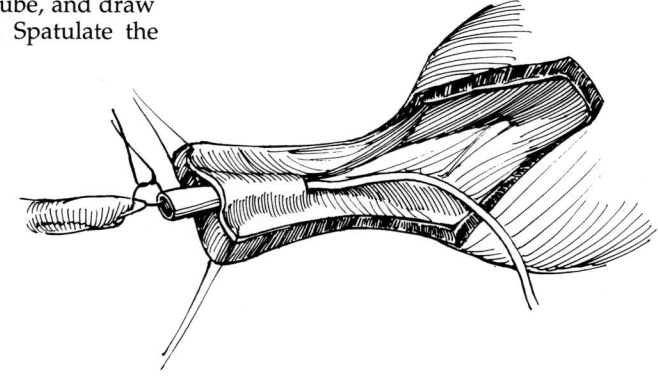

5 **A,** Fix the flap to the psoas minor tendon, avoiding the ilioinguinal and genitofemoral nerves.

B, Anastomose the ureter accurately to the flap. To provide ureteral fixation, the most distal suture should include the vesical subepithelium and muscularis. Complete the anastomosis with three or four more interrupted sutures to the vesical epithelium. Insert an infant feeding tube in the ureter as far as the renal pelvis. Tack it to the epithelium of the flap just distal to the anastomosis with 3-0 plain catgut. Bring the free end through a stab wound in the bladder and body wall, and fix it at once to the skin with 2-0 silk. Place a Malecot or silicone balloon catheter through the opposite bladder wall, to exit through a stab wound.

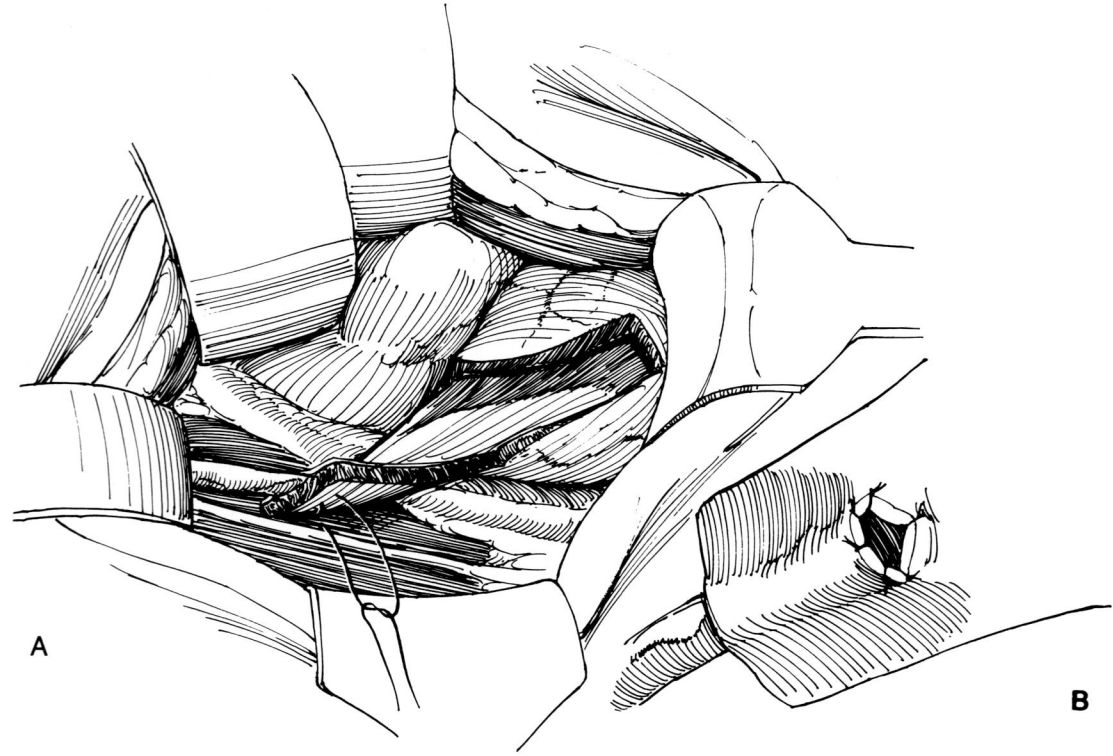

A

B

6 Close the tube and bladder with a running 3-0 plain catgut suture. Place a second row of interrupted 3-0 plain catgut or synthetic absorbable sutures through the adventitia and muscularis, excluding the epithelium. Place a few sutures of 5-0 chromic catgut to approximate the end of the flap to the adventitia of the ureter. Hitch the bladder at the base of the tube to the psoas muscle with 3-0 chromic catgut sutures. Place Penrose drains retroperitoneally, to exit through a stab wound. For the transperitoneal approach, close the peritoneum and drain the area extraperitoneally. Remove the stent on the 8th postoperative day and the bladder catheter 2 days later if no drainage occurs.

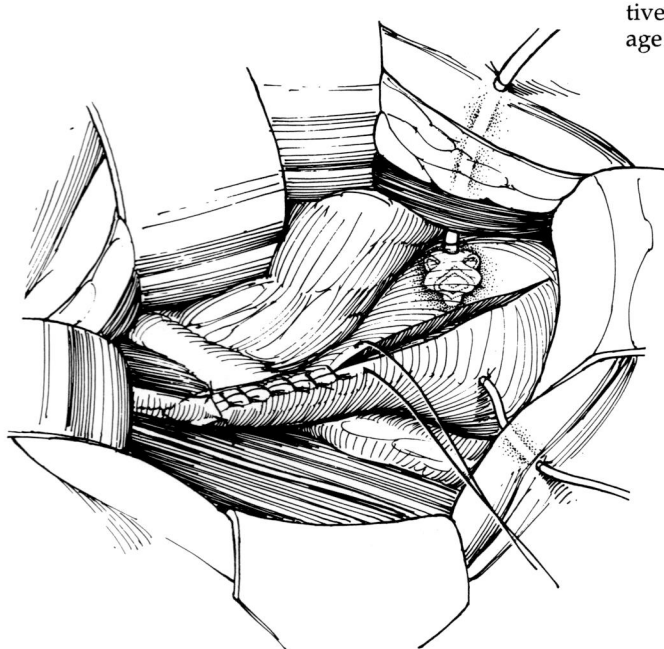

POSTOPERATIVE PROBLEMS

Injury to the opposite ureter should be thought of if the patient has pain or low-grade fever. Perform intravenous urography or sonography and do a bulb ureterogram.

Urinary infection with a febrile reaction may occur on removal of the stent and is treated with antibiotics. Only if it is severe and prolonged is ultrasonography followed by percutaneous nephrostomy indicated, because obstruction at the orifice must be bypassed. *Leakage* usually arises from the area of the bladder closure, rather than from the anastomosis. Leave the catheter indwelling until it stops. If it continues, make an intravenous urogram to locate the site of leakage. If the anastomosis is at fault, intubate it transurethrally, and leave the stent in place 5 or 10 days. In a few difficult cases, an ileal ureter may be constructed or a nephrectomy done. *Late stenosis*

from scarring can occur and requires revision or, if caught too late, nephrectomy.

Commentary by Kevin A. Burbige

Dr. Hinman is right to stress that most often a psoas hitch with or without a downward nephropexy will compensate for a long length of compromised ureter. My technique is essentially that illustrated herein. I generally outline an initial flap that is wider and longer than what one has measured, because excess tissue can be trimmed later, and the flap tends to contract with handling. Fixation of the posterior bladder wall and flap to the psoas is extremely important to prevent angulation and functional ureteral obstruction with bladder filling postoperatively. Although a nonrefluxing ureteral anastomosis is preferable, a direct end-to-end (refluxing) anastomosis of the ureter to the rolled flap may be needed if the ureter is very short. The postoperative complications of any type of ureteral reimplantation need to be kept in mind, because in any anastomosis, tension is to be avoided.

CHAPTER 45

Renal Displacement and Autotransplantation

RENAL DISPLACEMENT

Consider simple displacement of the kidney without transplantation of the renal artery as an alternative to ileal interposition or autotransplantation for defects in the mid or upper ureter if a bladder flap or psoas hitch is not feasible. The kidney can be moved down a significant distance by transecting the renal vein and reanastomosing it lower on the vena cava. Because of the greater length of the right renal artery, the right kidney can be moved farther than the left.

1 *Incision:* Use a midline or anterior subcostal incision, depending on whether the projected site for ureteral anastomosis is high or vesical implantation is necessary. Dissect the renal vessels and adjacent vena cava. Heparinize the child systemically. Occlude the renal artery with a vascular clamp. Give protamine in a dose suitable for size of the child. Consider cooling the kidney with slush. Place two Satinsky clamps on the side of the vena cava proximal to the renal vein. Use different-sized clamps to allow transection of the renal vein flush with the cava for maximum length and to provide an edge for easy closure of the cava. Transect the vein distal to the outer clamp.

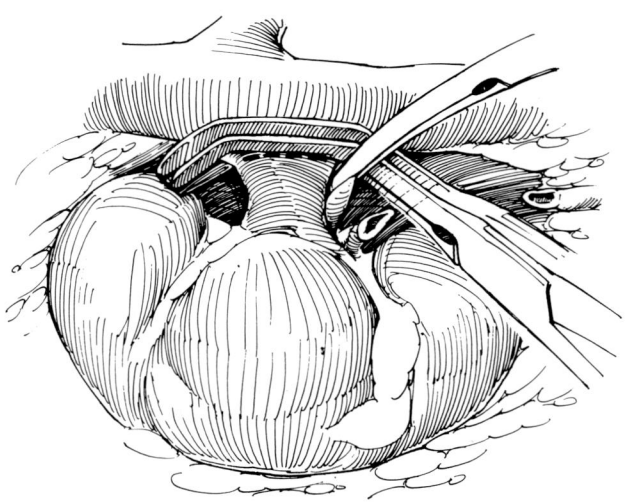

2 Remove the distal clamp, and close the cavotomy with a running 5-0 nonabsorbable suture. Remove the remaining clamp.

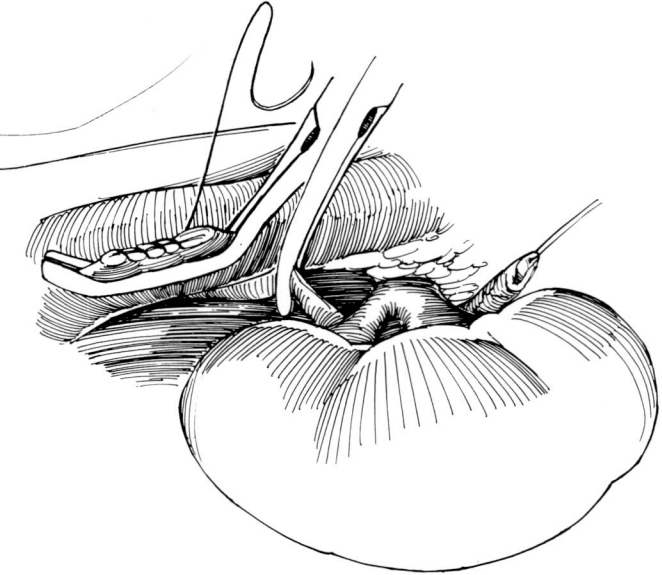

3 Reapply the Satinsky clamp to the vena cava at a lower level, selected to achieve a tension-free ureteral anastomosis. Greater length can be obtained on the right by ligation and transection of the lumbar vein that may tether the renal artery. Incise the vena cava a distance equal to the diameter of the renal vein. Anastomose the vein to the vena cava by an end-to-side technique. Begin posteriorly, working from the inside, because the kidney cannot be flipped over as in renal transplantation.

4 Fix the kidney to the psoas muscle and proceed with the ureteroureteral or other anastomosis.

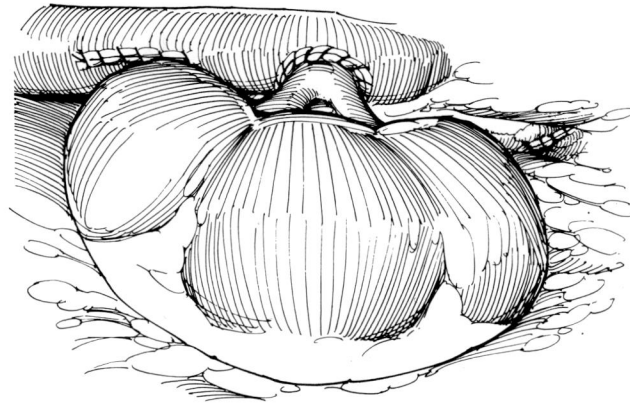

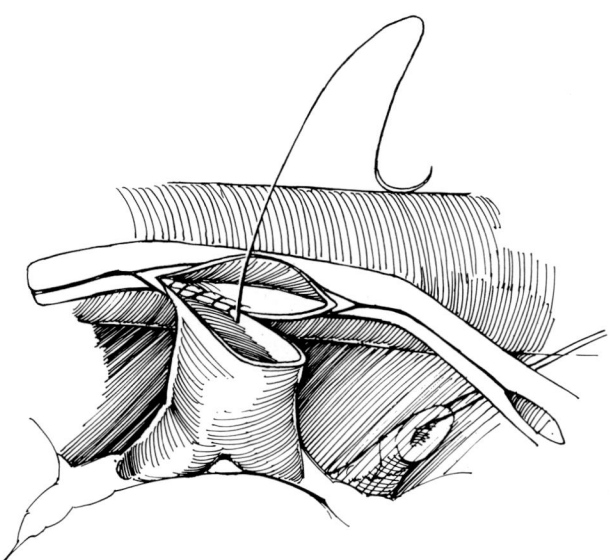

AUTOTRANSPLANTATION

Autotransplantation is used in cases of extensive ureteral loss, severe renal trauma, and complicated renovascular disease.

Incision: Use a long midline incision or a subcostal incision for freeing the kidney and a lower oblique extraperitoneal incision to implant kidney, to expose the iliac artery and vein.

Dissect between the vena cava and aorta to pull the artery out from under the vena cava. To obtain as much length as possible, divide the renal artery as close to the aorta as possible. Similarly, divide the renal vein very close to the vena cava. Dissect the adrenal gland carefully from the kidney. Preserve pelvic and ureteral blood supply by avoiding the adventitia of the pelvis and ureter. Transfer the kidney to the iliac fossa, and anastomose the renal to the iliac vein; then anastomose the arteries. Restore ureteral continuity with ureteroneocystostomy, pyelovesicostomy with or without a bladder flap, or ureteroureterostomy.

Commentary by Kevin A. Burbige

Renal displacement should be considered when significant upper ureteral loss is present and more conservative measures are inappropriate. However, certain maneuvers need to be assessed prior to vein transplantation. A downward nephropexy without disturbing the renal vasculature can close a 2- to 3-cm ureteral gap (page 244). The kidney should be displaced inferiorly after mobilization to determine if this alone will suffice. Likewise, the renal pelvis is often dilated because of obstruction from the diseased ureter, so that one should consider developing a pelvic flap. This can be accomplished in much the same way as a Boari bladder flap with its base at the most dependent area of the pelvis, rolled into a tube, and anastomosed directly to the distal ureter. If these maneuvers are not possible, one should proceed with dissection of the renal vein. In small children and infants, bulldog clamps can be substituted for Satinsky clamps, which can be cumbersome. Both intraoperative and postoperative blood loss should be anticipated, and donor-designated blood should be available. One must be careful not to attempt to displace the kidney too far inferiorly, because undue traction on a small renal artery can result in intimal damage and thrombosis. An external ureteral stent is preferable, because it allows for postoperative surveillance of urine production from the operated kidney. If urine output is not sufficient, one must be alert to vascular complications (*ie*, thrombosis of vein or artery), as well as urinary extravasation. Radioisotope imaging and prompt reexploration may be required if the problem is vascular.

Autotransplantation is useful in situations in which there has been almost complete ureteral loss and ileal interposition is not indicated. It also is advantageous after extracorporeal (bench) renal surgery. The major complications are vascular (thrombosis, hemorrhage) and may result in the loss of the kidney. Again, an external ureteral stent is preferable to monitor urine output from the transplanted kidney.

CHAPTER 46

Ureteroureterostomy

CROSSED URETEROURETEROSTOMY FOR NONDUPLICATED URETERS

Ascertain that the recipient ureter does not allow reflux and is not partially obstructed. Be sure that the child has not had pelvic radiation; if so, plan a high anastomosis away from the field. Provide antibiotic coverage.

1 **A,** *Incision*: Midline transperitoneal (page 83) unless the child has had extensive abdominal surgery, in which case an extraperitoneal approach may be easier. **B,** A left-to-right ureteroureterostomy is described. Hold the descending and sigmoid colon to the right, and pack the small bowel into the upper abdomen. Incise the parietal peritoneum lateral to the colon, and expose the damaged ureter, preserving all the adventitial tissue with its vasculature. Clamp the ureter just above the diseased portion. Place a 3-0 synthetic absorbable stay suture proximal to the clamp, divide the ureter, and ligate the distal stump with the same suture material. Free the donor ureter (for a distance of 9 to 12 cm in the adolescent) while preserving the adventitial vessels.

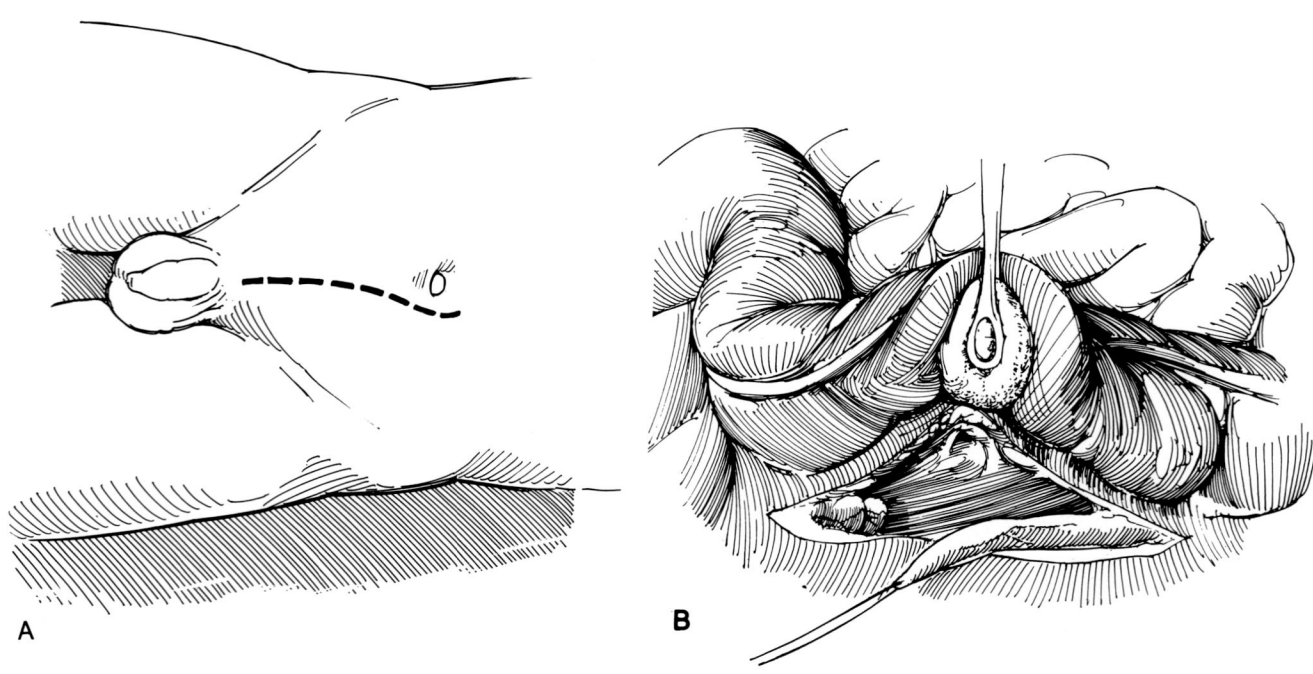

2 Incise the posterior peritoneum over the right, recipient ureter for not more than 3 to 4 cm, just above the pelvic brim. This should be at a level 4 to 6 cm above the level of transection of the donor ureter. Expose the recipient ureter, but barely dissect it from its bed, only freeing it enough to provide space for the anastomosis, ie, a few centimeters. Make a retroperitoneal tunnel by digital dissection, and draw the left ureter through it by its stay suture. It may pass over (preferably) or under the inferior mesenteric artery, depending on the length of ureter available, but it must not be wedged under the artery, where it may become trapped between the artery and the aorta to become obstructed from fibrosis. Be sure the ureter is not angulated and is under no tension.

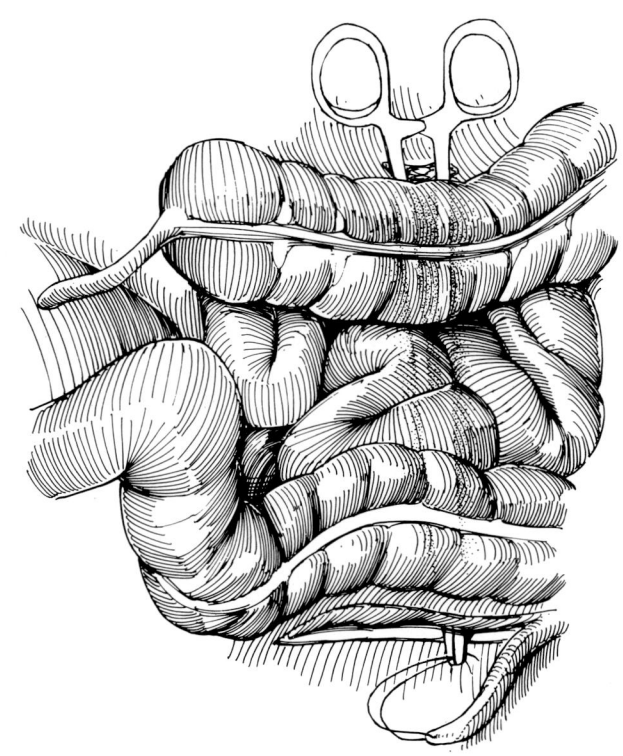

3 A, Trim the ureter obliquely to provide a 1.5-cm opening. Spatulation rarely is needed. With a hooked blade, incise the wall of the recipient ureter on its medial surface for a distance slightly longer than the opening in the donor ureter. Avoid inserting the ureter into the anterior wall because of the risk of angulation.

B, Place a 4-0 or 5-0 synthetic absorbable suture from outside in at each end of the incision in the recipient ureter and then through each extremity of the end of the donor ureter from the inside out. Tie both sutures.

C, Run the upper suture down the back wall from the inside, occasionally locking a stitch. Tie it to the lower suture, then run that suture up the front wall from the outside. Consider inserting a double-J stenting catheter into the recipient ureter prior to the anterior closure. It also is possible to use an infant feeding tube brought out retroperitoneally through a stab wound. A second stent into the donor ureter may be inserted. Place an omental wrap (page 292) if the quality of either ureter is questionable. This usually can be done without mobilizing the omentum merely by bringing it through the peritoneal defect. Tunnel a Penrose drain extraperitoneally from the site of the anastomosis through the body wall and skin of the flank. Close the peritoneal defects with 3-0 synthetic absorbable sutures. Drain the bladder with a suprapubic tube or urethral catheter. Close the wound. Instill contrast medium into the stents 10 days postoperatively; if you see no extravasation, remove the stents. Then remove the cystostomy tube or urethral catheter.

Alternatively, dissect extraperitoneally on both sides to expose the ureters, then pass one retroperitoneally over the great vessels for anastomosis to the other.

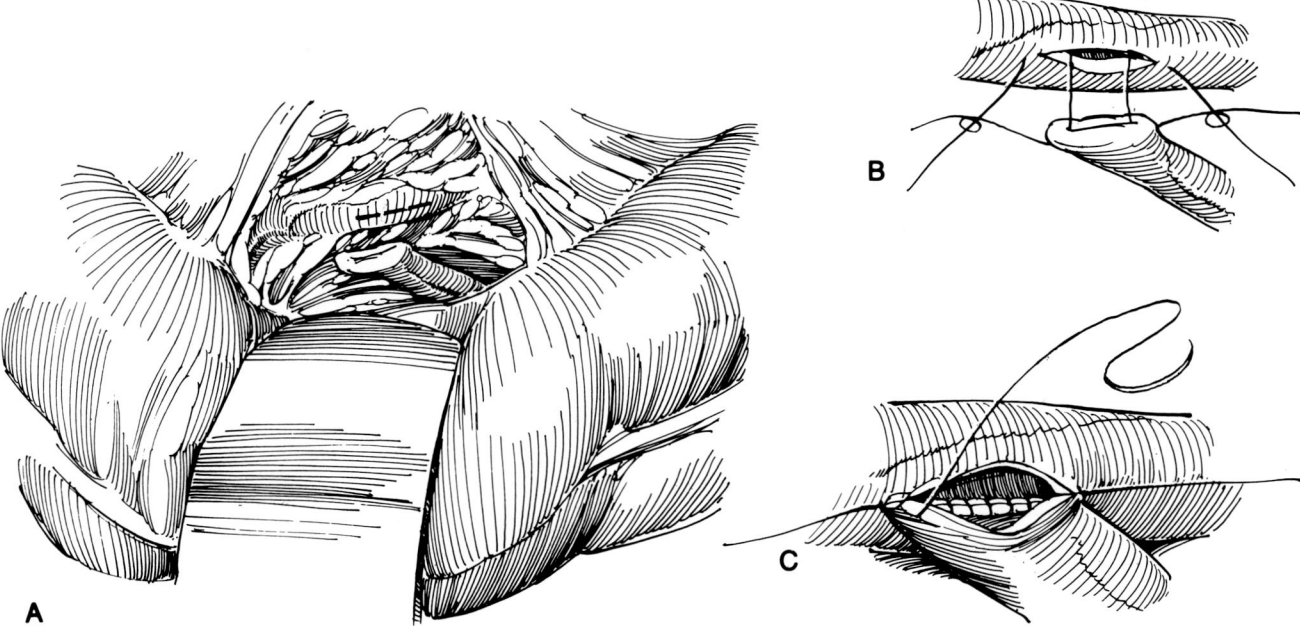

PEDIATRIC TRANSURETEROURETEROSTOMY WITH CUTANEOUS STOMA

Transureterostomy in conjunction with cutaneous ureterostomy can be a useful procedure in an ill child with one dilated ureter, but more recently, it has been applied for salvage of failed reimplantations and in undiversion procedures; in such cases, the better ureter often is implanted in the bladder accompanied by a psoas hitch or one ureter is implanted into an augmented bladder or a pouch.

4 Approach the donor ureter retroperitoneally and mobilize it carefully, preserving all the adventitial tissue, especially when it has been disturbed previously. Divide it distally and ligate the stump. Open the peritoneum over the recipient ureter, and create a wide, straight tunnel retroperitoneally from both sides with the fingers. Pass a large clamp to retrieve the stay suture on the donor ureter. Be careful that the ureter is not trapped at the takeoff of the inferior mesenteric artery from the aorta (consider passing the ureter above, or divide the vessel). Carefully mobilize the recipient ureter as high as is needed (even to the renal pelvis) to reach the skin. Divide and ligate it distally. Form an end-cutaneous ureterostomy (page 360). Anastomose the donor ureter to the recipient as high as is feasible by cutting the ureteral end obliquely and the recipient ureter vertically on the medial aspect. Use everting full-thickness 6-0 synthetic absorbable sutures. Be sure to leave the recipient ureter in its normal bed. Stent both ureters if the recipient ureter is large enough, or use only one stent if that ureter is normal. For stenting of transureteroureterostomies in complex reconstructions involving ureteroneocystostomy and nonrefluxing colonic anastomoses, place two 5 or 8 F infant feeding tubes, brought out retroperitoneally via stab wounds. In addition, insertion of nephrostomy drainage may be wise if the ureter has been mobilized or tapered. Place suction drain tubes from both sides.

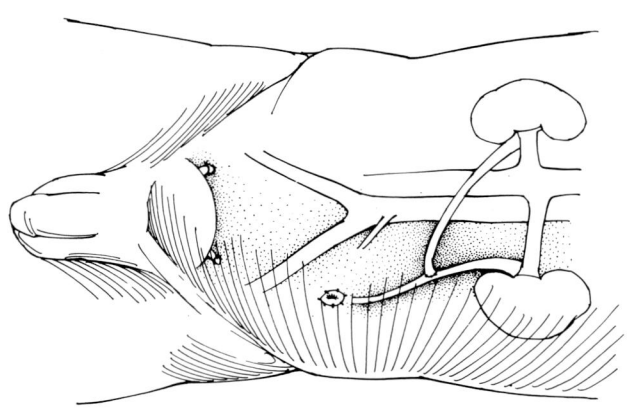

POSTOPERATIVE PROBLEMS

Obstruction at the site of anastomosis can be diagnosed by ultrasonography and a retrograde ureterogram. *Leakage* almost always will stop spontaneously. *Stenosis* at the stoma must be watched for. *Ileus* and *pelvic abscess* have been reported. *Intraperitoneal leakage* can result from tension on the anastomosis and will evidence itself as ileus from urinary ascites. Diversion by percutaneous nephrostomy may be needed. *Stricture* of the normal ureter is rare and probably can be treated by ureteroscopic techniques.

IPSILATERAL URETERAL ANASTOMOSIS

Reanastomosis of the ureter may be required for ureteral stricture, high-velocity projectile injury, intraoperative injury, and retrocaval ureter.

For ureteral stricture, determine the site of obstruction by a combination of antegrade and retrograde urography. Try passing a stent or attempt directvision ureterotomy.

5 **A**, Make an incision appropriate to the site of the lesion; a Gibson incision (page 270), which is shown here, may be adequate, but for lesions in the lower ureter, a midline extraperitoneal incision (page 263) gives better exposure, because the ureters lie close to the midline in the pelvis. The midline incision also allows cephalad extension if the kidney must be mobilized. For upper-ureteral lesions in children, the anterolateral approach is suitable (page 87).

B, Locate the ureter extraperitoneally, realizing that it will be displaced anteriorly during exposure, because it is adherent to the peritoneum. It crosses the bifurcation of the iliac artery and lies just under the obliterated hypogastric artery. Pinch it with forceps to elicit peristalsis for identification. A dilated ureter may be deceptive; aspiration with a fine needle will identify it. In difficult cases, transperitoneal exposure with subsequent extraperitoneal drainage is preferable. Isolate the ureter by careful sharp and blunt dissection, avoiding the adventitia. Place a Penrose drain or vessel loop around it. Identify the site of obstruction; a ureteral catheter placed previously on a stilet to keep it in place may help.

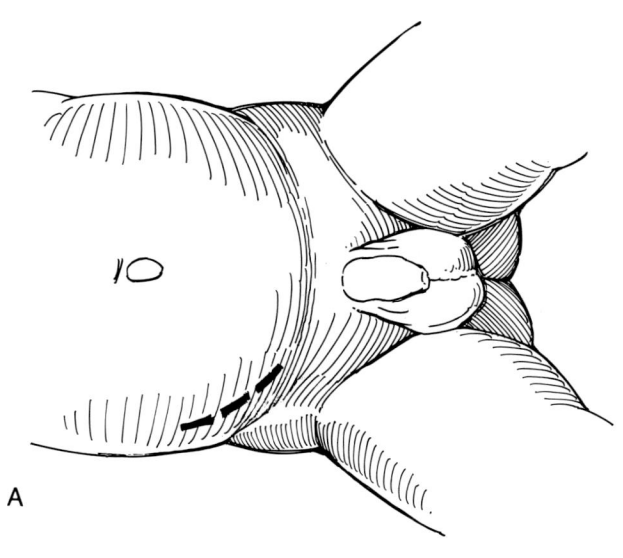

A

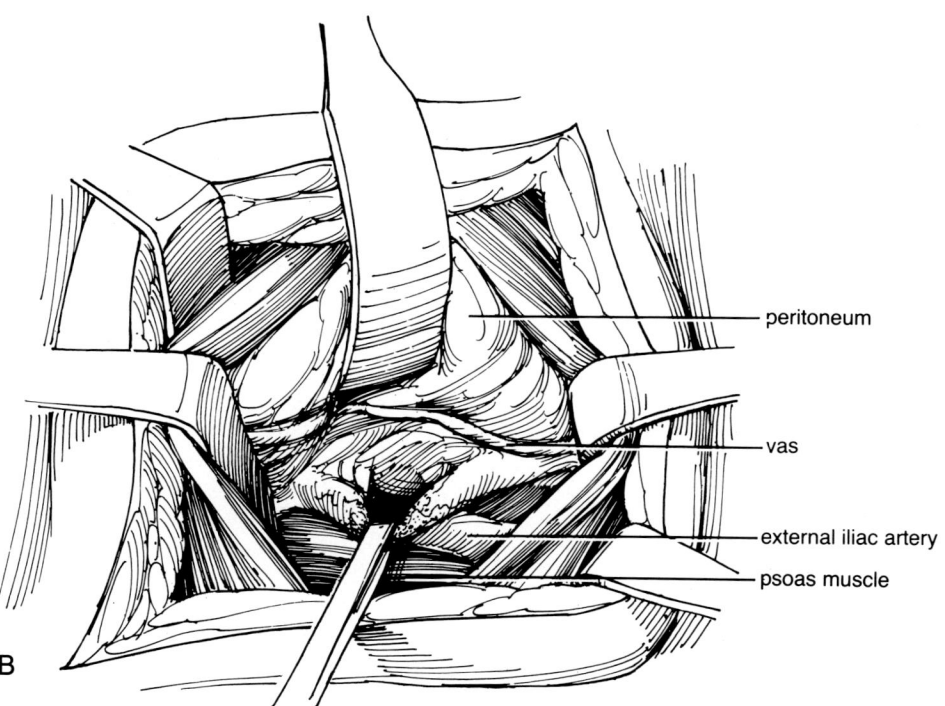

peritoneum

vas

external iliac artery

psoas muscle

B

6 Place stay sutures above and below the lesion and excise it, being sure that healthy ureter is reached. Débridement to normal ureter is important, especially in the presence of infection or after radiation. Replace the stay sutures with a fine traction suture in each end of the ureter on the medial aspect, and carefully dissect sufficient length for the anastomosis while avoiding the vessels in the adventitia.

Intubated ureterotomy is an alternative in long strictures with minimal periureteral involvement. Incise the stricture throughout its length, and insert a suitable-sized double-J stent, extending into the pelvis and bladder. Pad the area with fat or omentum (page 272). Leave the stent in place 6 weeks.

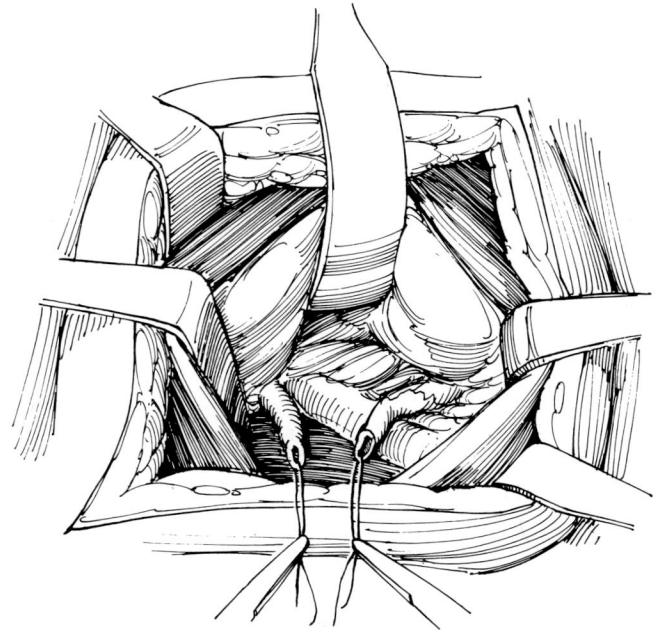

7 Transect the ureteral ends obliquely from the stay sutures, and spatulate each end for a distance of 2 to 3 mm, preferably on the lateral border. If one lumen is very small, gently dilate it to 8 F. Do not use forceps on the ureter; manipulate it with stay sutures.

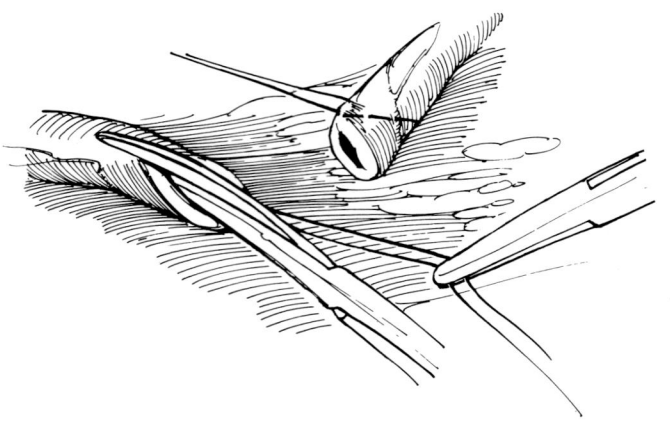

8 A, Insert two running 5-0 or 6-0 synthetic absorbable sutures in through the tip of the spatulated portion and out through the notch of the opposite ureteral wall. It helps to use a binocular loupe. Tie the sutures. Place a double-J stent if the vitality of the ureteral wall is in doubt. Be sure its upper end lies in the pelvis, and the lower end, in the bladder. Do not continue if the ureter is under tension—use an alternative method.

B, Run one of the apical sutures down one side of the defect with bites 2 mm apart, catching more serosa and muscularis than epithelium, working from inside the ureter. The suture may be locked every third or fourth stitch. Run the other suture from the outside. Tie each suture to the free end of the other suture. Place a Penrose drain to exit extraperitoneally by the long-suture technique (page 127), taking great care not to let it lie against the anastomosis, and fasten it to the skin. Replace the retroperitoneal fat around the repair, and close the wound as described elsewhere. An omental wrap (page 272) may aid healing by decreasing periureteral scarring and providing neovascularity. If there is urinary drainage postoperatively, leave the drain in place until leakage has ceased for 2 or 3 days, and then remove it gradually.

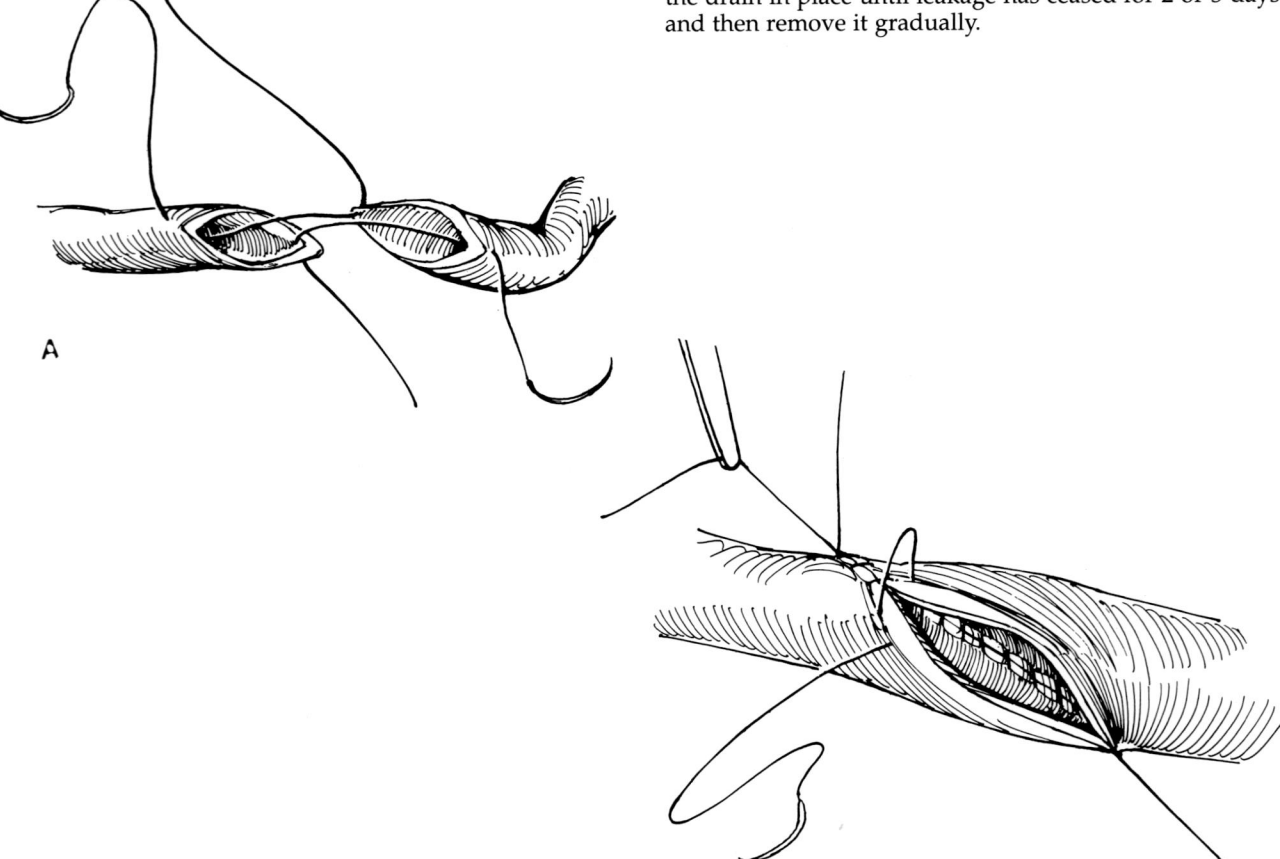

A

B

Renal Mobilization

9 When the ureteral length is inadequate for tension-free reanastomosis, mobilize the kidney. Reflect the colon medially, and continue the retroperitoneal dissection cephalad, inside Gerota's fascia. The peritoneum may need to be opened in some cases. Bluntly free the renal capsule from the perirenal fat. If it is extremely adherent, extend the incision in the gutter so that Gerota's fascia may be opened and the dissection carried out under vision, as for simple nephrectomy (page 155). Now the kidney will rotate downward on its pedicle, adding 3 to 5 cm of ureteral length. Fix it to the psoas muscle with two 2-0 synthetic absorbable mattress sutures, incorporating fat pads.

Alternatives would be a psoas hitch (page 236), Boari bladder flap repair (Chaper 44), transureteroureterostomy (page 240), ileal interposition (page 255), renal displacement by division of the vein (page 244), and renal autotransplantation.

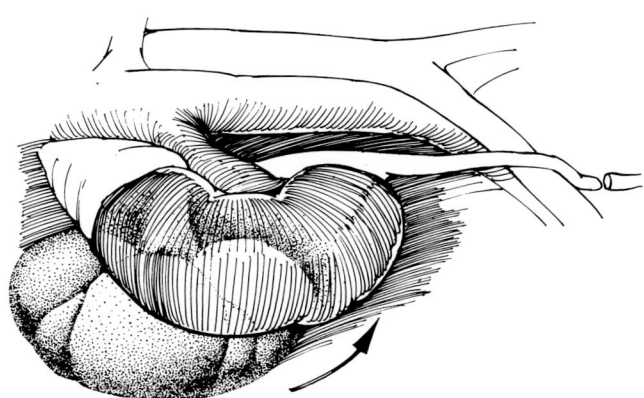

INTRAOPERATIVE INJURY TO THE LOWER URETER

To repair an intraoperative injury to the lower ureter, immediately extend the existing dissection to gain adequate exposure. Lack of exposure was probably what led to the injury. If the patient's condition does not allow repair, place a silicone tube or double-J stent up the ureter to the renal pelvis and bring it out extraperitoneally for temporary drainage.

POSTOPERATIVE PROBLEMS

Urinary drainage, if prolonged, suggests first that the drain may be in contact with the repair. Shorten the drain. Distal obstruction may be responsible. Pass a double-J stent to the renal pelvis, and leave it in place 2 to 3 weeks. A *urinoma* may form if the drain is removed before drainage has ceased. A *stricture* may develop later; follow-up intravenous pyelograms are important to detect silent obstruction.

URETEROURETEROSTOMY FOR RETROCAVAL URETER

If the diagnosis is in doubt, perform a venacavogram simultaneously with a retrograde pyelogram. Note on the intravenous urogram whether the ureter crosses behind the inferior vena cava at the level of the third lumbar vertebra (Type I), in which case a ureteroureterostomy is done, or at the level of the renal pelvis (the less-common and less-obstructive Type II), in which case a pyeloureterostomy is appropriate.

10 A, Approach the ureter through an anterior subcostal incision. It is advisable to look for a persistent postcardinal vein instead of the vena cava itself as the obstructing vessel, in which case it simply can be ligated and divided to free the ureter. With a retrocaval ureter, do not bother to dissect the ureteral segment from behind the vena cava, because it probably is secondarily stenotic, and the ureter always is elongated anyway. Expose the ureter below where it emerges from behind the medial side of the vena cava, and place a Penrose drain around it. Dissect it to the border of the vena cava, transfix it with a stay suture, and divide it. The proximal stump need not be ligated.

B, Moving laterally, identify the dilated pelvis and upper ureter. Dissect the ureter similarly to the lateral margin of the vena cava. Fix it with a stay suture, and divide it distally with an oblique cut. This end of the ureteral stump need not be ligated either, because the obstructive segment is now isolated. Anastomose the ureter to the pelvis by the Anderson-Hynes technique (page 223) or to the dilated upper ureteral segment by ureteroureterostomy, with or without a double-J stent. Drain the area with an accurately placed Penrose drain exiting extraperitoneally. Remove the stent after a week if the anastomosis is firm, and remove the drain several days after drainage has stopped.

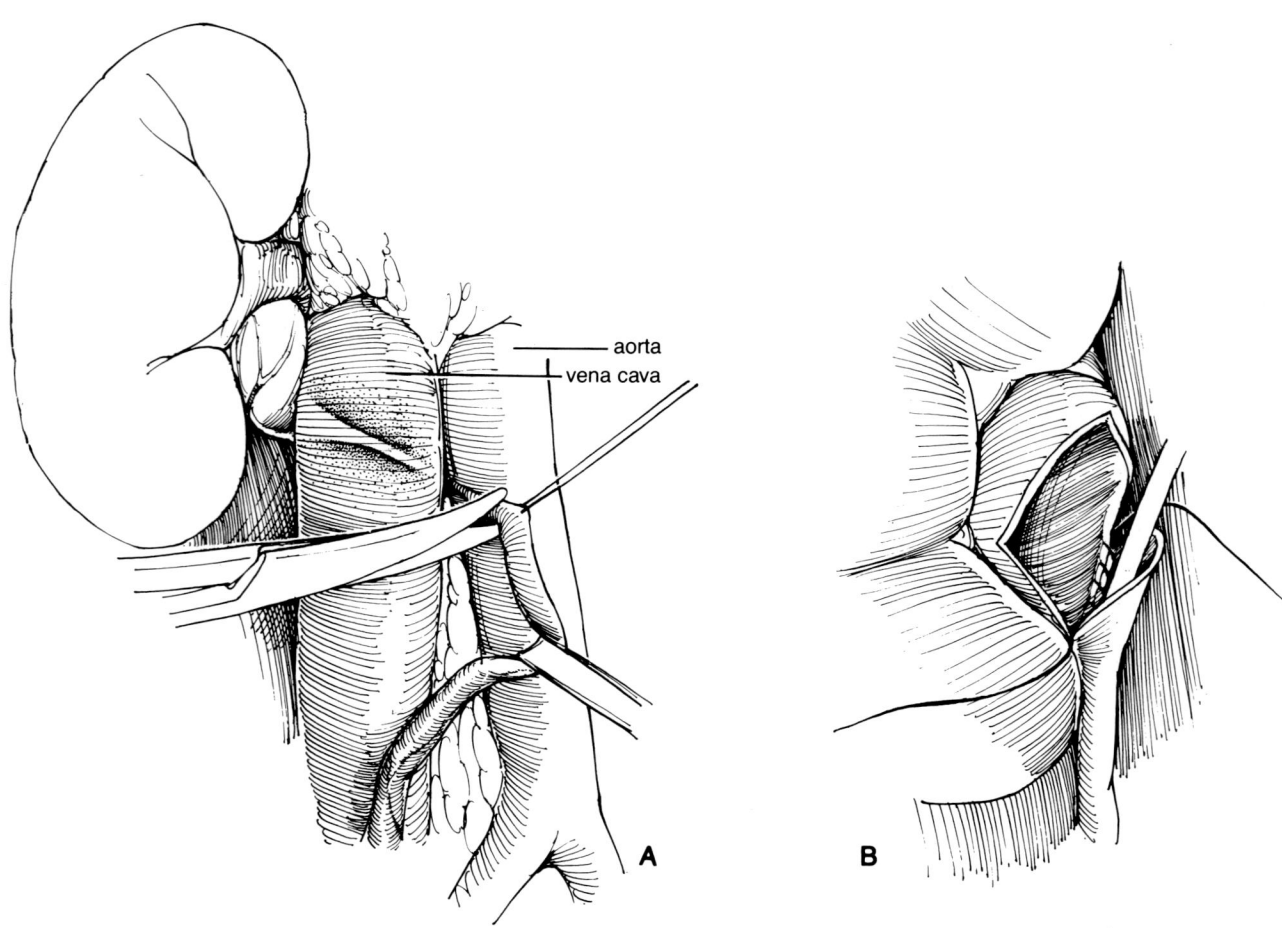

Commentary by Evan J. Kass

Ureteroureterostomy is an uncommon procedure in children, because the potential for anastomotic stricture is significant, given the small caliber of the undilated ureter in a child. We prefer to perform a Boari flap for most injuries of the lower third of the lower to mid-ureter and have been surprised at the length of ureter that can be bridged. Inferior mobilization of the kidney will reduce even further the need for primary ureteral anastomosis. If ureteroureterostomy is the only option, the anastomosis should be well spatulated and free of tension. We use a ureteral stent routinely and leave it in place for 6 weeks.

CHAPTER 47

Calycoureterostomy

First consider all other procedures for bridging a defect between pelvis and ureter, because this operation may be followed by ureterocalyceal stricture. Alternatives include the Davis intubated ureterotomy (page 131), autotransplantation (page 245), ileal ureter (page 255), and nephrectomy (page 155). The renal cortex over the involved calyx must be thin and have a dilated collecting system; otherwise, the parenchyma will contract around the ureter.

Incision. An anterior subcostal incision (page 87) usually is adequate, but an anterior transperitoneal incision (page 81) allows intestinal interposition if that proves necessary. Place a ureteral catheter cystoscopically if identification of the ureter may be difficult. Proceed as for pyeloureteroplasty (page 123). In addition to thoroughly mobilizing the kidney, it is important to be able to control the renal artery if the need should arise. Identify the normal ureter distally, and place a small Penrose drain around it. Continue ureteral dissection up to the scarred ureteropelvic junction. The ureter may be long enough after the diseased portion is resected, or an alternate procedure may be preferable. Place a fine traction suture in the ureter and a clamp just above it. Divide the ureter obliquely below the clamp, and ligate the stump on the pelvic side with a 2-0 synthetic absorbable suture.

1 Incise the capsule around the lower pole of the kidney in the frontal plane, and carefully peel it back. It probably will be quite adherent. Estimate the level of the upper-pole infundibulum from the pyelogram, and bluntly divide the renal parenchyma with the knife handle, cutting the arcuate vessels with scissors. Remove more parenchyma if necessary to expose the infundibulum of the lower calyx; excess parenchyma will contract around the ureter and constrict it. Control the bleeding by encircling the lower half of the kidney with the left hand while placing figure-eight sutures of 4-0 synthetic absorbable material, tied by your assistant, to control the arteries. Hemostasis must be complete. Free the calyx enough to hold sutures, or free the infundibulum of the calyx and cut it tangentially.

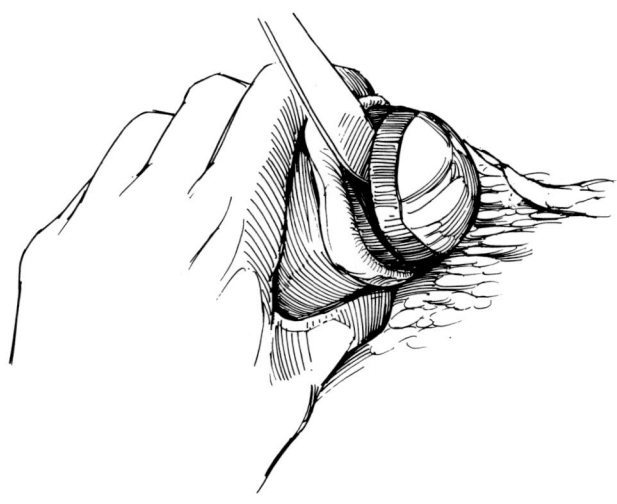

2 Spatulate the ureter on its lateral side for a distance equal to the length of the calyceal defect. Anastomosis is similar to that for pyeloplasty (page 126). Place two 4-0 synthetic absorbable sutures side by side through the capsule, then into the medial end of the calyx and out through the ureter at the notch of the spatulation. Tie them. Run one suture along the posterior to the opposite end, with each bite catching the capsule, ureter, and calyx. Lock an occasional stitch. Do the same with the anterior suture, here including, in order, the capsule, ureter, and calyx. Just before the defect is completely closed, insert a double-J stent that extends down the ureter to the bladder and up into the renal pelvis. Additionally, with a curved clamp, draw a small Malecot catheter through the cortex into a middle calyx, and fix it to the capsule with a 2-0 synthetic absorbable suture. Complete the ureterocalyceal anastomosis, and tie the two sutures together. Irrigate through the nephrostomy tube to be sure the closure is watertight. Place a nephropexy stitch, and drain the area well with a Penrose drain that exits retroperitoneally. Replace the perirenal fat with Gerota's fascia to encase the repair. However, if coverage seems inadequate, bring the omentum into the retroperitoneum and tack it about the anastomosis. Postoperatively, remove the stent, and test for pressure and flow through the anastomosis before removing the nephrostomy tube.

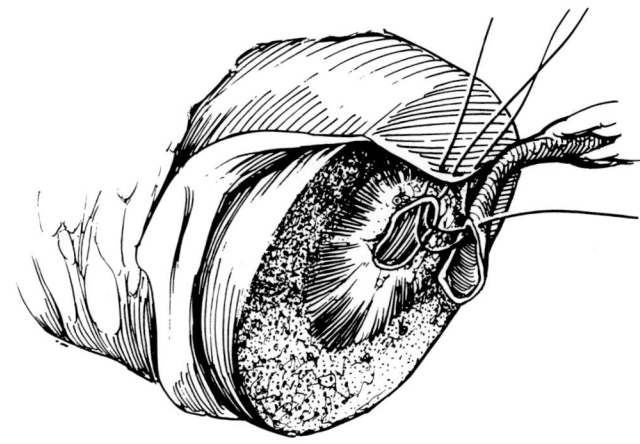

Commentary by Evan J. Kass

We have used calycoureterostomy primarily for ureteropelvic junction obstruction with massive hydronephrosis. In this setting, a primary pyeloplasty may not achieve dependent drainage, and because the lower-pole parenchyma usually is quite thin, no renal tissue needs to be excised. One simply chooses the most dependent calyx, excises a button of tissue, and performs a primary spatulated tension-free anastomosis.

Calycoureterostomy also may be necessary as a salvage procedure following a failed pyeloplasty or a complex stone operation. However, here there usually is thick parenchyma over the lower pole and considerable perirenal fibrosis. It is essential to mobilize the calyx sufficiently so that the anastomosis is epithelium-to-epithelium and free of tension. A ureteral stent is mandatory and usually is left in place for 6 weeks. We find it easier to pass a double-J stent before starting the anastomosis.

CHAPTER 48

Ileal Ureteral Replacement

Explore all alternatives that use tissue from the urinary tract before electing to use ileum. Determine that the bladder neck is widely open and that the patient empties the bladder easily; if not, consider a YV-plasty as part of the procedure. In boys, resection of the prostate transurethrally may be adequate. Be certain that the patient has adequate renal function; serum creatinine level should be 2.2 mg/100 dl or less. It is assumed that nephrostomy drainage is already in place.

Prepare the child as for an ileal conduit (page 371). Do not place a urethral catheter, but allow the bladder to fill. If the ureter is to be excised, insert a ureteral catheter cystoscopically.

1 *Position*: Place the child in a lateral position with the table flexed and the shoulder and chest held at right angles to the table. Allow the hip to fall back as far as is reasonable and place a sandbag under it. *Incision*: Palpate the 12th rib and begin the skin incision over its angle. Continue semiobliquely to the midline, then vertically to the pubis. Alternatively, use a thoracoabdominal incision for better exposure for the renal anastomosis; for bilateral cases, a long midline incision is best. Cut through the anterior part of the latissimus dorsi muscle onto the surface of the 12th rib. Place the index finger in an opening in the lumbodorsal fascia at the tip of the rib and work posteriorly, cutting the serratus inferior posterior muscle and intercostal muscles, if encountered. Divide the external and internal oblique and transversus muscles, and enter the peritoneum. Divide the rectus muscle and retract it laterally while continuing the incision down the midline, opening the peritoneum further at the same time.

Incise the peritoneal attachment of the terminal ileum to the sacral promontory, and divide the lateral attachments of the ascending colon in the white line of Toldt to mobilize it to the region of the duodenum and as far medially as the great vessels, as for retroperitoneal lymph node dissection. Let the bowel fall back. Now open the peritoneum, continuing anteriorly in the line of the incision.

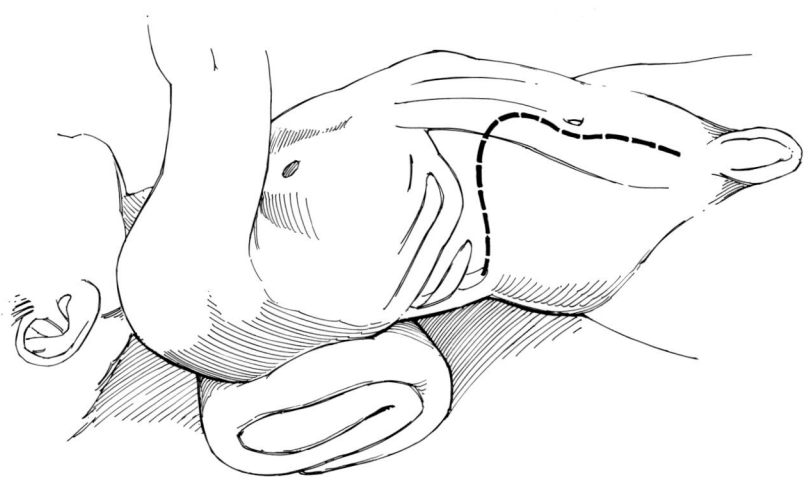

2 For an adolescent, select a 20- to 30-cm segment of ileum near the ileocecal junction; the length depends on the size of the child and on how much ureter is to be replaced. Choose sites of transection to allow for total mobilization of the segment of ileum by allowing for the cuts in the mesentery deep enough for the upper end to reach the renal area (this can be difficult) and the distal end of the loop to reach the bladder. Special care must be taken to get a good arterial supply and to make certain that two major branches of the superior mesenteric artery enter the loop.

On the *left* side, a segment of *descending colon* can be used instead of the ileum. Mark the bowel at each end with a stay suture; throw a loose tie onto the suture at the distal end as a marker to be sure that later the segment is placed isoperistaltically. Divide the mesentery deeply between the ileocolic artery and the terminal branches of the superior mesenteric artery. Divide it also at the proximal end deeply enough to allow that end to reach the kidney. Apply Kocher clamps and divide the bowel. Restore bowel continuity as described for ileal conduit (page 375). Irrigate the loop with a catheter and a 50-ml syringe containing saline solution, followed by 1 percent neomycin-bacitracin solution and, finally, by air. Close the mesenteric defect with 4-0 silk sutures.

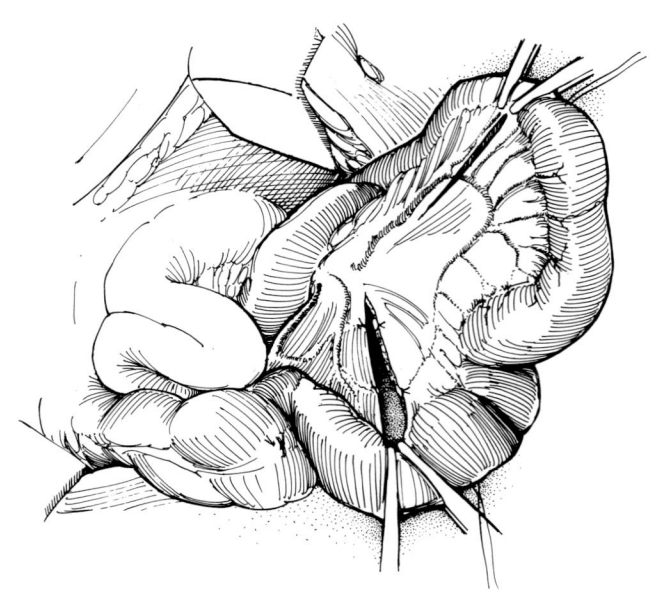

3 For replacement of the *right* ureter, the ileal segment should be placed extraperitoneally by lifting the cecum forward and exposing the retroperitoneal space. Make a small opening in the mesentery of the ascending colon near the cecum, and bring the ileum through it. On the *left* side, the descending colon is mobilized medially by incising along the white line. Make a window in the colonic mesentery, and push the isolated segment of ileum out through it so that it lies in an isoperistaltic manner in the left retroperitoneal space. Because the anastomoses to the pelvis and to the bladder are retroperitoneal, the ileum will lie behind the descending colon. Rotate the ileum 180 degrees counterclockwise to place the knotted stay suture marking the distal end near the bladder, ensuring isoperistaltic orientation. In either case, carefully close the opening through the mesentery to prevent internal herniation and at the same time avoid constriction. Grasp the end of the loop again with the Kocher clamp. For unilateral ureteral substitution, close the proximal end of the loop, spatulate the ureter, and anastomose it to the ileum, as described for ureteroileostomy. Connect the ureter end to side if it is dilated, even if tailoring is necessary. At this time, consider placement of a nephrostomy (page 140).

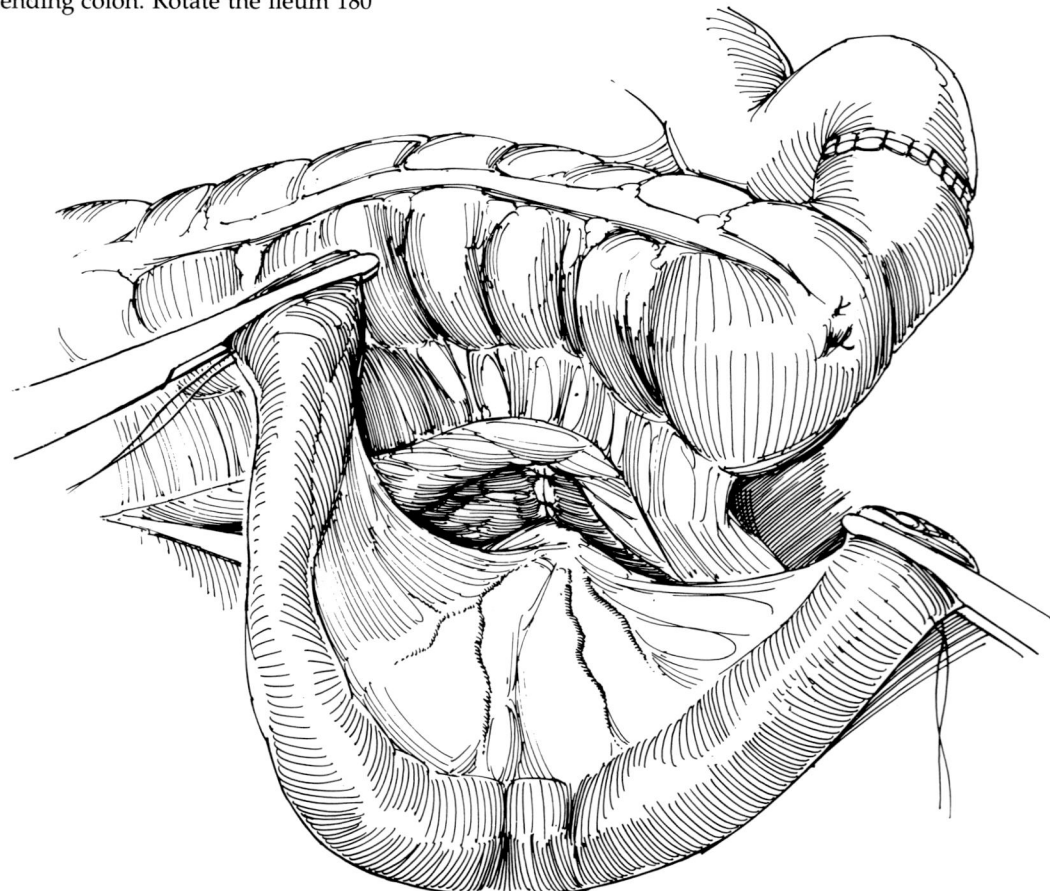

4 Direct pyeloileal anastomosis may be advisable for children with recurrent xanthine stone formation. The renal pelvis must be mobilized, often difficult after previous stone procedures. If the pelvis is obscured by scar, insert curved Randall forceps through the nephrostomy site and cut on its tip, staying away from the vascular pedicle. Leave the ureter *in situ*. Consider instillation of coagulum if small calculi are present. Open the renal pelvis widely vertically. Pass Randall stone forceps through the pyelotomy into the lower-pole calyx, and cut down on the forceps with the cutting current to open the entire lower collecting system. Place 3-0 chromic catgut sutures from the capsule to the calyx to control parenchymal bleeding. Remove persisting calculi with the aid of a nephroscope. Insert a small Malecot nephrostomy tube with two wings removed through the parenchyma via a middle calyx.

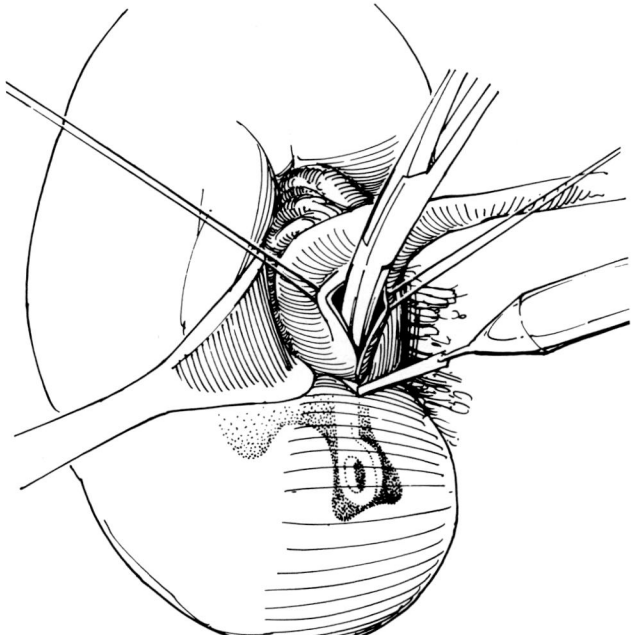

5 Spatulate the ileum to form an ellipse by opening its antimesenteric border, incising it until it is large enough to fit the pelvic defect. Place a 3-0 or 4-0 chromic catgut suture through all layers of the tip of the bowel, then through the upper margin of the pelvic defect, and tie it. Run the suture down the back wall; occasionally lock a stitch. Continue the suture up the anterior wall and tie it to the end of the original suture. Alternatively, use interrupted 3-0 or 4-0 chromic catgut sutures, placing the posterior row with the knots outside. Either suture line may be reinforced with serosa-to-adventitia sutures. Fill the pelvis through the nephrostomy tube, and reinforce the anastomosis at sites of leakage.

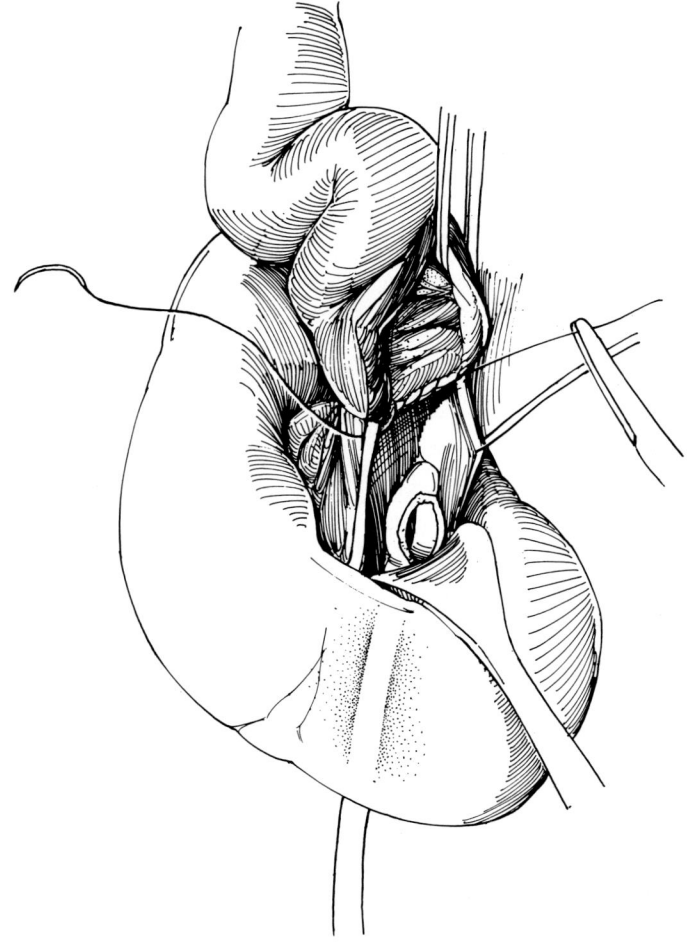

6 Mobilize the peritoneum from the upper and lateral margins of the bladder, and make a short incision in the dome extraperitoneally. Insert the index finger, and move the posterolateral wall of the bladder toward the psoas muscle. If the ileal loop is short, making it necessary to get greater vesical mobilization, carry the dissection down to include the superior vesical pedicle by incising the peritoneum in the cul-de-sac. Grasp the bladder with an Allis clamp at the site of the fingertip over the psoas muscle, and excise a small circle of bladder wall. Suture the posterior wall of the bladder to the psoas muscle with several 3-0 chromic catgut sutures. Move the ileal segment alongside to determine the length needed. Keep the loop as short as is feasible, but allow enough redundancy to permit formation of a nipple. If the operation is done for stone disease, omit the nipple. Excise the redundant portion of the ileum, first dividing its vessels close to the bowel to avoid interference with the major blood supply.

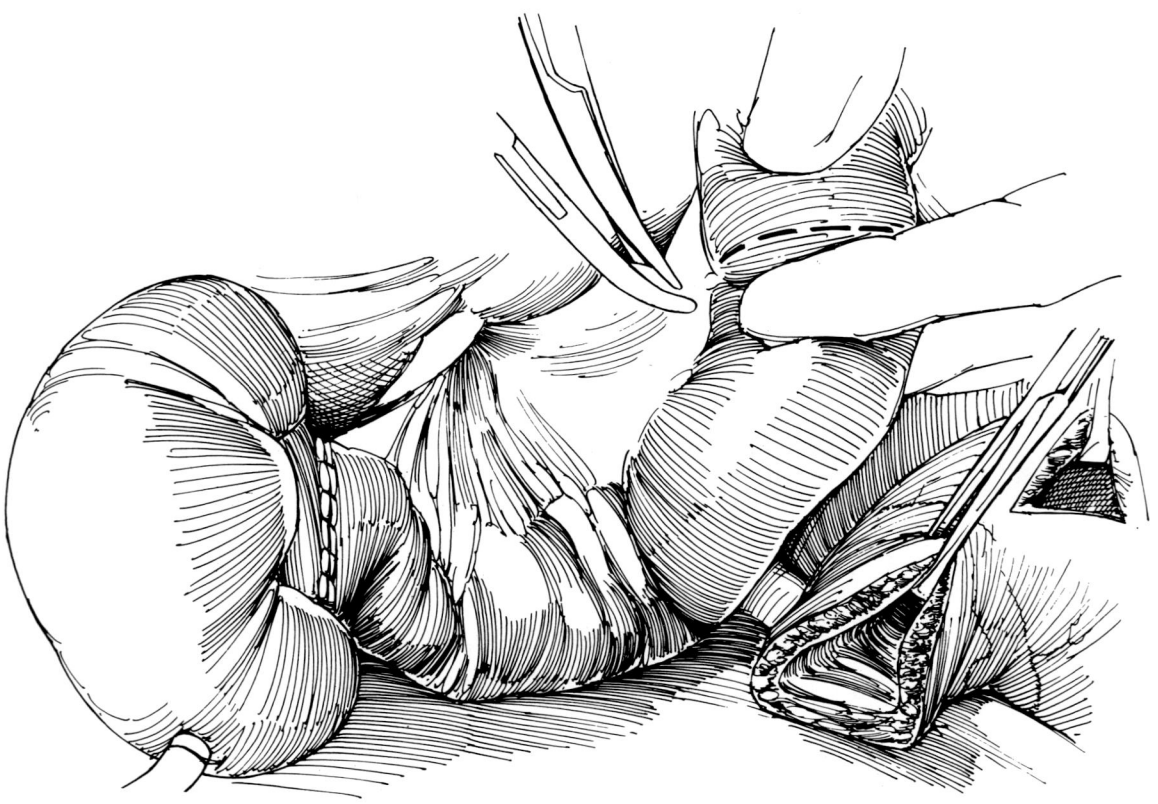

7 **A**, Pull several centimeters of bowel into the bladder. In children, taper the ileum and insert it in a subepithelial tunnel, as is done for large ureters (page 220).

B, Alternatively, turn the bowel back on itself as a cuff, and suture its mucosa to vesical epithelium, or perform an ileoileal intussusception. Suture the bowel to the bladder wall with interrupted 3-0 chromic catgut sutures. It often may be easier to open the bladder wide and anastomose the ileum by suturing from inside the bladder. Consider a YV-plasty on the bladder neck (page 298). Place a Malecot cystostomy tube through a stab wound, and close the bladder defect in two layers. Insert a small 5-ml silicone balloon catheter transurethrally. A stent in the ileum probably is unnecessary. Place a medium-sized Penrose drain near the pyeloileal anastomosis, and bring it out through a stab wound in the posterior axillary line. Place a second drain by the long-suture technique (page 127) near the vesical anastomosis, and bring it out anterolaterally. Adequate drainage is essential. Tack the colon laterally to the peritoneal edge to extraperitonealize the entire segment. Close the peritoneum and the wound. Finally, suture the nephrostomy and cystotomy tubes to the skin with heavy silk.

Remove the urethral catheter on the 5th postoperative day. The cystostomy tube may be clamped on the 7th day for a trial of voiding, but there is no hurry to do this. Perform a gravity nephrostogram and cystogram subsequently to check for leaks; if none are detected, remove the cystostomy and nephrostomy tubes. Remove the drains 24 hours later. Check the functional result by following the level of the serum creatinine and the anatomic result by an intravenous urogram at 6 weeks.

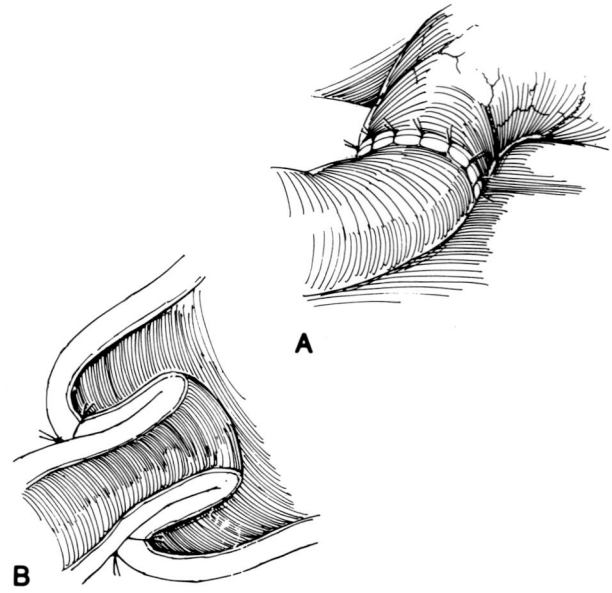

BILATERAL TOTAL URETERAL REPLACEMENT

8 **A,** Working anteriorly and intraperitoneally, anastomose the loop to the left pelvis end to end, and connect it to the right pelvis end to side.

B, Bring the ureters through the posterior peritoneum near the midline, and proceed intraperitoneally with anastomosis of the ureters to the loop and the loop to the bladder.

POSTOPERATIVE PROBLEMS

Anastomotic leakage with consequent urinoma or fistula can be picked up by the nephrostogram, in which case the nephrostomy is left for a longer time. *Obstruction* usually is caused by edema or excessive production of mucus. A kink in the ileum also must be suspected. Leaving the nephrostomy tube in place allows these factors to resolve. *Ischemic necrosis* of the segment requires immediate reoperation.

Electrolyte imbalance is rare if preoperative renal function is adequate and the segment is short and drains well. *Gross dilatation* of the segment with consequent hyperabsorption of electrolytes can be avoided if an open bladder outlet is provided or a valve is created at the ileovesical junction by forming a nipple or by tapering the ileum and creating a subepithelial tunnel or by intussusception. Long-term follow-up is needed to detect incipient outlet obstruction.

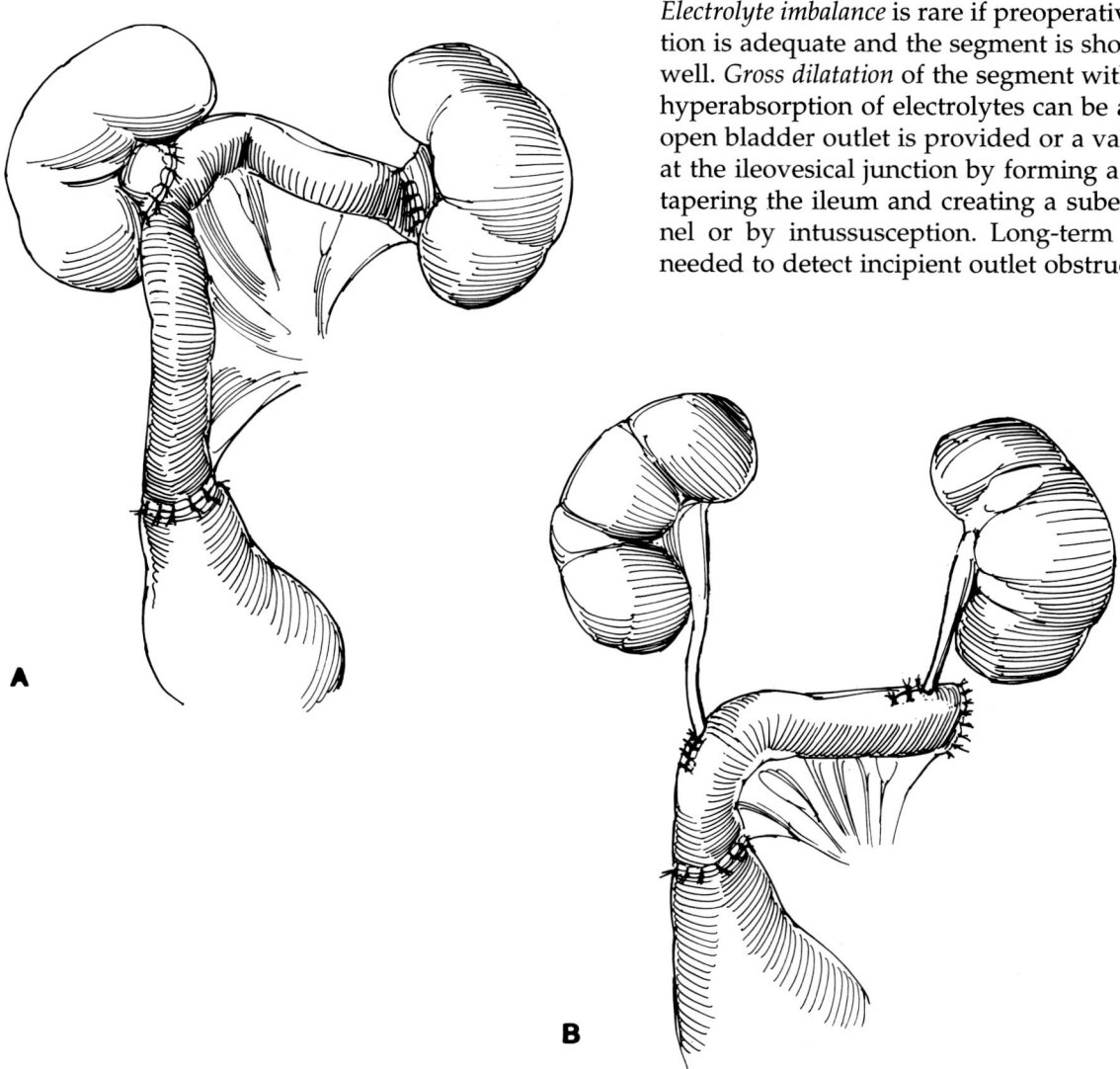

A

B

Commentary by Casimir F. Firlit

Use of the small bowel as an interpositioned conduit from the renal pelvis to the bladder represents a creative application for the substitution of the entire ureter. Although the procedure of ileal substitution of the ureter has become less and less applicable in modern times, it nevertheless represents an operative procedure that should be retained within the urologist's armamentarium. Modern-day approaches might suggest a renal autotransplant to bridge the renal pelvis directly to the bladder in the form of a pyelovesicostomy, or, if there is enough proximal ureter, to simply bring the kidney down as an autotransplant and reimplant the ureter into the bladder. However, expertise

in renal autotransplantation varies throughout the country and the world, and in situations where that expertise is not available, the use of ileal substitution for a stenotic, fibrotic, strictured or destroyed ureter represents a viable alternative to save functioning renal parenchyma. The illustrations are clear in the application of this modality for both pediatric and adult urologic patients. The ileal ureter itself represents a sluggish hypoperistaltic urinary conduit; nevertheless, it does serve to salvage a kidney that has had ureteral disease and now represents an operative procedure that will salvage such a renal unit.

The ileal ureter deserves to be preserved in the surgical armamentarium for application in situations where renal autotransplantation is not available.

CHAPTER 49

Ureterolithotomy

Unless combined with a reparative procedure, ure-terolithotomy currently is rarely performed. Because of the length of the ureter, a different incision is required for each level of involvement. Consequently, care must be used to prevent the stone from moving out of the area exposed by that incision.

A radiograph the morning of operation or on the way to the operating room is mandatory.

Commentary by Evan J. Kass

Today, ureterolithotomy rarely is necessary, because the majority of ureteral stones in children can be managed either by extracorporeal shockwave therapy or by endoscopic manipulation. The key to success is preoperative preparation. A radiograph should be taken on the operating room table just before induction of anesthesia to reconfirm the location of the stone. If the stone cannot be located at surgery, one should not make a ureteral incision. Radiographic localization intraoperatively may be frustrating but often is possible, and it permits the surgeon to direct the search for the stone appropriately.

SECTION 6
Bladder

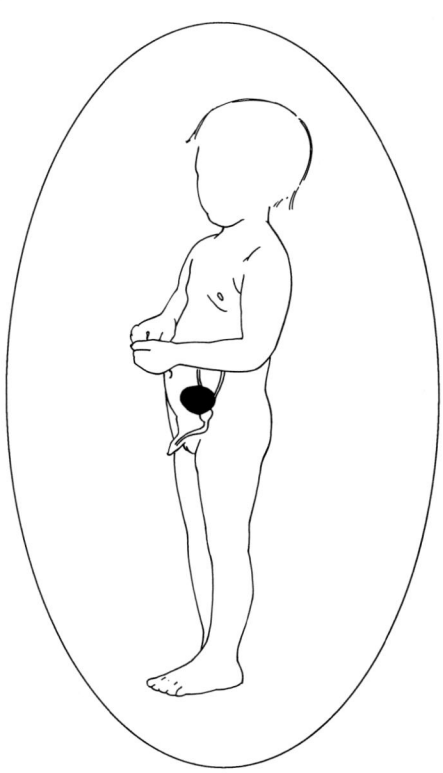

PART I

APPROACHES TO THE BLADDER

CHAPTER 50

Lower Midline Extraperitoneal Incision

The lower midline extraperitoneal incision provides exposure of the lower ureter and structures in the pelvis. Elevating the pelvis may help with exposure in a child. An extended midline extraperitoneal incision can give simultaneous access to both upper and lower retroperitoneal organs.

1 *Incision*: With the child supine and the buttocks over the kidney rest, make a midline paraumbilical incision to the left of the umbilicus, extending down over the symphysis pubis.

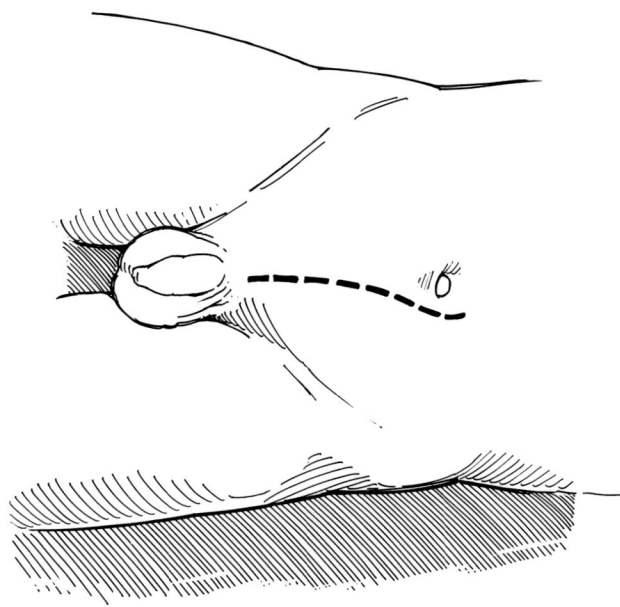

2 Incise the linea alba of the rectus fascia for a short distance. To be certain of the location of the midline, look for the edge of the rectus muscle on one side or the other. Continue the incision well over the symphysis pubis to the insertion of the fascia. This will allow the incision to open at the lower hinge to the fullest extent.

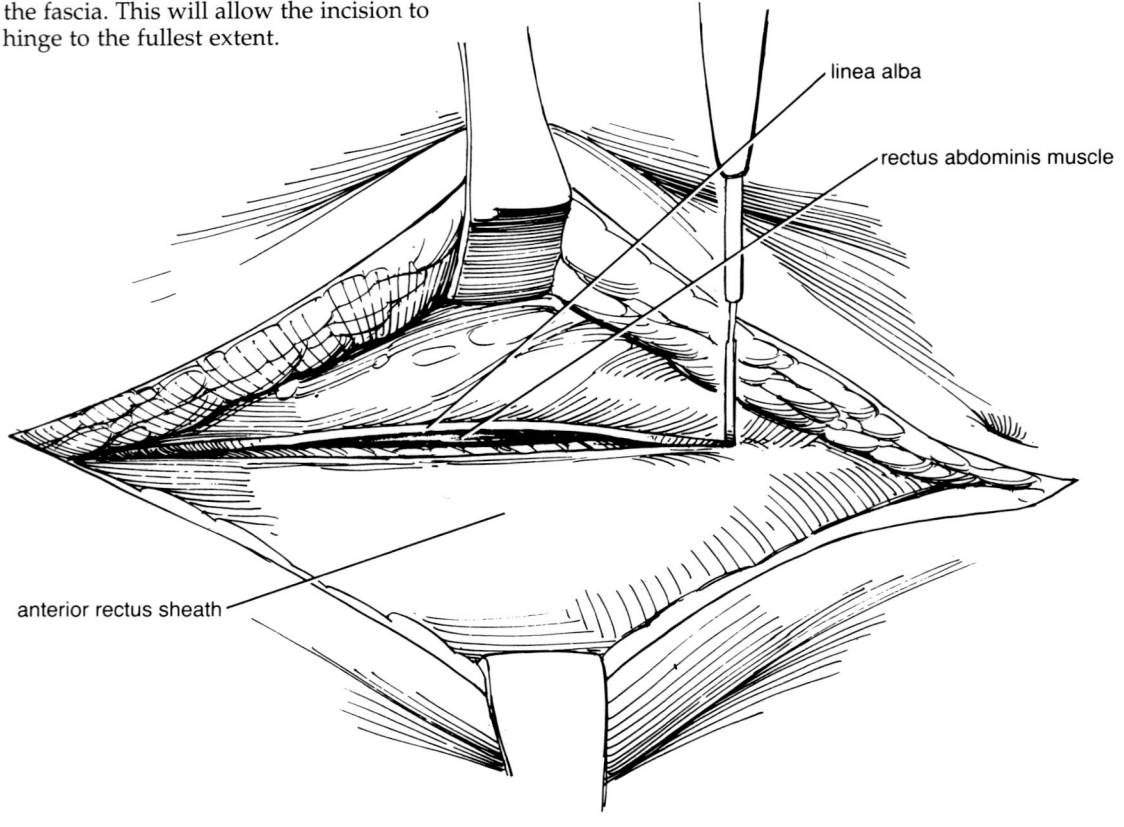

linea alba

rectus abdominis muscle

anterior rectus sheath

3 Retract the rectus muscles laterally, and incise their investing fascia. Sharply open the contiguous thinned transversalis fascia laterally where it lies beneath the rectus muscle to expose the retroperitoneal connective tissue.

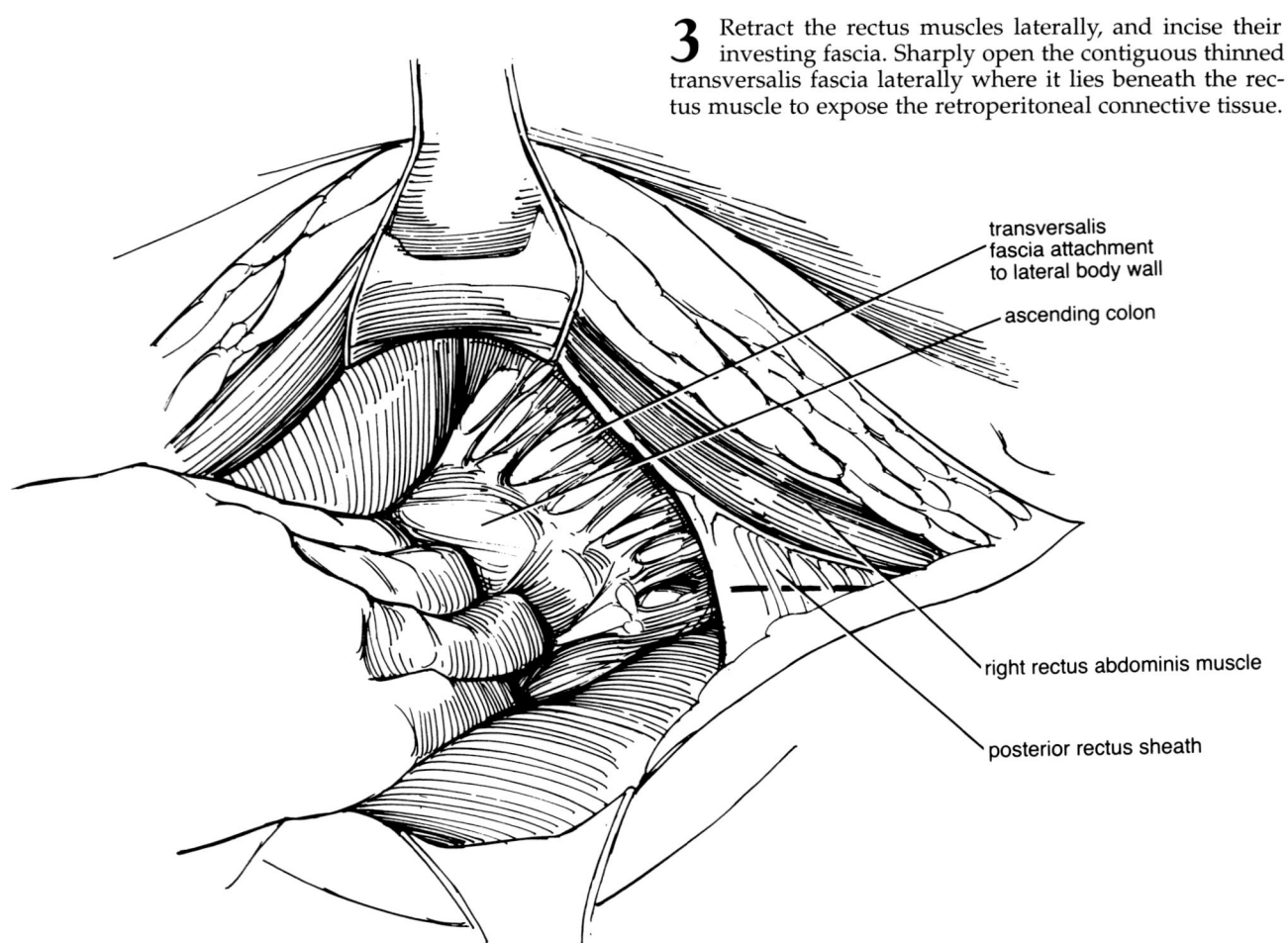

transversalis fascia attachment to lateral body wall

ascending colon

right rectus abdominis muscle

posterior rectus sheath

4 Dissect anterior to the retroperitoneal connective tissue inferiorly and laterally with a sponge stick, thus mobilizing the peritoneum medially but staying deep to the inferior epigastric vessels.

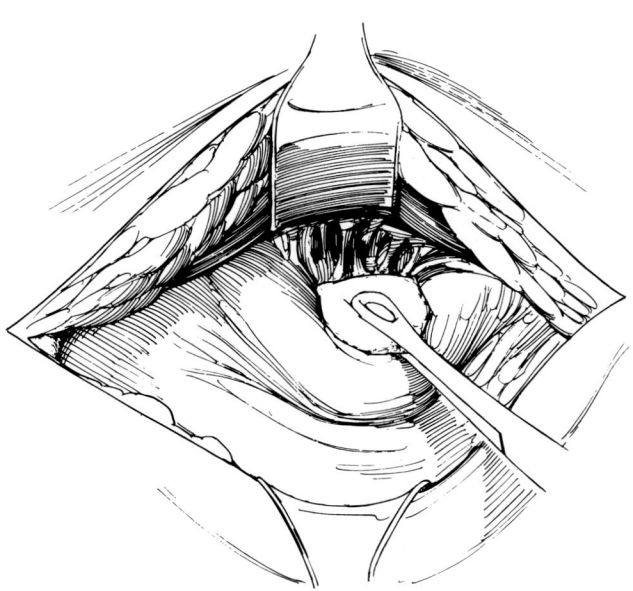

5 Follow the obliterated hypogastric (umbilical) artery to the superior vesical pedicle, if indicated, and follow the vas to the inguinal canal.

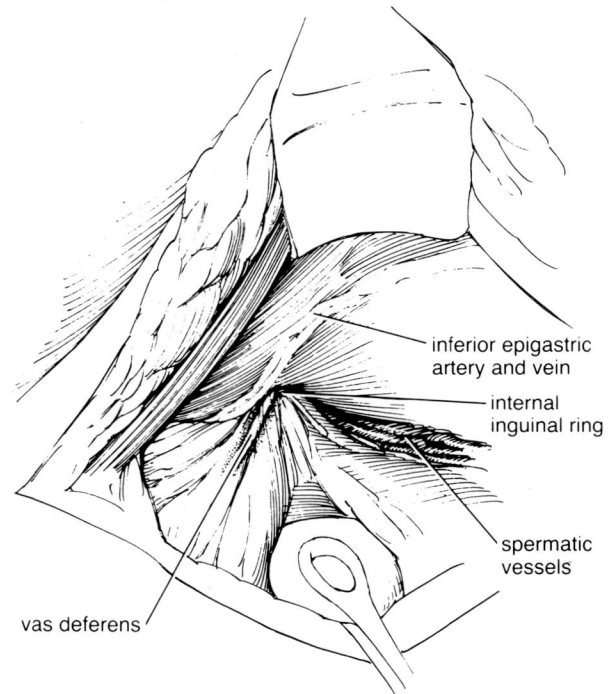

inferior epigastric artery and vein

internal inguinal ring

spermatic vessels

vas deferens

6 Identify the ureter attached to the peritoneum as it crosses the iliac vessels and encircle it with a small Penrose drain.

If the urinary tract has been opened, bring a Penrose or suction drain through a stab wound. Close the rectus fascia with a running absorbable (in infants) or nonabsorbable (in adults) suture or with interrupted sutures, and close the skin with a subcuticular 4-0 or 5-0 synthetic absorbable suture.

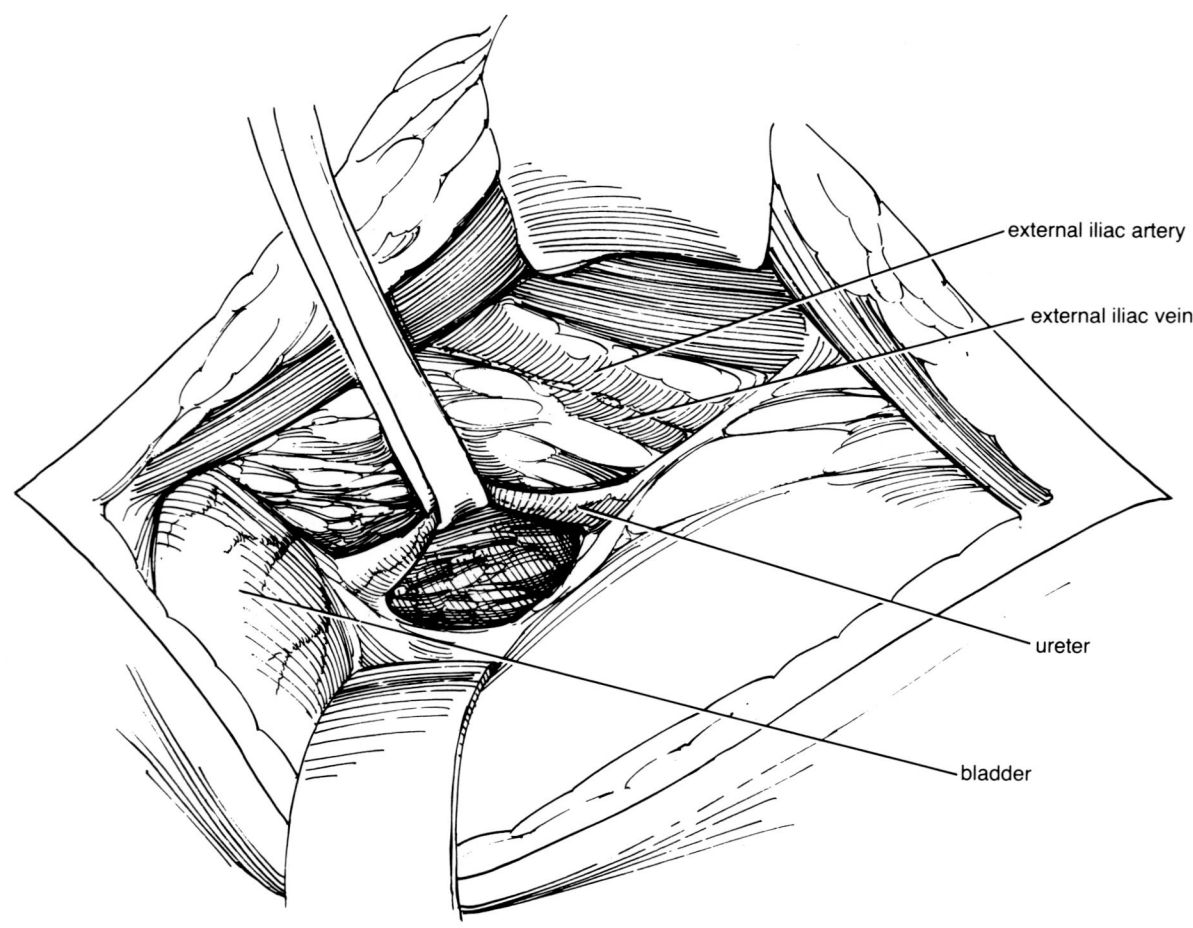

external iliac artery

external iliac vein

ureter

bladder

Commentary by Tom P. V. M. de Jong and Jan D. van Gool

General comments on opening and closing the wound and the bladder: we usually make only a superficial skin incision. The rest of the incision is done with cutting current exclusively, using a needle electrode. Bleeding vessels are coagulated.

Before opening the bladder, it is filled to capacity. This can be done at the end of a preoperative cystoscopic examination or with an indwelling catheter. We first identify and open the thin adventitial layer that surrounds the bladder. This is done by grasping the layer in two forceps and then cutting it in the midline with scissors. Then, the layer is swept laterally. The detrusor muscle is cut in the midline, with coagulating current, up to the mucosa. The mucosa is opened bluntly.

After closure of the bladder wall, the adventitial layer is closed separately with two or three approximating sutures, thus providing less adherence of the bladder scar to

the abdominal wall. This permits the bladder to move freely with filling and emptying. In adults, we also use absorbable sutures for closure of the abdominal wall. We never use Penrose drains for drainage but use minisuction drains instead. For retraction of ureters, we use silicone vessel loops. We try not to use any catheter or drain containing latex, especially in patients with spina bifida.

When extensive exposure of the urethra is needed, this easily can be done in patients approximately 7 years of age or younger by cutting the symphysis pubis in the midline with coagulating current and opening the symphysis with an orthopedic retractor. The pelvic floor is cut in the midline to the level of the urethra. This gives good access to the prostatic and bulbar urethra in boys and to the whole urethra in girls. After the pelvic floor is closed with one or two absorbable sutures, the symphysis is closed with two heavy absorbable sutures passing through the bony part; we take great care not to interpose urethral tissue.

Regarding the lower midline extraperitoneal incision, always pass the umbilicus at the left side.

CHAPTER 51

Lower Abdominal Transverse Incision

(PFANNENSTIEL)

The lower abdominal transverse incision is an incision useful for operations on the bladder and lower ureter, as well as for other pelvic operations. It is not appropriate for procedures such as ileocystoplasty.

1 *Incision*: Make a symmetric, semilunar incision through a point one fingerbreadth above the symphysis pubis. Carry it down to the rectus sheath, but again check the distance (one fingerbreadth) above the symphysis by palpation before incising the sheath.

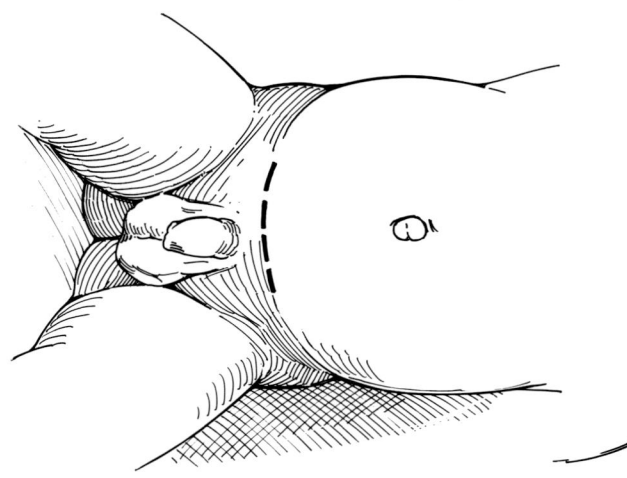

2 Incise the rectus sheath with a needle electrode in a semilunar arc to avoid the inguinal canals. Continue the incision laterally to divide some of the external and internal oblique and transversus abdominis aponeuroses and muscles at each extremity.

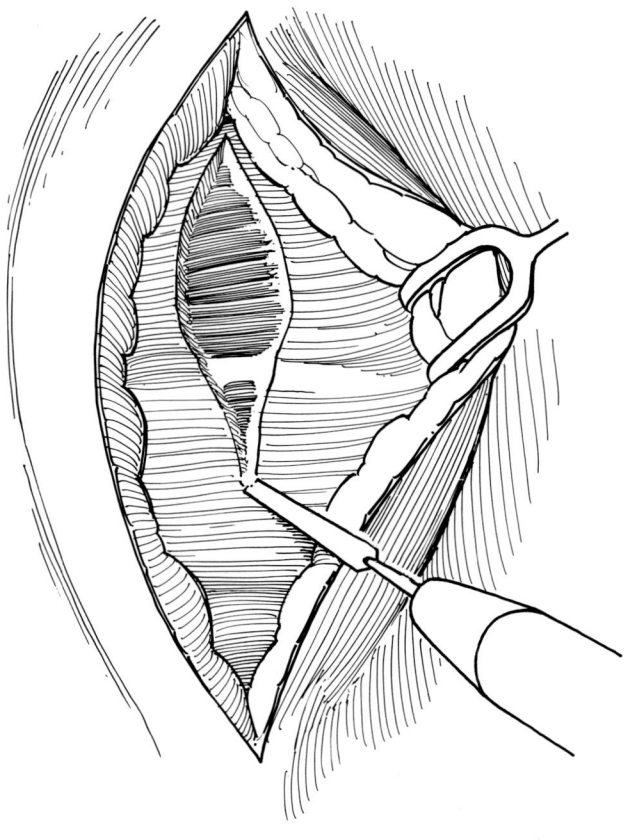

3 Grasp the upper edge of the rectus sheath with Kocher clamps, elevate it, and divide its midline attachment with the cutting current for at least 10 cm in the adolescent. Push down on the muscle with sponge sticks to free it from the sheath. Take care to avoid the two symmetric perforating branches of the inferior epigastric vessels, or coagulate and divide them.

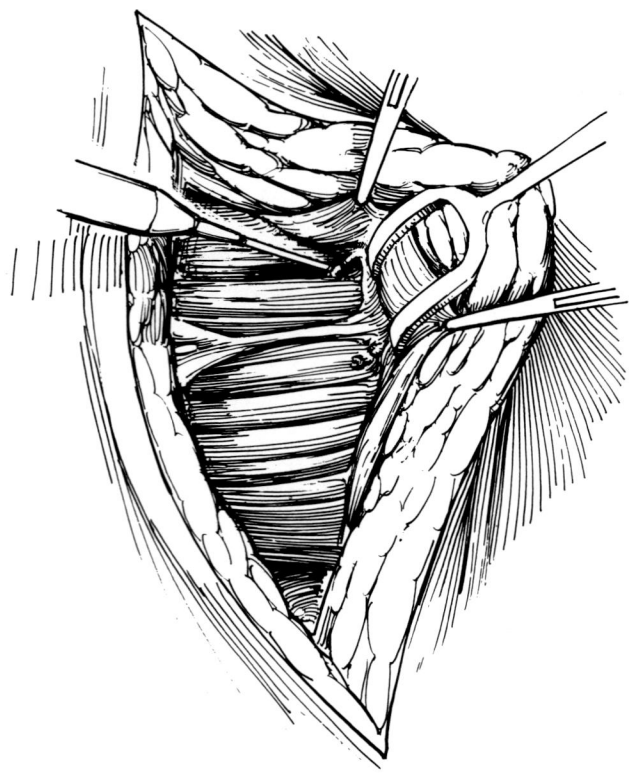

4 Free the lower flap similarly, elevating both pyramidalis muscles, if they are well developed, or leave them both attached to the rectus.

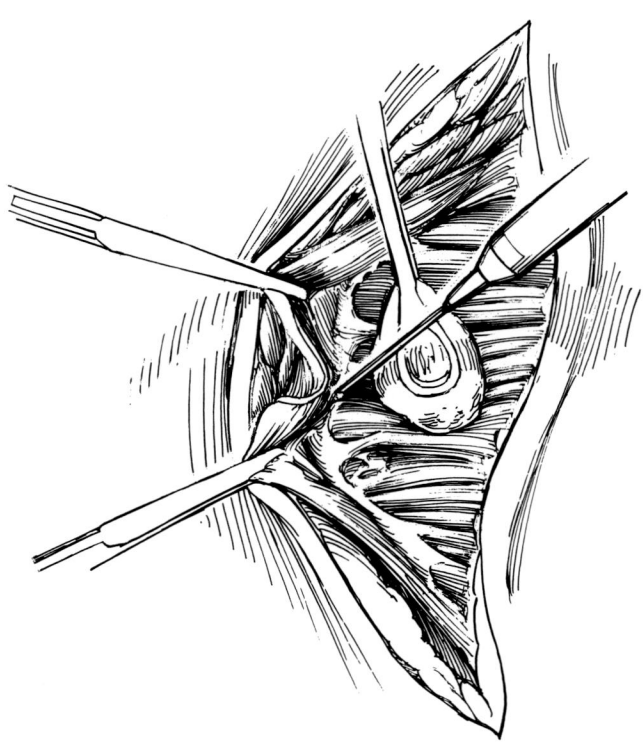

5 Cut in the midline to enter between the rectus muscles and between the pyramidalis muscles by sharp fascial incision of the transversalis fascia or by separation with a curved clamp until the preperitoneal and prevesical space is identified. The muscles may then be split with the fingers. If greater exposure is required, the tendinous insertions of the rectus muscles may be divided at the symphysis (Cherney incision), but the subsequent closure is less stable.

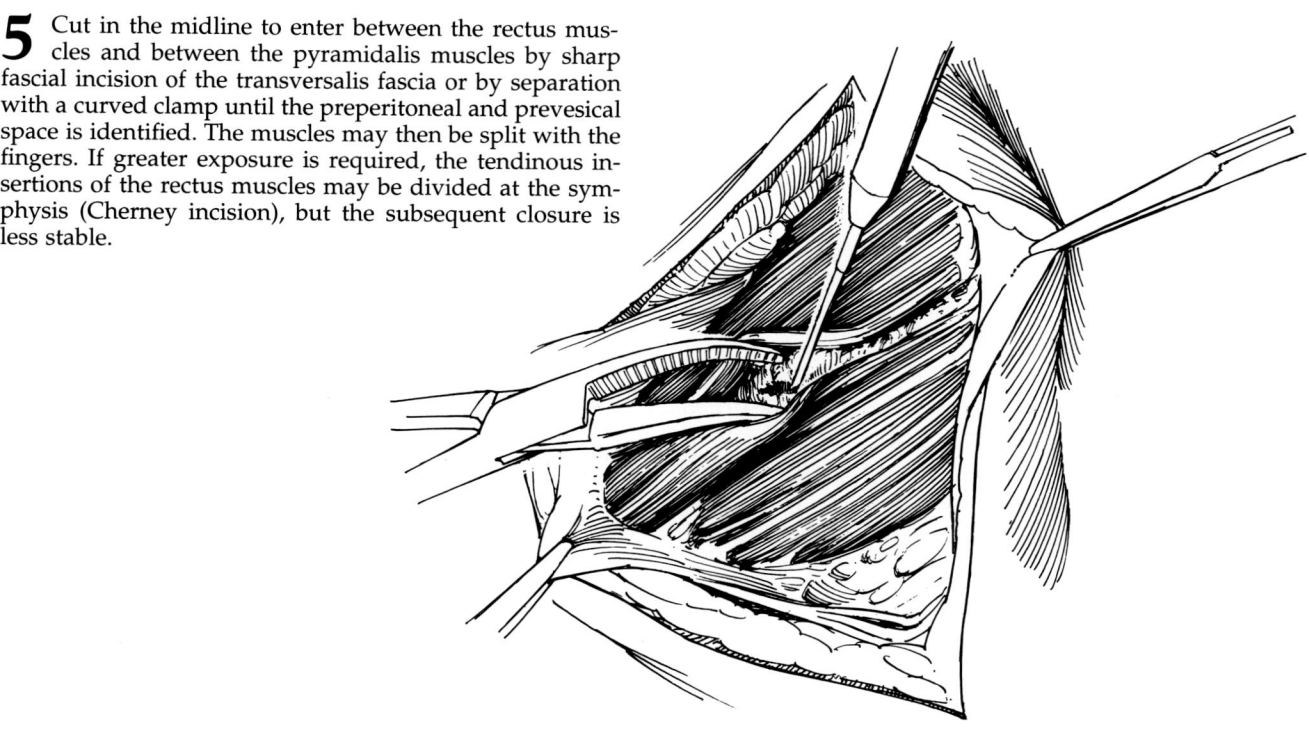

6 Separate the attenuated transversalis fascia in the midline to expose the anterior surface of the bladder and vesical neck. Closure begins with loose approximation of the rectus muscles and closure in layers of the transversus, internal, and, finally, the external oblique aponeuroses.

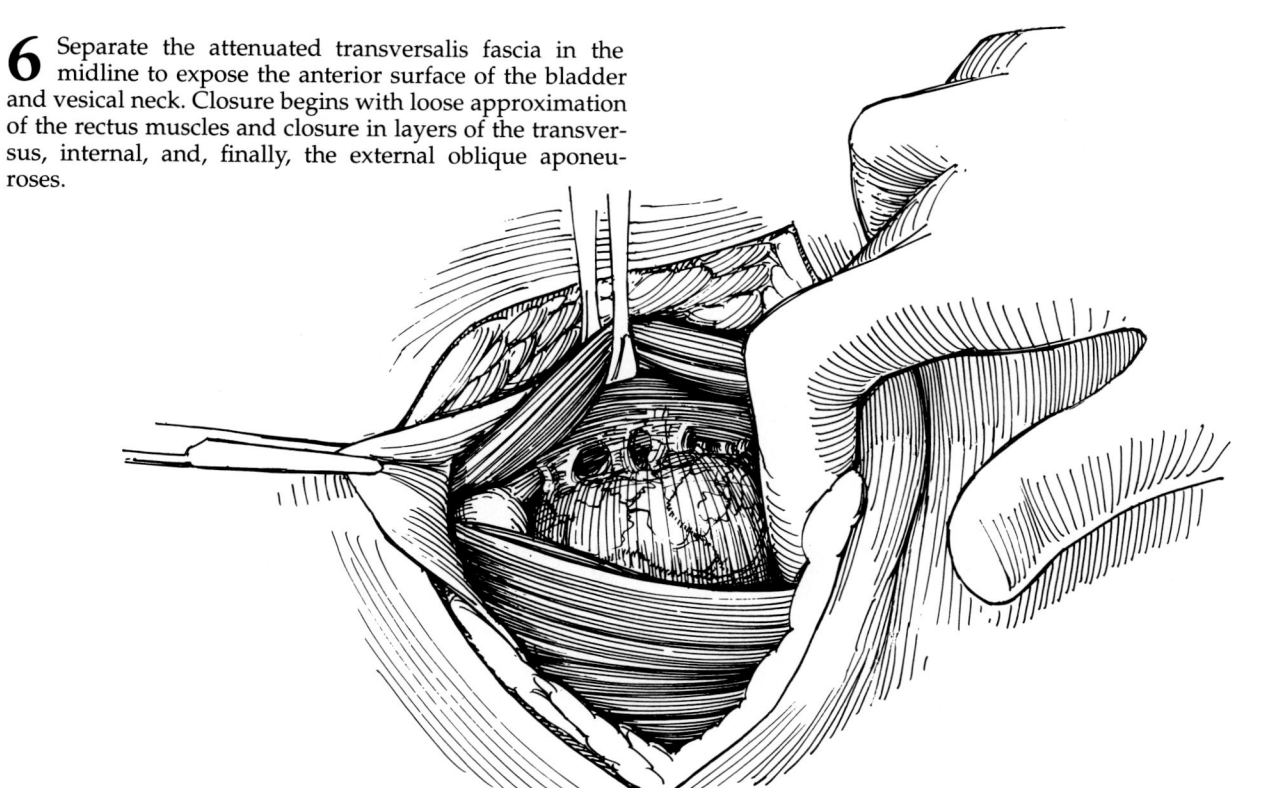

Commentary by Tom P. V. M. de Jong and Jan D. van Gool

The lower abdominal transverse incision can be a clumsy approach when an ileocystoplasty is being done through it. We use this approach only for autoaugmentation (detrusorectomy) and augmentations using megaureters. It also works well for an augmentation with sigmoid colon.

CHAPTER 52

Gibson Incision

Access to the lower third of the ureter can be obtained by a variety of incisions. Because the ureter terminates near the midline, an approach that is as direct as the midline incision is through an oblique incision in the right or left lower quadrant—the Gibson. In girls, a transverse incision is more acceptable cosmetically.

1 *Position*: Place the child supine in a partial Trendelenburg position. *Incision*: Make a hockey-stick incision extending from 2 cm medial to the anterior superior iliac spine, running 0.5 cm above the inguinal fold to the border of the rectus muscle.

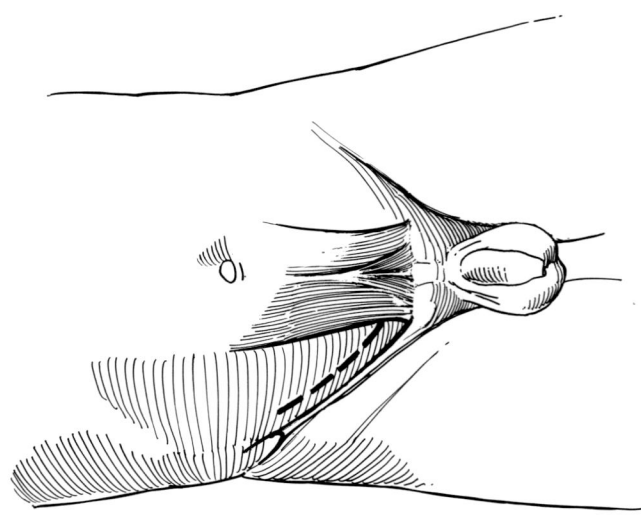

2 Divide the external oblique aponeurosis in the direction of its fibers.

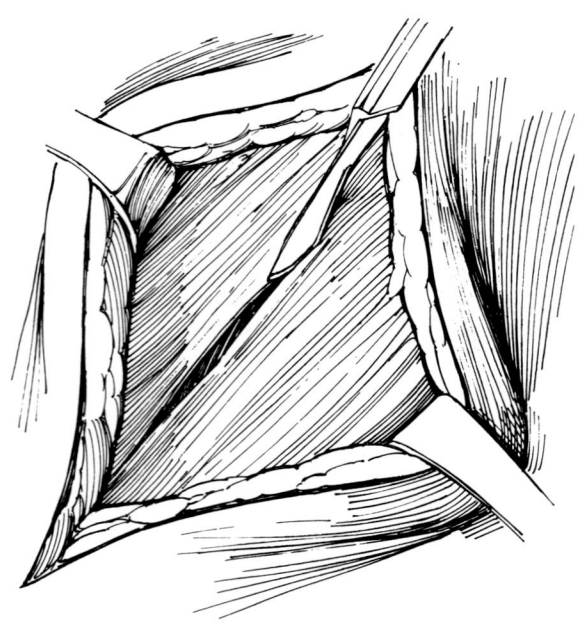

3 Separate the internal oblique muscle in the direction of its fibers, and open the transversus abdominis muscle layer. If greater exposure is required, the muscles may be divided.

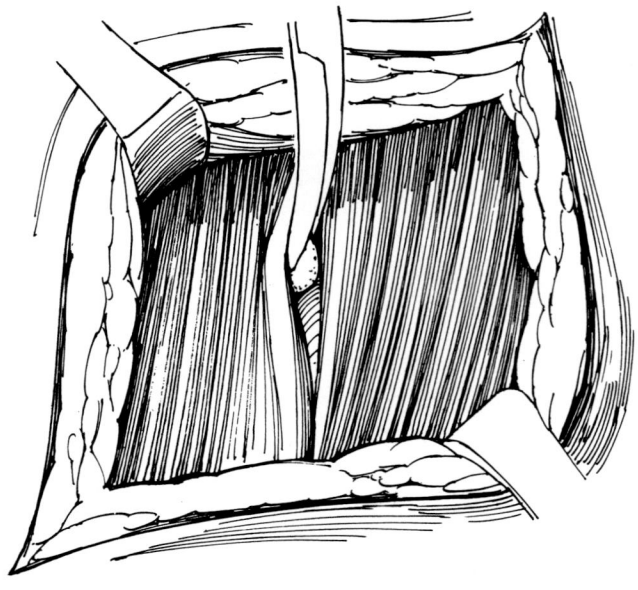

4 Draw the transversalis fascia medially (here it is a thin structure), carrying the peritoneum off of the vessels and the lateral body wall. Divide the residuum of the processus vaginalis at the internal ring (or the round ligament in girls), so that the peritoneum can be completely mobilized medially as the lateral subperitoneal spaces are opened and the iliac vessels exposed.

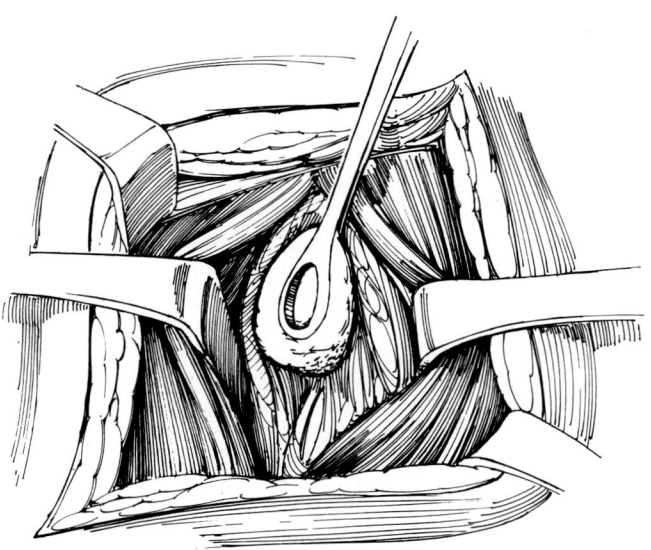

5 **A,** Identify the ureter against the peritoneum as it crosses the iliac vessels.

B, Grasp the ureter in a Babcock clamp or encircle it with a Penrose drain for further dissection.

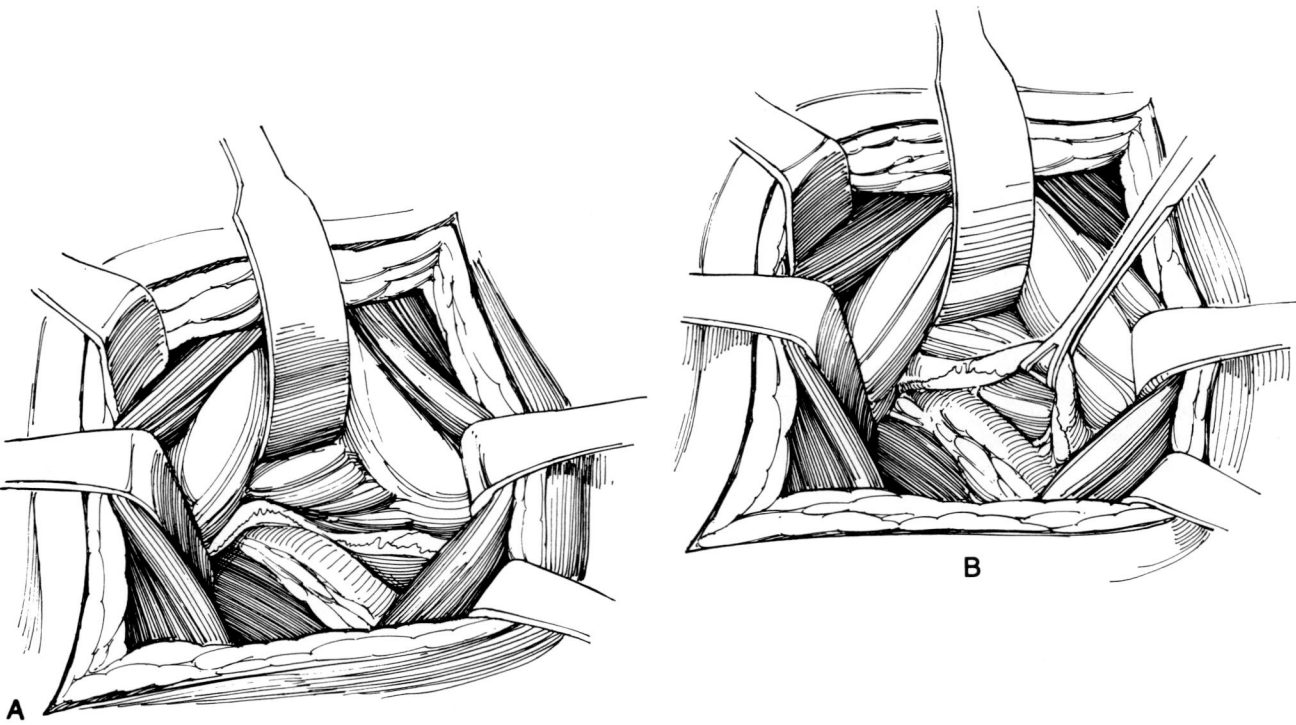

Commentary by Tom P. V. M. de Jong and Jan D. van Gool

Take care to identify the spermatic vessels when using the Gibson incision. When an open processus is present, divide it and ligate the proximal part.

CHAPTER 53

Mobilization of the Omentum

Unfortunately, in children there may not be enough omentum to supply the coverage needed so a vascular pedicle supplied by the inferior epigastric vessels, such as the gracilis or the rectus abdominis, may have to be used instead. However, plan to provide proper access to the omentum, using a midline abdominal wall incision, in case an omental graft, wrap, or interposition is needed. This planning is especially important before starting a complex reconstructive operation.

1 Mobilization of the omentum based on the right gastroepiploic vascular pedicle in a left-to-right fashion is preferred, because the right pedicle is larger and more caudal in origin than the pedicle on the left side, which arises higher in the abdomen. Transilluminate the omentum. Note that the blood supply to the omentum arises from both sides. The larger right gastroepiploic artery is a branch of the gastroduodenal artery. The relatively small

left gastroepiploic artery arises from the splenic artery. Together they form the gastroepiploic arterial arch.

Certain anatomic facts are important: (1) the right gastroepiploic branch of the gastroduodenal artery is always larger than that on the left, and it supplies two thirds to three quarters of the apron. For placement of the omentum into the pelvis, it is always best to base it on the right gastroepiploic artery, if it has not been damaged by previous surgery; (2) in 1 case in 10, the gastroepiploic arcade from left to right is deficient, usually near the origin of the left gastroepiploic pedicle, so basing a mobilized omentum on the smaller vessels of the left pedicle may result in deficient vascularization; (3) the often-illustrated arcade running across the lower margin of the apron is of small caliber and supplies minimal amounts of blood; (4) partial transverse division of the apron below the gastroepiploic arcade divides the vertical vessels and diminishes the circulation to the apron; and (5) the origin of the right artery is lower than the left, so a short apron mobilized on a full length of the gastroepiploic arcade will reach the pelvis. In one third of adolescents and adults, the lower margin of the omentum can be moved into a pelvic defect without mobilization. However, in these cases, the omentum should be separated from its natural adhesions to the transverse colon and mesocolic vessels to prevent its dislocation by postoperative intestinal distention. In another one third of cases, division of the left gastroepiploic is all that is needed. In the remaining cases, full mobilization on a right epiploic pedicle is required to achieve enough length.

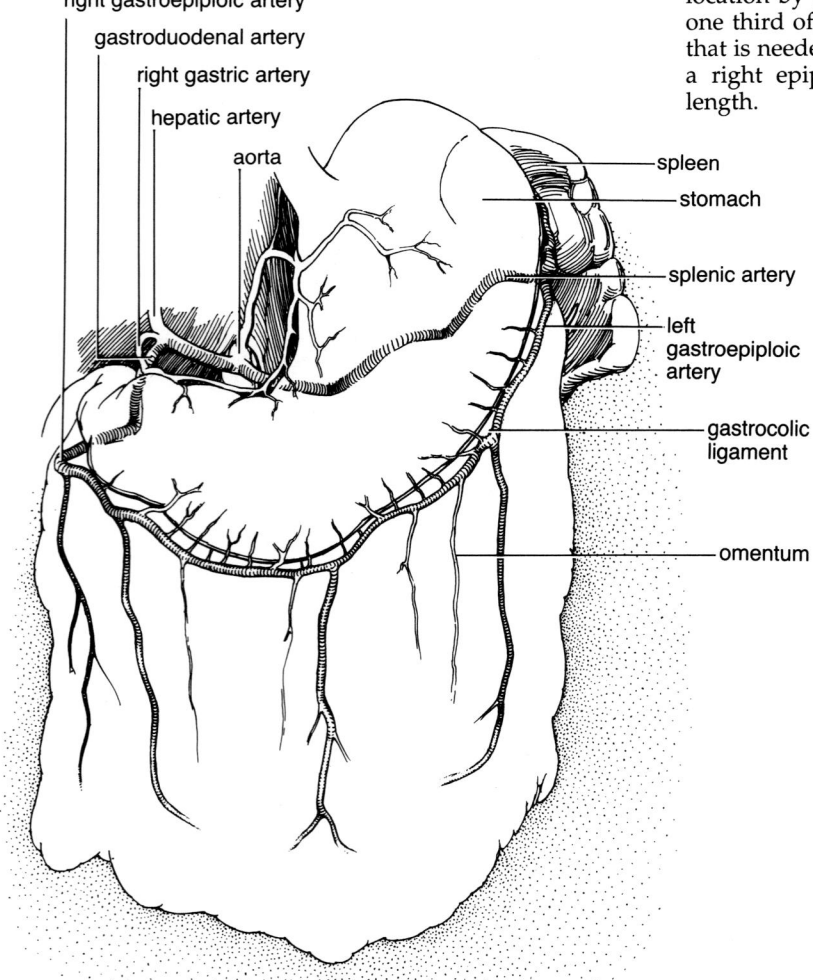

right gastroepiploic artery
gastroduodenal artery
right gastric artery
hepatic artery
aorta
spleen
stomach
splenic artery
left gastroepiploic artery
gastrocolic ligament
omentum

2 **A,** Palpate the right gastroepiploic artery. Free the omentum from the transverse colon and mesocolon by dividing its avascular adhesion.

B and **C,** Trace the exposed gastroepiploic arch to the left. When necessary to gain extra length, divide and ligate the left gastroepiploic vascular pedicle at its splenic origin. It is not necessary to divide it as high as is shown.

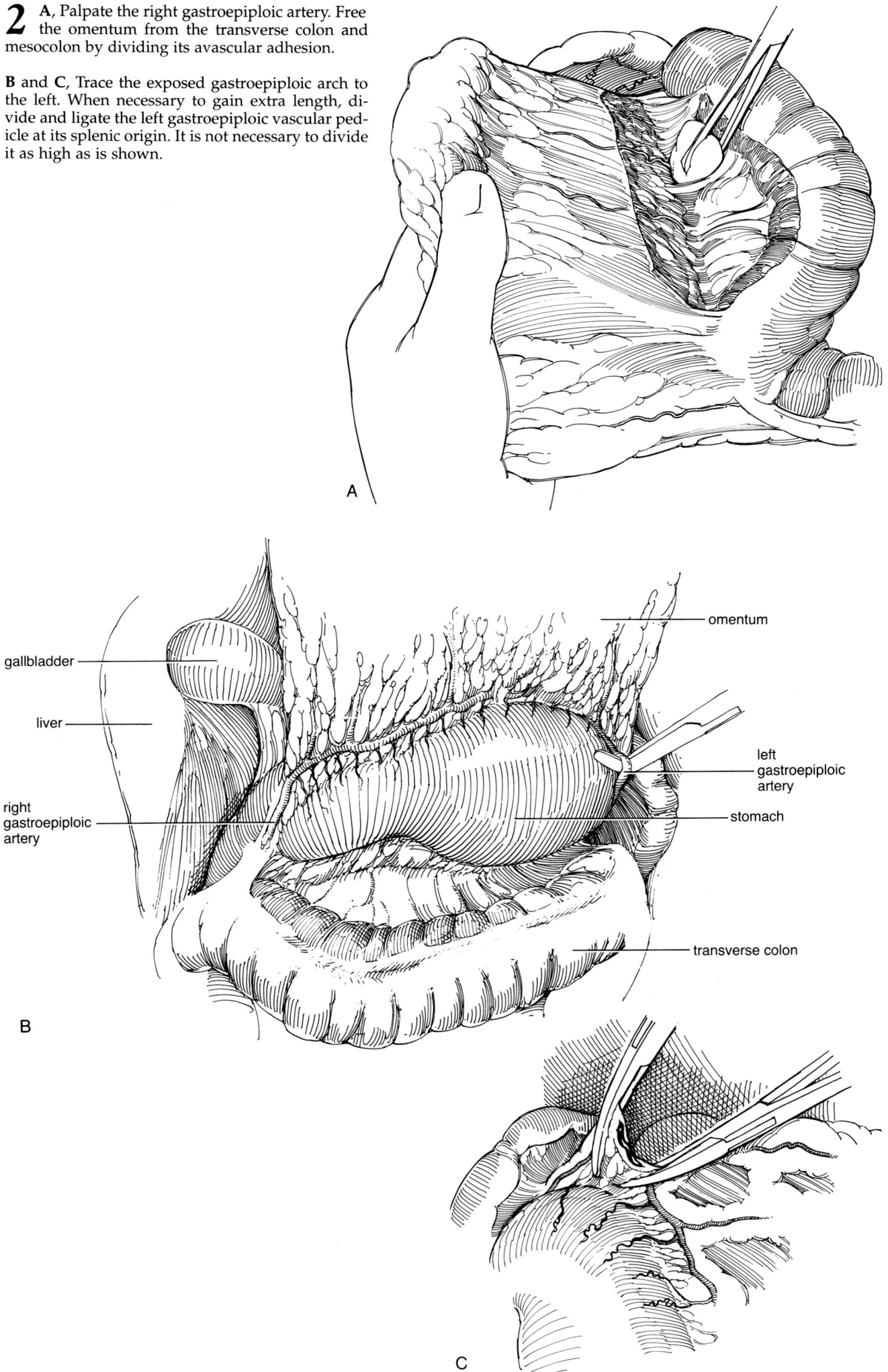

A

gallbladder

liver

right gastroepiploic artery

omentum

left gastroepiploic artery

stomach

transverse colon

B

C

3 **A**, Pass a Providence clamp through the omentum on each side of the first short gastric branch of the left gastroepiploic artery, elevate it, and draw a 4-0 synthetic absorbable suture under it (nonabsorbable sutures would foster infection and drainage in the recipient area). Tie the suture.

B, Clamp and divide the artery close to the stomach, then ligate the end of the vessel in the clamp. This technique of

ligation avoids retraction of the proximal (omental) end that occurs when a hemostat ligation escapes and quickly produces a potentially harmful interstitial hematoma. An alternative, and safer, method is to pass and tie two sutures without clamping the vessel.

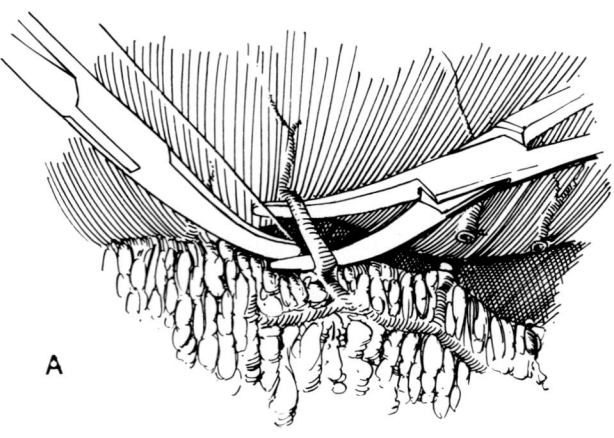

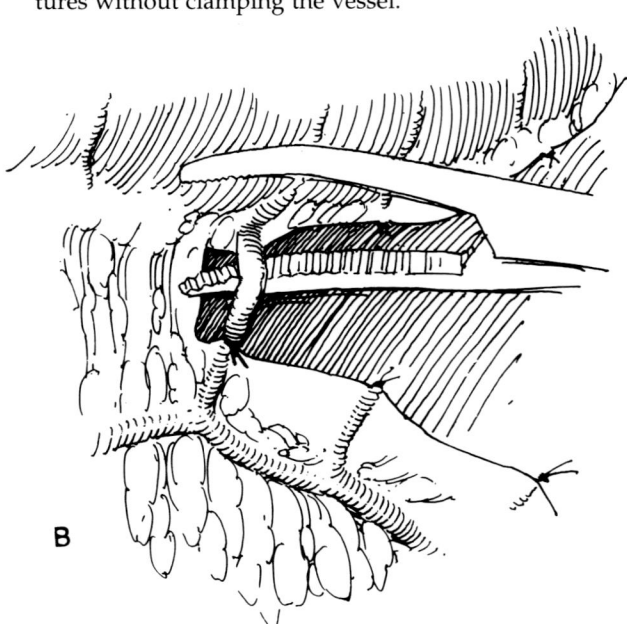

4 Continue dividing the remaining 20 or 30 branches individually to reach up to the gastroduodenal origin of the arch, carefully avoiding mass ligation that reduces the available length of the gastroepiploic arterial arch itself. An undivided branch is easily torn when the omentum is pulled into position. Preserve a 5- to 7-cm band of omentum at the right end intact to protect the vessels from avulsion.

5 For use as graft or for interposition in the pelvis, mobilize a section of the ascending colon and allow the omentum to lie behind its mesentery, in the paracolic gutter. In a complicated case with an extensively mobilized graft, place a nasogastric tube, or better, create a gastrostomy into the exposed stomach (page 400). Use Penrose drains rather than suction drains, which tend to be clogged by the loose omental surface.

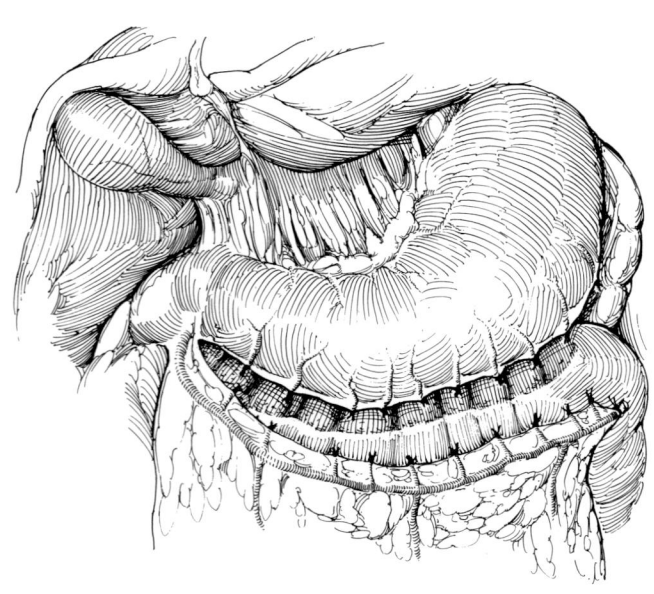

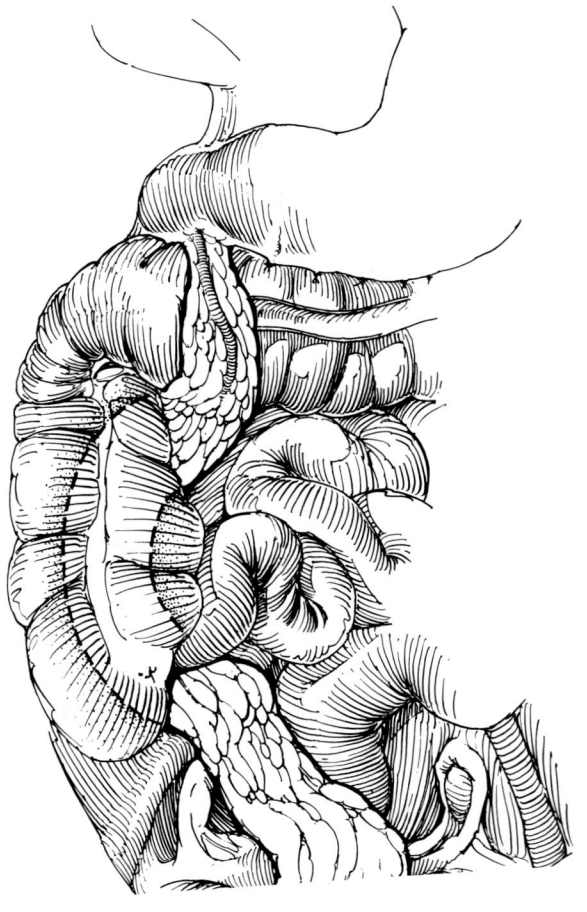

6 **A,** For use as a wrap about the kidney or upper ureter, mobilization may not be necessary.

B, It is easy to pass the omentum through a window in the colonic mesentery after vertical separation of the omental apron in the midline.

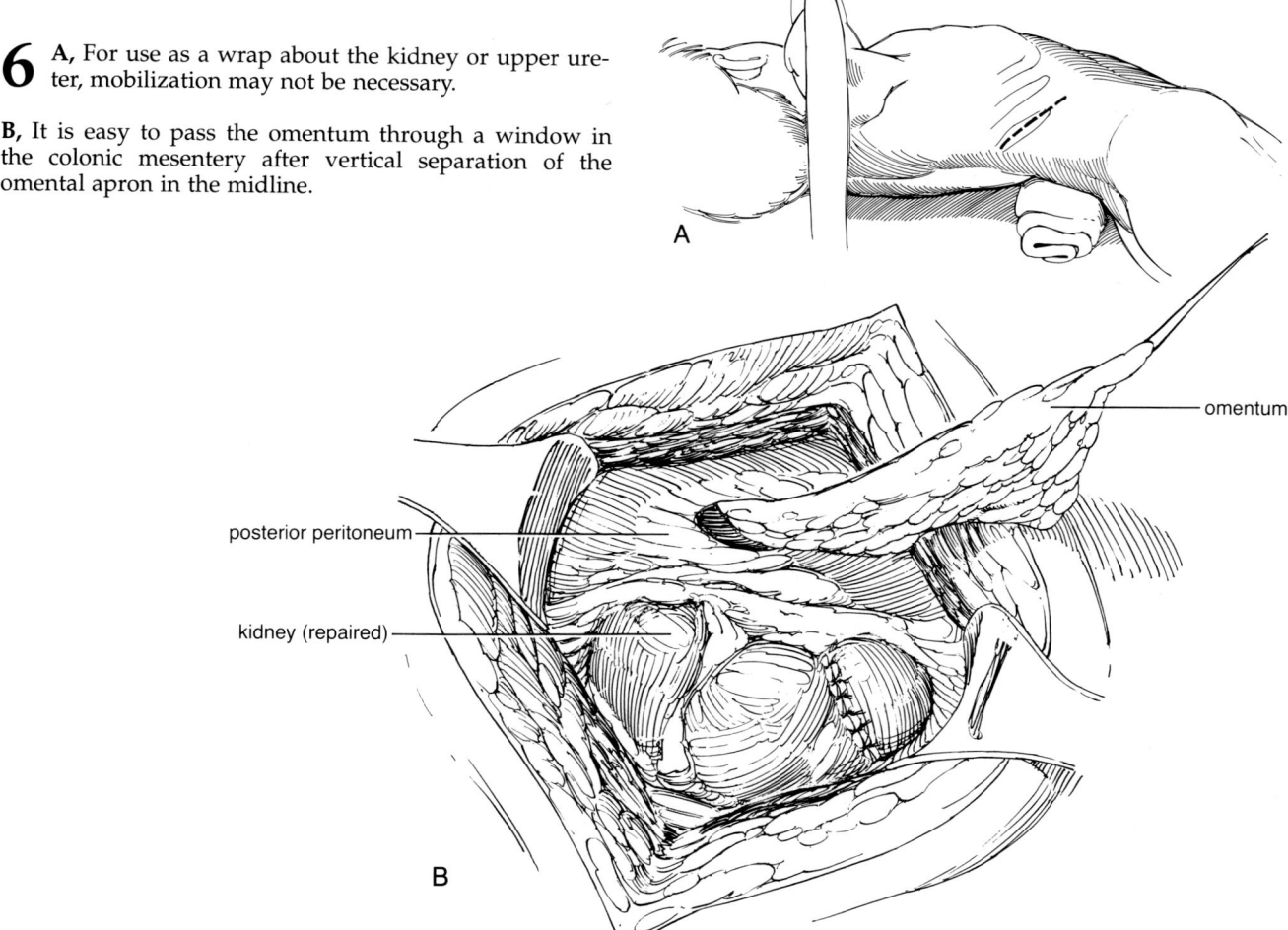

A

omentum

posterior peritoneum

kidney (repaired)

B

POSTOPERATIVE PROBLEMS

Infection, abscess, or *persistent leakage* at the site of the repair can occur as a result of technical errors that damage the blood supply during mobilization of the vascular pedicle, such as failure to make the tunnel behind the peritoneum large enough (which compromises the omental blood supply) or failure to provide enough bulk of omentum to fill and cover. Ileus and abdominal distention can interfere with circulation to the graft only if the graft passes anterior to the bowel; it always should pass behind the hepatic flexure, which is the shortest and most protected route. Gastric suction is important prophylactically; a temporary gastrostomy may be more humane.

Commentary by Richard Turner-Warwick

The omental apron of children is not fully developed; consequently, it tends to be relatively short. Therefore, full mobilization of its vascular pedicle more often is required to enable it to reach the pelvis than it is in the adult. Even full mobilization may not be sufficient, so that alternative pedicled support tissue, such as the gracilis muscle or a rectus abdominis supplied by the inferior epigastric ves-

sels, may have to be used. Complex reconstructive operations in the pelvis involve (1) replacement of a deficient bulk of pelvic septal or perineal tissue; (2) vascular support of tissues compromised by previous surgery, infection, or irradiation; (3) closure of complex fistulas; and (4) the preservation or restoration of the mobility of the urinary tract to allow it to perform its urodynamic function.

Proper access and planning is essential for complex reconstructive pelvic surgery—a midline abdominal wall incision is essential to enable the vascular pedicle of the omentum to be mobilized from the greater curvature of the stomach when this is necessary.

The "magic" of the omentum depends not only on its good blood supply but also on its excellent lymphatic drainage, which provides a "physiologic drain" for the macromolecular exudates and debris of an inflammatory response that otherwise can accumulate and result in abscess formation. In addition, unlike the fatty tissue of the retroperitoneal and retropubic areas, it retains its flexibility after an inflammatory response; consequently, it has a unique "urodynamic value" in preserving the functional mobility of urinary tract reconstructions when it is used as a supporting wrap for these.

Regarding Figure 1, in 30 percent of patients, the omental apron is long enough to reach the perineum without any mobilization of its vascular pedicle; however, it generally is advisable to separate its natural avascular adhesion to the transverse colon and mesocolic vessels to prevent its dislocation by postoperative gaseous distention of the bowel. In another 30 percent of cases, simple division of the left gastroepiploic vascular pedicle is sufficient to enable the omental apron to reach the pelvis.

Regarding Figure 2, when full-length mobilization of the omental pedicle is required to enable it to reach the pelvis, this should be based on the *right* gastroepiploic vessels because

1. The right gastroepiploic pedicle is larger than the left, and it directly supplies approximately three quarters of the omental apron.
2. Its origin from the gastroduodenal vessels is lower in the abdomen than that of the left gastroepiploic pedicle from the splenic vessels.
3. Mobilization of the full length of a normal gastroepiploic arch from the greater curvature of the stomach enables the omentum to be redeployed in the pelvis, but whether the bulk of this is sufficient for the intended purpose depends on the actual size of the omentum apron.
4. The vertical branches of gastroepiploic arch that supply the omental apron do not have the sizeable distal collateral arcade communications that are commonly illustrated in textbook diagrams; consequently, if the omentum is mobilized by horizontal incisions from the left side that transect its vertical vessels below the gastroepiploic arch, the extremity of its apron generally becomes imperfectly vascularized.

Regarding Figure 3, the mobilization of the full length of the main right gastroepiploic vascular pedicle of the omentum requires careful individual division of every one of its 20 to 30 branches to the stomach, using an absorbable ligature material and avoiding mass ligation, which can critically foreshorten the effective length of the gastroepiploic pedicle.

Regarding Figure 4, after full-length mobilization of the right gastroepiploic pedicle of the omentum, it generally is advisable to protect the extended route to the pelvis by mobilizing the ascending colon and laying its slender vessels behind it. A prophylactic appendectomy generally is advisable to avoid the possibility that the subsequent removal of the appendix as an emergency might jeopardize the omentum. Temporary gastric drainage generally is advisable after extensive mobilization of the right gastroepiploic omental pedicle from the stomach, and a temporary gastrostomy is a more humane procedure than a nasogastric tube. Because the fenestrations of a suction drain tend to become clogged by the supple mobilized omentum, a Penrose drain generally is preferable.

Postoperative problems resulting from the redeployment of the omentum are rare, provided the anatomic principles of the mobilization of its vascularization are carefully followed. It must be remembered that there is only one omentum, and its loss as a result of careless technique can be a disaster for a patient whose reconstruction partially depends on it.

A postoperative ileus lasting 1 or 2 days is not unusual after full-length mobilization of the gastroepiploic pedicle from the stomach—hence, the advisability of nasogastric or temporary gastrostomy drainage. The stomach has an abundant blood supply, and deprivation of its gastroepiploic vascularization does not cause problems.

Omental adhesions in the peritoneal cavity are the natural result of the resolution of any localized intra-abdominal inflammation, but, unlike direct bowel-to-bowel adhesions, they rarely cause intestinal obstruction.

PART II

BLADDER RECONSTRUCTION

CHAPTER 54

Pubovaginal Sling

Test the child urodynamically to be certain that the principal cause of incontinence is an incompetent urethra (usually following multiple surgical attempts, but also after pelvic trauma or radiation, or with some neurologic defects) and not detrusor hyperactivity or only vesicourethral malposition. Determine detrusor contractility, because its absence means that the patient will require perpetual intermittent catheterization. For children with meningomyelocele with poor compliance or intractable uninhibited contractions and incontinence, perform augmentation cystoplasty in addition to the sling procedure.

Exhaust medical approaches using α-adrenergic and anticholinergic medications. Caution the family about complications such as the need for intermittent catheterization, persistent untreatable detrusor instability, upper urinary tract damage, and urinary tract infection.

Arrange for two surgeons. *Position*: Low lithotomy with the legs suspended by the feet. Prep the lower abdomen, perineum, and vagina. Drape to provide access to the vagina. Place a balloon catheter in the bladder. One surgeon stands on the left side of the patient and the other, between the child's legs.

1 *Retropubic operator*: Make a transverse lower abdominal skin incision (page 267) and expose the rectus sheath. Incise the sheath transversely above the symphysis for 5 to 15 cm, depending on the size of the patient. Lift up both edges and separate them from the rectus muscles superiorly and inferiorly, as usually is done for this incision. Place a stay suture at each end of the lower flap, and cut a fusiform strip of fascia from it, the length determined by an estimation of the distance around the urethra and through and over the rectus muscle and fascia. The center of the strip should be almost 2 cm wide to provide broad urethral support. Cover it with moist gauze, and put it aside. Alternatively, the strip may be harvested after the retropubic dissection. A similar-sized rectus fascial strip could be harvested, following a midline skin incision and a vertical fascial incision.

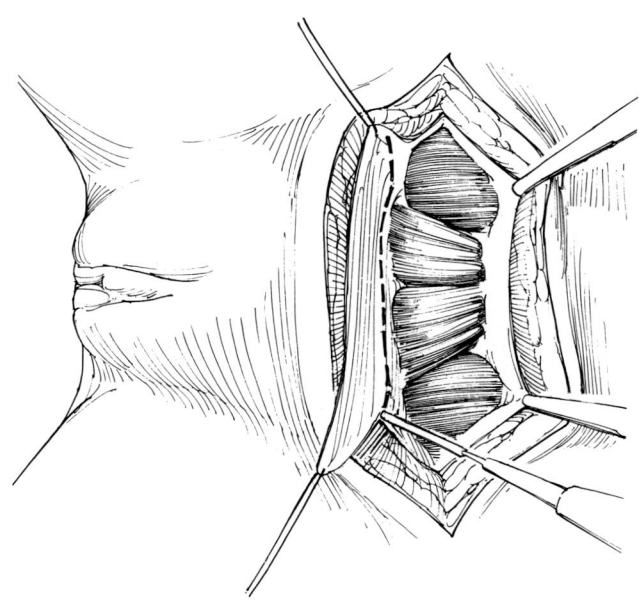

2 Bluntly, and alternately sharply, dissect the anterior bladder wall and urethra. Continue the dissection until the endopelvic fascia of the pelvic floor is reached. In difficult cases after multiple procedures, detach the rectus muscles from the symphysis for a short distance on either side of the midline, and dissect with the point of the scissors directly on the periosteum of the symphysis pubis to its lower margin while depressing the bladder posteriorly. Opening the bladder at this point can facilitate the dissection, but it usually is not necessary.

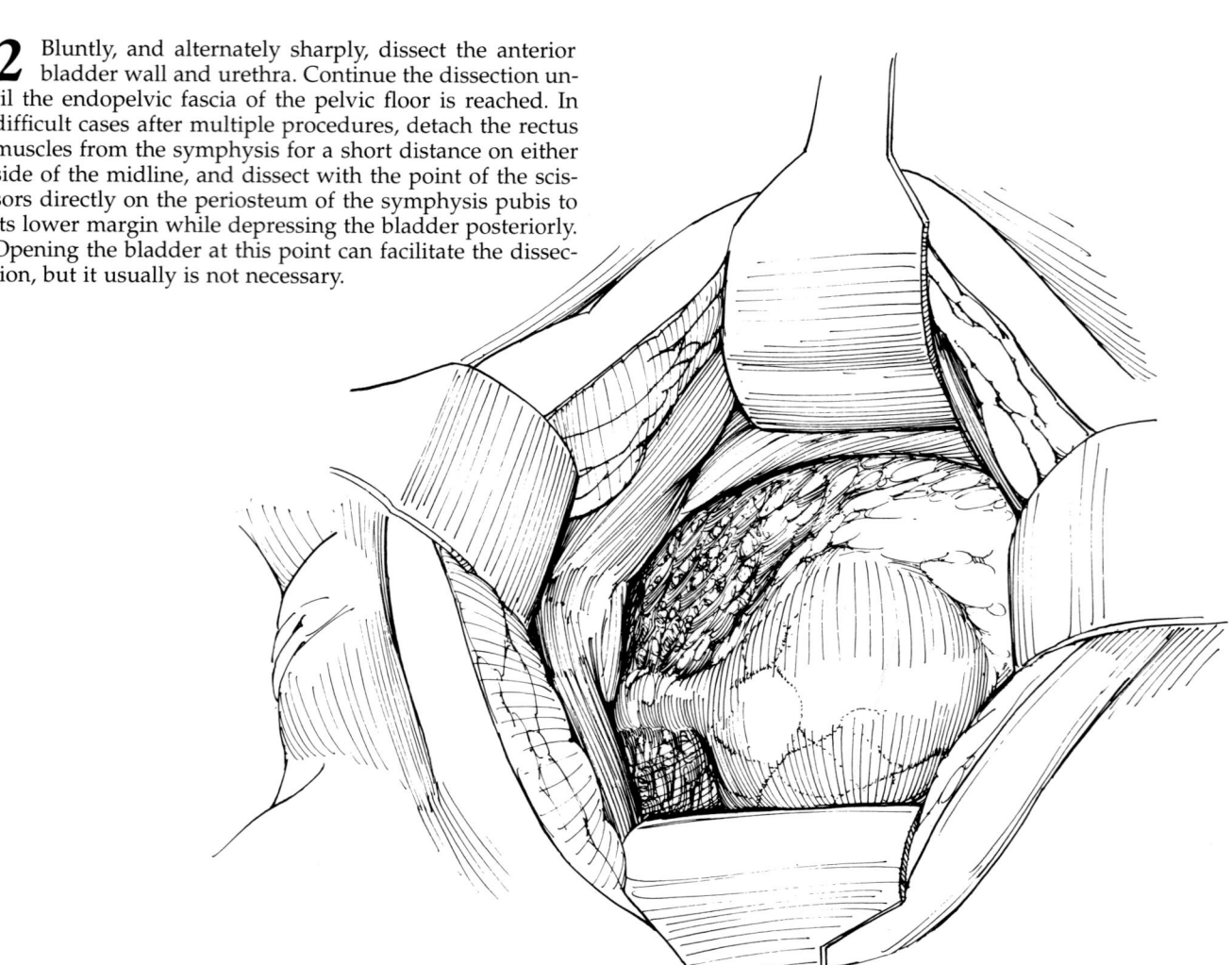

3 *Perineal operator*: Make a 2-cm vertical incision in the vagina, and dissect lateral to the urethra until the retropubic space is reached at the inferior margin of the pubic symphysis. Dissect only the vaginal epithelium free, leaving behind the white paraurethral fascia. As an alternative, incise the pelvic floor, and dissect with the fingers superiorly and laterally to develop the retropubic space. If not done earlier, open the bladder to help with orientation for creation of the tunnels for the sling and to allow detection of vesical injury.

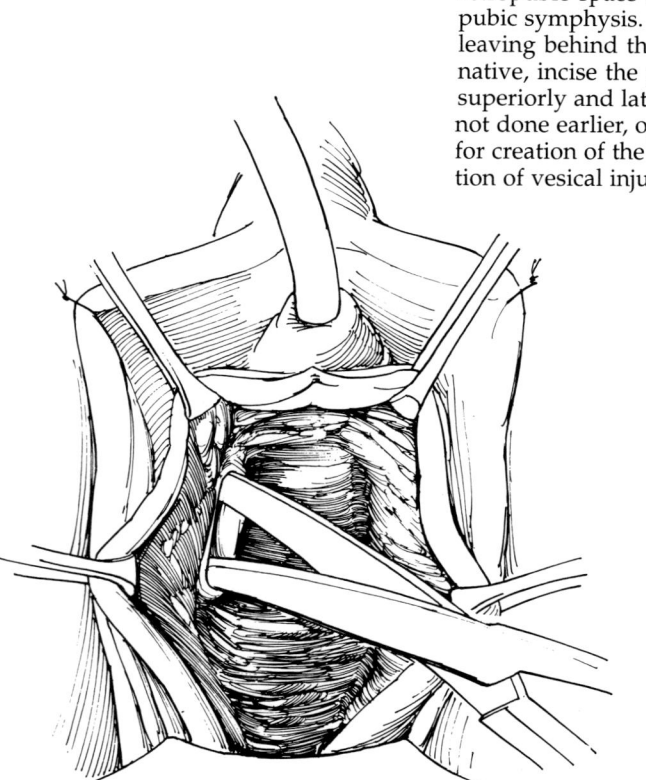

4 **A** and **B**, *Retropubic operator*: Free the urethra and insert the scissors lateral to it on both sides to make an opening in the pelvic floor where the pelvic floor attaches to the symphysis. Be sure that the points of the scissors are leading laterally and superiorly toward the anterior superior iliac crest. Enlarge the opening with a finger in this same direction. Insert one finger of the left hand in the vagina. Grasp a curved clamp in the right hand with the concave side up, and advance it down the right side from above, keeping the tip against the symphysis to avoid entering the bladder.

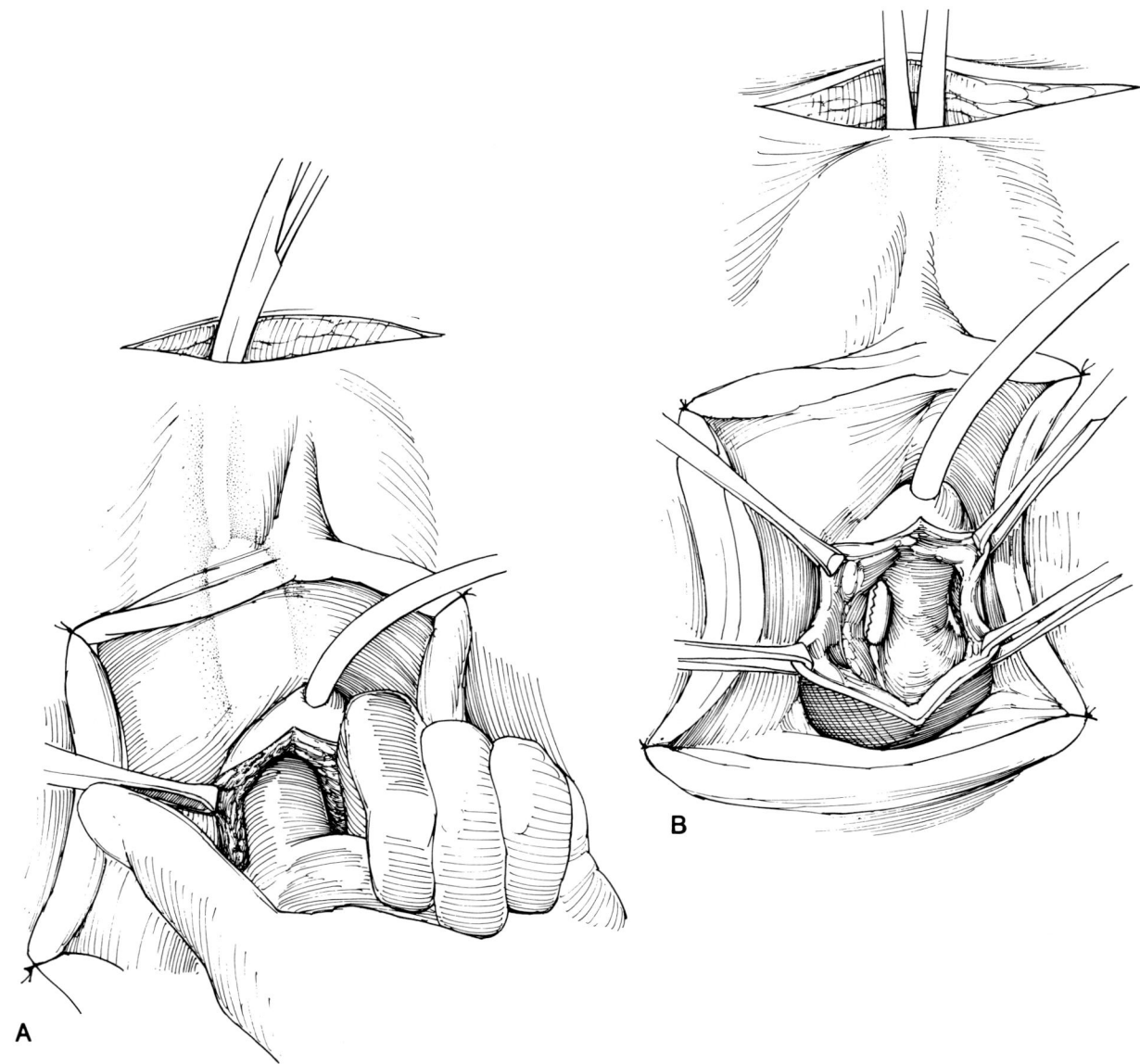

5 Grasp one end of the sling (or its stay suture) presented by the perineal operator, and draw it retropubically into the upper wound. Spread the middle of the sling and tack it to the paraurethral tissues and perineal fascia, smooth surface down, with an absorbable suture to obtain as broad a bearing as possible. Repeat the procedure on the left side, passing the clamp down that side and drawing up the other end of the sling. Suture one end of the rectus fascia with multiple interrupted 2-0 or 3-0 nonabsorbable sutures. Alternatively, pass a tonsil clamp through the belly of the rectus muscle on the right, and draw the end of the strip through it and the corresponding rectus fascia. Bring the other end of the strip through muscle and fascia similarly on the left side. Suture one end to the fascia with 2-0 or 3-0 nonabsorbable sutures, taking three bites of the fascial strip with the suture. Have the perineal operator close the incision in the vaginal mucosa before the retropubic operator tightens the sling. Alternatively, bring the strip through the fascia and muscle, and suture one end of the strip over the other on top of the rectus fascia for added strength. Also, suture the strip to the fascia at the point of exit. This allows the strip to have an ovoid shape, which keeps better tension on the urethra.

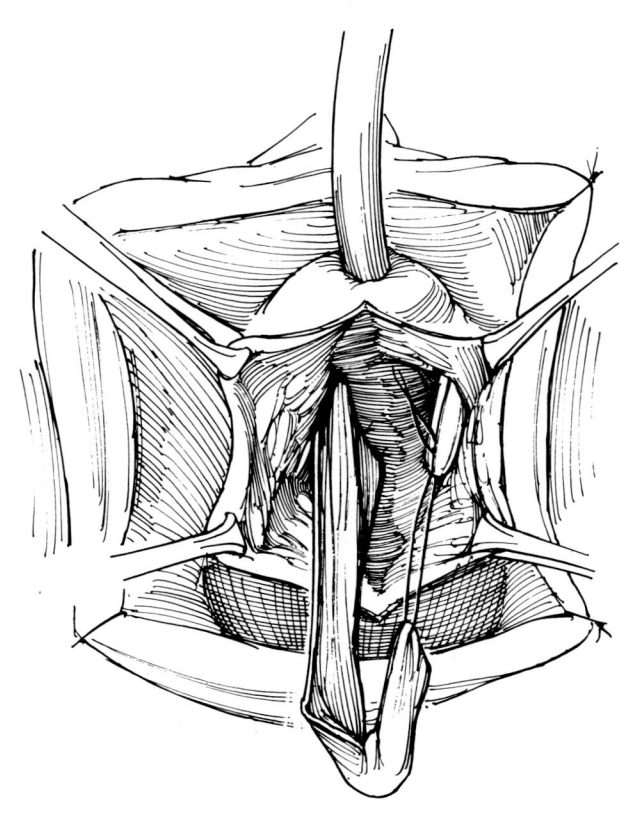

6 **A,** Draw the other end of the sling until approximately 6 to 7 cm H_2O pressure is exerted on the urethra (this can be checked by endoscopic inspection or by profilometry). A good way to check is to insert the endoscope and adjust sling tension to slightly compress the proximal urethra under the sling.

B, Trim any excess from the strip, and suture the free end to the fascia with 2-0 or 3-0 nonabsorbable sutures. Another way to fix the sling is to place the sutures in each end using multiple stitches, then tie them together over Teflon bolsters. *Note*: obtaining correct tension requires considerable judgment, because no exact criteria can be

used. Place a catheter through the bladder wall, and close the bladder and suprapubic wound. Place a vaginal pack, then remove it and the catheter after 3 days; at this time, start intermittent catheterization if the child is unable to void.

Alternatively, in children with neurologic incontinence, a short (1- to 3-cm) strip of rectus fascia can be placed perineally under the urethra and held by 2-0 monofilament sutures inserted over nonabsorbable pledgets. Advance the sutures retropubically, checking endoscopically for correct routing and tension.

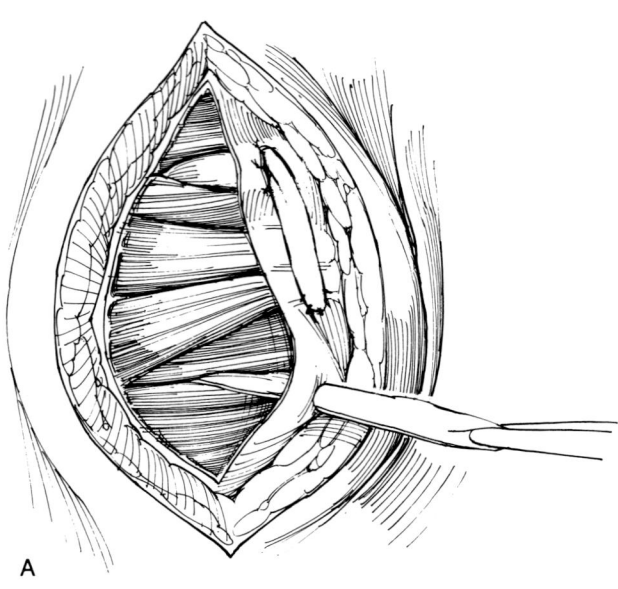

A

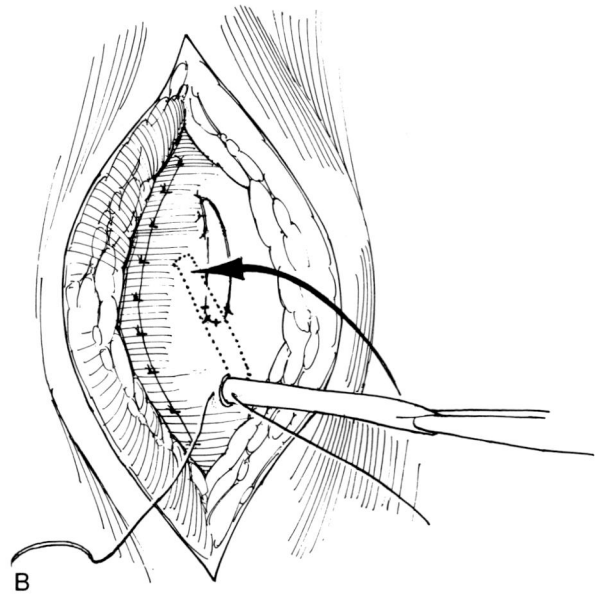

B

POSTOPERATIVE PROBLEMS

Urinary retention is the greatest concern and usually is the result of too much tension at the urethrovesical junction. Straining to void only tightens the sling, so the child must learn to void by perineal relaxation with its accompanying detrusor contraction. The options are intermittent catheterization or removal of the fascial sutures (as a come-and-go procedure), placing dependence on the fibrosis that has developed. Expect a third of patients to void at least by 7 days and one third, within 3 months; the remainder will require longer-term intermittent catheterization. In one fourth of the patients, uninhibited detrusor contractions may persist postoperatively, but these usually respond to anticholinergic medication.

Other Problems. The sling may erode into the urethra or bladder, obliterating the lumen or producing a urethrovaginal fistula, or the sling may not sufficiently compress the urethra because of excessive scarring from previous procedures.

Commentary by Stuart B. Bauer

A fascial sling seems to work best in those patients in whom urethral tension fails to increase in response to increases in abdominal pressure or actually diminishes as the bladder fills to capacity, because the bladder neck area opens with filling, or when there is a paradoxic relaxation in resistance following a Valsalva or Credé maneuver. It is ideally suited for patients with neurogenic bladder dysfunction who are already on intermittent catheterization because they cannot empty on their own but are wet with any activity in between times. As with any operation designed to increase outlet resistance, one must ensure that detrusor compliance is adequate and that intravesical pressure does not rise above 40 cm H_2O.

The sling achieves continence by increasing bladder outlet resistance in a number of ways. The posterior aspect of the bladder neck area is compressed by the strip of fascia; the bladder neck and proximal urethra are positioned more intra-abdominally; and the bladder neck is buttressed against the undersurface of the pubis. Although urethral resistance may not be raised dramatically at rest following the sling procedure, any sudden increase in abdominal pressure transmitted to the bladder is counterbalanced by the same forces acting on the compressed and repositioned bladder neck and proximal urethra, now that they are located more intra-abdominally. Finally, because the sling is tied to itself over the rectus fascia, the forces that tend to push the bladder neck inferiorly during any increase in abdominal pressure are prevented from doing so by the reflex tightening of the rectus abdominis muscle in response to any increase in abdominal pressure.

CHAPTER 55

Trigonal Tubularization

(GUY LEADBETTER)

By urodynamic studies, determine that the child's incontinence is caused by low urethral closure pressure, usually with scarring and fixation of the urethra from previous operations, and that the detrusor is compliant.

1 Proceed as described for vesical neck tubularization (page 285), except that the more posterior aspects of the bladder and urethra need not be mobilized. Open the bladder in the midline all the way into the deep urethra. Insert 5 F silicone catheters into the ureters. Mobilize the ureters extravesically, taking care to bring them under the vas or uterine vessels. Implant each ureter 3 to 4 cm more cephalad, using a tunnel technique. Transtrigonal implantation is a good choice.

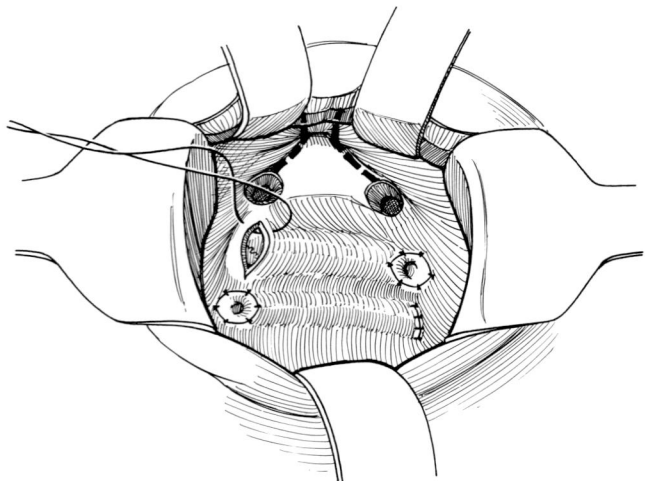

2 Place a stay suture in the anterior urethral wall at the apex of the initial cut. With curved scissors, cut through the entire thickness of the urethra and bladder wall, beginning just lateral to the stay suture and continuing through the site of the previous orifice and 1 to 2 cm beyond. Alternatively, it may be easier to start the incision at the trigone and cut distally. The entire trigone must be tubularized. This leaves a posterior segment 1.5 to 2 cm wide and 4 to 5 cm long. Place an 8 or 10 F silicone catheter up through the urethra.

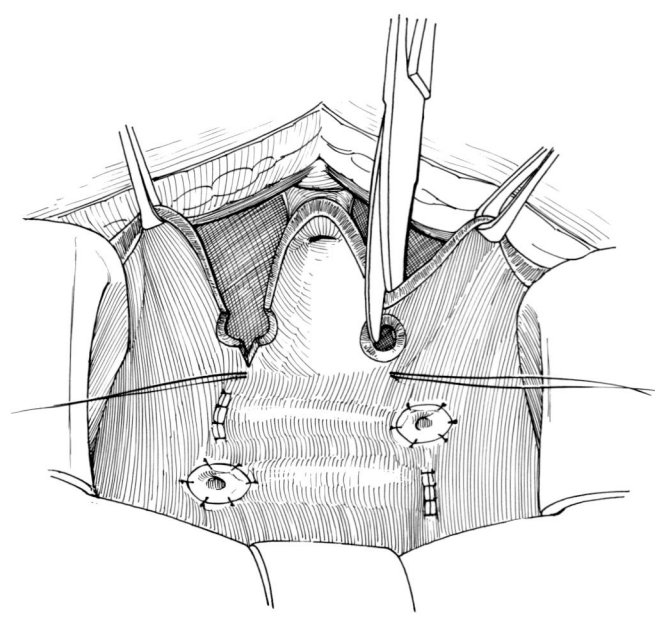

3 **A,** Approximate the epithelium of the edges of the neourethra with interrupted sutures of 5-0 chromic catgut, making the strip snug around the catheter. In fact, it is difficult to make it too tight. If placing the distal sutures is difficult, spread the symphysis with a pediatric rib spreader.

B and **C,** Imbricate the detrusor muscle in the neourethra by suturing one edge firmly to the undersurface of the opposite edge and then lapping that edge back to the first side. If the resulting bladder capacity is small, consider augmentation followed by intermittent catheterization.

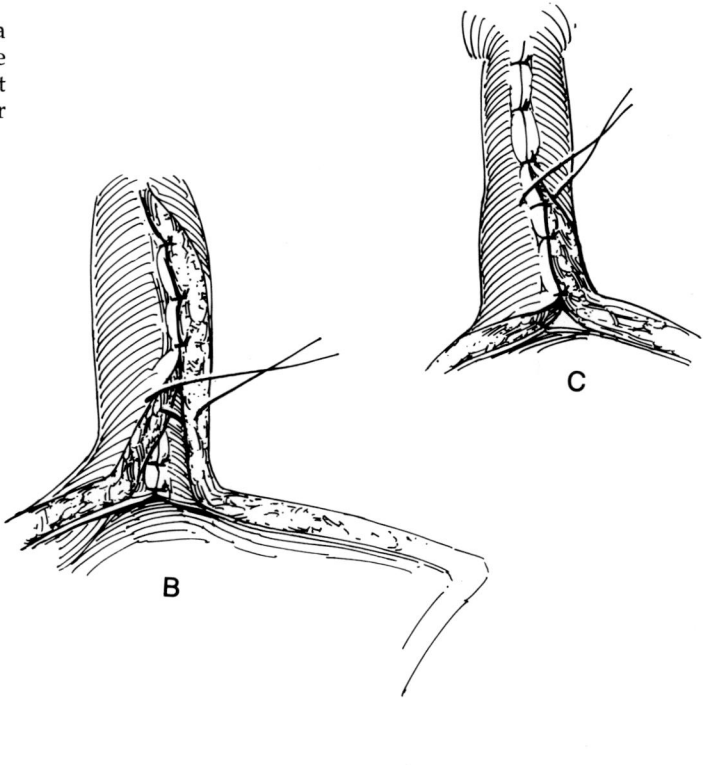

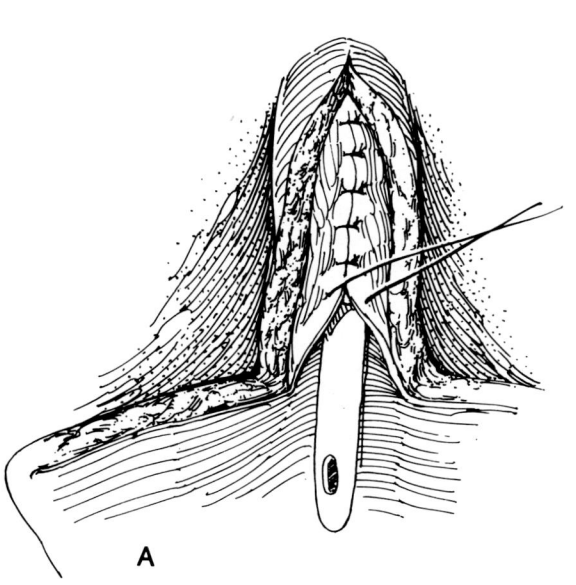

4 Draw a 14 or 16 F Malecot or balloon catheter through the bladder and body walls and fasten it to the skin with a nonabsorbable suture. Have the catheter from each ureter exit through stab wounds. An 8 or 10 F balloon catheter may be left as a urethral stent if desired. Close the bladder defect with a running 4-0 or 5-0 chromic catgut subepithelial suture, with interrupted 3-0 or 4-0 chromic catgut sutures to the muscle and adventitia. Close the wound around a Penrose drain. Remove the stents in 1 to 2 weeks, and the suprapubic tube in 2 weeks.

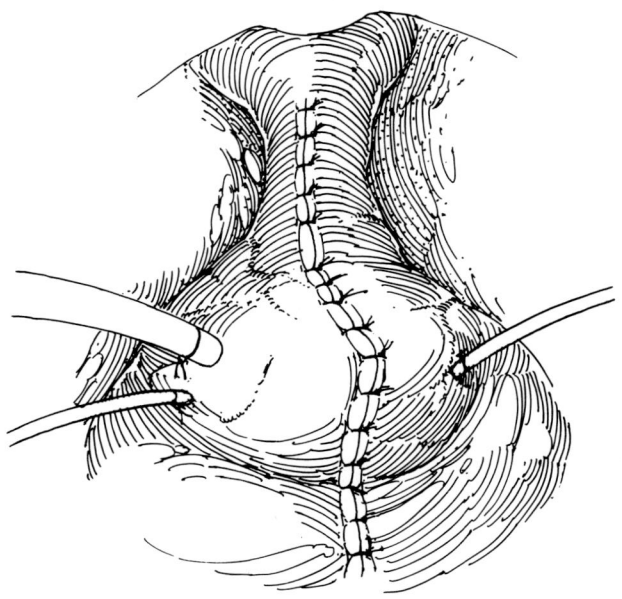

POSTOPERATIVE PROBLEMS

Urinary retention is rare; patients who undergo this procedure always seem to be able to void unless the bladder has been augmented. In that case, intermittent catheterization may be needed. Incontinence may persist and require bladder augmentation if it is from poor vesical compliance. If outlet resistance is low, a sling procedure or implantation of an artificial sphincter may be needed. Ureteral obstruction can occur, as with any ureteroneocystostomy. Failure of the cystostomy site to close indicates stenosis in the new urethra.

Commentary by Guy W. Leadbetter, Jr.

Some comments and tips gained from 30 years of experience with this operation are as follows: First, the procedure often is long and arduous and tests one's equanimity.

In a child, splitting the symphyseal cartilage and spreading the symphysis with a pediatric rib spreader may give better exposure and room for suturing, but never spread an adult symphysis, because this will cause severe pain in the sacroiliac area postoperatively. In adults, it is better to remove a portion of symphysis if necessary. This trigonal flap method is contraindicated in adult men unless total prostatectomy has been done.

It is important to place sutures at the sites of the ureteral orifices to mark where the trigone is to be tubularized. It is essential for continence that the trigone be tubularized to make the new bladder neck.

Do not remove dog-ear flaps from the bladder after the urethral bladder incision has been made, because this would cause a decrease in bladder capacity. When reimplanting the ureters, it is important to be certain that they are brought out from under the vas or uterine vessels. This then allows a straight entrance into the bladder. If this is not done, the ureters, as the bladder fills, will be obstructed by the vas or vessels.

Ureteral and suprapubic catheters are left in place for 7 to 14 days. This allows healing to occur in a urine-free field. I believe this prevents possible fibrosis or fistula formation, which may occur if urine should leak into the reconstructed bladder neck area.

CHAPTER 56

Vesical Neck Tubularization
(TANAGHO-FLOCKS)

Vesical neck tubularization is suitable for both boys and girls with epispadias, short urethra, and selected cases of high urogenital sinus or urethral trauma. If reflux is present, use the technique of trigonal tubularization (page 282).

Clear (or suppress) bacteriuria. Panendoscopy may show a treatable bladder-neck stricture or residual obstruction, and cystometrography may show treatable detrusor hyperreflexia. Children with hyperactive neurogenic dysfunction are not candidates for this operation, but those with compliant bladders do well if intermittently catheterized. The wall of an atonic bladder is not suitable material for a tube, nor is that of a bladder subjected to previous cystostomies and anterior incisions.

Position. Place boys supine with pelvis slightly elevated; for girls, use a modified lithotomy position, and for infants, the frog-legged position. After prep-

ping and draping, insert a 16 F 5-ml balloon catheter and instill sterile water into the bladder to partially fill it.

Incision. Use a lower midline extraperitoneal (page 263) or lower transverse (page 267) incision.

1 Reflect a limited area of the peritoneum from the anterior bladder surface, and dissect carefully in the space of Retzius to expose the proximal two thirds of the prostate. In girls, expose the urethra to the level of the endopelvic fascia. In a girl who has had previous procedures, take care not to disturb the vessels on the anterior bladder wall.

Dissect laterally around the vesicourethral junction, identified by the balloon on the catheter, avoiding the rectum or vagina and neurovascular bundle. Place four stays to outline a flap on the anterior surface of the half-filled bladder, marking a 1-inch square beginning exactly at the internal meatus. The two distal sutures will be in the prostate in boys and in the urethra in girls.

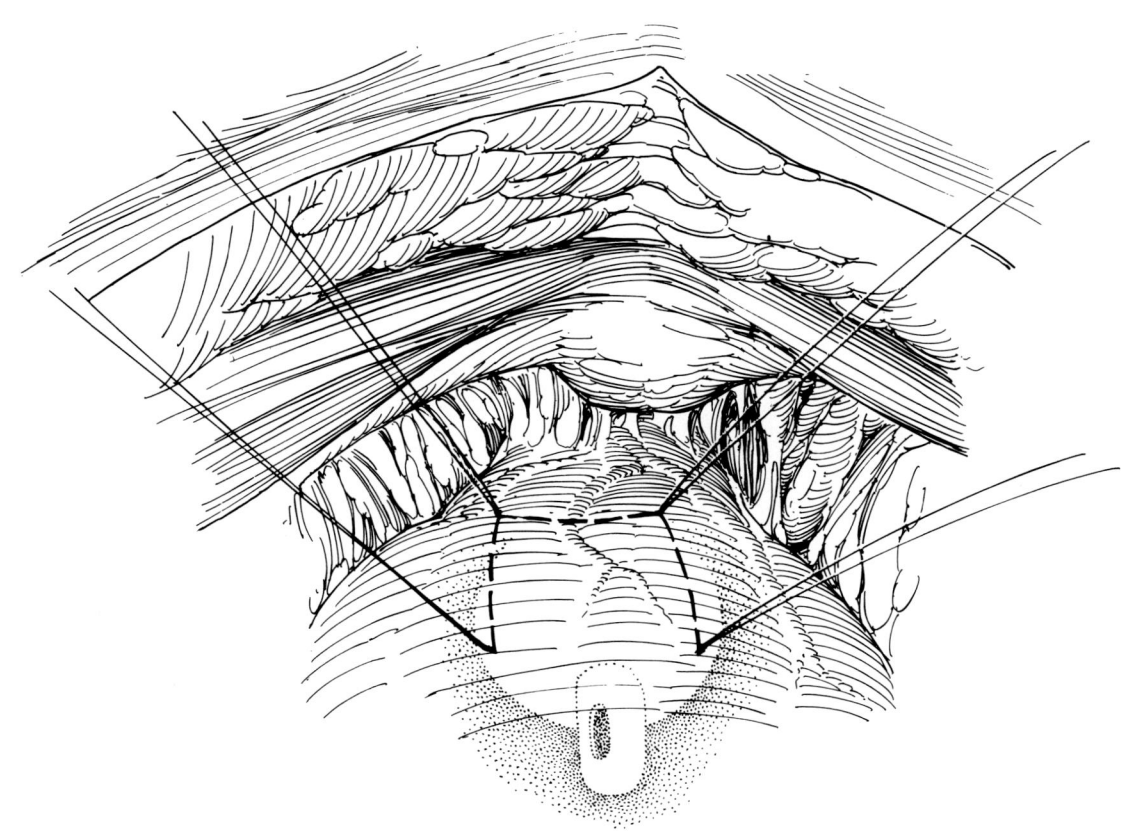

2 Make a full-thickness transverse incision across the bladder neck with the cutting current just below the distal sutures of the flap. Once in the bladder, extend the initial transverse incision at the vesical neck, cutting laterally inside the bladder. Identify the trigone and ureteral orifices. Cut deeply at the apex of the trigone through the full thickness of the bladder to expose the seminal vesicles and ampullae in boys, sufficient to allow the base of the bladder to slide upward for 1 or 2 cm.

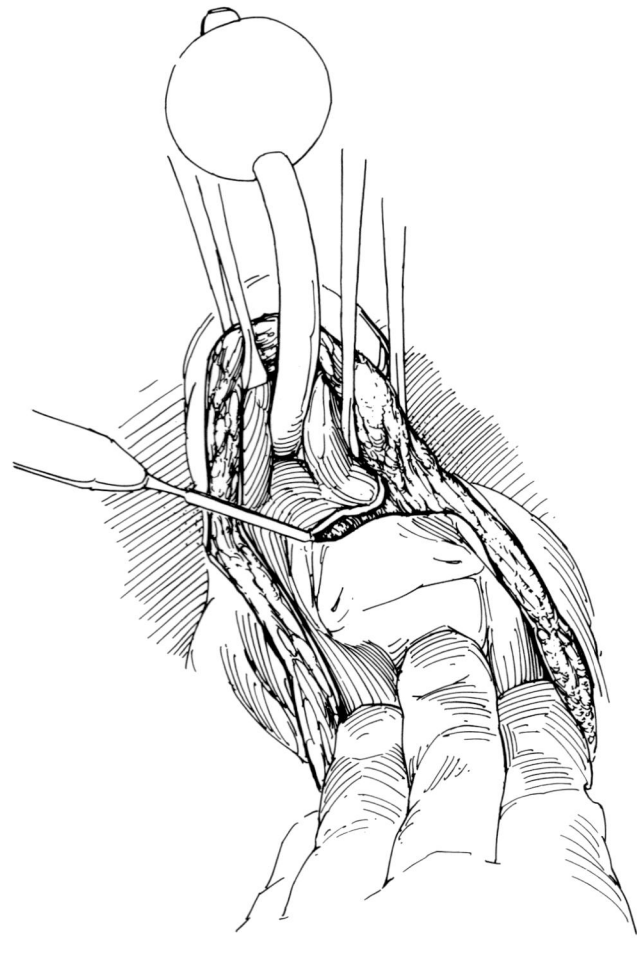

3 Make two parallel cuts running from the lower to the upper stay sutures. Reflect the flap upward. Insert a Malecot catheter as high as possible and to one side through the dome of the bladder, and lead it out through one lower abdominal quadrant. Anchor it to the skin with a nonabsorbable suture. Roll the bladder flap into a tube around the balloon catheter, and suture the sides together with full-thickness stitches of 3-0 or 4-0 synthetic absorbable sutures. Be sure to catch the retracted middle layer of the detrusor in each stitch. Start by putting one suture at the base of the flap and one at the apex, and then fill in between.

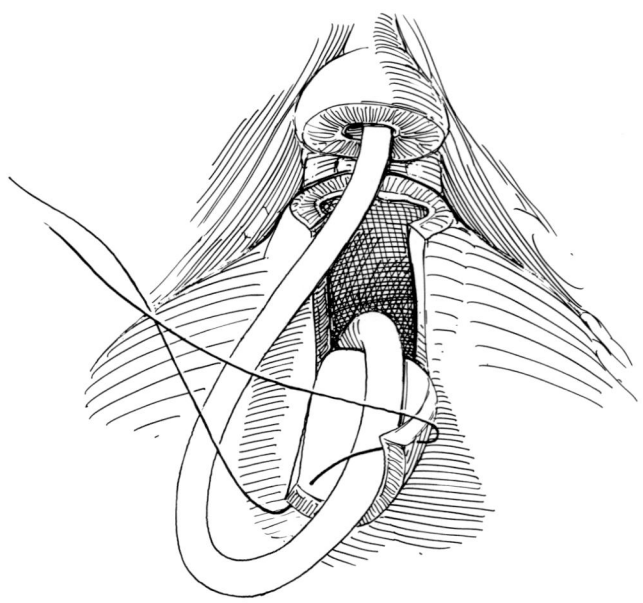

4 Attach the apex of the trigone to the base of the tube with a mattress stitch, and close the remainder of the defect in the bladder transversely.

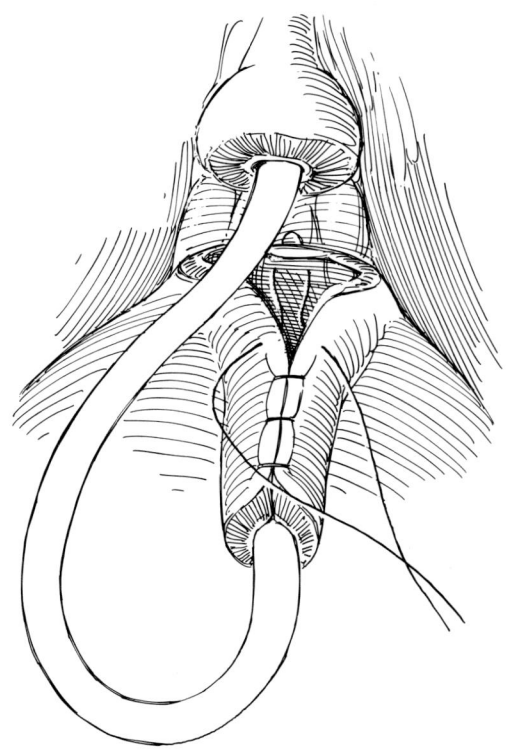

5 Anastomose the tube to the cut end of the urethra with five or six 3-0 or 4-0 synthetic absorbable sutures. Place all the sutures first, then pull them down and tie them successively. In boys, insert two 3-0 or 4-0 chromic catgut sutures into the anterior bladder wall close to the base of the tube, and bring them through the lower rectus fascia. In girls, use sutures in the vaginal wall as in a suprapubic vesical suspension.

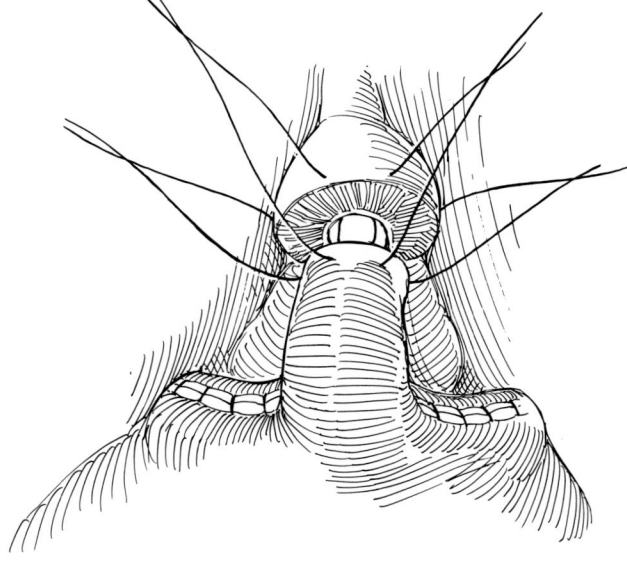

6 **A** and **B**, Alternatively, raise a transverse flap and suture it to the urethra in a corkscrew fashion (Flocks and Boldus, 1973). Another option is that the bladder can be transected, and a tube formed from the distal portion, which is then tunneled under the trigone to move the vesical neck into the bas-fond. Insert Penrose drains to the posterior suture line. Close the wound. Maintain cystostomy drainage for 3 to 4 weeks, then test for residual urine before removing the tube.

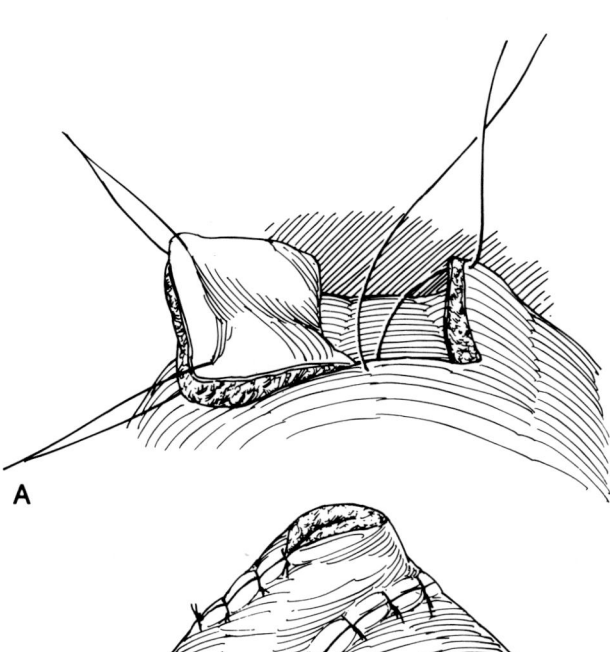

POSTOPERATIVE PROBLEMS

Persistent incontinence can occur in children with noncompliant bladders or in those with tubes constructed from bladder wall of poor quality. *Strictures* can develop between the tube and the prostatic fossa, requiring internal urethrotomy. Postoperative instrumentation and catheterization can be difficult and must be done under direct vision.

Commentary by Emil A. Tanagho

Formation of an anterior bladder tube is a useful reconstructive procedure that enables regaining of continence in boys and girls born with epispadias. It also is beneficial in girls with a short urethra (significant hypospadias) or a high urogenital sinus with a short urethral segment, which might have to be mobilized independently of the urogenital sinus and brought down to the vaginal vestibule. The technique also can be used in cases of trauma in which the urethrovesical segment is disrupted, especially in girls, and in selected cases of flaccid neurogenic bladder.

The rationale of the procedure is to incorporate in a bladder flap the ventral condensation of circular fibers that extends above the internal meatus for approximately 1 inch on the anterior bladder wall. Normally, if this area has not been violated before by surgery or trauma, the condensation of circular fibers raised in a flap and turned around into a tube will have enough tonus to provide an occlusive effect and sphincteric function that can replace a nonexistent or traumatized normal sphincteric segment. Do not try to make the tube too long; it should be confined to the condensation of circular fibers in the anterior bladder wall; if this is less than an inch in length, the tube should be made shorter. It is the quality of the muscles in the tube rather than the length that is important. The tube should not be occlusive; it should be of adequate diameter to wrap easily around a 16 F catheter, although in pediatric cases we usually wrap it around a 10 F catheter. Bring the apex of the trigone to the base of the tube, and re-create the bladder neck configuration, providing for a sharp transition from the big cavity of the bladder to the adequate lumen of the reconstructed tube. Extreme care should be taken in mobilizing the anterior bladder surface, keeping all the adventitial layers and blood vessels on it. During exposure, aim at the urethrovesical junction. Do not try to free too much of the anterior bladder wall, because this might interfere with the blood supply to the flap. Mark the flap with the bladder half distended before starting the incision to avoid losing orientation. The flap consistently looks narrower after it has been delineated and cut because of the contraction of the circular fibers in it; this is a good sign.

It is essential to handle the tissue with the utmost care to avoid devitalizing any of the critical delicate muscle tissue. Accurate coaptation of epithelium to epithelium with full-thickness muscle-wall sutures is essential in both constructing the tube and establishing the anastomosis between the tube and the urethra. The procedure is suitable for both female and male patients. In cutting the bladder neck completely from the urethra, extreme care should be taken posteriorly not to enter the vaginal wall in girls and not to injure the seminal vesicle and vas in boys. However, a full-thickness cut into the bladder muscle wall is essential to permit the bladder to slide upward.

Closure of the rest of the bladder will leave two small dog-ear flaps; do not attempt to smooth these, because they will round themselves and become absorbed into the bladder cavity with time to provide additional capacity. If there is a midline incision in the bladder from a previous cystostomy and if conditions are favorable, a one-sided tube can be used; the site of the midline incision can be one lateral margin, and the flap can be taken more from one side. Extensive previous surgery on the anterior bladder wall will doom the operation to failure. Proper suspension and support should be provided without putting tension on the tube and on the suture line between it and the urethra. Mobilize the bladder base and trigone upward to prevent formation of a sharp posterior angle, which can be obstructive. Suprapubic drainage should be adequate for at least 3 weeks and tested for adequate voiding with minimal residual urine before removing the suprapubic tube. Temporary stenting of the reconstructed tube and site of anastomosis by urethral catheter is desirable for 10 days.

In selected patients with a flaccid neurogenic bladder, a tube also can be most effective. Its purpose is not to act as a sphincter but to provide resistance to permit continence between intermittent catheterization. Emphasis is on supporting the tube after its reconstruction to prevent it from being telescoped or crushed by the weight of the bladder above it. Thus, some kind of suspension is created using either the vaginal wall in girls or the anterior bladder wall in boys and in small girls if the vaginal wall is not appropriate for suspension.

The surgeon must be extremely aware of the major potential causes of failure of this technique: a devascularized flap leading either to contracture or sloughing and fistulization, a too-wide flap becoming funneled and absorbed into the bladder cavity, a too-narrow flap becoming a precursor for ischemia once it is wrapped into a tube around the catheter, inaccurate apposition of epithelium to epithelium sutures at the site of an anastomosis, and lack of proper suspension of the bladder after tube reconstruction.

CHAPTER 57

Intravesical Urethral Lengthening
(KROPP)

Consider simultaneous bladder augmentation in children with poorly compliant bladders, because a low-pressure reservoir is essential. In older boys, an artificial sphincter or continent diversion should be considered as an alternative, especially because catheterization through the male urethra generally is not well accepted.

1 Insert a 24 F balloon catheter transurethrally. *Incision*: Lower midline (page 263). Expose the bladder neck and posterior urethra.

A, Mark a rectangular bladder flap with stay sutures with the base at the bladder neck. The length should be that required for the new urethra (4 to 6 cm), and the width should be the proposed circumference (knowing that 20 F equals 2.0 cm).

B, Incise the flap with the cutting current, and continue the incision posteriorly around the bladder neck. (An alternative to separating the tube from the bladder, leaving it attached only by the rectangular strip, is to preserve the outer posterolateral musculoadventitial fibers.) The midline posterior bladder muscle must be incised completely, so that the bladder neck–anterior bladder flaps can be converted into a tube.

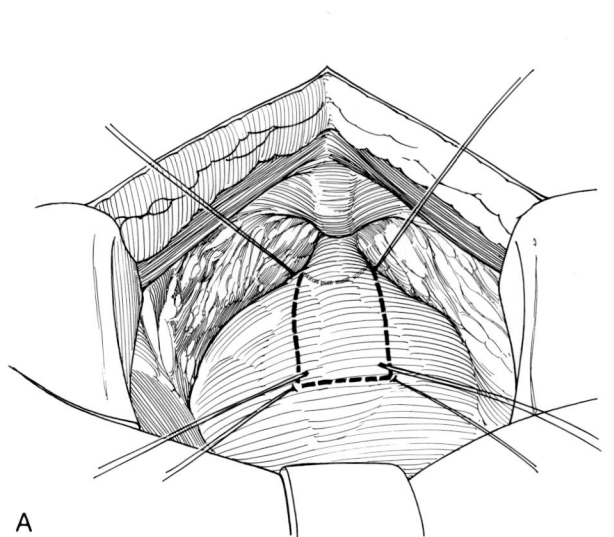

A

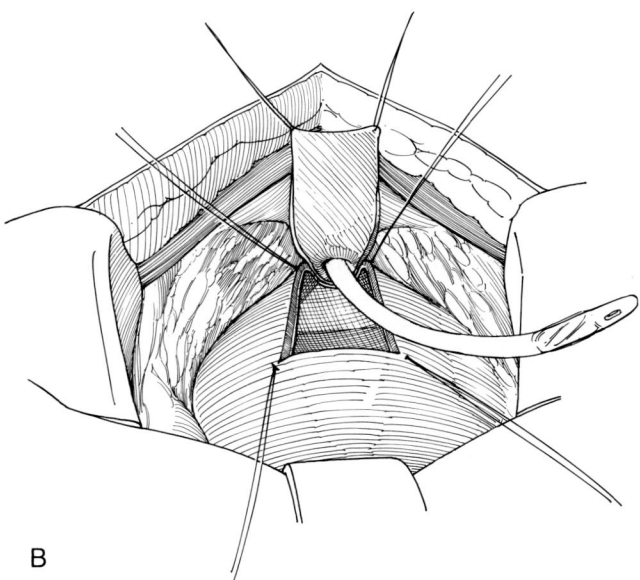

B

289

2 Roll the flap into a tube over a 20 F balloon catheter, and close it with a continuous subepithelial plain catgut suture and interrupted sutures of 4-0 chromic catgut, starting at the distal end.

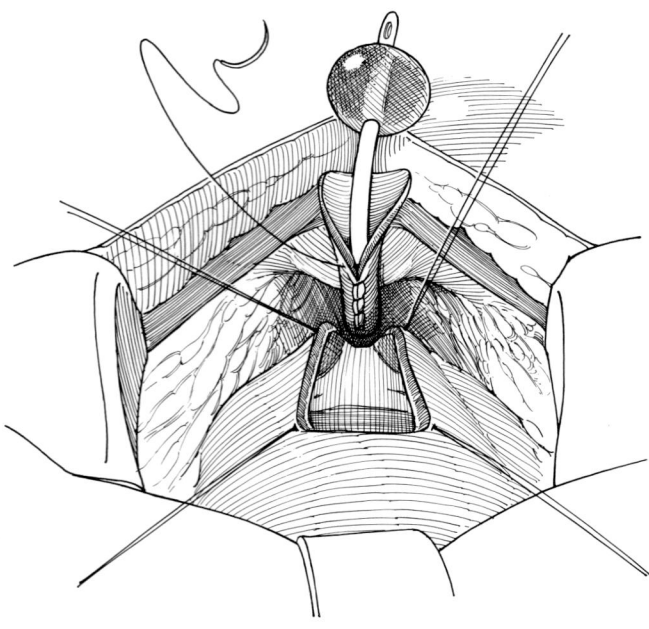

3 With scissors, make a wide tunnel beneath vesical epithelium and over the trigonal musculature that extends between the urethral orifices, using blunt and sharp dissection. An alternative is merely to create a channel in which to place the new urethra and then cover it with the adjacent epithelium.

Insert the end of the new urethra into the flange of a Robinson catheter, and insinuate it up through the tunnel. At the same time, pull the bladder down over the new tube to reach the former bladder neck.

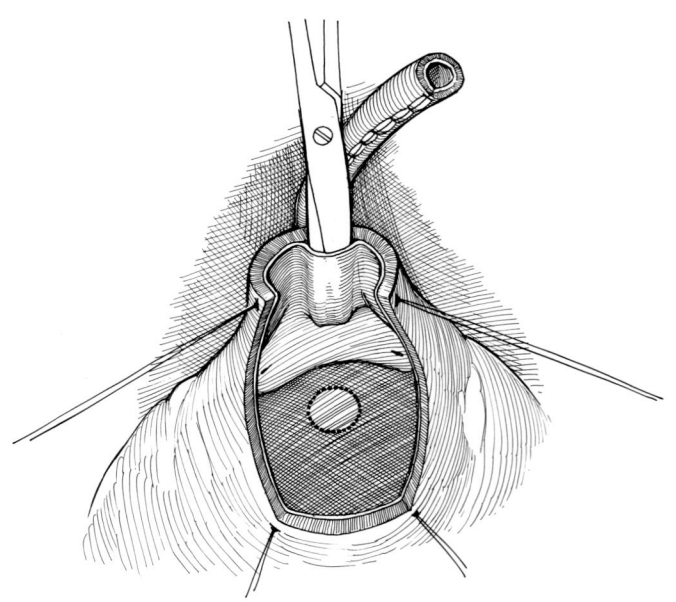

4 Fasten the tube to the bladder wall in the fundus with interrupted 4-0 chromic catgut sutures and to the former bladder neck with similar sutures.

Close the anterior bladder wall, starting distally around the urethra with a running plain catgut subepithelial suture, and reinforce the suture line with interrupted 4-0 chromic catgut sutures. Alternatively, the closure may be started proximally.

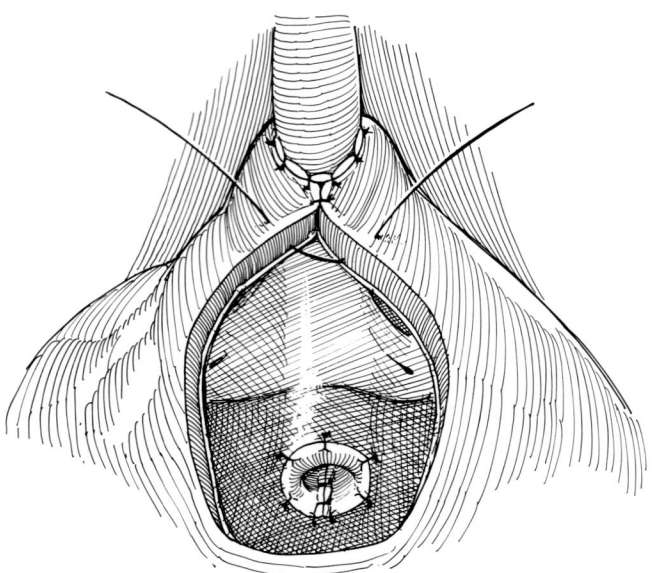

POSTOPERATIVE PROBLEMS

Difficulty with catheterization may require cystoscopic manipulation. In boys, a perineal urethrostomy may be required. Leaving the stent in place 5 to 6 weeks reduces the problem. *Reflux* may develop postoperatively. It may not require correction if catheterization is done frequently.

Commentary by Kenneth A. Kropp

Prior to making the skin incision, a Foley catheter of a size that will be used for intermittent catheterization is placed. The bladder is filled to capacity. A midline incision is made from umbilicus to pubic symphysis, but the peritoneal cavity is not entered at this time. The anterior bladder wall and bladder neck–proximal urethra are exposed. The bladder neck is identified via position of the Foley balloon. The rectangular strip is outlined approximately 6 × 2 cm, and stay sutures are placed at the cephalad corners of the rectangular strip. The bladder is opened using the needle-tipped coagulating current. Once the bladder is open, the catheter is withdrawn into the bladder and placed up over the pubic symphysis.

Both ureteral orifices are catheterized, and these catheters are sutured into position, because they will remain for approximately 4 days. The incision around the bladder neck is then completed with a needle-tipped coagulating current, completely separating the bladder from the bladder neck, except for outer posterolateral musculoadventitial attachments. These posterolateral attachments are left, so that the bladder does not completely separate from the bladder neck. Further dissection is carried downward underneath the bladder neck posteriorly, so that when the suturing of the bladder neck–tubular strip begins, there will be a smooth transition. Occasionally, a wedge will be taken out of the posterior bladder neck to effect such a transition.

Once the rectangular strip has been tubularized around the Foley catheter, the bladder is bivalved in the midline back to approximately 3 to 4 cm from the interureteric ridge. Subepithelial tunnels are started with sharp dissection, making two parallel tunnels, each of them just medial to either ureteral orifice. The two tunnels are then joined by placing the blades of the scissors in each of the tunnels and cutting. When the tunnel has been developed down to the interureteric ridge, we find it easier to develop a submuscularis tunnel from bladder neck back up to the interureteric ridge. This tunnel is really between the superficial and deep trigonal musculature, and the tunnel from above is then reentered. This tunnel must be wide enough to easily accommodate the tubularized bladder strip. We find that pulling the flanged end of a red rubber catheter through the tunnel with ease usually means that the tubularized bladder also can be pulled easily through the tunnel. The previously placed stay sutures are threaded onto Keith needles; these are threaded through the inside to the outside of the flanged end of the red rubber catheter, so that the flanged end can act as a guide for bringing the tubularized bladder strip up through the subepithelial tunnel.

Sutures are placed through the bladder musculature on either side of the tunnel at the bladder neck area; these are sutured to the bladder neck–proximal urethra and tied. This effectively brings the bladder neck back down to the original bladder neck. The length of the tubularized strip need not be much longer than 1 or 2 cm cephalad to the interureteric ridge. The excess of the tube, if any, is amputated, and the bladder epithelium is tacked to the epithelium of the bladder tube. Ureteral catheters are brought out through stab wounds in the bladder, and a suprapubic tube is brought through another stab wound. At this point, the peritoneal cavity is opened, and the bowel augmentation is done in the usual manner.

The ureteral catheters are removed on the 4th postoperative day. The suprapubic and Foley catheters are irrigated alternately every 4 hours to make sure that the family is familiar with the irrigation technique and no mucus buildup occurs, causing plugging of the Foley and suprapubic catheters. The child usually is discharged on the 6th or 7th postoperative day and is seen weekly on an outpatient basis. Between 4 and 6 weeks postoperatively, the child is readmitted for a short stay. The Foley catheter is removed, and the suprapubic tube is clamped. If catheterization is being performed easily, the suprapubic tube is removed, and the child is discharged. We initially recommend catheterization every 1 to 1½ hours, with the frequency decreased over the next 3 to 4 weeks to 4 to 6 times per day.

CHAPTER 58

Insertion of Artificial Sphincter

Perform uroflowmetry to detect outlet obstruction and check residual urine. Do a cystometrogram to rule out uninhibited contractions. In some cases, urethral pressure profilometry is indicated. Obtain a cystogram or perform cystoscopy to look for structural vesical abnormalities and to help select the best site for cuff placement. Avoid placing a cuff around a reoperated bladder neck. If used around bowel, add extra fluid, because the wall will shrink.

Have the patient shower preoperatively with organic iodine soap solution. Treat urinary tract infection and give perioperative cephalosporin. Shave the adolescent patient in the operating room. Prep for 10 minutes with iodophor, including the perineum and external genitalia (and vagina in girls). Restrict traffic through the operating room, and reduce room contamination to a minimum (most prosthetic infections are caused by airborne *Staphylococcus epidermidis*). Spray the wound throughout the operation with a dilute antibiotic solution.

Instruments. Provide a basic set, a genitourinary fine set, a Scott retractor with small and large stays, a baby Deaver retractor, skin hooks, Babcock clamps, Lahey clamps, large right-angle dissecting scissors, four curved and four straight mosquito clamps shod with silicone tubing, a DeBakey forceps, two pairs of Cushing forceps (smooth and toothed), Hegar dilators, a headlamp, a soft adjustable stool, penile prosthesis (AS 800) in three sterile packages (pump, prep package with sizer and blunt needles, and connectors), one bowl for 11.5 percent Cysto-Conray II, one bowl for dilute antibiotic solution (50,000 units bacitracin, 1 g neomycin, 300 ml saline), dilute methylene blue solution, two basins with 1500 ml of water to wash gloves, nonpenetrating towel clips, a silicone sheet to block the anus, a 14 F 5-ml silicone balloon catheter with syringe, lubricant and a plug, a scrotal supporter, 2-0 Prolene sutures for connectors, 4-0 chromic catgut with RB-1 needle, two half-inch Penrose drains, and vacuum suction and tubing. Be sure to flush all air from the components of the system.

BLADDER NECK PLACEMENT

The bladder neck is the site used for children, who have small bulbar urethras. This technique has the advantages of being more physiologic than bulbar urethral placement, less prone to erosion, and less irritating with intermittent catheterization.

1 *Incision:* Make a vertical incision; a transverse lower abdominal incision often is more suitable for children. Insert a 5-ml balloon catheter of suitable size. After previous retropubic operations or trauma, insert a rectal tube or vaginal pack to help identify the tissue planes. Open the bladder if necessary. Incise the visceral extension of the endopelvic fascia, and establish a plane bluntly between the bladder neck and the underlying vagina or rectum, pushing the tissue containing the neurovascular bundle laterally. Stay cephalad to the parietal endopelvic fascia and below the level of the trigone. With the thumb and index finger, palpate the catheter and trigone anteriorly and the vas deferens posteriorly. Pinch the trigone anteriorly to separate it from the vasa. Use a right-angle clamp and scissors on the finger to dissect between the bladder neck and the ejaculatory mechanism. Pass an umbilical tape through the tract for traction exposure to allow control of any venous bleeders. (Clips are inadvisable where metal could erode into silicone rubber.)

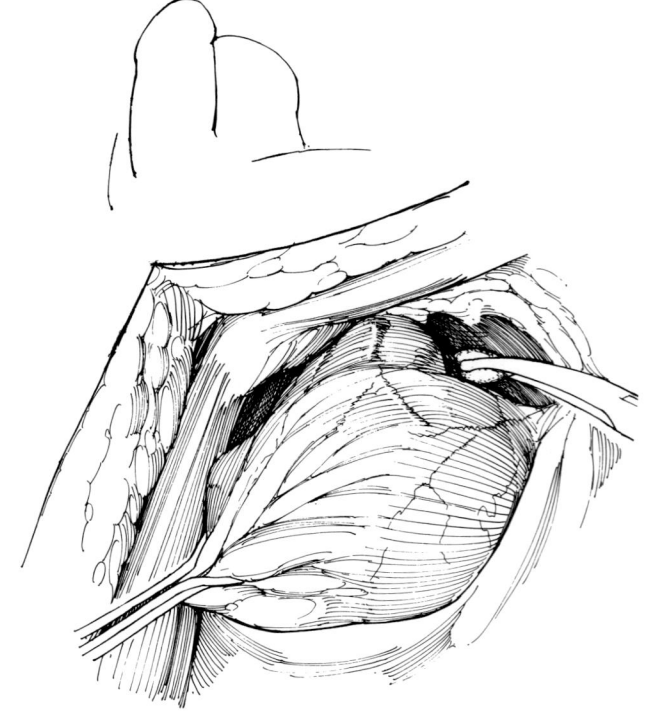

2 Remove the balloon catheter. Pass a large right-angle clamp beneath the bladder neck, and draw the sizer tape through.

3 Measure the circumference with the markers on the tape while drawing it against the bladder neck. In boys, the caudal edge of the tape should be at the top of the prostate; in girls, the cephalad edge should lie just above the bladder neck, as previously determined by palpation of the catheter balloon.

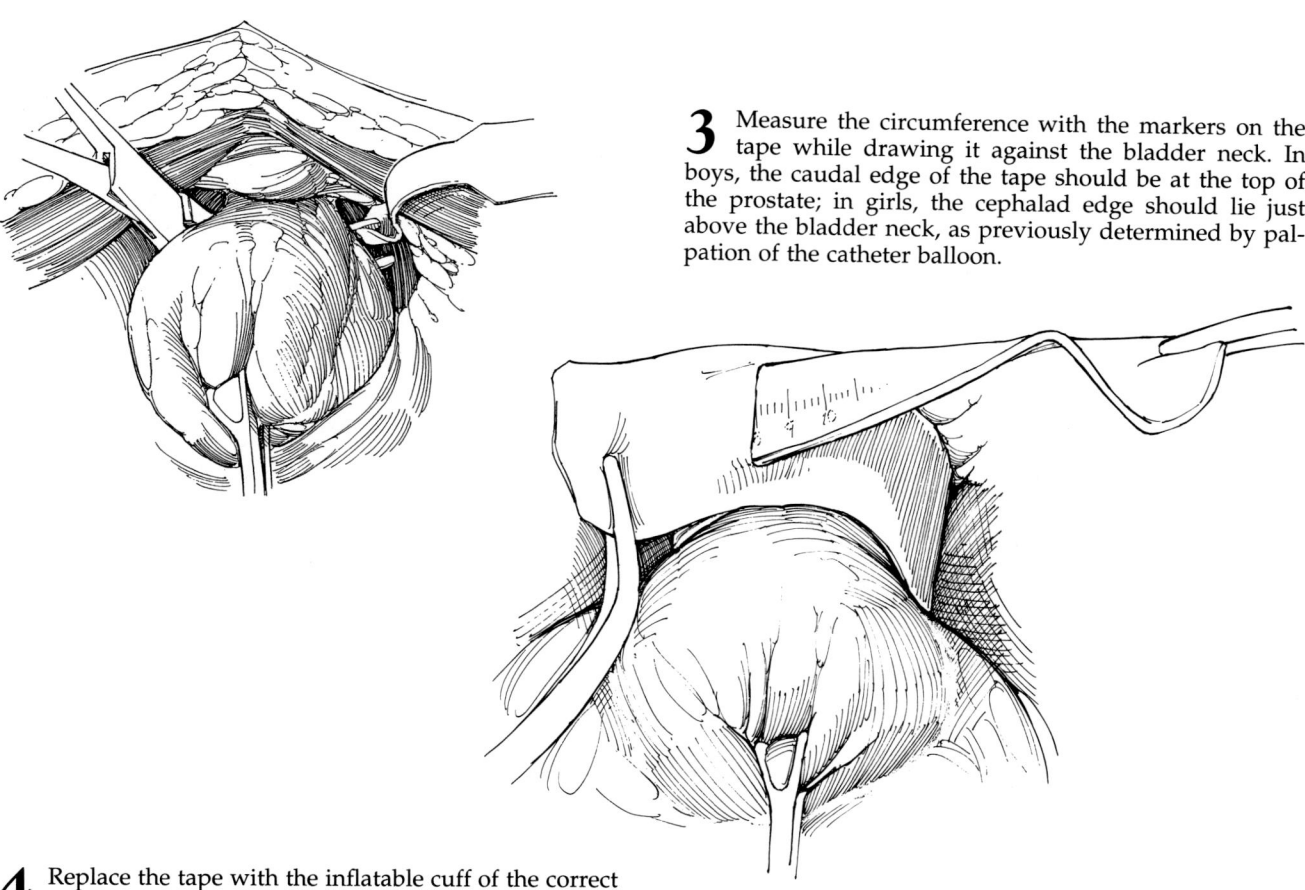

4 Replace the tape with the inflatable cuff of the correct size, and snap it into place. Pass a large clamp through the inguinal canal, and draw the tubing from the cuff and reservoir through the canal. Alternatively, use the blunt tubing needle supplied and work from inside out.

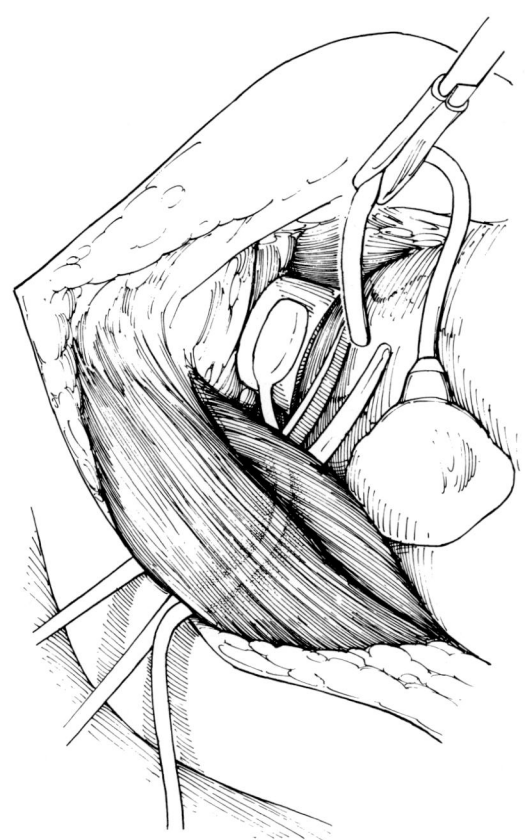

5 Run a Hegar dilator or large curved clamp down into the scrotum. Insert the pump and milk it into position. Select the pressure reservoir that will just maintain continence. Although methods are described to determine the pressure required, none are reliable. Fill the reservoir with 18 ml of isotonic contrast medium (11.7 percent Cysto-Conray II) or physiologic saline, and connect its tubing to the cuff tubing. Clamp both tubes with rubber-shod hemostats (one click only). Withdraw the fluid from the reservoir. If it contains less than 16 ml, the cuff size is too big and should be replaced (see previous step). If it is the correct size, refill the reservoir with 20 ml of solution, and connect the tubing with stainless steel connectors. Test for continence. Close the wound in layers without drainage. Continue parenteral antibiotics for 4 days and oral antibiotics for 2 weeks. Six to 8 weeks postoperatively, activate the cuff by firm pump pressure to displace the poppet valve and thus allow the fluid to flow through the pump to fill it.

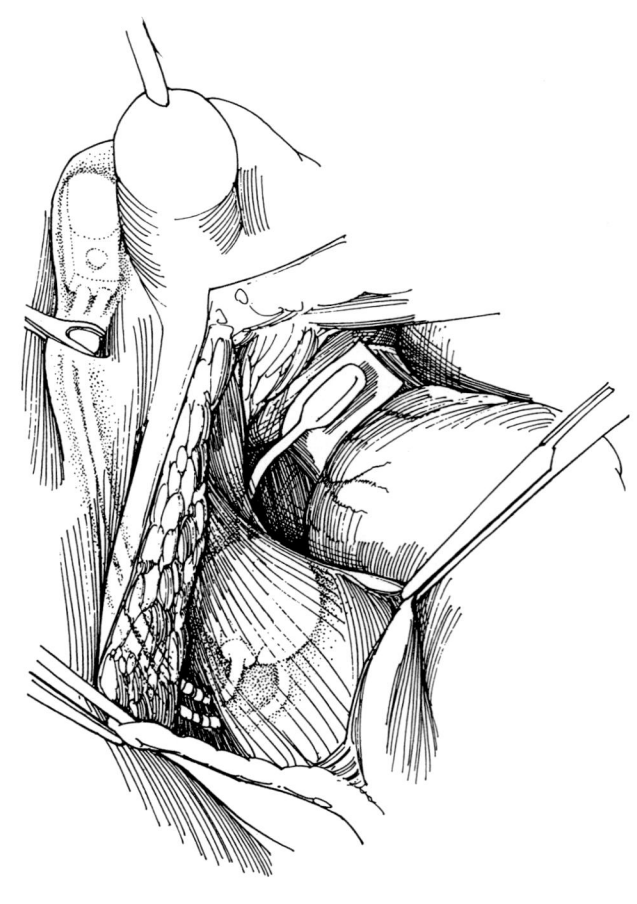

POSTOPERATIVE PROBLEMS

Persistent *incontinence* may arise from failure of the prosthesis because of leakage or may result from pressure atrophy under the cuff. If particulate matter was left in the system, its action may be intermittent and suggest a leak. Kinks in the tubing may do the same. Incontinence also may come from reflex bladder activity or poor detrusor compliance.

Infection is the greatest hazard. Preoperatively, the urine must be cleared of bacteria. Infection of the device usually requires its removal. For this reason, maintain strict asepsis postoperatively. Culture the urine if doubt exists or if for any reason, catheterization is necessary. Myelomeningocele patients have a high rate of infection of the prosthesis with both gram-positive and gram-negative bacteria; they require assiduous attention to clear bacteriuria. Should a dental procedure be required in any patient, prophylactic coverage is essential. When the devices become infected by bacteria carried by the bloodstream, it usually is at the area of least vascularity, that is, at the cuff. In an occasional case, prompt evacuation and irrigation of the infected area with antibiotic solutions can save the device.

Cuff erosion into the urethra is heralded by burning perineal pain and swelling in the scrotum at the site of the pump. Check with cystoscopy, and if cuff erosion is present, proceed with removal. In an occasional case, evacuation of the collection in the periurethral area, diversion of urine, and irrigation with antibiotic solutions can save the device.

Commentary by J. Keith Light

The artificial sphincter is designed to substitute for an inadequate sphincter mechanism and not to control abnormal detrusor function. As such, it is important to determine the status of bladder function and the presence or absence of outflow obstruction preoperatively. The urodynamic test that provides the most information regarding the lower urinary tract is video urodynamic evaluation. Following careful urodynamic testing, the surgeon will know whether to perform an augmentation cystoplasty and, if the patient is not to perform self-intermittent catheterization, ablate outflow resistance.

The surface-treated, narrow-back design cuff is now routinely implanted. These two modifications have significantly diminished the incidence of cuff leaks and tissue pressure atrophy. The cuff preferably should be placed around the bladder neck in the prepubertal child, because the prepubertal bulbar urethra usually is too small for the 4.5-cm cuff. Proper cuff sizing is still the key to a successful procedure. This is facilitated if the bladder is opened first. The cuff sizer should be tightened just sufficiently to allow the tip of the fifth finger, introduced into the opened bladder, to pass through the bladder neck. A cuff size 9 cm or larger around a pediatric bladder neck indicates inaccurate measurement or excess tissue introduced during the dissection. A 61- to 70-cm balloon significantly increases the incidence of pressure atrophy, resulting in recurrent urinary incontinence. I no longer pressurize the cuff as a separate procedure. Twenty-two milliliters of the appropriate solution is placed in the balloon, with an associated empty cuff. The deflation characteristics of the balloon still allow ample fluid to accommodate any tissue atrophy, while still maintaining the appropriate balloon pressure. Care should be taken that the balloon does not slide down the pelvic wall to impinge on the cuff. Silicone rubbing on silicone creates the "creep" phenomenon, predisposing to early leakage. Placement of connectors in an accessible subcutaneous plane allows for easy access, should revision be required, because exposure of the connectors is the first step to establish the cause of device malfunction. The development of incontinence within the first 6 months postoperatively in a patient who had reliable preoperative urodynamic evaluation and the standard surgical approach, as described in this chapter, is most likely to be secondary to either an alteration in detrusor function or an inefficient cuff.

CHAPTER 59

Female Urethral Construction

(HENDREN)

1 Place the girl *prone* in the "skydiver" position with the legs apart, the knees flexed, and the feet suspended from a stirrup holder fixed to the table. This unusual position gives ideal exposure of the anterior vaginal wall, from which a urethra or urethral extension will be constructed. An inverted U-shaped incision is made to roll into a tube, which will be the urethra. Its width depends on the size and age of the patient. It must be wide enough to roll in and close without tension.

2 Roll the strip into a tube with a running synthetic absorbable suture over a straight catheter of size appropriate for age. There is ample tissue at the level of the introitus to close two or three layers over the distal end of the tube, which will be brought close to the base of the clitoris. The technical problem is that there usually is insufficient tissue to cover the proximal tube. Hence, a buttocks flap will be used. A flap of skin and subcutaneous fat is raised from the buttocks. It must be long enough to reach high into the vagina and wide enough that good blood supply is present at the end of the flap.

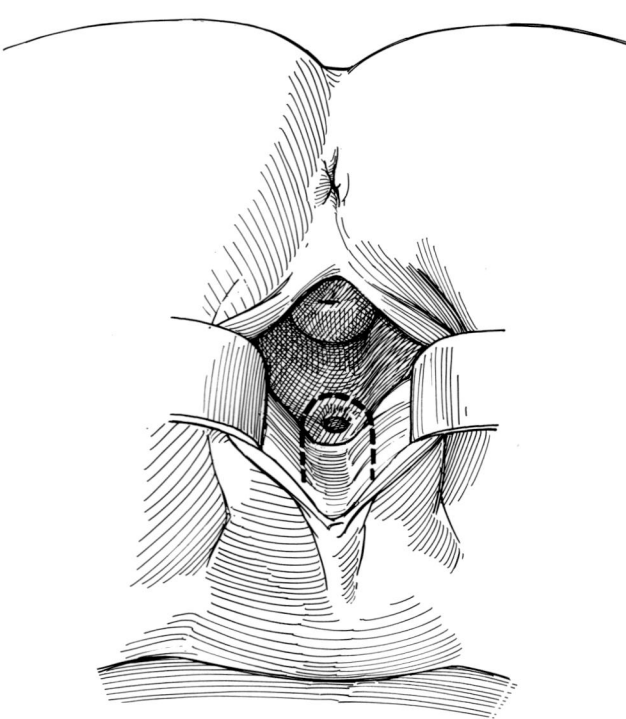

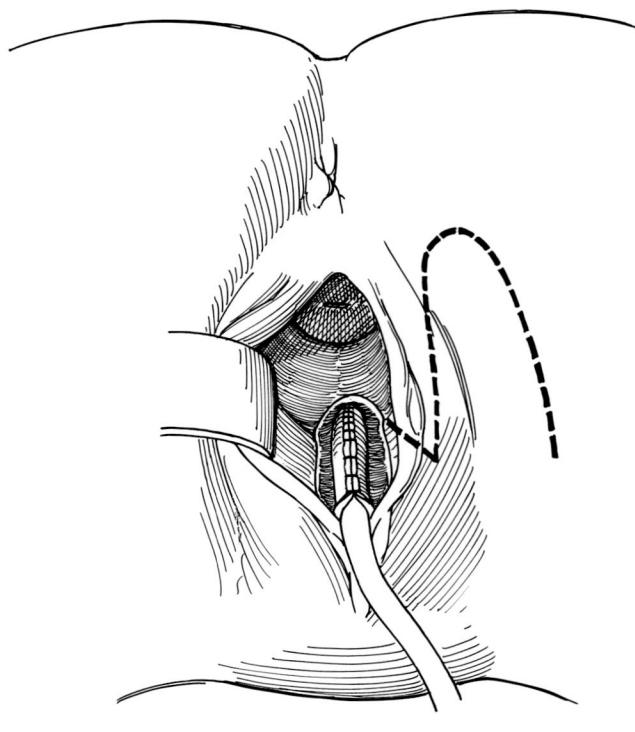

3 Open the introitus to lay the flap in place. Overlying suture lines should be avoided. Therefore, the end of the flap should be at least 2 cm higher in the vagina than the beginning of the urethral tube. Suture the flap in place with interrupted sutures. A loose dressing is applied, because a tight dressing can compress the blood supply in the base of the flap.

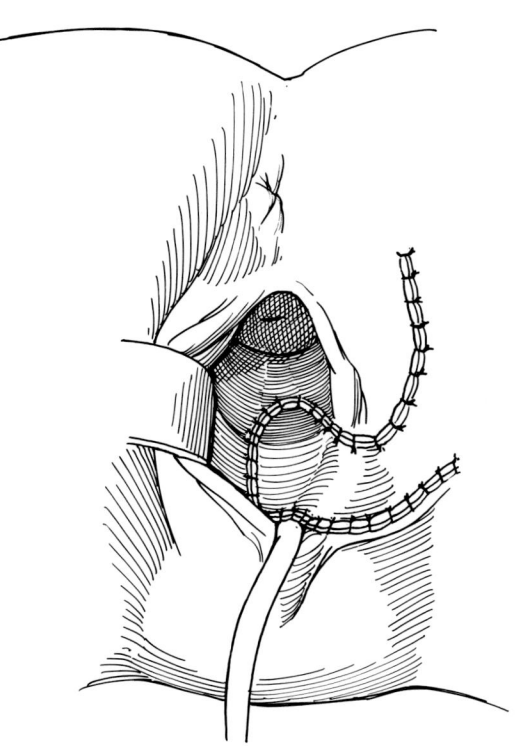

4 Several months later, the base of the flap can be divided and returned to where it came from on the buttock.

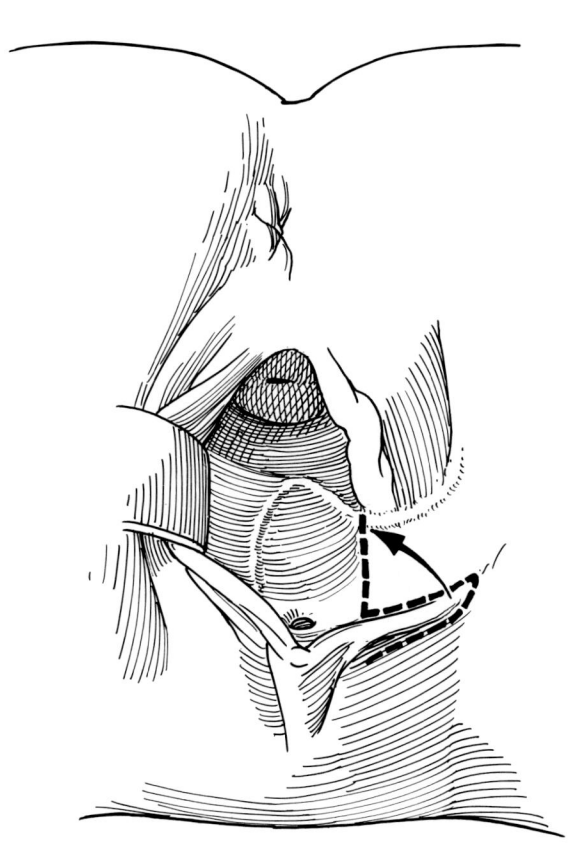

5 The introitus is then closed appropriately, giving it a normal appearance once again, with the isolated end of the flap becoming the anterior vaginal wall.

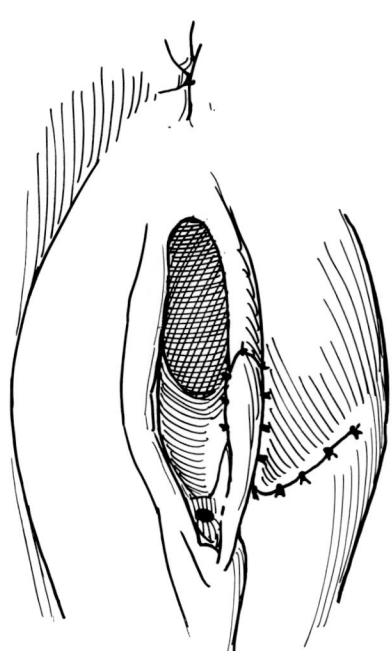

Commentary by W. Hardy Hendren

I first used this operation in 1975 to close a urethral fistula, which resulted from paucity of local tissue when a urethra was made by tubularizing the vaginal wall in this fashion. The fistula was closed and covered with a buttocks flap to prevent its reopening. The buttocks flap was substituted for the vaginal wall to create a urethra. This worked well. Since then, the operation has been used in more than 35 patients whose urethras were too short from a variety of causes, including congenitally deficient urethras, bilateral single ectopic ureters with a short urethra, severe pelvic trauma with urethral destruction, cloacal cases, myelodysplasia with short urethras, and (in one adult patient) following radical hysterectomy-vaginectomy. The average age of the patients was 13 years, with the youngest being 3 and the oldest 30 years of age. There were two fistulas requiring closure. One was caused by a dressing that was too tight on the base of the flap, resulting in necrosis. The operation was repeated 6 months later. The second fistula was caused by having the tip of the flap too close to the urethral closure. This serves to emphasize that overlying suture lines should be avoided. All of the patients originally had been incontinent. The majority were dry after having one or more operations to narrow the bladder neck and lengthen the urethra upward, with urethral lengthening from below. In some patients, urodynamic study demonstrated additional outlet resistance created by the distal urethra, which is surrounded by introital musculature.

CHAPTER 60

Retropubic YV-Plasty
(BONNIN)

Retropubic YV-plasty has few applications, so be certain of the indications (obstruction exists and it is at the vesical neck, caused by muscular dysfunction there) by performing urodynamic studies. At the same time, ascertain the competence of the distal passive sphincter by cystography, cystoscopy, and urodynamic studies. Look for trabeculation, residual urine, or both. Rule out neurologic disease and strictures, and exhaust conservative measures. Moreover, determine that the urethra is of adequate length and is free of cystocele.

Make a transverse lower abdominal (page 261) or midline (page 263) incision. Displace the prevesical fat laterally with cherry sponges and smooth forceps to expose the anterior bladder neck and urethra. Fulgurate or ligate the exposed vessels. Apply a little traction to the balloon catheter and palpate the urethra. The bladder neck now can be located accurately. The balloon is felt immediately above it, and a ring of thickened muscle is felt against the catheter. Begin the V-incision with a hooked blade, and complete it with curved scissors. Avoid a sharp angle at the apex. Incise the urethra vertically far enough to sever the thickened circularly oriented fibers of the bladder neck, but do not extend this incision any farther down the urethra. Insert a Malecot cystostomy tube of appropriate size, and bring it through the body wall via a stab wound. Suture the V-flap into the Y-extension with interrupted 2-0 chromic catgut sutures that include all layers. Pass the first stitch through the anterior urethral wall just beyond the end of the vertical incision and back through the tip of the flap. Ignore the disparity in thickness of flap and bladder neck.

Hold the ends but do not tie them. Insert stitches at the end of each arm of the V to hold up and align the wound edges. Place the next pair of sutures 4 mm away. When the sutures are all in place, starting distally, tie first one side and then the other, but tie the central suture last. Note that the flap must advance into the V. It may need to be

lengthened by rotating the ends of the bladder incision medially. Place the remaining sutures obliquely so that they draw the flap a little distally, thus removing any tension from its apex. Alternatively, place a running subepithelial layer of 4-0 plain catgut and a muscle layer of 3-0 synthetic absorbable suture. Using 4-0 chromic catgut sutures, fix a pedicle of any available extravesical fat between the suture line and pubis. Suture the cystostomy tube to the skin with a heavy silk suture. Place a Penrose drain and close the wound. Remove the urethral balloon catheter after dressing the wound. Leave the suprapubic tube in place for 10 days.

POSTOPERATIVE PROBLEMS

Persistent drainage suprapubically usually will clear if the urethral catheter is reinserted. Incontinence can result if the flap is advanced too far or if the distal passive sphincter is incompetent.

Commentary by Jeffrey Wacksman

The indications for YV-plasty of the bladder neck in children are few; this is a very limited procedure. We rarely advocate this procedure for neurovesical dysfunction. Most of the cases I have done have been on patients who have had previous bladder neck or urethral reconstructions (eg, exstrophy).

An important part of the initial procedure is to adequately mobilize the bladder by the lateral pelvic walls. In patients who have had previous surgery, this can be tedious. The flap to be cut should be broad based to preserve vascularity. The incision through the bladder neck needs to be long enough to carry through the strictured area. When possible, I prefer to accomplish a two-layer anastomosis with a running fine absorbable suture in epithelium as well as muscularis.

298

CHAPTER 61

Closure of Female Vesical Neck

Provide continent diversion or place a cystostomy at the end of the procedure. Clear the urine of infection, if possible, and provide antibiotic coverage.

The simplest method (and an effective one if well executed) to close the female vesical neck is to open the bladder, make a circumferential incision around the bladder neck to remove a divot of epithelium, and then close the muscularis and subepithelium with two layers of pursestring absorbable suture. More security may be obtained by inverting the urethra, as is done with the combined approach. The key to success is to be sure that all of the epithelium has been removed, so that the surfaces in contact are bare.

VESICAL APPROACH WITH URETHRAL INVERSION

1 Through a lower transverse abdominal or lower midline incision, enter the retropubic space, and free the urethra by dividing the pubourethral ligaments superficial to the dorsal vein complex. Dissect the urethra distally from the vagina with the aid of a finger in the vagina. Elevate the urethra from the vagina by sharp dissection with a knife to include the adventitia. The longer the segment freed by sharp dissection, the easier the procedure. Divide the urethra and ligate both ends, leaving the proximal suture long.

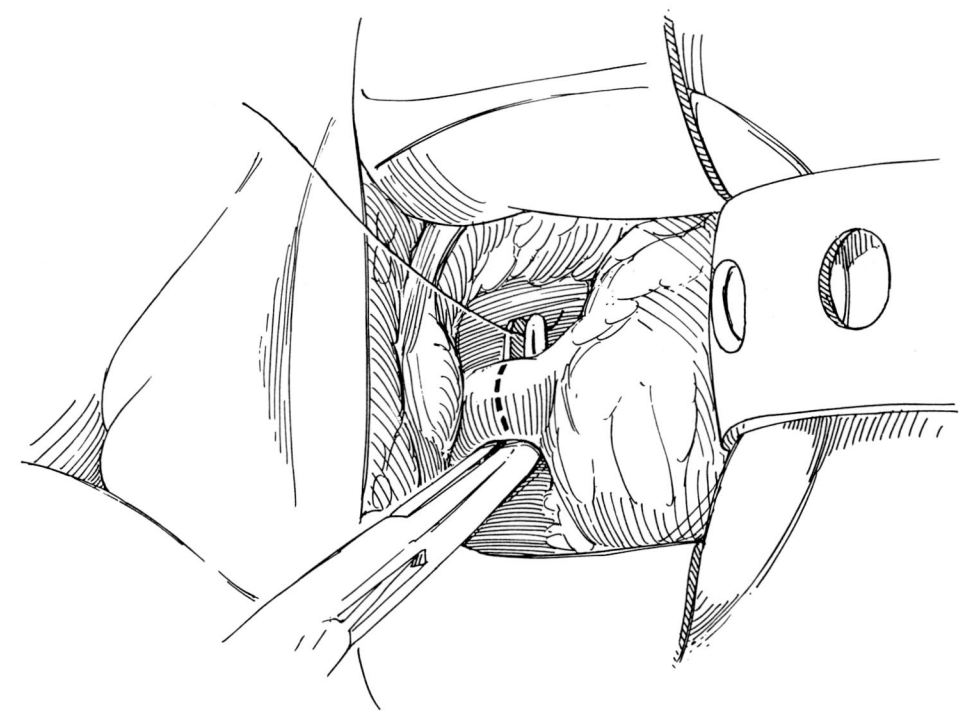

2 Open the bladder and visualize the outlet. Insert ureteral catheters for safety. Place four 3-0 synthetic absorbable traction sutures through the epithelium, closely surrounding the vesical neck. With a hooked knife, cut through the epithelium circumferentially 1 to 2 cm away from the outlet, and free up the epithelial margins with scissors.

3 Trim the freed epithelium flush with the outlet, being certain that all the lining of the outlet is removed.

Insert a curved clamp into the cut-off urethra, grasp the suture on the end of the proximal suture, and invert the urethra into the bladder. Trim the urethra.

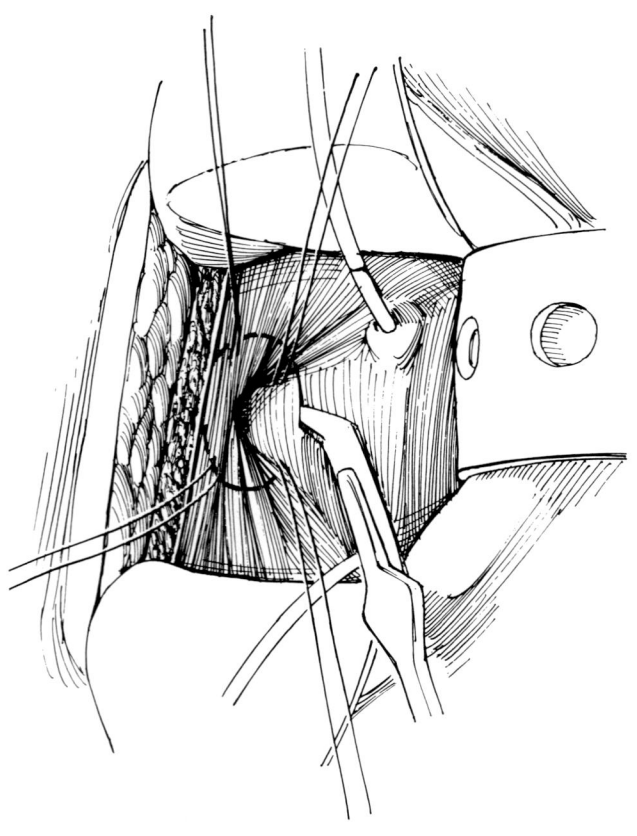

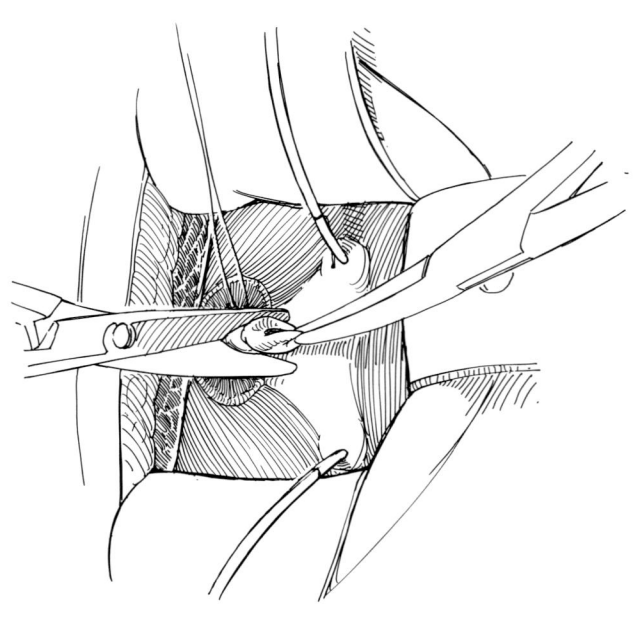

4 **A**, Close the end of the trimmed urethra with inverting sutures, and tack it to the surrounding detrusor.

B, Place a 3-0 or 4-0 synthetic absorbable pursestring suture 1 cm from the urethra that inverts the urethral epithelium as the suture is tied. Place a second circumferential suture 1 cm outside the first and tie it. Close the epithelium of the bladder over the repair with interrupted 4-0 plain catgut sutures. Insert a Malecot catheter to exit through a stab wound. Close the bladder and the wound. Further security may be had by excising the urethral epithelium perineally and obliterating that space.

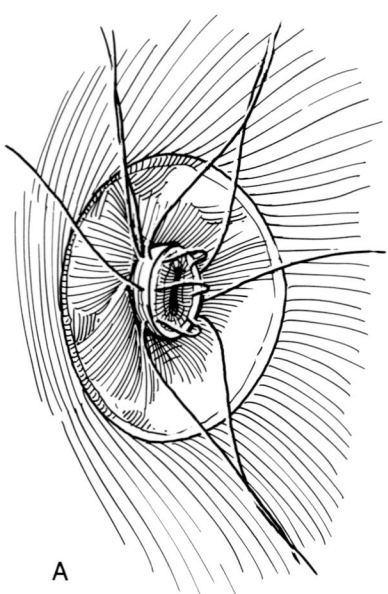

A

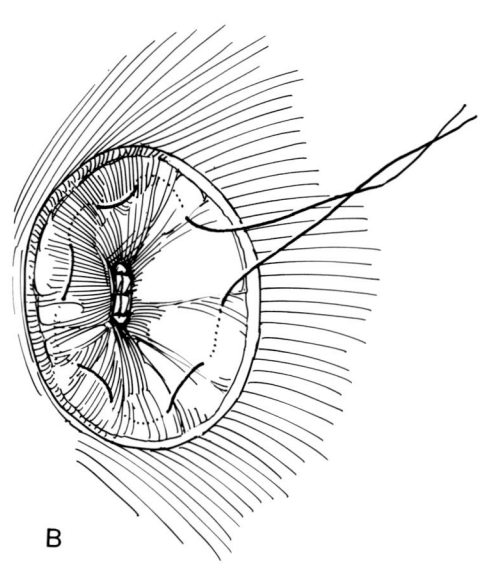

B

URETHRAL APPROACH

This approach avoids an abdominal incision yet inverts the urethra into the bladder.

5 With the child in the dorsal lithotomy position, place four traction sutures about the meatus that extend through the urethral subepithelium. Incise the meatus circumferentially. Free the urethra from the vagina and from the retropubic tissue to the level of the bladder neck by dividing the endopelvic fascia laterally and entering the retropubic space. It is necessary to divide the pubourethral ligament to expose the base of the bladder.

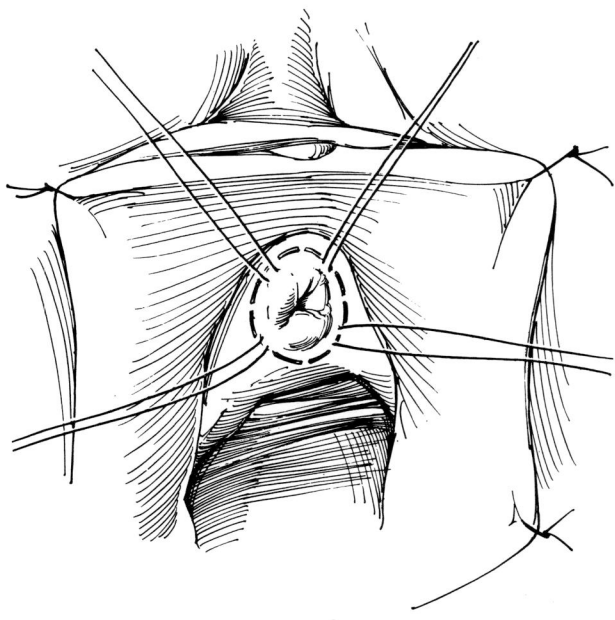

7 Approximate the periurethral fascia with several 4-0 synthetic absorbable sutures, and close the epithelium vertically with interrupted 4-0 chromic catgut sutures. Pack the vagina to reduce the chance of formation of a hematoma.

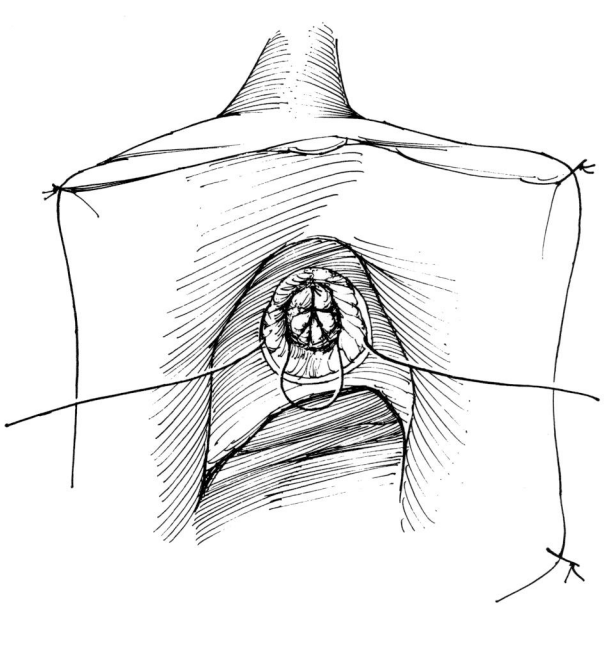

6 Place three end-on 4-0 synthetic absorbable mattress sutures in the urethral wall to invert the meatus. Alternatively, the urethra may be trimmed and closed with an inverting pursestring suture.

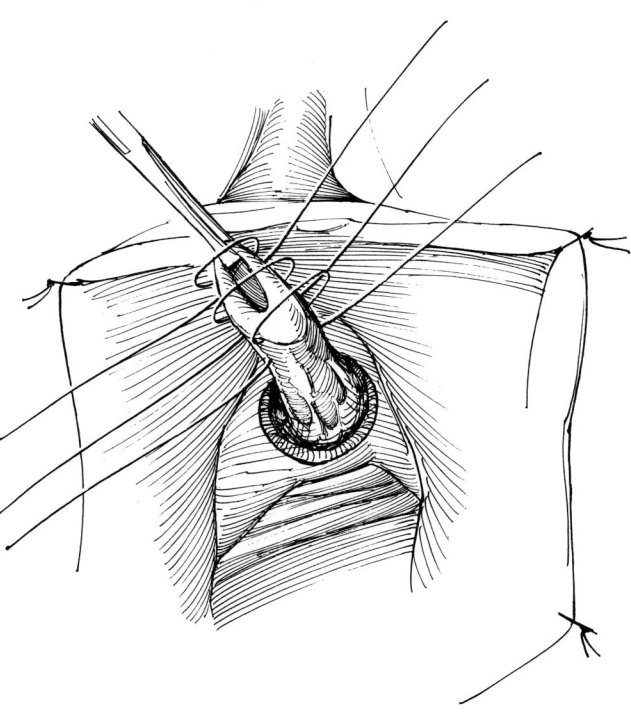

TRANSVAGINAL APPROACH
(ZINMAN)

The method may be appropriate for adolescents, especially if paraplegic.

8 With the child in the dorsal lithotomy position, fix the labia laterally with stay sutures, and place a small posterior retractor in the vagina. Incise widely around the urethra, as far as the introitus, and continue the wings of the incision into the vagina beyond the bladder neck as an inverted U.

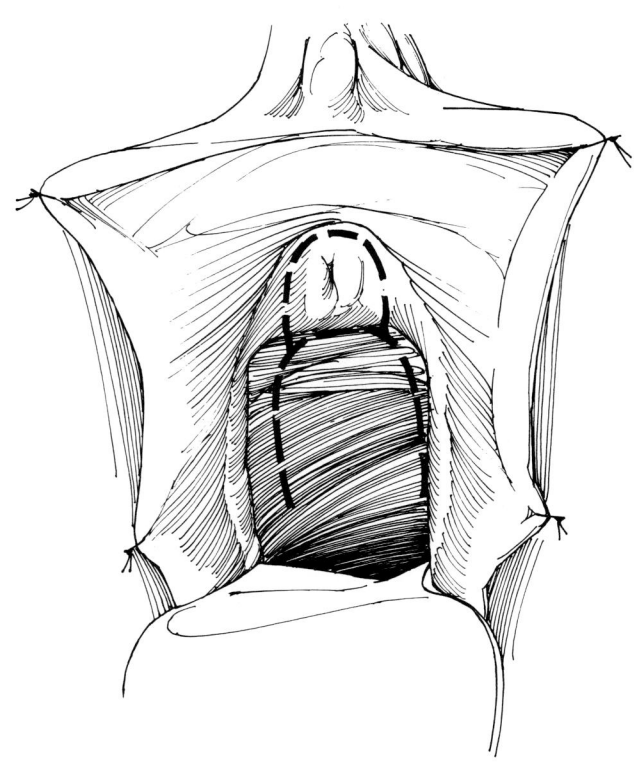

9 Free the vaginal flap from the urethra and posterior bladder neck after injecting normal saline beneath the anterior vaginal wall to help delineate the plane.

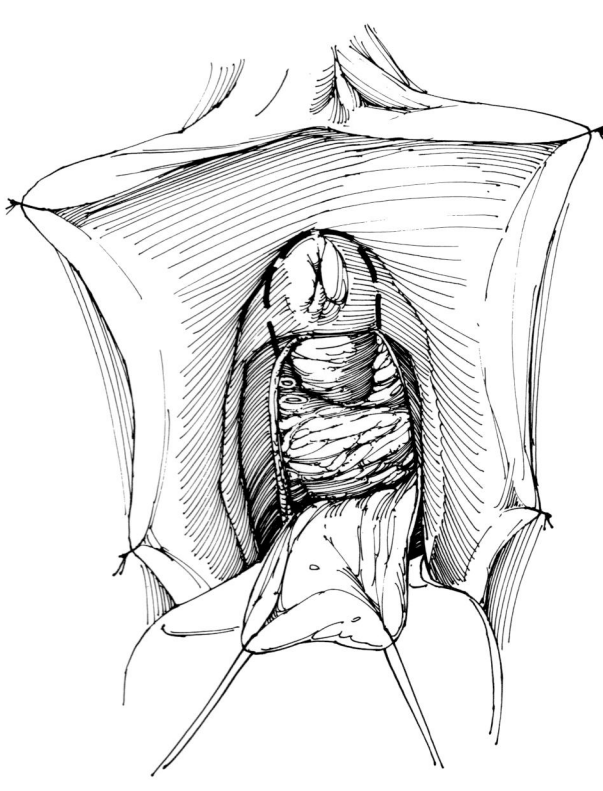

10 Continue the dissection around the urethra and bladder neck. Separate the bladder from the endopelvic fascia and from its retropubic attachments, including the pubourethral ligaments, staying close to the vesical wall. Give 5 ml of indigo carmine intravenously to identify the ureteral orifices, then trim the urethra flush with the vesical neck.

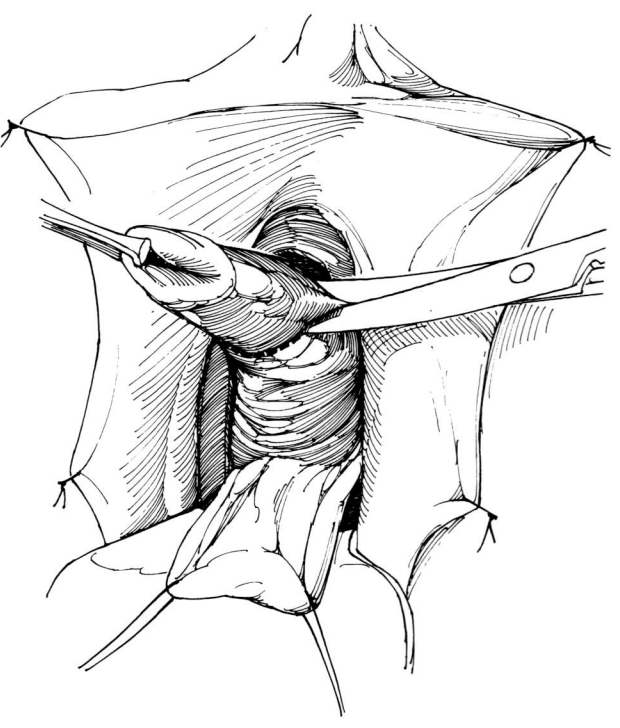

11 Close the vesical neck with a running 3-0 plain catgut suture placed subepithelially in a vertical direction. Over this, place a running 3-0 synthetic absorbable suture.

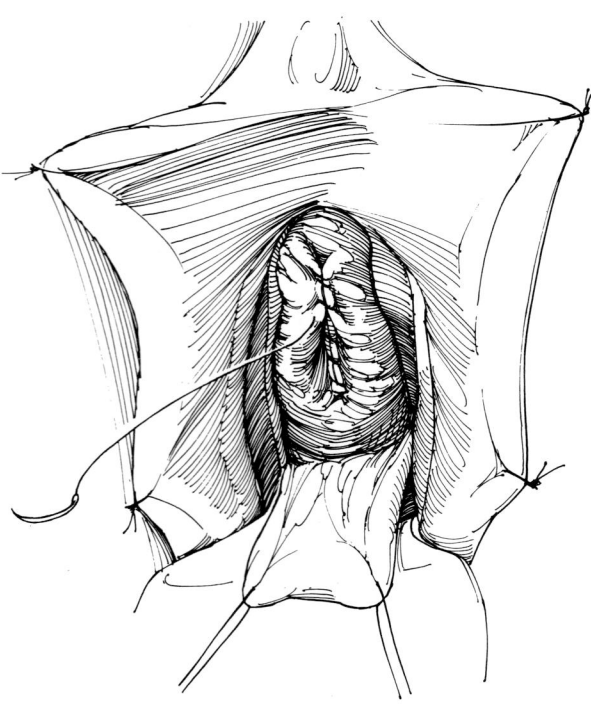

12 Reinforce this suture line with a transversely placed running 3-0 synthetic absorbable suture to the perivesical fascia and superficial layer of the bladder wall, which will move the repair behind the symphysis.

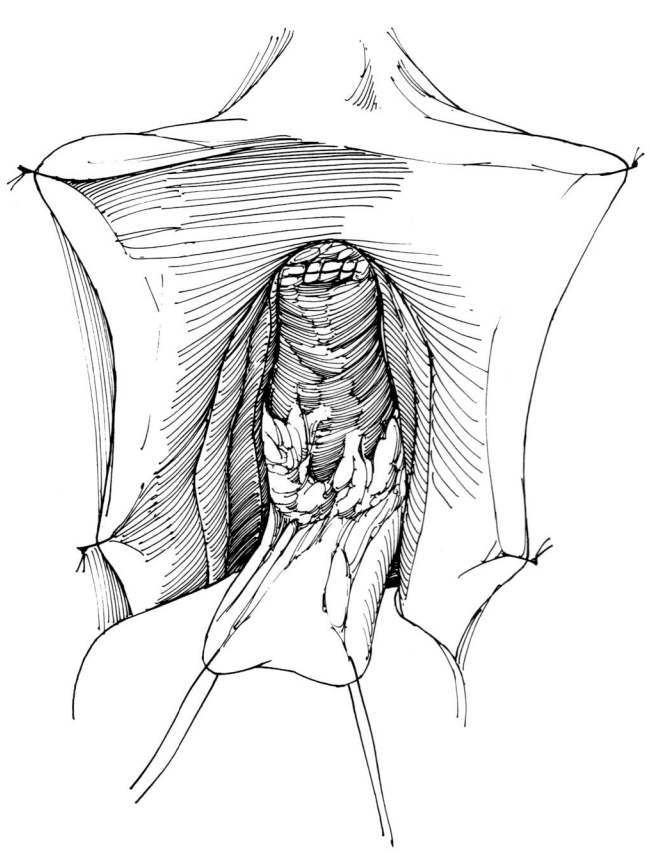

13 Bring the vaginal flap forward to cover the urethral defect, and tack it in place with four or five 3-0 synthetic absorbable subcutaneous sutures. Run a 3-0 synthetic absorbable suture with occasional lock stitches to fasten the flap to the defect. Alternatively, bring a vascularized labial fat pad into the defect before suturing the flap (page 668–670). Test for watertightness. Pack the vagina over strips of petroleum jelly gauze. Perform a continent diversion procedure, or install a suprapubic cystostomy.

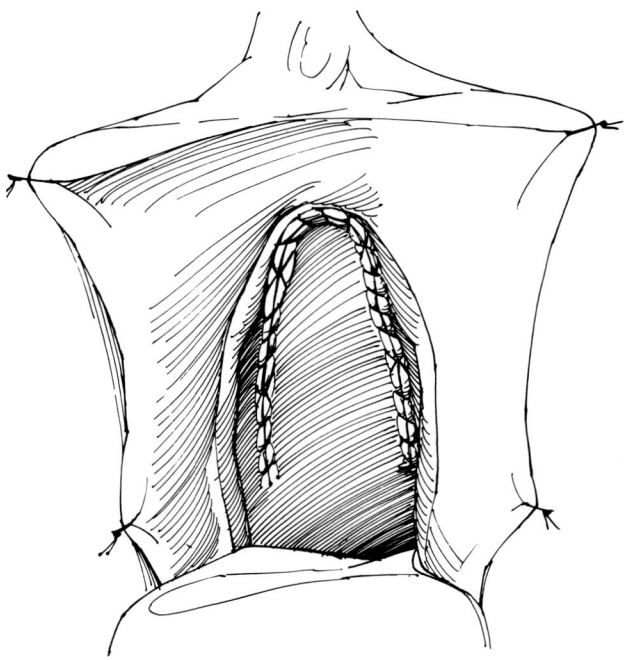

POSTOPERATIVE PROBLEMS

Leakage may appear immediately if the bladder has not been continuously decompressed. It may occur later as the sutures are resorbed and areas of injured tissue break down. Providing prolonged suprapubic drainage sometimes will allow the fistula to close.

Commentary by John M. Palmer

These drawings show the several techniques for permanent interruption of the urethra in girls and really require little comment, because the illustrations are superb, and the methods are fully and efficiently described. The procedure, however, is deceptively easy to contemplate and, unless properly performed, will suffer a high failure rate. Complete exposure is the key. This often is difficult to obtain by the retropubic approach because of anatomy distorted by previously failed surgical attempts at achieving continence. For that reason, I tend to prefer the transvaginal approach.

The key aspect of any of these well-illustrated methods is the complete division of the urethra with inversion of the proximal remnant, along with dependable vesical or supravesical urinary diversion. As long as the urothelium is fully interrupted, the surgeon can depend on a high degree of patient satisfaction with any of these techniques.

The major risk from either the vaginal or retropubic approach is a vesicovaginal fistula, which creates a situation profoundly worse than the original state. Despite meticulous dissection, complications occur and may require several additional procedures before they are corrected. Because neighboring tissues often are too flimsy for multilayered interposition closure, I try to mobilize a pedicled labial flap pad placed between the bladder and vaginal suture lines when operations are from below. The major advantage of the retropubic approach is the ready access to the omentum, which can be interposed as an additional layer to fortify the bladder neck closure and buttress any areas of weakness in the repair.

CHAPTER 62

Reconstruction for Vesical Exstrophy

IMMEDIATE STAGED RECONSTRUCTION (ANSELL-JEFFS)

Protect the vesical epithelium with coated gauze. Assess maximal bladder size with the finger, rule out hydronephrosis by intravenous pyelogram, estimate the adequacy of the rectal sphincter, and consider the state of the external genitalia (with inadequate penile length, sex reversal may be advisable). If the bladder is large enough, perform sacral osteotomy, and close the bladder. If the infant is seen within the first 48 hours after birth, osteotomy may not be necessary. Proceed with staged functional reconstruction by either the Ansell-Jeffs or the Arap technique, keeping in mind that exstrophy ranges all the way from superior vesical fissure to cloacal exstrophy. Plan the reconstruction in a series of stages, timed to take advantage of conditions at each age.

In the Ansell-Jeffs approach, the first stage creates an incontinent epispadias. It is essential that this initial bladder closure does not fail, because subsequent attempts at reconstruction will be more difficult to perform and prone to failure. In the second stage, both antireflux and continence mechanisms are formed. In the third stage, the urethroplasty is completed. The Arap technique requires a colonic or ileocecal conduit as the first stage, vesical neck construction as the second, anastomosis of the conduit to the tubularized bladder as the third, and closure of the stoma as the last stage.

First Stage: Osteotomy and Vesicourethral Closure

Perform a "pinch test" in the neonate to assess the need for iliac osteotomies. Squeeze the greater trochanters between the thumb and forefinger of one hand. If the index finger of the other hand is pinched between the pubes, osteotomy probably is not necessary. Infants older than 1 or 2 days probably will require osteotomies.

1 *In boys,* prep the lower trunk and legs after anesthesia, and place the child on sterile drapes. Wear wide-field loupes with 2.5 or 3.5× magnification.

A, Make bilateral curved sacral incisions over the sacroiliac regions.

B, Divide the iliac bones exactly vertically, with the chisel close to the sacroiliac joints, so that both tables of the ilia are divided. Close the incisions.

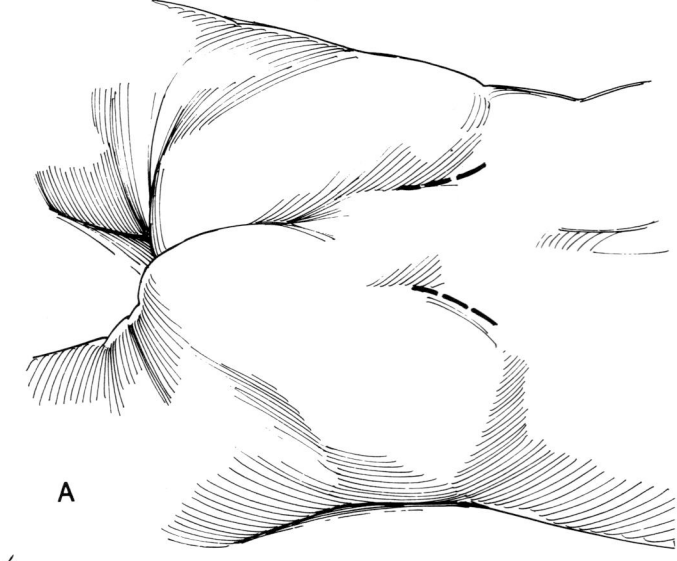

A

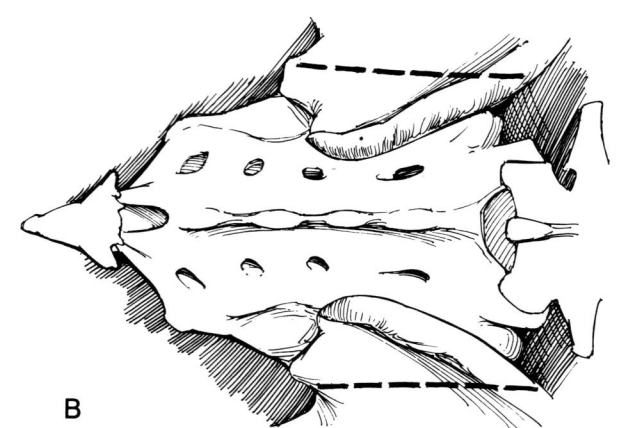

B

304

2 Turn the child over. Remove the excess umbilical cord in neonates to prevent contamination of the wound. Place a traction suture in the glans. Mark and incise around the mucocutaneous junction, including the prostatic urethra, and form two flaps lateral to the vesical neck in the paravesical skin. Free the bladder enough to be able to obtain a two-layer bladder closure. Make a circular incision through the skin and subcutaneous tissue at the proper site for an umbilicus. Incise around the umbilicus itself.

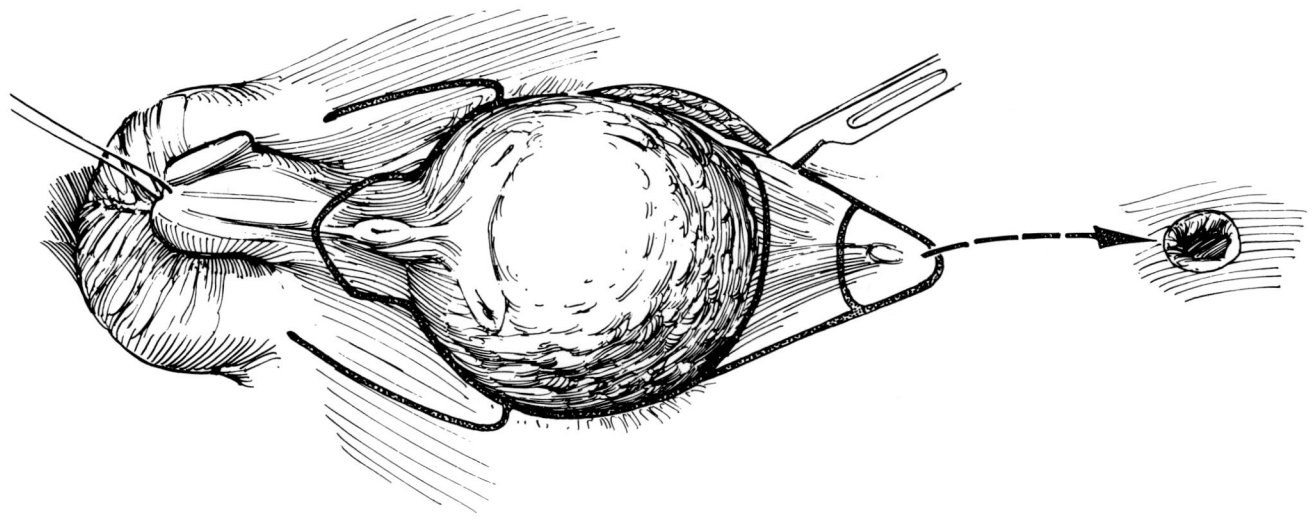

3 Start the dissection at the vesicourethral junction, and expose the subcutaneous fat. Palpate and dissect directly down on the edges of the separated pubes, which become the key to all the other important structures and will become the critical anchors for the stability of the entire closure. The rectus tendon and sheath, the perineal musculature, and the corpora cavernosa all attach to the pubis or to the adjacent ischial rami.

Clear the subcutaneous fat from the rectus fascia and muscle bellies, and remove the mucocutaneous scar. Elevate the urethral segment with small hooks to expose successively the bifid suspensory ligament, corporal bodies, and crura. Carefully dissect their medial borders, and avoid the neurovascular bundle. Place traction on the penile suture to open the space between penis and prostate, then approximate the corporal bodies for a short distance with 4-0 synthetic absorbable sutures. Close the penile skin over the joined corpora.

4 Expose and grasp the urachus and obliterated hypo-gastric arteries below the umbilicus to allow sharp and blunt dissection of the peritoneum from the dome of the bladder. Excise the rudimentary umbilicus, while preserving its deep attachments. Carefully burrow upward subcutaneously to the site where the button of skin had been excised. Move the umbilicus to the new site, and fix it with interrupted 4-0 nonabsorbable sutures. For alternative methods of umbilicoplasty, see page 321.

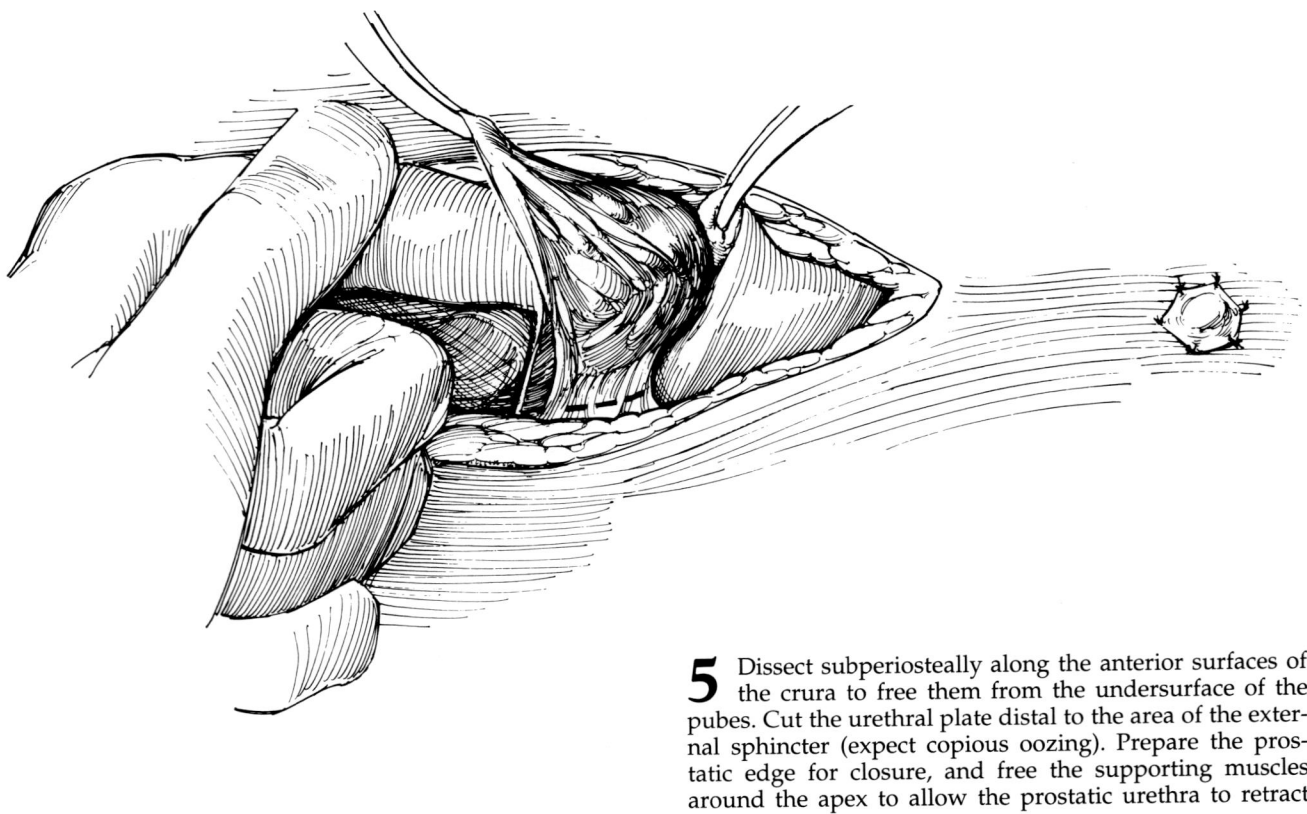

5 Dissect subperiosteally along the anterior surfaces of the crura to free them from the undersurface of the pubes. Cut the urethral plate distal to the area of the external sphincter (expect copious oozing). Prepare the prostatic edge for closure, and free the supporting muscles around the apex to allow the prostatic urethra to retract cephalad.

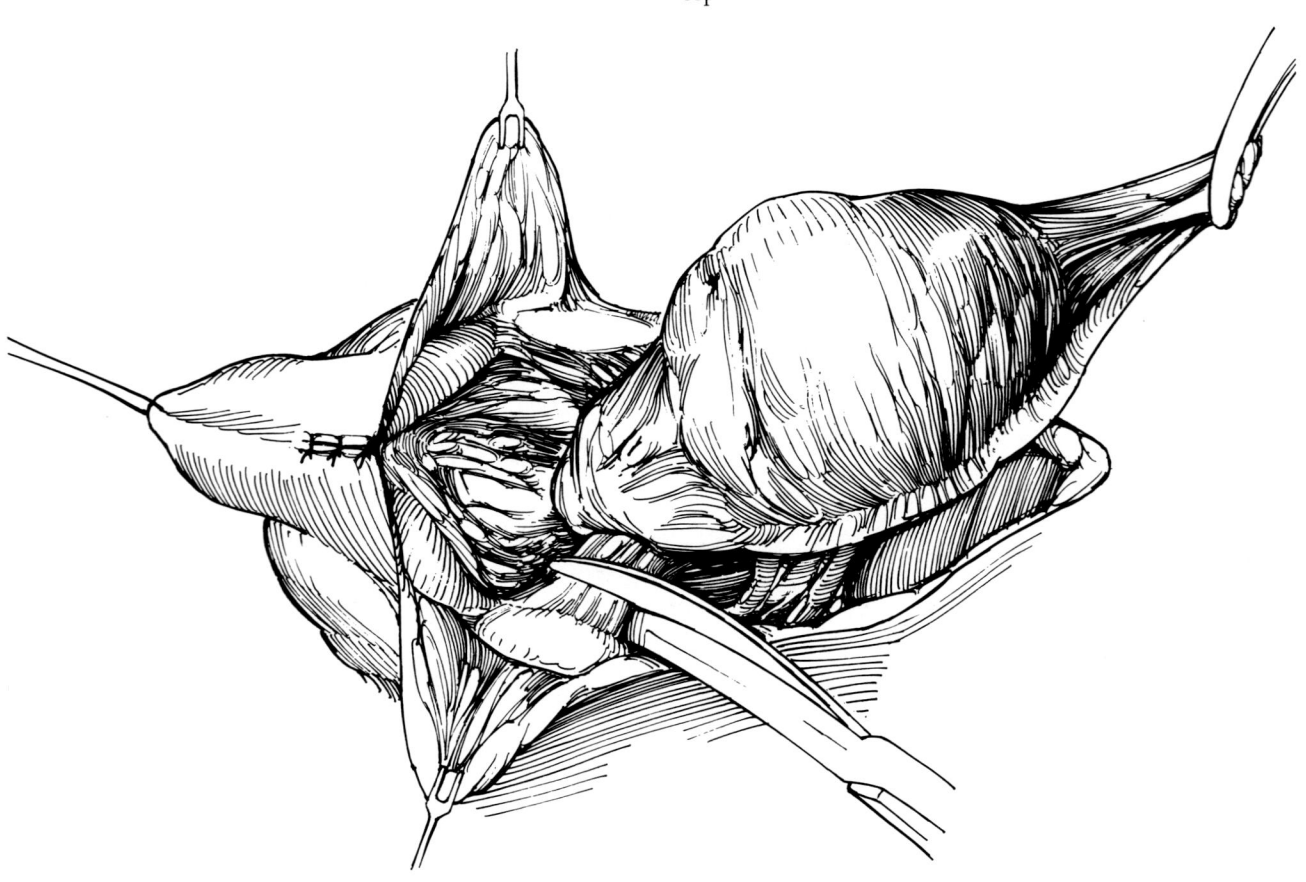

6 Place a small Malecot catheter (or, in infants, a 5 or 8 F feeding tube) in the dome of the bladder. Approximate the corpora cavernosa as far cephalad as possible without undue tension. Close the overlying pair of exstrophy skin flaps over the corpora to lengthen the urethra. Bring the distal edge of the prostatic urethra down, and suture it with both subcutaneous and skin sutures to the proximal edge of the skin flaps.

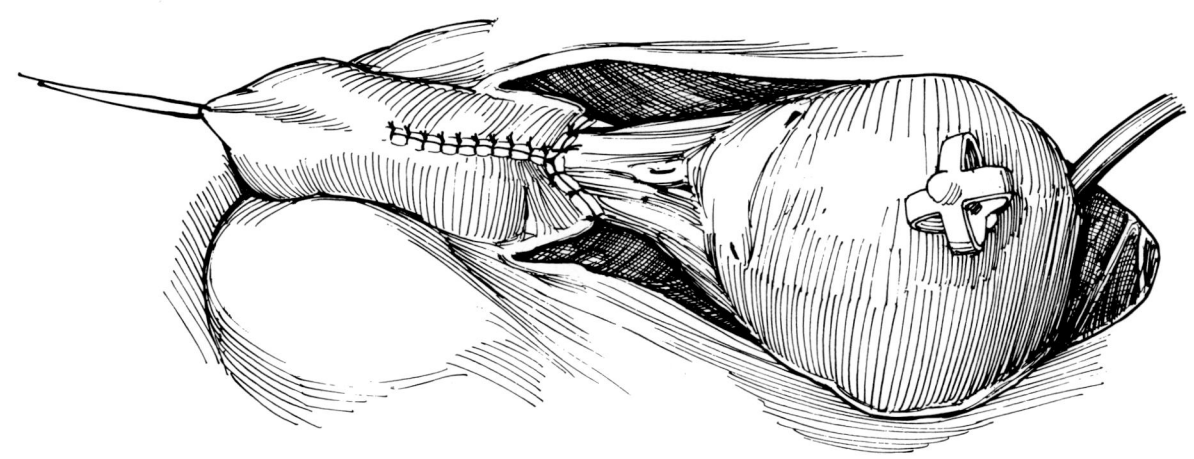

7 Insert 3 F infant feeding tubes into both ureters as far as the lumbar spindles. Lay a 10 F Robinson catheter along the proposed urethra. Approximate the prostatic urethra with 4-0 synthetic absorbable sutures, grasping the full thickness of the tissue. Draw the ureteral tubes through the bladder wall in either side, and suture them in place. Trim the attenuated epithelial edges from the bladder, and close with 4-0 synthetic absorbable sutures. Continue closure until tension limits further approximation.

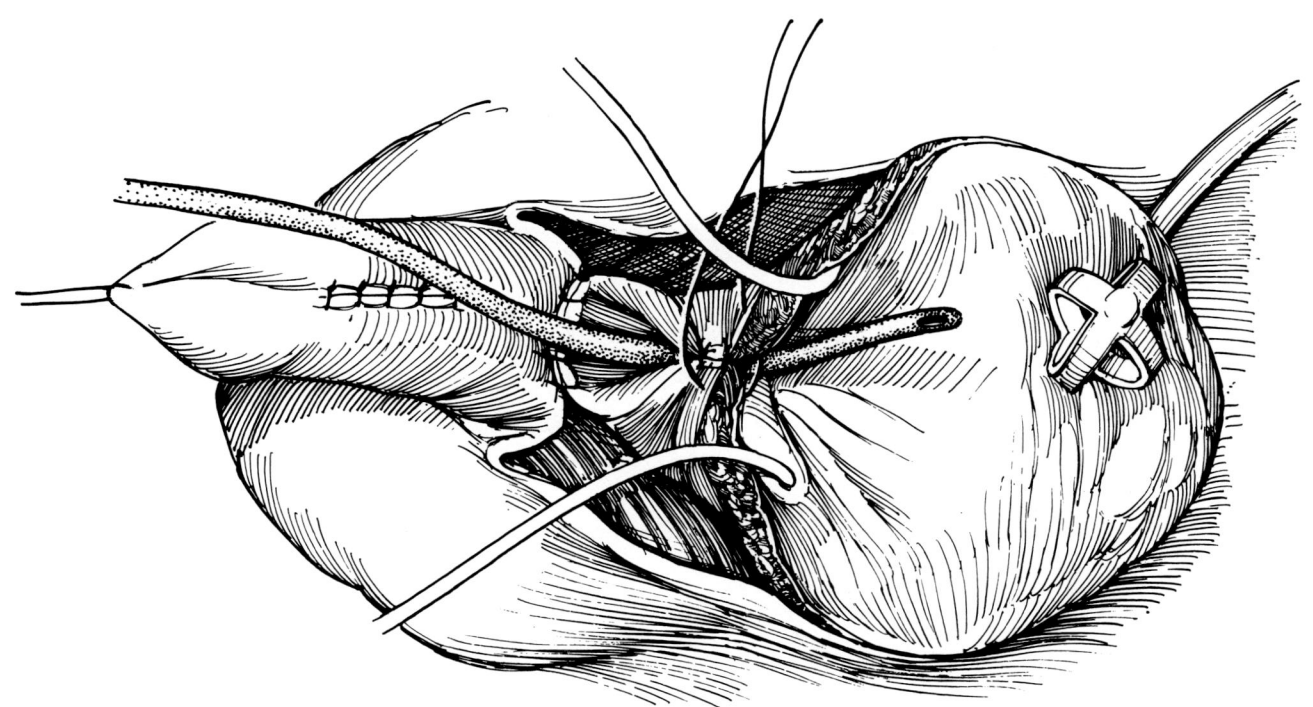

8 *In female neonates,* for primary closure use paraexstrophy flaps for urethral construction (Spindel *et al.,* 1988). Mark and elevate strips of skin 2 cm in length lateral to the bladder, carefully preserving the blood supply from below.

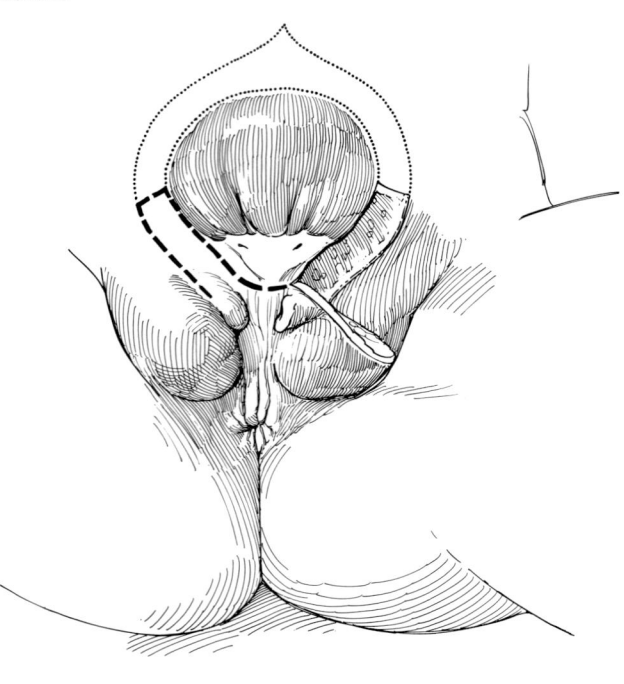

9 Divide the urethral plate, and allow the bladder to move intra-abdominally.

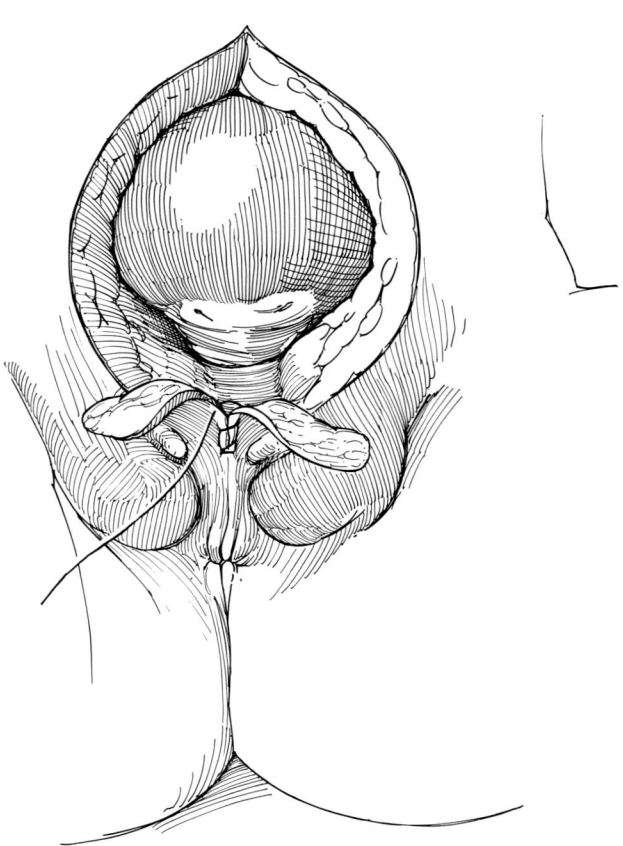

10 Approximate the medial edges of the skin flaps with running full-thickness synthetic absorbable stitches. Place ureteral and urethral stents to exit through the urethra and a Malecot catheter through the bladder wall before closing the bladder neck.

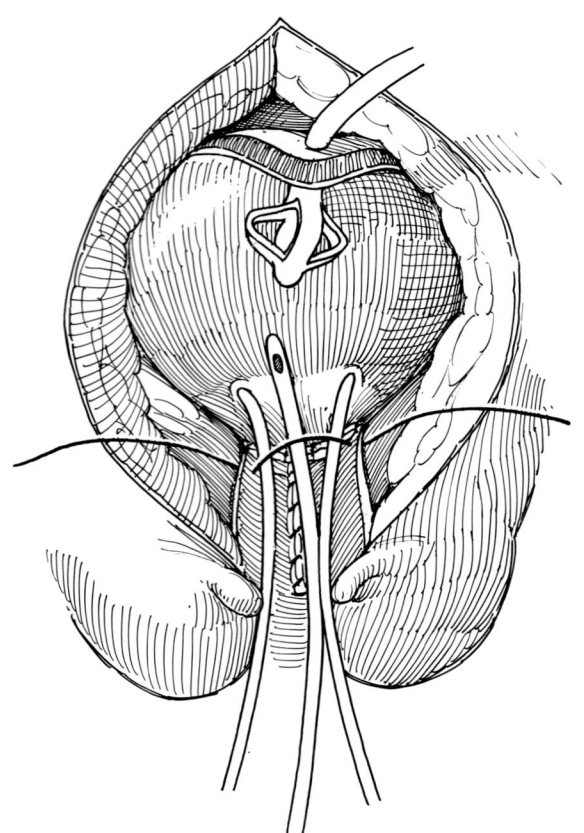

11 Close the flaps anteriorly with a running absorbable suture, and anastomose the new urethra to the bladder neck with interrupted sutures. Approximate the pubic rami and join the bifid clitoris. Place the infant in Bryant traction for 4 weeks, and remove the suprapubic tube a week later if the bladder empties.

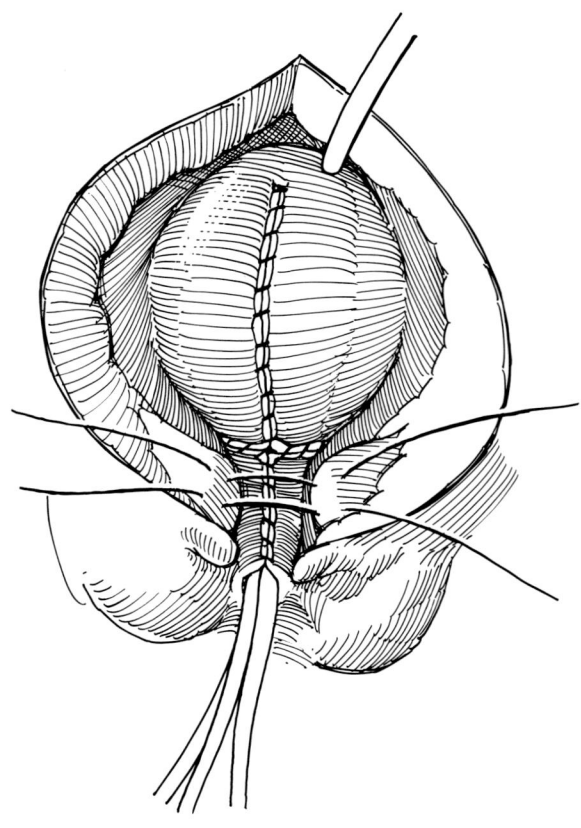

12 *In boys* (continued), place a second row of sutures in the bladder wall extending into the prostatic urethra.

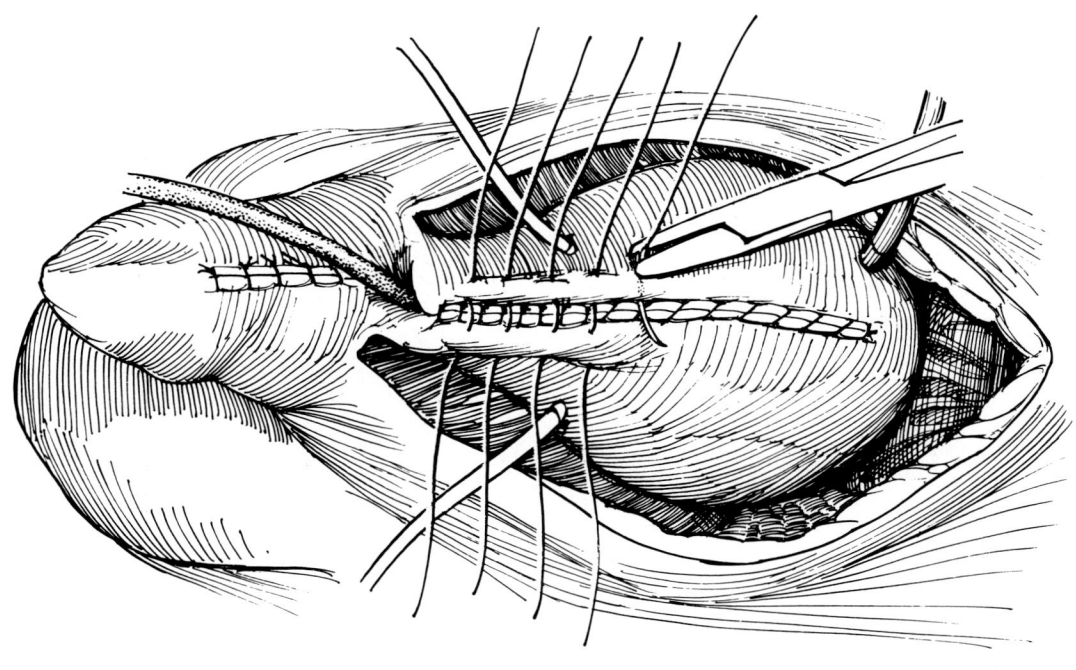

13 Suture the edges of the muscle and the fascial layers together over the urethra, so that closure of the bladder can be continued without undue tension. It may be necessary to tie these sutures while the symphyses are being held together by internal rotation of the legs.

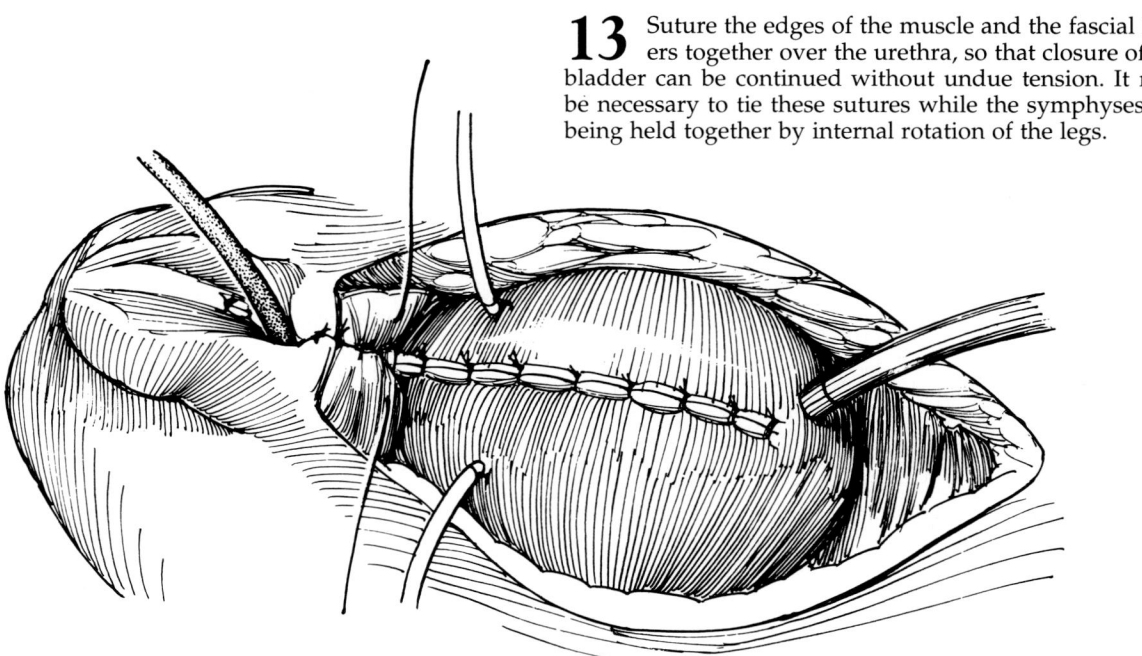

14 Place two #1 polyglactic acid sutures as a horizontal mattress suture deeply in the periosteum through all layers of the anterior surface of the symphysis on each side, avoiding the pudendal bundles. While your assistant compresses the pelvis and rotates the legs inward using the greater trochanters as levers, tie each suture with five square knots. An alternative is to insert a plastic electrician's strap (Tygon-tie) and cinch it down during the trochanteric compression. Bring the ureteral and vesical catheters to the surface through stab wounds, and sew them to the skin with nonabsorbable sutures. Check for leakage with saline in a 30-ml syringe. Remove the urethral catheter.

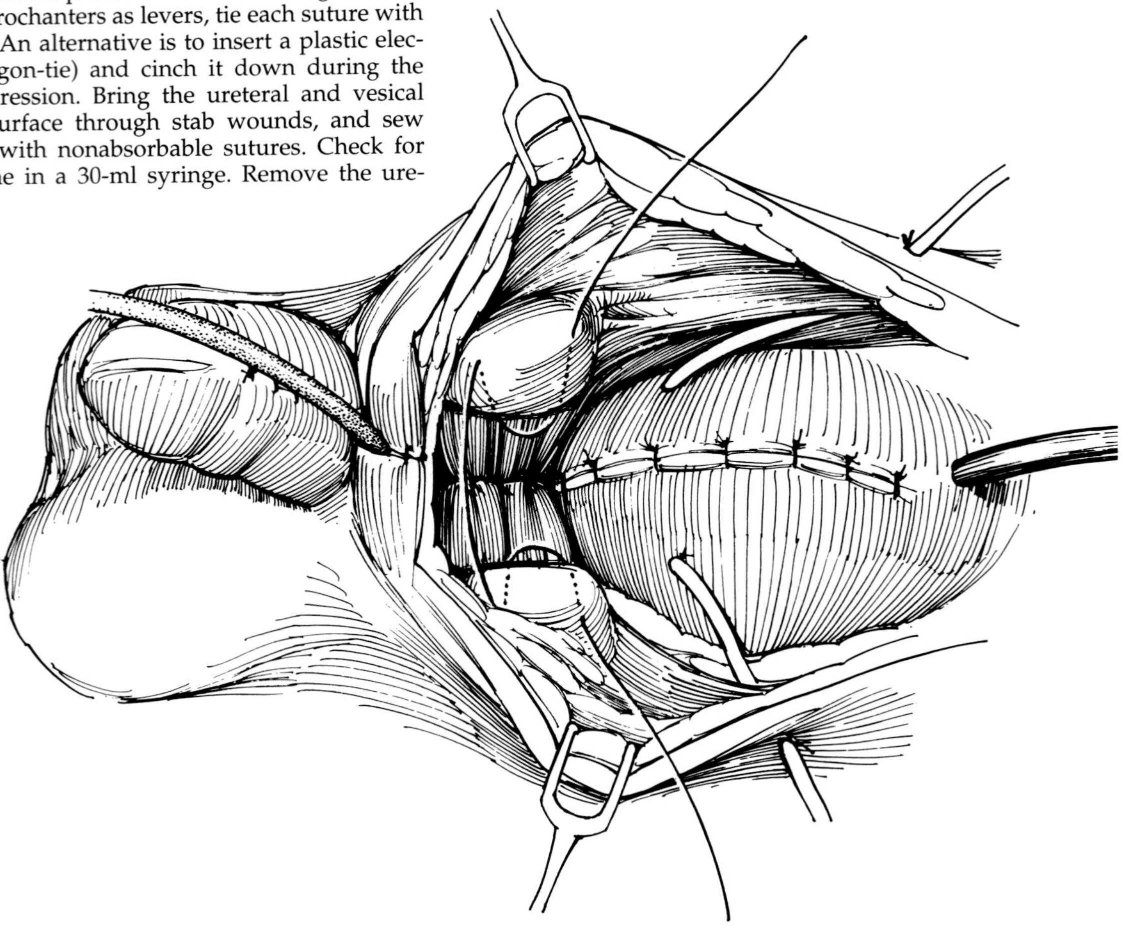

15 Approximate the laterally displaced edges of the rectus muscles. A rectus abdominis muscle flap divided at the costal margin and rotated on the inferior epigastric vessels may be placed over the bladder and its neck to fill the defect and reduce scarring (page 52). Avoid superimposition of suture lines. Close the skin with fine interrupted nonabsorbable sutures.

Either bind the lower thighs, knees, and calves together with elastic bandage for several weeks, or place the child in modified Bryant traction. Maintain the child on intravenous antibiotics (ampicillin and gentamicin) for 7 days. Remove the ureteral catheters in 8 to 10 days and the suprapubic tube in 3 weeks.

At 4 weeks, calibrate the urethra with a catheter or cystoscope to verify its adequacy. Obtain intravenous urograms. Check for residual urine, and clear any infection with antibiotics. Continue regular follow-up of upper and lower tracts. Dilate the urethra if residual urine and backpressure develop. At 3 to 5 years of age, measure bladder capacity during distention. It should be at least 60 ml; if it is less, delay bladder neck reconstruction until capacity improves, but proceed with epispadias repair.

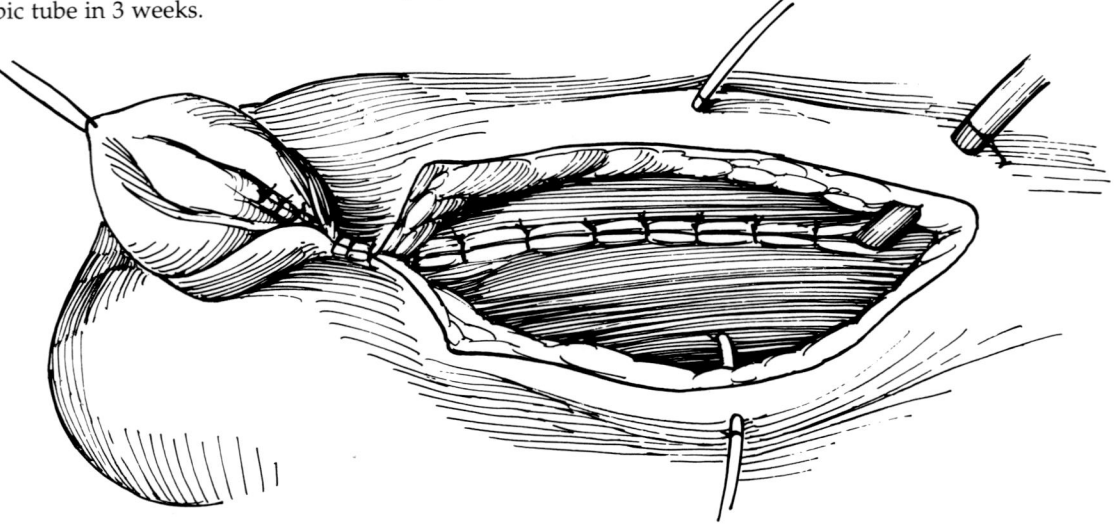

Second Stage: Antireflux and Incontinence Procedures

Make a low transverse incision, and perform a transtrigonal ureteroneocystostomy (Cohen technique) (page 208). Place stents. Construct the posterior urethra over a catheter. Remove the catheter.

16 A and B, Place several suspension sutures in the urethral wall, and pass them through the tissue at the upper margin of the symphysis to elevate the urethrovesical junction. Insert a 10 F Malecot catheter above the upper end of the suture line. In children with large bladders, the stents and cystostomy can be omitted. Attach a container of normal saline to the catheter, and check for urethral leakage as it is raised to 60 cm. Elevate the suspension sutures until leakage stops. Although visual judgment may be best, urethral pressure profiles, if measured, need to show an effective length of 2.5 to 3.5 cm and a closure pressure between 50 and 60 cm H_2O. Close the incision in layers, bringing the catheters through stab wounds.

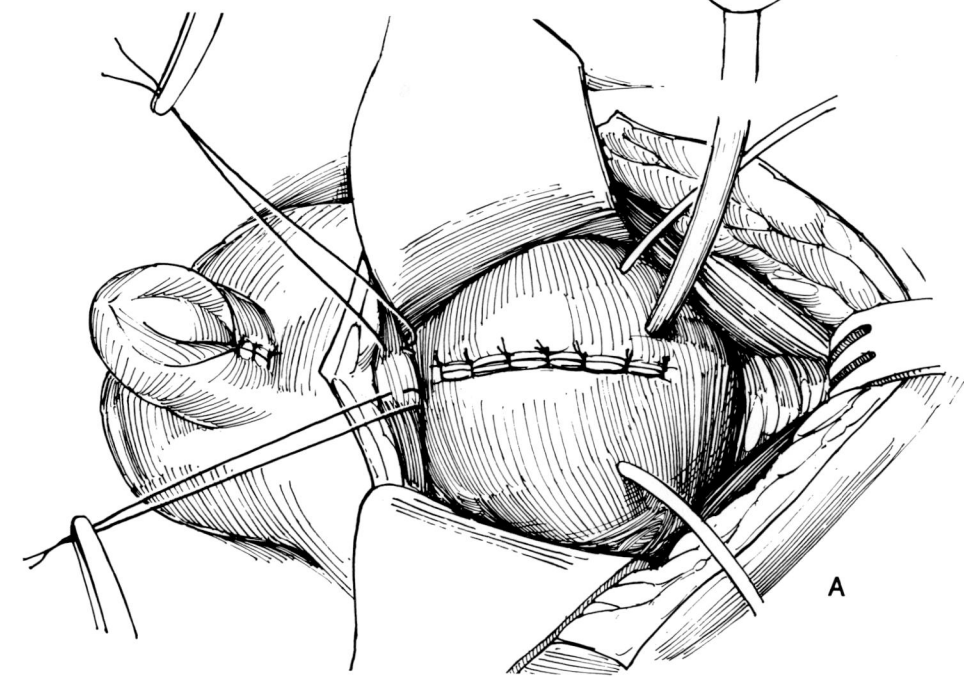

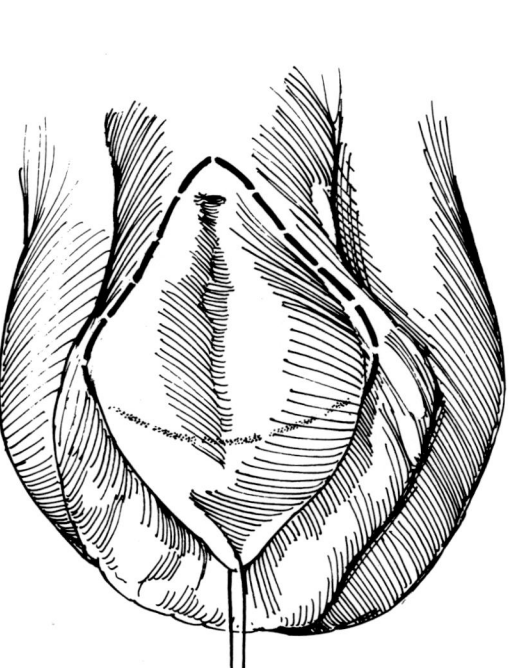

Third Stage: Epispadias Repair

17 Insert a traction suture in the glans. Mark and incise the skin, beginning around the urethral meatus and continuing around the coronal sulcus, degloving the shaft.

18 **A**, Make a Z-incision in the urethral plate.

B, Free the flaps from the groove between the corpora cavernosa, and suture them in tandem to lengthen the shaft. Be prepared for considerable oozing. If chordee persists, as shown by inflating both corpora (use two needles), consider inserting patches of dermis. Incise the glans on either side of the urethral groove.

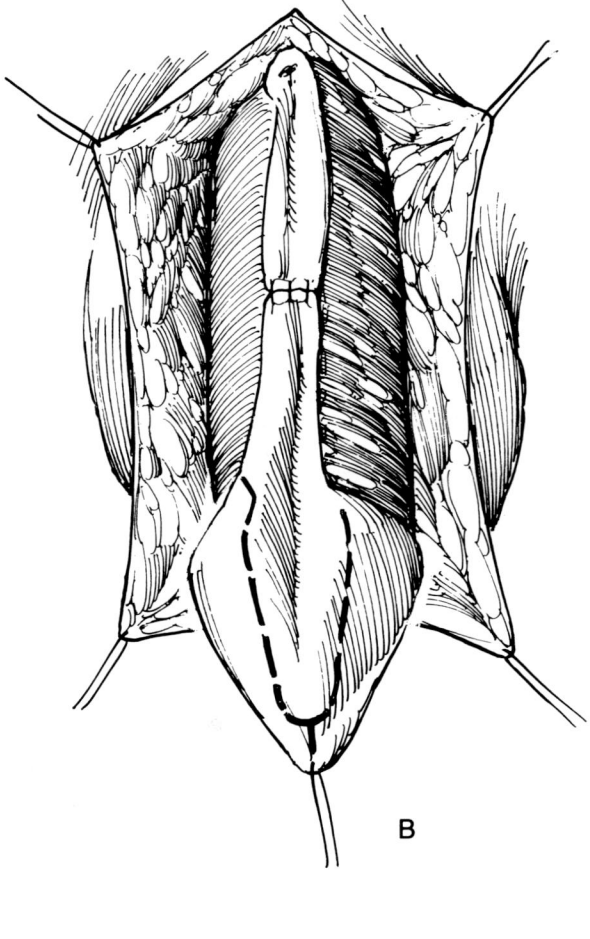

B

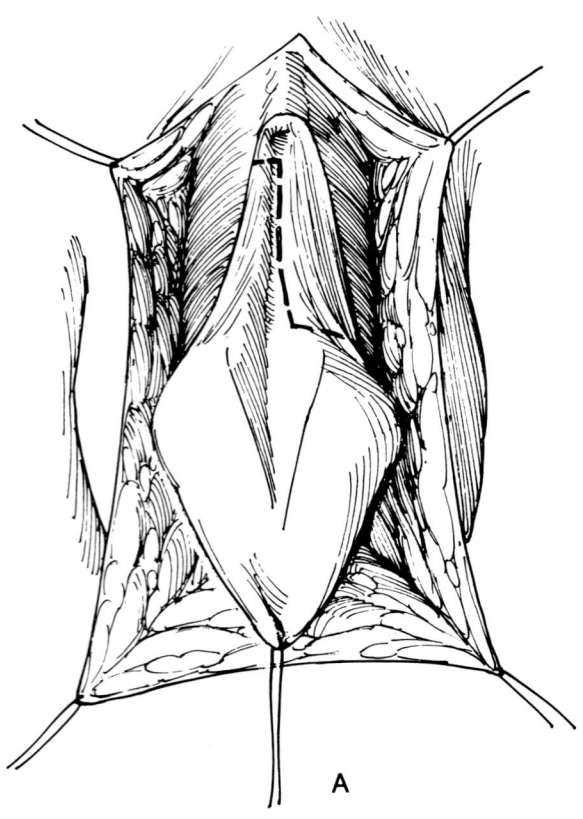

A

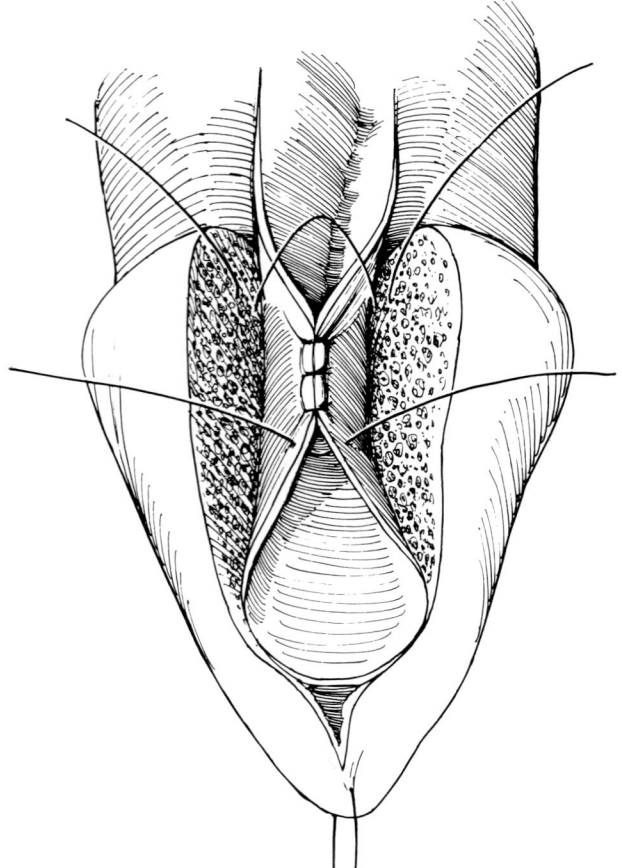

19 Raise the epithelium and subepithelium on one side to form a tube; close it with 5-0 synthetic absorbable sutures. Partially divide the glans vertically, and pass the neourethra between the denuded surfaces. Suture the glans over the tube in two or three layers, and fasten it around the new meatus. Close the Z-plasty end to end.

20 Obtain a preputial island flap (page 588), and form the roof of the urethra up to the site of the old meatus.

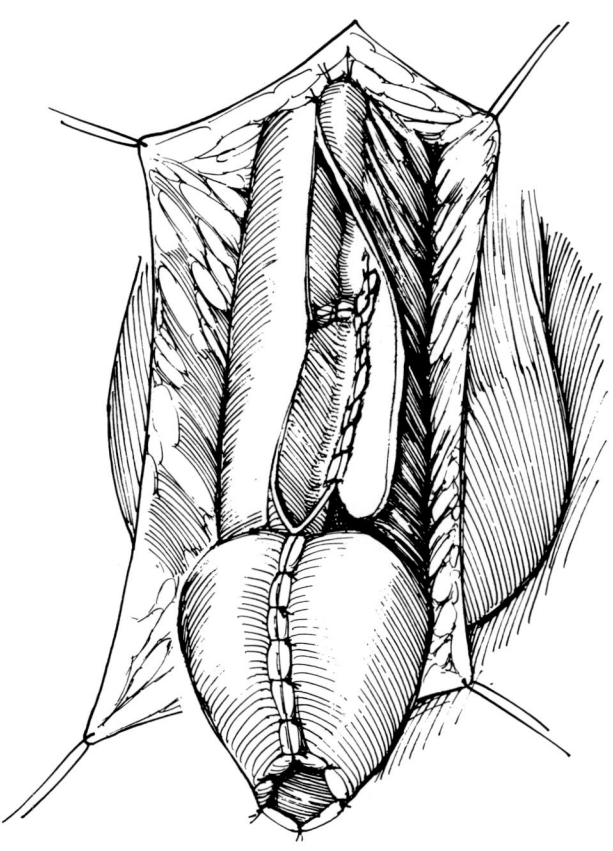

21 Apply the skin originally degloved back onto the shaft. Transpose the remainder of the ventral prepuce after unrolling it.

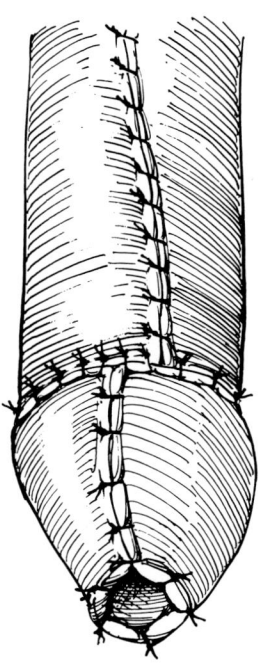

POSTOPERATIVE PROBLEMS

Dehiscence after bladder closure, or at least fascial separation, will make subsequent operations to obtain a continent bladder virtually impossible. A *stricture* may form at the bladder neck or in the neourethra, resulting in poor emptying and stone formation. A vesicostomy may be required. It may be advisable to delay closure of the bladder neck until a time when the child can be managed with intermittent catheterization. Upper-tract obstruction must be watched for assiduously.

Eventual adequate bladder capacity is jeopardized by failure to perform initial osteotomy, repeated closures of the bladder, recurrent infections, prolapse of the bladder and dehiscence (because of too short a bladder neck and posterior urethra, presence of a urethral catheter after repair, or an insecure closure of the pelvic ring, as well as abdominal distention and inadequate provision for urinary drainage), calculi, and the formation of a vesicostomy (Gearhart and Jeffs, 1991). The new outlet may be compromised by having too large or too small a caliber (14 F is ideal), less than 6 weeks of suprapubic drainage, less than 2 weeks of diversion through ureteral stents, failure to stent a concomitant epispadias repair, lack of adequate antibiotic coverage, and failure to calibrate the new urethra before and after the suprapubic tube is removed.

Failed closure of exstrophy can be managed by urinary diversion and removal of the bladder, by waiting 6 months and trying again, or by closing the bladder with temporary urinary diversion and subsequently arranging some form of continent diversion. Vesicostomy is to be avoided.

Commentary by Lowell R. King

Bladder exstrophy remains one of the most challenging problems in urology. Closure usually can be achieved, but continence remains somewhat ethereal, and male patients often need several procedures to lengthen the penis and move enough skin to the dorsum to make it dependent. In the past two decades, several principles that have evolved for the management of exstrophy have helped to standardize the treatment, and continence rates gradually have increased. Even more important, because the great need to prevent reflux has been recognized, the upper tracts are now less likely to suffer hydronephrosis and deteriorate following closure (Jeffs, 1987).

A consensus exists that there is an advantage to closing bladder exstrophy in the neonate. For the most part, this advantage results from the cartilaginous nature of some of the pubic bones at birth and to the relative relaxation in the sacroiliac joints. Most pediatric urologists prefer to use osteotomies to facilitate closure of the pelvic girdle; however, as this lessens pressure on the abdominal incision after closure and makes healing *per primam* more likely. This primary closure is proving to be important, because a much lower percentage of patients gain urinary control after secondary or tertiary bladder closures than in instances in which the bladder is successfully closed at the first operation.

Historically, approximation of the pubic symphysis over the bladder neck and urethra never has been considered important in itself. However, if the distance between the pubic rami can be reduced, the bladder assumes a more normal position deeper in the pelvis, and the subsequent production of an angle between the bladder and posterior urethra may make subsequent continence more likely. Much attention has been addressed to the short, stubby penis in the boy with exstrophy after closure. An important principle is to lengthen the penis by detaching it from the pubic rami, in whole or in part, before the epispadias is repaired.

The kidneys can be protected after the continence procedure by ascertaining that the tubularized bladder forming the muscular portion of the neourethra is fairly uniform and approximately 10 F in caliber, as described. The upper tracts also are protected by routine antireflux implantation of the ureters into the bladder above the trigone.

The development of urinary control subsequent to the procedure to provide continence takes time, often years. If the patient retains some urine in the bladder and voids intermittently, even at very short intervals, that is a good prognostic sign. When urethral resistance is adequate, the bladder usually will enlarge gradually, and the intervals between voiding become longer. Many patients remain enuretic after reasonable social daytime control is achieved. Some boys with continued incontinence after healing will gain urinary control at puberty with growth of the prostate. If a patient remains wet but unobstructed, an array of further adjuncts, ranging from an artificial urinary sphincter to bladder augmentation, are available to improve continence or bladder capacity.

Although patients with exstrophy pose a surgical challenge, and several operations usually are needed, the child who gains urinary control repays these efforts handsomely, because most patients with exstrophy do not have other significant congenital abnormalities and can function normally in society after successful treatment.

Commentary by Julian S. Ansell

The concept needs to be emphasized that exstrophy is a spectrum of congenital anomalies, ranging from superior vesical fistula/fissure, through continent epispadias and classical exstrophy, to the almost monstrous deformities of cloacal exstrophy. A subtitle for this chapter could be "Correction of Representative Types of the Exstrophic Spectrum/Syndrome." Another important principle needing emphasis is that in all but the least-involved variations of the spectrum, closure is carried out in a series of stages, months and years apart.

Superior vesical fissure (or fistula) is the most minor manifestation of the exstrophy complex. The bladder neck and urethra are intact, so only simple closure of the bladder is needed.

Cloacal exstrophy is a form we now are seeing as often as the classic type in the northwestern United States probably because infants with this condition are not being considered hopeless but are referred for tertiary care. In these cases, the symphyses usually are more widely separated, and osteotomies probably will be required. A decision as to sex of rearing may be hastened by the need to intervene urgently to correct the omphalocele or other acute intestinal problems. Regardless of sex assignment, the ultimate genital appearance, male or female, is likely to be abnormal. Therefore, contrary to several authorities, we tend to accept the existing chromosomal and gonadal sex if in a full-term, neonatal, potential male, the phallic structures are over 3.5 cm in length from pubis to midglans, even if the phallus is bifid and partially embedded in the abdominal wall or groin. We have nine cloacal exstrophy patients with 46XY karyotype being raised as males in Seattle.

The early dominating problems are the omphalocele and intestinal obstruction due to atresia, duplication, intussusception, or some combination of these. If the intestinal problems are easily corrected, the bladder may be closed at the same sitting; if not, the bladder halves can be united in the midline as part of the abdominal wall closure and then freed at a later date and closed as in classic exstrophy. Reflux is a less-common problem in cloacal than in classic exstrophy, but in some cases initially, and in others over time, ureteral stenosis will occur and needs to be watched for. Bilateral, prevesical, lower ureteral stenosis was the source of infection and sepsis and contributed significantly to the deaths of two of our neonates with cloacal exstrophy.

The short-gut syndrome has been such a problem in our series that we work hard to save a portion of the colonic plate and roll it into a tube to serve as a terminal colonic conduit and colostomy, rather than leave the child with an ileostomy. Even a short segment of colon appears to have a remarkable effect in cutting down the massive fluid loss that some of these children with ileostomies experience. In general, all intestinal mucosa is incorporated into the gastrointestinal tract.

Because the cloacal bladder is more superficially located than the classic exstrophic bladder, cloacal exstrophy is technically easier to close. However, the pubes are farther apart, and most will require osteotomies to allow pubic approximation without undue tension. The bladder halves usually are generous. The tailgut, which usually has an orifice in the colonic plate in the midline at the level of the caudal edges of the bladder halves, is extremely useful and must not be discarded. From it we have constructed urethra, vagina, and colon conduit. In some children, it is long enough to consider as a terminal colon, which in a few of these children with functional anal muscle around the imperforate dimple might be pulled through as a rectum and anus. If you cannot figure out what to do with the tailgut at the time of the initial closure, leave it *in situ* attached to the bladder halves as a bladder-augmenting tube of bowel.

With a lot of support from pediatric medical and surgical colleagues, nurses, social workers, psychologists, physical therapists, and ancillary health workers, surprising results can be achieved. In Seattle, we (Ansell, Mitchell, and Burns) have primarily closed 24 neonates with cloacal exstrophy. With the surgical techniques available today, we feel that acceptable toileting and continence should be obtained in all.

DEFERRED STAGED RECONSTRUCTION (ARAP)

First Stage: Sigmoid Conduit

22 Select a segment of sigmoid colon at least 20 cm long, and divide the mesentery and the colon. Reanastomose the colon on the right side of the proposed loop. Close the distal end (Figure 4 in Chapter 76) of the loop, and tack it to the peritoneum covering the bladder. Anastomose the ureters to the center of the loop by the Politano-Leadbetter technique (page 202). Alternatively, in small children use the Kelalis technique (see page 430), which does not require a subepithelial tunnel. Bring the proximal end of the loop through the body wall at a suitable site in the left lower quadrant and form a stoma. Lengthen the penis at this time. In follow-up, perform loopograms after 3 months.

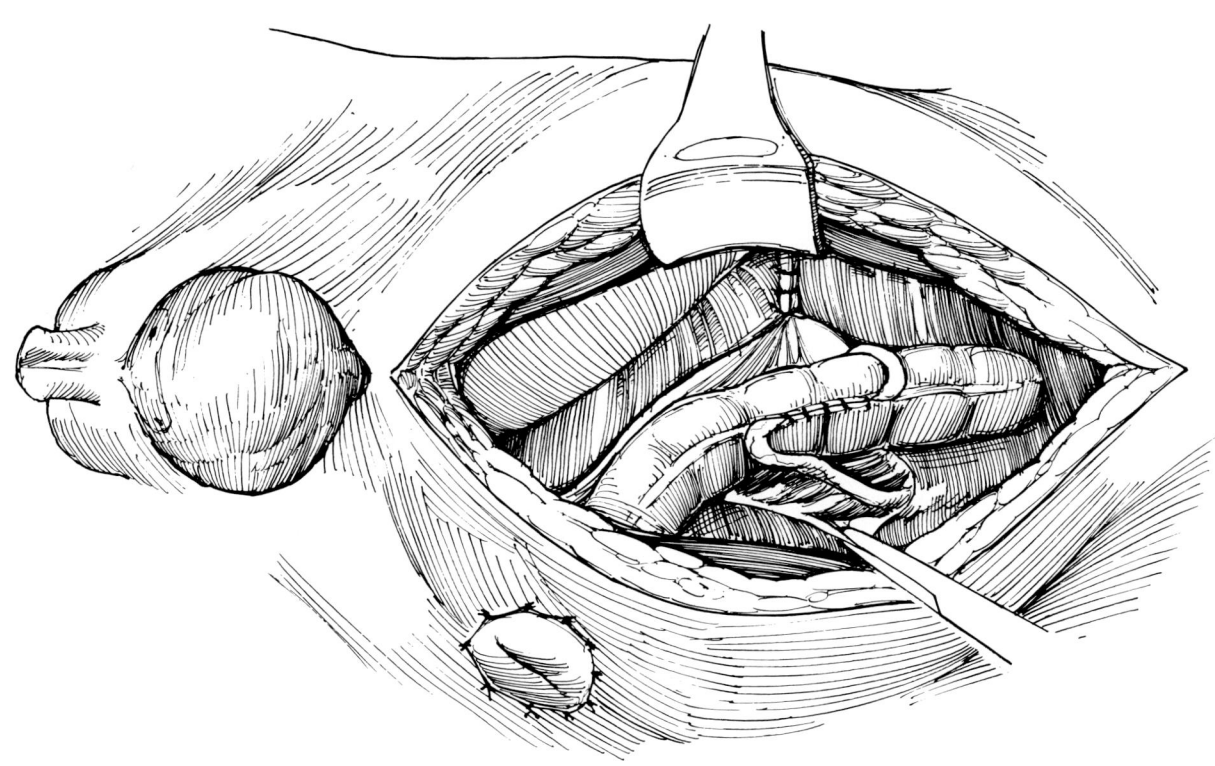

Second Stage: Urethrovesical Tubularization and Vesical Neck Reconstruction

23 Make a circumferential incision at the junction between the bladder epithelium and abdominal wall. With the cutting current, free up the superior and lateral walls of the bladder. Take care posteroinferiorly not to damage the area of the superior vesical pedicle.

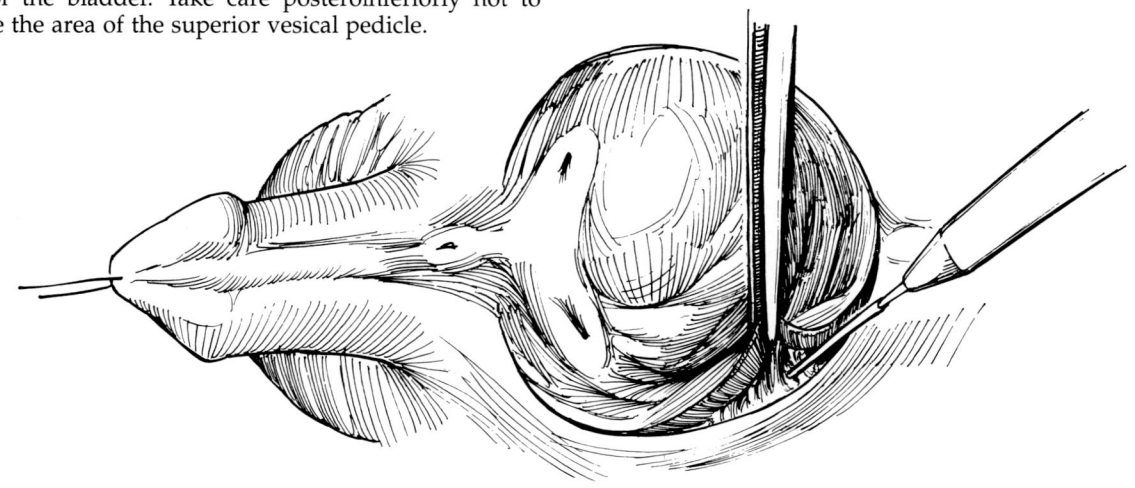

24 Cut two parallel incisions through the epithelium 5 to 6 cm long (in a 1-year-old boy) and 1.5 cm apart, beginning at the site of the vesical neck and continuing up across the trigone and well onto the bladder. Remove the epithelium lateral to these incisions, but leave it intact in the dome.

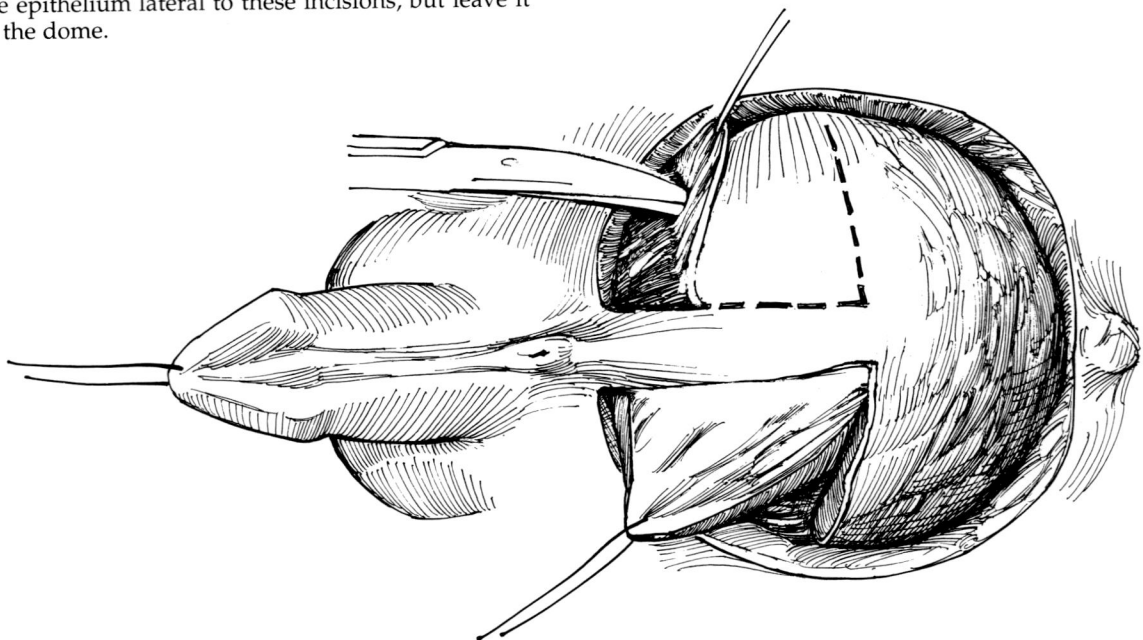

25 Place an 8 or 10 F Robinson catheter on the epithelial strip, and fasten the strip as it is rolled over the catheter with interrupted 4-0 synthetic absorbable sutures that catch a little of the underlying muscle. Fold the vesical muscularis on the left side over the tube, and secure it to the muscular bed on the opposite side with interrupted 4-0 synthetic absorbable sutures.

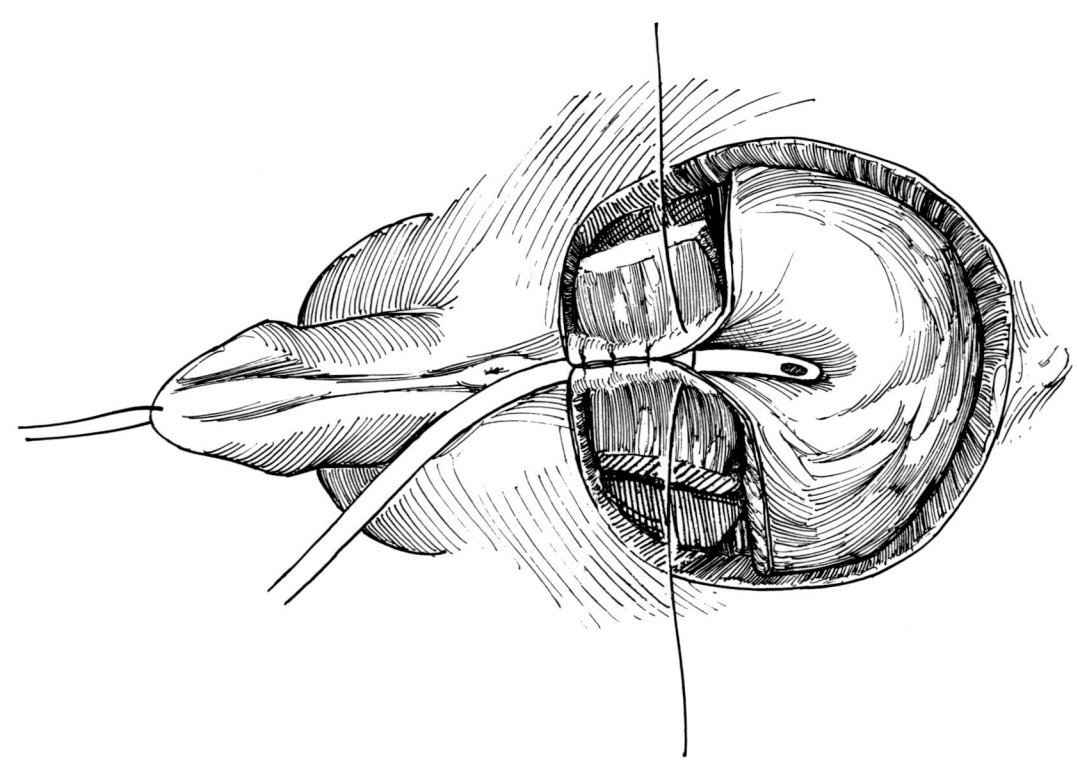

26 Overlap the muscularis from the right side, and suture it on the left.

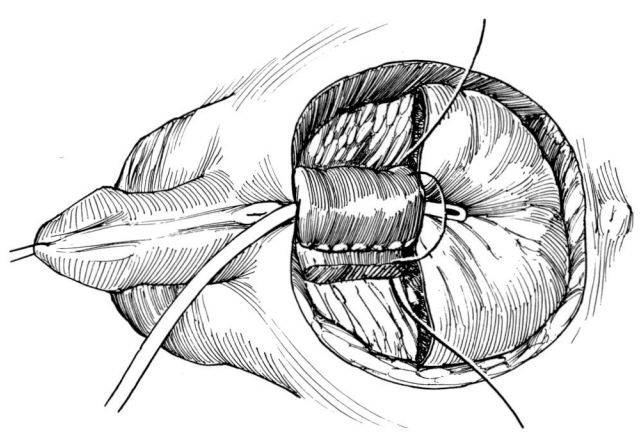

27 Close the dome of the bladder in two layers to make a small cavity for later anastomosis to the conduit. Extraperitonealize the bladder. Construct the urethra as described for epispadias repair (page 610). Remove the catheter. Close the abdominal wall defect. Raise two flaps from the rectus sheaths with the hinges oriented medially. Rotate the flaps to the midline, and join them with interrupted 3-0 synthetic absorbable sutures. Correct inguinal hernias or cryptorchidism at this stage. Wait 3 to 4 months for healing to occur. Test the urethrovesical tube by cystography.

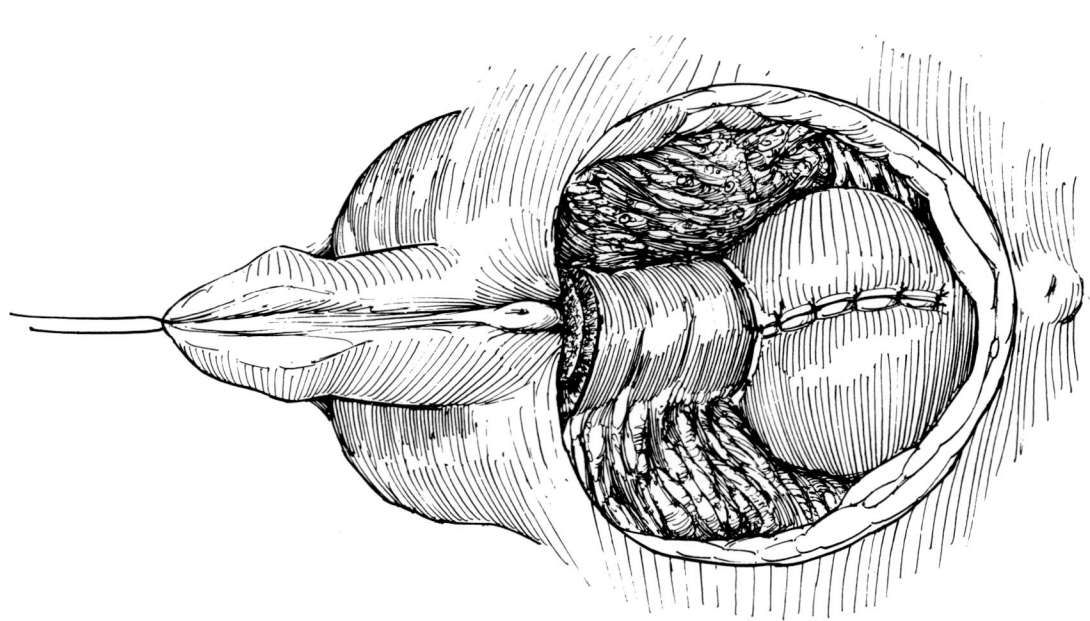

Third Stage: Colovesicostomy

28 Place a 10 F urethral catheter and leave the end available for instillation. Open the midline incision, excising any scarred skin. Identify the colonic conduit and the bulge at the end of the vesical tube. Dissect and open the colon conduit, and turn it back on itself to form a pouch. Anastomose the bowel to the opened bladder with two layers of 4-0 synthetic absorbable sutures. In older children, proceed with the next step, closure of the cutaneous stoma; in small children, mucus may obstruct the obligatory catheter if the stoma is closed before the suture line is healed (10 to 14 days).

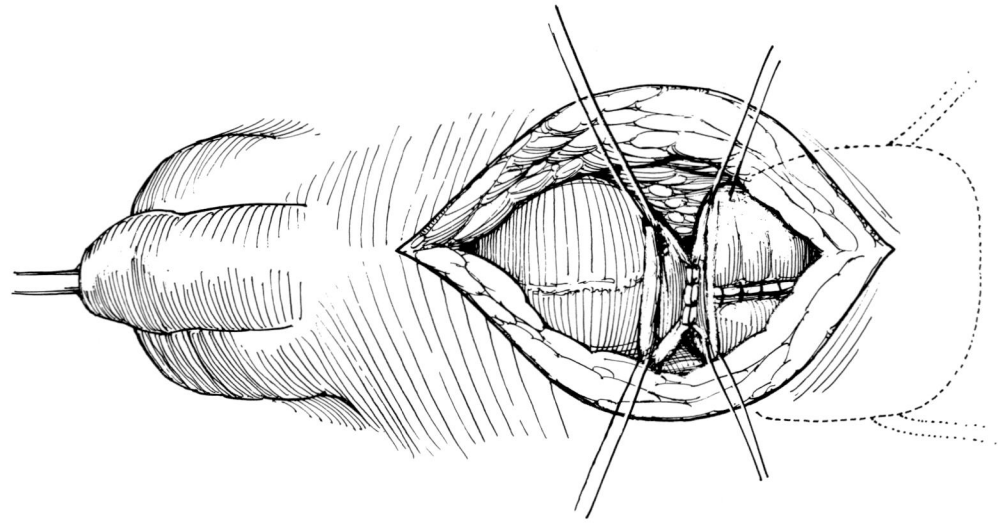

Commentary by Sami Arap and Amilgar M. Giron

The important aspect of reconstruction for vesical exstrophy consists of its conception itself. It proposes the creation of a urinary reservoir, where continence is maintained through the tubularization of the bladder, turned into a muscular urethra. The principle is the same as the one widely applied today for continent urinary diversion. Selection of patients is more strict today, and the results of the functional bladder reconstruction have restricted the use of this operation. It is useful, however, when the bladder does not attain adequate capacity, following its initial closure.

Since its introduction in 1968, several improvements have been perfected. Today, the operation is performed in one surgical step, because anesthesia and technical conditions have improved in our hospital. Intestinal bladder replacement routinely consists of detubularized intestinal loops.

The examination of complications after the reconstruction indicates that the failures can be handled in two ways: either the detubularized intestinal loops are anastomosed to the sigmoid (thereby creating better pressure conditions in the sigmoid) after transecting the urethra; or an artificial urinary sphincter may be used, although the risk of erosion is greater in these cases. Whenever its use is indicated, consideration should be given to the use of omentum enveloping the urethra to improve blood circulation and employment of a delayed activation of the sphincter, which minimizes the risks of erosion.

In conclusion, deferred staged reconstruction (Arap procedure) has been modified, incorporating new developments. It now is considered an alternative program, because most bladder exstrophies today are treated surgically with staged functional bladder reconstruction. Continence is maintained through the neosphincter, that is, the tubularized bladder. The tubularized bladder acts as a sphincter for the intestinal bladder, which should have large capacity and adequate compliance.

The evacuation of this intestinal bladder is not always possible through the Valsalva maneuver; intestinal mucus also can bring about problems in this situation. Several patients are continent with the help of intermittent catheterization; some of them sporadically need to have their bladders catheterized to evacuate mucus. Late failures can be handled either by separating the colonic conduit again and anastomosing it to the sigmoid or by employing an artificial sphincter.

THE BOYCE-VEST PROCEDURE

The *Boyce-Vest procedure*, although it passed out of favor with the advent of more anatomically acceptable techniques, has merit over simple ureterosigmoidostomy in case the infant cannot be sent to a highly trained team. At 5 years of age, do a permanent colostomy at the level of the rectosigmoid, and close the distal stump. Irrigate the distal segment with antibacterial solutions. In 2 weeks, make a 4-cm incision through the base of the bladder into the cul-de-sac over the rectum, dividing the trigone. Superiorly, suture the serosa of the bladder to that of the rectum to achieve extraperitonealization. Make a second 4-cm incision in the anterior wall of the bladder opposite that made in the trigone. Anastomose the two structures with fine chromic catgut. Circumscribe the base of the exstrophic bladder, and close it over with a continuous suture of chromic catgut. Excise the remainder of the vesical epithelium , and imbricate the detrusor to act as a buttress in the anterior abdominal wall; reinforce it with flaps from the adjacent fascia. Proceed with penile repair.

PLASTIC CORRECTION OF THE SUPRAPUBIC DEFECT (OWSLEY-HINMAN)

29 Preliminary skin expansion may be helpful. Mark two curved incisions for rotation flaps beginning just below the vaginal introitus in girls or at the margin of the excised bladder in boys and ending just medial to the anterior superior iliac spine. Mark a back cut just above the inguinal crease, leaving a triangular piece of skin to be excised at the outer end of each incision.

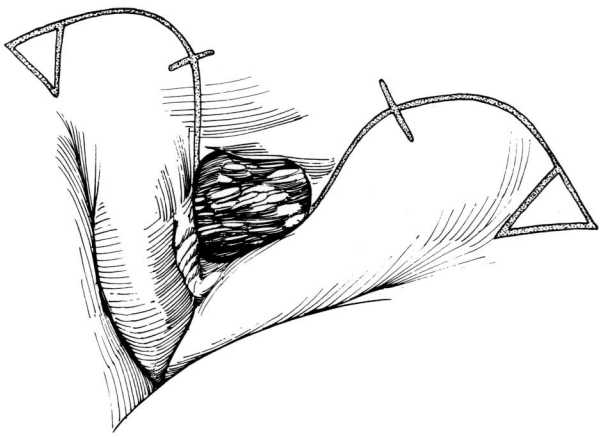

30 Elevate and widely undermine the skin flaps. Join the tips in the midline with subcutaneous 3-0 synthetic absorbable sutures. (In girls, mobilize the vagina posteriorly, start suturing in the midline just above the introitus, and bring the bifid clitoris and the preputial hood together.) Continue suturing to bring the hair-bearing pubic skin together in the midline using 3-0 synthetic absorbable sutures subcutaneously and interrupted 4-0 nonabsorbable sutures for the skin.

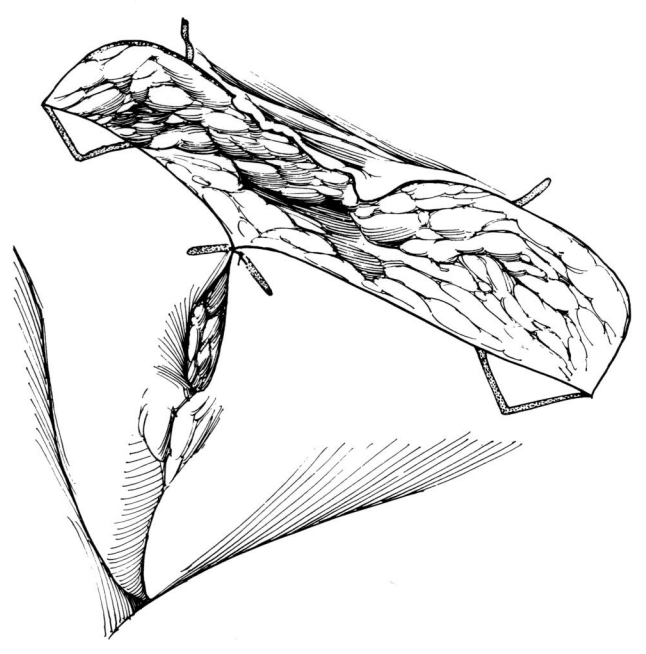

31 Approximate the skin in the superior transverse portion in the same way after an appropriate adjustment at the extremities of the incision. Insert two multiperforated drainage tubes beneath the flaps.

The abdominal wall defect can be reinforced by raising aponeurotic flaps from the rectus sheaths and overlying skin, tissue that is supplied by the superficial circumflex iliac and inferior superficial epigastric vessels. Such flaps are formed by extending the lateral incisions 5 cm into the groin line to facilitate medial rotation (Arap-Giron). In addition, because the former site of the bladder is represented by a depression and the mons veneris is absent, a more cosmetic result may be obtained by inserting skin expanders on either side that generate enough tissue to allow formation of a tube of de-epithelialized skin that is buried to fill the defect and to provide skin for cover (Marconi *et al.*, 1993).

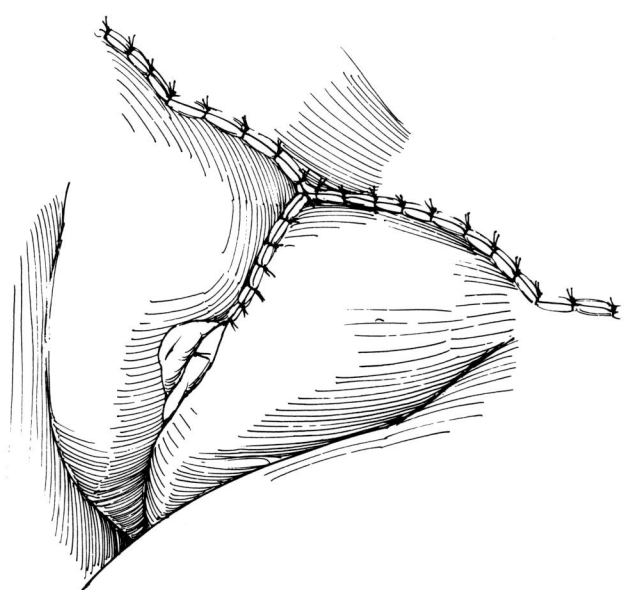

ALTERNATIVE CORRECTION OF SUPRAPUBIC DEFECT

32 Mark and incise two flaps on either side of the defect with bases posteriorly.

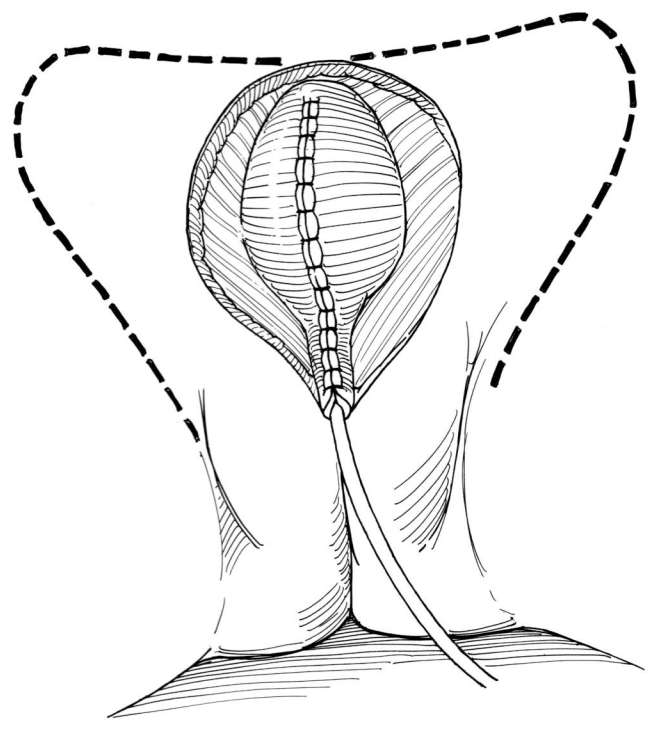

33 Incise the fascia laterally and bring the flaps together in the midline.

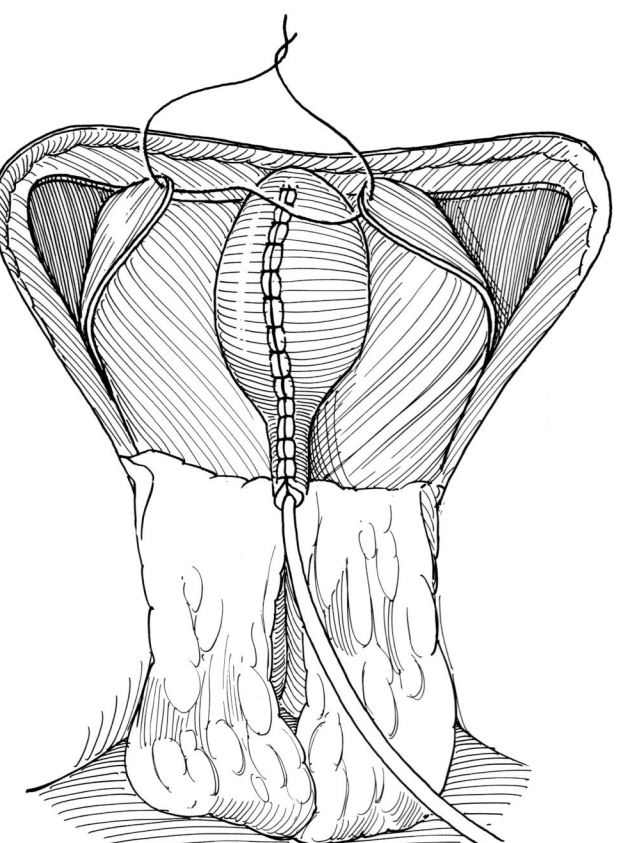

34 Close the apices and suture the skin flaps in the midline.

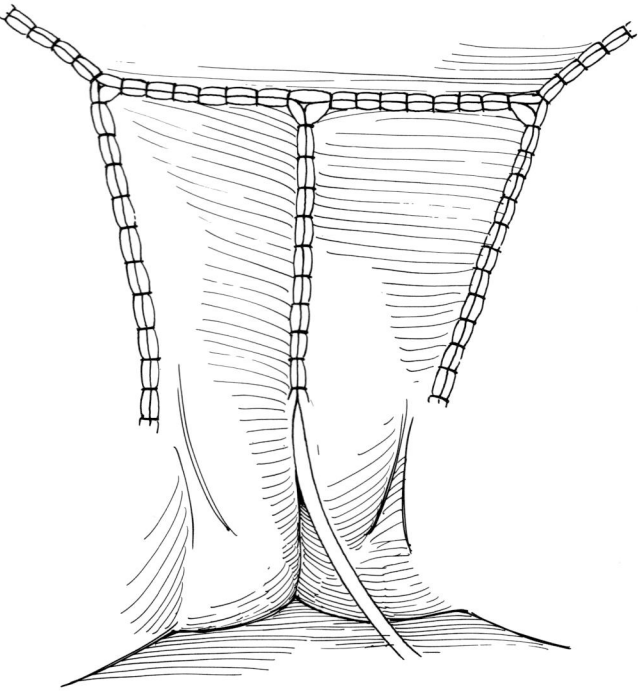

UMBILICOPLASTY, SKIN DISK METHOD

35 A, Remove a disk of skin and subcutaneous tissue 1.5 cm in diameter at the projected site for the umbilicus, deep enough to expose the rectus fascia. Defat the skin disk. Excise the fat and subcutaneous tissue under the edges of the circular defect.

B, Suture the skin edges to the underlying fascia with fine monofilament sutures.

C, Apply the disk of defatted skin and suture it in place. Apply a bolster dressing.

UMBILICOPLASTY, BURIED SKIN METHOD (HANNA AND ANSONG)

36 A, Site the umbilicus midway between xiphoid and pubis. Mark and create a Y-incision with its center at the site.

B, Elevate the V-flap and excise enough of the underlying subcutaneous tissue to expose the rectus sheath.

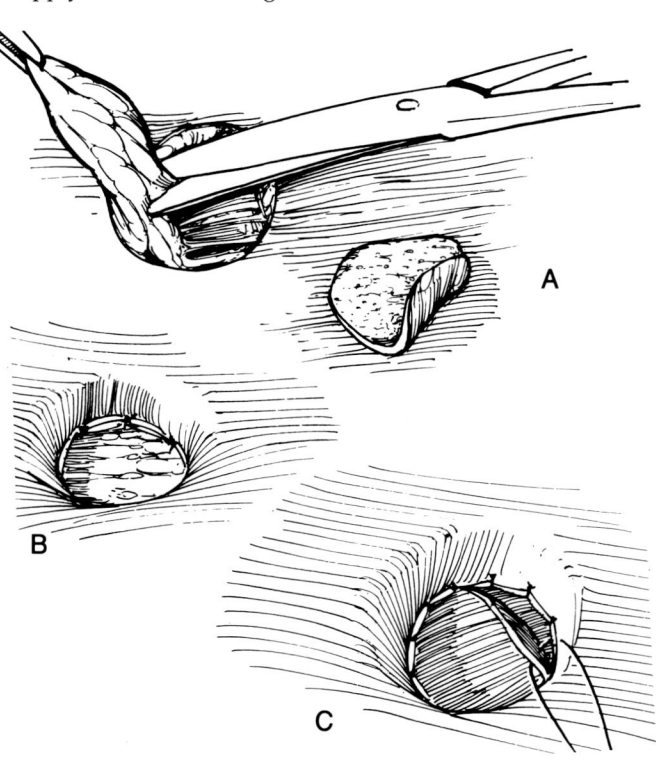

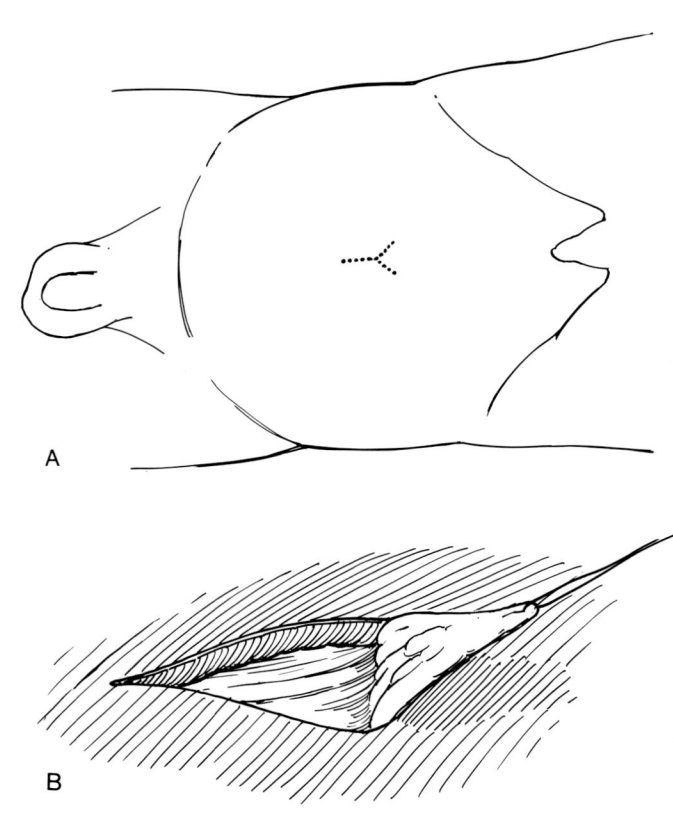

37 A, Suture the V-flap to the rectus sheath with three 3-0 synthetic absorbable sutures.

B, Bring the edges of the Y together over the flap, and suture them with two layers of sutures. Pack the wound with iodoform gauze, and cover it with a transparent dressing to allow inspection. Change the gauze as necessary, but keep the pack in place for several weeks until granulation tissue has formed and epithelialization is underway.

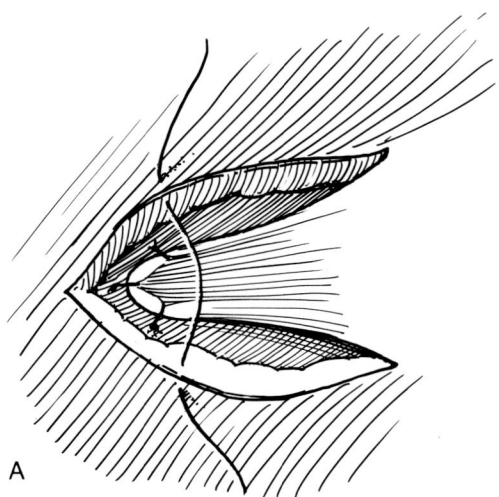

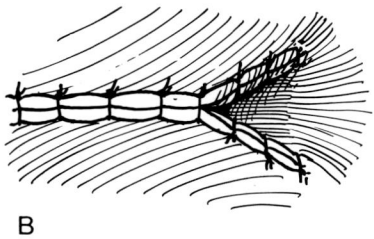

CHAPTER 63

Cloacal Repair

(PEÑA)

The child already will have had a colostomy. Hold the child up by the heels and prep the entire lower body, because the child may need to be turned from prone to supine to prone.

Position: Prone with the pelvis elevated. Locate the parts of the anal sphincter by electrostimulation, and make a transverse mark on the skin at that level.

Incision: Make an incision extending from the sacrum to the cloacal orifice.

1 Keeping exactly in the midline, divide the muscle layers, including the external anal sphincter and its complex on both the anterior and posterior aspects. Use a needle tip on the electrosurgical unit. Stimulate the muscle with direct current to maintain the dissection in the midline. Divide the fine midline sagittal fascia to leave it to contain the perirectal fat. Insert two Weitlaner retractors superficially, above the muscle layer. Split the coccyx in the midline to expose the levator ani, which is divided in the midline to expose a yet to be identified visceral structure.

2 Open the visceral structure in the midline and hold it open with stay sutures. Within it will be found the rectum, vagina, and urethra. Dissect a plane between the rectum and vagina (the two will be densely bound together at first). Dissection will be time consuming but is aided by injection of dilute epinephrine.

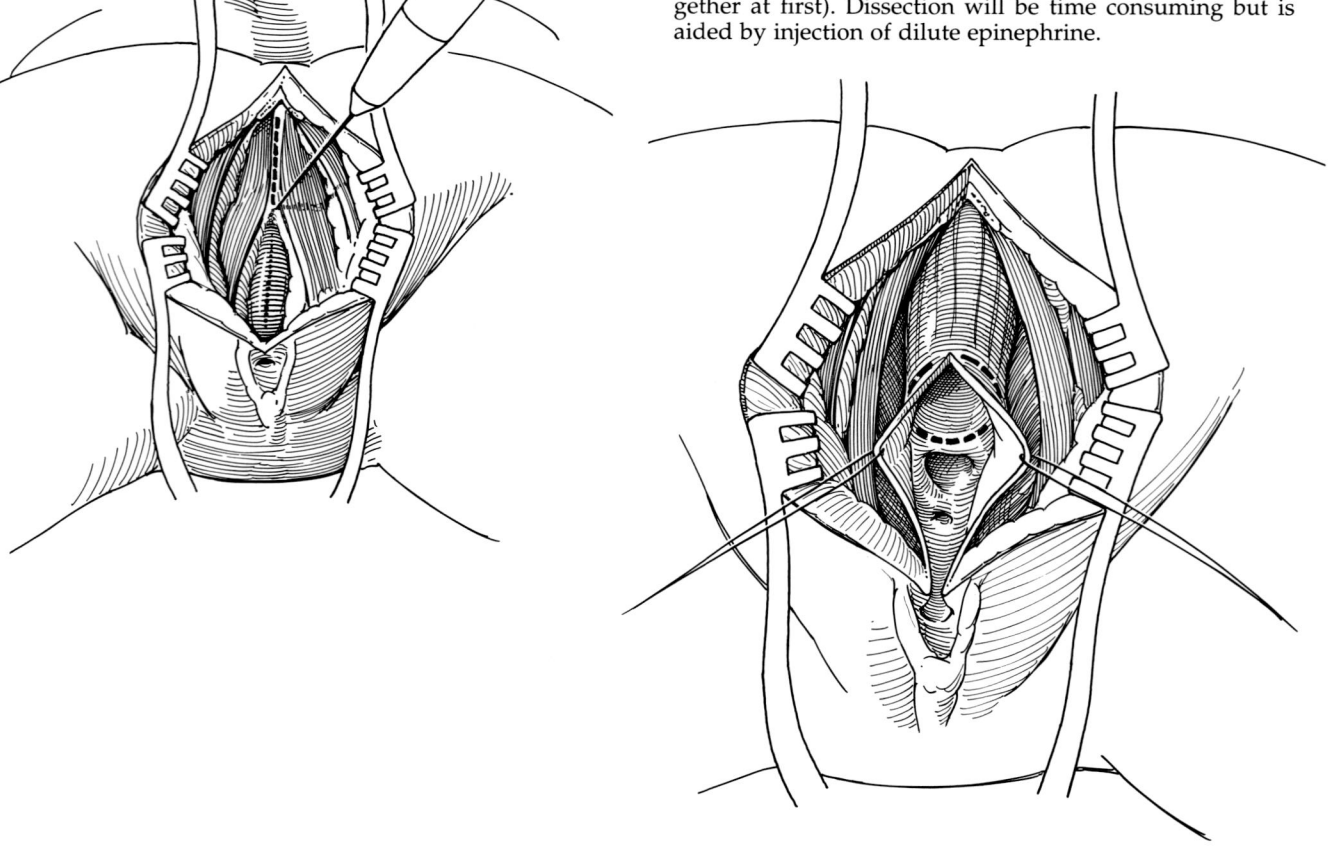

3 Separate the vagina from the urinary tract, keeping as close as possible to the heavier vaginal wall. The tissue here is extremely friable. Close the urethra using tissue from the cloacal channel.

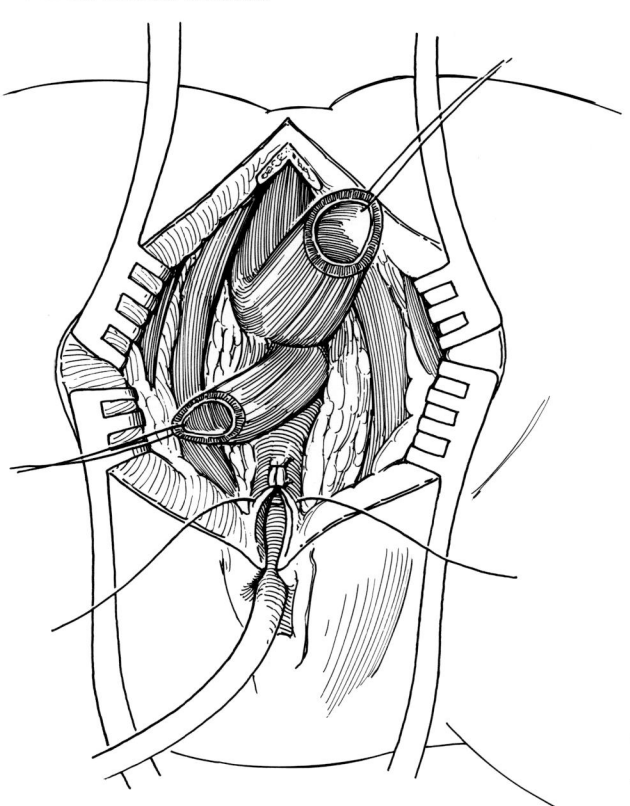

4 Suture the vagina to the perineum with interrupted synthetic absorbable sutures. With the stimulator, identify the anterior and posterior limits of the sphincter mechanisms, and approximate the anterior layer with interrupted sutures.

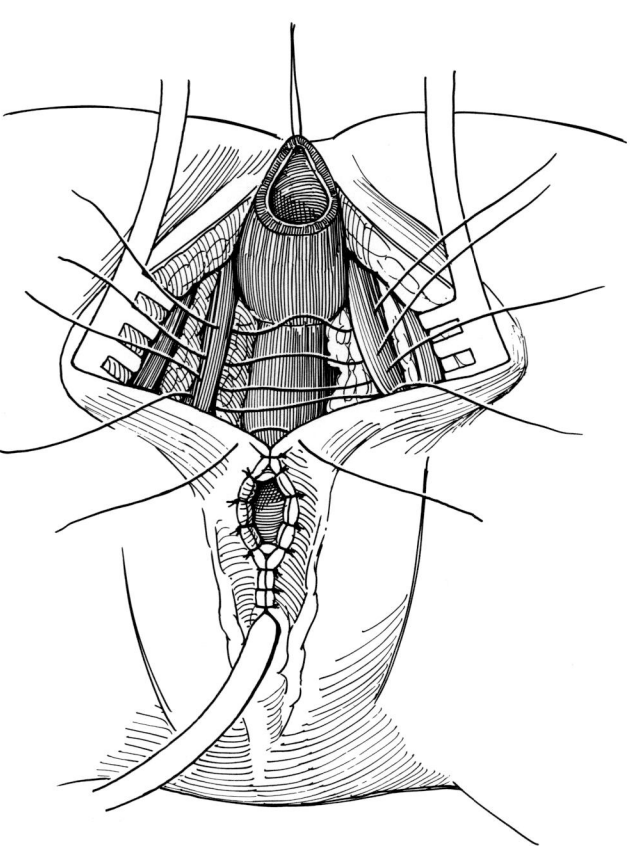

5 Because the rectum must fit between the two sphincteric layers, reduce its caliber by resecting a segment of the posterior wall and reapproximating the edges with two layers of interrupted sutures. Incorporate a bite of rectal wall in each stitch that is used to close the posterior layer of the sphincteric complex.

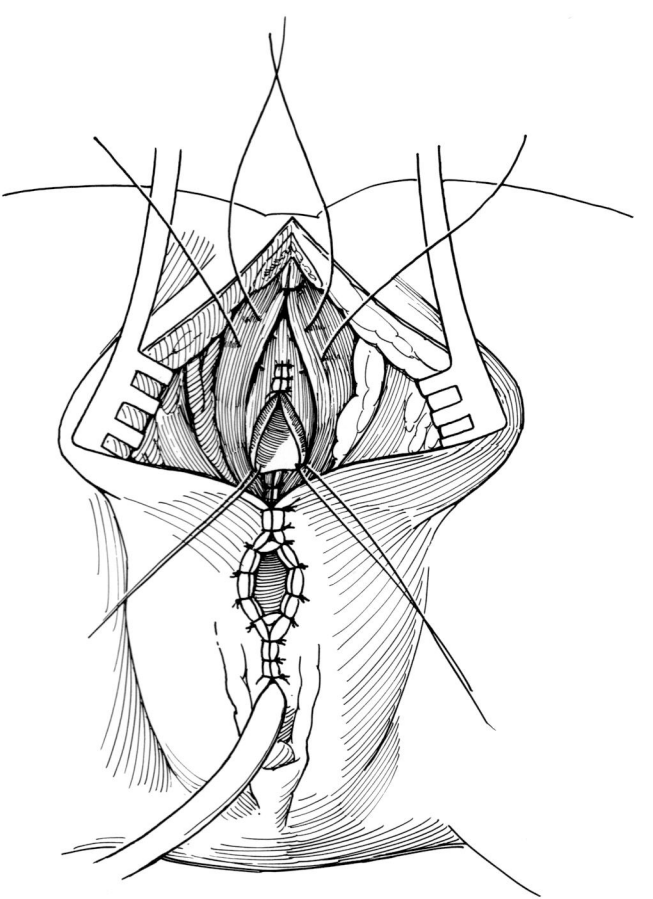

6 Fasten the rectal margin to the perineal skin with interrupted sutures, and place a balloon catheter to remain 1½ to 2 weeks.

Postoperatively, begin twice-daily anal dilations to gradually increase anal size. The vagina does not require dilation.

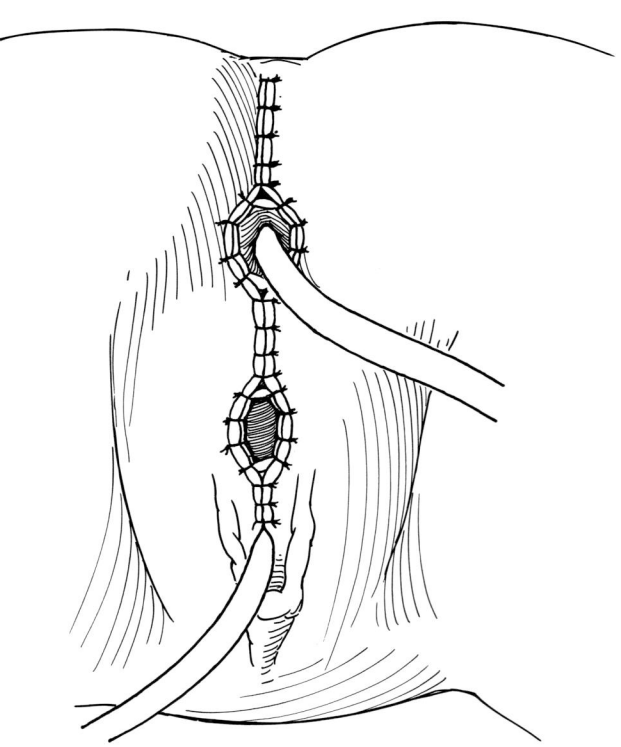

CHAPTER 64

Prune Belly Syndrome: Abdominal Repair and Umbilicoplasty

EHRLICH TECHNIQUE OF ABDOMINAL REPAIR

1 **A**, Make a midline incision from the xiphoid to the pubis, passing around the umbilicus on either side. Add a short transverse extension at the lower end. Proceed with orchiopexy or urinary tract reconstruction, as needed.

B, Sharply separate the skin and subcutaneous tissues from the attenuated abdominal muscles and fascia on each side to the midaxillary line, but preserve an anterolateral pedicle of fascia, so that the umbilicus is suspended on a vascular stalk. Avoid injury to the fascia itself during the dissection. Achieve hemostasis.

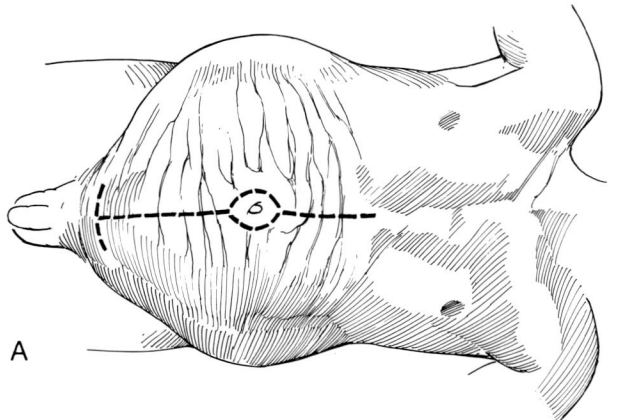

A

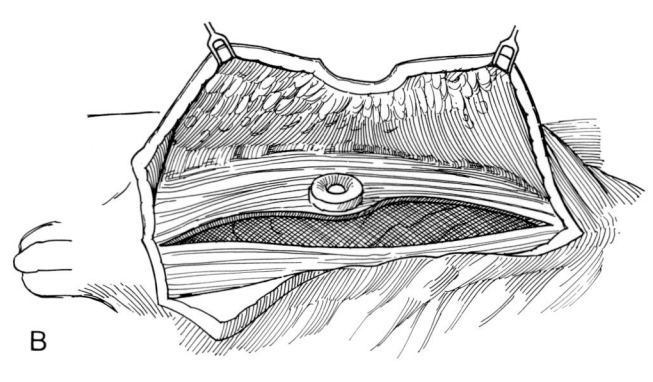

B

2 In a double-breasted fashion, advance one flap of fascia across the midline under the other flap with the umbilical pedicle attached. Insert a row of through-and-through 1-0 polyglactin sutures to approximate the edge of the deep layer to the surface of the overlying fascial layer. Place a second row of sutures to fasten the edge of the upper flap to the basal surface of the lower flap. Insert a few of the lower sutures through Cooper's ligament and the pubic tubercle to stabilize the lower end of the repair.

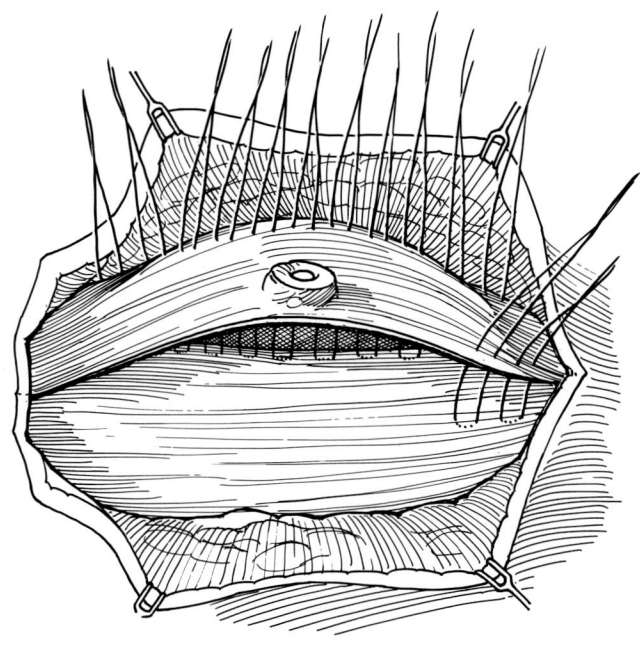

3 Hold the ends of the sutures in clamps and tie them successively.

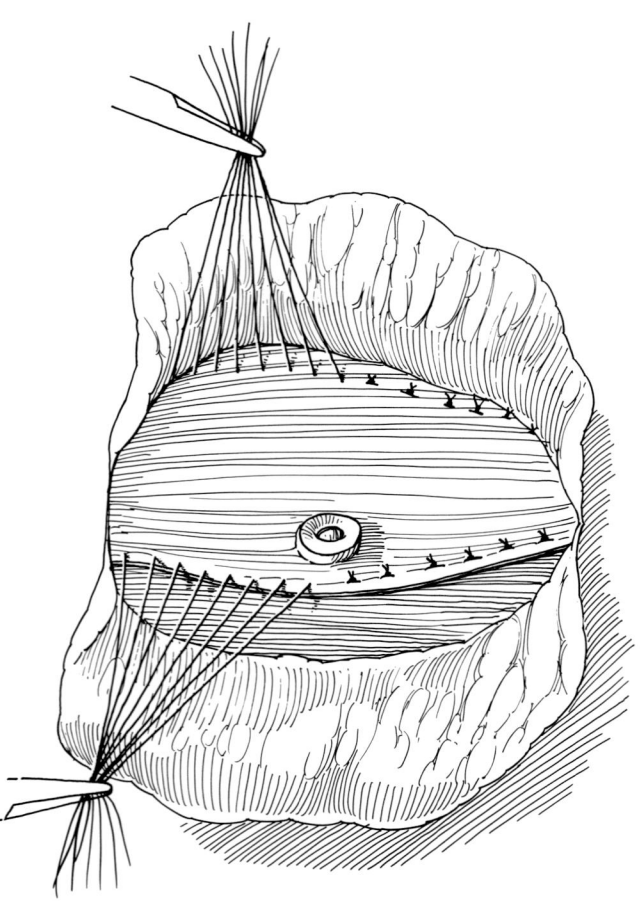

4 A, Excise the excess skin from the sides of the defect. Position the pedicled umbilicus in the appropriate position, trim the skin to fit around it, and fasten it with both subcutaneous and cutaneous sutures.

B, Close the rest of the subcutaneous tissue with interrupted chromic catgut sutures, and approximate the skin with upper and lower running subcuticular 4-0 synthetic absorbable sutures after inserting two small drains under the flaps.

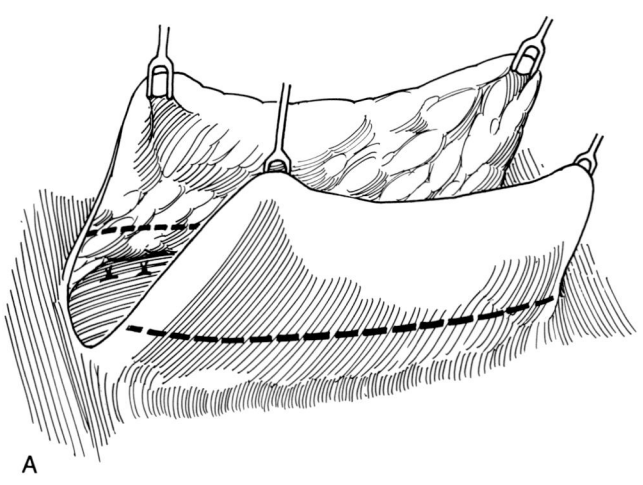

A

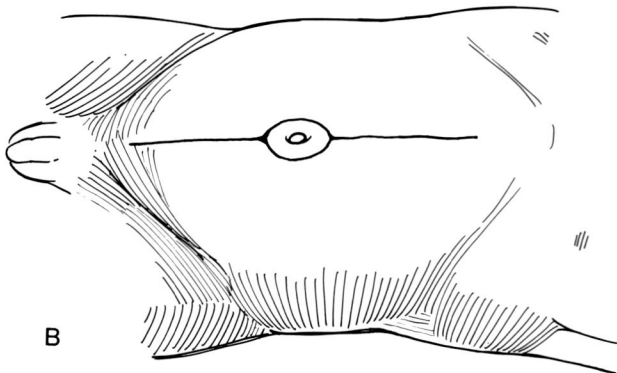

B

MONFORT TECHNIQUE

5 **A,** Estimate the amount of excess abdominal wall by grasping it with both hands.

B, Mark the skin at the margin of the raised wall (dashed line), and also mark it closely around the umbilicus to leave it as an island (dotted line). Start an incision near the xiphoid, following the skin marks, leaving an acute angle at either end. Incise the full thickness of the skin, and excise it, including the subcutaneous tissue with the electrocautery, but leave some fat on the fascia to avoid devascularization. Hemostasis must be meticulous. Leave the umbilicus in place. The excision will leave an asymmetric defect and expose the degenerate abdominal plate that is composed of the aponeuroses of the external and internal oblique muscles, the rectus fascia, and the peritoneum.

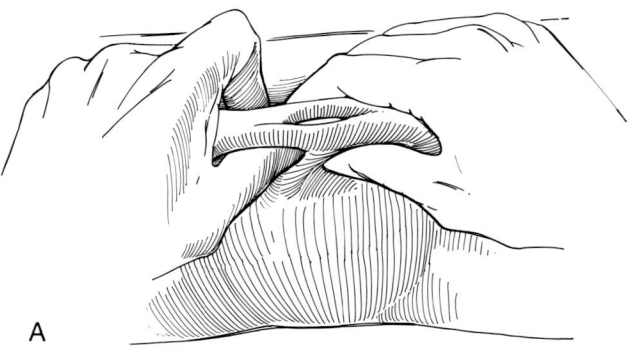

A

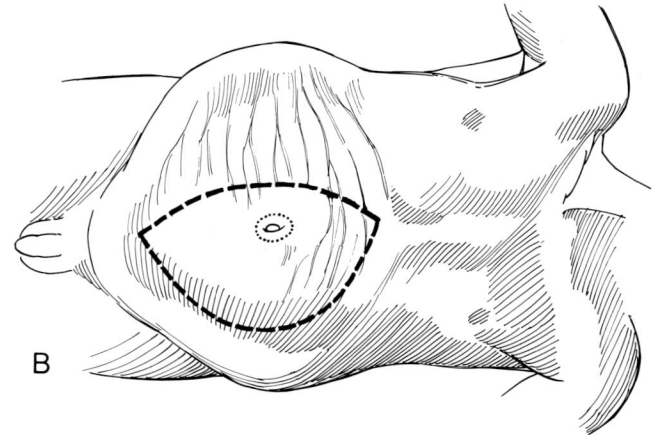

B

6 **A,** Incise the abdominal fascia and musculature lateral to the rectus muscles on either side for the length of the skin incision, and enter the peritoneal cavity. The incision extends from the superior to the inferior epigastric vessels, which can now be seen from the inside. Leave these vessels intact to supply the central musculofascial plate. Perform any intra-abdominal procedures at this point.

B, Make a vertical incision through the peritoneum of the lateral colonic gutters on each inside aspect of the body wall to bare a strip of the inner surfaces of the lateral abdominal wall muscles.

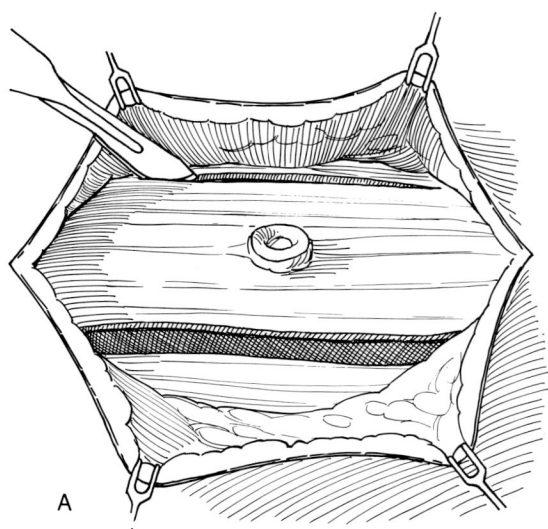

A

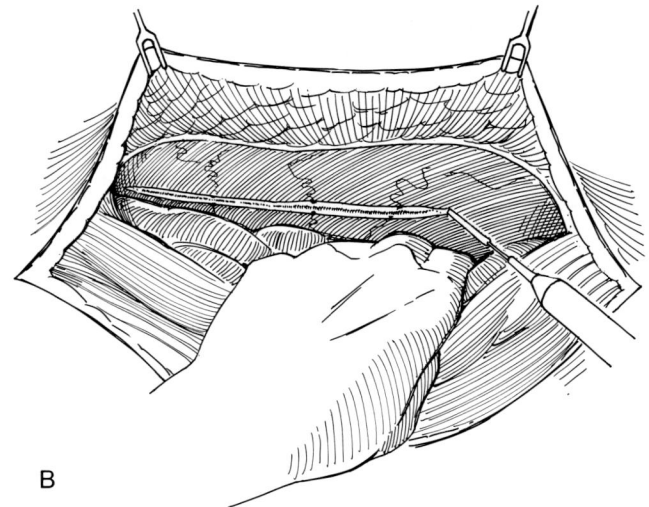

B

7 **A,** Suture the lateral margins of the central plate to the lateral body wall musculature through the peritoneal incisions on each side.

B, Trim the skin flaps to fit, provide notches for the umbilical island, and bring the flaps over the plate. Trim any excess skin and close it around the umbilical island.

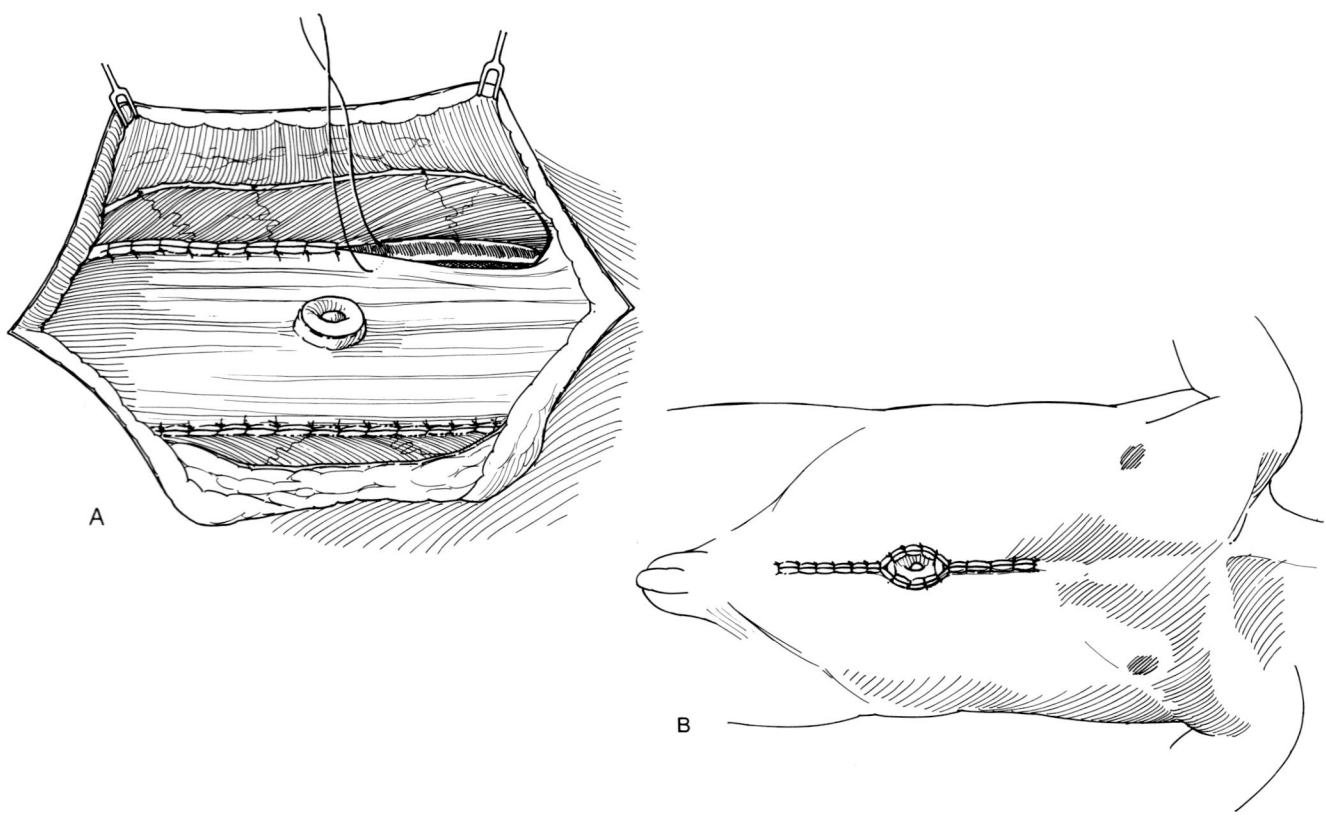

Commentary by Richard M. Ehrlich

In 24 patients treated since we first reported our technique, we have been impressed with the ease of performance and satisfactory long-term results. Our youngest patient was 7 months of age, and the oldest, 14 years. We know of one early case in which minor one-sided weakness developed 4 years after surgery, but the cosmetic deformity has not been severe enough to require reoperation.

For interest, we performed one Monfort procedure, and although we obtained a satisfactory result, we were struck by the attenuation of the midline plate, which was of concern for long-term strength and holding power. Accordingly, we still maintain that our double-breasted wrap technique provides superior abdominal wound tensile strength. Many other surgeons employing our technique have achieved similar satisfactory results.

One child developed renal failure and underwent renal transplantation, and another underwent an emergency appendectomy. In both instances, restoration of the abdominal repair was readily performed and did not result in return to laxity.

Caution must be exercised in the use of the Bovie coagulating current when separating the skin from the underlying muscle to prevent postoperative skin necrosis of the margins.

Ever since our technique was modified to preserve the umbilicus, superior cosmetic results have been achievable.

Numerous parents have volunteered that their children after surgery have had fewer respiratory difficulties, with a decrease in upper-respiratory infections due to facilitation of coughing. Although we never made this claim as a justification for proceeding, we also have noted this finding.

We continue to be impressed that these operations improve the cosmetic and, thus, psychologic well-being of these unfortunate children. The technique has withstood long-term scrutiny and deserves to be offered with enthusiasm.

CHAPTER 65

Closure of Rectourethral Fistula

POSTERIOR SAGITTAL APPROACH (PEÑA)

The posterior sagittal approach is used for imperforate anus with rectourethral fistula after a colostomy has been formed.

Consider a team approach involving a pediatric surgeon. Obtain plain films with coned views of the lumbosacral spine and an abdominal ultrasound study looking for other urinary-tract anomalies. A voiding cystourethrogram is indicated, especially if the results of the ultrasonography are abnormal. Renal scanning with diethylenetriamine penta-acetic acid or an intravenous pyelogram may be needed. Prior to forming the colostomy, it is not necessary to visualize the fistula; do so during convalescence. If abnormalities require it, intervene with a vesicostomy for significant reflux with the VATER complex or persistent cloaca. In some cases, cutaneous pyelostomy may be preferable to immediate tapering and reimplantation.

Prepare the bowel, including the colostomy, and administer antibiotics.

1 *Position and Incision*: Insert a balloon catheter into the bladder, and turn the child into the prone jackknife position. Make a midline incision extending from the midsacrum through the center of the anal sphincter into the perineum past the site of the anus. For imperforate anus, use an electrostimulator to identify the components of the residual pelvic and sphincteric musculature, so that the incision can be made exactly in the midline.

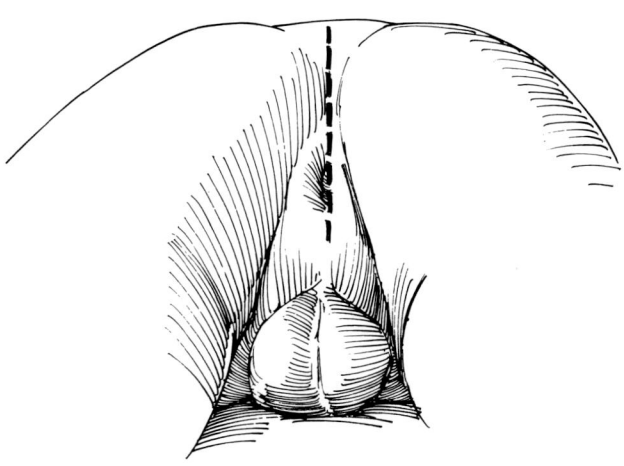

2 **A,** Divide the deep external sphincter into halves, then split the coccyx. Separate the parasagittal fibers of the external sphincter, and continue the incision down to the levator ani muscles and muscle complex. Open the levator muscle; the rectum will bulge through the edges. Continue the incision exactly in the midline onto the longitudinal smooth muscle coat of the rectum.

B, Place stay sutures in the rectal edges, and mobilize the rectum with sharp dissection, performed as close as possible to the rectal wall to avoid nerve damage to the urinary structures. Elevate the rectal wall with 5-0 silk stitches, and make a small opening in it with a needlepoint cautery in the midline. Through the opening, one can identify the fistula site in the lowest part of the rectum.

Open the rectum further, over the site of the fistula. Circumscribe the fistula, and dissect behind the prostate. It is important to dissect submucosally from the site of the fistula toward the proximal part of the rectum for at least the 5 mm or so in which only a common wall separates them. This avoids injuring the prostate, seminal vesicles, and vas deferens. At first, the common wall is very thin, but it becomes thicker as the dissection is continued in the cephalad direction. Use multiple 5-0 silk sutures placed in the mucosal edge for traction. Excise the fistula into the urethra, bladder, or urogenital sinus. Approximately 5 mm above the fistula, it becomes possible to mobilize the full thickness of the bowel from the full thickness of the urethral wall. For rectoprostatic fistulas, go as high as the peritoneal reflection (even opening the peritoneum if necessary) to have enough bowel to bring down using traction on the sutures in the rectum. Close the defect in the urethral (or vesical) wall with full-thickness 5-0 synthetic absorbable sutures. Close the defect in the rectal muscosa and muscularis similarly. It is now necessary to divide the rectum distally (dashed line) to mobilize it, so that it will reach the perineum without tension. Careful dissection is aided by making traction in silk mucosal sutures. Only a moderate amount of dissection is needed with bulbar fistulas, but for high prostatic fistula, the dissection will be much more extensive and difficult.

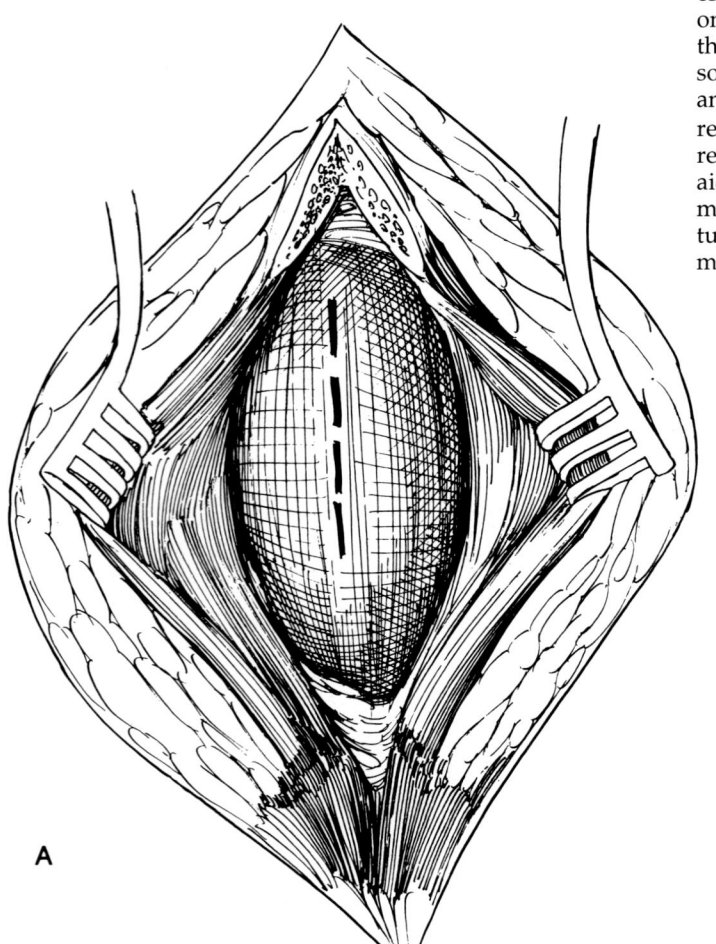

A

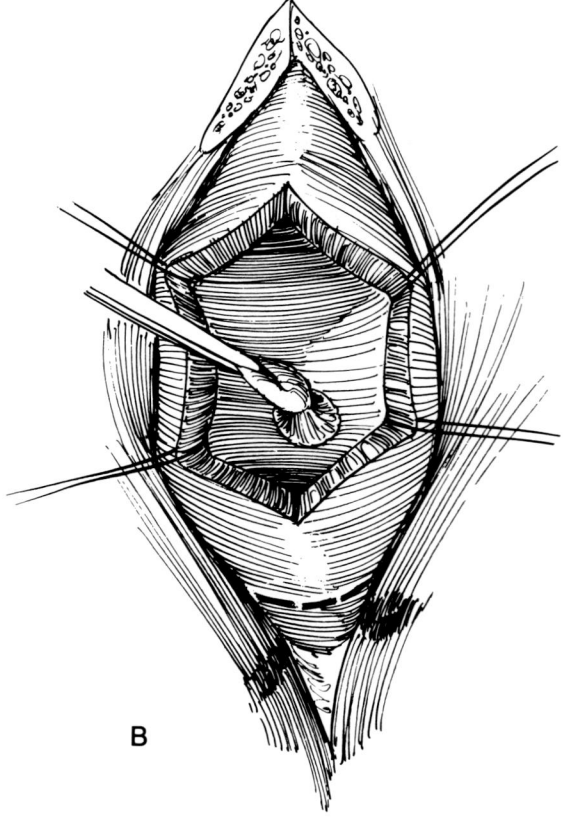

B

3 **A,** Close the rectum. It will be dilated and may require tailoring; this is done by placing two layers of interrupted 5-0 monofilament synthetic absorbable sutures.

B, Reapproximate the anterior margin of the muscle complex, as well as the margin of the external sphincter, with interrupted 5-0 synthetic absorbable sutures. Stitch both levator muscle edges together with the same suture material. Pass the rectum in front of them, and suture the remaining portion of the levator muscles together. Reapproximate the posterior edge of the muscle complex behind the rectum with stitches that include the muscle complex edge and the rectal wall. Next, reapproximate the posterior edge of the rectal external sphincter, the puborectalis portion of the levator, and split the coccyx over the rectum. Suture the muscular coat of the bowel circumferentially to the corresponding external sphincter portion of the striated muscle complex.

C, Complete the anoplasty by trimming the mucosa to fit. Irrigate the wound well, and close the subcutaneous tissues and skin around a small Penrose drain with a 5-0 nylon subcuticular suture. Remove the drain in 3 days and the catheter in 8 days. Close the colostomy after 2 months.

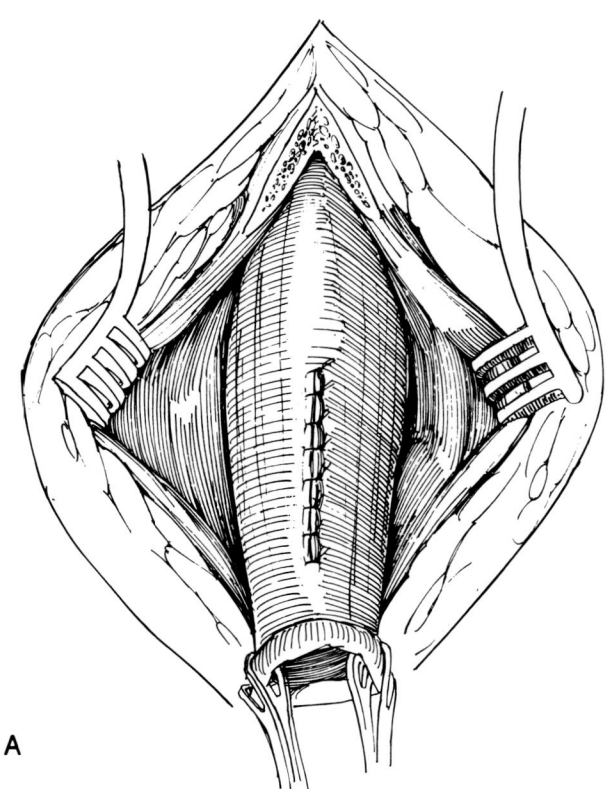

A

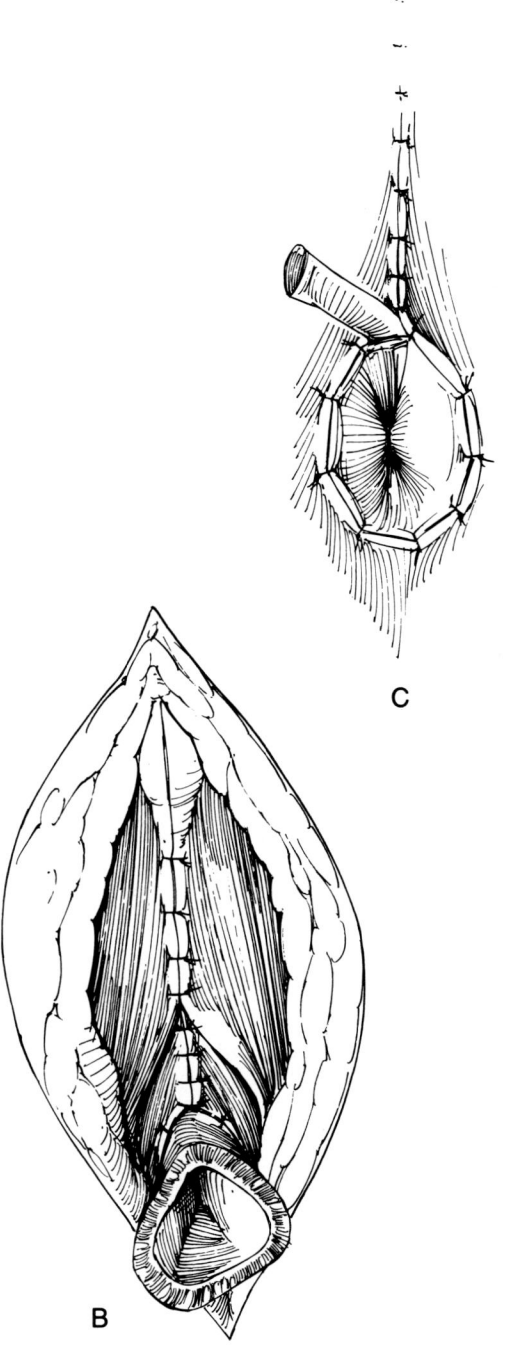

B

C

POSTOPERATIVE PROBLEMS

If the fistula is not closed initially, a descending colostomy is constructed. This prevents contamination of the urinary tract, which puts these infants at greater risk, because vesicoureteral reflux is common. Recurrent *epididymitis* is not rare, but it is less frequent with prophylactic antibacterial therapy.

Hyperchloremic acidosis from colonic filling may be found after transverse colostomy, but a colostomy formed in the descending colon allows the urine to escape through the mucous fistula and avoids stagnation. Treat hyperchloremia with oral bicarbonates, at the same time looking for urethral obstruction.

Commentary by Alberto Peña

A protective colostomy is done prior to repair. A Foley catheter is inserted into the bladder before the operation is started. A full posterior sagittal anorectoplasty is done through a midsagittal incision that runs from the middle portion of the sacrum down to and through the center of the external sphincter. In patients with rectoprostatic fistulas, one may try to preserve the anterior limit of the external sphincter. However, with rectobulbar fistulas, it is more convenient to continue the incision a little beyond the anterior limit of the external sphincter. The parasagittal fibers of the external sphincter are separated, and one continues deepening the incision down to the levator muscle and muscle complex. Once the levator muscle is opened, the rectum is then tented with two 5-0 silk stitches and opened with the needlepoint cautery in the midline. Once the rectum is opened, one can identify the fistula site in the lowest part of the rectum.

The posterior sagittal approach allows a direct exposure of the anatomy of the rectum and levator ani. The most conspicuous impression that I have had in my experience is that there is no way to identify the structures, such as "puborectalis," because the striated sphincteric mechanism is represented by a continuous striated funnel-like piece of muscle. Also, there is no way to identify the "ganglia." Thus, it is necessary to mobilize the rectum with sharp dissection, performed as closely as possible to the rectal wall to avoid nerve damage to the urinary structures.

Remember that the rectum and urethra share a common wall immediately above the fistula site. The best way to avoid damage to the vas deferens, seminal vesicles, and prostate is to perform a submucosal dissection from the fistula site toward the proximal part of the rectum for at least 5 mm, using multiple 6-0 silk stitches at the rectal mucosal level for traction. The reason is that immediately above the fistula, there is a common wall between the rectum and urethra that extends for approximately 5 mm. By submucosal dissection, we can guarantee that we will not damage the underlying structures. Once the dissection has reached the 5-mm distance, we can continue our dissection full thickness, because at that point, the rectal wall and urethral wall become fully and completely separated. There are no recognizable neurovascular bundles between rectum and urethra.

Closure of the fistula site must be done by full-thickness 5-0 absorbable sutures through the urethral wall, because one cannot visualize the separation of mucosa from muscle.

A meticulous rectal dissection is then carried out while making traction on the silk sutures to gain sufficient length to be able to suture the rectum to the perineal skin without undue tension. The dissection aimed to gain rectal length usually is an easy affair when dealing with a bulbar fistula, but it sometimes entails rather complex maneuvers with rather high prostatic fistulas. The amount of circumferential dissection required to mobilize the rectum varies from case to case, so that it is not always necessary to dissect to the peritoneal reflection. In rectourethral bulbar stricture, it is unusual to see the peritoneal reflection; whereas, in prostatic fistulas, frequently we must go as high as the peritoneal reflection and even open the peritoneum to be able to mobilize the peritoneum down.

The rectum usually is ectatic and distended, and frequently it is necessary to tailor it to make it fit within the muscular structures. Not every patient will need rectal tapering; the decision is made on an individual basis, depending on the size discrepancy existing between the rectum and the enclosing structures. The goal is to reconstruct the levator muscle behind the rectum and to locate the rectum within the limits of the muscle complex and external sphincter. The tapered rectum is reconstructed in two layers with 5-0 Vicryl sutures. The anterior limit of the muscle complex, as well as the limit of the external sphincter, is reapproximated with similar stitches. The same suture material is placed in both levator muscle edges, and then the rectum is passed in front of them. The remaining portion of the levator muscle is sutured together with the same suture material. The posterior edge of the muscle complex is then reapproximated behind the rectum with stitches that include the muscle complex edge and the rectal wall. The anoplasty is done, and the skin is closed with subcuticular 5-0 nylon. The urethral catheter usually is left in place for 5 to 7 days.

Urinary contamination is not a problem. Approximately 80 percent of male patients have a rectourethral or bladder neck fistula. The opening of a colostomy during the neonatal period, with separated stomas and irrigation of the distal stoma prevents it, in my experience. As for hyperchloremic acidosis, it is true that urine may pass from the urinary tract to the rectum, and it could be absorbed in the rectum. In real practice, this situation is extremely unusual. I specifically recommend the opening of a descending colostomy. The hyperchloremic acidosis phenomenon may occur more when one opens a right transverse colostomy, because then the urine sits in the rectum and has time to be reabsorbed. A descending colostomy allows the escaping of urine through the mucous fistula; therefore, we do not see hyperchloremic acidosis. Urinary tract infections only are conceivable in cases that have a defective colostomy—namely a loop colostomy—that allows the passing of stool from the proximal into the distal colostomy.

TRANSANORECTAL REPAIR (GECELTER)

If the fistula is small and below the peritoneal reflection, as it usually is, a colostomy is not necessary, but if the case is complicated, a colostomy should be done weeks before the operation. Provide bowel preparation and antibiotic coverage.

4 **A,** Place the child in the lithotomy position. Insert a suprapubic cystostomy. Make a vertical incision anterior to the anus, from the anal verge as far forward as needed for exposure.

B, Divide both rectal sphincters exactly in the midline to avoid injury to nervous or vascular structures, and continue to open the rectum itself longitudinally. Pack the rectum with roller gauze, so that blood and irrigant will not pool there. Continue the incision in the rectum until the fistula is reached. Transect the fistula and excise the scar tissue from both the rectal and the urethral walls.

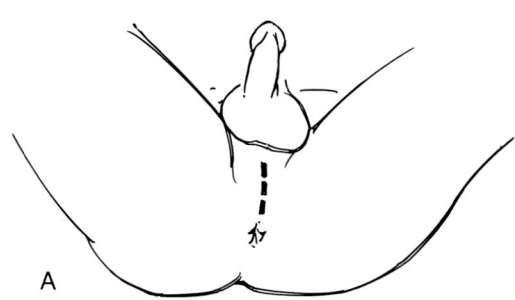

A

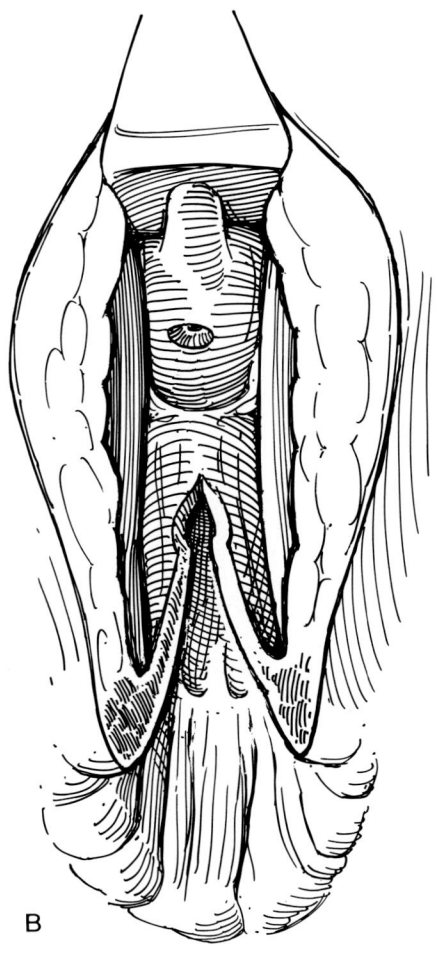

B

5 Close the urethral opening with a 4-0 synthetic absorbable continuous suture under a layer of similar interrupted sutures. If that is not possible, insert a dermal graft. Close the rectum and anal canal first with a running 4-0 synthetic absorbable suture to the mucosa-submucosa.

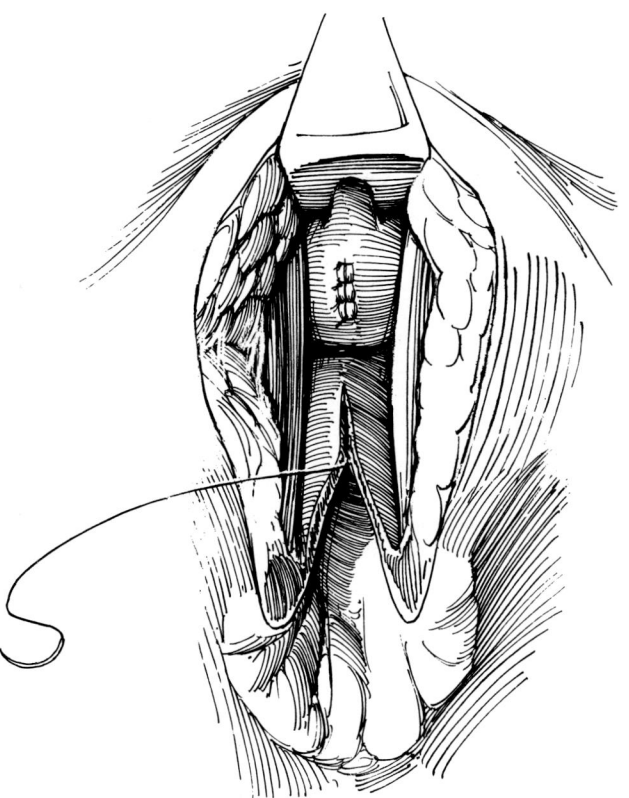

6 **A,** Place interrupted sutures to approximate the muscularis.

B, Interpose any available soft tissue, and mobilize the levator ani muscles to approximate them in the midline. Place a Penrose drain, to be removed in 3 days. Continue suprapubic drainage for at least 14 days—longer if the tissues appeared compromised. Obtain a voiding cystourethrogram before removing it.

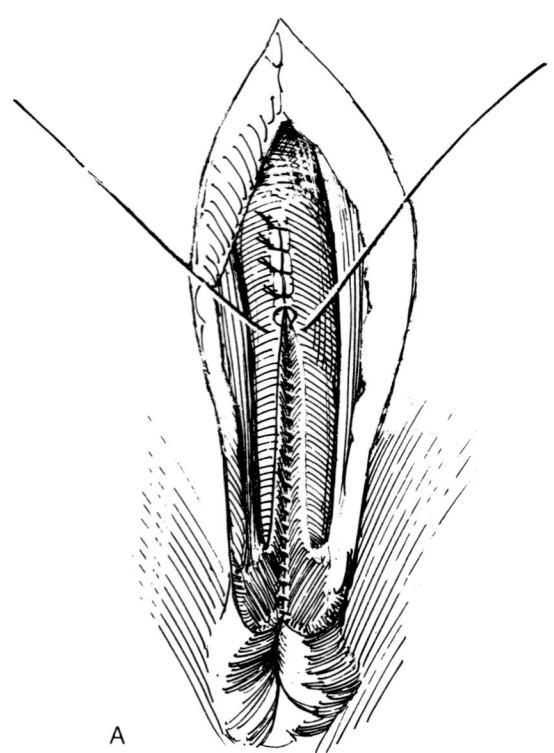

A

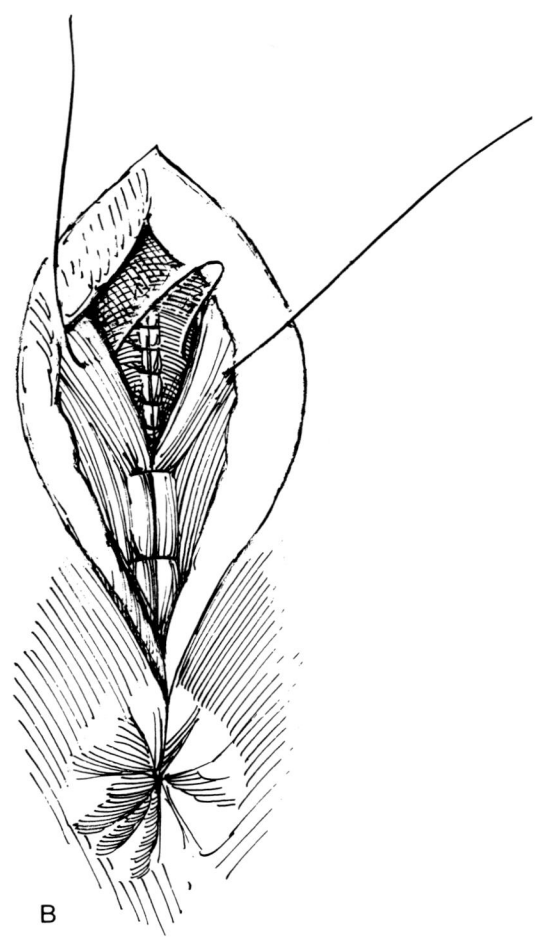

B

Commentary by Louis G. Gecelter

The natural aversion that surgeons may have for incising the anorectal canal to gain exposure to the lower genitourinary tract should not be a serious contraindication to this procedure with modern aseptic and antiseptic techniques.

Function of the anorectal canal is in no way compromised by this incision, and anal tone and function are rapidly regained after surgery.

Closure is simple, and the exact apposition of the main muscles, although ideal, is not always mandatory. Colostomy is not always indicated when the fistula is small and below the peritoneal reflection, as it usually is.

My incision is always strictly in the midline without any lateral skin or deep muscle extensions and extends from the anorectal verge as far forward as necessary, extending it the whole length of the penis if so required. Do not make any lateral extensions, being careful to remain strictly in the midline. The vascular and nerve supply does not cross the midline, and the perineal and pudendal structures are not damaged. This eliminates the possibility of impotence, as with perineal prostatectomy.

Anterior transanorectal repair of a urethrorectal or prostatorectal fistula is the most direct approach to the problem and also gives excellent exposure for high urethral strictures, which may be repaired by a variety of free or pedicled skin inlay grafts using this technique.

It is not always necessary to incise the anorectal mucosa and submucosa, and an attempt should be made to strip this layer off the deeper incised muscles. The anus is easily kept open by a Parks retractor, assisted by a mastoid self-retaining retractor in the perineum, as required.

CHAPTER 66

Excision of Urachus

PATENT URACHUS

First test for outlet obstruction.

1 *Position*: Have the child lying supine. Place a fine tube into the bladder through the urachus, although this may not be possible because of narrowed areas. Try a stiff 3.5 F polyethylene pediatric feeding tube, a pigtail ureteral catheter, or even a lacrimal duct probe. If nothing will pass, stain the tract by instilling somewhat dilute methylene blue for subsequent identification. Insert a small balloon catheter through the urethra, and partially fill the bladder.

Incision: Place a lower transverse incision in a skin fold well above the symphysis. In infants, because of the high position of the bladder, the incision can be placed nearer the umbilicus. A midline incision is an alternative.

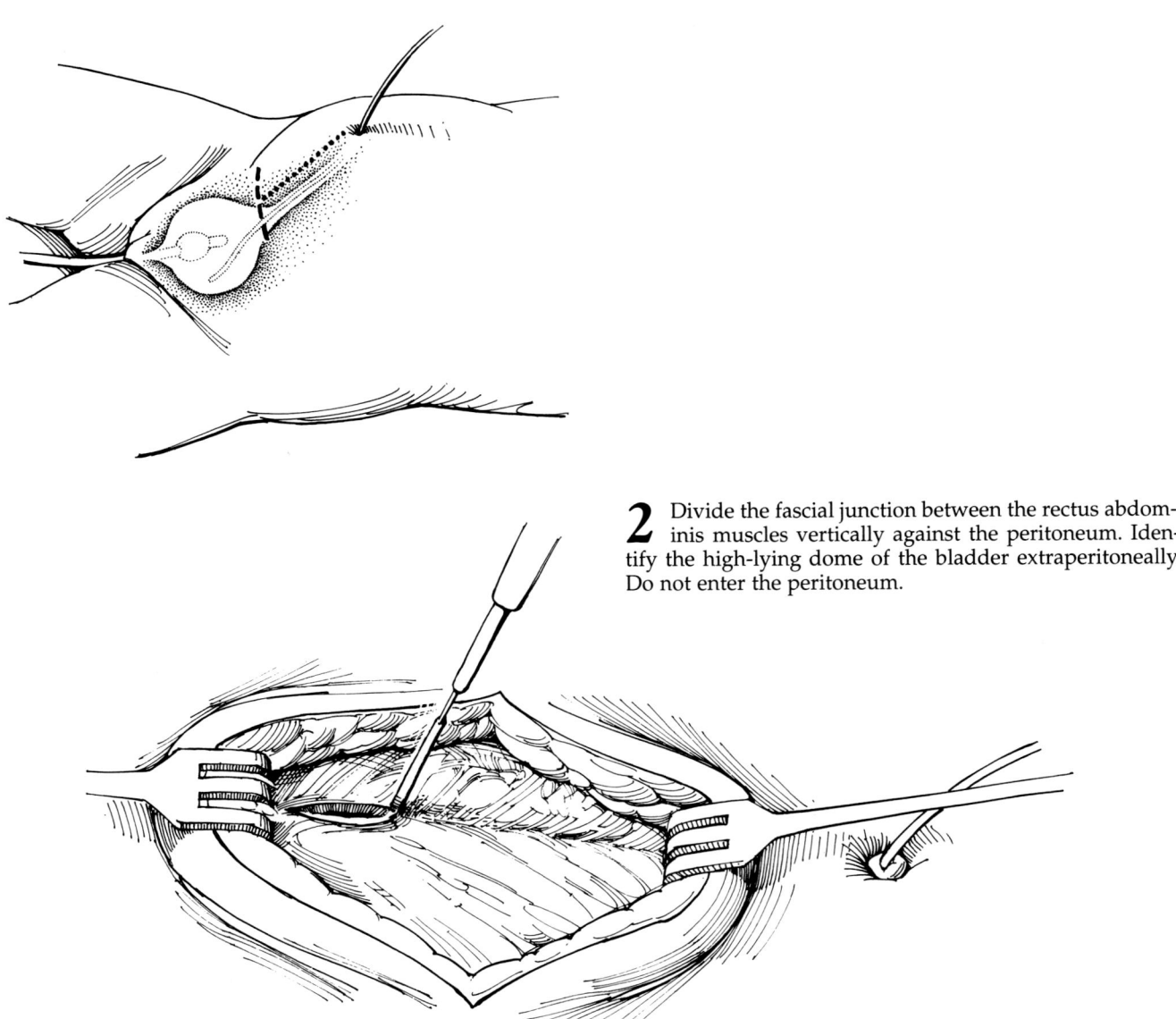

2 Divide the fascial junction between the rectus abdominis muscles vertically against the peritoneum. Identify the high-lying dome of the bladder extraperitoneally. Do not enter the peritoneum.

3 At the bladder dome, carefully free the connective tissue between the vesical adventitia and the peritoneum to expose the two obliterated umbilical arteries with the urachus lying between. Bluntly dissect the urachus free at a convenient level, and encircle it with a vascular tape or Penrose drain. Continue to sharply dissect the urachus down to the bladder. Place two stay sutures in the adjacent bladder wall.

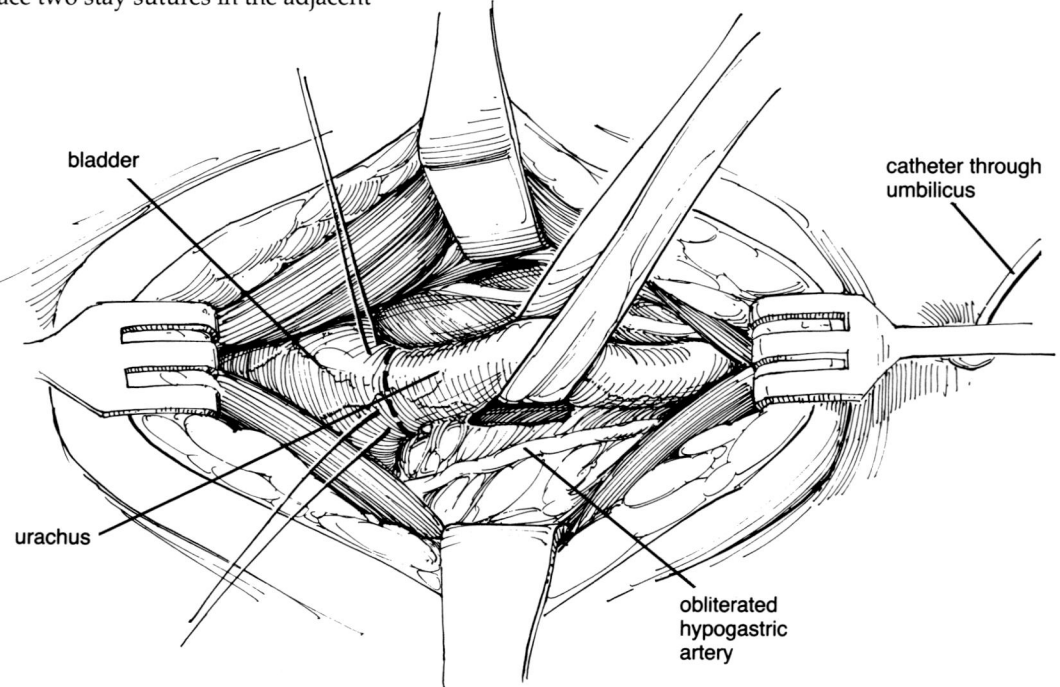

bladder

catheter through umbilicus

urachus

obliterated hypogastric artery

4 Divide the urachus within the bladder wall to remove a small cuff. Use progressive cuts, so that a 4-0 plain catgut continuous suture can be inserted to invert the epithelium while the area is suspended by the urachus. Add interrupted 3-0 or 4-0 synthetic absorbable sutures to approximate the muscularis. Elevate the upper end of the wound, and dissect the urachus from the closely adherent peritoneum, as far as the umbilicus. Excise the urachus, along with the ends of the umbilical arteries, and remove the specimen. It is not necessary to remove the last bit of the urachal stoma. Close the umbilical defect in two layers from inside, preserving as much of the umbilicus itself as possible for cosmetic reasons.

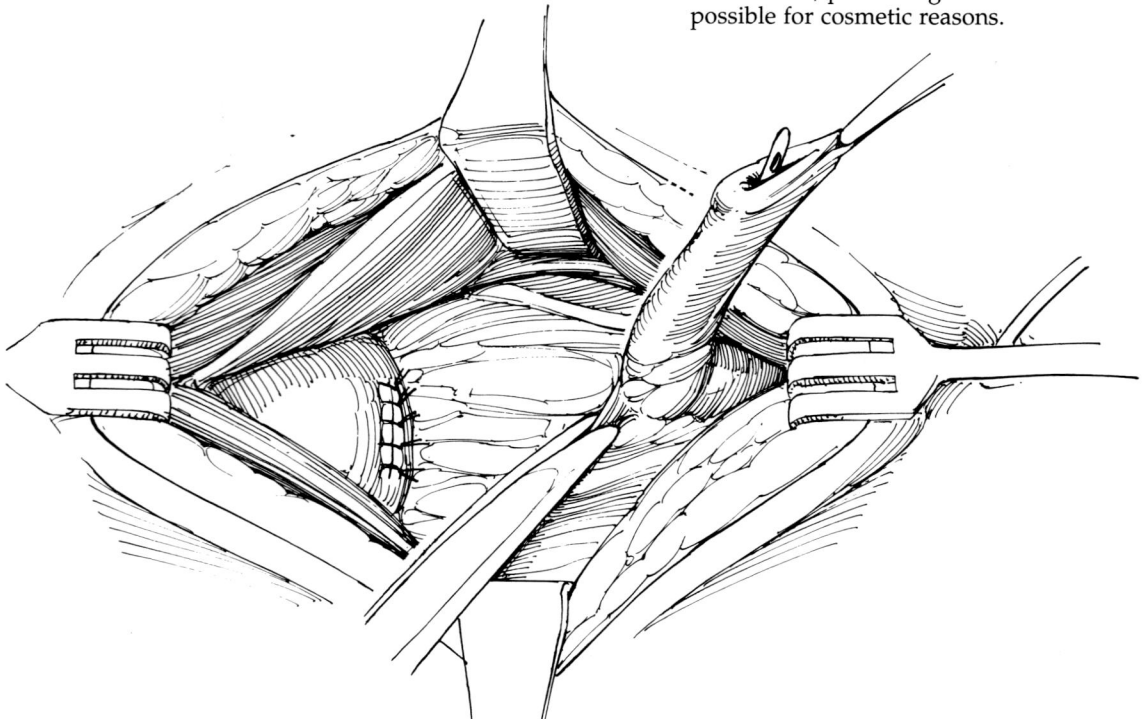

5 Place a drain through a stab wound to the bladder region. Approximate the rectus muscles loosely, and close the incision in layers. Remove the drain in 3 days if the wound is dry. Leave the catheter indwelling for 7 days.

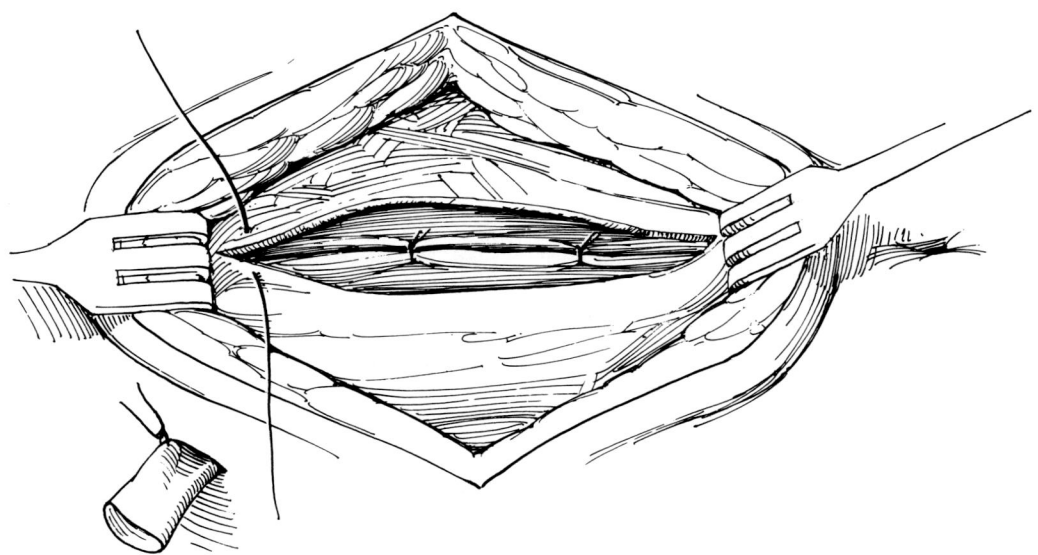

A large acontractile *urachal diverticulum* at the apex of the bladder is resected in the same way as the caudal end of a patent urachus.

LARGE URACHAL CYST

For a large urachal cyst, use the same technique as for the patent urachus, but dissect the bulging cyst from the surrounding tissues and from the peritoneum behind it. Divide its attenuated attachment to the bladder, and ligate it. Dissect the upper end from the umbilicus.

URACHAL SINUS

6 *Incision*: Make a circumferential cut around the stoma of the sinus to preserve as much of the umbilicus as possible, although it may be necessary to remove the entire umbilicus, as shown here. (For umbilical reconstruction, see page 321). Place Allis clamps on the stoma, and sharply dissect the tract to its termination. Ligate the obliterated hypogastric arteries as they are encountered. Drain the area, because a sinus tract usually is infected. For urachal carcinoma, proceed as for patent urachus, but leave wide margins, especially at the upper end, by excising the umbilicus.

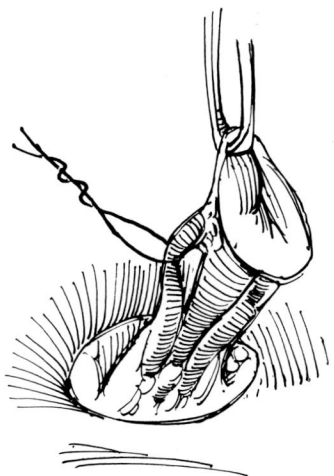

POSTOPERATIVE PROBLEMS

Persistent *urinary drainage* may require replacement of a catheter to drain the bladder. *Wound infection* about the umbilicus usually is superficial.

Commentary by Anthony A. Caldamone

The urachus is a vestigial structure connecting the umbilicus to the bladder. The urachus may be the source of four underlying pathologic entities: patent urachus, urachal cysts, urachal diverticulum, or alternating urachal sinus. Most of these entities will require surgical excision. The only exception is the patent urachus in the neonate, because some of these may close spontaneously in the absence of bladder outlet obstruction. The excision of an uninfected urachal remnant is nicely delineated in the text accompanying the figures. Although a transverse incision will result in excellent exposure, alternatively, a vertical midline incision along the course of the urachus may be more direct and can allow for extension to the umbilicus in a cosmetic fashion, should this be required because of difficulty in procuring the umbilical end of the urachus. Whenever possible, it is helpful to place a stent or probe through the patent urachus and into the bladder. It also is advantageous to have the bladder distended as well as possible to bring the anterior bladder wall up to the abdominal wall and, in doing so, to push the peritoneum cephalad. The operation is facilitated by identifying the proper plane of dissection between the peritoneum posterior to the urachus and the posterior rectus fascia, which is anterior to the urachus. In this same plane will lie the obliterated umbilical arteries. The obliterated umbilical arteries may be ligated proximally on the bladder wall or distally at the umbilicus. It is advisable to take a small cuff of bladder wall with the urachus to prevent a residual diverticulum.

A two-layered bladder closure in the pediatric population generally will allow for a short period of bladder catheter drainage, if at all. It most often is sufficient to drain the bladder for less than 24 hours.

Infected urachal remnant structures, such as an infected urachal cyst and an infected urachal sinus, may present a much more challenging dissection. In fact, it sometimes is advisable for a large infected urachal cyst to drain the cyst initially percutaneously and allow a period for antibiotic therapy to reduce the inflammation. Smaller infected urachal cysts or urachal sinuses, however, can be managed safely as a single procedure. With these infected remnants, it may be impossible to dissect the urachus away from contiguous structures. For instance, a larger portion of the bladder may need to be removed with the infected urachal cyst. Similarly, one may find it impossible to separate the infected cyst or sinus from the underlying peritoneum. One should be extremely careful in identifying adherent loops of bowel that may have been involved in the inflammatory process, which can extend through the peritoneum.

CHAPTER 67

Radical Cystectomy for Rhabdomyosarcoma

Plan chemotherapy, biopsy, and extirpative surgery. For lesions that are incompletely resected, add radiation therapy to postoperative chemotherapy.

1 Select a site for a stoma with the child in sitting and standing positions, and mark it with a needle scratch. Begin intravenous hydration with lactated Ringer's solution or 5 percent dextrose in 0.5 percent normal saline solution the afternoon before surgery. Use polyethylene glycol–electrolyte solution (GoLYTELY) as a mechanical bowel prep, and add fluconazole to the prophylactic antibiotics to avoid yeast overgrowth.

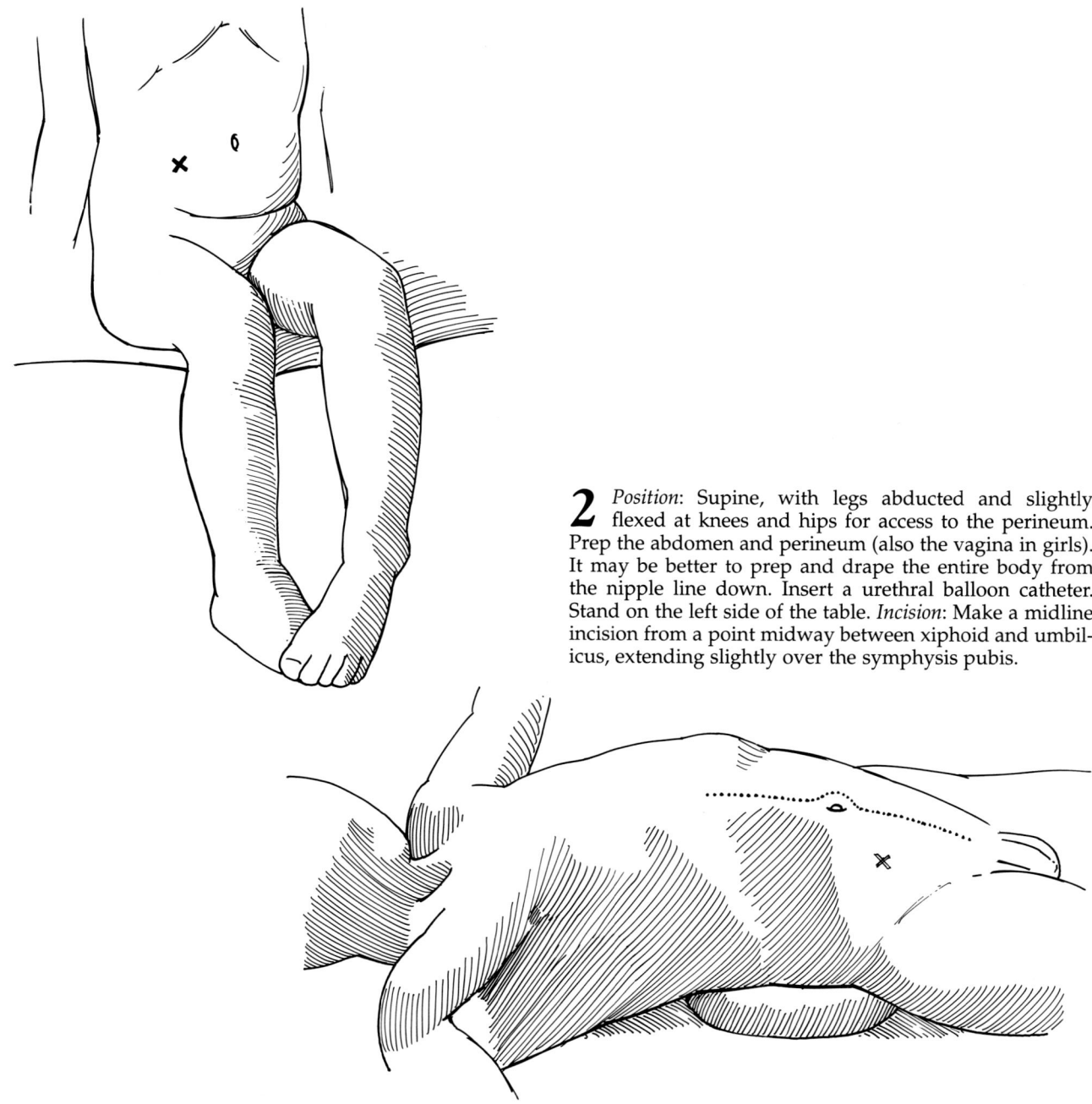

2 *Position*: Supine, with legs abducted and slightly flexed at knees and hips for access to the perineum. Prep the abdomen and perineum (also the vagina in girls). It may be better to prep and drape the entire body from the nipple line down. Insert a urethral balloon catheter. Stand on the left side of the table. *Incision*: Make a midline incision from a point midway between xiphoid and umbilicus, extending slightly over the symphysis pubis.

3 **A** and **B**, Open the peritoneum in the line of the incision in the upper half, but cut the lower portion in a V shape toward the iliac vessels to provide a peritoneal cuff on the bladder. Check the mobility of the tumor with a thumb in the preprostatic space and fingers in the cul-de-sac. Explore the abdomen, palpating especially the liver and pelvic nodes. Send any suspicious nodes for pathologic frozen-section examination.

Open the parietal peritoneum along the right common iliac artery, starting just above the bifurcation. Free the right ureter with its adventitia as low as possible, clamp it with a right-angle clamp, insert a stay suture proximally, and divide it distal to the suture. Send a segment for frozen-section examination. On the left, incise the lateral perito-

neum along the white line of Toldt, and reflect the sigmoid colon and rectum to the right side. Transect the left ureter similarly. Burrow with the fingers from one retroperitoneal opening to the other, insert a curved clamp, and pass the left ureter through by traction on the suture. Be sure the ureter is not twisted and runs in a smooth curve. It probably is unnecessary to insert infant feeding tubes; if used, tack them to the end of the ureters with 4-0 synthetic absorbable sutures and arrange for their connection with a drainage bag. Open the parietal peritoneum over the external iliac artery, and carry this incision anteriorly to the free peritoneal edge near the symphysis. Divide and ligate the vas deferens. Proceed with pelvic lymphadenectomy, exposing the iliac and hypogastric arteries and carrying the dissection into the obturator fossa.

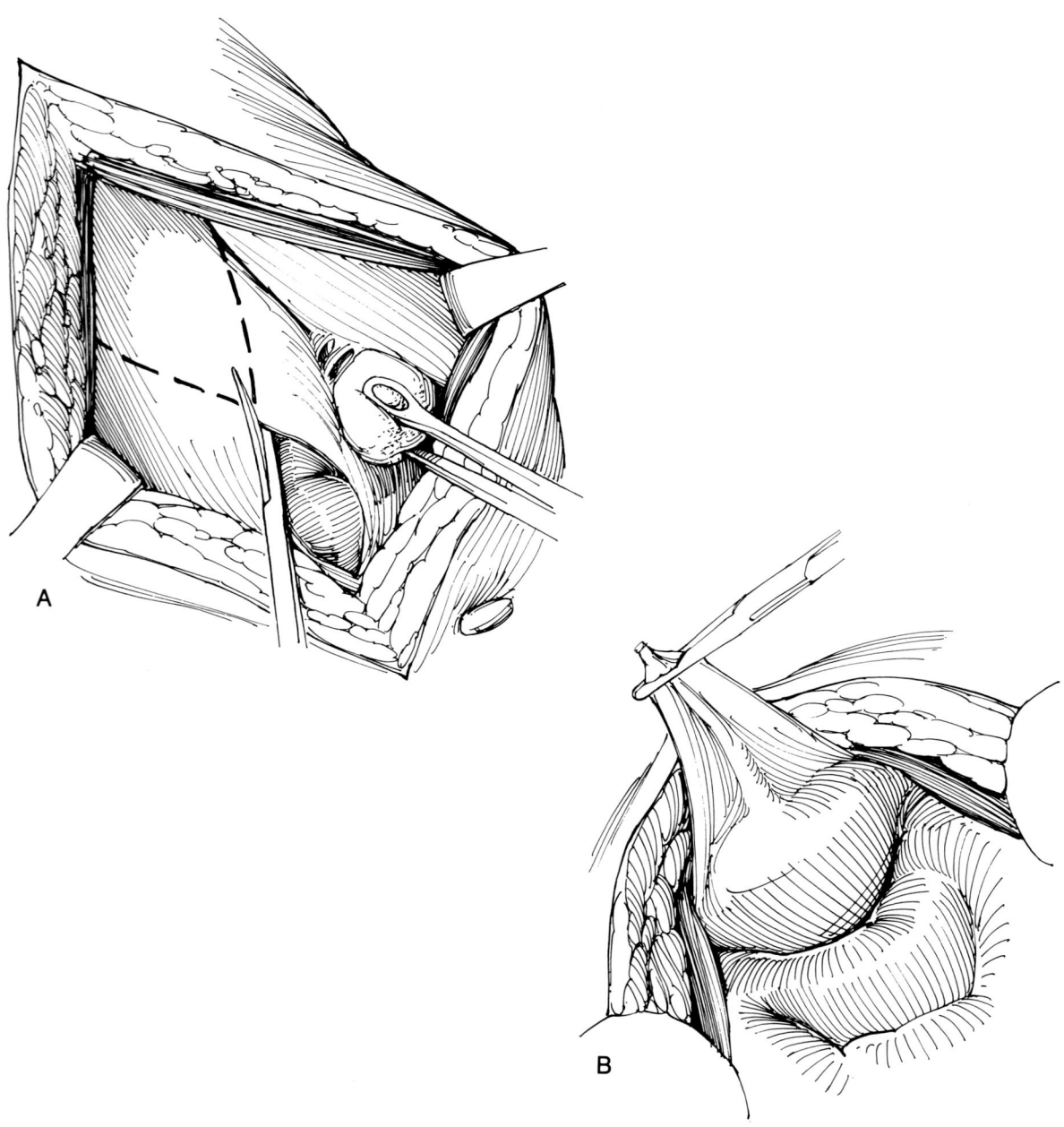

DIVISION OF ANTERIOR PEDICLE

4 **A** and **B**, Insert the index finger of the left hand behind the internal iliac (hypogastric) artery while the rest of the fingers retract the bladder. Sweep the finger parallel to the sacrum down to the endopelvic fascia to separate the pedicle to the bladder from that to the rectum. Clear the hypogastric artery and identify its first branch, the superior gluteal. Tie the obliterated umbilical artery and the superior vesical and middle vesical arteries, and clip the specimen side, clipping the vesical pedicle with large clips on right-angle appliers down to the endopelvic fascia, using the index finger to develop the plane and protect the rectum. Be sure enough tissue (0.5 to 1 cm) projects beyond each proximal clip to avoid dislodgment. Do not ligate the hypogastric artery to preserve the neurovascular bundle, but, if necessary, put a bulldog clamp on it. Dissect with care, and use clips on the large veins under the superior vesical arteries.

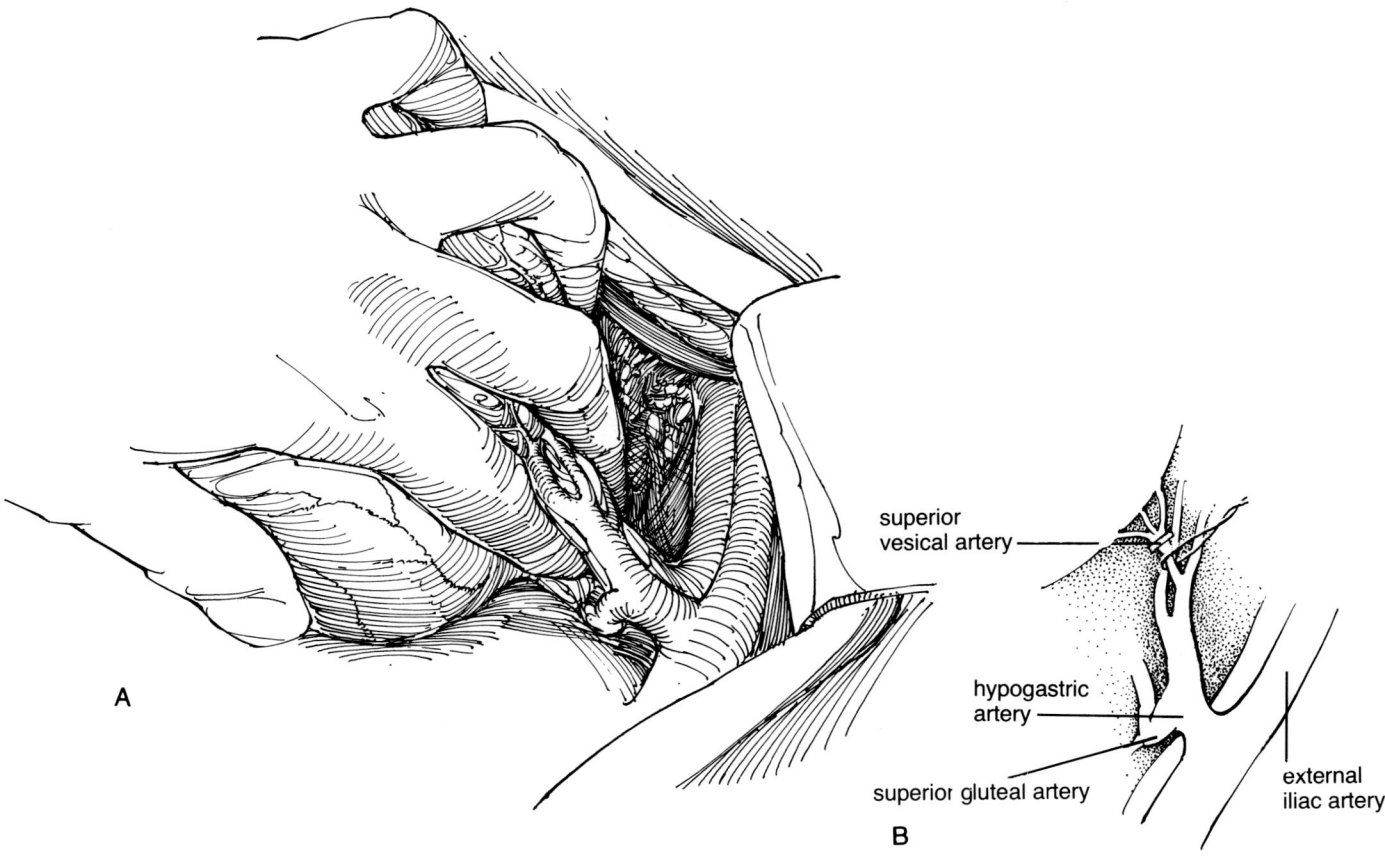

superior vesical artery

hypogastric artery

superior gluteal artery

external iliac artery

B

DIVISION OF POSTERIOR PEDICLE

5 Draw the bladder (uterus) up to be able to view the cul-de-sac. Incise the peritoneum beginning on either side of the rectum, and join the incisions in the cul-de-sac exactly at its junction with the anterior rectal wall, leaving the fused fascial fold (Denonvilliers' and rectal fascia) anteriorly.

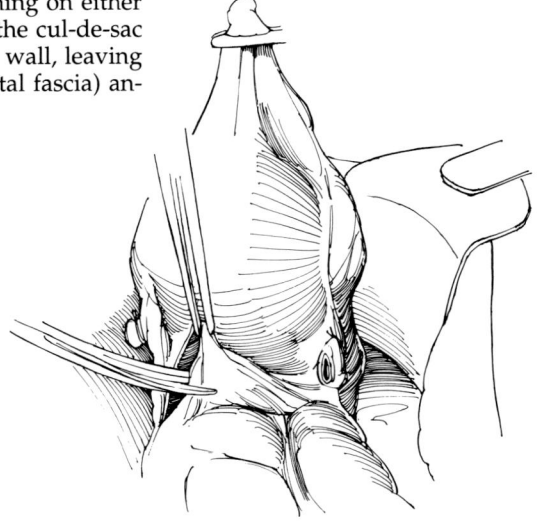

6 **A**, Sweep the rectum back off the bladder, seminal vesicles, and prostate (posterior vaginal wall) to develop the posterior pedicles. Take the pedicles lateral to the seminal vesicles to avoid the neurovascular bundle.

B, Clip and divide them. The bundles will be seen on the dorsolateral surface of the rectum.

In Girls

Clip and divide the right posterior pedicles along with the cardinal ligaments 4 to 5 cm below the cervix. Proceed with total hysterectomy. Open the vagina posteriorly just below the cervix, and divide it circumferentially. Free its anterior wall from the bladder as far as the urethra. Clip and divide the distal pedicles so formed.

Note: The dissection on the left side is easier if the surgeon stands on the right side of the table and returns to the left to clip and divide this pedicle.

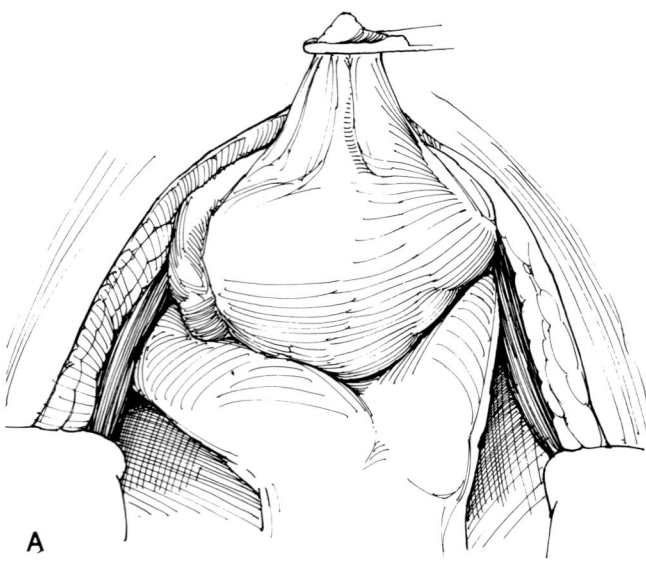

A

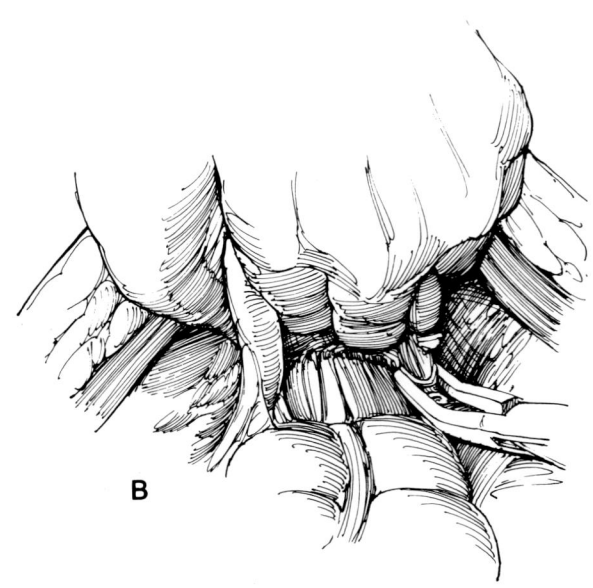

B

URETHRAL DIVISION

7 Free the prostate from the pubis. *Note*: If there is concern with extension of the neoplasm, open the periosteum with the cutting current, and develop a subperiosteal plane to the level of the urethra. Cut the puboprostatic ligaments (they will not bleed).

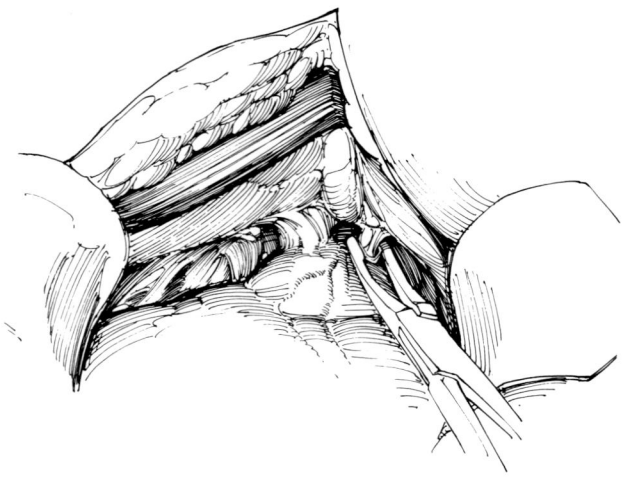

8 Pass a right angle clamp between the urethra and the dorsal vein complex and clamp and tie these with synthetic absorbable sutures. Clips or nonabsorbable sutures may migrate through the urethra when a continent diversion is connected. Stretch the urethra and transect it near the prostate. Do not clamp it, because this will jeopardize the anastomosis for continent diversion. Cut the anterior wall first, then pull the catheter into the incision and cut the posterior wall. Clamp and cut the catheter, and use the proximal part as a tractor to elevate the specimen. Be careful not to compromise the external urethral sphincter or injure the rectum. If the rectum is penetrated, coat the area with organic iodine solution. Close the injured site, and subsequently dilate the anus. Consider colostomy only if there has been extensive radiation. Pass the left index finger behind the urethra, and divide it and the indwelling catheter. Try to leave a good stump of urethra to facilitate the anastomosis with continent diversion. Pass a right-angle clamp between the urethra and the dorsal vein complex, and clamp and tie these with synthetic absorbable sutures. Clips or nonabsorbable sutures may migrate through the urethra when a continent diversion is connected.

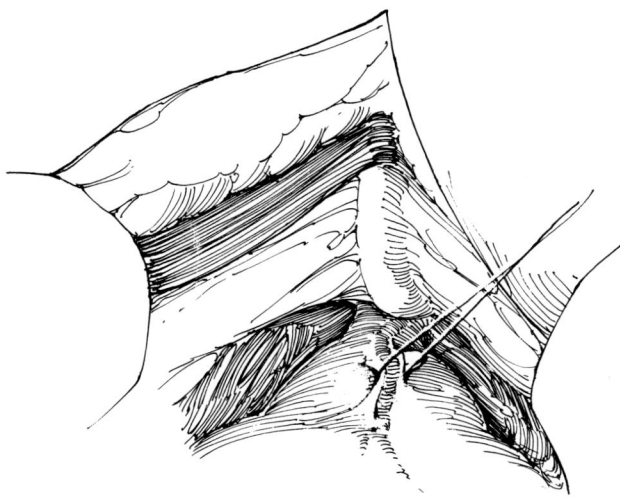

9 Divide the remaining lateral connections while avoiding the neurovascular bundles, at least on one side. Remove the specimen. Replace the bowel carefully, and pull the omentum down. Place drains. Maintain serum protein at normal levels subsequently.

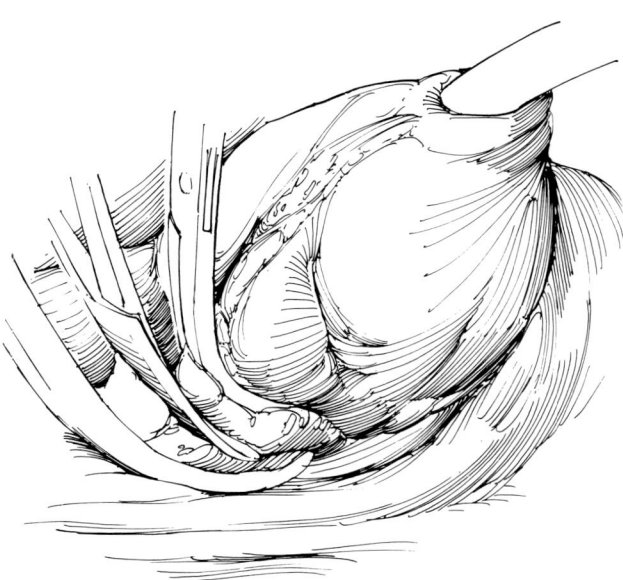

In Girls

Divide the urethropubic tissue. Place a curved clamp on the urethra. Open the anterior vaginal wall distally, and incise it around the urethral meatus. Close the cuff with interrupted 3-0 synthetic absorbable sutures. Use the same sutures to tack the previously closed vagina to Cooper's ligament to prevent its descent. Approximate the levators for hemostasis. Place a figure-eight 3-0 synthetic absorbable suture through both levators anteriorly just behind the pubis. Check for bleeding elsewhere. Drainage (suction) usually is needed for protection of the diversion. A two-team approach in older children allows removal in continuity. Pack the pelvic space, and proceed with urinary diversion or substitution if indicated. Drain and close the wound appropriately.

Commentary by Allan M. Shanberg

The addition of continent urinary diversion in boys has revolutionized, in our view, the care of rhabdomyosarcoma of the prostate. There has been a great reluctance on the part of pediatric hematology/oncology physicians to submit these children to cystectomy because of the psychologic disfigurement of making them wear a bag for an ileal conduit. The use of continent diversion has completely eliminated this reluctance, and as proved in the literature, radical cystoprostatectomy with adjunctive chemotherapy and radiation therapy still results in the highest cure rate.

In boys, we have found that the preoperative bowel prep using GoLYTELY is quite important to adequately clean the intestine prior to construction of the continent urinary diversion. We also use 72 hours of prophylactic antibiotics postoperatively, which obviously is the reader's choice. However, we strongly encourage adding the antifungus drug fluconazole in children because of the high risk of fungus overgrowth that we have found with continent urinary diversions, prophylactic antibiotics, and indwelling tubes in the reconstructed urinary tract. The techniques of the actual cystectomy itself are well described in the diagrams with appropriate commentary. We have tried to preserve the hypogastric vessels because of the obvious desire to try to preserve the neurovascular bundle, when possible, in children. Depending on the size of the tumor, this sometimes is not feasible, but if this can be done, it obviously makes the procedure more successful for children. It is quite important to avoid permanent sutures and hemoclips in the area of the urethra. Unfortunately, these have a habit of migrating through the anastomosis into the continent urinary diversion, and, as such, we use absorbable sutures and tie these areas where ties are necessary. If the rectum is opened inadvertently during the procedure, we see no problem in doing a primary closure of the rectum after cleansing the area with povidone-iodine (Betadine) paint. However, we do use a three-layer closure of the rectum using one layer of Dexon material, followed by two separate layers of imbrication, generally with polydioxanone or Maxon sutures, which are long-acting monofilament absorbable sutures, and we have not found it necessary to do a colostomy in any of our children or adults when this injury has occurred. Naturally, if the patient has had extensive pelvic radiation and there are fears of closure, doing a colostomy is always a safe decision.

PART III

NONCONTINENT URINARY DIVERSION

CHAPTER 68

Introduction to Noncontinent Urinary Diversion

NEITHER URETHRA NOR URETEROVESICAL JUNCTION PRESENT

Because most diversions are potentially reversible, it is no longer as necessary to distinguish between temporary and permanent diversion.

Diversion From the Bladder. A *cystostomy* provides direct drainage for the bladder, especially after open operations on the bladder, but for long-term drainage, the catheter may be irritating, and continuous drainage and infection may result in a small bladder. For temporary drainage, a *perineal urethrostomy* diverts the urine effectively from the urethra, but usually if a urethral catheter is inadvisable, a cystostomy is preferable in children. For more permanent diversion, a *vesicostomy* provides effective drainage at the price of poor stomal position and a tendency for stomal stenosis, infection, and stone formation.

Diversion for the Upper Tract. *Percutaneous nephrostomy* drainage and *indwelling ureteral stents* can allow relief of obstruction without formal surgical intervention, but in infants and children, the need for good drainage is imperative, and quality of the endodrainage often is inadequate. A *nephrostomy* is most effective but is associated with so much infection and concomitant renal damage that it is used for more extreme circumstances and is seldom considered, even for short-term diversion. A percutaneous nephrostomy usually is better. Because the ureter and pelvis are dilated, a cutaneous ureterostomy or cutaneous pyelostomy is feasible. *Cutaneous (end) ureterostomy* is a simple form of urinary diversion but is more often permanent, unless done in the distal ureter. A prerequisite is a ureter dilated to at least 1 cm in diameter, thick walled and well vascularized. Be certain that a cutaneous ureterostomy is made low enough in the ureter so that it will not interfere with later reconstruction. This procedure can be appropriate for temporary diversion in infants but is seldom applicable in adolescents with normal ureters because of the high incidence of stricture from ischemia of the cutaneous portion of the nondilated ureter.

Pediatric loop nephrostomy has the advantages of good drainage and ease of closure when no longer needed. If situated high in the flank, drainage is optimum, but appliances are hard to maintain. If lower, drainage may be satisfactory for less-compromised renal units, and maintenance of appliances is simplified, but later reconstitution may be more difficult. An end-cutaneous ureterostomy may be preferable.

During a difficult operation on the lower ureter, a *ureterostomy in situ* may be used as a last resort. Intubate the ureter and bring the tube retroperitoneally to the skin. After a tract has formed, the tube may be changed, but it must be done quickly or the tract will be lost.

Urinary conduits formed from intestine have the advantage of relative freedom from stenosis, but late complications (especially stricture at the site of ureteral anastomosis, as well as stomal problems) have reduced their use. They largely have been replaced by forms of continent diversion, avoiding the necessity of wearing an appliance. Whether the ileum makes a better conduit than the sigmoid or the transverse colon has not been determined. Colon conduits do have the advantage of allowing formation of a nonrefluxing ureteral anastomosis.

Ureteroileostomy is a standard procedure with good short-term results, although reflux can occur with stasis. The stoma can be a problem, and a device must be worn. A *high ileal conduit* may be useful in children. The *colon conduit*, whether the usual sigmoid conduit or the transverse colon conduit, is associated with few stomal problems, and the ureteral anastomosis can be made antirefluxive. It may serve well for the long run. The *sigmoid conduit* has certain advantages: it provides a greater length for high positioning of the stoma; it need not be isoperistaltic; it allows formation of a nonrefluxing ureteral anastomosis; and it results less frequently in stomal stenoses.

Although a sigmoid or transverse colon conduit can be constructed so that reflux with renal deterioration is less than with other systems, it is less acceptable for social, rather than medical, reasons than those procedures that produce continence. For temporary diversion before major vesical augmentation, the sigmoid conduit is useful. It is only after extensive pelvic irradiation, rarely seen in children, that the transverse colon conduit is preferred. It does have the additional advantage of requiring shorter lengths of ureter obtained away from the radiated field.

Follow-up. No matter what form diversion takes, long-term surveillance is essential to catch dysfunction before the kidneys are irreversibly damaged. Intravenous urograms and sonograms, urine cultures, retrograde loopograms, and repeated determinations of serum electrolytes are indicated at regular intervals.

Complications. (For further discussion of complications, see pages 286, 287.) *Bacteriuria* is common, but symptomatic *infection* requiring treatment is less frequent. A normally functioning system will keep itself free of infection; the corollary is that recurrent infection suggests malfunction of the conducting structures. *Pyocystis* is an extreme form of infection, restricted to the totally diverted bladder, most commonly occurring in girls. Antibiotics and lavage of the bladder with saline solution with or without an antiseptic usually suffice, especially because the condition is usually self-limiting. Overdilation of the urethra with a Kollmann's dilator can be effective, but opening the bladder into the vagina may be necessary in a few stubborn cases. *Stomal problems* begin with improperly fitting appliances. This often is associated with encrustation and stomal stenosis, the latter less often seen if skin is incorporated in the stoma. *Parastomal hernia* from too large a fascial defect usually requires taking the stoma down, repairing the defect, and making a new site for the stoma, preferably on the opposite side. *Residual urine* in the conduit may be secondary to a narrow stoma, but usually it appears later, caused by reduced peristaltic activity in the loop. Replacement of the segment may be required.

CHAPTER 69

Suprapubic Cystostomy

Alternatives to suprapubic cystostomy include perineal urethrostomy (page 350) and trocar cystostomy.

1 *Position*: Supine. Fill the bladder with sterile water until it is just visible or palpable suprapubically. *Incision*: Make a short vertical or transverse incision through the skin and subcutaneous layers slightly above the symphysis pubis.

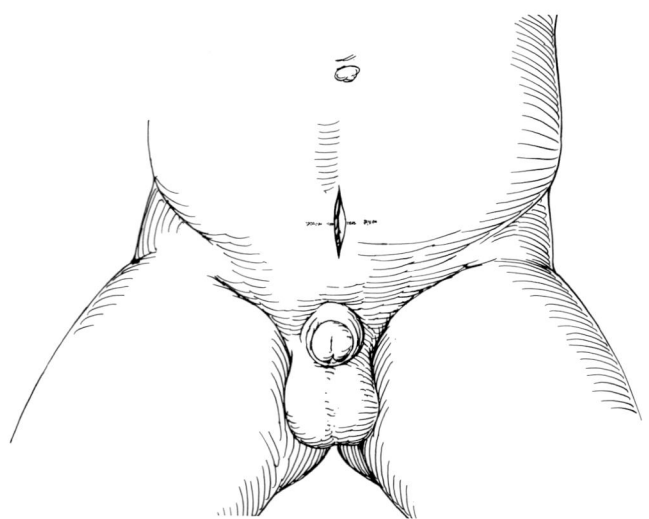

2 Expose the rectus fascia in the midline by pushing back the covering fat. Incise the fascia transversely.

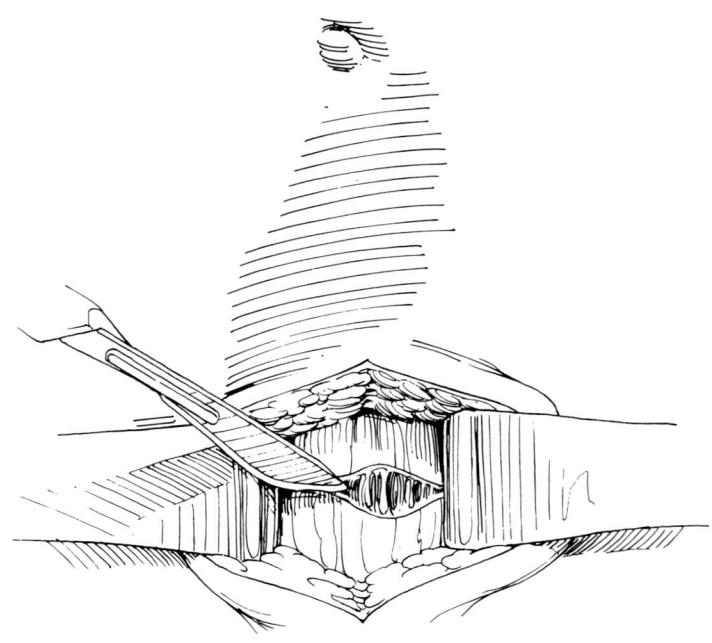

3 A, Separate the recti bluntly. Hold the muscles back with two retractors and expose the prevesical fat.

B, Push the peritoneal fold upward. Expose minimal bladder surface. The vascular pattern and tissue characteristics of the bladder usually are unmistakable. If in doubt, insert a fine needle and aspirate, or pass a curved sound through the urethra and palpate the tip.

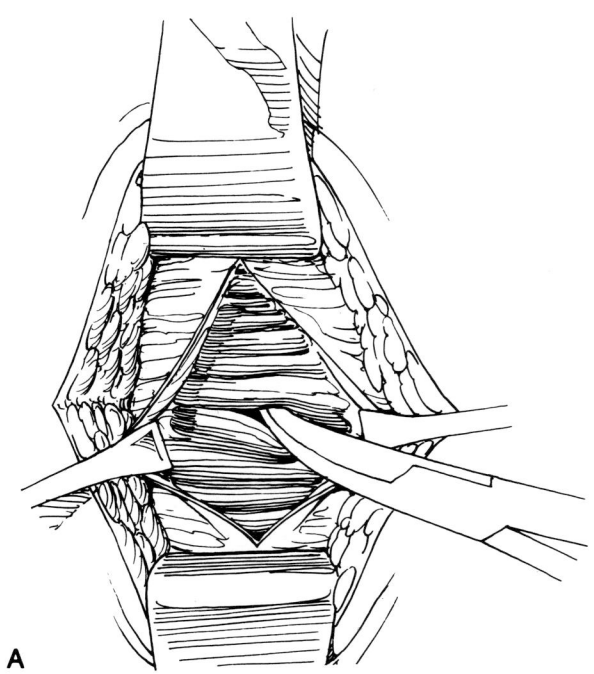

A

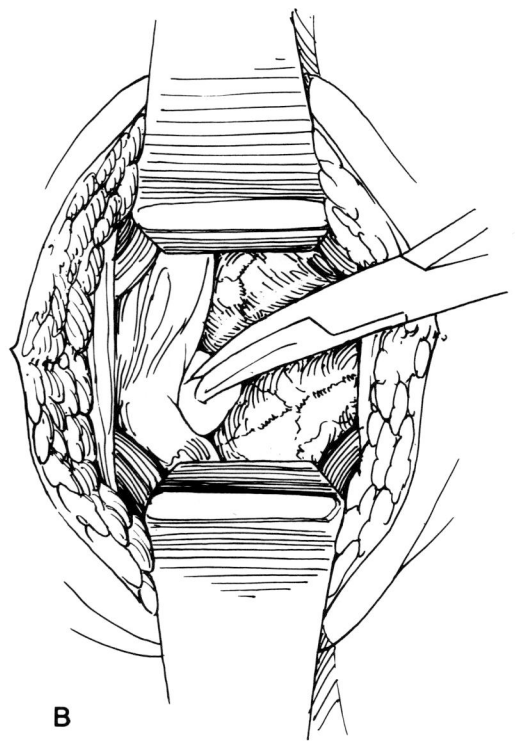

B

4 Place two 3-0 chromic catgut stay sutures into the bladder wall. (Alternatively, grasp it with two Allis clamps.) Fulgurate obvious crossing vessels. Incise vertically between the sutures with the cutting current, and enter the bladder.

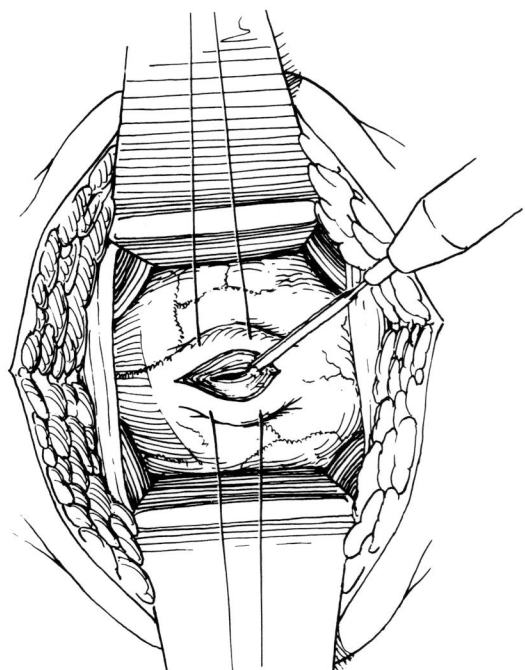

5 Reposition the Allis clamps to grasp the full thickness of the wall. Insert a silicone Malecot catheter stretched on a Mayo clamp while the urine is still running out. Alternatively, insert a balloon catheter and inflate it. Withdraw the catheter slightly to be sure the catheter tip does not touch the trigone.

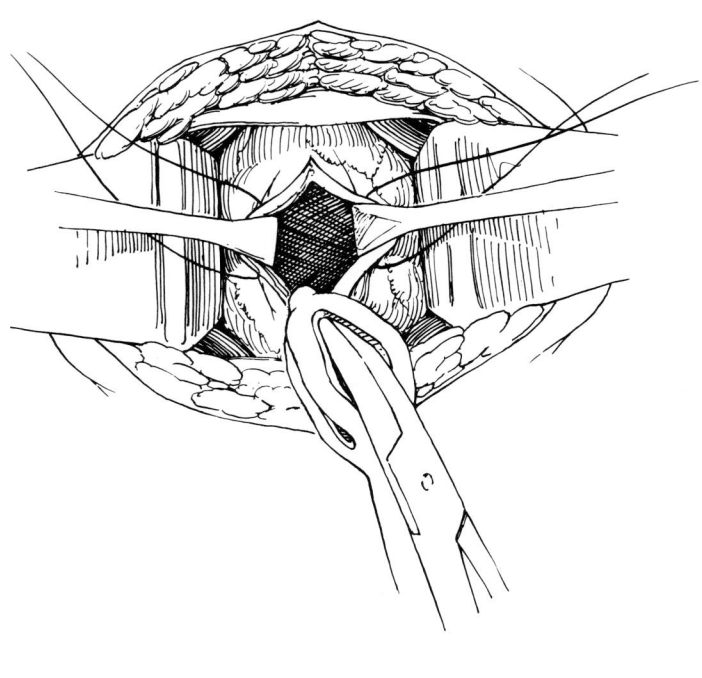

6 Close the bladder tightly around the catheter with 3-0 chronic catgut sutures. If the bladder wall is thin, use mattress sutures. Fasten the catheter to the bladder with the ends of one of the sutures.

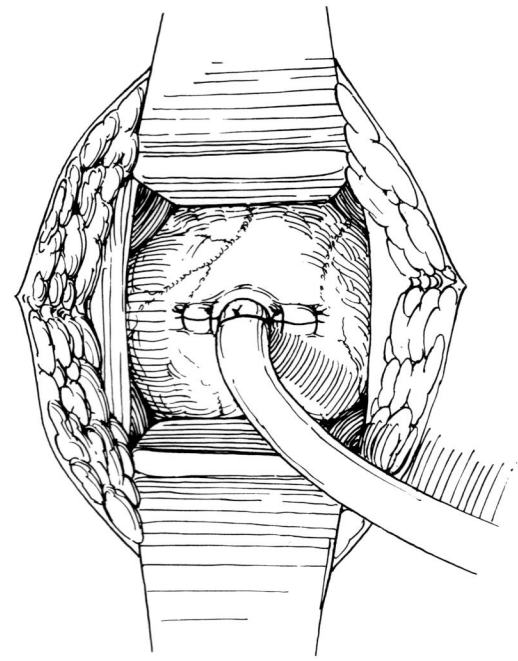

7 Make a stab wound in the skin near the incision well above the symphysis, and force a curved clamp through it to emerge beneath the rectus muscle. Trim the catheter end obliquely to shape it for pulling through the body wall. Grasp the apex and pull the catheter out.

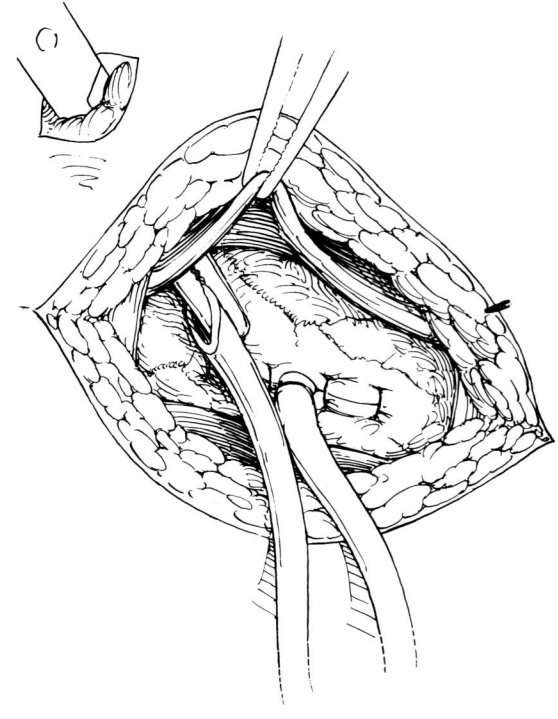

8 Close the fascia and skin around a Penrose drain with 3-0 chromic catgut sutures. Fasten the catheter to the skin with a heavy silk suture, and tape it to the abdomen with waterproof tape over tincture of benzoin. Connect the catheter at once to sterile drainage. For a more permanent cystostomy, suture the bladder to the rectus fascia, and bring the catheter through the wound.

One way of inserting a cystostomy tube in the exposed empty bladder is to pick up the double thickness of the bladder between thumb and forefinger and stretch the wall. Insert a curved clamp through both layers. Grasp the tip of a balloon catheter, draw it through the first layer of the wall, and inflate the balloon inside the bladder.

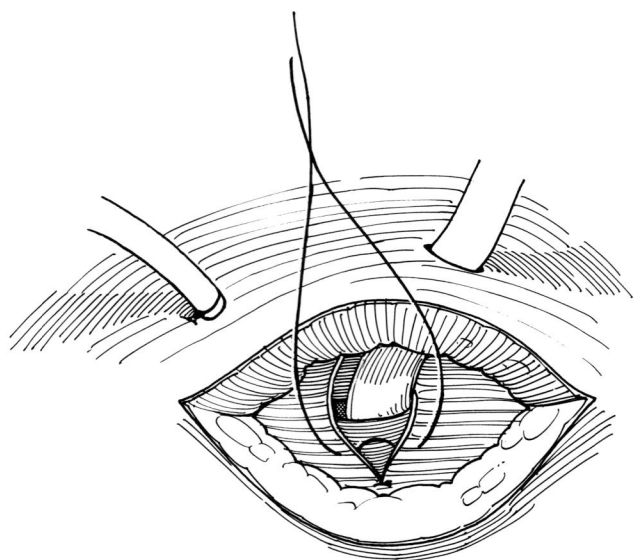

RETROGRADE APPROACH IN OLDER GIRLS

Insert a curved Lowsley retractor (or curved sound with a hole near the tip) through the urethra until it can be palpated suprapubically. Cut down on the tip of the retractor or sound to let it emerge suprapubically. Insert a heavy suture through the solid tip of a Malecot or balloon catheter, and run it through the eye of the retractor or sound and tie it. Draw the retractor and catheter out of the urethra, grasp the catheter tip with a Mayo clamp, and cut the tie at the meatus. Position the catheter in the bladder by countertraction suprapubically. Test the position by irrigation. Suture the catheter to the skin with heavy silk. Release the clamp from the catheter tip. Tape the catheter to the body wall.

Vesical lithotomy is used for those stones that cannot be removed by shock wave or instrumentally, especially in those cases associated with neurogenic bladder. Proceed as for suprapubic cystostomy, but insert a Mayo clamp into the opening, aspirate the contents, and insert two fingers to make the opening somewhat larger. Insert a Malecot catheter that exits through a stab wound. Because infection may cause problems, drain the prevesical space with a Penrose drain that also exits from a stab wound.

POSTOPERATIVE PROBLEMS

Obstruction requires irrigation. If that fails, make a cystogram to see if the end of the catheter is displaced. *Urgency* and pain, caused by contact of the catheter with trigone, can be distressing. Retract the tube and refasten it to the skin. *Inadvertent removal* of the tube will occur if it is not stitched to the skin and retaped regularly with fresh tape over tincture of benzoin. *Urinary infection* is delayed, but not prevented, by maintaining closed drainage and giving suppressive antibiotics. *Peritonitis* is a rare complication, secondary to puncture of the bowel during introduction of the tube.

Persistent drainage after removal of the tube usually will respond to urethral catheter drainage. If the tract has epithelialized, it will not close until the surface has been denuded with a silver nitrate stick, curette, or new wood screw.

Commentary by Victor Braren

In performing a suprapubic cystotomy, the smallest incision possible should be made. In neonates, this often can be 1.5 to 2 cm; conversely, in older children, especially those who are fat, a longer incision may be required. I much prefer to use a Malecot-type catheter than a Foley, because even when a Foley is pulled up securely to the dome, the tip of the Foley will always irritate the trigone somewhat as it drains the bladder. I also prefer to suture the catheter to the skin where it emerges, using a silk suture wrapped several times about the catheter; the size of the suture will depend on the size of the child. This prevents family and inattentive nurses from pulling the catheter out. Removing the stitch at the time of removal of the catheter is extremely simple. When one is using the retrograde approach, as described for older girls, it is important to hold the tip of the sound in such a way so that it is lying as inferior as possible in the midline, just above the symphysis pubis. Otherwise, one inadvertently may cut down through the perineal cavity to the bladder if the tip of the sound is too high.

CHAPTER 70

Perineal Urethrostomy

GROOVED SOUND TECHNIQUE

Provide a biopsy set, curved grooved (Gouley) sounds (12 to 14 F for boys and 18 to 24 F for adolescents), three small Allis clamps, 3-0 plain catgut sutures, and a balloon catheter already mounted on a lubricated stilet (10 to 12 F for boys).

1 Insert a grooved sound of suitable size until its tip rests in the prostatic urethra. Have your assistant press the curved portion caudad toward the perineum (arrows).

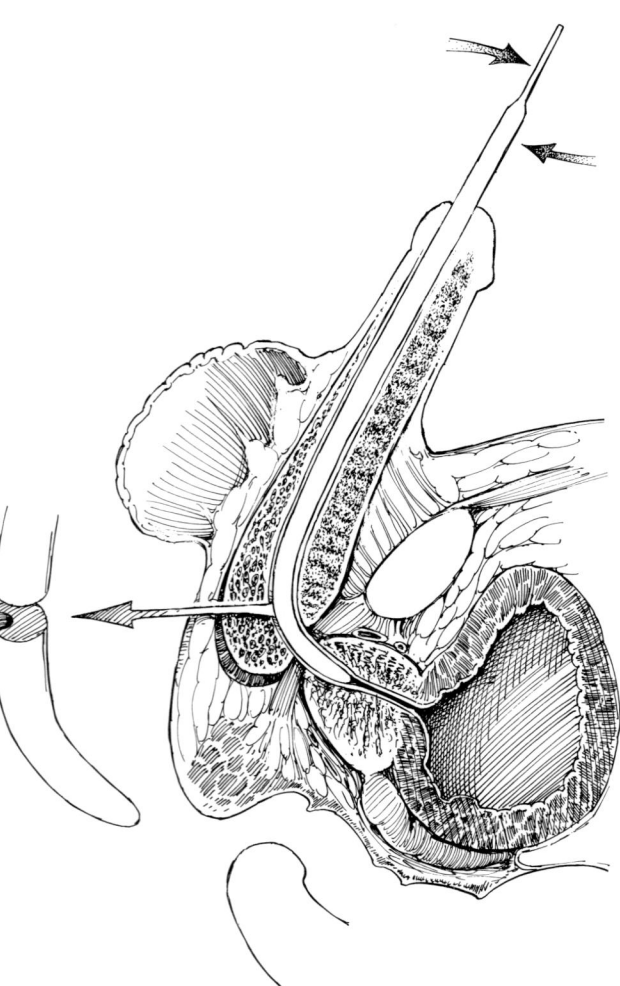

2 Grasp the sound through the perineum with the left thumb and index finger. Do not let go.

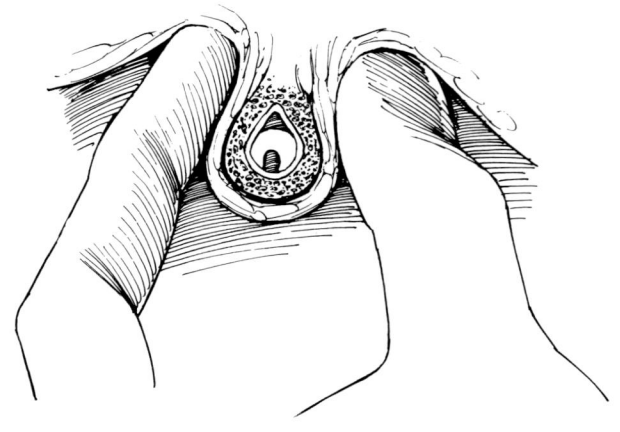

3 Incise the perineum into the groove over the curve of the sound with a #15 blade. Lengthen the stab wound anteriorly, then invert the knife to extend it posteriorly. Compress the urethra between the thumb and index finger to evert the urethra.

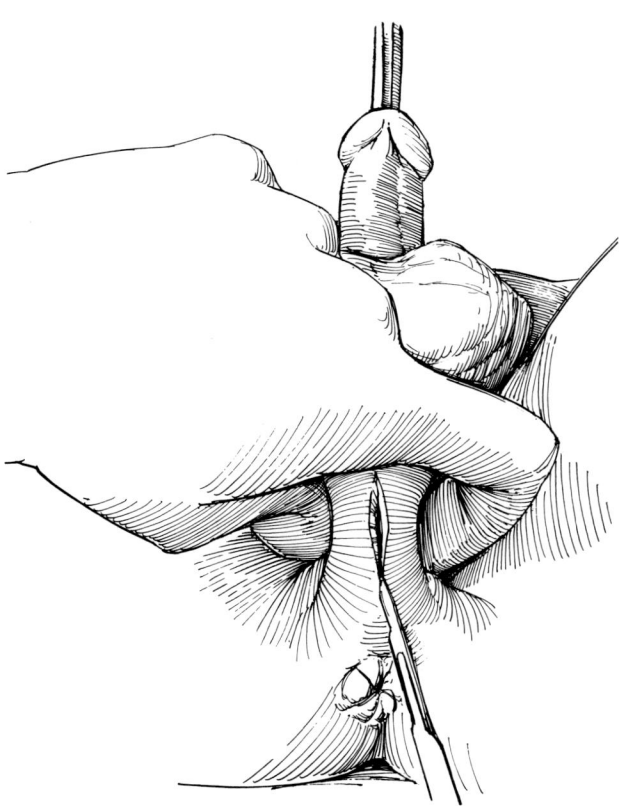

4 **A** and **B**, Secure the epithelial edge by inserting one blade of an Allis clamp into the groove of the sound to catch the epithelium and some of the spongy tissue; with the other blade, catch the skin as you close the clamp (in infants, use loupes). Secure the opposite edge in the same way with a second clamp. Substitute a third clamp if the epithelial edge is not caught cleanly the first time on either side.

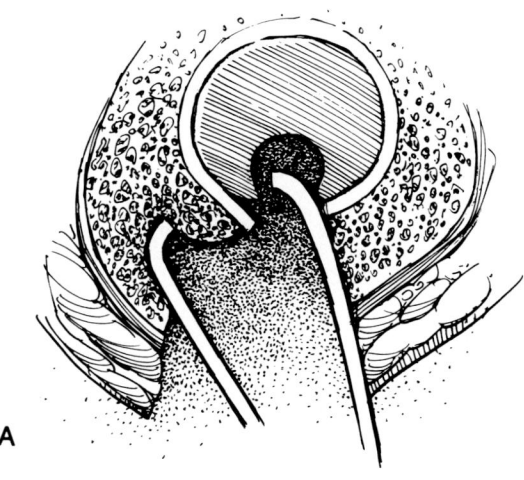

A

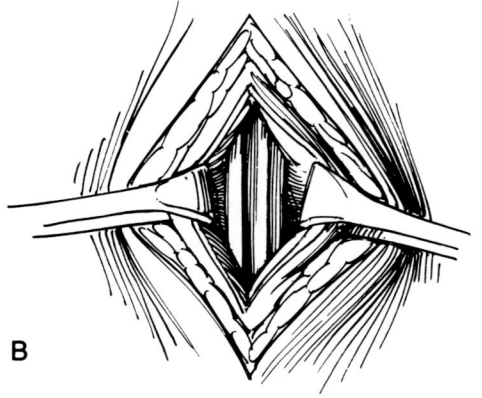

B

5 Release the grip on the sound and urethra. Have your assistant slowly withdraw the sound. As its tip clears the incision, insert the tip of the inverted catheter on its stilet into the urethra. Once it has entered the urethra, rotate it 180 degrees, and pass it up into the bladder.

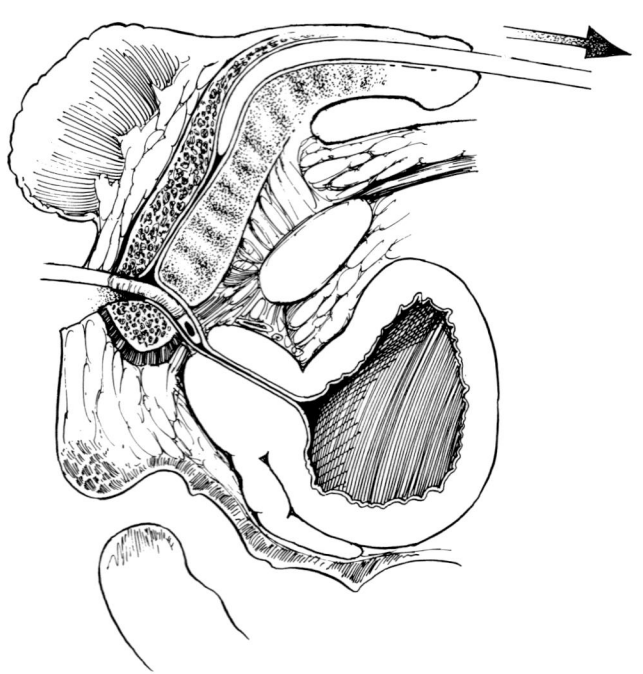

6 If the urethrostomy is to be permanent, place one or two plain catgut sutures to close the urethral wall and corpus spongiosum. Place these *proximal* to the exit site of the catheter, so that the urethral lumen cannot be compromised. Close the skin similarly. If the urethrostomy is to be temporary, place a 3-0 plain catgut suture through the epithelium and spongiosum on each side in place of the Allis clamps. On closure, tie these together or place additional 3-0 plain catgut sutures. In older children, be sure to place a small rubber drain (a piece of rubber glove is suitable) to the area. Close the skin around it with 3-0 plain catgut sutures. Remove the drain in 24 hours.

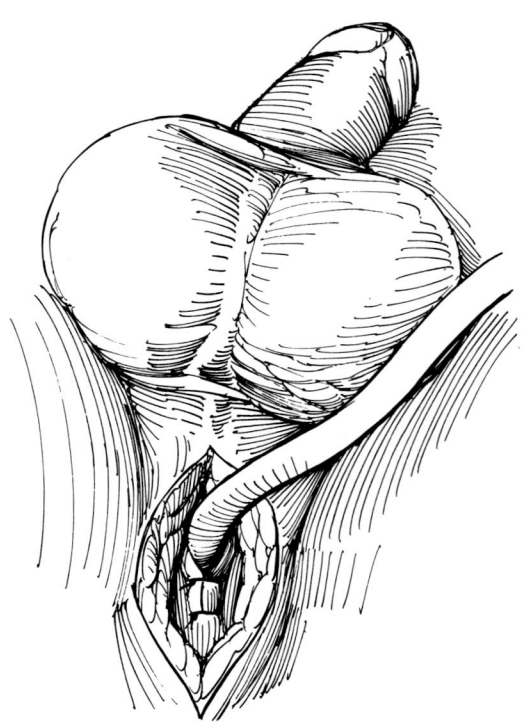

PEDIATRIC SOUND AND CATHETER TECHNIQUE

7 **A,** Insert a 10 F silicone balloon catheter into the bladder just beyond the point where it starts to drain urine. Tie a suture around it at the meatus as a marker. Cut off the flared segment.

B, Insert an 8 F sound into the lumen.

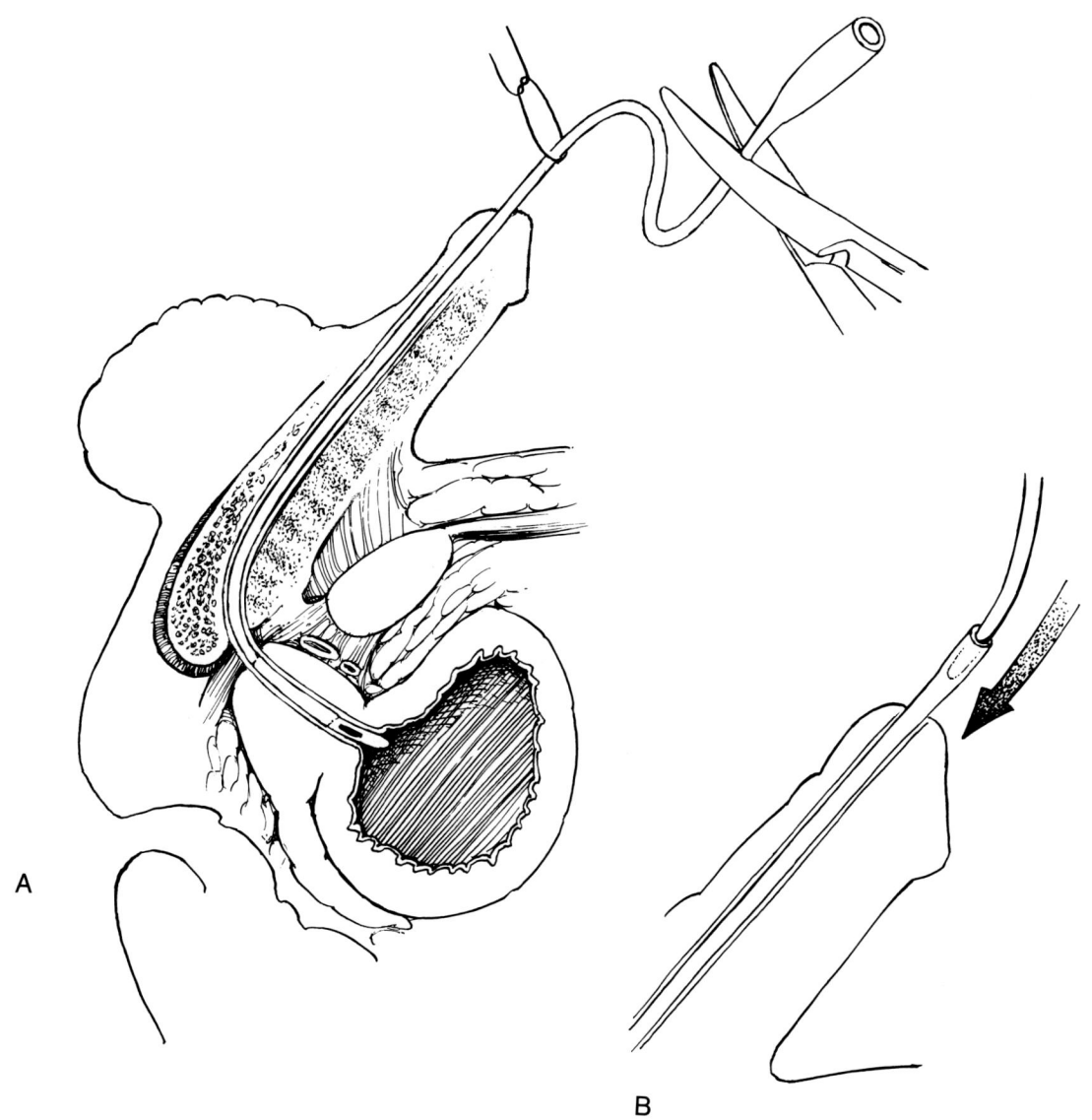

A

B

8 Advance the sound and catheter up the penile urethra, and rotate them 180 degrees to tent up the perineum. Cut down on the tip of the sound and catheter.

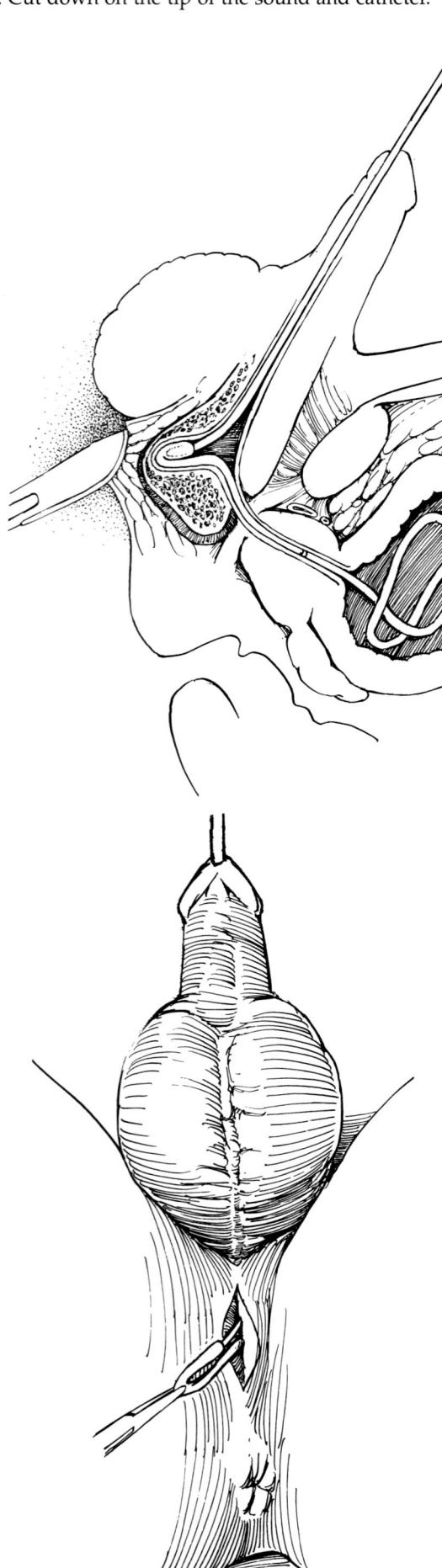

9 **A**, Push the sound and catheter out through the incision to grasp the distal end of the catheter in a clamp and extract it from the sound, which is then withdrawn.

B, Pull the distal end of the catheter out until the marking suture appears. Suture the catheter in place, or fill the balloon through a blunt-tipped needle inserted into the filling lumen of the catheter. Clamp the catheter, and plug the filling hole with a round toothpick that has been dipped in silicone glue. Attach the drainage tube with a Christmas-tree adapter.

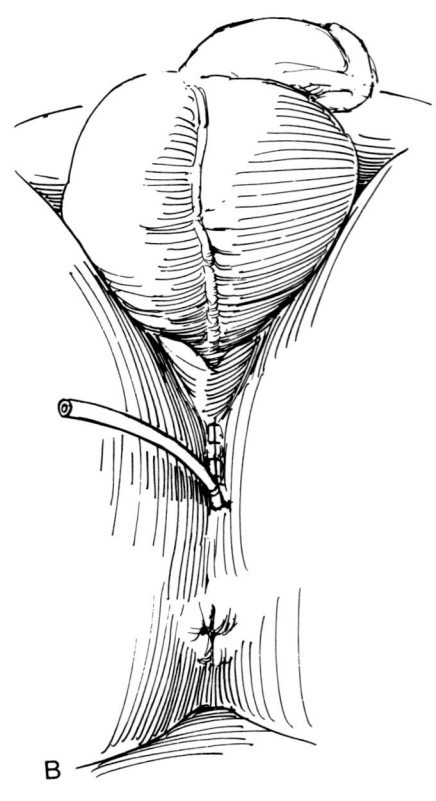

A

B

POSTOPERATIVE PROBLEMS

Abscess in the perineal wound is common if a drain is either not placed or removed too soon. The wound can be drained by insertion of a clamp. *Leakage*, if it occurs, will be temporary unless a distal stricture is present. In some children with very thin perineal layers, formal closure may be needed.

Commentary by Victor Braren

Considerable experience was gained with perineal ure-throstomy in the beginning of my practice, when I rou-tinely used it as a method of diversion proximal to hypo-spadias repair; I rarely use this procedure now. Some help-ful tips of positioning are to get the child in a slightly exaggerated lithotomy position so that the perineum is flat and slightly extended. It is extremely key that when the incision is made that one stay in the median raphe/midline throughout. This greatly decreases the amount of bleeding. I also have found it helpful to use silk temporary traction stitches when the urethra is entered to secure the edges thereof, instead of using Allis forceps, but this is a personal preference.

CHAPTER 71

Vesicostomy

PEDIATRIC VESICOSTOMY (BLOCKSOM)

Vesicostomy continues to be used frequently as a form of temporary urinary diversion in infants who are in need of urinary tract rehabilitation and delayed reconstruction. Consider vesicostomy in ill infants in whom reconstruction must be delayed and in neonates with posterior urethral valves, severe reflux, or a neurogenic bladder associated with meningomyelocele.

Insert a small catheter, and fill the bladder until it is quite full and palpable.

1 *Position:* Supine. The operation often is done in children with neurologic disorders, who require particular attention to avoid pressure sores.

Incision: Make a short (2-cm) transverse incision midway between the symphysis and umbilicus, over the dome of the bladder (stay at least 2 cm above the symphysis). The incision should be just large enough to admit the little finger; too large or too low an incision encourages vesical prolapse. Incise the rectus fascia transversely, and separate the muscles bluntly.

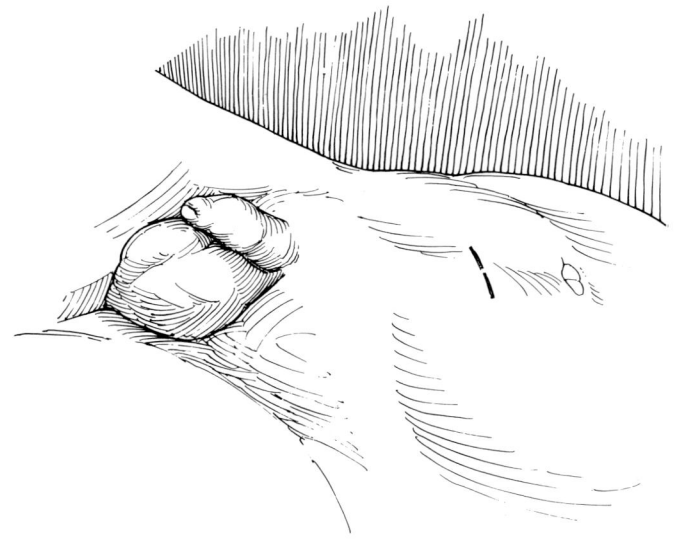

2 Remove small triangles from the fascia, and trim some of the muscle to make an opening for the stoma.

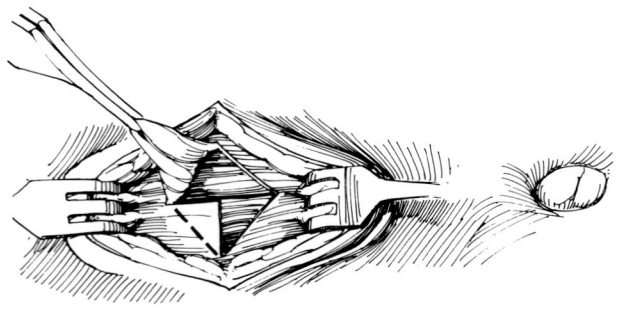

3 Expose the bladder, and place several traction sutures in the anterior wall to draw it inferiorly. Peel the peritoneum from the dome, mobilizing it until the obliterated umbilical arteries and urachus are identified, marking the end of the dissection.

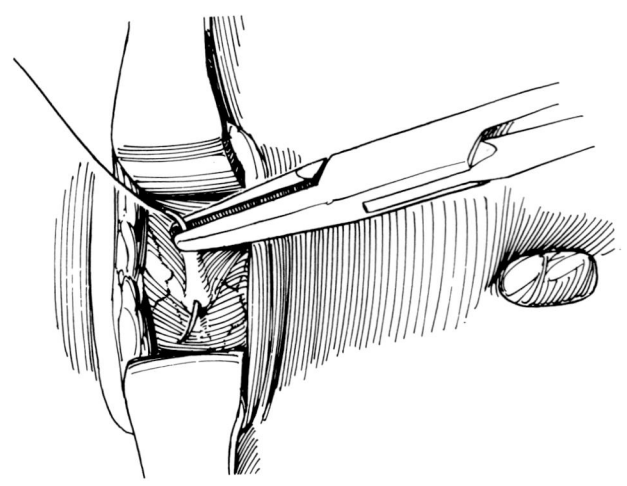

4 **A,** Pull the bladder into the wound so that the posterior wall is at skin level.

B, Open the bladder by excising the urachus.

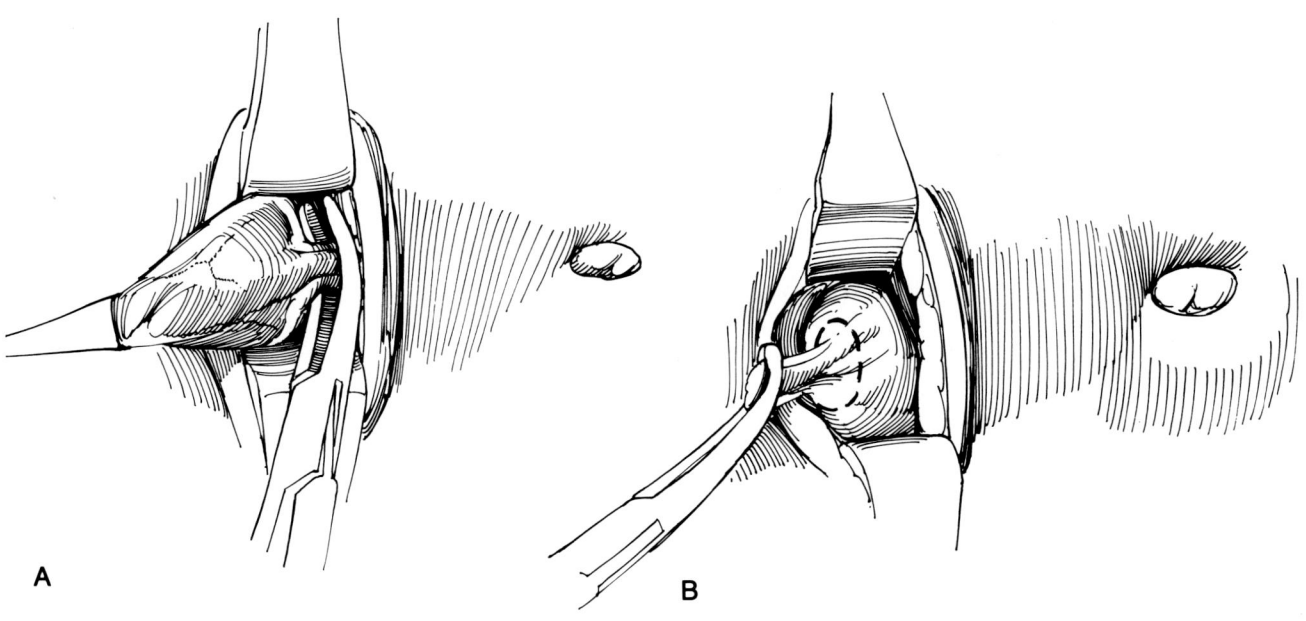

A

B

5 Suture the anterior and posterior walls of the bladder to the rectus fascia with at least six 3-0 synthetic absorbable sutures to tubularize the stoma. Close the lateral fascial defects around the outside of the bladder to achieve a 24 F lumen at the internal stoma. Too wide a stoma in a child with normal thickness of the bladder wall will allow prolapse. The thick bladders associated with myelomeningocele do not tend to prolapse. The thick-walled bladder in children with prune belly syndrome requires a larger stoma because of its tendency to stenose. Approximate the subcutaneous tissues.

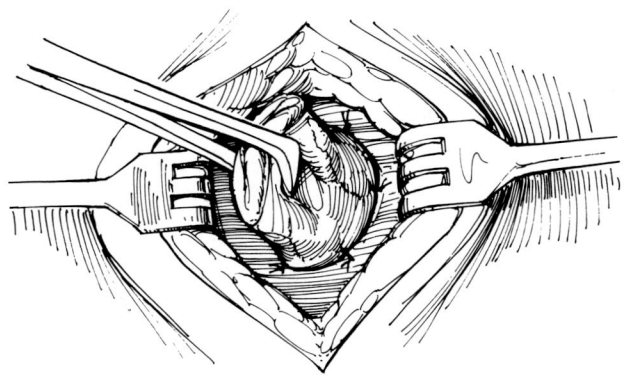

6 Suture the full thickness of the bladder to the subcuticular layer with 5-0 synthetic absorbable sutures. The stoma should not admit the fingertip but should calibrate to 24 F so that the fascial defect will be narrow enough to avoid prolapse of the posterior wall of the bladder through the stoma, except in cases of prune belly. Close the remainder of the incision. Apply petroleum jelly gauze and diapers.

Closure of the Vesicostomy: Excise the vesical epithelial tract. Place a cystostomy tube to exit through a stab wound. Close the bladder in two layers (5-0 plain catgut subepithelially, 4-0 synthetic absorbable to the wall). Approximate the fascia and the skin around a Penrose drain. In infants with valves, it may be expedient to fulgurate the valves through the vesicostomy stoma prior to its closure, thus using the same anesthetic. In these cases, place a urethral catheter for a few days to avoid stricture of the urethra from the absence of urine flow.

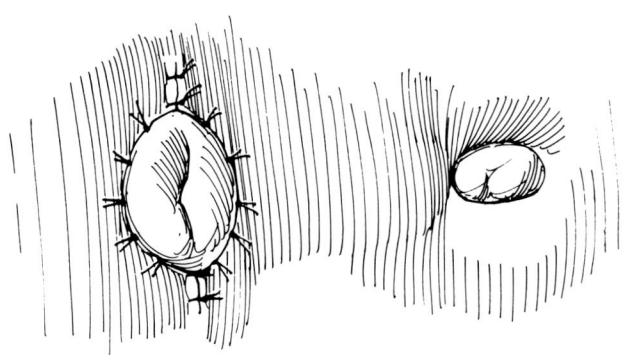

BLADDER TUBULARIZATION FOR CONTINENT ABDOMINAL STOMA (KLAUBER)

A large bladder with or without a vesicostomy may be converted into a continent reservoir with a catheterizable stoma. The tube, constructed from bladder wall, may be developed posteriorly beginning at the trigone or formed from the anterior wall. Tube length and coaptation of the tube to the bladder (flap valve) are responsible for continence.

7   **A,** Expose and mobilize the bladder and vesicostomy tract through a subumbilical incision, and open its anterior wall. Make two parallel incisions 2.4 cm apart and 13 cm long through the exposed posterior wall from the stoma to a point above the trigone, and free the strip.

B, Insert a 24 F silicone balloon catheter, and form a tube from the strip of bladder with a continuous 3-0 chromic catgut suture. Close the defect remaining in the posterior wall of the bladder with a similar suture.

C, Approximate the anterior bladder wall. Tack the new tube to the fascia during wound closure, so that it will neither prolapse nor recede, and suture the new stoma to the skin.

D, Complete the closure of the abdominal wall. Remove the catheter and start clean intermittent catheterization in 12 days.

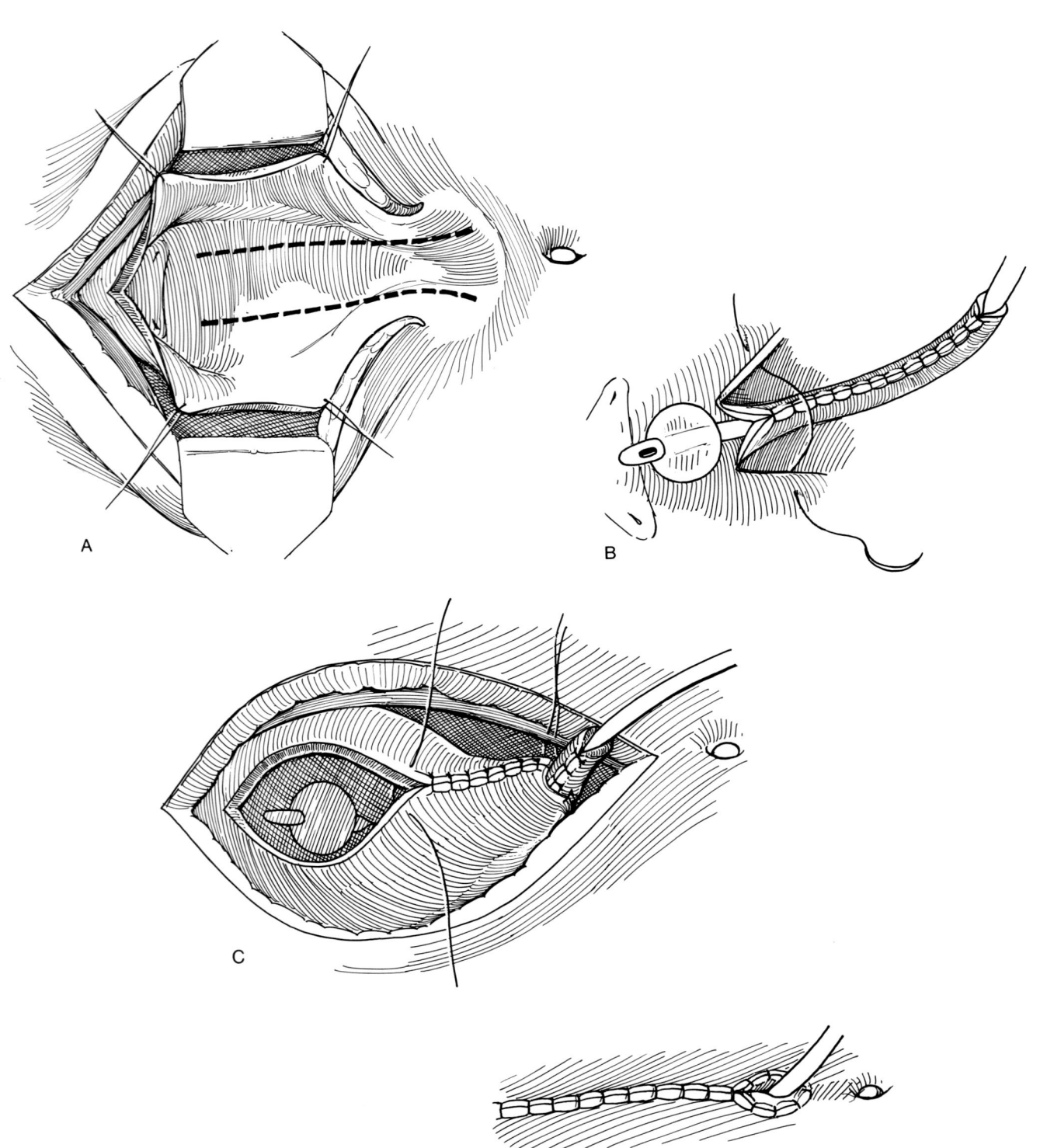

POSTOPERATIVE PROBLEMS

Watch for *inadequate decompression* of the upper tracts. The trial of catheter drainage preoperatively will have shown what to expect immediately after operation, but the ureteral orifices may become obstructive from edema, inflammation, or spasm of the detrusor, requiring percutaneous nephrostomy. If that fails, consider loop ureterostomy.

Dermatitis, when it occurs, is treated with antifungal and antibacterial agents, urinary acidification, and protective skin coatings. *Prolapse* of the posterior wall of the bladder is caused by placing the bladder incision too low and not fixing the dome. Revision is necessary to make a new opening in the most cephalad part of the dome and narrow the fascial defect. Vesical epithelial eversion and squamous metaplasia are managed at the time that the vesicostomy is closed.

Stomal stenosis seldom is a problem, because an opening of 8 F is actually large enough, but obstruction may occur in some thickened bladders, evidenced by residual urine, infection, and signs of backpressure on the upper tracts. Dermatitis also may narrow the lumen. Sometimes the stoma can be kept open by dilation with an eyedropper, but revision may be necessary. *Bladder capacity* usually increases after vesicostomy. Finally, advise the child to stay thin.

Commentary by Moneer K. Hanna

Vesicostomy is a simple and safe form of tubeless urinary diversion. Blocksom vesicostomy takes advantage of the abdominal position of the bladder in infants and the fact that the infantile bladder is highly mobile.

Before the skin incision is made, the bladder is distended with saline. Palpation of the dome of the bladder determines the incision site for the stoma. In our experience, the stoma usually is positioned 3 to 4 cm below the umbilicus.

Complications of this operation are uncommon and can be avoided by careful technique. In the past, the complication rate of vesicostomy was approximately 20 percent. These complications included bladder prolapse and stomal stenosis. The former can be prevented if the highest part of the bladder is exteriorized. Vesical epithelial eversion is not uncommon, but this is more of an esthetic nuisance rather than a serious problem. Stomal stenosis may occur if (1) the fascial opening is too small; (2) there is incomplete bladder mobilization, resulting in undue tension on the vesicocutaneous anastomosis; or (3) there is repeated postoperative dermatitis and scarring. The first two conditions can be prevented by careful attention to operative details. To avoid delayed stenosis, we instruct the parents to calibrate the "mature" stoma with a 14 F Mentor female catheter once a week and report to us if there is any resistance to passage of the catheter, or if there is significant residual urine (more than 10 percent of bladder capacity). Bladder stenosis still may occur in 5 percent of stomas draining the markedly thick fibrotic bladders, which are seen in some children with posterior urethral valves or neurogenic dysfunction.

When the bladder capacity is very large, an alternative to Klauber's posterior bladder tube (Figures 6 and 7) would be Lapides-Koff continent vesicostomy, constructed from the anterior wall of the bladder. A 10-cm-long, 2-cm-wide bladder flap is raised, and the lateral edges of the epithelium are trimmed. The epithelium is tubularized over a 12 F catheter, and the muscle wall is wrapped in an overlapping fashion. The abdominal neourethra is brought through the rectus muscle striated sphincter to the skin cephalad to the bladder. The mechanisms for continence are the detrusor muscle tube and the rectus muscle tone at rest and its contraction in response to sudden increase in intra-abdominal pressure.

CHAPTER 72

Cutaneous Ureterostomy and Pyelostomy

Ureterostomy In Situ. Ureterostomy *in situ* is a simple, quick way to provide temporary upper-tract diversion from a dilated ureter until a more definitive procedure can be completed.

Make a small incision above the anterior superior iliac spine, and identify the dilated ureter through the retroperitoneum. Make a small puncture wound in the ureter, and immediately insert a 6 F infant feeding tube or a single pigtail catheter before the ureter collapses and pass it to the renal pelvis. Make a stab wound in the flank below the incision, and draw the catheter through it. Fasten it securely to the skin with a silk suture. After 2 weeks, the stent can be replaced, but this must be done quickly after removing the initial catheter or the tract will be lost.

Cutaneous Ureterostomy. Before it is brought to the skin, the ureter should have been dilated, because the blood supply to the free end of a normal ureter becomes tenuous after passage through the abdominal wall. The ureter in obese adolescents sometimes will not reach the skin surface, and if it does, it will exit so far posteriorly under the rib cage that a collecting device will not remain adherent. Because cutaneous ureterostomy often can complicate subsequent surgical procedures, it should not be considered as first choice. The midportion of the ureter should not be disturbed. Before operation, select one or two sites on the abdomen suitable for retaining a collecting device.

DISTAL-END CUTANEOUS URETEROSTOMY

A distal-end ureterostomy, in contrast with a loop ureterostomy, may avoid a double procedure later.

Select a proper site in the lower quadrant for the stoma.

Incision: A transverse lower abdominal (page 261) or Gibson incision (page 270) is suitable. Approach the ureter extraperitoneally, but in large adolescents, it may be necessary to have the ureter traverse the abdominal cavity; however, intraperitoneal disease may make an intra-abdominal approach more difficult. Dissect extraperitoneally to reach the ureter over the sacral promontory. Free the ureter well toward the bladder, enough to bring the proximal end to the surface after division. Mobilize the ureter very carefully, keeping well outside the adventitia to preserve as much as possible of the blood supply coming from the upper end. Free the ureter all the way to the bladder to enable the end to reach the anterior abdominal wall, but do not attempt to straighten it by adventitial dissection. Clamp and divide it. Ligate the stump, and insert a stay suture in the free end.

1 A, Select a site for the stoma.

B, If both ureters are involved, consider a double stoma (Figure 5A to E).

C, A ureteroureterostomy with a single cutaneous opening (Figures 3 and 4). A cutaneous pyelostomy (Figures 6 and 7) is available for temporary diversion with a dilated pelvis.

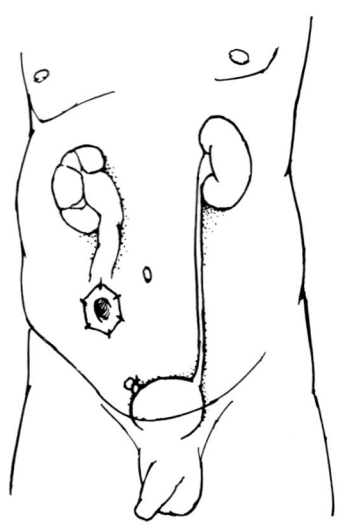

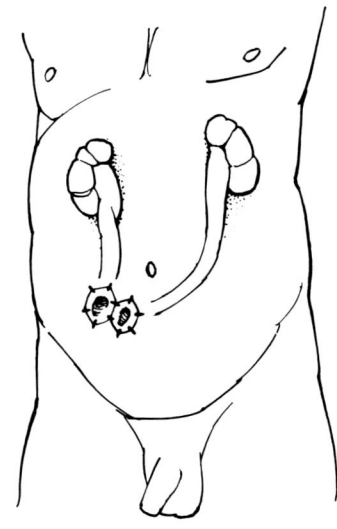

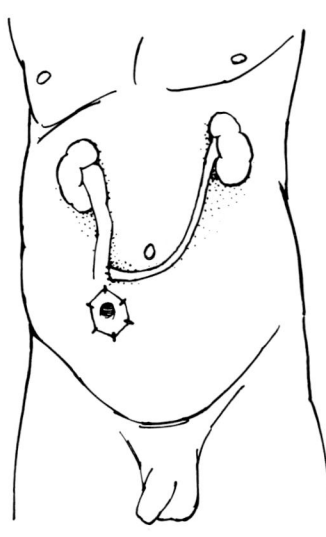

A

B

C

2 **A,** For the surface connection of the ureter, incise the skin in the shape of a U or V. Make a direct tract through subcutaneous tissue, rectus sheath, and peritoneum, as for an ileal conduit (pages 378, 379), taking care to keep the body layers lined up. Draw the ureter through the opening without tension for at least 3 cm. Incise the lateral, less-vascular side to spatulate it.

B, Insert a 4-0 synthetic absorbable suture through the apex of the skin flap into the apex of the ureteral slit and tie it. Pass a similar suture through each angle of the skin incision, then through the free corners of the ureter and tie them.

C, Place five or six everting sutures around the circumference, tie the sutures, then complete the attachment to have the end of the ureter at the level of the skin, or better, to form a little nipple, so that appliances will stay on better. Stenting is not necessary.

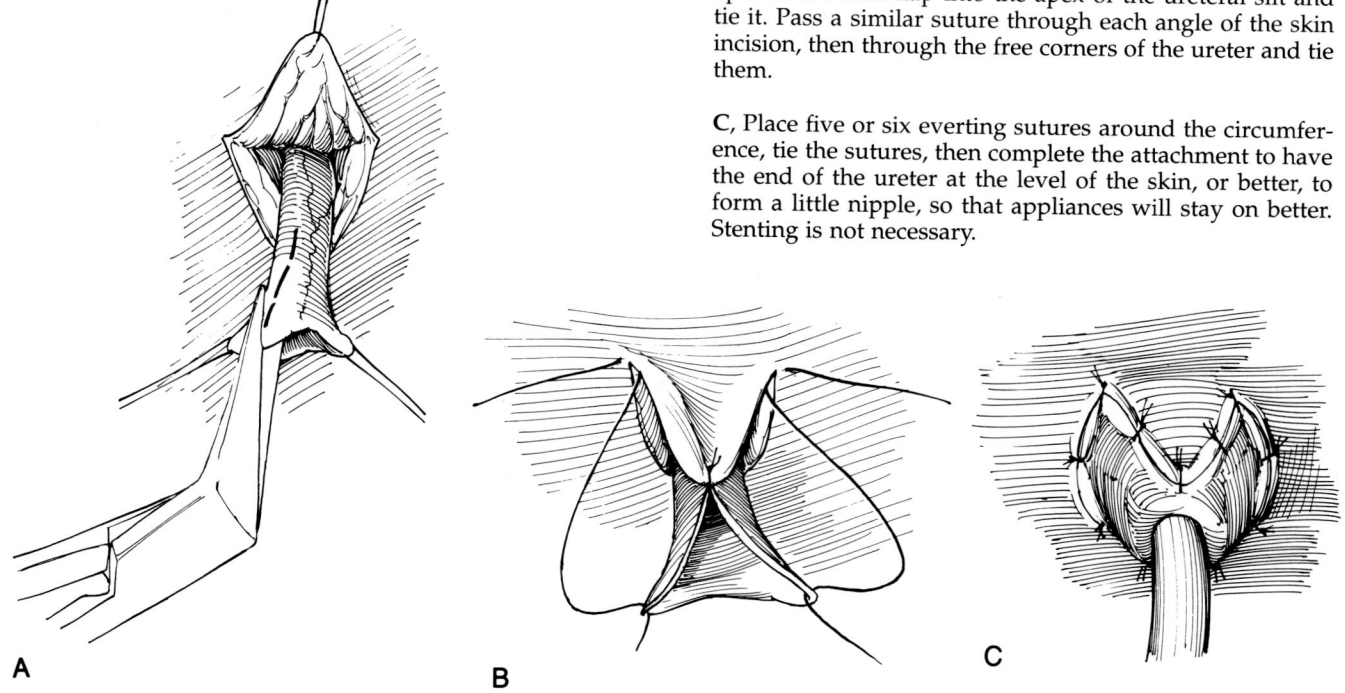

A

B

C

TRANSURETEROURETEROSTOMY WITH CUTANEOUS STOMA

If two ureters are involved, rather than forming a double stoma, bring the more dilated one to the skin and perform transureteroureterostomy (page 246) on the other, transabdominally or extraperitoneally, as shown in Figure 1C.

3 *Incision:* Make a midline transabdominal incision. Open the peritoneum, and pack the intestine into the upper abdomen. Lift up the parietal peritoneum over the more normal ureter near its crossing of the iliac vessels, and open it with Lahey scissors as far caudally as possible. Encircle the ureter with a small Penrose drain, well outside the adventitia, free it distally, and clamp it. Place a traction suture through the proximal end before cutting and ligating the distal stump with an absorbable suture.

Now open the peritoneum over the more dilated ureter, and expose a section of it. Under vision, digitally dissect a channel from one retroperitoneal incision to the other, and draw the smaller ureter through it with a curved clamp.

Dissect the larger ureter to the bladder; cut, place a stay suture, and ligate the stump. Continue the retroperitoneal dissection that was begun over the larger ureter around the lateral and anterior body wall to the site selected for the stoma.

Form the stoma as described previously but only through the subcutaneous tissue and muscles. Instead of entering the peritoneum, connect the stoma with the previous retroperitoneal dissection by freeing the peritoneum adjacent to it, working through its opening. Pass a large clamp through the stoma beneath the peritoneum to grasp the stay suture on the larger ureter, and bring it out through the skin. Be sure the ureter is not angulated.

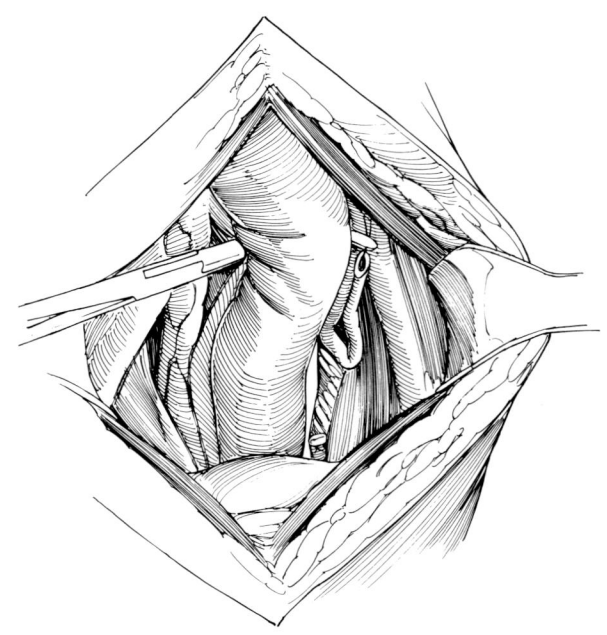

4 Trim the smaller ureter to the proper length to meet the more dilated one, cutting it obliquely. Make a 2-cm longitudinal incision in the dilated ureter, and proceed with transureteroureterostomy (page 246). Bring a Penrose drain extraperitoneally from the site through a stab wound in the skin below the stoma. Close the parietal peritoneal incisions and the abdomen. If necessary, spatulate the protruding ureter, then suture it to the skin as described in Figure 2. Stents are not necessary.

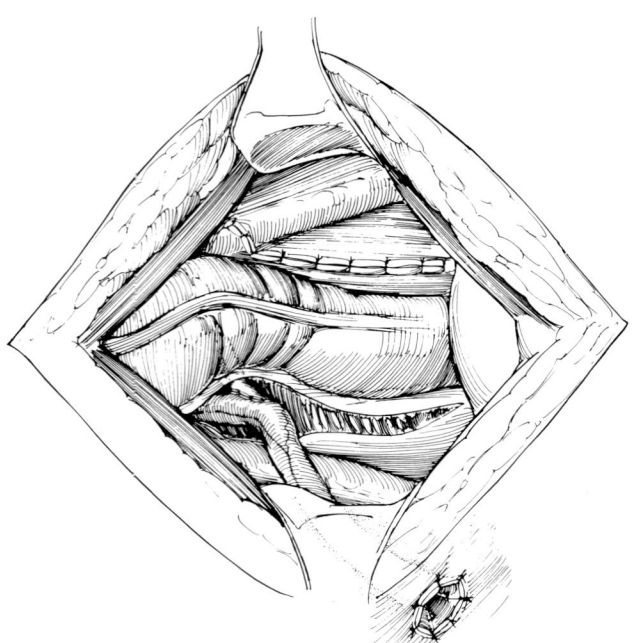

SINGLE-STOMA CUTANEOUS URETEROSTOMY

5 If both ureters are dilated, they may be combined into a single stoma with a Z-plasty (Straffon *et al.*, 1970).

Approach the ureters extraperitoneally. **A**, Make a Z-shaped incision in the skin in a previously selected site.

B, Trim the subcutaneous fat from the flaps.

C, Remove a minimum of fat to avoid inversion of skin at the site of the stoma, and excise a button of anterior rectus sheath. Make an X-shaped incision in the transversalis fascia and peritoneum.

D, Draw the ureters through the opening, and trim them to length. Spatulate each ureter by incising its lateral border.

E, Suture the flaps into the Vs with 3-0 synthetic absorbable sutures.

Alternatively, make a simple stoma by suturing the incised ureters together, everting them, and suturing them to the skin as shown in Figure 1*B*).

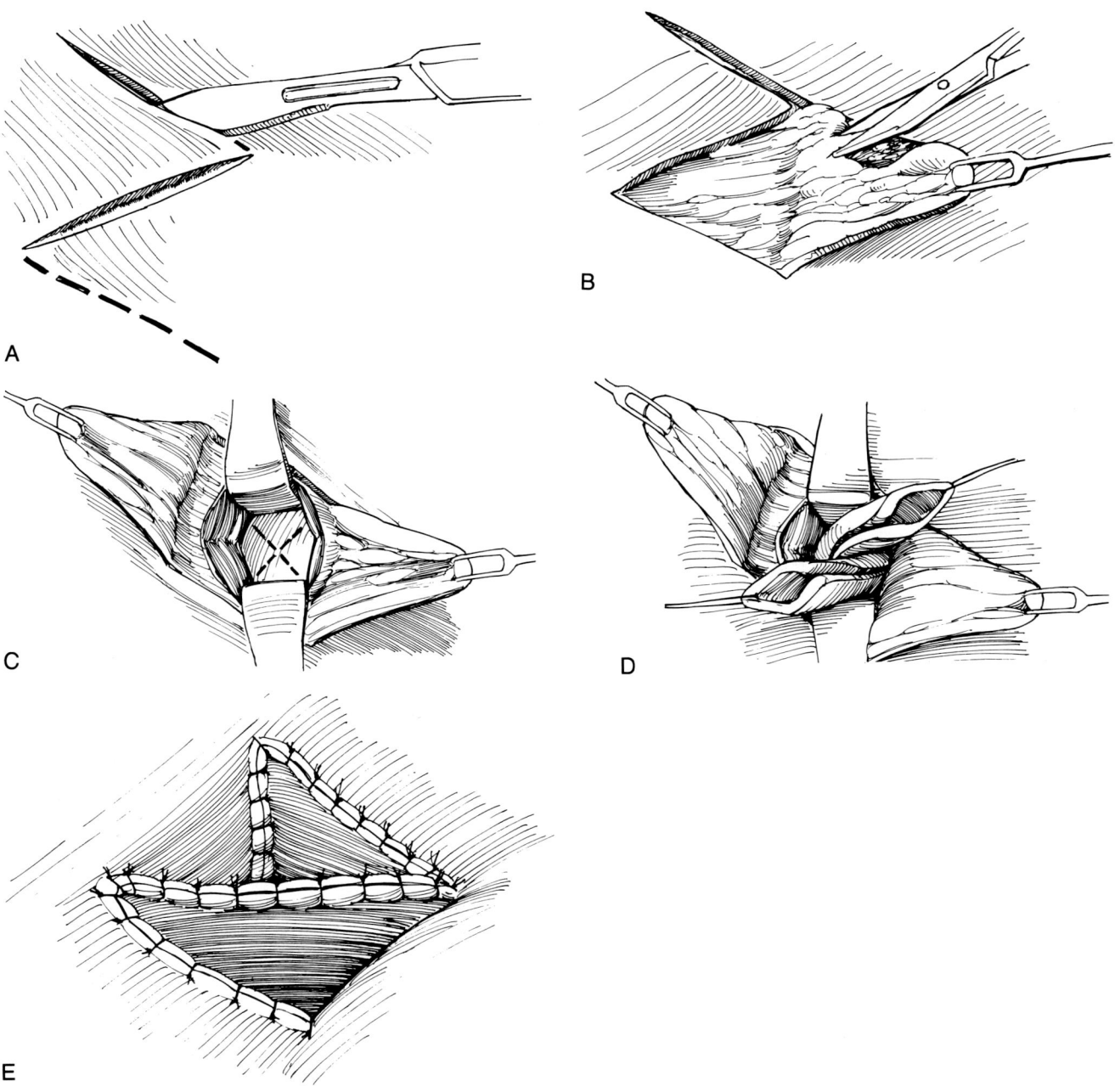

A

B

C

D

E

CUTANEOUS PYELOSTOMY

Cutaneous pyelostomy is a sometimes-useful temporizing procedure in the presence of obstruction and severe infection. It requires a large extrarenal pelvis but does not disturb the ureteral circulation, preserving it for later procedures.

Incision and dissection are done as described for ureterostomy, except that instead of actually mobilizing the proximal ureter, merely trace it to the renal pelvis. Rotate the kidney anteromedially.

6 Place two traction sutures in the posterior surface of the dilated pelvis, well above the ureteropelvic junction. Incise the pelvis with a hooked blade for 3 cm.

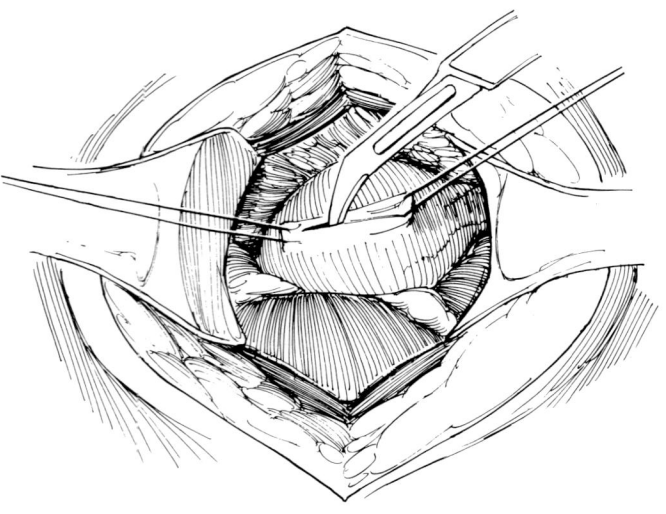

7 Place several 3-0 or 4-0 synthetic absorbable sutures between the pelvis and body wall to relieve tension. Suture the full thickness of the pelvis to the skin with interrupted sutures.

Closure of cutaneous pyelostomy: Encircle and dissect the redundant pelvis, staying clear of the ureteropelvic junction. Trim the edges, and close the defect with a running 4-0 synthetic absorbable suture, with occasional locked stitches.

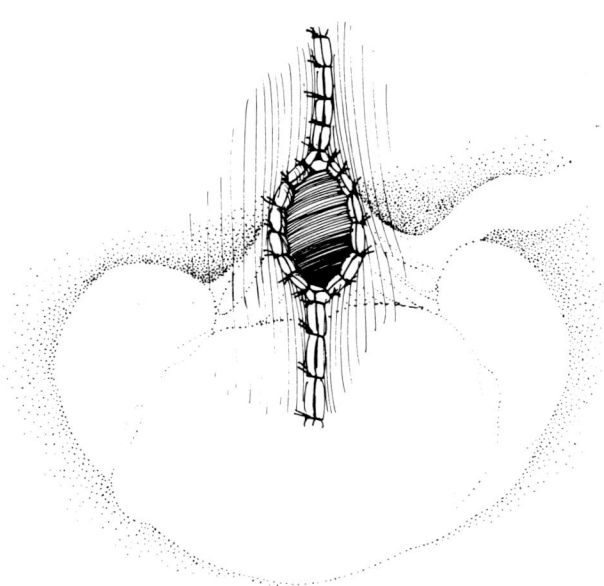

POSTOPERATIVE PROBLEMS

Stenosis is almost the rule because of relative ischemia of the ureteral tip. Try dilation, then treat the stenosis with intubation with a round-tipped silicone tube. A plastic meatotomy can be done. Surgical revision seldom helps, because the 3 cm of extra ureteral length necessary to achieve it seldom is available; rather, an alternate form of supravesical diversion must be applied. *Pyocystis* (empyema of the bladder) occurs not infrequently after diversion, especially if the bladder is denervated. Overdilation of the urethra followed by regular catheterization and irrigation often will provide long-term relief. In girls, the urethra may be split. If these measures are not successful, cystectomy may be advisable, unless continent diversion with intermittent catheterization is not planned.

Commentary by Joseph Y. Dwoskin

Ureterostomy *in situ* has been changed somewhat by endourologists to a percutaneous nephrostomy, which does not cause ureteral scarring and an aperistaltic segment—conditions that, in the long term, are deleterious. Cutaneous ureterostomy is an occasional procedure—one not often done. I have found that a short ileal conduit is superior in a few cases, especially in children with thicker abdominal walls.

Distal end cutaneous ureterostomy is a useful technique for few situations. These are fairly final procedures that commit the child to a stoma and collection device for a long period. Most ureteral drainage procedures, as I see them, are to decrease intrarenal pressure that causes progressive hydronephrosis. Pressures within the pelvis of the kidney change the growth aspects of the child, and when one is trying to allow as normal growth as possible, it is better to aim for more normal intraureteral and intrarenal pressure.

The techniques described are the standard techniques, but in the cases that I am familiar with, Z-plasty stomas cause much cutaneous scarring and are not necessary on the initial try. For the most part, making the stoma and just sewing the end of the ureter to it is sufficient. A nipple is unnecessary with the type of adhesives for the drainage appliances that are available today. Everting the ureter is obstructive and causes more problems, as I see it.

A transureteroureterostomy with cutaneous ureterostomy is an alternative in some situations, resulting in only one stoma. This procedure does work, but the goal in each of these procedures must be clearly defined before it is done.

Loop cutaneous ureterostomy and pyelostomy, as described in this chapter, may be obsolete at this point. Some work was done a long time ago to study the use of these procedures in adults, and because there were significant problems with stomas, this currently does not seem to be the best procedure. Pyocystis is a rare complication if the bladder is irrigated with gentamicin at the time of the procedure. It is more common in girls than in boys.

CHAPTER 73

Pediatric Loop Ureterostomy

Pediatric loop ureterostomy is an operation that was designed for infants with congenital posterior urethral valves, although it rarely is used at present. Treat the infant for shock and sepsis. If the infant's condition warrants, start catheter drainage using a 5 or 8 F feeding tube with a coudé tip. If the child does not respond, consider cutaneous pyelostomy (page 364). Those children who respond to catheter drainage but reach a nadir creatinine level require vesicostomy (page 356). Some may be managed by intermittent catheterization plus anticholinergic medication for their high-pressure bladders secondary to detrusor sphincter dyssynergia and their lack of feeling the need to void. After augmentation, these children will be in urinary retention and will require intermittent catheterization for a while.

Alternatives to high loop ureterostomy include low loop ureterostomy, Y-ureterostomy (in which the ureter is divided, one end is brought to the skin, and the distal end is anastomosed to the renal pelvis), cutaneous pyelostomy, and end-cutaneous ureterostomy (pages 360, 361). The loop from the upper ureter provides better drainage and easy closure, but that from the lower ureter is easy to form and can readily be anastomosed to the bladder at a later time.

HIGH LOOP URETEROSTOMY

1 *For mobilization of the ureter*, place the child in the lateral position over a bolster. *Incision:* Make a short subcostal incision (page 87). This will give the best exposure but does require rolling the child over and reprepping to do the other side. The supine position does allow for a bilateral operation; the prone position with lumbotomies also can be used.

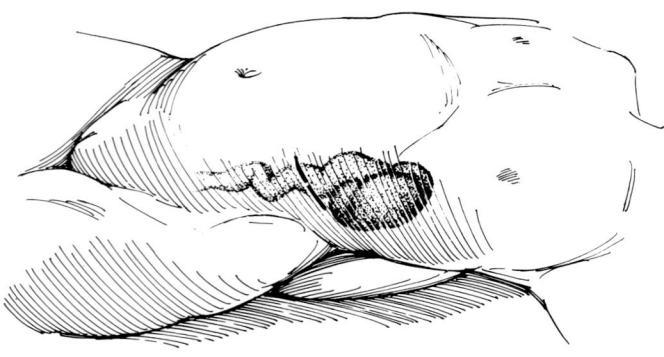

2 Mobilize the peritoneum medially near the psoas muscle (in infants, the peritoneum extends well posteriorly), and dissect the ureter retroperitoneally. Remember that it will be thick and redundant, so it will look like small bowel. If in doubt, aspirate it through a 26-gauge needle. Preserve all the adventitial blood supply, and encircle the ureter with a small Penrose drain. Clear the upper ureter so that it makes a loose curve to reach the incision. Be able to visualize the ureteropelvic junction, and keep as high on the ureter as possible after straightening any kinks.

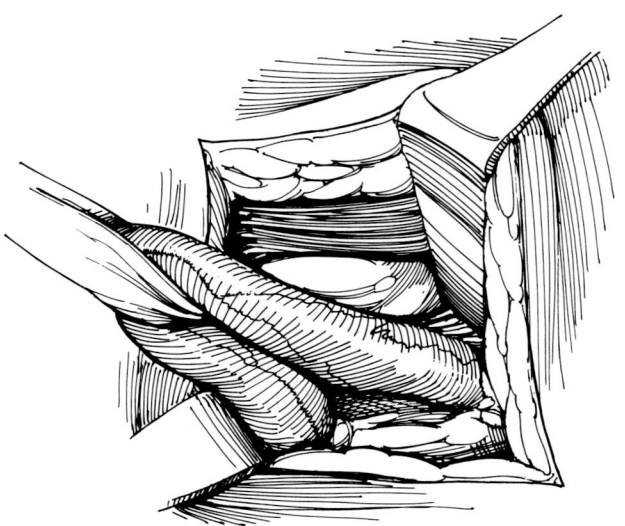

3 *For securing the ureter,* the classic method is as follows:

A, Close the flank muscles loosely beneath the loop with 4-0 synthetic absorbable interrupted sutures to prevent retraction.

B, Alternatively, close only the flank muscles caudad to the loop.

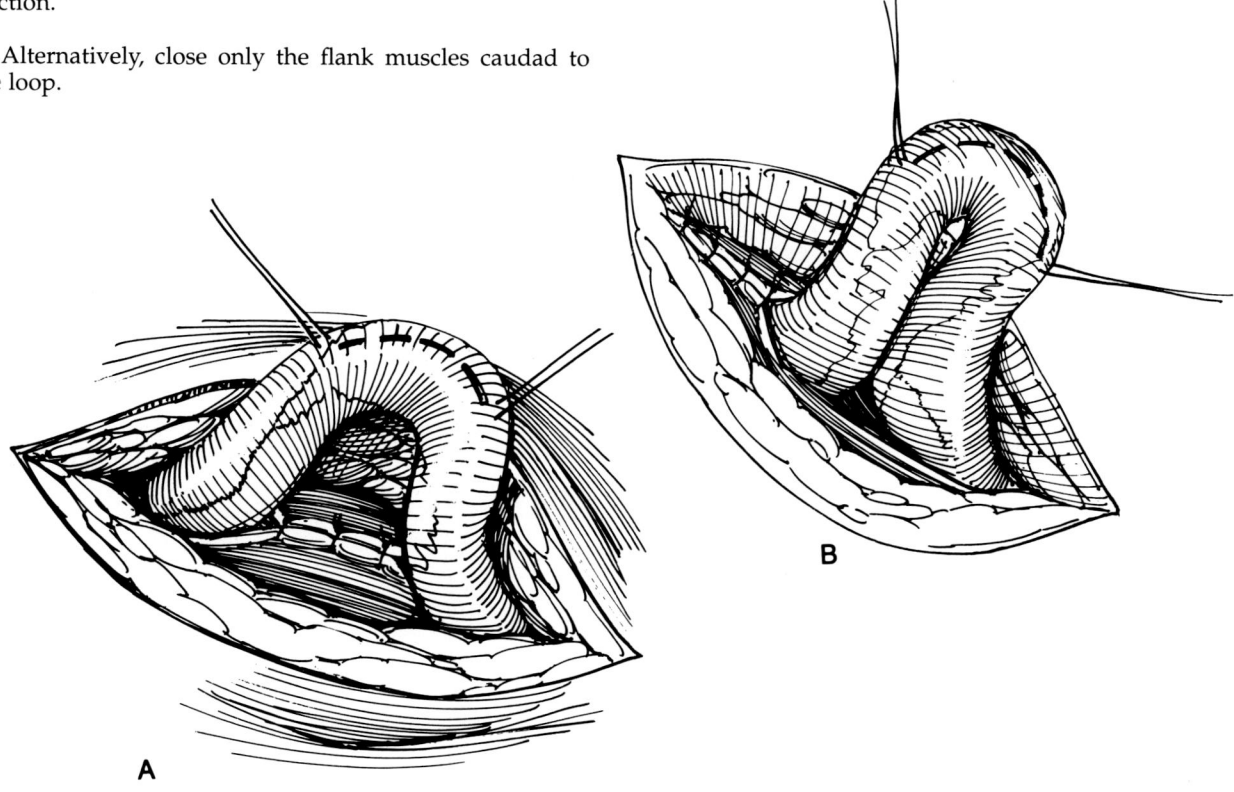

4 **A,** Place stay sutures and incise the loop longitudinally for 2 to 3 cm.

B, Insert an 8 F infant feeding tube to the renal pelvis. Suture the full thickness of the ureter to the adjacent skin edges with interrupted 4-0 chromic catgut sutures. If the ureter is duplicated, consider ipsilateral ureteroureterostomy, pyelopyelostomy, or ureteropyelostomy.

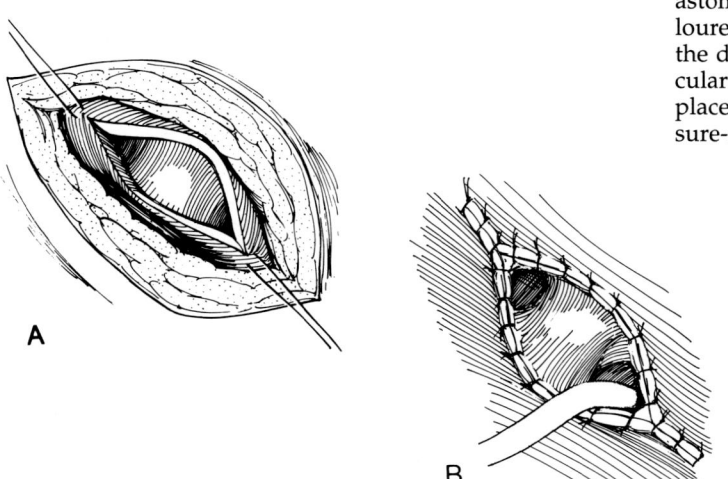

Closure of Loop Ureterostomy: Dissect the loop free from the skin and muscle layers, excise the involved segment, and anastomose the two ends. Place a ureteral stent into the kidney through a short incision in the ureter below the anastomosis for temporary drainage. Alternatively, dissect the ureter from the wound and divide it obliquely just below the stoma. Continue the ureteral dissection to the renal pelvis. Cut the ureter from the pelvis obliquely. Anastomose the ureter to the pelvis as in dismembered pyel(oureteroplasty (page 123). It may not be wise to reimplant the distal end of the ureter at this time, for fear of devascularization. If continued distal obstruction is possible, place a nephrostomy so that it may be evaluated by pressure-flow studies.

Low Loop Ureterostomy

Approach the ureter through a McBurney incision, splitting the muscles to reach the peritoneum. Secure the ureter with Babcock clamps to dissect it free, so that it will reach the surface without tension. Open the ureter for a short distance longitudinally, and pass an 8 F infant feeding tube to be sure the ureter is not kinked. Suture the opening to the skin with everting sutures as a nipple. It is best not to close the muscles or anchor the loop.

Closure is done by resection of the incised segment and end-to-end anastomosis. Alternatively, it may be done as part of a definitive operation if that is needed. Incise around the stoma, and free the underlying ureter. Open the bladder through a Pfannenstiel incision, and dissect the ureter intravesically to the level of the previous ureterotomy. Discard the terminal portion, and anastomose the proximal portion to the bladder by a nonrefluxing technique.

Alternatively, the dilated ureter can be approached through a midline incision and brought to the surface as an end ureterostomy. After a year or more, when the ureter and bladder are more normal, the ureter may be reimplanted, usually without tailoring (Belman and King, 1972).

RING URETEROSTOMY

The advantages of the ring ureterostomy are that it avoids kinking and diverticular ureteral protrusions, interference with the ureteral blood supply during closure, and reconstruction in compromised tissue.

5 **A,** Expose the ureter as described previously. Leave an adequate length of ureter between the ureteropelvic junction and the skin, so that as the kidney enlarges, it will not place traction on the ureter with resulting kinking and obstruction. Make a 3-cm longitudinal incision into the anterior aspect of the two limbs of the loop.

B, Suture the two openings together side by side with 4-0 or 5-0 synthetic absorbable sutures. The opening should be at least 2 cm long. Open the ureter longitudinally at the top of the ring.

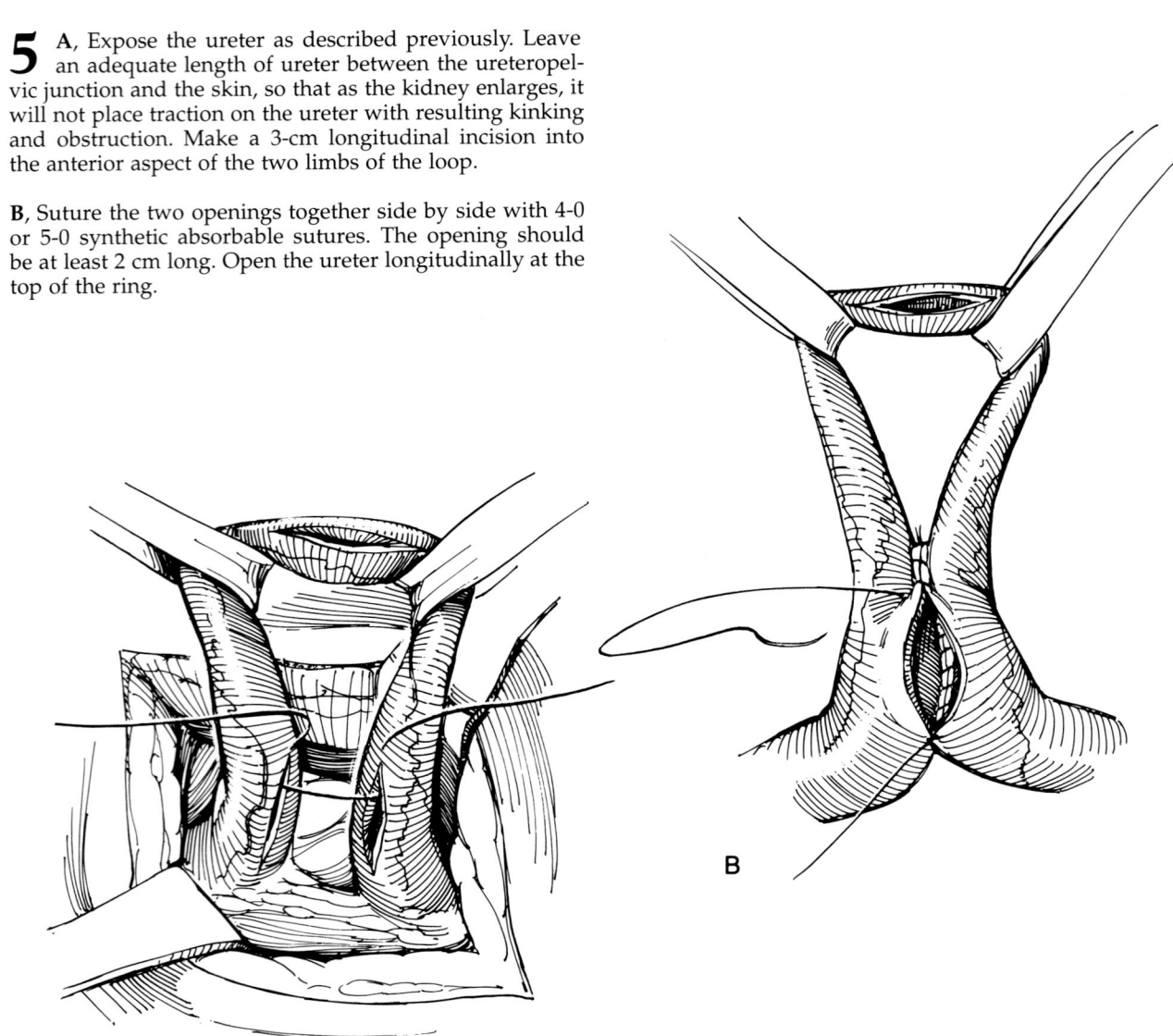

A

B

6 Close the flank muscles behind the loop, distal to the anastomosis. Excise a 2-cm button of skin, and suture the ureteral opening in the loop to the skin with 3-0 chromic catgut suture. Place an adhesive appliance.

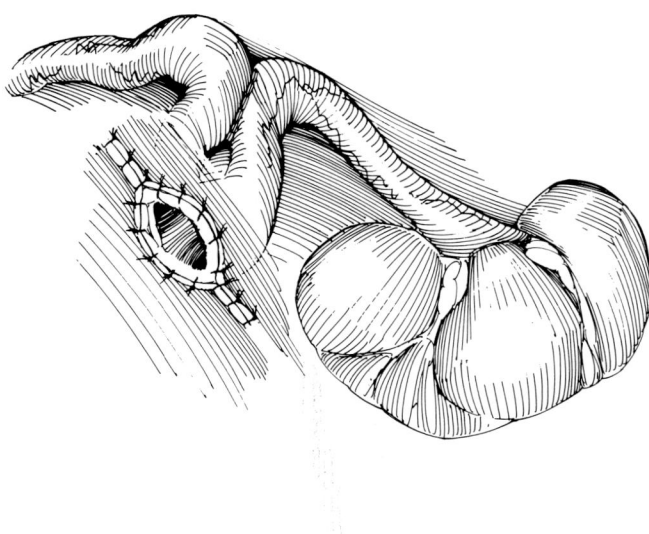

POSTOPERATIVE PROBLEMS

Ureteral devascularization and slough may occur if the adventitia has been overly dissected. Bleeding is not usual, and pressure will control it.

More serious is failure of the ureterostomy to drain the kidney, usually a result of selecting an unsuitable segment of the ureter, so that kinking or obstruction results. Intubation will take care of the immediate problem, but the loop must be revised if it is to remain.

Stomal irritation can be a problem. Local agents and urinary acidification are helpful. Stenosis is rare.

Commentary by Joseph Y. Dwoskin

Obstruction in many infants today will be diagnosed prenatally with sonograms and be uninfected at the time of birth. The work up can be done within 24 hours and appropriate drainage instituted quite rapidly.

Because the dilated ureter is very edematous and aperistaltic, drainage from below often is ineffective, especially if ureterovesical junction obstruction is present. Bladders with thick walls, such as those in children with posterior urethral valve, are a classic example of those that will not drain well with catheters.

Vesicostomy is a poor alternative, because it destroys a good bit of the bladder that will be useful later. The amount of scarring that occurs in the bladder that is open to the skin decreases the amount of useful bladder significantly, especially if it is thickened.

Prolapse also is a major problem, as is the scarring that occurs around the stoma. Reconstruction becomes much more difficult, especially if a reimplantation is necessary.

Bladder growth occurs in spite of the fact that the bladder is not used. For mobilization of the ureter, position the child in the lateral position with a towel under the opposite waistline, so that the infant is flexed; a short subcostal incision is correct. The other alternatives are difficult for the anesthetist.

The important aspect of loop cutaneous ureterostomy is that it allows drainage of the obstructed kidney from as high a point as possible in the drainage system. My experience with these cases is that the ureters are not only edematous but tortuous and almost totally aperistaltic. The pressures required to force urine through these systems into the lower urinary tract gradually cause the kid-ney to deteriorate at a time when normal pressures would facilitate normal growth. For that reason, I would like to emphasize that very high loop cutaneous ureterostomies or cutaneous pyelostomies should be done to decrease the pressure in the renal pelvis to facilitate growth during the early portion of the infant's life.

Many of these patients are now found prenatally and can be decompressed shortly after birth; the urinary tract will clear itself relatively rapidly.

Functional tests, such as renal scans, are quite useful. The Mag-3 scan, a relatively recent innovation, is quite useful in determining the degree of obstruction in these systems.

My technique is slightly different than the one described in the text. I have found that the ureter or pelvis can be brought to the skin's surface through a small incision and small ellipses of skin removed, so that the edges of a 1- to 1½-cm opening can be sewn to the skin with nylon. The reason for using 6-0 nylon is that these tissues are quite friable and do not heal well initially. By leaving the sutures in for a couple of weeks, we are assured that there will not be retraction of the ureter, because synthetic material may disintegrate earlier than healing occurs. This is especially so in this wet environment, with urine leaking over the sutures all the time. Closing the muscles underneath the ureter only causes obstruction, in my experience. Therefore, a small incision that is stretched with small Ruh retractors usually is all that is necessary. The skin can be closed on either side to shorten the incision down to the point of the ureterostomy.

A small piece of 5 F feeding tube is left proximally as a stent for 2 to 4 days until the swelling of the ureter recedes and the stoma functions satisfactorily from its proximal opening. The distal opening is quite useful in assessing the ureter prior to reconstruction.

Bring the child back for fluoroscopy periodically, insert a 5 F feeding tube, and instill diluted (50-50) contrast medium to see if the ureter is peristalsing and whether there is ureterovesical junction obstruction and retrograde peristalsis. A voiding cystourethrogram should be done prior to reconstruction to determine whether reflux is present.

When the ureter performs peristalsis satisfactorily and does not have large kinks in it, which will straighten out with growth, then reconstruction is possible. This may take as long as 4 years. Most patients, however, can be reconstructed within 18 months.

My technique for closure is to do the reimplant first, push the tube out of the distal opening in the flank, and then complete the reimplant. If both ureters have to be reimplanted, it is advisable to do both at the same time. Closure of the ureterostomies requires excision of a section of the loop and a ureteroureterostomy or ureteropyelostomy, depending on the anatomic findings. Insert the tube from below if sufficient for drainage of both the ureteroureterostomy or pyelostomy, and the reimplant. Size 5 F feeding tubes usually are sufficient. For closure of the flank, close the muscles over the repair, and leave a small polyethylene drain through the edge of the incision. This usually is removed within a week or so after a tubogram is done to determine whether the ureteroureterostomy or ureteropyelostomy is leaking into the retroperitoneum.

Long-term results have been quite good, although there is an occasional teenage patient who needs a ureteroureterostomy because of kinking.

This procedure also has been effective in situations where only one kidney functions and the other has to be removed at the time of reconstruction.

When doing a ureteroureterostomy, the incision should not be made too large, muscles should not be closed underneath the ureters, and the opening in the ureters should be relatively small—1 to 1.5 cm maximum. Using nonabsorbable sutures is important, and these can be taken out simply by using an Adson forceps and a #11 blade.

One of the major problems that can occur is when a patient is reconstructed too soon. These ureters take a good deal of time, in some cases, before they regain peristalsis. Peristalsis is easily visualized fluoroscopically, which is why the child is brought back periodically, at 2-, 3-, or 4-month intervals, to have their status checked.

Taking care of these children is quite easy when a diaper is used as a cummerbund around their flanks.

CHAPTER 74

Ureteroileostomy

(BRICKER)

A day or two before surgery, have the child sit and stand, so that you can select a site on the surface of the abdomen for the stoma where the skin is not rolled into folds. The stoma should not be near the umbilicus (unless it is through it), the edge of the rectus muscle, a bony prominence, or an abdominal scar. Mark the site with a ballpoint pen or scratch it with a needle. An even better plan is to have the patient wear the partially filled appliance for 1 or 2 days preoperatively to be sure the placement is optimum. The standard location for a stoma is just below the center of a line between the umbilicus and the anterior superior iliac spine. This often is too low, especially in children with myelodysplasia, in whom an umbilical stoma, or even an epigastric one, is easier to manage. An enterostomal therapist can be helpful, especially by counseling the child and allaying fears. Prepare the bowel.

Instruments

Provide four Kocher clamps, curved mosquito (Providence) clamps, a Kelly clamp, an Adson forceps, a tenotomy scissors, a Balfour retractor, 5 F and 8 F infant feeding tubes, a plastic rod, 4-0 silk sutures with detachable needles, 4-0 and 5-0 chromic catgut ureteral sutures, 2-0 and 3-0 synthetic absorbable sutures, and a Penrose drain.

URETERAL MOBILIZATION

1 *Position*: Place the child supine. After the operation has begun, ask the anesthetist to place a nasogastric tube. *Incision*: Make a midline transperitoneal incision (page 83). Make a vertical incision lateral to the sigmoid mesocolon where it joins the parietal peritoneum to expose the left ureter. Dissect medially over the left iliac vessels to locate the ureter where it is lifted up with the peritoneum.

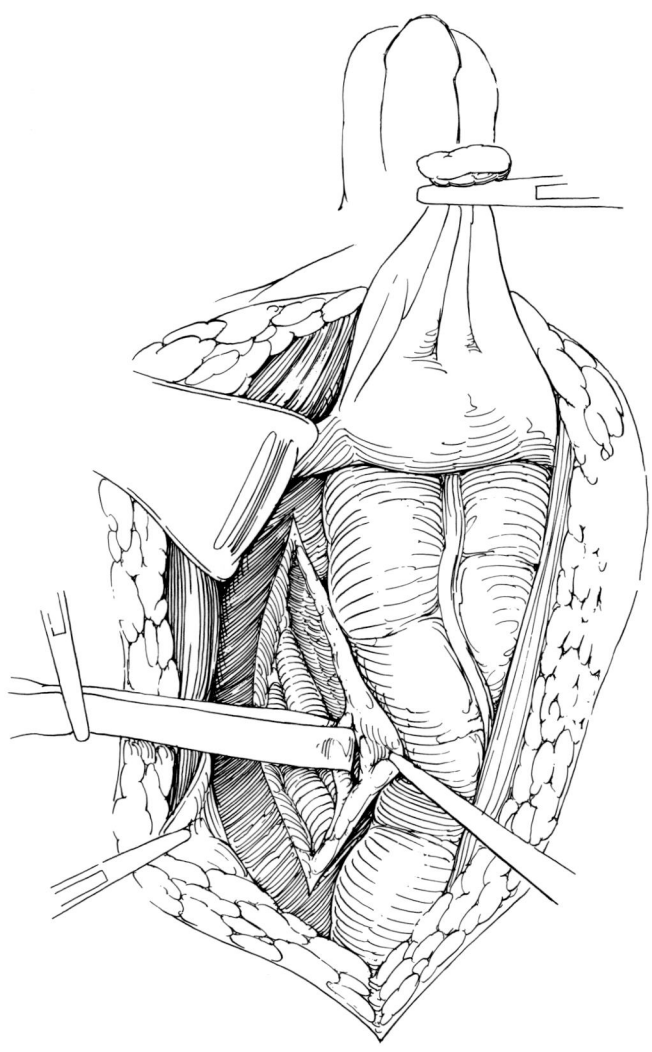

2 Free the left ureter with a right-angle clamp, followed by a Penrose drain for traction. Dissect it well down into the pelvis without disturbing its adventitial circulation. Clamp the ureter distally, place a fine traction suture in it on its anterior proximal surface, and divide it with a knife against the clamp. Ligate the distal stump with a 2-0 or 3-0 chromic catgut suture, cut long so it may later be identified. Now dissect the ureter proximally, so that approximately 8 cm is free. Repeat the procedure on the right side. Here, the ureter lies retroperitoneally just over the iliac vessels and so is easier to find. Also, less mobilization is needed on this side.

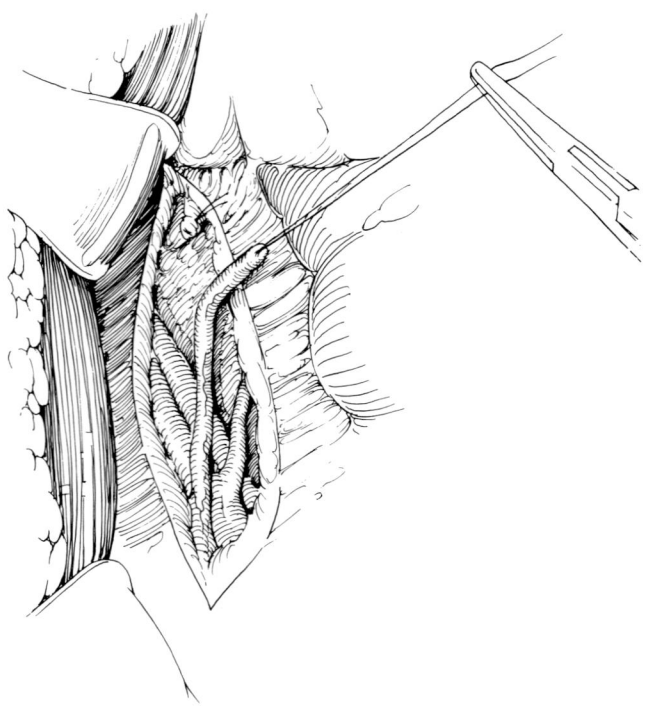

3 Tunnel gently with the index and middle fingers of each hand between the two peritoneal openings, staying beneath the superior hemorrhoidal vessels to create a channel for the left ureter, so that it can sweep over in a smooth arc from the left to the right side. Draw it through by its stay suture with a Péan forceps. Take great care that the ureter is not angulated or twisted.

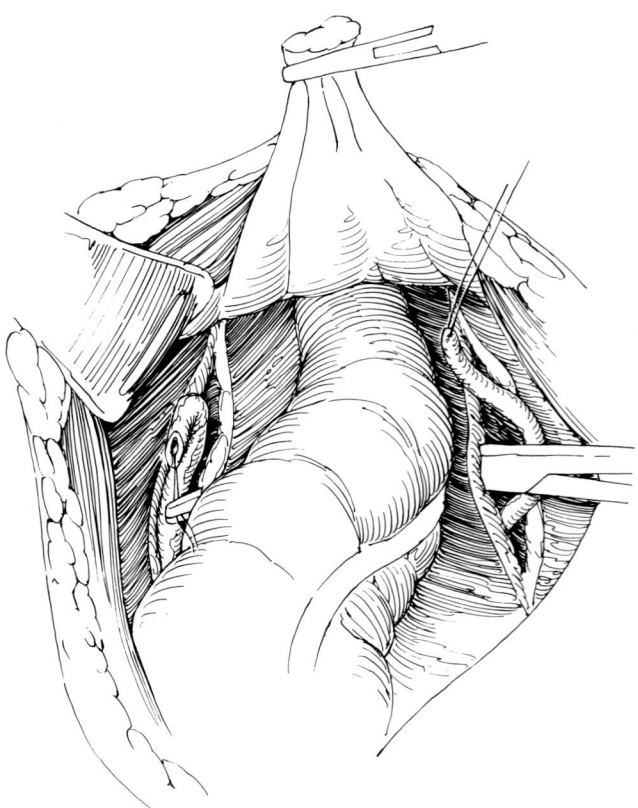

PREPARING THE LOOP

4 Select a suitable segment of ileum near the ileocecal junction by transilluminating its mesentery and visualizing the contained vessels. An avascular area of mesentery usually is found slightly more proximal than shown in the figure. If a suitable segment is not found, use the more proximal ileum or jejunum, or consider a transverse colon conduit (page 365). Place a temporary stay suture of 4-0 silk with a detachable needle in the bowel 10 to 15 cm from the ileocecal valve and beyond the ileocecal arcade, the distance depending on the size of the child. Select a loop of ileum that contains one or two distinct vascular arcades, as shown in the figure. Move the stay suture if necessary. It will mark the distal end of the segment, so tie a knot in the end to identify it and thus prevent later reversal of the loop. Measure the segment. It should be long enough to reach the skin level, plus another 2 cm. In an adolescent, the length of a Kocher clamp is about right. If a Turnbull loop stoma is to be formed, add 8 to 10 cm more. Place a second stay suture to mark the proximal end. Reexamine the loop and its arcades, moving the stay sutures as necessary to provide an adequate segment containing one (or preferably, two) major vascular arcades. Hold both stay sutures in clamps.

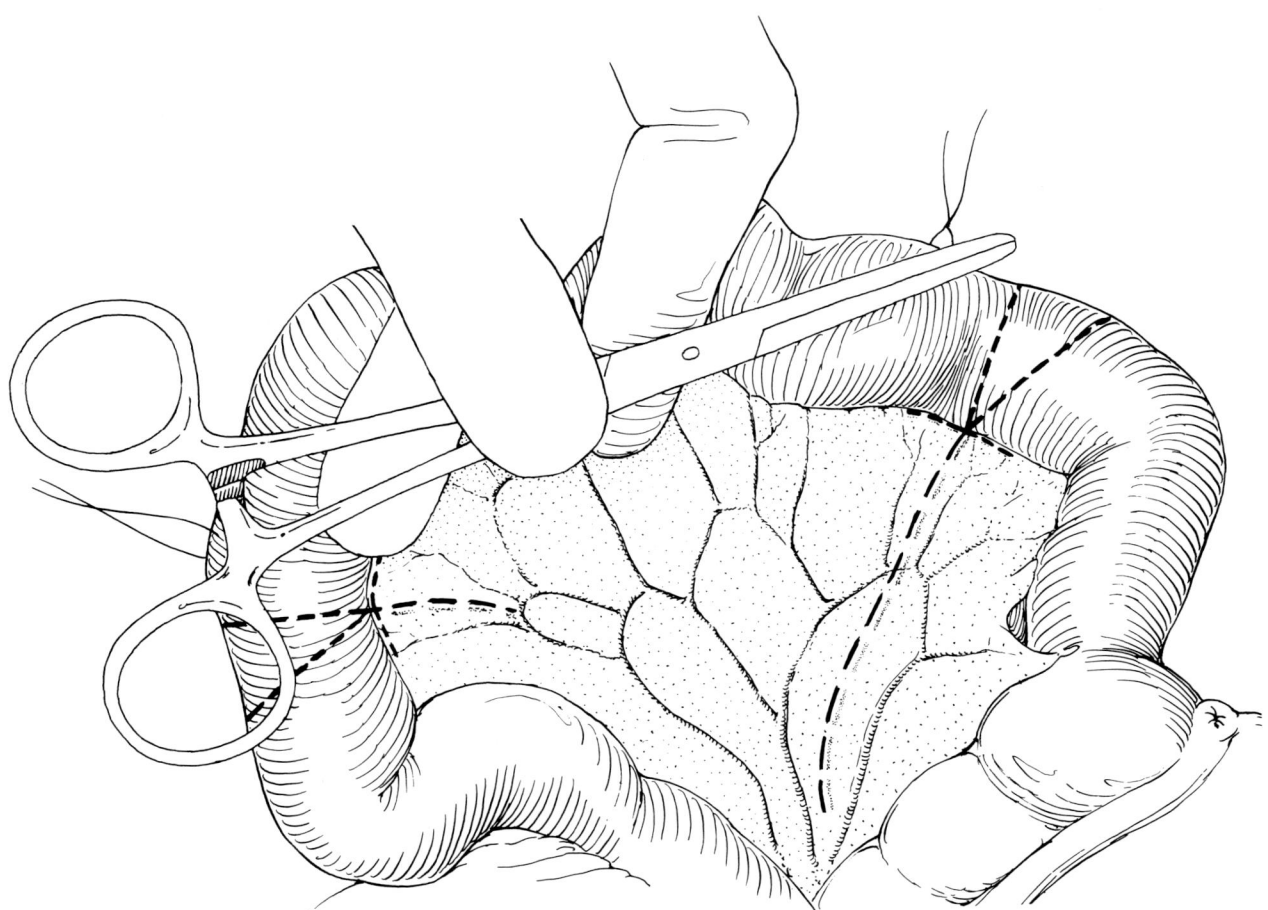

5 Divide the thin peritoneal layer of the mesentery on each side perpendicular to the bowel with a sharp #15 blade for 6 to 10 cm on the distal and 3 cm on the proximal end. Incise the peritoneum parallel to the bowel for a short distance with the handle of the knife, and gently retract the underlying fat away from the bowel wall to expose the straight vessels running from the arcades to the bowel. Insinuate mosquito clamps under each exposed vessel. Apply them in pairs very close to the bowel wall, divide between them, and immediately ligate each vessel with a 4-0 silk tie. Continue the process of sharply incising the peritoneum and clamping the vessels on the bowel margin for a distance of 1.5 cm each way from the proposed line of division. Place Kocher clamps at 45 degree angles on the bowel ends that will be reanastomosed; place them at right angles on the ends of the proposed loop. Divide the bowel with the cutting current, leaving a protruding 2-mm edge, which is then fulgurated (be sure to keep the adjacent bowel against the wound to ground it during fulguration). Discard the excised wedges; a sterile pan technique is not necessary, because the ileal contents are essentially sterile. Drop the isolated segment into the pelvis, and cover it with a moist laparotomy pad.

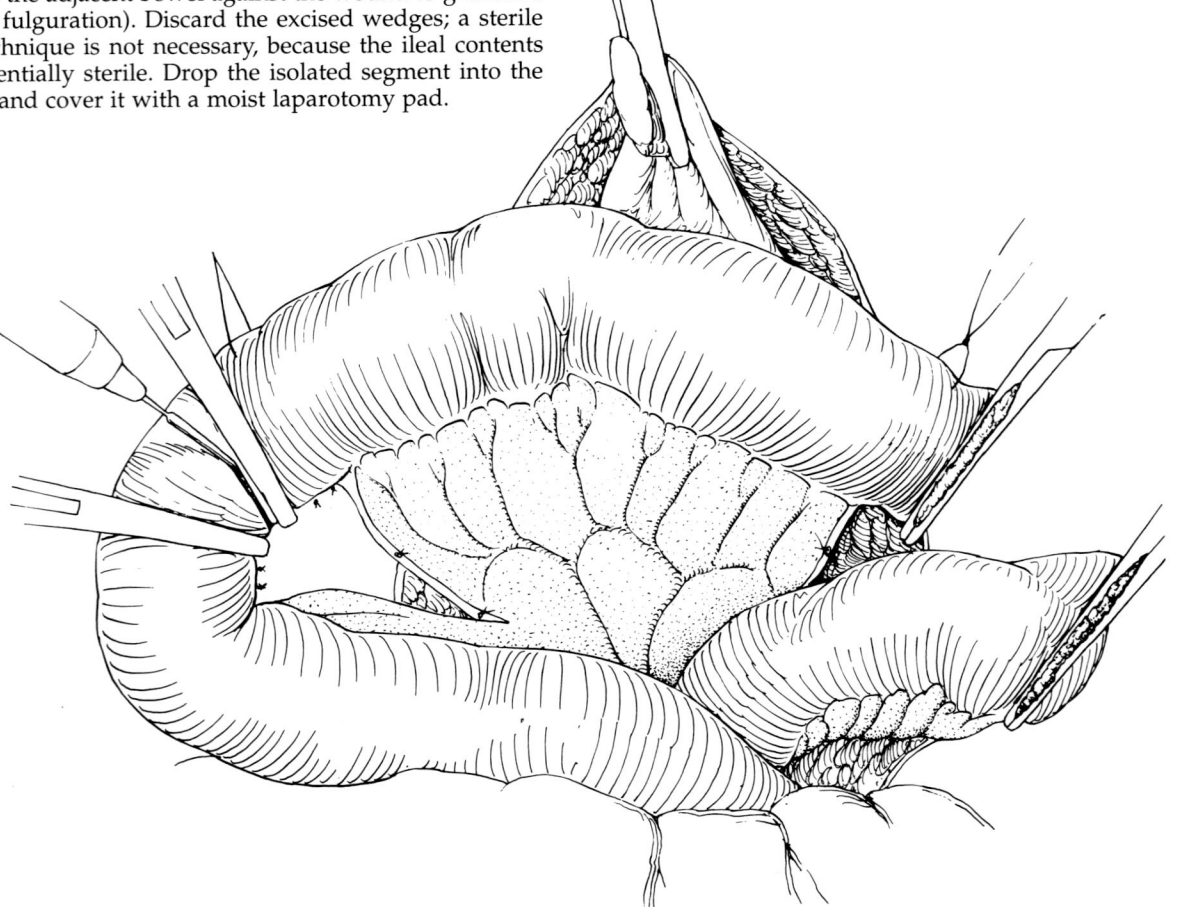

ILEOILEAL ANASTOMOSIS

Single-Layer Closed Technique

6 Hold the clamps so that the cut ends are apposed. Place 4-0 silk detachable sutures into, but not through, the submucosa approximately 3 mm apart. The wall will blanch when the submucosa is penetrated. If the sutures are placed too deep, they will catch the sutures on the opposite side and occlude the lumen. When one side is completed, bundle the sutures into a clamp, turn the bowel over, and place the sutures in the opposite side. Be certain that the sutures at the mesenteric angles are well placed; this is where leakage occurs. Again, bundle the sutures in a second clamp. Slowly manipulate and withdraw the clamps on the bowel as your assistant gently supports the ends of the sutures.

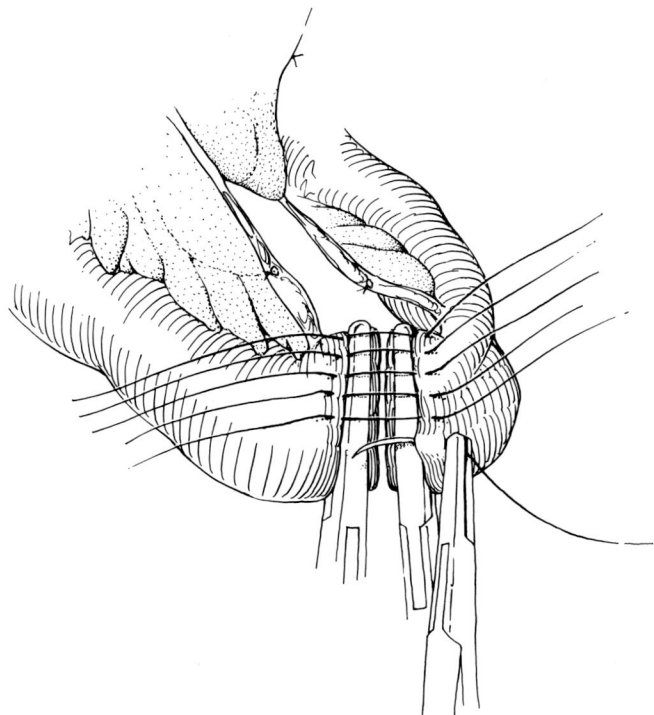

7 Tie the sutures successively as your assistant presents them in pairs lifted on a clamp. Do not cinch them too tight. If the edges do not automatically invert, have the assistant hold a clamp under the suture loop pressed against the bowel edges as the knot is tied. Do not hesitate to put in extra sutures.

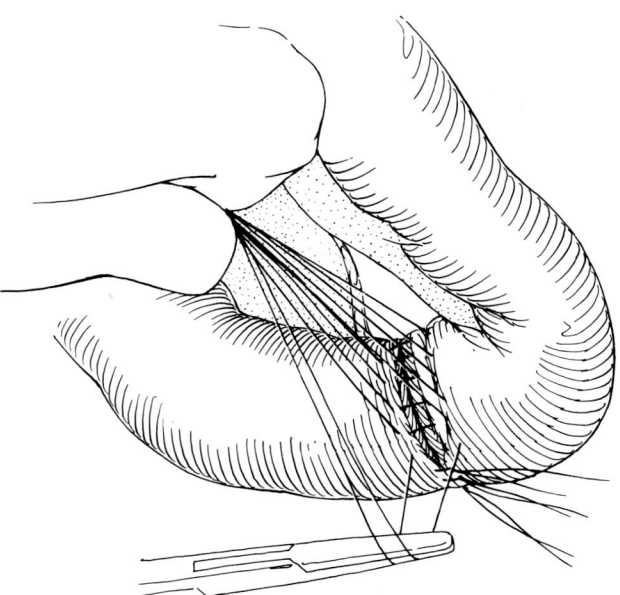

8 Check the patency of the anastomosis, first by inspection as the two bundles of uncut sutures are drawn apart, and then by palpation of the lumen with the thumb and forefinger. If in doubt, remove a few sutures and look inside, cut the offending sutures, and replace them. Cut the ends of the remaining sutures.

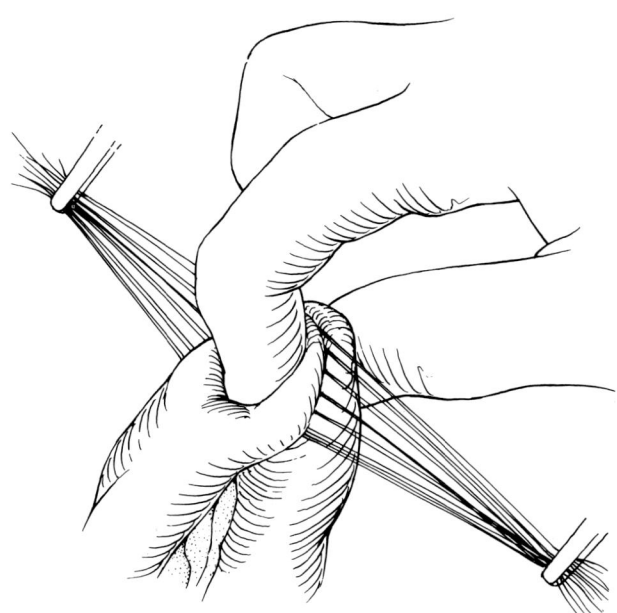

Single-Layer Open Technique

9 **A** and **B**, Appose the ends of the ileum with vertical mattress sutures of 3-0 silk, placed in four quadrants to catch 3 mm of serosa and submucosa and a little mucosa. Tie these sutures and add interrupted sutures that catch the submucosa between.

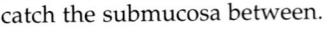

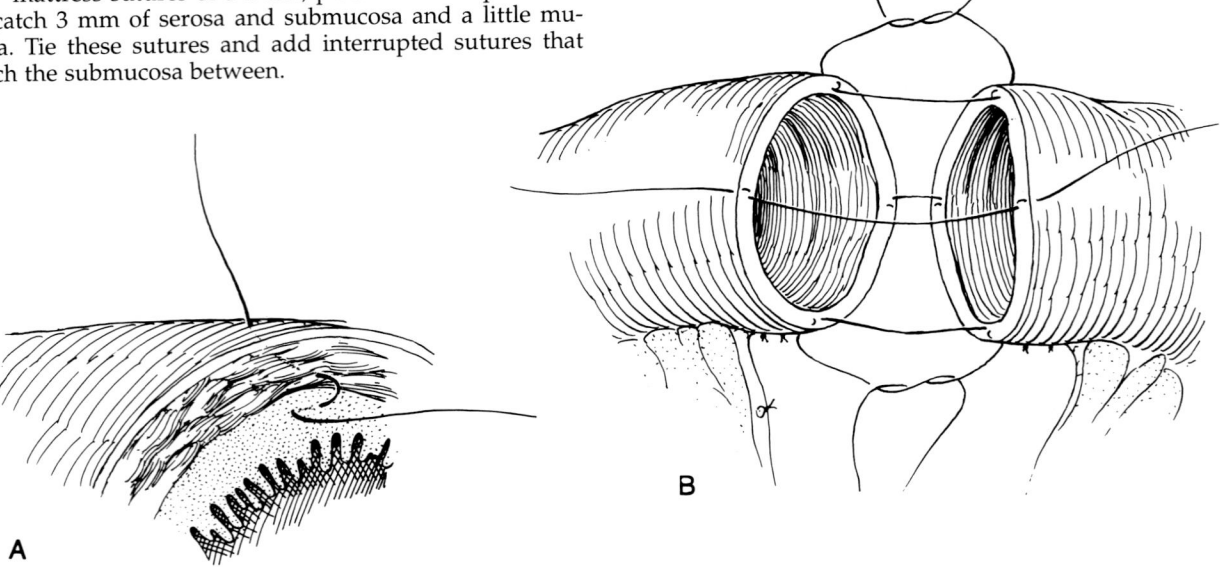

A

B

Two-Layer Closure

10 Approximate the posterior bowel wall with interrupted seromuscular sutures of 3-0 silk. Turn the bowel over. Place full-thickness continuous sutures of 3-0 or 4-0 chromic catgut to invert the mucosa of the posterior wall.

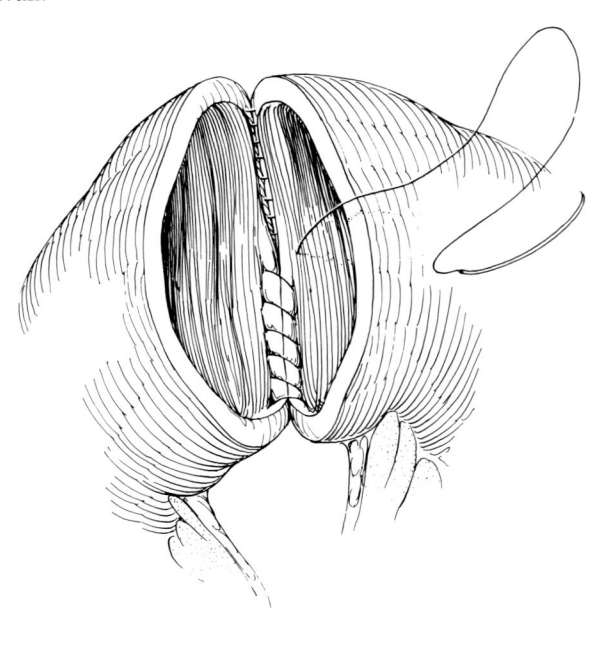

11 Continue this suture on the anterior wall and corners with a Connell stitch.

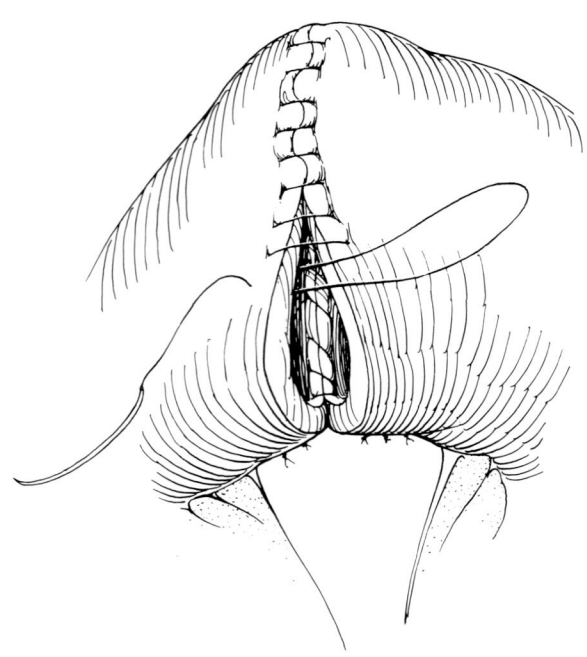

12 Complete the anastomosis with interrupted 3-0 silk sutures on the anterior seromuscular surface. For stapling closure, proceed as described on pages 32–36.

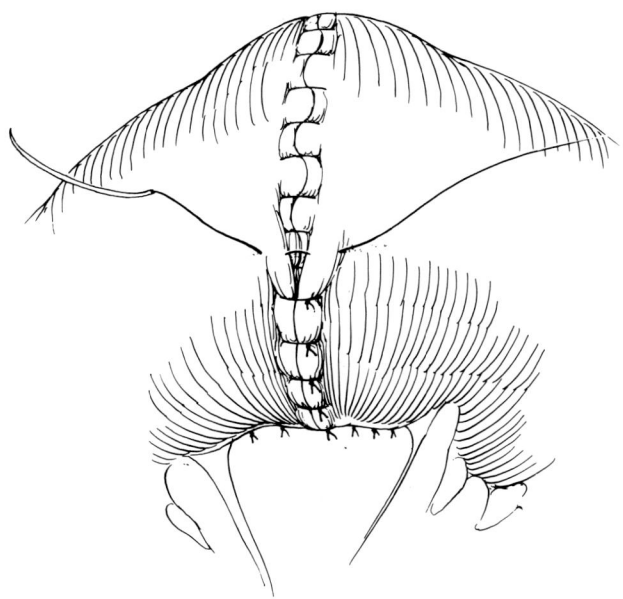

13 Close the mesentery on both sides with fine silk, taking care to incorporate only the delicate peritoneal surface. Annoying hematomas occur if a vessel is caught and breached. Test the anastomosis for patency (Figure 8).

The ileal conduit procedure follows the sequence (1) formation of the stoma, (2) implantation of the right ureter, (3) implantation of the left ureter, (4) resection of excess length from the proximal end of the loop, and (5) closure of the butt end of the loop. The stoma is formed before anastomosing the ureters to allow them to be placed in an optimum position.

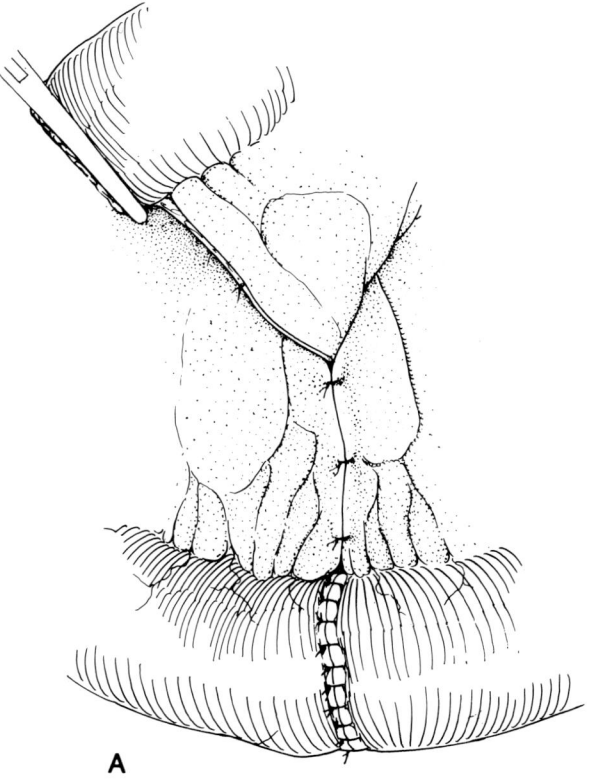

A

FORMATION OF STOMA

14 **A,** On the right side of the incision, draw the fascia and peritoneum in line with the skin using Kocher clamps. Alternatively, place heavy sutures through all layers of the abdominal incision. At the site marked previously, grasp the skin with a Kocher clamp, lift it, and sharply cut off the elevated mound with a knife, removing a circular piece slightly smaller than the diameter of the ileum.

B, Grasp the subcutaneous fat with a Kocher clamp and circumscribe it with the electrosurgical blade, taking care to angle the cut inward to remove a long but narrow core. Avoid undermining, because the subcutaneous tissue stretches; removing too much fat allows inversion of the stoma.

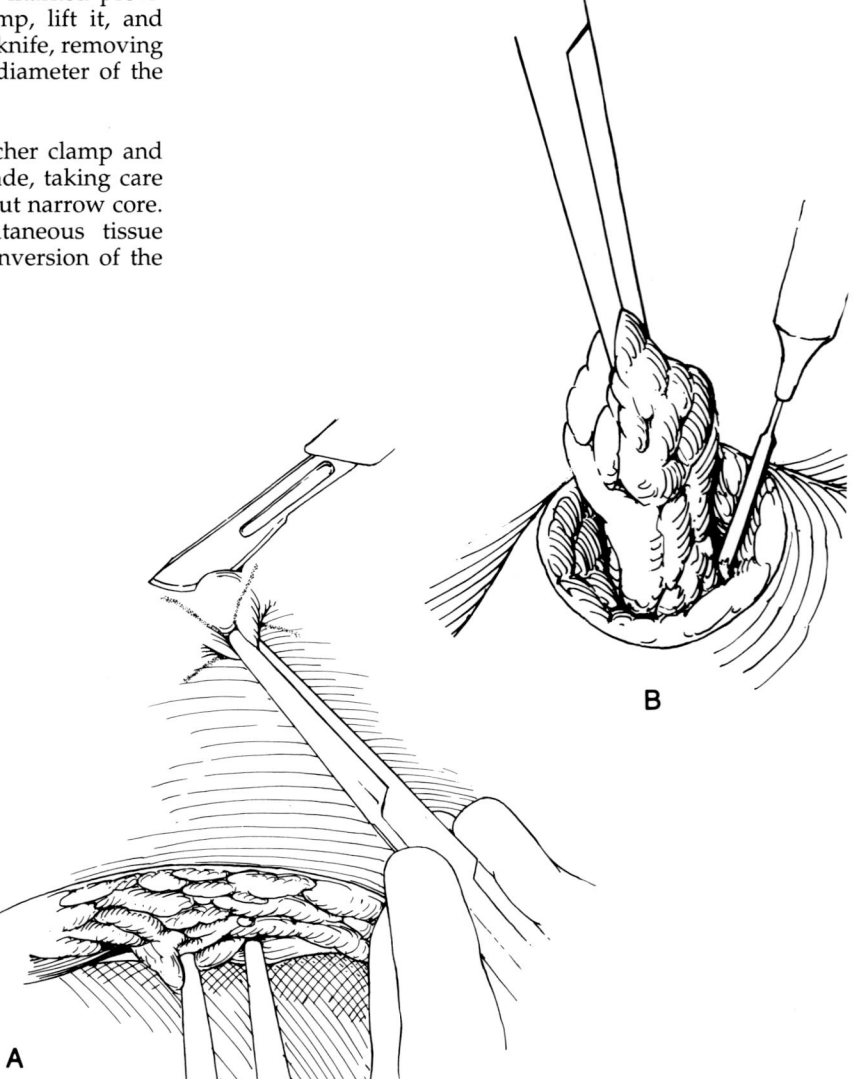

15 Incise the anterior rectus fascia with a cruciate cut with the cutting current, or preferably, remove a disk of fascia. Divide as little of the muscle as possible to help avoid parastomal hernia. Separate the rectus muscle bluntly, and hold it apart with US retractors to allow removal of a disk of the posterior fascial layer and the peritoneum, or incise in a cruciate fashion. Hold the left hand inside the abdomen to prevent injury to the bowel. A finger should now readily pass through all layers. Insert a

Kocher clamp into the stoma, grasp and clamp the traction suture on the end of the loop as it is simultaneously released from its clamp, and draw it out. Be sure it lies without tension 2 to 3 cm above the skin surface. Suture the adventitia of the loop to the peritoneum and underlying rectus fascia from inside the abdomen with five or six synthetic absorbable sutures to prevent peristomal herniation.

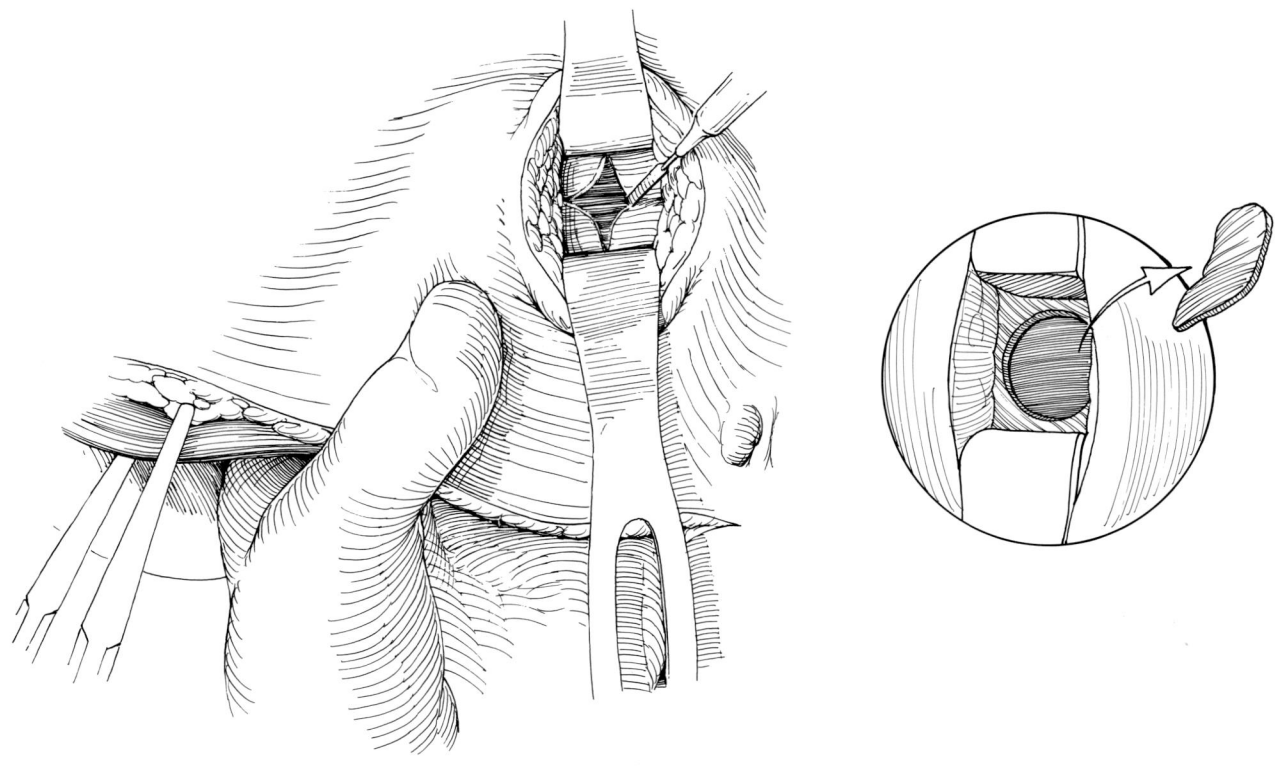

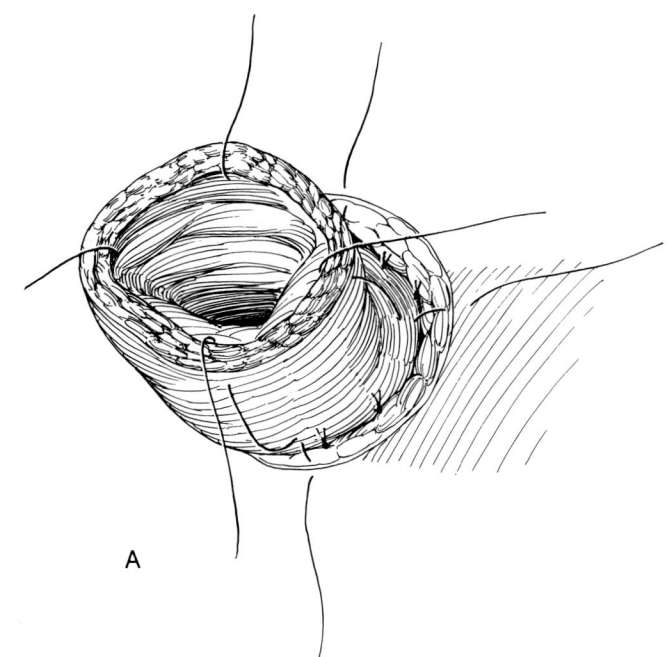

A

16 A and B, Suture the adventitia of the bowel to the fascia to prevent parastomal hernias. Suture the opened bowel to the skin with four quadrant sutures of 3-0 synthetic absorbable material, catching the bowel well below the level of the skin to evert the stoma. Place two more sutures through skin and bowel edge between each pair of quadrant sutures. Invert the suture, so that the knots will be buried. If the loop seems too short (tension), make the stoma flush. Anchor the loop to the peritoneum and posterior rectus fascia with three 4-0 silk sutures (avoid sutures about the mesenteric border).

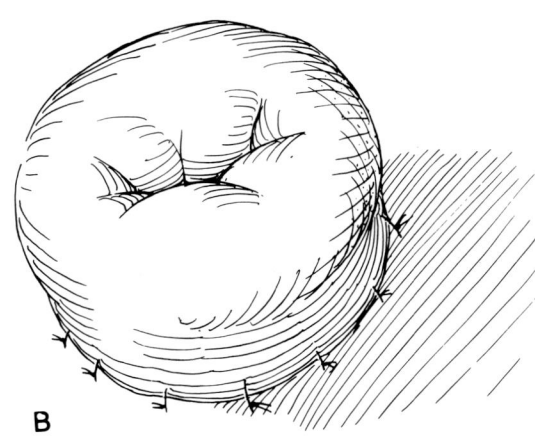

B

Nipple Variations

Nipple variations can be used to reduce stomal stenosis. This technique is more useful when redoing the stoma.

Z-Incision

17 A, Make a Z-incision in the skin at the stomal site.

B, Raise two flaps. If too large, trim them (dotted line).

C, Incise the mucosa and submucosa of the bowel on either side.

D, Insert the flaps in the defects, and suture them in place with 3-0 synthetic absorbable sutures.

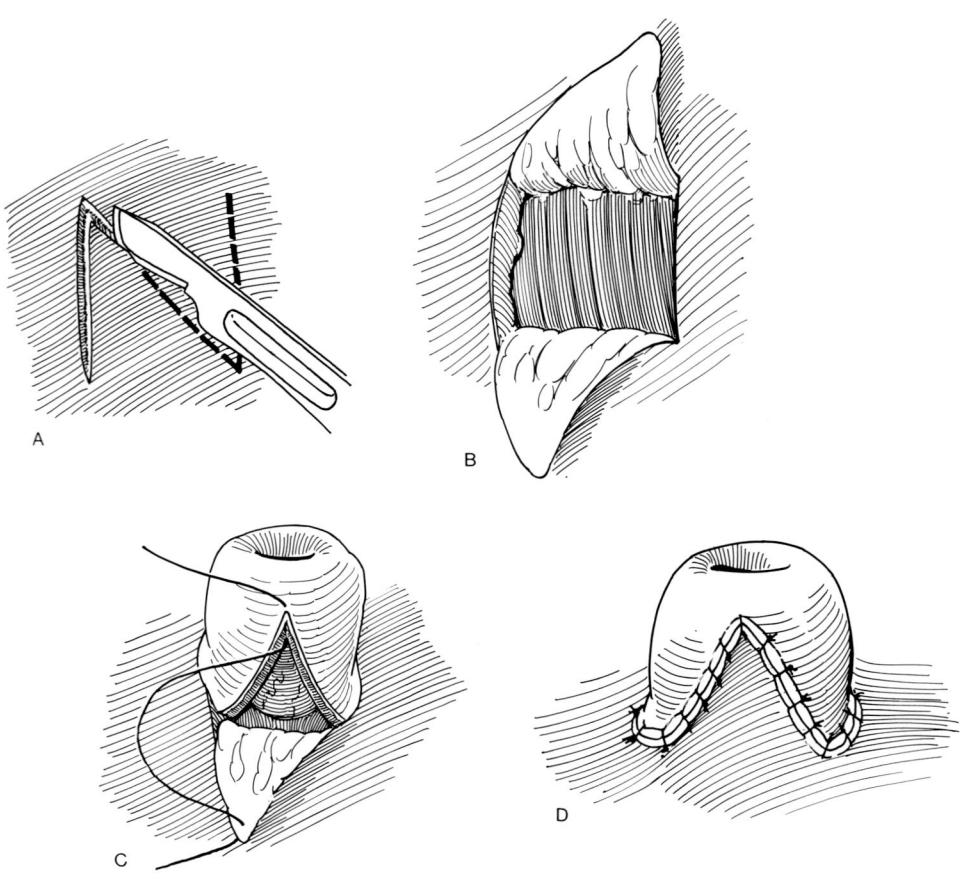

Alternate, Loop Stoma
(Turnbull)

For obese adolescents with a short mesentery, provide an ileal segment that is 8 to 10 cm longer.

18 A, Close the distal end of the conduit, as described previously for the proximal end. In obese children,

carefully undercut the mesentery of the distal end to obtain adequate mobility. Pass a clamp bluntly through the most mobile and well-vascularized part of the mesentery to loop it with a Penrose drain.

B, Draw the bowel loop through the body wall for at least several centimeters without tension or twisting.

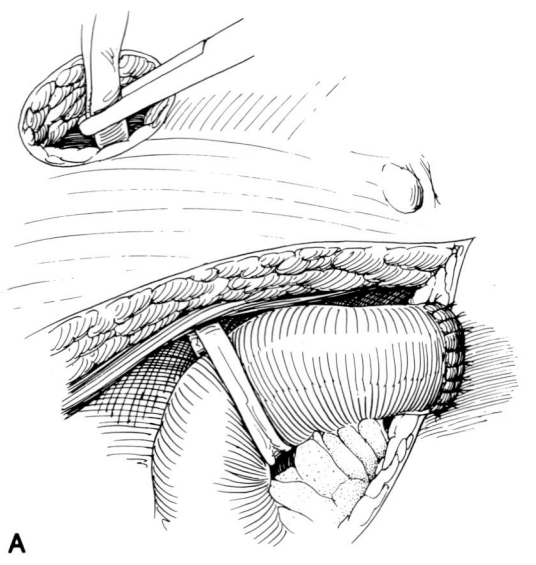

A

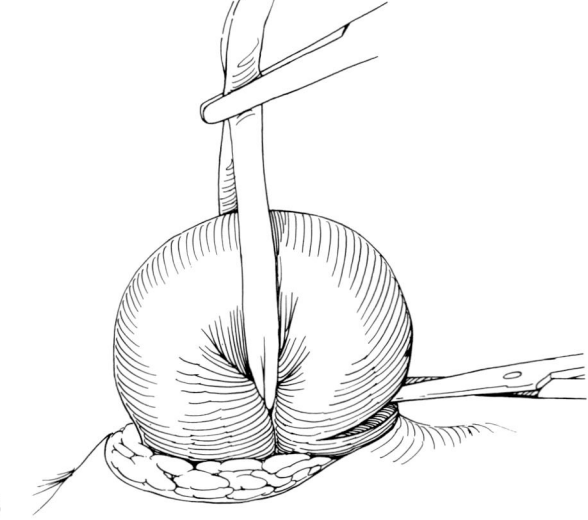

B

19 **A**, Replace the Penrose drain with a plastic rod. Open the loop transversely four fifths of the distance along the exposed bowel nearest the defunctionalized (distal) limb. Reach inside the opening with an Allis clamp, and pull out the mucosa.

B, Suture the mucosa to the subcuticular layer of skin with interrupted 4-0 synthetic absorbable sutures, catching the seromuscular layer of the bowel to evert the stoma. The defunctionalized portion requires only superficial sutures. Fasten the rod in place with two silk sutures; it can be withdrawn 1 to 2 weeks postoperatively.

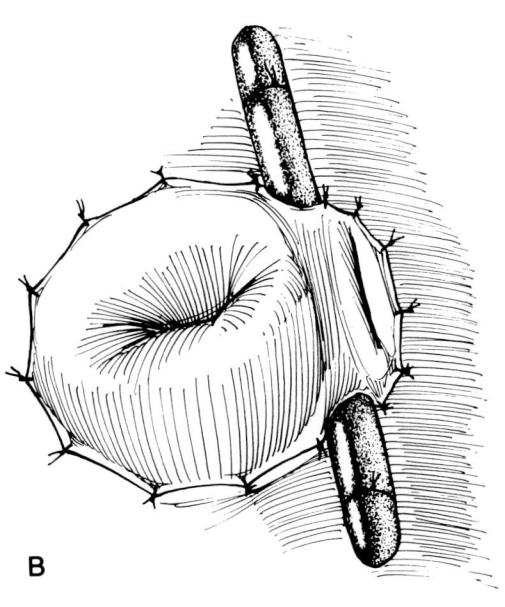

B

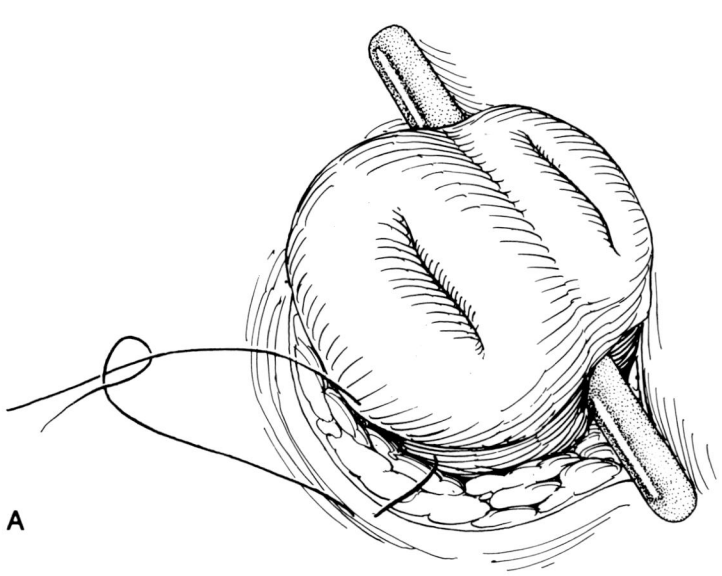

A

URETERAL ANASTOMOSES

Direct Anastomosis, Right
(Cordonnier)

Close the left parietal peritoneal opening with 4-0 silk sutures.

20 Cut the right ureter obliquely to freshen the end, and spatulate it to provide a larger lumen for anastomosis.

21 Place a 4-0 synthetic absorbable suture through the adventitia and muscularis of the ureter 2 cm from the end, and fasten it on the antimesenteric border.

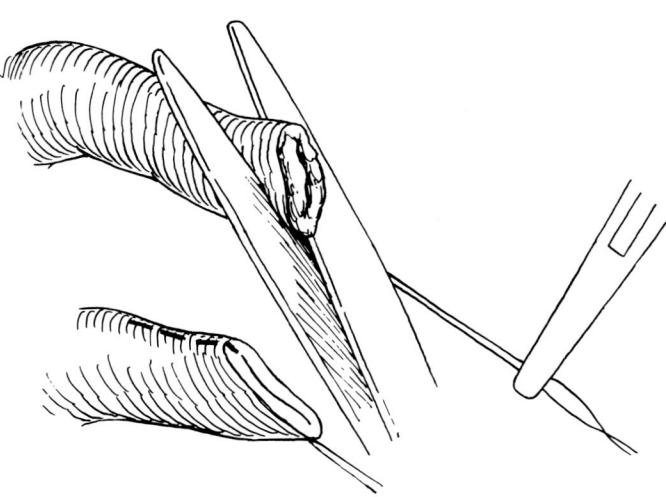

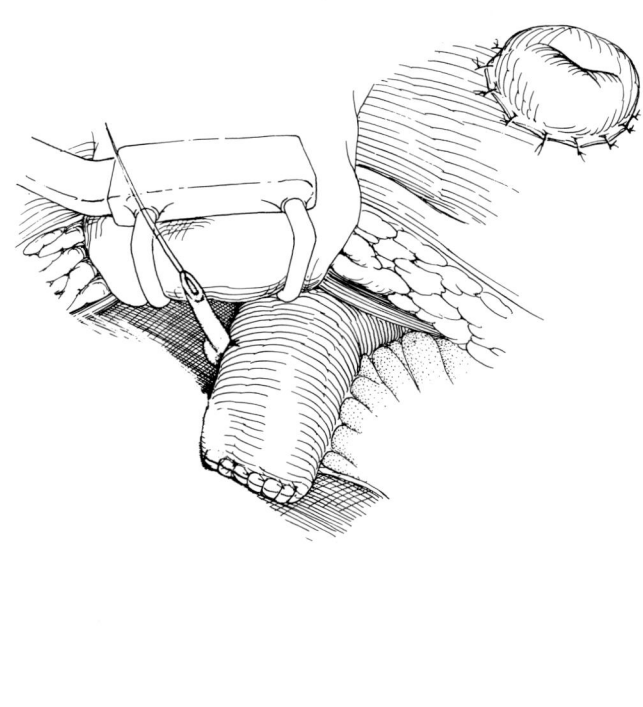

22 Pinch the bowel between the thumb and forefinger of the left hand, and incise through the muscularis with a #15 blade, exposing the fine vessels of the submucosa.

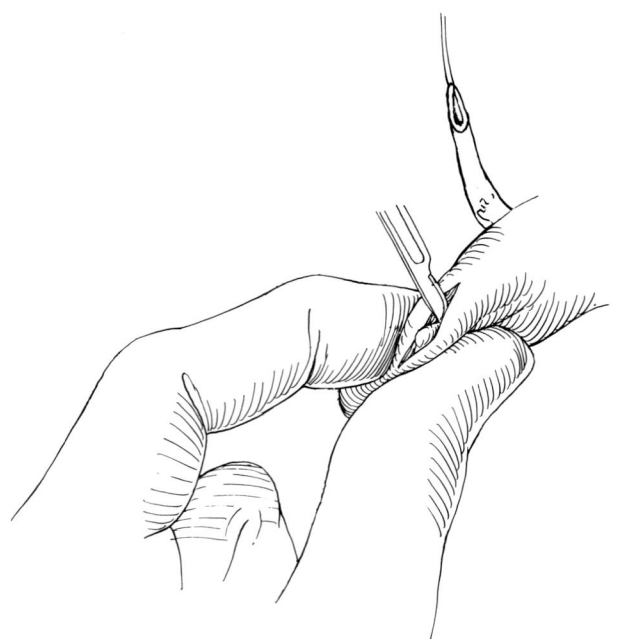

23 Grasp a bit of the extruding submucosa with smooth Adson forceps, and trim it off, along with the underlying mucosa, with tenotomy scissors. Remove as little as possible. Insert the tip of a mosquito clamp into the bowel lumen to check the opening.

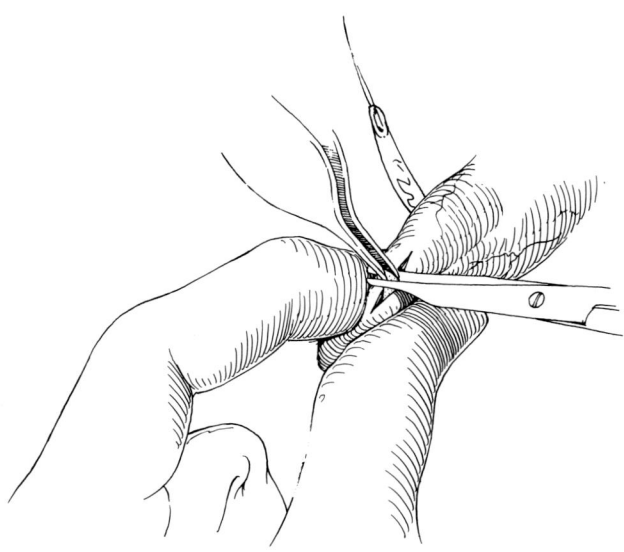

24 **A,** Place a 4-0 or 5-0 synthetic absorbable suture or chromic catgut through the apex of the bowel opening (from outside in), then through the apex of the ureter (from inside out), using the stay suture for manipulation (do not grasp the tissue with forceps). Incorporate a little mucosa, more muscularis, and adequate serosa in the stitch. Tie the suture.

B, Place and tie a suture similarly halfway along each side. A stent now may be inserted if you are concerned about the quality of the tissues. However, stents can be obstructive, take time to insert, and may come out too soon. Without them, leaks are uncommon. If a stent is to be used, mount a 5 or 8 F infant feeding tube on a Péan clamp, and pass it through the ileal stoma and out through the opening in the bowel. Irrigate it clear of mucus. Take it up in a Kelly clamp and introduce it into the ureter until resistance is felt as it reaches the kidney. Irrigate again to test

the position of the tip. Immediately fasten the tube to the skin with a silk suture; later, it will be cut short to fit within the collecting bag. Alternatively, a double-J stent may be inserted. Place a fourth suture through the bowel and the tip of the ureter, which is manipulated on its stay suture. Cut the stay suture.

C, Place three more sutures from the muscularis of the ureter to the serosa of the bowel to invert the anastomosis slightly into the bowel and provide a double layer for watertightness.

Perform the same maneuvers with the left ureter. Make certain that it passes beneath the colon in a smooth curve. Insert it 1 to 2 cm more proximally on the loop than the right, at a site where it is easily accommodated and not angulated.

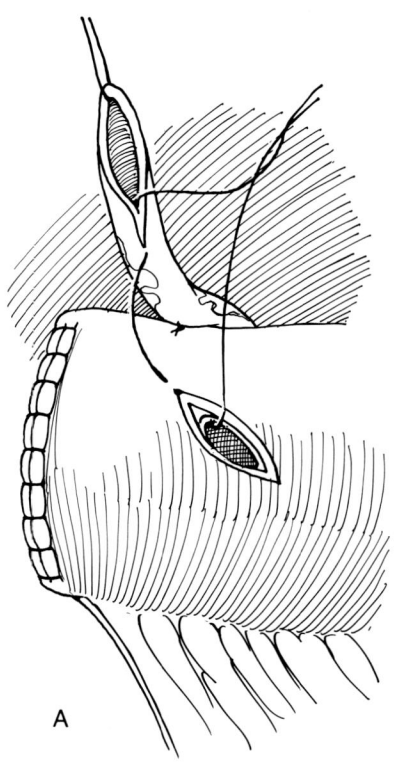

A

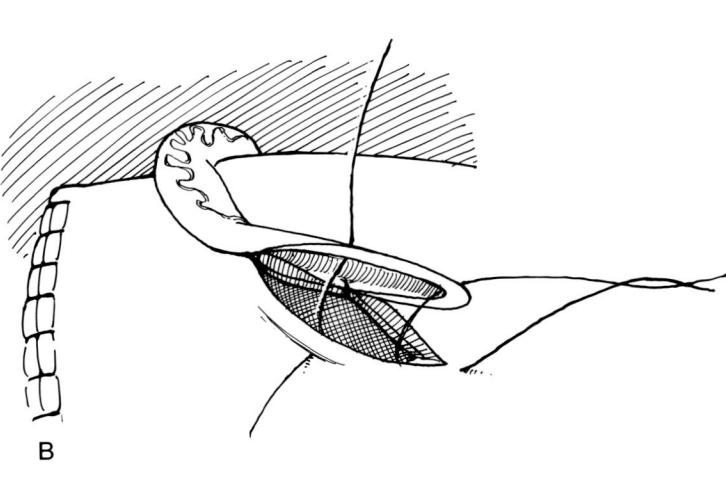

B

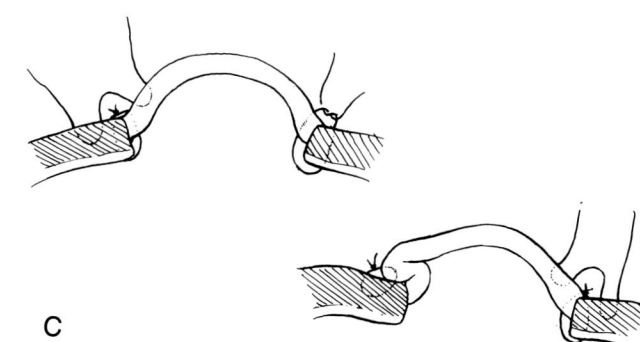

C

TRIMMING AND CLOSURE OF THE PROXIMAL END OF THE LOOP

Spread the loop so that it makes an easy curve from the stoma to the area from which the ureters emerge. Apply a second Kocher clamp proximal to the one placed initially, and trim any excess of bowel.

25 Insert stay sutures in the mesenteric and antimesenteric margins. Over the clamp, place a row of detachable 4-0 silk sutures. These pass through the serosa and muscularis and incorporate the submucosa. Slightly open, then withdraw the clamp, while keeping traction on the stay sutures.

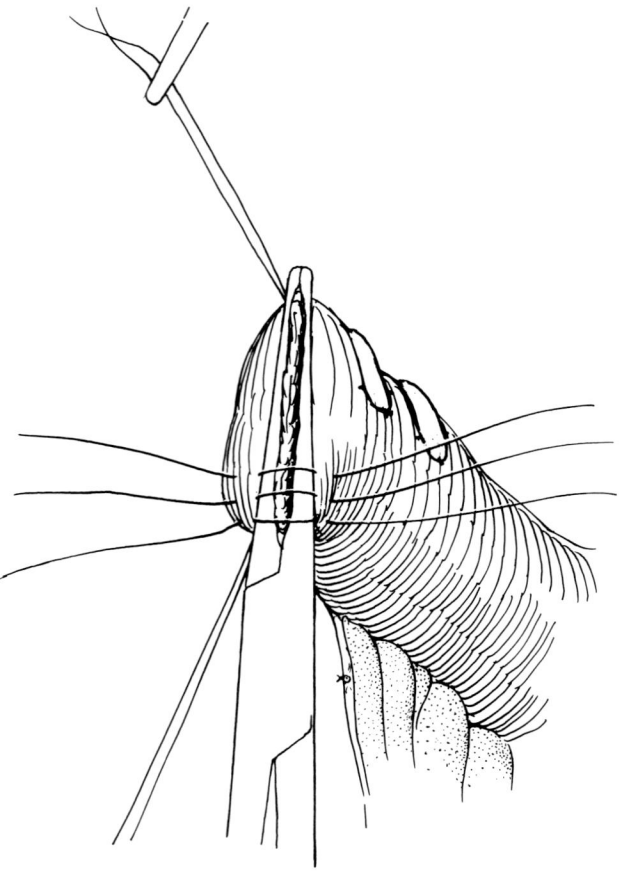

26 Tie the end sutures first to invert each end. A mosquito clamp is used to lift the crossing suture and, at the same time, depress the two edges of the bowel.

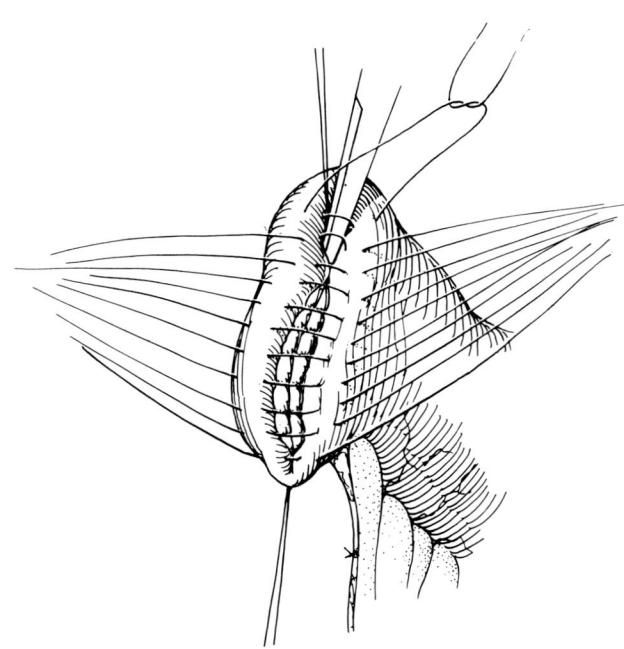

27 The loop is shown of the proper length, with the two ureters emerging from beneath it from the parietal peritoneal defect.

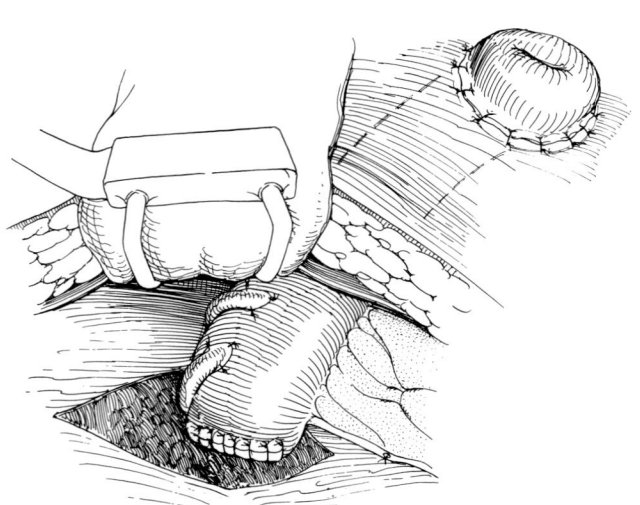

28 Pull the medial peritoneal flap over the ileal stump and ureters, and fix it with interrupted 4-0 silk sutures; continue these up along the mesentery to avoid an internal hernia. Survey the conduit. If it is dusky, apply warm packs. If in doubt, excise it and start over.

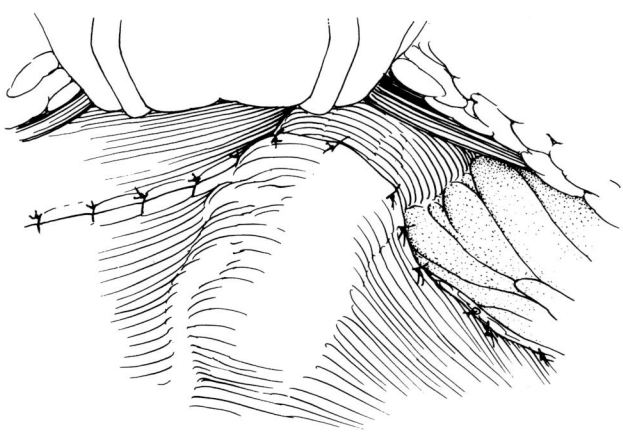

CONJOINED URETER TECHNIQUES

Side by Side

29 A, Do not close the proximal end of the loop. Spatulate each ureter for a distance equal to the diameter of the ileum. Join their posterior edges side by side with a fine running absorbable suture.

B, Anastomose the joined ureters to the open bowel with two running 4-0 synthetic absorbable sutures, placing an occasional lock stitch.

C, Reinforce the anastomosis with a second layer of five or six interrupted sutures. Proceed with closure. Trim the stents, and apply a collection appliance in the operating room. Drain the wound with suction drainage, and remove the drains as soon as the wound is dry.

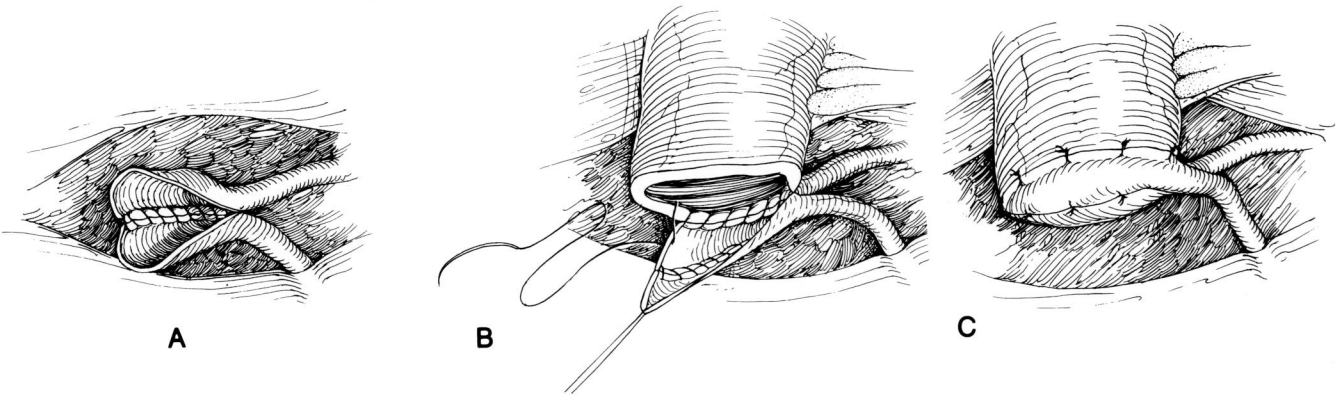

A   B   C

End to End
(Wallace)

30 A, Spatulate each ureter for a distance slightly more than the diameter of the ileum.

B, Join their posterior edges with two running 4-0 chromic catgut sutures, starting in the middle and continuing around each end.

C, Continue the sutures to join the backwalls of the bowel and ureter, taking care to invert the angles; then complete the closure anteriorly.

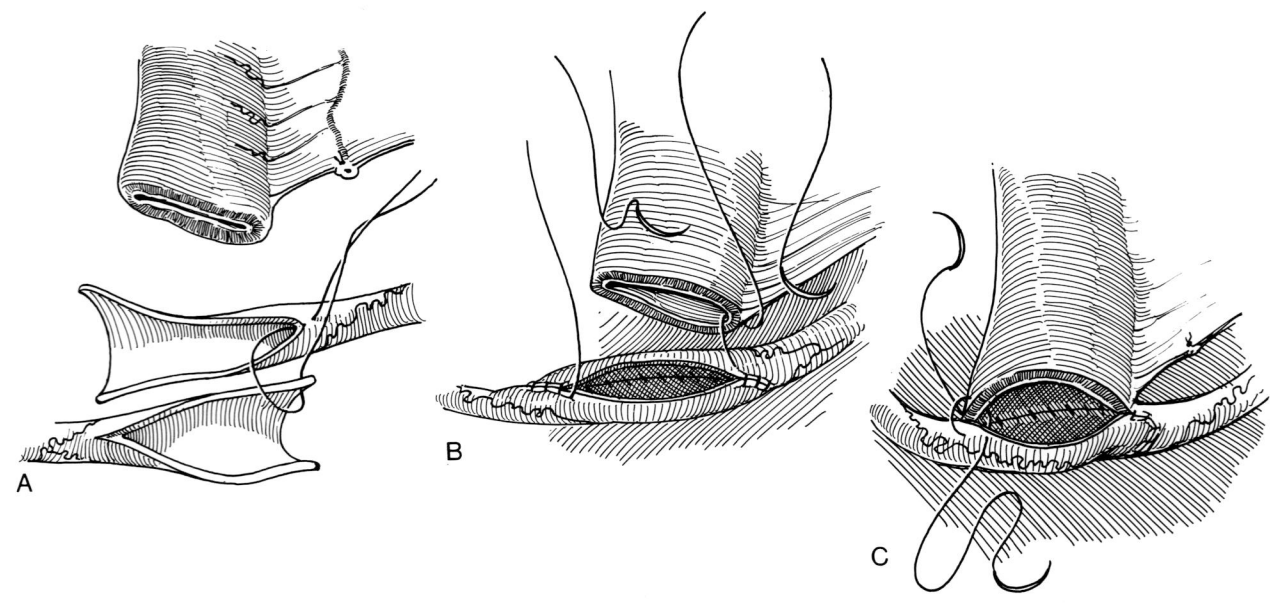

POSTOPERATIVE PROBLEMS

Anuria after surgery usually is secondary to operative fluid shifts, so a challenge with mannitol is the first step. *Obstruction* at the site of anastomosis is rare; this need not be considered if stents are in place and can be irrigated. Place a catheter in the stoma to check for obstruction at the level of the body wall. If all fails and no urine is recovered, place percutaneous nephrostomies.

Hyperchloremic acidosis, similar to that consequent to ureterosigmoidostomy, may occur infrequently. It usually is associated with obstruction at the stoma, either from stenosis or from infrequent emptying of the drainage bag with the associated backpressure. Catheterization of the conduit is immediately corrective; revision of the stoma or shortening of the loop may be needed for the long term. Jejunal conduits have greater problems with electrolyte imbalance, characterized by azotemia and hyponatremic hypochloremic acidosis, and should be used only if no other bowel is available.

Wound infection or dehiscence is uncommon in children. Malnutrition, which should have been corrected preoperatively, can be an important factor.

Running monofilament sutures with adequate bites of rectus fascia can prevent disruption.

Paralytic ileus is usual and resolves quickly if gastric decompression is maintained, but intestinal obstruction may occur from herniation of the bowel into the mesenteric "trap." Continuation of decompression with a long (Baker) tube usually permits resolution, but reoperation occasionally is necessary.

Intestinal fistulas can occur from the site of the ileoileal anastomosis as a result of local ischemia from interference with the mesenteric arcades, and the whole segment can become necrotic if the mesentery is carelessly tacked to retroperitoneum or if it is subjected to too much tension. The vascular supply can be judged by the color of the stomal mucosa. Leakage at the ileoileal anastomosis usually is caused by tension and rough handling of the tissue. Leakage also can occur at the suture line closing the proximal end of the loop. Leakage from the ureteroileal anastomosis is uncommon. The source can be determined by testing the fluid from the drains, because urine has a higher urea content than blood. Intraperitoneal absorption causes the blood urea nitrogen level to rise relative to the creatinine. Do a loopogram. If the leakage is minimal, place a double-lumen suction tube (a Malecot catheter containing an infant feeding tube connected to low suction) to allow healing. Alternatively, insert a tube into the kidney percutaneously or place stents antegradely. If an appreciable urinoma has formed and the child is ill, reoperation with resection of the anastomosis and reimplantation at a new site is required. This is not an easy procedure, but attempts at resuturing seldom succeed. Prompt reoperation with insertion of a gastrostomy and replacement of the loop usually is required. *Redundancy* of the segment usually is secondary to obstruction at the stoma or at the body wall. For correction, not only should the loop be shortened but the cause of the obstruction must be corrected.

Obstruction at the ureteroileal anastomosis usually develops within the first 2 years, but it may occur late. It is caused by devascularization of the terminal ureter and usually is unsuspected. Regular follow-up is necessary to avoid this complication, with sonograms, scans, or intravenous pyelography, and loopograms at regular intervals. Before reoperation, an attempt may be made at balloon dilation of the anastomosis through a percutaneous nephrostomy tract, but this seldom is successful because of the fibrous cause of the stricture. Repair entails an approach through a modified Gibson incision or transperitoneally. Dissect retroperitoneally, but stay away from the stoma. Incise the ureter and bowel at the site of the anastomosis, and perform a Heineke-Mikulicz transverse closure. Alternatively, take an ellipse from the ureter, incise the ileum above the stricture, and suture the defects side to side. It also is possible to detach the ureter and either reanastomose it or do a ureteroureterostomy.

Stomal problems are very common and often are directly related to the quality of stomal care. *Peristomal dermatitis* is common and may lead to stenosis. The cause may be an improperly located or constructed stoma, an appliance that does not fit, poorly tolerated adhesive, alkaline urine, or inadequate stomal care. It starts with skin inflammation and progresses to ulceration and encrustation. Hyperkeratosis, scarring, and stenosis are the final result. *Stomal ischemia* usually is temporary, but if it persists, it will require stomal revision with resection of a short segment. If the whole loop is ischemic, remove it, ligate the ureters, and place percutaneous nephrostomies. Wait 3 months and repeat the whole operation. *Stomal stenosis* occurs at the circular mucocutaneous junction. A Z-flap technique or an end-loop stoma lessens the chance of stenosis. Everted (nipple) stomas have a lower incidence of stenosis. It usually occurs at the skin level, secondary to the effects of dermatitis, but can result from fascial angulation or ischemia of the terminal portion of the bowel. Alignment at the time of formation and prevention or correction of peristomal dermatitis are the remedies. Correction is needed if the stoma will not admit a 30 F catheter, the residual urine is more than 10 ml, or luminal pressure is greater than 20 cm H_2O.

Revision of the Stoma. The stoma usually can be circumscribed close to the mucosa and excised, because the redundant bowel is readily mobilized through the defect. Free the bowel for 10 to 12 cm through the body wall by dissecting intraperitoneally and dividing adhesions, resect the terminal portion with its mesentery, and tack the bowel to the fascia. Form a new nipple stoma by interposing a V-flap of skin to prevent further circular contraction. If the adjacent skin is badly scarred, form several Z-plasties or insert a spiral flap (David, 1976). Most important is improved care with the help of an enterostomal therapist. *Stomal prolapse* results from inadequate fixation of the loop to the peritoneal and fascial layers, and the treatment is similar to that for stenosis. *Parastomal hernias* usually occur on the mesenteric side secondary to inadequate fixation of the conduit at the peritoneal opening. They can make fitting the appliance difficult and may lead to incarceration of the bowel. Repair them by freeing the stoma and distal loop, as done for stomal stenosis, excising the peritoneal sac, fixing the loop internally, and closing the defect in the fascia. If this is not feasible, relocate the stoma to the opposite side, which can be done without opening the abdomen by passing the end of the loop from the old stoma to the new one on ring forceps. It can be corrected using the same technique as for stomal stenosis. *Excessive length* of the loop can be resected through the stomal site by progressively dividing the mesenteric arcades as they join the bowel.

Appliances. If it becomes impossible to keep an appliance attached because of body configuration, move the stoma up or down on the same side, place it at the umbilicus, or move it across the abdomen. Sometimes, the entire loop must be mobilized or a new conduit constructed to reach the new site.

Ureteral dilation may result from *ureteral stenosis* from technical error or may appear late, cause unknown. Revision is necessary unless the ureter is atonic, in which case, a new anastomosis will not help.

Renal calculi appear later, usually in alkaline urine, harboring urea-splitting bacteria. Shorten the loop, increase water intake, give thiazides, add bicarbonate, and inhibit the infection with antibiotics. Removal usually is reserved for stones that are obstructive. *Pyelonephritis* occurs with increasing frequency the longer diversion is present, as a result of a combination of backflow and bacteriuria. Antibacterial therapy for symptomatic attacks and attention to better drainage may help.

Commentary by Lowell R. King

Because of stomal problems, an ileal conduit seldom is the optimal choice for cutaneous urinary diversion in children. As the child grows, the stoma, surrounded by scar tissue, does not. This means that stomal revision is required approximately every 4 years until full growth is achieved.

Additionally, ileal stomas in children are prone to squamous metaplasia and inflammation, which may quickly result in obstruction. Erythromycin or penicillin may be useful in preventing, and even reversing, such changes, but stomal irritation is a common, and often chronic, complication. Additionally, stones in the kidneys also become common in adolescence, possibly forming on a nidus of refluxed mucus. Because the ureters are anastomosed end-on, the potential for such reflux is virtually always present.

Large bowel–colonic stomas are much more satisfactory in children, in part because the stoma is larger, but mainly because stomatitis and stenosis are rare. The ileocecal or Zinman conduit confers the advantages of a colonic stoma with the simplicity of an ileal loop—the ureters are anastomosed end to side to the ileum, and the ileocecal valve serves as a partial antireflux mechanism. A formal colon conduit should utilize a segment of sigmoid, so that muscle flaps may be separated from the mucosa with relative ease to facilitate an antirefluxing ureteral anastomosis.

Finally, a cutaneous ureterostomy with transureteroureterostomy is a reliable form of supravesical diversion when the ureter that is brought to the skin is at least 1 cm in diameter in its collapsed state. Such stomas occasionally become stenotic, but on the average require revision only every 4 to 5 years until the child is grown. An ileal conduit may be preferred as the long-term form of supravesical diversion, because undiversion, anastomosing the proximal portion of the conduit carrying the ureters to ileum above a nipple valve, is then a simple and standardized procedure that can be used when the bladder is augmented or a continent reservoir is formed, perhaps when the child is old enough to reliably do intermittent catheterization to empty. An ileal conduit also is versatile. The loop may be turned upward and the proximal end anastomosed to the renal pelvis, bypassing very dilated or tiny ureters. An end-on anastomosis of the ureter to the antimesenteric border of the ileum is simple and relatively easy technically. Postoperative obstruction is rare. The ileum is mobile enough that the stoma can be placed anywhere, important in patients with severe lordosis and scoliosis, who often are confined to wheelchairs.

Technique is important in ileoconduit surgery. Ideally, one would like to make the stomal incision first. If the optimal location has been selected, excision of successive disks of abdominal wall tissue guarantees that the incision will not be partially obstructed by fascial or muscular baffles.

The ileal loop itself should be as short as possible, with a minimum of "dead space" between the site of left ureteral implantation and the closed end of the conduit. The Wallace technique of end-on anastomosis of the ureters to the proximal end of the conduit avoids stasis in the loop completely and is recommended. Usually, the stoma is formed first. The right ureter is anastomosed, and then the left. Proximal excess conduit length is resected before the butt end of the conduit is closed.

Ileal loop stomas are prone to inflammation in children, and stomal stenosis can occur relatively quickly. The stoma should be calibrated frequently and revised promptly to prevent renal damage if partial obstruction occurs.

CHAPTER 75

Pediatric High Ileal Conduit

In a child with bilateral hydronephrosis, large extrarenal pelves, and ureters of such extreme tortuosity and fibrosis that urine conduction would be poor, a high ileal conduit may be a form of diversion of last resort. If decompression of the lower tract by vesicostomy is not adequate, temporary cutaneous ureterostomy can provide additional improvement. A transureteroureterostomy is the next-best solution for chronically dilated ureters, if accompanied by straightening and shortening of the ureters. The single ureter may be placed to open on the skin or, if function permits, may be implanted in the bladder.

1 *Incision*: From the right side of the table, make a long midline transperitoneal incision (page 83), extending to the xiphoid.

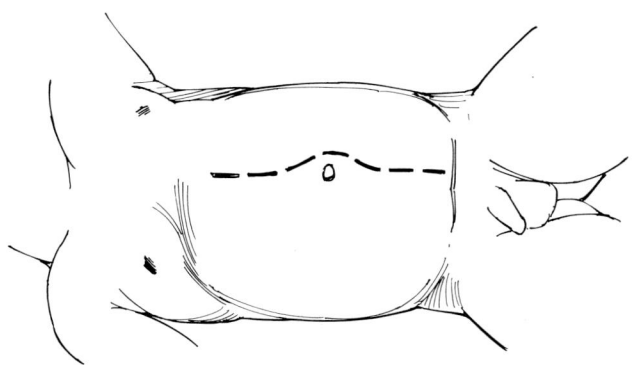

2 Reflect the splenic flexure of the colon medially and inferiorly by incising along the line of the lateral peritoneal reflection, and bluntly dissect the peritoneum toward the midline. Open Gerota's fascia, and clear the perirenal fat from the lower pole and pelvis of the left kidney. Pass a Penrose drain around the ureter to aid in freeing it.

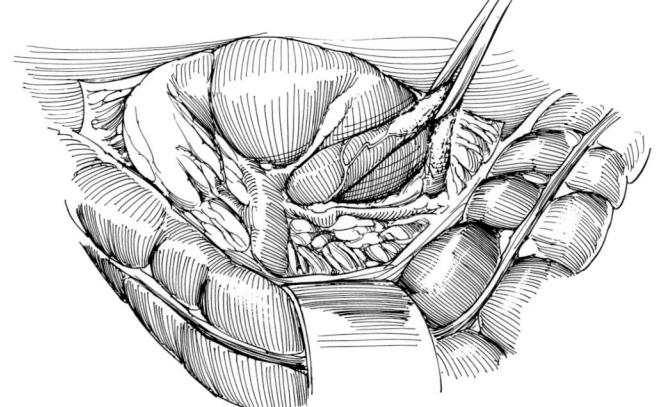

3 Reflect the hepatic flexure medially. Expose, clear, and tag the upper right ureter.

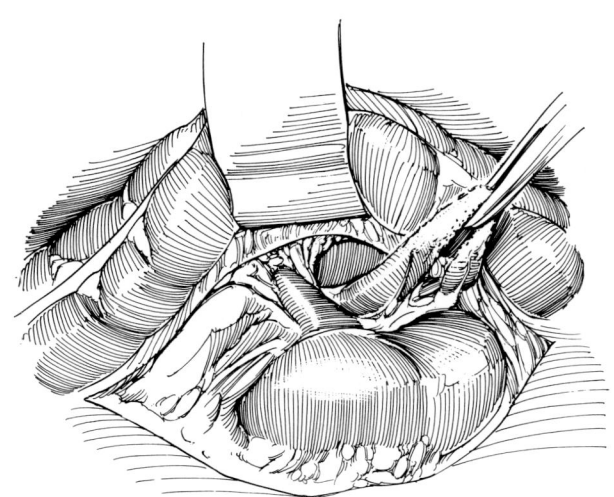

389

4 Create a tunnel bluntly with the fingers from one opening to the other, just beneath the peritoneum, keeping the track below the level of the superior mesenteric artery and above the inferior mesenteric artery. Widen it digitally, so it will accommodate the loop of bowel. Pass an umbilical tape through it on a long clamp.

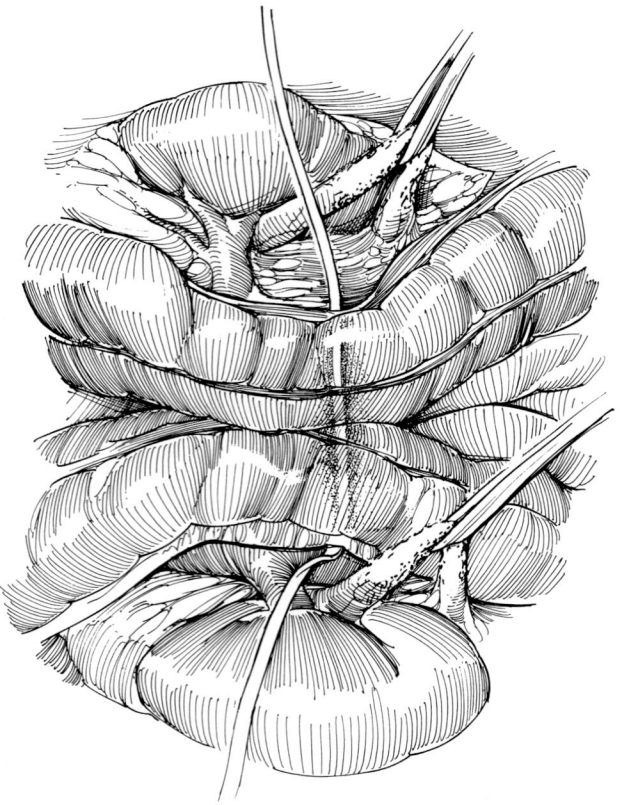

5 Select a loop of ileum that must be longer than that used for a standard conduit. The jejunum, instead of the terminal ileum, can be resorted to if the bowel mesentery is short or fatty. Provide for two arteries long enough to allow a 6- to 8-cm cut in the mesentery at both ends. Tag the proximal end of the proposed segment with a fine silk suture. Incise the mesentery, divide the bowel between clamps, and restore continuity, as described for ileal conduit (page 377). The loop must lie above the restored ileum. Close the mesentery with 4-0 silk detachable sutures, taking care not to catch the fine terminations of the straight arteries and produce a mesenteric hematoma.

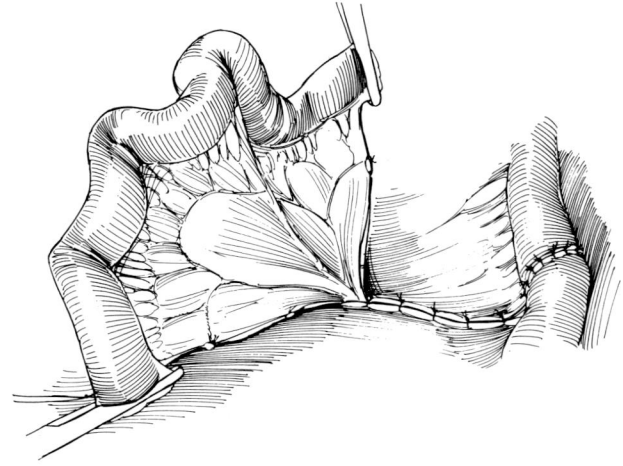

6 Identify the right renal pelvis through the posterior peritoneum medial to the hepatic flexure, and incise a window just below it. Grasp the left end of the previously placed umbilical tape in a clamp to draw the first clamp through the tunnel to the window. Now, use it to grasp the stay suture on the bowel and to gently draw the loop through the window, then through the tunnel. Be sure that the mesentery of the loop is not compressed; if you have doubts, enlarge the tunnel.

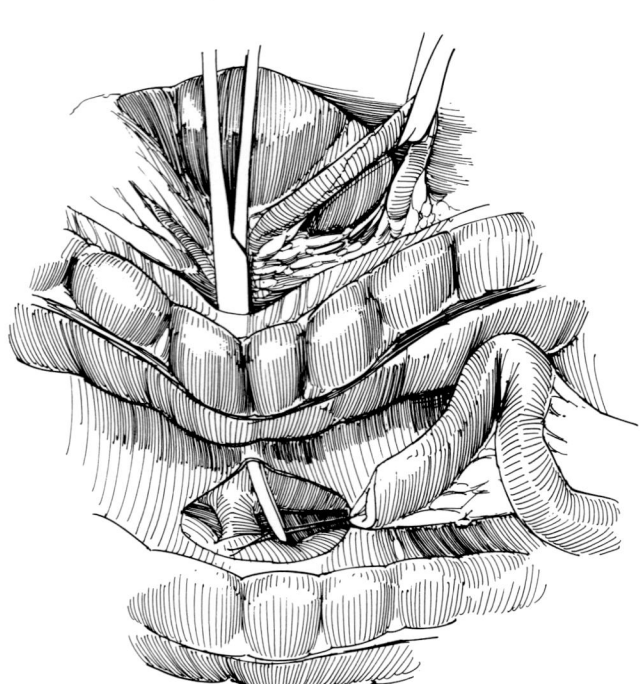

7 Transect the left renal pelvis where it is 3 or 4 cm in diameter. Place a 4-0 synthetic absorbable stay suture through both bowel and pelvis at either end of the proposed anastomosis, and run one suture up the posterior wall, tying it to the other suture. Then, run the second suture down the anterior wall and tie it to the first. The suture line may be reinforced with interrupted sutures. Make a stab wound through the flank, and draw a Penrose drain to the surface extraperitoneally. It may be tacked near the anastomosis with 3-0 plain catgut to prevent displacement.

Trim the right pelvis with a transverse cut. Excise a full-thickness button of bowel opposite the pelvis. Place 4-0 synthetic absorbable stay sutures through the bowel and pelvic wall at either end of the proposed anastomosis, and run a posterior layer with one suture and an anterior layer with the other. Place a second retroperitoneal Penrose drain through the flank.

If only the ureter is available for anastomosis to the bowel because the pelvis is intrarenal, close the end of the loop and cut the ureter obliquely. Place two stay sutures in the bowel on the antimesenteric border, and make a full-thickness opening the same size as the dilated ureter. Place two 4-0 synthetic absorbable sutures side by side at the apex of the proposed anastomosis, and run each down each side; tie them together.

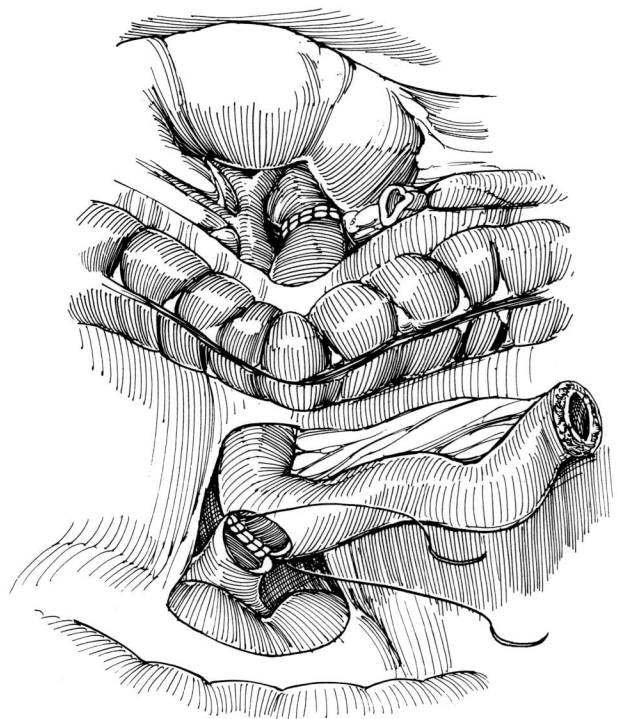

8 Select a stoma site, usually in the right upper quadrant or at waist level, so that the loop takes a straight course without tension. Complete the stoma. If the bladder is normal, the loop may be anastomosed directly to its fundus, forming a bilateral ileal ureter (see page 255). Check the anastomoses for leaks by injecting very dilute methylene blue solution through a fine needle into one renal pelvis. Close the peritoneal window around the loop, and suture the colonic mesentery to it to hold it in place. Tack the hepatic and splenic flexures back into position. Close the wound securely in layers.

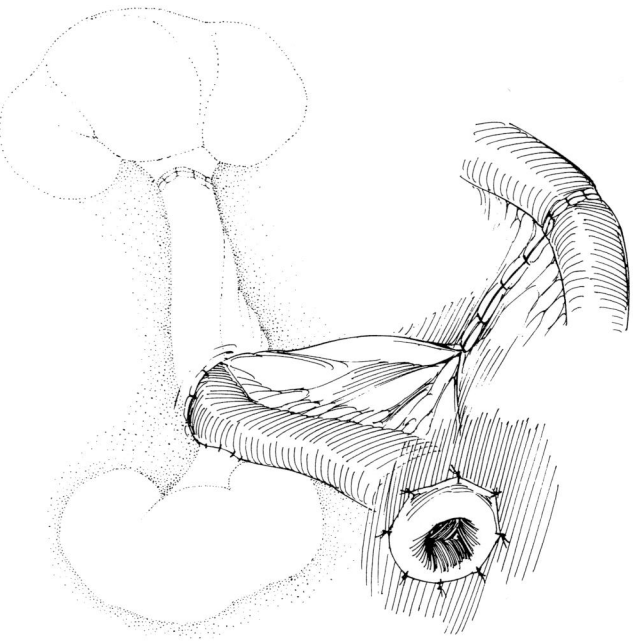

Commentary by William A. Brock

There are few current indications for an ileal conduit urinary diversion in children and almost none for this particular procedure. The choice of a high ileal conduit would require almost complete loss of both ureters as well as the bladder. In adults, this is occasionally seen with bilateral ureteral involvement with transitional cell carcinoma, after multiple open procedures for recurrent stone disease or secondary to tuberculosis or schistosomiasis. The field of endourology and use of extracorporeal shock wave lithotripsy have decreased the need for recurrent stone procedures but have added a new set of complications from endoscopic ureteral injury. The most likely indication for a high ileal conduit in a child would be after a failed total reconstruction for prune belly syndrome, posterior urethral valves, or bilateral obstructive megaureter, complicated by almost complete loss of both ureters and bladder. Combinations of inferior nephropexy, bladder flaps, and a vesicopsoas hitch can replace surprisingly long segments of ureter. I also would rather remodel (using the Hendren or Hanna technique) wide ureters than abandon them. Even if wide ureters are atonic, I believe they make a better choice for cutaneous urinary diversion by means of a transureteroureterostomy plus an end-cutaneous ureterostomy of the recipient ureter. With the newer techniques of continent diversion now available, this incontinent form of urinary diversion seems dated and truly useful only as a last resort.

Technical points that should be emphasized include the need for extended cuts into the mesentery of the isolated loop of bowel, especially at the proximal end, to allow passage of this end beneath the peritoneum to the left renal pelvis. I prefer isoperistaltic placement of the loop, if possible (left to right to skin). I also would prefer to place the isolated loop caudal or beneath the reconstituted small bowel, rather than above it.

If the renal pelvis is small, scarred, and intrarenal, the medial border of the lower pole of the kidney can be divided in continuity with the pelvis to provide a wider anastomosis between the bowel and the pelvis and calyces (ileopyelocalycostomy). Finally, I would place nephrostomies and/or use large-caliber stents to drain this conduit for 1 to 2 weeks.

CHAPTER 76

Sigmoid Conduit

For obese adolescents, a transverse colon conduit (page 395) performed by a technique similar to that for a sigmoid conduit may be preferred, especially if the ureters have been shortened.

1 **A,** *Incision:* Midline (page 83). Usually, place the stoma on the left, except when replacing an ileal conduit with the previous stomal site available. Perform an appendectomy, unless it will be used later as a conduit. Isolate and divide the ureters below the pelvic brim.

B, Incise the lateral attachment of the sigmoid colon along the white line. Choose a segment of sigmoid colon longer than will be needed, because it shortens after division (6 to 8 in usually is enough). Be sure it has a broad-based blood supply. Place a double set of stay sutures in the bowel at each end, above and below the sites of division. Incise the peritoneum on the anterior surface, and divide and individually ligate the crossing mesenteric vessels. Mobilize the sigmoid colon from its lateral and posterior attachments as far as the sacral promontory medially and the inferior mesenteric artery superiorly. Release the splenic flexure if greater length is required, because it

must be possible to rotate the loop 180 degrees after it is created and to be able to reanastomose the sigmoid colon. Divide the superior hemorrhoidal branch of the inferior mesenteric artery to give increased mobility to the distal end of the loop. Make the proximal mesenteric cut very short. Clear the ends of the bowel of appendices epiploicae and mesenteric fat. Divide the bowel with a knife; clamps are not needed. Wash out the lumen.

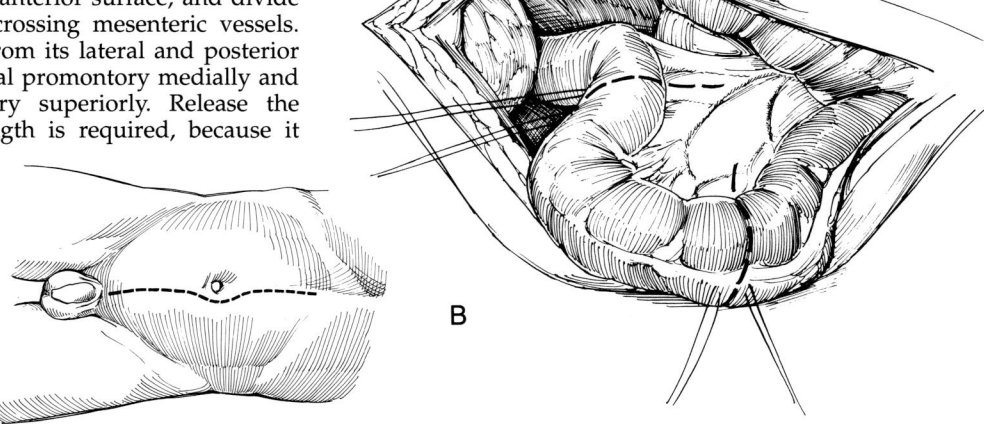

A

B

2 Place the bowel segment to the left of the sigmoid colon. (If the stoma is to be on the right, leave the segment on that side.) Rotate the segment 180 degrees counterclockwise.

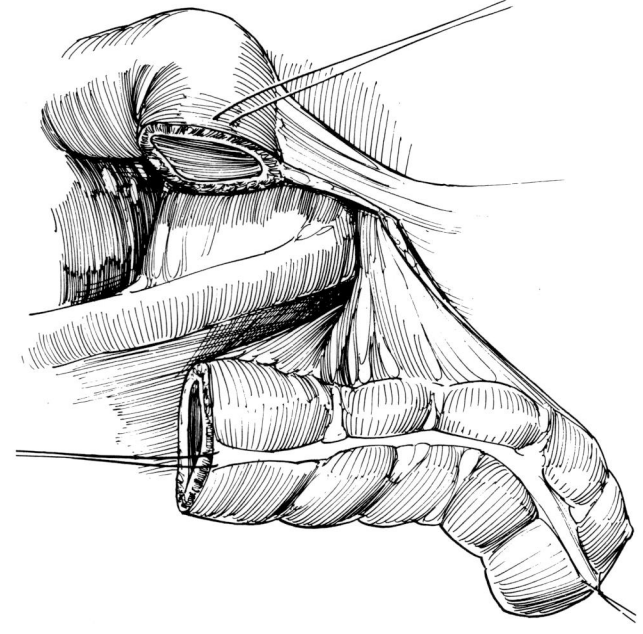

3 Close the proximal end with a Parker-Kerr stitch of 3-0 chromic catgut plus a layer of 4-0 silk Lembert sutures (page 32). Alternatively, use staples (page 36).

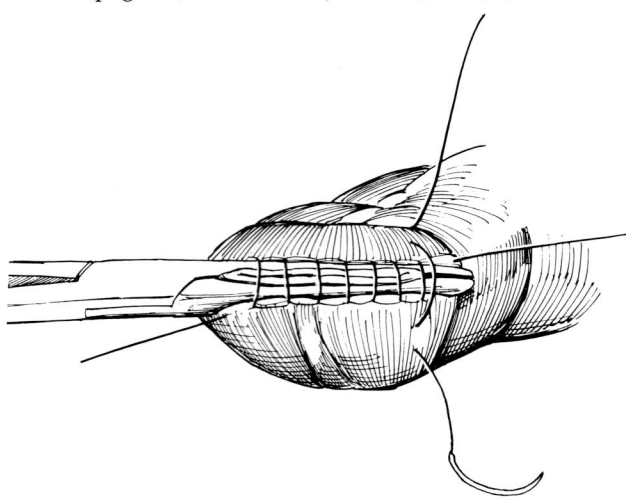

5 Construct a stoma by everting the end of the colon as a short nipple. Bring the right ureter under the sigmoid colon through a tunnel under the parietal peritoneum. Anastomose the ureters to the colon by the method described for ureterosigmoidostomy (pages 427–434), making long (6- to 8-cm) tunnels and undermining well laterally for each. Place 5 F infant feeding tubes as stents. Take care not to constrict the ureter; be able to insert a right-angle clamp after closure of the tunnel. Taper large ureters (page 220). If both are very dilated, consider ureteroureterostomy (page 227) with implantation of a single tapered ureter into the bowel.

Suture the segment firmly to the anterior peritoneum at the site of exit to prevent prolapse. Suture the mesentery and the stump of the sigmoid to the posterior parietal peritoneum to prevent twisting. Extraperitonealize the conduit with the lateral peritoneal flap. Close the wound with or without drainage.

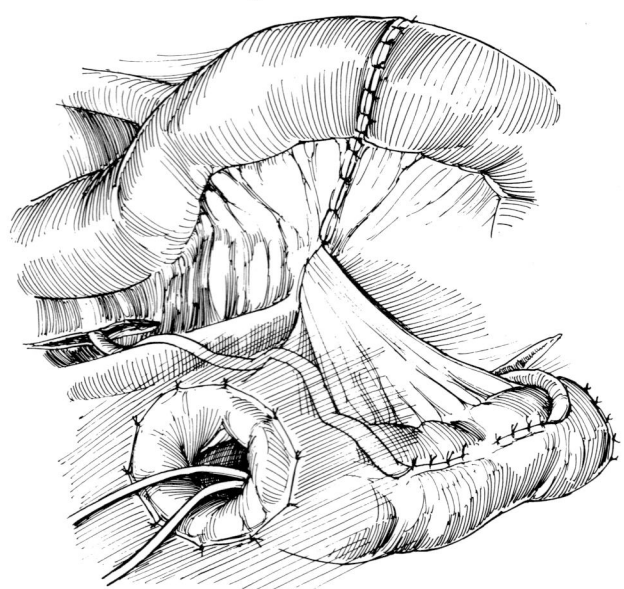

4 Reanastomose the sigmoid colon with a running 3-0 chromic catgut Parker-Kerr stitch and interrupted Lembert sutures. Alternatively, use staples.

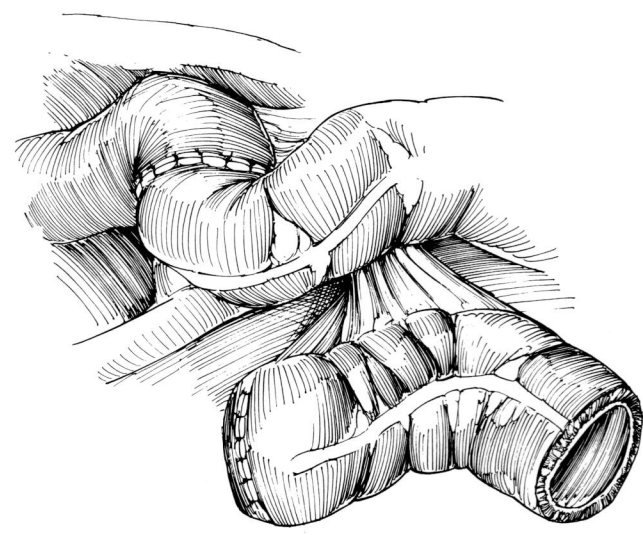

POSTOPERATIVE PROBLEMS

Compared with the ileal conduit, one formed from the sigmoid colon has fewer complications. Although *early leakage* is less common, *ureteral stenosis* is more likely to occur; therefore, stenting is advisable. Compared with ureteroileal strictures, those at the ureterocolic anastomosis are more easily dilated endoscopically. *Stomal problems* are seen less often, but the *antireflux mechanism* of the ureteroileal anastomosis may fail, accelerating renal deterioration.

CHAPTER 77

Transverse Colon Conduit

A transverse colon conduit, performed with a technique similar to that for a sigmoid conduit, may be preferred for obese adolescents, especially if the ureters were shortened previously. It is especially useful after pelvic irradiation.

Prepare the bowel, and sterilize the urine, if possible. Provide high-calorie and protein supplements. Mark the preferred stomal site with the patient in a sitting position. Instruments and postoperative problems are the same as those for ileal conduit (page 371) and sigmoid conduit (page 393).

1 **A,** *Incision:* Make a midline incision (page 83). **B,** Transilluminate the transverse mesocolon to choose a suitable 10- to 15-cm segment, and place stay sutures to mark it. Dissect the greater omentum from the superior surface of the transverse colon. Incise the mesocolon, making the cut longer on one side (left side shown) for increased mobility.

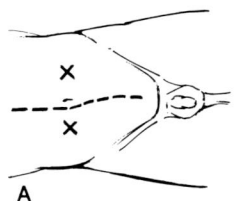

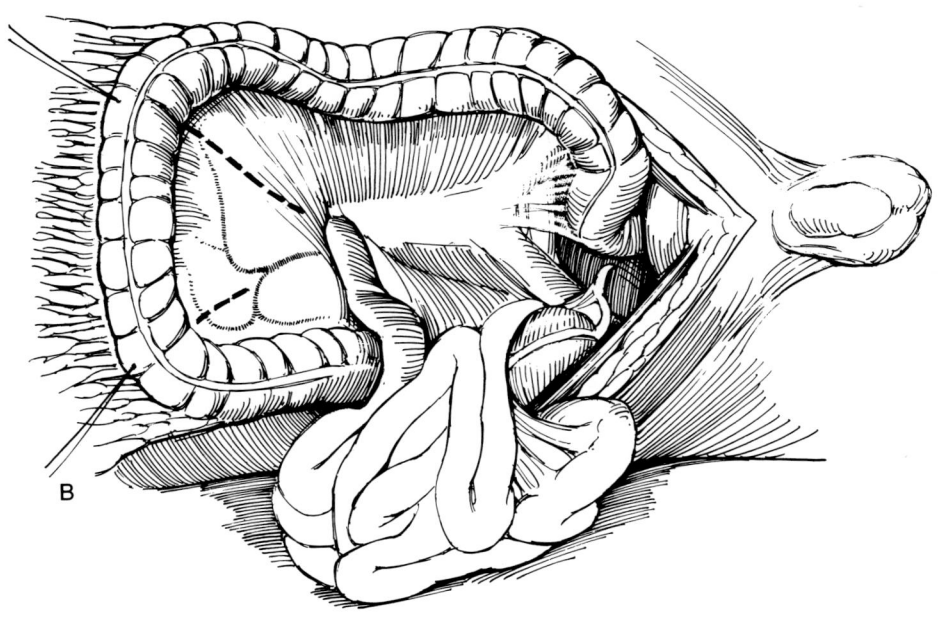

2 Divide the colon, and reanastomose it superior (or inferior) to the segment. Approximate the mesentery with a few 3-0 silk sutures. Choose the portion of the conduit that appears better suited as the stomal end, and close the opposite end of the conduit (page 6). Fix it securely to the adjacent parietal peritoneum near the midline. Incise the retroperitoneum, and mobilize the ureters. Lead them into the peritoneal cavity together through a suitably sited peritoneal incision. Trim the ureters obliquely to the proper length, and spatulate them.

3 Incise the conduit along a tenia, and anastomose the ureters directly with 4-0 chromic catgut sutures, using a submucosal tunnel technique (pages 427–429). Place stents if the ureters are small, if they are large and aperistaltic, or if the quality of the tissue is in doubt. Bring up the inferior peritoneal flap to cover the anastomoses.

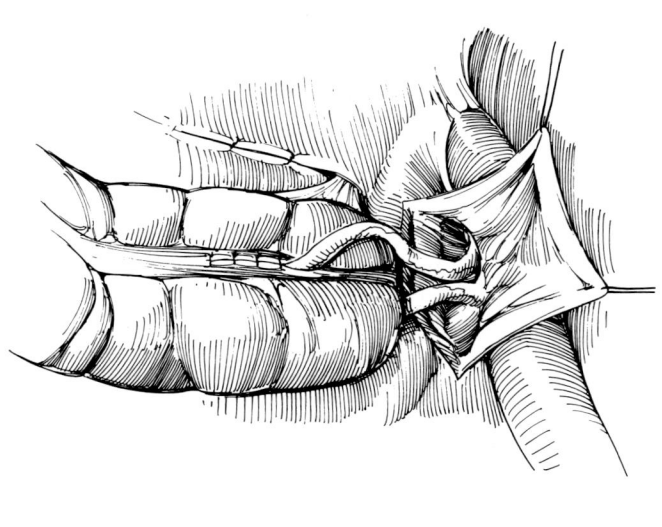

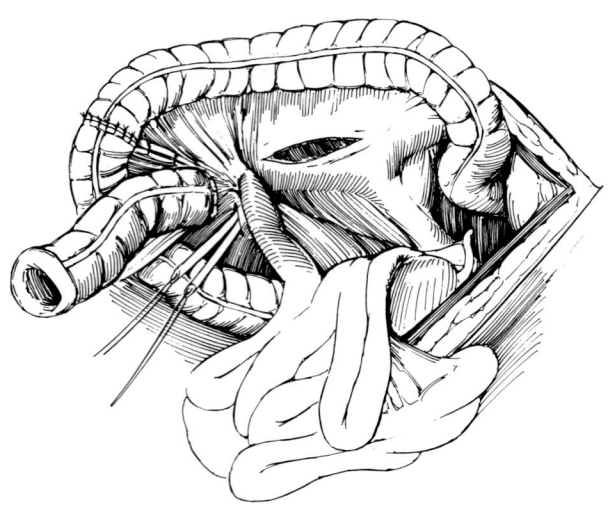

4 Situate the stoma in either upper or lower quadrant, whichever provides the easiest egress for the segment. Fashion a stoma (page 394). Close the wound and place a temporary appliance.

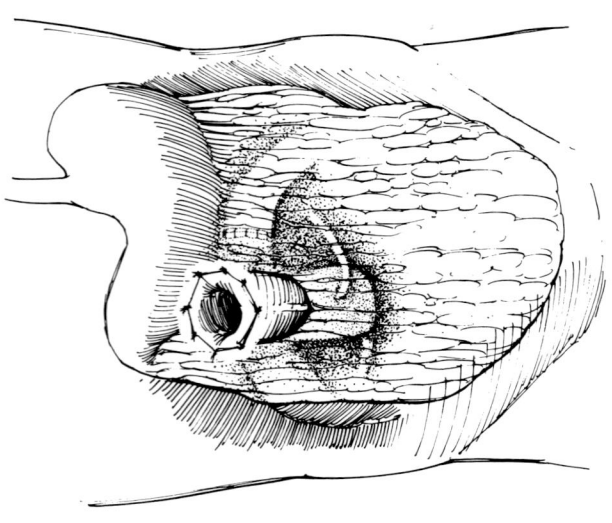

Commentary by Bernard M. Churchill

Colon conduits have a distinct advantage over ileal conduits, because nonrefluxing ureteroenteric anastomosis can be fashioned. We have noticed a significant difference in the risk of upper tract deterioration in patients undergoing colon conduits versus ileal conduits. Eighty-two percent of patients undergoing ileal conduit diversion had evidence of renal damage versus 22 percent in patients with colon conduits. This well-known risk of chronic pyelonephritis and parenchymal loss caused by freely refluxing ureteroileal anastomosis makes nonrefluxing colon conduits a better option over ileal conduits in patients who will require long-term cutaneous urinary diversion.

However, in this age of continent diversion, few patients will require long-term diversion. With the varied forms of continent diversion available, children may be able to undergo continent diversion and never need conduit diversion. Those who initially undergo a temporary incontinent diversion could undergo subsequent undiversion within a few years. Because the deleterious effects of ileal diversion take several years to materialize, and because undiversion usually can be performed a few years after diversion, there is no real advantage to colon conduits in most patients.

A midline incision should be made coursing around the umbilicus to the left side. This will preserve the vascularity of the umbilicus for later appendicovesicostomy. Similarly, we would not recommend performing a routine appendectomy. If undiversion is later performed, the appendix would be needed for a Mitrofanoff procedure. We now use staples for most of our bowel work. We find that even in small children, stapled anastomosis leads to good enteroenterostomies and reduces operative time. The blind end of the conduit should be closed with absorbable sutures, however, to prevent stone formation.

CHAPTER 78

Transverse Colostomy and Closure: Loop Ileostomy

If primary anastomosis is inadvisable, rather than make a colostomy, resect the colon for obstructing tumors or diverticulitis, and leave a mucous fistula and an end colostomy. If an anastomosis is done and it appears tenuous, a colostomy may be the safest course.

TRANSVERSE COLOSTOMY

1 Make a short oblique incision in the left (or right) upper quadrant through all layers of the body wall.

2 **A,** Expose enough of the transverse colon to be able to select a mobile portion. Pass a fine clamp through the mesentery close to the colon in the center of the selected portion. **B,** Draw a narrow Penrose drain through to loop the colon in a sling. Grasp the ends of the drain in a clamp and gently pull on them, while coaxing the colonic loop through the opening. Grasp the protruding colon with a moist sponge and pull it out until the mesenteric slit is seen. **C,** Run a plastic rod through the mesenteric defect. Fix the colon to the parietal peritoneum with two silk sutures that pass successively through the colonic serosa, the parietal peritoneum, and the posterior fascia. Suture the bowel at either end with silk sutures through the tenia and the skin edges. Tack the rod to the skin with braided silk sutures.

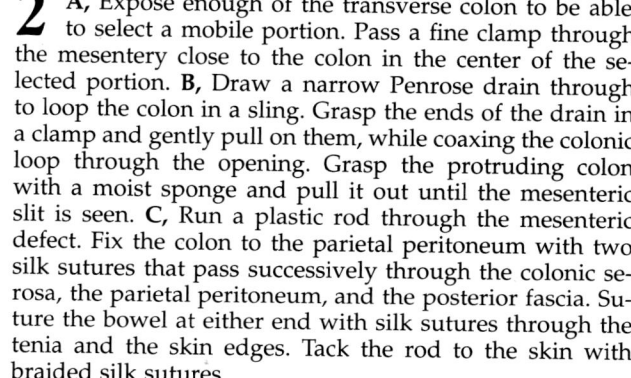

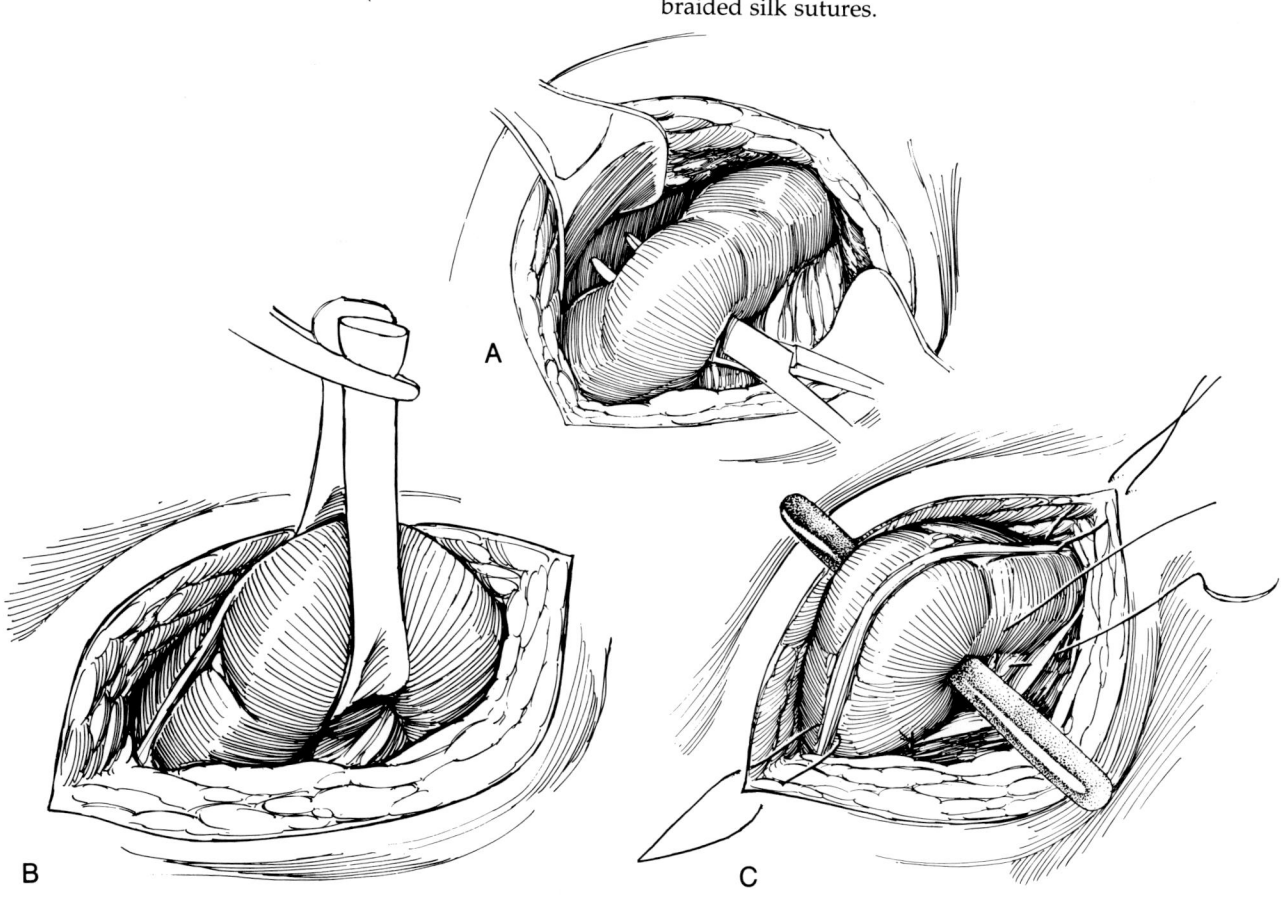

A

B

C

3 Open the colon longitudinally immediately after deep wound closure, and fasten the mucosal edges to the skin with interrupted 3-0 synthetic absorbable sutures. A more conservative approach is to wait 2 to 3 days, and then open the bowel longitudinally, first with a knife and then with electrocautery, because entering intact bowel with a cautery may spark an explosion of colonic gas. No further sutures are needed; the bowel is now adherent. In either case, leave the bridge in place for 5 to 6 days.

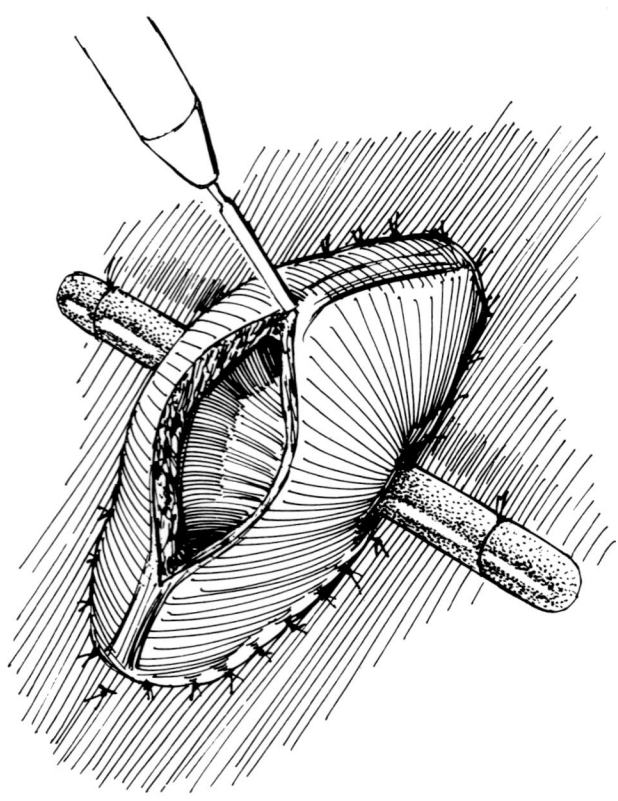

CLOSURE OF COLOSTOMY

Cleanse the defunctionalized distal portion by copious lavage, using saline first and then antibiotic solution.

Provide noncrushing intestinal Doyen clamps and Kocher clamps.

4 Place a running suture to close the lumen of the colon. Incise the junction of the skin and the bowel, and free the colostomy edges. Enlarge the skin opening at either end for 1 or 2 cm. Separate the two limbs of the colostomy from the subcutaneous layers by sharp dissection, while maintaining traction on the loop with a Penrose drain passed through the mesentery. Locate the fascia and free the colon from it with a spreading motion of the scissors; incision of the fascia seldom is necessary. Identify the mesocolon and lyse its adhesions to the parietal peritoneum.

Apply a noncrushing intestinal clamp and a Kocher clamp to each limb. Divide the colon below each Kocher clamp (dashed line). Proceed with end-to-end anastomosis. As an alternative, merely freshen the edges of the colostomy opening, and close it with a two-layer technique, without excising a segment. Remove the Doyen clamps. Close the mesocolic defect, and drop the colon into the abdomen.

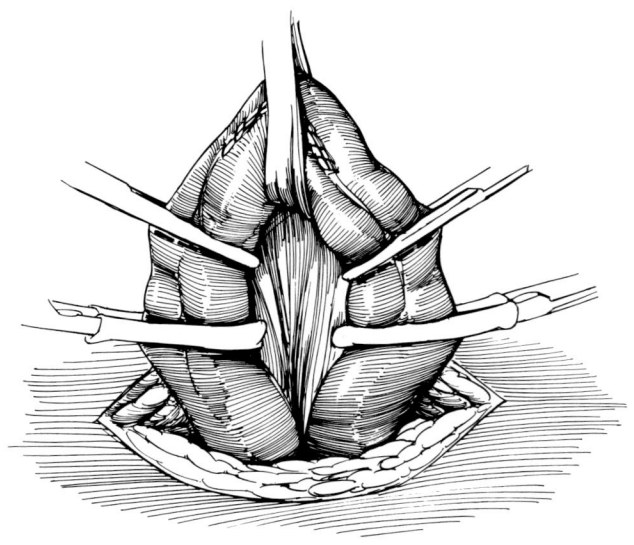

5 Start closure of the abdominal wound by placing a #0 polypropylene suture at each end of the wound to include the peritoneum and deep fascia and tying it. Run each suture to the center and tie them; make the knot with seven square throws.

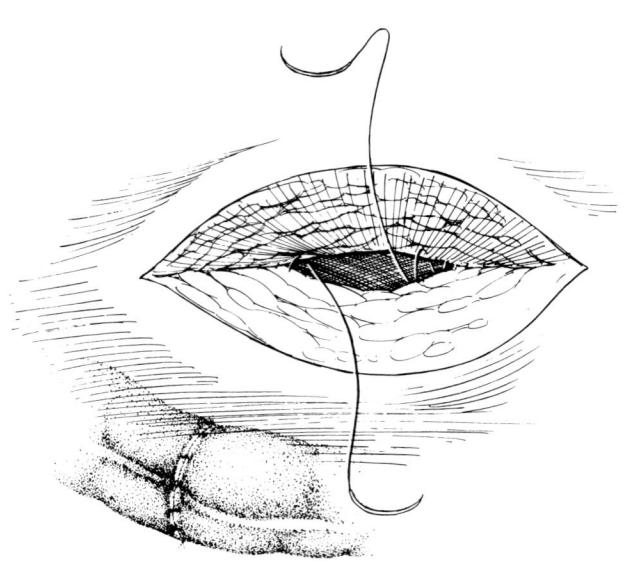

6 Place interrupted #0 synthetic absorbable sutures to close the anterior fascial layer. Insert three or four vertical mattress sutures of 3-0 polypropylene through the skin and subcutaneous tissue; cut them to a length of 15 cm, and tie the ends together, leaving them loose. Dress with petroleum jelly (Vaseline) gauze and a dry dressing.

Alternatively, omit the skin sutures and use only sterile skin strips.

On the 5th postoperative day, cut the knots from the ends of the skin sutures and tie them. The delayed closure reduces the chance of a wound infection; if there is any inflammation, do not close the wound, but allow it to heal by second intention.

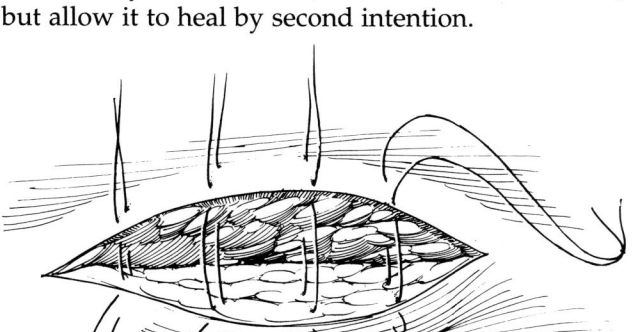

LOOP ILEOSTOMY

This often is a good substitute for transverse colostomy. The bowel is smaller, the procedure simpler to perform and take down, and the stoma easier to cover with a bag.

With the patient sitting, mark a stomal site at the summit of the infraumbilical fat mound, overlying the middle of the rectus muscle.

7 **A,** Approach the ileum through a midline incision, usually already created. Make an opening for the stoma, as described on pages 378–381. Pass a small Penrose drain through the mesentery of the ileum approximately 15 cm from the ileocecal junction, and draw the loop through the opening. A plastic rod may be substituted for the Penrose drain but is not essential.

B, Incise the ileum for four fifths of its circumference on the distal end, 1 cm above the skin. Place 4-0 chromic catgut sutures through the full thickness of the ileum, and then through the subcutaneous tissue, and tie them. Remove the Penrose drain or rod in 5 days.

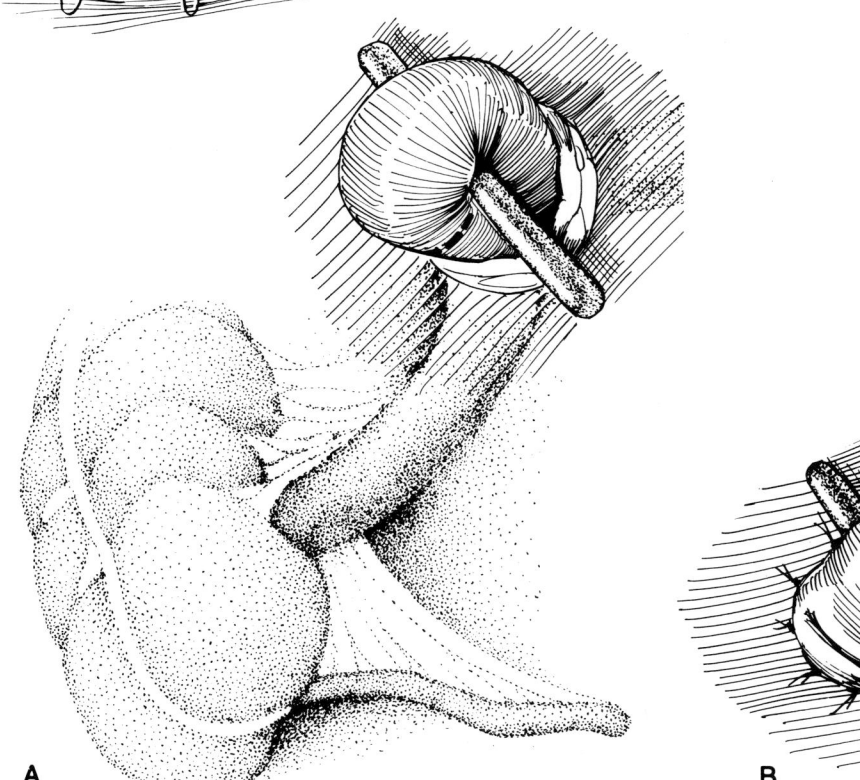

A

B

Commentary by George T. Klauber

Transverse colostomy, although less commonly performed than a decade or two ago, always should be considered if an unprepared rectum or distal colon is entered during pelvic surgery. Certainly, construction of a colostomy remains the safest and most conservative course of action under such a circumstance. I would, of course, advise any urologist to utilize preoperative bowel preps prior to undertaking major pelvic surgery, such as an anterior exenteration of a bladder for prostatic rhabdomyosarcoma. Primary closure of a prepared rectum, with a rectal tube placed proximal to the injury site and triple antibiotic therapy, can be an alternative to a diversionary colostomy in some cases.

I would like to emphasize the need to begin opening the bowel with a knife before using the electrocautery because of the risk of explosion. Use of absorbable suture, such as Vicryl, obviates the need for suture removal later and, in my experience, causes less skin reaction. In neonates with imperforate anus or cloacal malformations, complete division of the colon into an end colostomy and a distal mucous fistula is preferable to loop colostomy because of the propensity for stool to enter the distal limb of a loop colostomy. Many children with imperforate anus have coexistent hydronephrosis or a multicystic dysplastic kidney, so that a preoperative abdominal/renal sonogram is mandatory. Coexistent pathology can and should influence stomal placement.

CHAPTER 79

Gastrostomy

Select a dependent area of the stomach that is nearly free of vessels, not near the pylorus, and as high on the anterior wall as is convenient. Place one pursestring suture of 2-0 chromic catgut 1 cm distant from the proposed site and a second pursestring suture concentrically 2 cm from the site. Make a stab wound incision with a #15 blade. A short incision with a small opening is best. The opening in the mucosa always enlarges to admit the catheter. Insert a suitable size Malecot catheter stretched on a curved clamp. Tie the inner suture as you pull the wings of the catheter up against the stomach wall. Have your assistant gently depress the catheter, but not so hard that the catheter slides further in, while you tie the outer suture.

Lift the omentum up, and fold it back to cover. Pass a clamp through it to grasp the tube and bring it through the opening. Let the stomach fall back to its normal position, and anchor the tube at the skin level so there is no undue tension between stomach and abdominal wall. The path of the tube intra-abdominally will be sealed off quickly by adjacent tissues. It is not necessary to bury the catheter in the wall of the stomach beyond the pursestring or to try to anchor the site of the pursestring to the undersur-

face of the abdominal wall. This only distorts the normal anatomic relationships. Cut the end of the catheter obliquely so it can be drawn through the body wall, or grasp the very end of the catheter transversely in a clamp and pull it through a stab wound on the anterior abdominal wall. Suture it in place with a 2-0 braided silk suture.

Commentary by George T. Klauber

I prefer constructing a gastrostomy rather than maintaining prolonged nasogastric intubation for some children, especially those who are uncooperative, those who cannot tolerate a nasogastric tube, and those undergoing major abdominal surgery, such as radical cystectomy or creation of a catheterizable urinary reservoir or bladder augmentation. Children with gastrostomy tubes can ambulate sooner and have less discomfort than those with nasogastric tubes.

It is not absolutely necessary to interpose omentum, which can be quite rudimentary in young children, between the stomach and the abdominal wall; the stomach can be sutured directly to the abdominal wall, thus reducing the risk of intraperitoneal leakage when the gastrostomy tube is pulled. I personally like to use a Foley or a Pezzer catheter, rather than a Malecot, because it is less likely to be inadvertently dislodged.

CHAPTER 80

Appendectomy

In the past, appendectomy was a common procedure with bowel diversionary procedures because of the fear of later appendicitis, but now that the appendix has uses in diversion procedures, appendectomy is rare, except when the appendix is inflamed.

Commentary by Barry A. Kogan

Appendectomy is almost outmoded. Because of the versatility of the appendix in reconstructive surgery, considerable thought should be given before performing an incidental appendectomy.

Unless the appendix is acutely inflamed, a Babcock clamp is safer for retraction than a single clamp on the most distal vessel. The Babcock also provides good exposure of the vessels.

To save time, the appendiceal side of the vessels usually is left clamped and not tied. Also for security, the surgeon may wish to tie the vessels with silk suture (probably 4-0 in a child). Even a good bowel prep may not clear the appendix. Hence, it probably is safer to treat the appendiceal stump with povidone-iodine (Betadine) or alcohol before burying it. Although it is wasteful to staple the stump under normal circumstances, if the base is acutely inflamed or friable, another approach is to staple across the base of the cecum and then bury the staple line.

PART IV

CONTINENT URINARY DIVERSION

Incorporation of intestine into the urinary tract can achieve a larger bladder capacity; it is done when both the urethra and the ureterovesical junctions are present (augmentation), it can replace the entire bladder down to the urethra (substitution), it can provide a urinary conduit if both urethra and ureterovesical junctions are gone (noncontinent diversion), or it can provide a continent reservoir (continent diversion).

Urinary reservoirs for vesical augmentation and substitution, as well as for continent urinary diversion, require adequate capacity at physiologic pressure.

In selection of a segment, other factors to be considered, in addition to capacity and pressure, are (1) tolerable electrolyte reabsorption and loss, (2) accessibility of the segment, (3) simplicity of the procedure, (4) need for an antireflux mechanism, (5) carcinogenic risk, and (6) special requirements and age of the patient.

Selection of a particular bowel segment for bladder augmentation depends on the preference of the surgeon, because we have no objective data indicating that one region is better than another. The colon allows implantation of a normal ureter using an antireflux technique. Combining ileum with cecum based on the ileocecal artery allows formation of a mobilizable reservoir of good capacity free from mass contraction and an ileal arm to substitute for any loss of ureteral length. However, exclusion of the ileocecal segment from the intestinal tract in children with neurogenic bladders who rely on constipation for rectal continence may result in loose stools and fecal incontinence, as well as later vitamin deficiency. After extensive pelvic radiation, a transverse colon conduit may have to be resorted to. A segment from the stomach can be useful, especially in a child with compromised renal function in whom electrolyte reabsorption would exacerbate the problem. The stomach is elastic; half of it can provide a reservoir with a 300- to 500-ml capacity.

The objectives in any case are to make a low-pressure, compliant system during the filling phase (best achieved when the tubular organization of the bowel is disrupted to protect the upper tracts from backpressure during spontaneous mass contractions, which in turn may induce incontinence) and to provide adequate capacity to relieve the patient of inconvenient frequent voiding or catheterization. In addition, protection from reflux must be provided, and incontinence, prevented.

CHAPTER 81

Introduction to Continent Urinary Diversion

NEITHER URETHRA NOR URETEROVESICAL JUNCTION PRESENT

Continent diversion requires a reservoir, an antireflux mechanism, and a stoma that will not leak but can be catheterized. Continence can be achieved by forming a conduit by ileal intussusception, plicated terminal ileum, or tunneled ureter or appendix. Different parts of the bowel, including the stomach, can be used as the reservoir, and selection of the antireflux mechanism depends on the site of implantation.

Detubularized bowel segments provide a greater capacity at lower pressure and require a shorter length of intestine than do intact segments. The function of bowel as a reservoir is determined by its geometric configuration, accommodation, compliance, and contractility (Hinman, 1988). Geometric capacity depends on the fact that the volume of a reservoir rises with the square of the radius. Thus, folding the bowel once doubles its capacity, and folding it twice increases it four times. Accommodation follows the Laplace relation: as the viscus fills, the stress on the wall increases, which permits the pressure to remain constant. Because the bowel is viscoelastic, it demonstrates compliance as it fills. Contractility is reduced by folding, because the several components no longer contract synchronously.

The purpose of continent diversion is to improve the quality of life of patients who have lost a usable bladder. It may well not improve renal function or prolong survival. Ultimately, the patient must make the choice between ileal diversion and more-complicated continent procedures, with older patients favoring the former and younger ones, the latter.

Continent urinary diversion is contraindicated in (1) children who have insufficient bowel secondary to intestinal or mesenteric adhesions, previous resection, or disease of bowel; (2) those who would experience adverse effects of loss of bowel length, especially children with neurogenic bladders, in whom resection of the ileocecal region can result in loose stools with fecal incontinence; (3) those who have had prior radiation to the intestine; and (3) those who are inadequately motivated and skilled to take care of the new system, which may require intermittent self-catheterization.

Spontaneous rupture of continent reservoirs in children is not a rare event, especially if the conduit is leakproof. It probably occurs during overdistention in the presence of peritoneal adhesions that induce a seromuscular tear. The parents and child must be told of the virtue of frequent emptying and the dangers of overfilling. It is advisable that the child not only wear a medical alert bracelet that states the situation but also have access to an 18-gauge needle to allow direct vesical puncture in an emergency. Malignancy may occur in bowel interposed in the urinary tract.

Undiversion to a continent reservoir is appealing, but it is not suitable for very young children (even though their parents may desire it) and for those without adequate motivation. Poor renal function is not an absolute contraindication, because undiversion not only may provide a better life but may delay the time for renal transplantation.

Preoperatively, the function of the bladder must be assessed with a voiding cystourethrogram followed by cystoscopy under anesthesia. A small catheter can be placed percutaneously, so that the child can fill his or her bladder and report on volume, sensation, and continence.

A definitive procedure should be done at the first attempt, preferably through a very long midline incision, including transureterostomy with stenting. Use an omental wrap to prevent adhesions, place a cuff if an incontinence device is going to be needed later, and remove all abnormal tissue except the bladder, which later may be used for a bladder neck,

for the formation of a new urethra, or for future mucosal grafts. It is advisable to take the original diversion completely apart and then put it together using all your talents. The greatest error is not doing enough. For conversion from an existing conduit, take down the peritoneal adhesions, and dissect the conduit from the abdominal wall. Excise the previous small bowel anastomosis, including the site of the mesenteric division. Be familiar with more than one technique, so that you can adapt to the circumstances found at surgery.

Several choices are available for continent reservoirs. One constructed entirely of ileum, such as the Kock pouch, has the advantage of avoiding use of the ileocecal region but is technically more difficult. Some form of cecoileal reservoir, despite its functional disadvantages, is the technique most often selected, especially after cystectomy, whether for malignancy or congenital vesical abnormality. The Mainz pouch uses ileum to gain capacity at low pressure, whereas the more easily constructed Indiana pouch must incorporate most of the ascending colon; however, an ileal patch can reduce the amount of colon needed. The appendix interposed for a catheterizable stoma, as is done in the Penn pouch, is an alternative to using intussuscepted or plicated ileum. Ureterosigmoidostomy, which may be an alternative in adults with short life expectancies, seldom is suitable for children.

The stoma of a continent pouch, because it will not require coverage with an appliance, may be placed in a lower position, below the belt (bikini) line, but not so low that it cannot easily be catheterized by the patient while sitting. Do not be concerned about skin folds. The umbilicus may be preferable, because that area of the abdomen is thinner, there is less chance for parastomal hernia, and the stoma is easier to catheterize, especially if the child is in a wheelchair. It may be advisable to mark the standard site as well before undertaking the operation and also warn the patient, in case a ureteroileostomy is all that can be done.

COMPLICATIONS

Select children willing and able to assume responsibility for care of the diversion and complications will be fewer. *Bacteriuria* is the rule after pouch diversion involving intermittent catheterization, but clinically important infections are the result of increase in the bacterial population from infrequent or incomplete emptying or from refilling from reflux. Training is necessary to teach the child how to empty to the last drop, by aspiration if necessary. *Mucus collection* requires vigorous irrigation in the immediate postoperative period but becomes less of a problem with time. Daily irrigation is then usually sufficient. *Calculi*, usually struvite stones, result from stasis, but some may form on staples. It is possible to manipulate or fragment the stones though the stoma, albeit with some risk to the mechanism; direct puncture into the reservoir is an alternative. *Electrolyte imbalance* with hyperchloremic acidosis is especially prevalent in those children with initially poor renal function and requires bicarbonate supplements, at least for the first 6 to 12 months. Unfortunately, *spontaneous perforation* of the neobladder is not rare and also is often overlooked until the child is gravely ill. Voluntary overfilling may lead to repeated ischemia at a weak point in the bladder. *Malignancy* may occur.

Intussusception following abdominal or retroperitoneal surgery on the intestinal tract in children is a rare complication and presents as prolonged ileus followed by symptoms of small bowel obstruction. The pain is not colicky, and a mass is not felt, perhaps because the site of intussusception postoperatively is high (ileoileal or jejunojejunal). Immediate reoperation is required.

Vitamin B_{12} deficiency may appear after the terminal ileum is harvested. The disorder needs to be detected by obtaining Vitamin B_{12} levels at regular intervals, so that life-long parenteral supplement may be given if needed.

Enuresis is a common, very distressing complication, probably resulting from an obtunded sensation of fullness of the bladder, combined with perineal relaxation.

CHAPTER 82

Ileal Reservoir
(KOCK)

Evaluate the upper urinary tract by ultrasonography and intravenous urography. Determine renal function, because children with deteriorated tracts are not candidates for this type of diversion. Treat existing urinary tract infection, and start prophylactic antibiotics. Prepare the bowel carefully. The measurements in the text are those for adolescents.

Instruments. Provide a PI-55 stapler with 4.8-mm staples, removing the six staples nearest the straight arm before; a 30 F Medina tube; polyglycolic acid (PGA) mesh cut in 2-cm strips; Marlex mesh; two 8 F infant feeding tubes; 3-0 synthetic absorbable sutures; and #1 nylon, #1 PGA, and 2-0 chromic catgut sutures.

1 **A,** *Position:* Supine, slightly hyperextended. *Incision:* Make a midline incision, leaving the umbilicus on the side opposite the site for the proposed stoma. **B,** Divide the mesentery in the avascular plane of Treves between the terminal branch of the superior mesenteric artery and the ileocolic artery, carrying the division up to the base of the mesentery to provide adequate mobility for the efferent limb of the reservoir. Divide the bowel. With a sterile flexible centimeter tape, measure four segments along the bowel, and mark each with a silk suture: 17 cm for the efferent conduit, two 22-cm segments for construction of the pouch, and a 17-cm segment for the afferent limb (13 cm for patients with existing ileal conduits). Err on the side of taking too much ileum, because a large volume is essential. In an obese patient, make the efferent segment longer than 17 cm. Tie these stay sutures loosely and trim the ends.

Divide the mesentery for a short distance, and divide the bowel between clamps 5 cm apart. Resect and discard the 5 cm of ileum proximal to the segment, along with a wedge of mesentery to provide separation of the pouch from the small-bowel anastomosis. Close the proximal end of the segment (page 384). If there is an existing ileal conduit, leave the end of the ileum open for anastomosis to the proximal end of the conduit. Anastomose the ileum to restore continuity (pages 375–377).

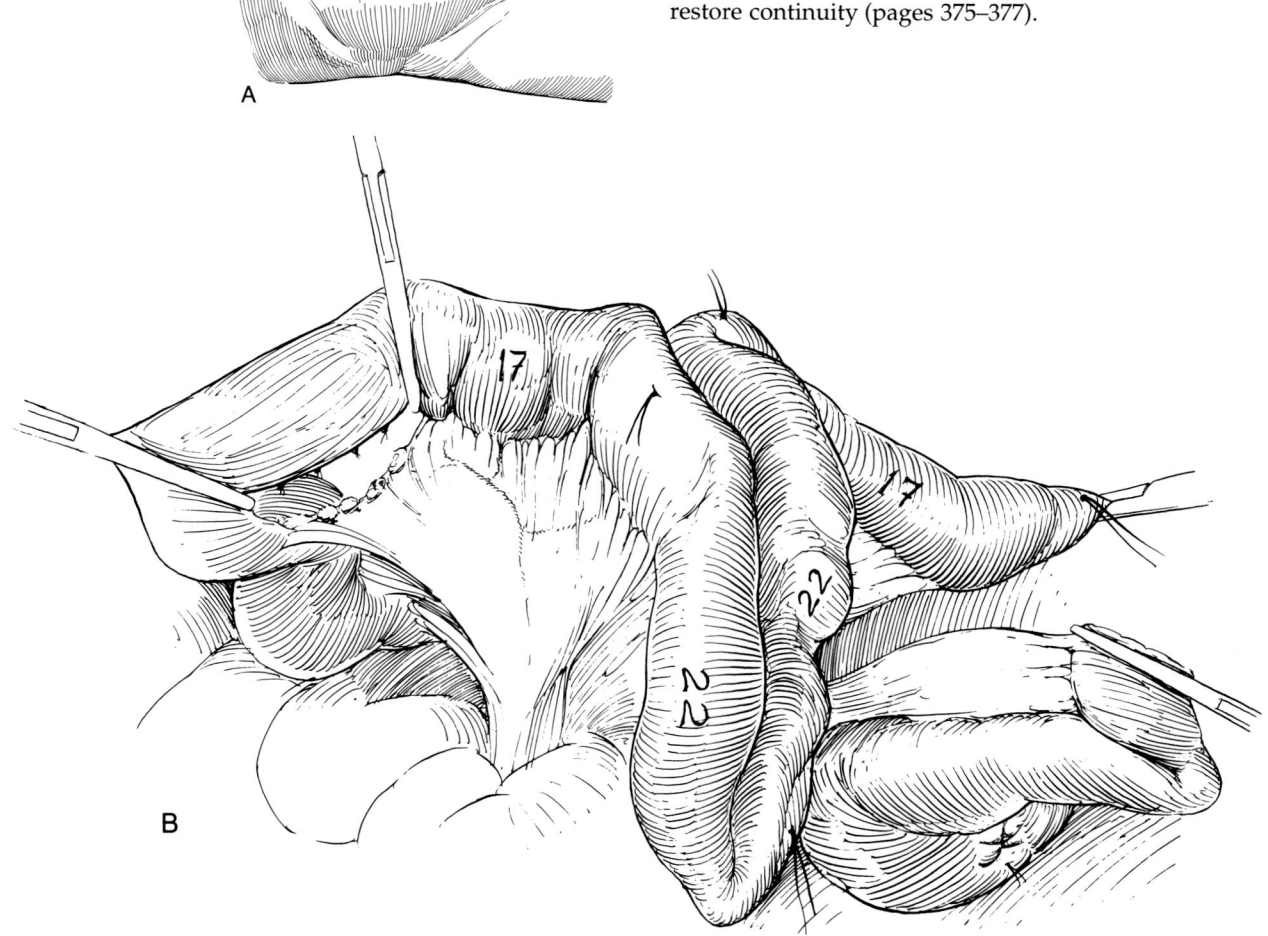

2 Lay the isolated segment on a moist lap tape in the shape of a U pointed caudally. The bend of the U should coincide with the marking suture that was placed between the two 22-cm segments. A second surgical team may now enter the field. Sew the two sides together with a running locking 3-0 synthetic absorbable suture so that the serosa 2 to 3 cm lateral to the mesentery is apposed. With the coagulating current, incise the bowel just lateral to this serosal suture. Extend the incision into the efferent loop for 3 cm and for approximately 2 cm into the afferent loop. (This allows the nipples to be staggered and prevents the staples from involving the posterior suture line.)

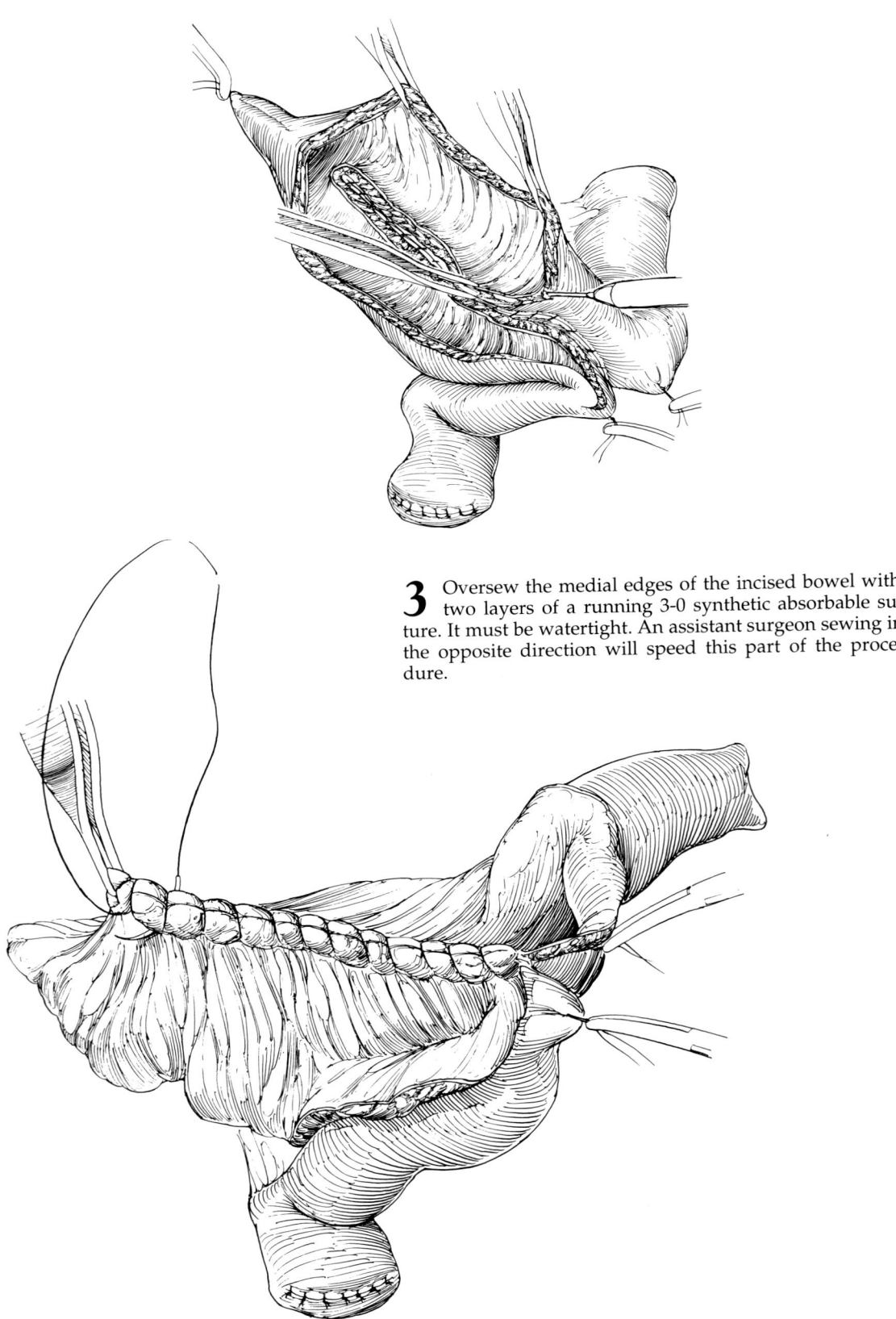

3 Oversew the medial edges of the incised bowel with two layers of a running 3-0 synthetic absorbable suture. It must be watertight. An assistant surgeon sewing in the opposite direction will speed this part of the procedure.

4 Clear the mesentery cleanly from the proximal end of both limbs for a distance of 7 to 8 cm using Adson forceps and electrocautery; leave a little fat on the mesentery. Pass a Mayo clamp through the mesentery at a point one arcade beyond this opening in the mesentery, and draw a 2.5-cm strip of PGA mesh through it. Do the same on the other limb.

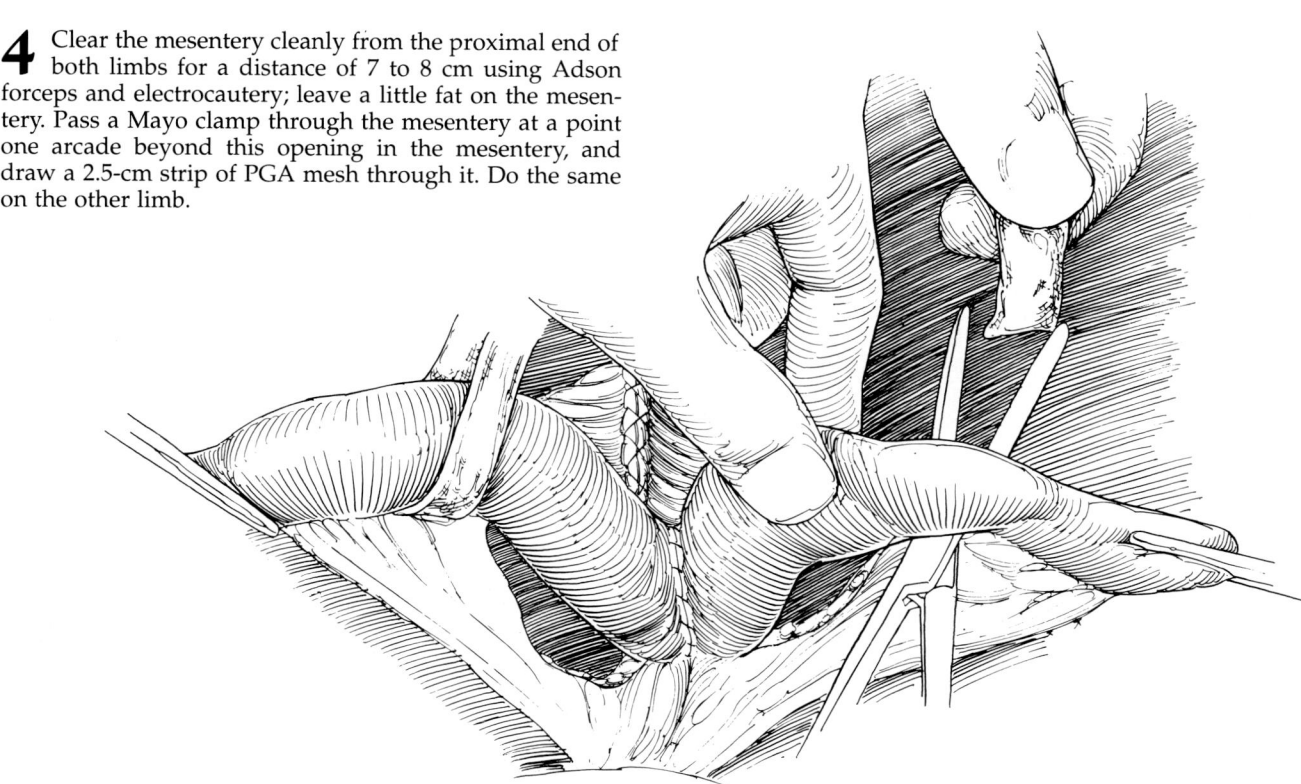

5 **A** and **B,** Insert two Allis clamps up the lumen two thirds of the way to the mesh, and grasp the mucosa to intussuscept the ileum into the open pouch to form a nipple.

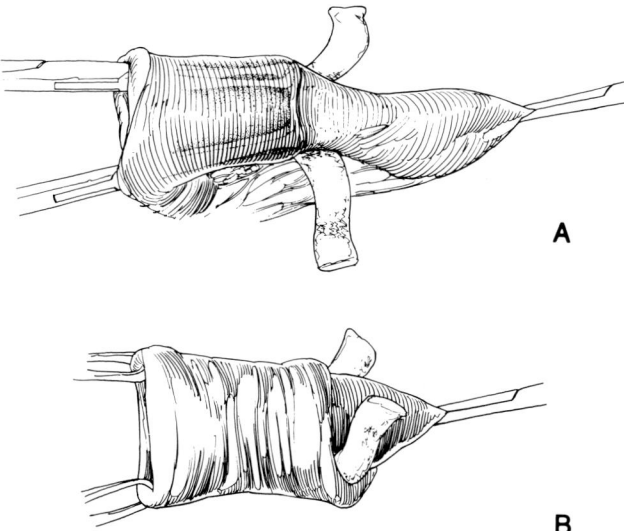

A

B

6 Use the PI-55 stapler with 4.8-mm staples (the six staples lying adjacent to the straight arm having been removed by the scrub nurse before the operation) or with a Mueller custom staple cartridge in which the six staples have been removed at the factory. Use the pin in the stapler to provide alignment. After stapling, be sure to close the pinhole with 3-0 synthetic absorbable sutures. Place two parallel rows of staples around the anterior 180 degrees while suspending the nipple with an Allis clamp. Insert the stapler to its full 5.5-cm length, thus ensuring a nipple at least 5 cm long. At the same time, be sure the last staple is not so close to the edge of the pouch that the pouch cannot be closed.

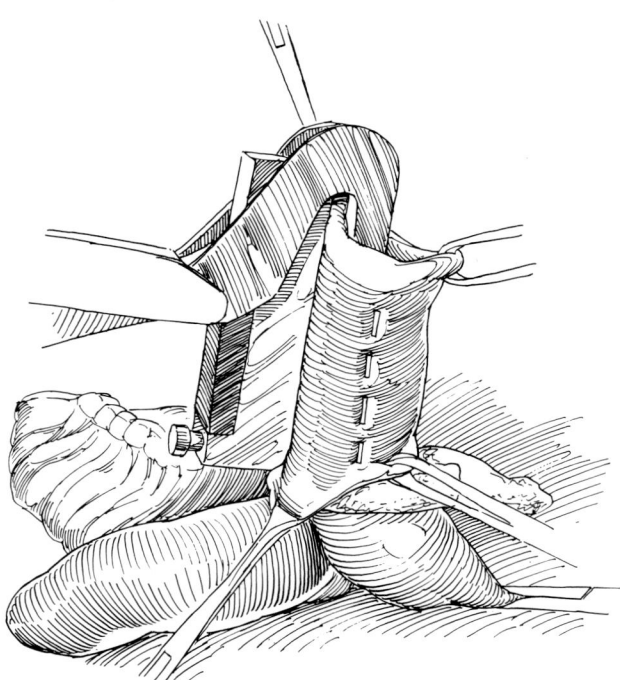

7 A third row of staples should be placed posteriorly to fix the nipple to the back wall of the pouch. This can be done by inserting the anvil up the inside of the nipple near the mesentery from outside the pouch, thus fixing one wall of the nipple to the back wall of the pouch.

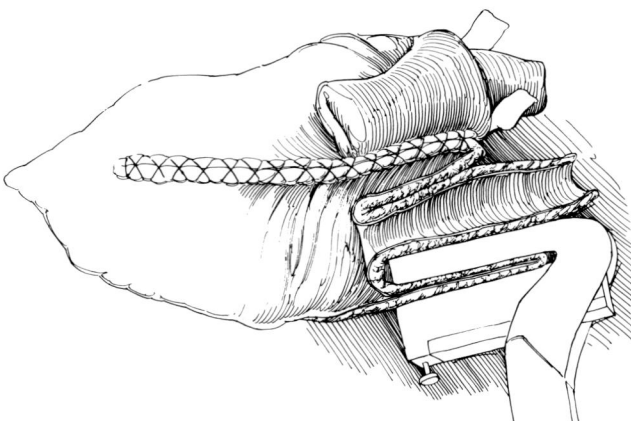

8 Another method is to make a hole in the back wall at the site to which the nipple should extend, insert the anvil from outside the bowel, extend it up the nipple, and then staple its full thickness to the back wall of the pouch.

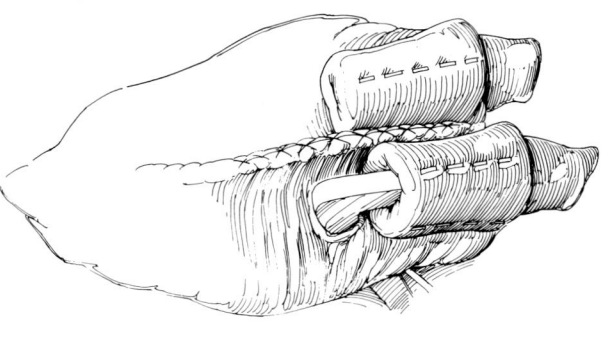

9 Insert a 30 F Medina tube through the nipple. Sew the PGA mesh strip that has been soaked in tetracycline solution (250 mg in 10 ml normal saline) circumferentially to the serosa of the pouch and the respective limb of ileum with interrupted figure-eight 2-0 chromic catgut sutures. The tube will prevent the collar from being too tight. Trim the redundant PGA mesh. Suture the tip of the nipple to the bowel wall for extra stability.

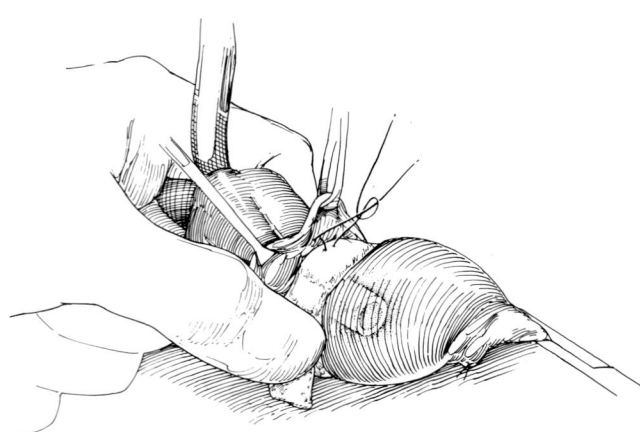

10 Complete the fixation with a distal row of similar sutures. Do the same for the other limb.

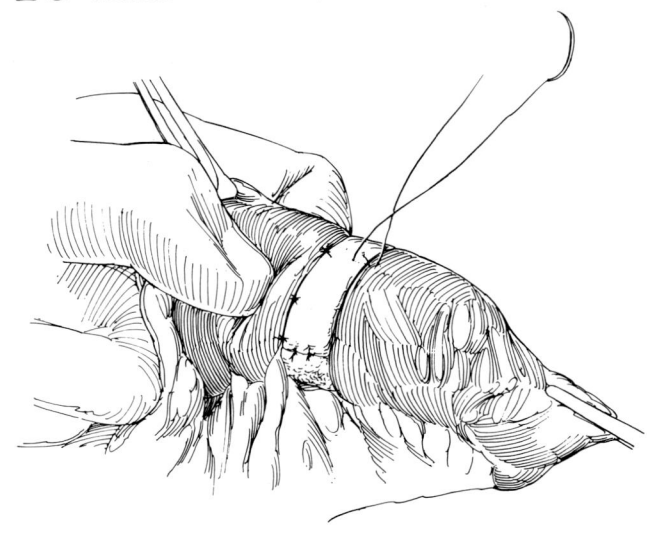

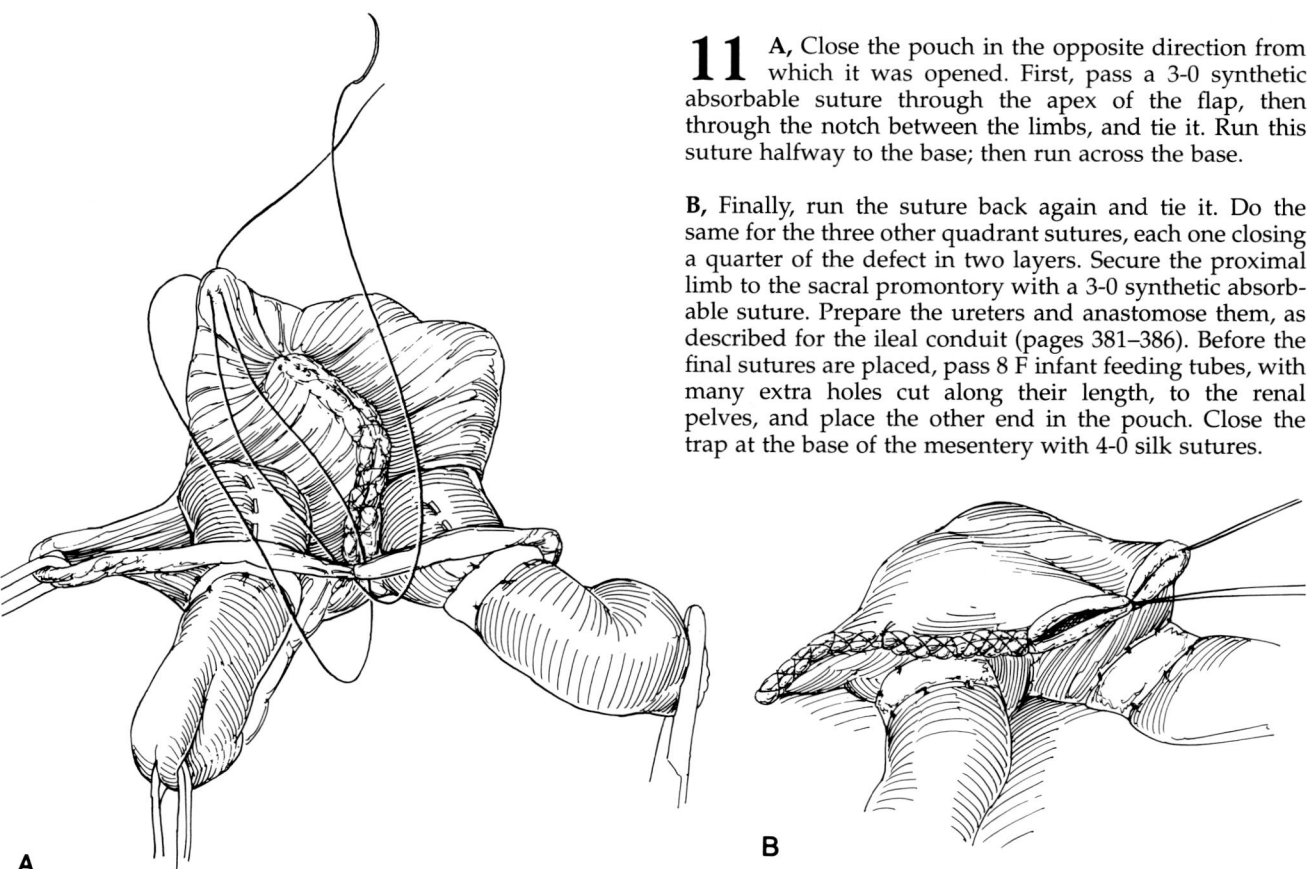

11 **A,** Close the pouch in the opposite direction from which it was opened. First, pass a 3-0 synthetic absorbable suture through the apex of the flap, then through the notch between the limbs, and tie it. Run this suture halfway to the base; then run across the base.

B, Finally, run the suture back again and tie it. Do the same for the three other quadrant sutures, each one closing a quarter of the defect in two layers. Secure the proximal limb to the sacral promontory with a 3-0 synthetic absorbable suture. Prepare the ureters and anastomose them, as described for the ileal conduit (pages 381–386). Before the final sutures are placed, pass 8 F infant feeding tubes, with many extra holes cut along their length, to the renal pelves, and place the other end in the pouch. Close the trap at the base of the mesentery with 4-0 silk sutures.

A

B

12 **A and B,** Remove a plug of skin smaller than for ureteroileostomy at the stomal site. Make a vertical incision in the fat and anterior rectus fascia, split the muscle, and incise the peritoneum sufficiently to admit two fingers. Pass a #1 synthetic absorbable suture through the rectus fascia medial to the pouch, then through the width of the PGA mesh strip and back through the strip at a distance of one quarter of the circumference; finally, pass

the suture through the rectus fascia of the corresponding quadrant. Repeat the procedure on the lateral side of the stoma.

Secure a 2-cm strip of Marlex mesh to the posterior abdominal fascia, lateral and slightly cephalad to the opening in the fascia. Bring this strip through the window of Deaver in the pouch mesentery adjacent to the PGA mesh. Pull up on the two #1 synthetic absorbable sutures to embed the PGA mesh in the rectus muscle. Test for a straight run into the pouch with the index finger. Fix the Marlex strip to the abdominal wall medial to the pouch with a #1 nylon suture. This permanent mesh acts like a strut to prevent a parastomal hernia and fixes the base of the efferent nipple to the abdominal wall, which also greatly facilitates catheterization.

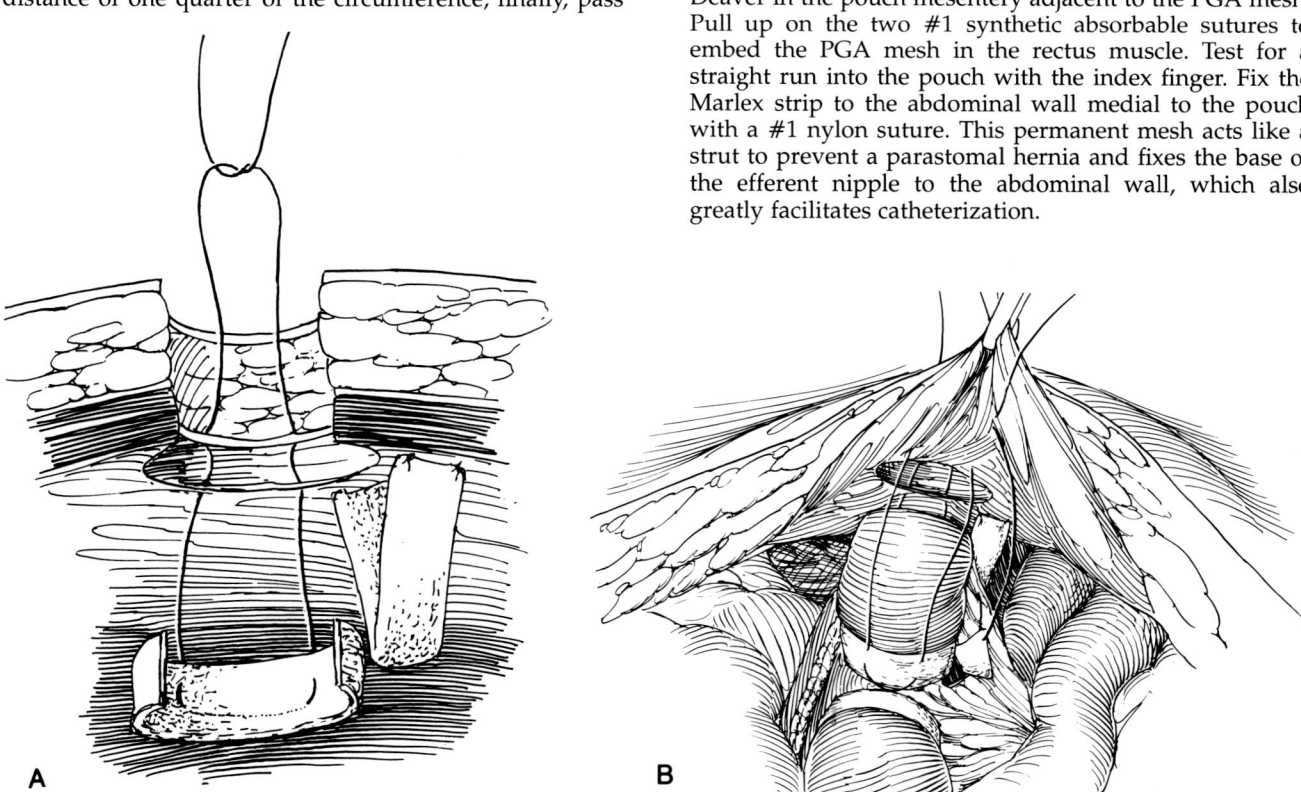

A

B

13 Trim any redundant ileum, and make a flush stoma by suturing the mucosa to the subcuticular layer with interrupted 3-0 synthetic absorbable sutures.

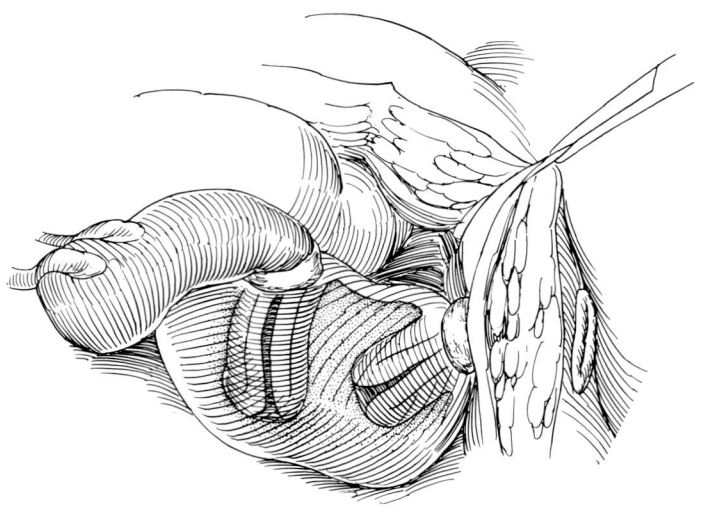

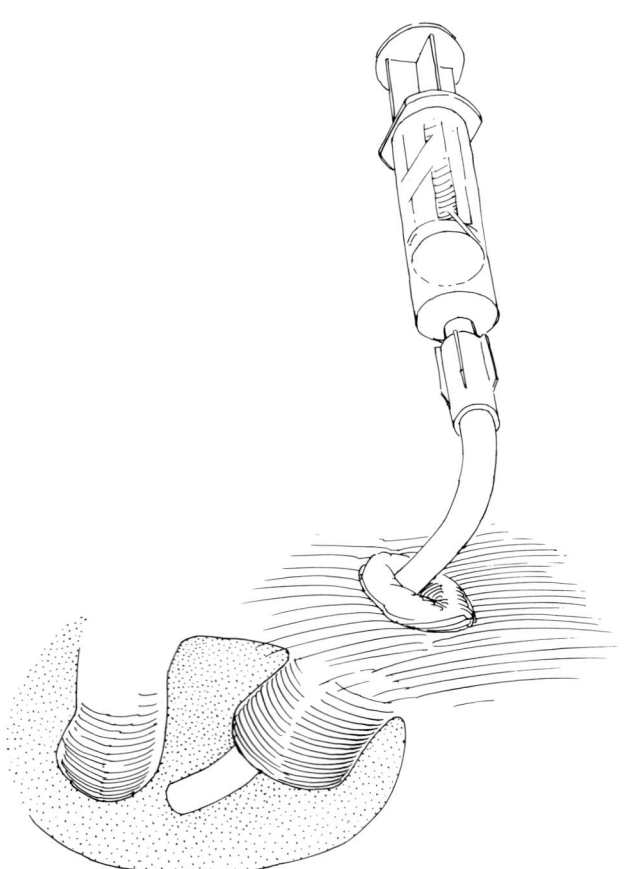

14 Insert a 30 F Medina tube into the stoma, keeping the drainage holes away from the efferent nipple and the end of the tube away from the suture line. Test it for free irrigation and free exchange of water during respiration. Suture it to the skin with two #1 nylon sutures. Insert a 1-in Penrose drain through a stab wound, and fasten it to the psoas muscle a few centimeters from the pouch with a 3-0 chromic catgut suture. Close the wound in layers.

Postoperatively, have an experienced nurse irrigate the Medina tube every 4 hours with 60 ml of normal saline to prevent obstruction from mucus. The patient can soon learn self-irrigation. After 2 days, remove the sutures holding the Medina tube and place an ileostomy flange to hold the tube in place, so that it can be rotated by the nurses to prevent it from pressing against just one portion of the reservoir wall and producing ischemia and necrosis. Have the patient readmitted to the hospital at 3 weeks, and administer aminoglycosides parenterally. Remove the Medina tube. Inspect the pouch with a cystoscope, and remove the stents. Fill the pouch with contrast medium for a cystogram. Obtain an intravenous urogram. Teach the patient self-catheterization beginning at 2- to 3-hour intervals and provide instruction to always keep the catheter at hand. Continue oral antibiotics for another month or two, and consider suppressive medication thereafter. Treat urea-splitting colonization aggressively. The catheterization interval can be extended 1 hour per week until intervals of 6 hours during the day and 8 hours at night are reached. For *substitution*, the Kock pouch can be anastomosed to the urethra after it is rotated 90 degrees, so that it will reach the urethra at the end of the suture line. Make sure it is firmly attached to the periosteum of the pubis.

POSTOPERATIVE PROBLEMS

Efferent valve malfunction causes the most trouble from this operation, occurring in one fourth of the patients. It results in incontinence and difficulty with catheterization. The *incontinence* results from a fistula secondary to ischemic erosion between the valve and the pouch. The goal of treatment is to create a new efferent limb and valve after rotating the pouch, because direct closure of the fistula usually is not feasible.

Incontinence even more commonly arises because the intussusception fails to be maintained. Correction involves intussuscepting the nipple again and fixing it with more rows of staples, a new sling, and refixation to the abdominal wall. The valve also may prolapse, but this may be corrected through the stoma.

Difficulty with catheterization occurs when the pouch becomes loosened from the abdominal wall and migrates to one side. The entering tip of the catheter impinges on the fascial edge and cannot be advanced. In an emergency, if a soft coudé catheter cannot be manipulated through the angulation, the pouch must be aspirated with a needle or the body wall relaxed by general anesthesia. Later, the pouch must be reattached to the abdominal wall.

Afferent valve malfunction is less frequent, so reflux into the upper tracts is not a common complication. However, *ureteroileal stenosis* does occur, producing upper tract obstruction. Stenosis of the nipple has not been seen.

Urinary tract infection is not common, although bacteriuria is the rule. *Calculi* have been a problem on exposed staples. *Hyperchloremic acidosis* can occur, especially in patients with impaired renal function. Loose bowel movements may persist for a while. Vitamin B_{12} deficiency has been rare, but supplements should be provided at 5-year intervals.

Commentary by Alan B. Retik

We rarely employ the Kock pouch in children. Most of the children who require continent diversion have myelodysplasia with its attendant bowel problems. Resection of a large segment of ileum may wreak havoc on bowel function in this setting. A number of our other children who are candidates for continent diversion have cloacal extrophy where there is a bowel shortage. Simpler forms of diversion are better suited for this group.

We feel that other forms of continent diversion employing the Mitrofanoff (flap valve) principle or the Indiana pouch are satisfactory methods of continent diversion with a much lower complication rate.

CHAPTER 83

Cecoileal Reservoir

MAINZ POUCH

Urologists who know more than one technique are equipped to adapt to unanticipated findings. Locate the stomal site before operation. For children, it may be preferable to catheterize the penis, perineum, or umbilicus, the last being especially suitable for obese or wheelchair-bound children.

1 **A,** *Incision:* Make a midline incision (page 83). Stand on the right side of the table. Mobilize the cecum and ascending colon all the way to the hepatic flexure. **B,** Starting from the cecum, measure 10 to 15 cm on the ascending colon, and mark that point with a stay suture. Measure and mark three segments on the ileum, starting at the ileocecal valve: 10 to 15 cm, 10 to 15 cm, and 20 to 25 cm (measurements given are for adolescents). Divide the mesentery of the ascending colon above the ileocolic artery and the mesentery of the ileum at the most proximal stay suture, then divide the bowel at each end.

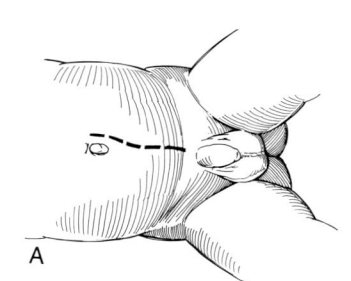

A

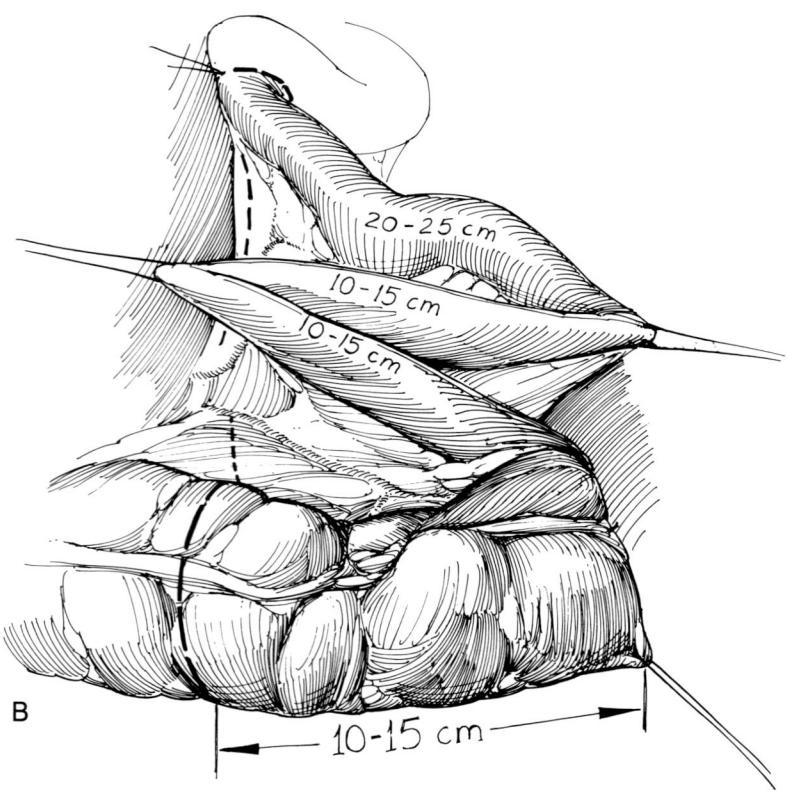

B

2 Spatulate the antimesenteric border of the ileum, and anastomose it to the cecum with staples, using the EEA and TA-55 staplers with 3.5-mm staples (page 34). Let the loop drop behind the anastomosis (do not leave it anterior to the anastomosis, as is done with ureteroileostomy).

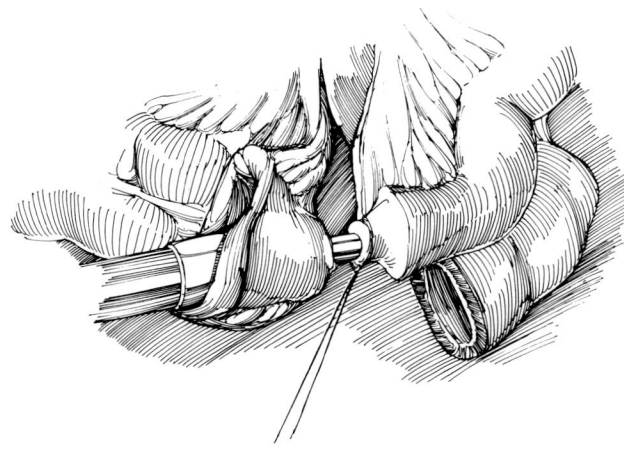

3 Open the bowel segments with scissors on the antimesenteric border, but leave the proximal 20 to 25 cm of ileum intact to provide for the construction of nipple and stoma.

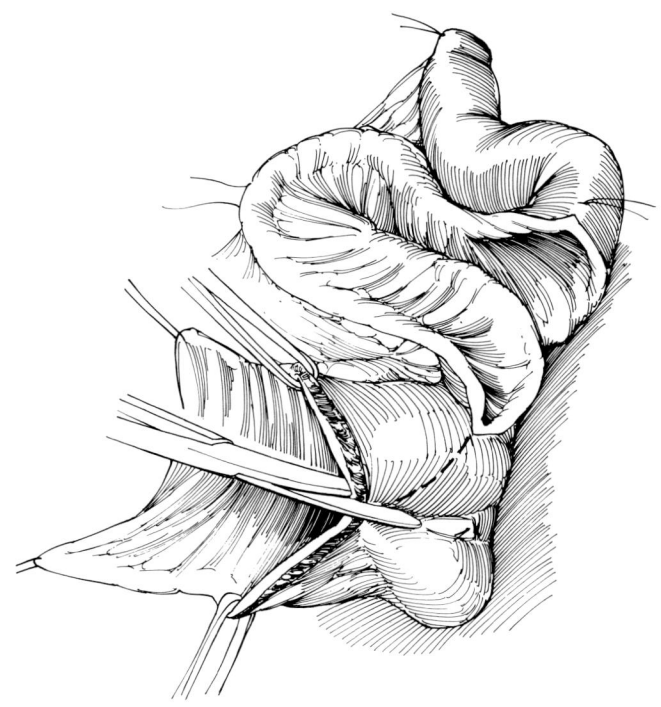

4 Suture the medial edge of the ascending colon to the first part of the ileum, then suture that first ileal segment to the second, as identified by the marking stay sutures. Use a single row of through-and-through running 4-0 synthetic absorbable sutures swagged on a straight needle. Mobilize the left ureter to the level of the lower pole of the kidney, and pull it through retroperitoneally below the duodenum. The right ureter needs less dissection.

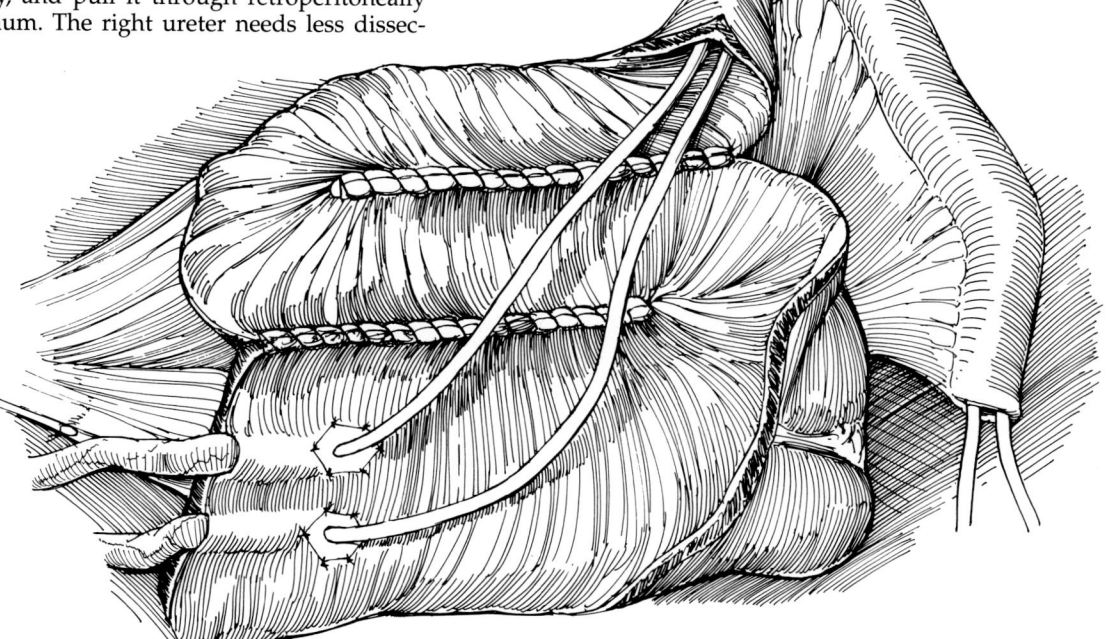

Ureteral Implantation: Mark the site of implantation with four stay sutures through the mucosa and sub-mucosa to tent up the mucosa. Enter the free edge between submucosa and mucosa with blunt-tipped scissors, and form a 4- to 5-cm pocket. Cut down on the tip of the scissors, insert a clamp back to the free edge, and draw the ureter into the tunnel. Spatulate it, fasten the tip to the submucosa and muscularis with a stitch, and approximate the edges mucosa to mucosa. Tack the ureter at its site of entry into the tunnel. Repeat the procedure for the second ureter. Place a 6 or 8 F infant feeding tube in each, and bring the ends of the tubes out through the intact segment of bowel.

5 *Create an intussuscepted ileal valve.* First, form a 6-cm window in the mesentery midway on the unopened segment, and make a smaller window halfway out from the midpoint.

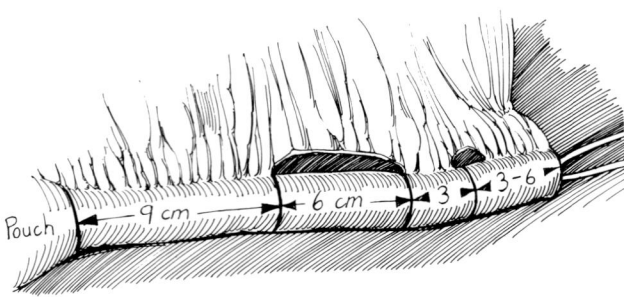

6 Invaginate the bowel with two Allis clamps, and place three or four rows of 4.8-mm metal staples by inserting the TA-55 stapler from outside the pouch at the base of the intussusception into the space between the inner and outer walls.

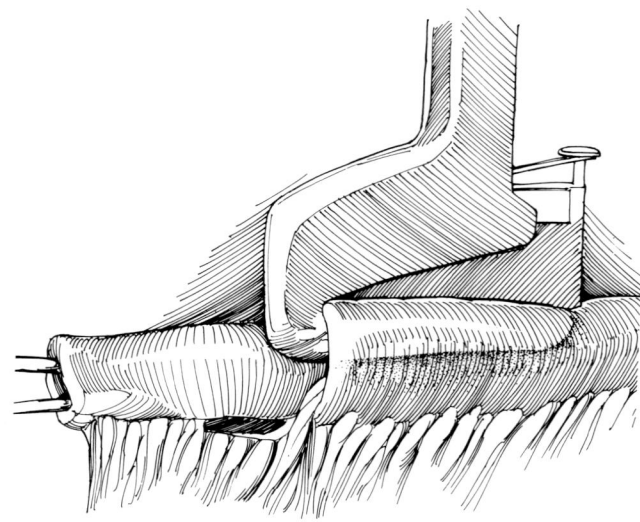

7 Close the anterior wall of the pouch in a single layer with a running suture. At the sites of ureteral exit, take care to close only the mucosa and to use interrupted sutures.

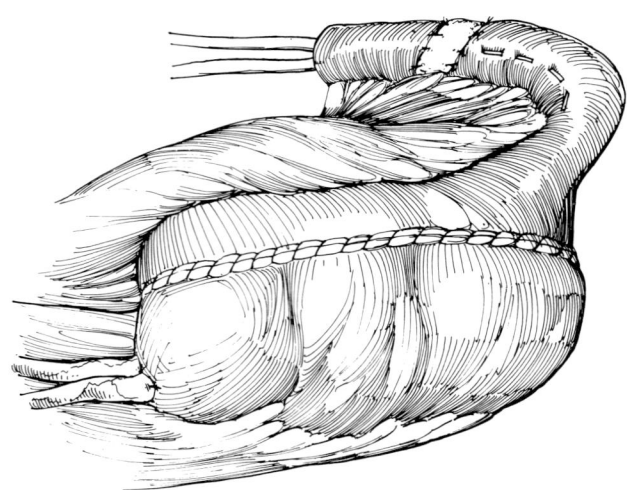

8 Stretch the ileal spout lengthwise; it will have contracted during the operation. Run a 2-cm strip of polyglycolic acid mesh through the second mesenteric window and around the ileum. Fix it in place with multiple interrupted 3-0 synthetic absorbable sutures on both sides. Make an opening in the body wall (page 379) at the umbilicus or in the right lower quadrant within the future hairline. Place three mattress sutures in the mesh, and fasten them to the external oblique or rectus fascia. Trim excess ileum, and suture the ileum flush with the skin with sutures that include mucosa and submucosa, then some muscularis proximal to the edge, and, finally, the skin edge. Remove the retractor after the intussusception has been sutured in place to allow the abdominal wound to assume its normal alignment for a trial of catheterization of the new stoma.

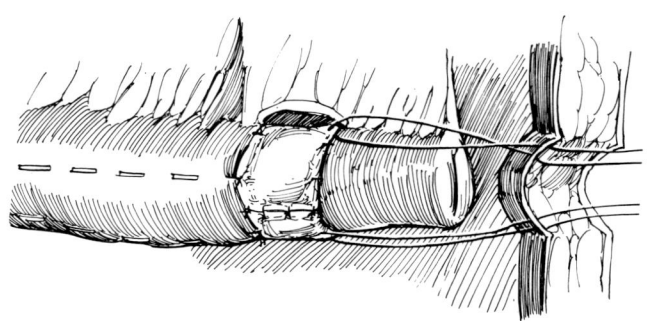

9 Irrigate, test for leaks, drain the pouch with a 26 F 5-ml balloon catheter, and drain the site of ureteral anastomosis with a Jackson-Pratt drain on gravity drainage. Cycle the reservoir with 20 to 30 ml of saline three times a day while the patient is in the hospital. Remove the stents one at a time in 10 days and the catheter in 2 to 3 weeks. If a suprapubic tube is used, be sure to keep it clamped when the urethral catheter is removed, so that urination will prevent the anastomosis from sealing.

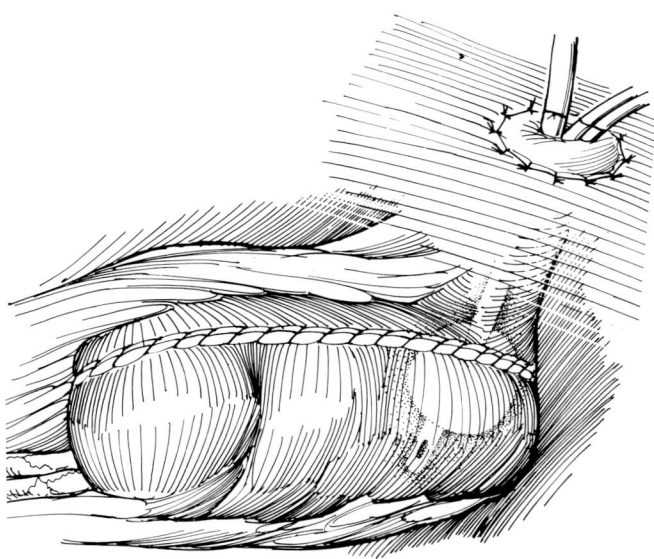

MAINZ POUCH WITH APPENDICEAL STOMA

Form a Mainz pouch, but keep the cecal end intact. Form a tunnel in the tenia to the base of the appendix to form a submucosal bed. Clean the mesentery of the appendix to skeletonize the vessels while preserving the appendicular artery and a branch of the anterior or posterior cecal artery.

Bury the appendix in the tunnel for 4 cm, and close the pouch. Make a V-plasty in the umbilicus to cutaneous stoma in the umbilicus to form a funnel for connection to the appendix. Attach the pouch to the anterior abdominal wall to keep the course of the appendix straight.

INDIANA POUCH

10 **A,** For an adolescent, take a 25-cm segment of cecum and ascending colon with 15 to 18 cm of terminal ileum. Be sure not to make the reservoir too small. If the cecum and ascending colon are short or especially narrow in diameter, take an additional 15- to 20-cm segment of ileum, open it, and place it as a patch over the open cephalad end and lateral margin of the cecum to augment the reservoir. (Alternatively, the appendix tunneled in the tenia can serve as the conduit, releasing the terminal ileum to be applied as the patch.)

B, Split the ascending colon and cecum down its antimesenteric border to within 2 cm of the caudal tip. Proceed with appendectomy. **C,** Close the U-shaped defect by folding the distal portion of the colon into it with a running 3-0 synthetic absorbable suture to the mucosa and some of the muscularis and a serosal Lembert stitch with occasional lock stitches, leaving the ileum to form the conduit. Anastomose the ileum to the ascending colon.

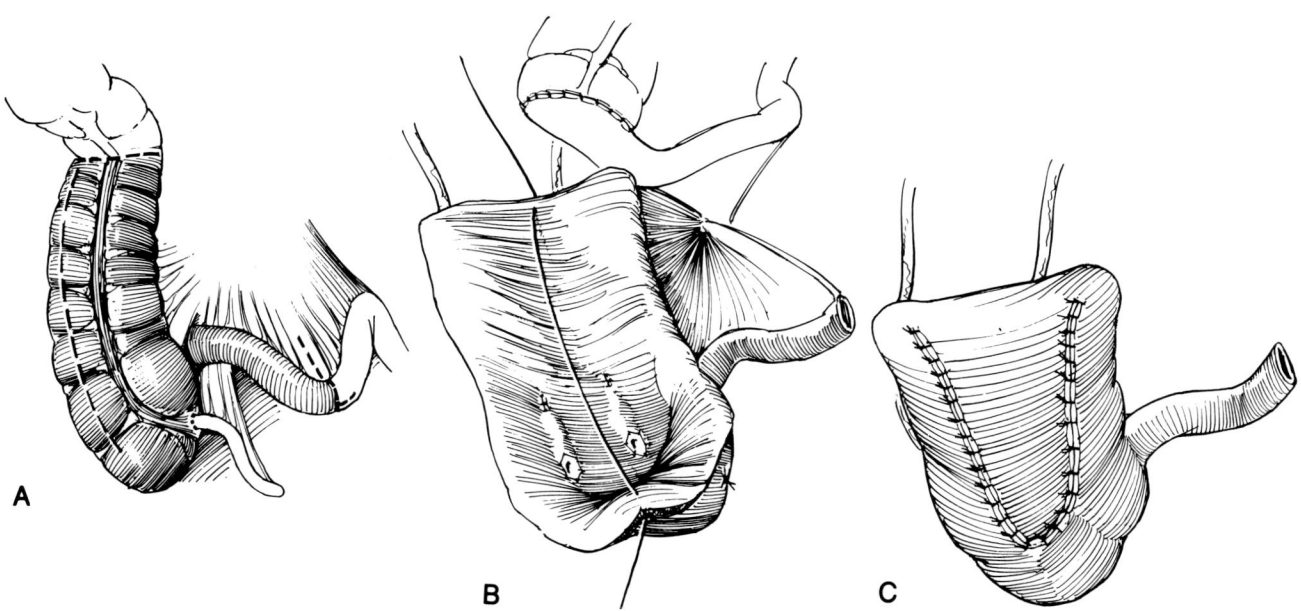

A   B   C

11 To form a conduit from the terminal ileum, use the GIA 90-mm stapler placed firmly against an indwelling 14 F Robinson catheter on the antimesenteric border. The staple line should extend right down to the ileocecal valve. This should create a very straight and smooth catheterizable channel. During the stapling process, make traction along the long axis of the terminal ileum to make sure the catheterizing channel is straight and without folds. With the catheter in place, several interrupted sutures may be inserted at the ileocecal junction to maintain the continence mechanism of the ileocecal valve, not necessarily to "nipple" the terminal ileum into the cecum. Remove the catheter after filling the reservoir. There should be no leakage into the terminal ileum. Tunnel the ureters into the cecum through the tenia. Tack the ureters to the bowel wall outside the anastomosis, and fix the adjacent cecum to the pelvic wall. Stents may be placed.

Insert a 22 or 24 F Malecot catheter as a cecostomy tube to drain the pouch for 3 weeks. Secure the pouch to the abdominal wall with 3-0 synthetic absorbable sutures, so that the tube has a straight run through a stab wound. Bring the terminal ileum into the urethral remnant or, better, the umbilicus, although it may be placed in either the right or left lower quadrant. Make sure that after final positioning, catheterization can be done with no difficulty, so repeatedly try catheterization throughout the final steps and after closing. Ease of catheterization is essential. Bring the cecostomy tube through the abdominal wall, and tack the cecum to the peritoneum about it. Also, bring the ureteral stents and a Penrose drain (led behind the pouch) out through stab wounds, and fasten them internally to the fascia. On the 9th day, before discharge from the hospital, have the patient practice catheterization.

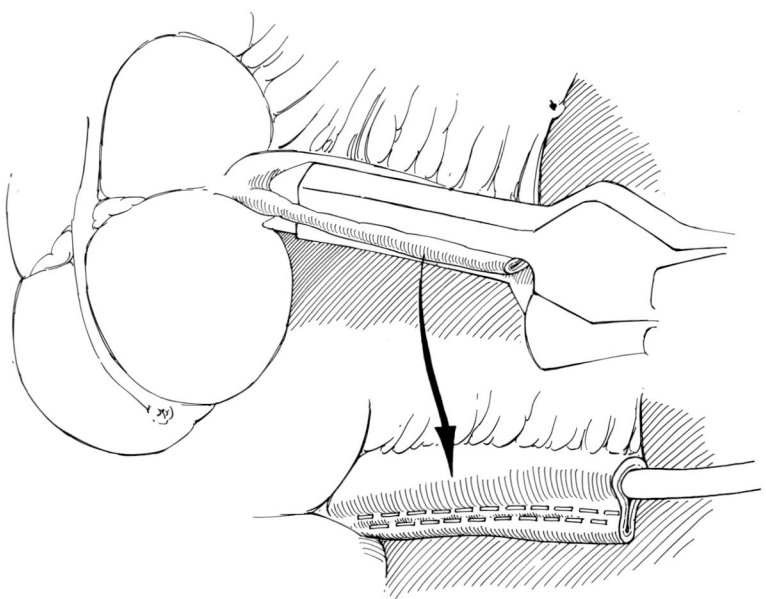

Commentary by Michael E. Mitchell

The Indiana reservoir initially was developed from the Gilchrist procedure as a means of reconstruction of exstrophy in pediatric and young adult patients who previously had a cystectomy. The procedure subsequently has been successfully applied to the adult cystectomy population. We now have experience with more than 80 patients and have been quite satisfied with the results.

There are advantages to the procedure. It is not technically difficult to perform. The reservoir, antireflux mechanism, and continence mechanism are dependable and do not require an extensive learning curve. Furthermore, we believe the principles used are solid. Reflux is prevented by a submucosal tunnel. The reservoir is large and approaches a spheric configuration. The catheterizable channel is straight, without nipples or extensive surgical modification, to ensure ease of catheterization. No staples or nonresorbable sutures ever should be placed in the reservoir.

Errors made in the construction of the reservoir are (1) improper selection of patients; (2) making a reservoir that is too small, because not enough bowel was used (it is easy to make a reservoir too small but difficult to make one too big); and (3) making the catheterizable channel too short or too large, so that the catheter cannot easily be passed. Repeated trial catheterization must be made throughout the final stages and after closing. Ease of catheterization is a primary objective. Proper patient selection and attention to surgical detail remain the important factors for success.

PENN POUCH

(DUCKETT)

12 Prepare a cecal pouch by opening 30 cm of colon on the mesocolic tenia and 20 cm of ileum on its antimesenteric border. Fold the ileum into a U, and suture the edges with 3-0 synthetic absorbable running sutures. Insert the ileal patch into the cecal defect. Fold the distal end of the cecum to complete the pouch.

If the mesoappendix is mobile and vascularized, excise the base of the appendix, taking a generous disk of cecum, while preserving the mesentery of the appendix. Close the cecal defect in two layers. Implant the ureters into the cecum by an antireflux method (pages 427–429).

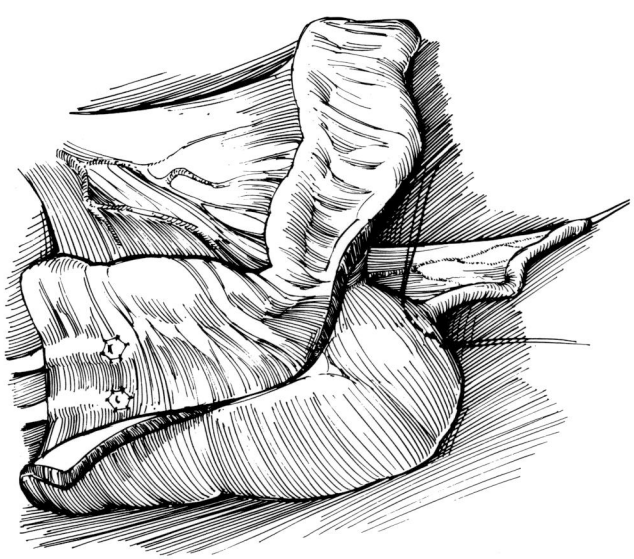

13 Rotate the appendix on its mesentery, and trim its tip until an adequate lumen is reached. Calibrate it with a *bougie à boule*, continuing to trim the end as necessary. Create an 8-cm trough in the most accessible tenia of the seromuscular wall of the ascending colon, laying back flaps and exposing submucosa for a width of 2 or 3 cm. The trough can be widened by grasping the bowel wall on either side and gently pulling it open. Open the mucosa at the distal end of the groove, and anastomose the opened tip of the appendix with interrupted 4-0 synthetic absorbable sutures. Close the lateral seromuscular flaps over the appendix with 3-0 synthetic absorbable sutures, taking care not to constrict its mesentery in the tunnel. Three to 4 cm within the tunnel is sufficient to produce continence. Lead the base of the appendix through the body wall in an appropriate site in the left lower quadrant, and suture it to the skin. Alternatively, the appendix may be shortened and placed with a V-flap in the umbilicus to hide it. Hitch the cecum and ascending colon to the retroperitoneum, so that the appendix and its mesentery are not kinked. If this procedure is used for bladder augmentation, fix the bladder to the psoas muscle, so that the appendiceal mesentery does not move during bladder filling. Place a Moreno tube (not such a large one that it stretches the appendix) to drain mucus from the pouch. Close the wound appropriately.

The appendix may be buried without detachment from the cecum, as described in the section "Mainz Pouch with Appendiceal Stoma," although then it may be more difficult to catheterize.

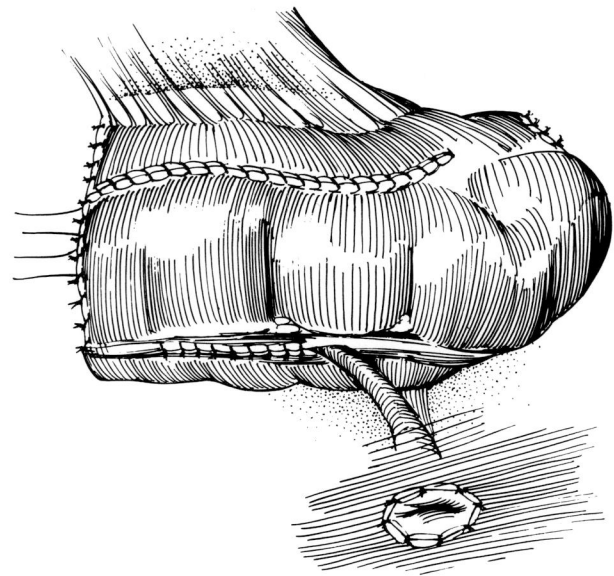

Commentary by John W. Duckett

The ureterocecoappendicostomy, or Penn pouch, uses the Mitrofanoff principle, although Mitrofanoff did not describe this arrangement. We would, therefore, like to take credit for it. The Penn pouch was designed to simplify the construction of a continent urinary reservoir in patients with cancer of the bladder. Fisch, Wammach, Müller, and Hohenfellner have adapted this procedure instead of the Mainz pouch I, with its ileal nipple continence mechanism. They have not detached the appendix but folded it back *in situ*. Obviously, the normal anatomy must be complete—that is, the ileum, cecum, and appendix. A standard bowel prep should precede the procedure. Any refluxing implants of the ureter into the colon have been quite successfully corrected with either the Goodwin or Leadbetter techniques. The same principle applies to the placement of the appendix into the tenia. Surprisingly, the mesentery of the appendix can be engulfed in the seromuscular layer of the bowel without compression and still maintain a continent flap valve. Care must be taken to arrange the mesentery of the appendix in such a way that it is not stretched as the pouch is filled with urine. The appendicocecostomy avoids the complexity of ileal intussusception.

Florida Pouch. This is similar to the Indiana pouch but has a greater capacity, because it involves more colon and is more spheric. Incise the parietal peritoneum and gastrocolic ligament to mobilize the right colon, hepatic flexure, and the right half of the transverse colon. Leave the middle colic artery within the left portion of the transverse mesocolon. Reconstitute the colon by a lateral anastomosis between ileum and transverse colon.

Fold the colon into a U shape. Open it on the antimesenteric border, and suture the inner edges with a running locking 3-0 synthetic absorbable suture, followed by suture of the outer edges to form a large tube. Anastomose the ureters by a standard technique. Taper the ileum (page 220), and bring it through the abdominal wall.

The end of an ileal loop may be opened on the antimesenteric border and applied to a Florida pouch to convert the child to continence.

POSTOPERATIVE PROBLEMS FROM URINARY RESERVOIRS

Urinary tract infection (bacteriuria) is inevitable in systems requiring self-catheterization, but pyelonephritis is rare. *Mucus secretion* is greater in reservoirs of cecum than of ileum, and it persists longer. In contrast, the ileal mucosa atrophies. Mucus often is obstructive and requires weekly irrigations with sterile water or bicarbonate solution. Occasional obstruction during catheter drainage may be overcome

if the patient coughs. *Stone formation* is secondary to residual urine and may be managed by direct-vision litholapaxy. The *metabolic changes* of increased serum chloride and decreased bicarbonate occur frequently. Some patients must be managed by ingestion of bicarbonate, more frequent emptying of the reservoir, and continuous drainage at night. Loss of potassium is not a problem. Renal function must be monitored. *Urinary fistulas* can occur around the valve in an ileocecal reservoir and require reconstruction. If the leak is from an ileal pouch, continuous catheter drainage usually will allow it to close.

Commentary by Alan B. Retik

Although we much prefer the Mitrofanoff, or flap-valve, principle for continence, we occasionally do not have this option and require a nipple for continence. In this situation, it is preferable to employ the Indiana rather than the Mainz Pouch, because less bowel is used. This is of major importance in the myelodysplastic population. It is preferable to incise the antimesenteric portions of isolated segments of bowel with cautery rather than scissors.

When constructing an Indiana pouch, we employ staples rather than sutures. This ensures a more uniform caliber of the conduit. Babcock clamps grasp the antimesenteric portion of the ileum, which is catheterized with a 12 F red rubber catheter, and a 6-cm GIA stapler is applied to the terminal ileum. The excess bowel wall is removed by the stapler, and the remaining bowel will cover the catheter smoothly. In addition, the GIA stapler is used at the ileocecal junction to create a funnel-shaped segment of the terminal ileum. This area is then plicated with 3-0 silk Lembert sutures; in effect, this also plicates the ileocecal valve.

We have found the Heineke-Mikulicz principle in the formation of the Indiana pouch quite effective; for the most part, it eliminates the necessity for additional ileum as a patch. When we are converting a preexisting ileal conduit to an Indiana pouch and the capacity of the cecum is marginal, the preexisting ileum can be used to augment the colon.

No matter what technique is employed, when performing continent diversion, it is extremely important that one ensure at the operating table that the continence mechanism is effective and that the conduit can easily be catheterized with suitable catheters at various degrees of reservoir filling. If there is any difficulty catheterizing a conduit in the operating room, it will be that much harder afterward! Therefore, I usually test the conduit with various types of catheters that will be employed postoperatively, and I leave the conduit catheterized with an indwelling Silastic catheter, which is tied off and sutured to the skin. I leave this in for approximately 7 to 10 days.

CHAPTER 84

Gastric Reservoir
(MITCHELL)

1 Harvest a wedge from the stomach (for details, see pages 468–470). Remove the staples. Partially close the edges.

2 With curved tenotomy scissors, form 2-cm oblique tunnels in the plane under the gastric mucosa on the posterior wall, and draw the ureters through them. Place a deep suture at the apex of each spatulated ureter, and suture the edges of the ureter to the gastric mucosa.

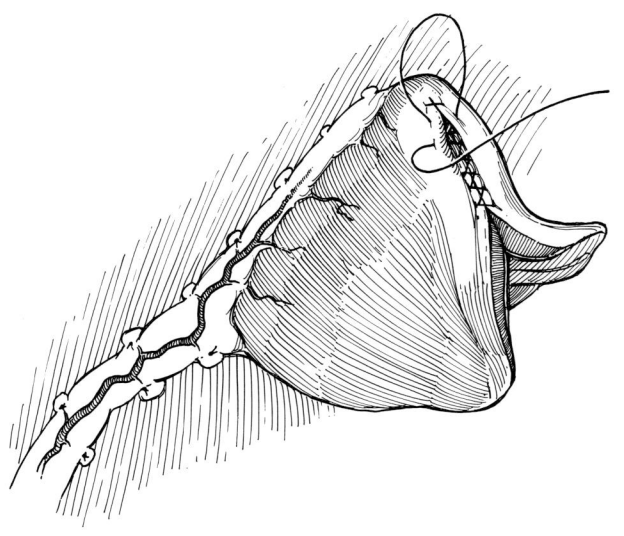

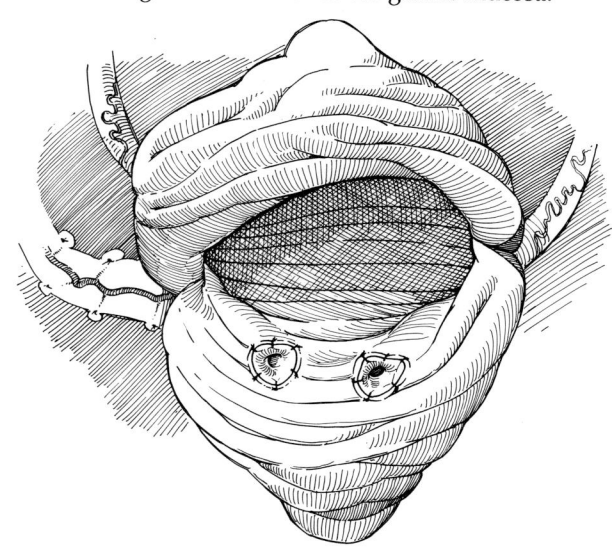

Stomach Tube Conduit

3 Construct a conduit from a portion of the stomach. Mark and cut a strip 2-cm wide from the anterior arm of the flap. Form it into a tube over a 10 F catheter.

4 Slightly intussuscept the base into the reservoir to increase resistance. Close the reservoir. Bring the open end of the tube to the skin of the anterior abdominal wall, and fix it in place. Fill the reservoir to make absolutely certain that it will be catheterizable.

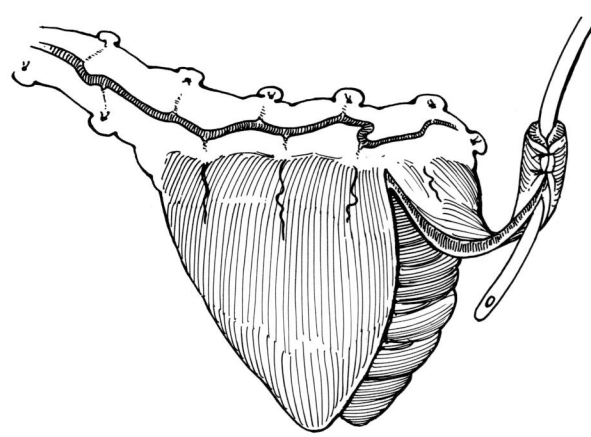

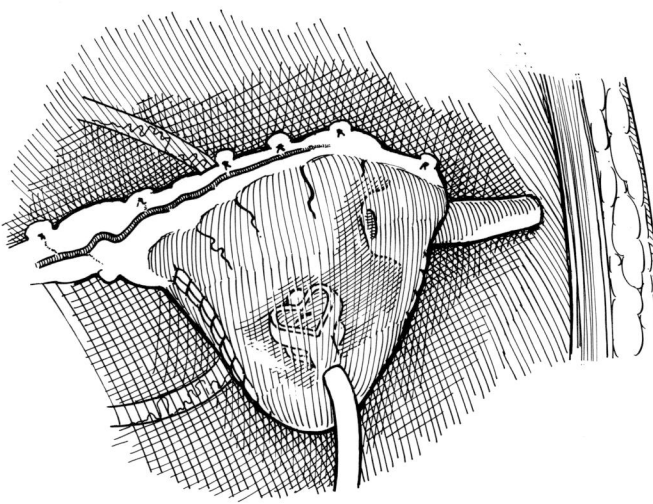

Mitrofanoff Adaptation

5 Continue the closure of the edges of the flap after insertion of a Malecot catheter into the reservoir. Form a Mitrofanoff valve by tunneling the appendix (the

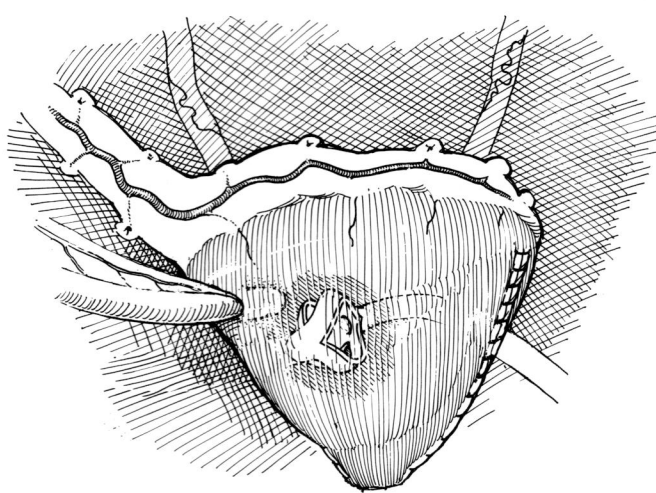

residual ureter could be used as well) through the wall obliquely from the outside, and fix it to the neobladder wall at the site of entrance. Bring the end of the appendix through the body wall, and fix it to the skin. Suture the wall of the stomach to the abdominal wall, as for a gastrostomy, to avoid leakage when the cystostomy tube is removed. Complete the closure.

POSTOPERATIVE PROBLEMS

Painful urination and perineal pain are managed with an H_2 receptor antagonist. For low urinary pH levels and irritative symptoms, irrigate the bladder with phosphate buffer. In children with renal failure, severe salt loss may occur during episodes of diarrhea and vomiting, requiring intravenous replacement.

Appendicovesicostomy

APPENDICOVESICOSTOMY

(MITROFANOFF)

Access to a continent reservoir for intermittent catheterization may not be possible through the urethra. The submucosal implantation of the appendix provides continence and furnishes a catheterizable stoma. Alternatives using the same principle include tapered ileum, ureteral remnants, and uterine tube. The technique for use of the ureter is simpler and the complications fewer, making that tissue preferable to appendix if it is available. Because these stomas will not leak, even with high intravesical pressure, the risk of spontaneous perforation is appreciable unless another route is present that responds to a lower leak pressure. For that reason, closure of the vesical neck may not be advisable unless the child has stress incontinence.

Prepare the bowel. Insert a balloon catheter transurethrally.

1 *Incision:* Make a midline lower abdominal incision (page 263). Before opening the peritoneum, prepare the lateral vesical space generously on the right. Divide the spermatic cord, vas, and obliterated hypogastric artery to gain adequate exposure.

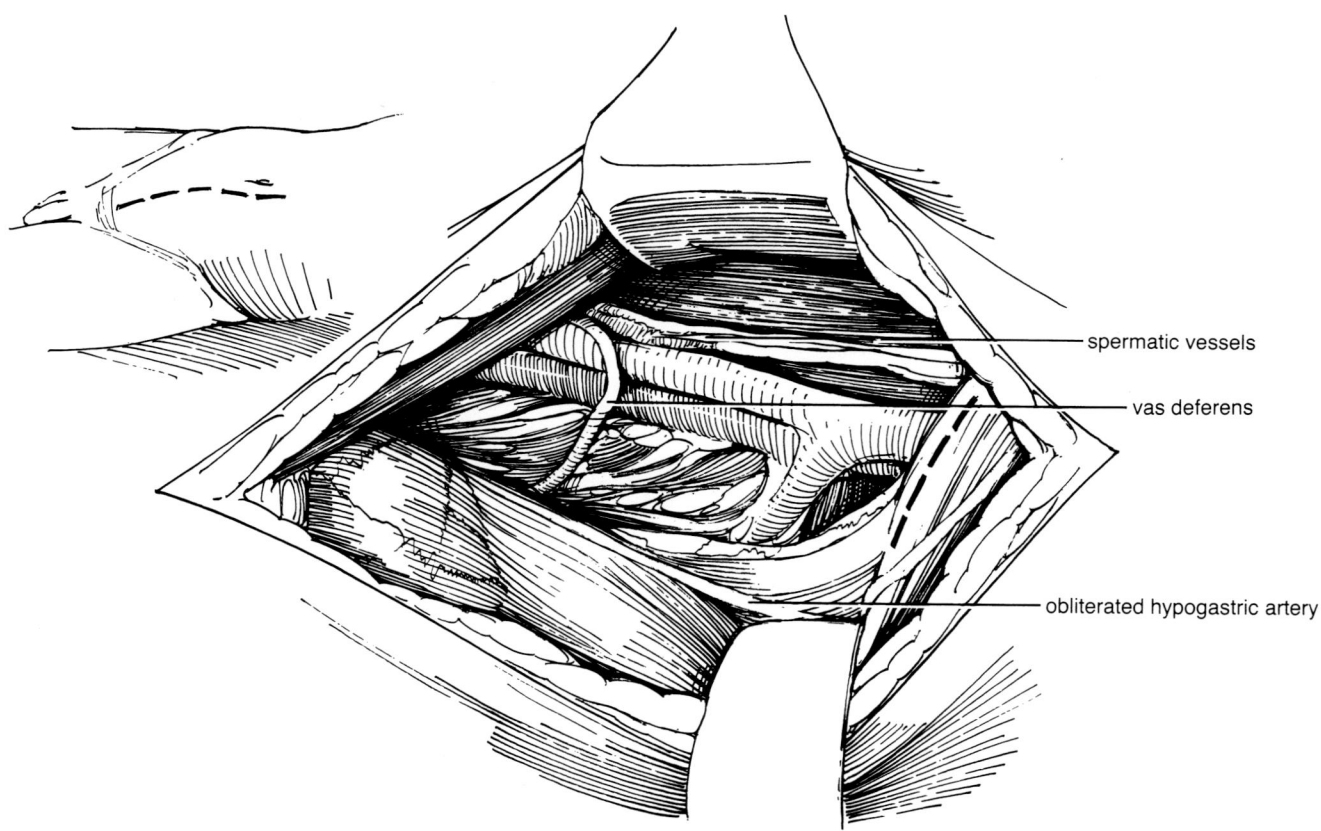

spermatic vessels

vas deferens

obliterated hypogastric artery

2 **A,** Open the peritoneum. At the base of the appendix, insert stay sutures and incise the wall circumferentially to take a cuff of cecum. Separate the appendiceal mesentery for a short distance from that of the cecum, preserving all the blood supply to the appendix. Close the cecal defect left by the appendix with an inner running 3-0 synthetic absorbable suture and an outer layer of interrupted Lembert 3-0 synthetic absorbable sutures (page 31). **B,** Alternatively, secure a broad base for the appendiceal conduit by applying a stapler across the cecum a short distance from the base, taking care to preserve the vascular pedicle to the appendix. If needed, this cecal portion can be fashioned into a tube to lengthen the appendix.

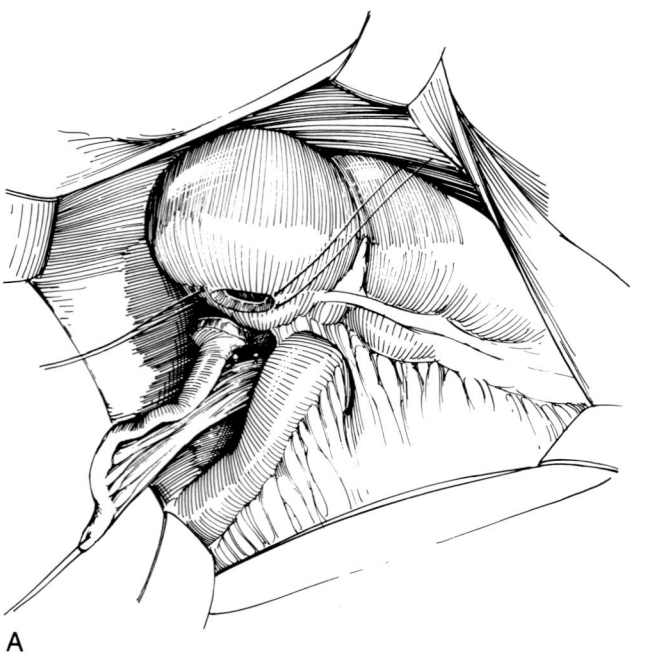

A

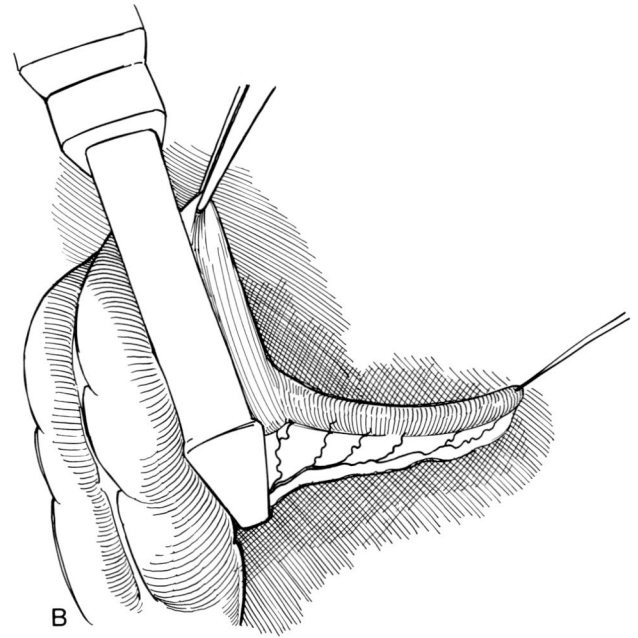

B

3 Extraperitonealize the appendix through a small opening in the peritoneum behind the ileocecal junction. Close the peritoneum with a running suture. Trim back the appendiceal tip successively with Mayo scissors until an adequate lumen is exposed.

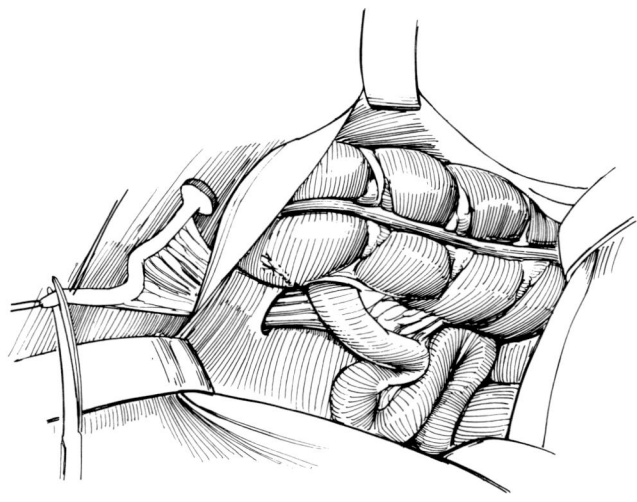

4 **A,** Open the bladder in the midline down to the vesical neck and extend the incision transversely so as to completely transect the neck. Close it solidly (pages 299–303). Invert the urethra distally with 3-0 synthetic absorbable sutures.

B, In the posterolateral wall of the bladder, develop a wide submucosal tunnel beginning well above the right ureteral orifice, as in the Cohen procedure (page 208). Implant the appendix and its mesentery in the tunnel. Proceed with bladder augmentation.

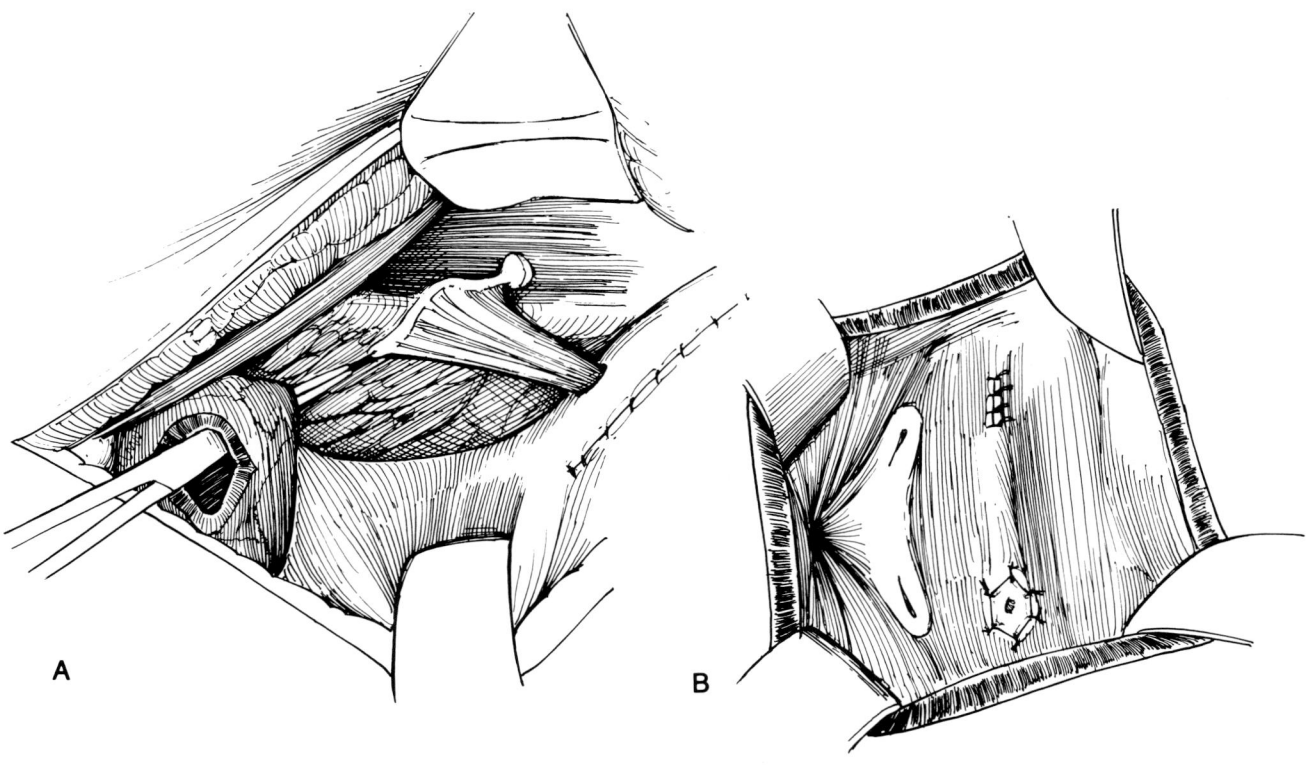

A

B

5 Pass the appendiceal base through a large opening in the abdominal muscles and a small opening in the skin in the edge of the future hairline in the right lower quadrant. Alternatively, it may be placed in the umbilicus. Hitch the bladder to the anterior abdominal wall around the hole to prevent kinking of the appendix and to compensate for its limited length. Protect the appendiceal mesentery. Suture the appendiceal base to the skin with 3-0 chromic catgut sutures. Leave a balloon catheter (10 or 12 F) through the appendix for 2 or 3 weeks, at which time the child is taught intermittent catheterization. Drain the bladder with a suprapubic Malecot catheter. Irrigate it with saline to eliminate mucus if an enterocystoplasty has been performed. Do a cystogram at 4 weeks at the time the tube is removed.

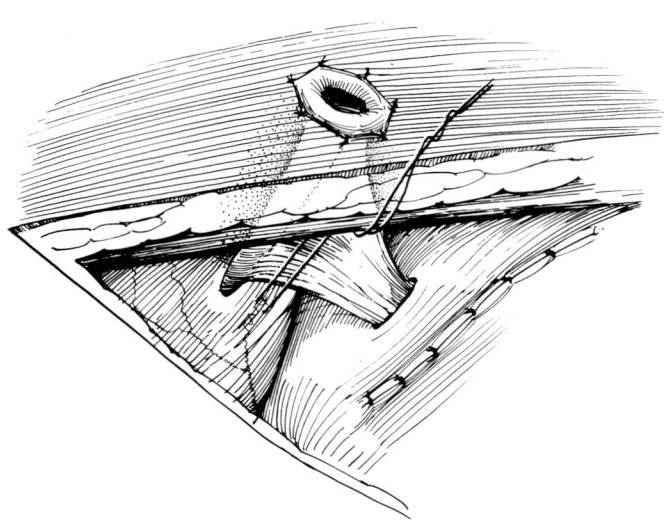

Other structures such as ureter, uterine tube, and tailored small bowel may be implanted into the bladder or into an intestinal reservoir using the Mitrofanoff principle. For implantation into the large bowel, make a 5-cm incision in the tenia down to, but not including, the submucosal vessels. Make a trough by undermining the edges, and cut the longitudinal muscle of the tenia transversely at the proximal end. Open the mucosa at the distal end, and perform a mucosa-to-mucosa anastomosis of the tubular structure that was selected for the conduit. Cover the ureter with the reflected muscle and serosa.

POSTOPERATIVE PROBLEMS

Necrosis of the base of the appendix requires revision but usually is limited to the cecal cuff. *Urinary fistulas* pose a larger problem, either from leakage into the urethra at the site of vesical neck closure or at the vesical suture line anteriorly. *Reflux* also can be a problem and should be corrected at an earlier stage. If reflux begins after operation, the incidence of upper tract dilatation can be reduced by vesical augmentation. *Mucus* is a problem, even if the bladder has been augmented with stomach. Mucus from the appendix falls into the base of the bladder, where it is not completely evacuated by intermittent catheterization; it fosters infection and obstructs the catheter.

Commentary by Paul Mitrofanoff

If there is reflux after appendicovesicostomy, it requires correction in a preliminary stage, but it usually is a symptom of bladder hypertonicity that requires bladder augmentation. The decision to perform an enterocystoplasty to enlarge the bladder must be made at the first stage if the bladder is too small and hypertonic or later if reflux or upper tract dilatation appears. Thus enterocystoplasty seems to be necessary in approximately one half of the cases of neurogenic bladders that are retained for urinary storage.

Specific Technical Points. A large peritoneal dissection of the right lower quadrant is necessary to best place the appendix and its mesentery under the peritoneum. This dissection is easier to perform before opening the peritoneum. Good vascularization of the appendix of course is essential. If it appears jeopardized during the operation, another solution must be used: ureterovesicostomy or intestinal stoma associated with an enterocystoplasty.

I believe that the bladder should be opened for three reasons: (1) for bladder neck closure, (2) to select the best place to implant the appendix, and (3) to help accomplish the bladder hitch to the anterior abdominal wall. This hitch is useful to avoid kinking of the appendix between the abdominal muscles and bladder and also if the appendix is short.

The closure of the bladder neck is necessary in almost all the cases, the neck being left open only if it appears to be totally continent (self-catheterization being impossible because of an orthopedic situation). In girls, this closure easily could be carried out in a later stage using a perineal approach. It is better to carry out the enterocystoplasty in the same stage as the vesicostomy, but sometimes the symptoms of the bladder hypertonicity develop with the passing years after the closure of the bladder neck. The bladder must then be enlarged without delay.

Complications. Different types of complications can occur, such as those with the appendix (stenosis of the cutaneous stoma or appendicular kink blocking the catheterizations). A limited reoperation is sufficient to resolve these problems. Urinary leakage by the cutaneous stoma requires a more difficult reoperation to lengthen the submucosal tunnel of the appendix and to restore continence. However, it is essential to check if this leakage is not due to a high bladder pressure requiring an augmentation.

Vesicourethral fistula, urinary infections, dilation of the upper tract, or reflux are possible. They almost always are symptoms of too small a bladder with too high a pressure. Anticholinergic drugs usually are insufficient, and enterocystoplasty is necessary.

Bladder lithiasis is caused by the presence of the intestinal mucus. Such stones often are well tolerated, and their removal usually is easy to perform. Prevention should involve increased diuresis and catheterizations with a large catheter, 14 F when possible, with the goal of having the child perform complete emptying at each time by siphoning. A weekly bladder wash can be useful.

More severe is the occurrence of a spontaneous rupture of an enteroplasty. It probably is caused by too-infrequent catheterizations leading to an overdistended bladder. Therefore, it is essential to teach the patients to follow a timetable with at least four catheterizations a day.

URETEROVESICOSTOMY

The ureter may be a good substitute for the appendix. To use the lower end of the ureter requires a transureteroureterostomy and an antireflux procedure performed in two stages. A ureteral conduit is especially suitable when one end of the ureter is well vascularized, as after cutaneous ureterostomy.

6 Divide the ureter that was implanted in the skin in its midportion. Insert the proximal end of its distal segment in the bladder or bladder substitute and the distal end of its proximal segment in the contralateral ureter, which, in turn, is implanted in the bladder (or into an augmentation) with an antireflux technique. A pedicle graft of ureter can be formed by preserving the branch from the internal iliac artery. Divide the distal end, place a rubber-shod clamp on the proximal end, and check for viability (a Doppler stethoscope helps). Place (or leave) one end of the ureter on the skin for intermittent catheterization and the other end in the reservoir as a nonrefluxing valve with a tunnel of the same proportions as for ureteroneocystostomy. Placing one end of the ureter in the perineum allows the urogenital diaphragm to be used for continence.

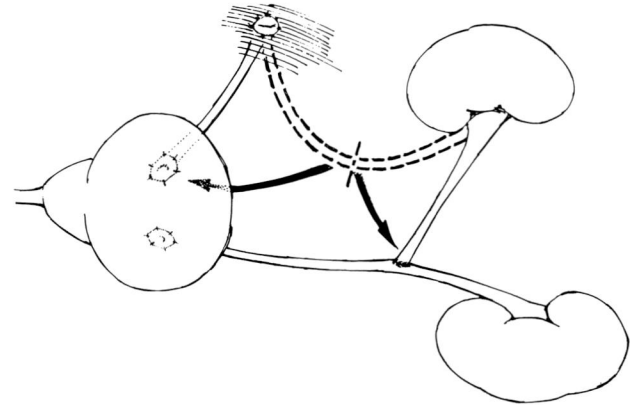

POSTOPERATIVE PROBLEMS

Bladder calculi are not uncommon, perhaps secondary to mucus that passes down into the pouch from the appendix and is not reached by the catheter. *Disruption* may occur from traumatic catheterization or acute or chronic overfilling. *Fistulas* may occur in the early postoperative period.

CHAPTER 86

Ileonipple Conduit

(BENCHEKROUN)

After formation of a reservoir, secure a separate 14-cm segment of ileum with its mesentery proximal to the 8-cm terminal portion that is left attached to the cecum in the formation of the pouch.

1 **A,** Insert two Allis clamps in the lumen from the distal end and grasp the rim of bowel at the proximal end. Pull this end into the lumen to invaginate it, forming a double-walled tube (inkwell). **B,** Suture the mucosa of

the inner and outer bowel edges together with a running 3-0 synthetic absorbable suture that extends on the ventral side halfway around the circumference. Reinforce this with a serosomuscularis suture. Place a single full-thickness mattress suture halfway between the terminations of the running suture, leaving two distinct openings between the layers of the inverted ileum, opening on either side, that allow the sac between the two layers of ileum to fill with urine from the reservoir and shut the valve.

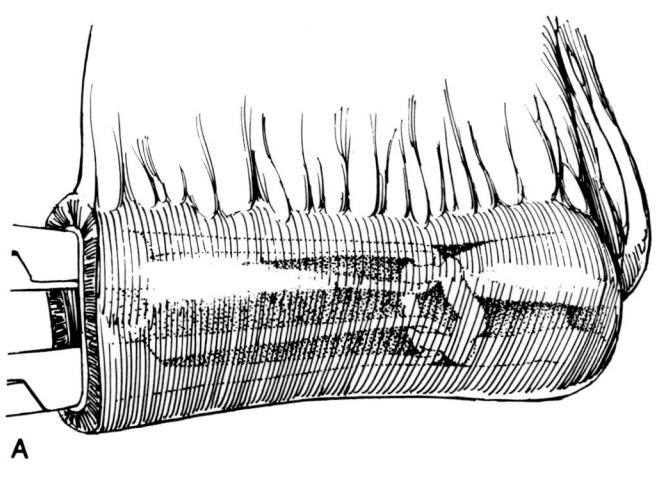

A

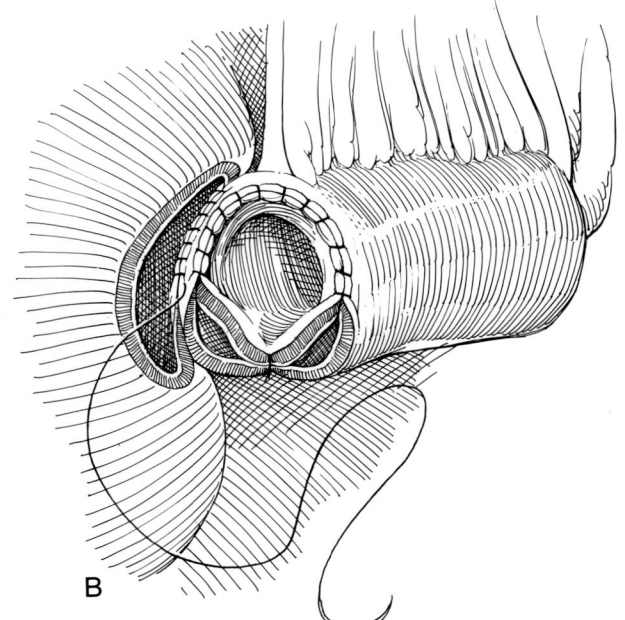

B

2 Suture the double end to the opening in the bladder or bladder augmentation in two layers with 3-0 synthetic absorbable sutures. Place a Levine tube through the stoma, to remain for as long as 3 weeks.

The same principle may be used as an afferent limb to prevent reflux by spatulating and joining the ureters side by side to form a large opening, anastomosing this opening to the end of the ileal segment, and, finally, intussuscepting the ureters into the ileum (see Dr Benchekroun's description in his commentary.)

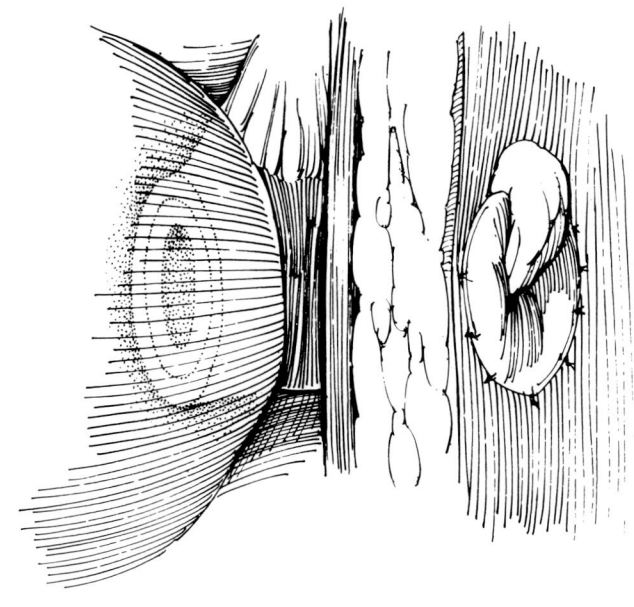

POSTOPERATIVE PROBLEMS

Fistulas between the conduit and the skin may occur if more than the serosa is sutured to the fascia and skin. An indwelling catheter may allow healing, but the valve usually must be replaced. *Stomal stenosis* results from poor stomal care and infrequent catheterization. It may be relieved by dilatation and prolonged catheterization; it can be mitigated by inserting a V of skin at the time of construction but may require refashioning the stoma. *Pouch overdistention* causes the Benchekroun valve to overfill and distort the mechanism., resulting in inability to catheterize the stoma. It can be relieved by needle aspiration of the pouch and a period of catheterization to restore the valve to normal. *Deintussusception,* resulting in difficulty with catheterization or incontinence, is secondary to poor fixation of the invaginated ileum.

Commentary by Abdellatif Benchekroun

The ileal valve can be adapted to all types of reservoirs, according to the indications in the patients involved.

Ileocecal Reservoir. The "hydraulic valve" can be inserted in an ileocecal reservoir by placing it over the distal end of the cecum (ascending colon) and using the terminal ileum for ureteral implantation.

Detubularized Ileocecal Reservoir. A valve-in-continuity can be formed in a Hautmann pouch by inverting the 16-cm efferent loop and converting it into a hydraulic valve. This is done through a transverse ileotomy made 12 cm from the end and by exteriorizing the valve in the right iliac fossa. The ureters are implanted into the reservoir by the LeDuc-Camey method.

Sigmoid Bladder. The loop is isolated and closed distally. The ureters are implanted by the Leadbetter antireflux technique. The ileal valve is placed on the proximal end of the segment and exteriorized. There are few indications for this procedure, but we did it in two cases to transform a wet colostomy into a continent sigmoidostomy and colostomy and in one case for a man with right colonic agenesis.

Rectal Bladder Bypass. The valve also can be used for bypassing the rectal bladder. After the rectum is sectioned, the valve is attached to the margins of the proximal rectotomy and the stoma placed in the left iliac fossa.

Transverse Colonic Reservoir. In one case with a short cecum, we used the transverse colon as the reservoir after closing one end and putting the valve on the other.

Continent Cystostomy. This technique consists of preserving the vesical reservoir, excluding the bladder neck, and apposing the ileal valve on the bladder dome. The cutaneous stoma can be either median or pararectal.

Ileocecal Continent Reservoir. For implantation into the cecum, the Leadbetter technique is used. The ureters are implanted into the ileum that is attached to the cecum by one of three techniques: (1) eversion of 1 cm of ureter in a flap; (2) the LeDuc-Camey method; (3) an antireflux valve. For the formation of an antireflux valve, the ureters are spatulated and conjoined and then fastened to the end of the ileal segment. The end of the segment is inverted by making a transverse ileotomy 8 cm from the end and drawing the end with the attached ureters into the body of the segment, as is done for an ileal hydraulic valve. The end is attached to the proximal lip of the ileotomy by a three-quarter circumferential continuous 3-0 polyglycolic acid suture. Finally, the ileotomy is sutured with the distal lip on one side and the proximal edge of the ileotomy–ureteral anastomosis on the other side.

With this ureteral implant technique, we constructed a hydraulic valve antireflux system while retaining a large ureteroileal anastomosis. Opacifying the continent urostomy enabled us to observe the integrity of the ileal valve, referred to as the "crab claw."

During the past 18 years, we have performed successfully 250 cases of continent urinary diversion, of which 30 were children younger than 15 years of age. The incidence of most complications such as disinvagination, fistula of the valve, and ureteroileal stenosis has decreased.

Cautions and Pitfalls. Concerning the abdominal fixation of the valve, your needle must take only the serosa. Ureteral stents must be exteriorized through the reservoir and not through the stoma. When the hydraulic valve is made, the two posterior openings must be loose to allow free passage of urine between the reservoir and the valve. Sometimes you need to excise a cuneiform part of the inner layer to enhance the passage outside this layer.

CHAPTER 87

Ureterosigmoidostomy

Techniques for urinary storage after loss of the bladder should be directed at providing continence, while at the same time preserving renal function and maintaining normal electrolyte balance. Ideally, the patient should be free of appliances, should be able to empty the urine, and should remain continent. Either a substitute bladder can be placed, or a reservoir can be devised for intermittent catheterization. Options include reservoirs formed from ileum, cecum, sigmoid colon, or stomach that provide antireflux and continence mechanisms. Ureterosigmoidostomy probably is the oldest (and certainly, the technically easiest) means of continent diversion. Despite its limitations of electrolyte imbalance, potential for upper tract damage, and association with later development of adenocarcinoma near the ureteral anastomosis, it still has a place in certain cases.

An alternative that may produce better long-term results at the cost of a permanent colostomy is the Boyce-Vest operation, in which the base of the closed exstrophic bladder is anastomosed to the adjacent bladder wall.

Determine if the anal sphincteric mechanism is intact digitally by anal stimulation and by having the child hold warm water for a couple of hours. Perform an intravenous urogram to be sure there is absolutely no ureteral dilatation (a contraindication to this operation). Provide both mechanical and antibacterial bowel preparation. This procedure is most successful in terms of achieving urinary continence when performed in children who have attained fecal continence prior to ureterosigmoidostomy

Place the child on a liquid diet for 24 hours, and prepare the bowel with polyethylene glycol–electrolyte solution (GoLYTELY). Provide two cleansing enemas with neomycin solution the day before the operation. Give intravenous cephalosporin 6 hours preoperatively and continue for 72 hours. It may be advisable to install a central venous line.

CLOSED TECHNIQUE FOR URETEROSIGMOID ANASTOMOSIS (LEADBETTER)

1 *Position:* Supine, in slight Trendelenburg position. Insert a large rectal tube as high as possible, and tape it near the anus with waterproof tape placed over tincture of benzoin. If a straight rectal tube is used, cut extra holes and suture it para-anally. The right-handed surgeon will stand on the right side of the patient. **A,** *Incision:* Make a midline transabdominal incision. In exstrophy patients, the incision must be well off the midline over one belly of rectus muscle. Excise the bladder first, leaving the transected ureters to drain freely. Have a nasogastric tube inserted, and palpate it in the stomach. Free any adhesions. Pack the small bowel in the upper end of the abdominal cavity. Determine the sites of the incisions in the parietal peritoneum. Move the rectosigmoid junction to the right, and incise the parietal peritoneum where it touches the tenia to be sure that the anastomosis can be reperitonealized. **B,** Elevate the left peritoneal flap and expose the left ureter. Carefully mobilize it sharply and bluntly from its bed, preserving the adventitial vessels. Watch for vessels entering laterally below the pelvic brim and medially above it; clamp, cut, and ligate them. Continue releasing the ureter to as close to the bladder as possible to provide a long ureter for a low anastomosis. Place a 4-0 silk stay suture in the ureter; clamp it distal to the suture with a right-angle clamp, and divide and ligate it. If the ureter is small, it may be ligated just proximal to the site of division to allow it to dilate before anastomosis. Repeat the procedure on the right side by moving the sigmoid colon to the left. Incise the adjacent peritoneum at the site of contact with the colon; here, the retroperitoneal incision can be made somewhat more medially. Expose and free the right ureter, as was done on the left.

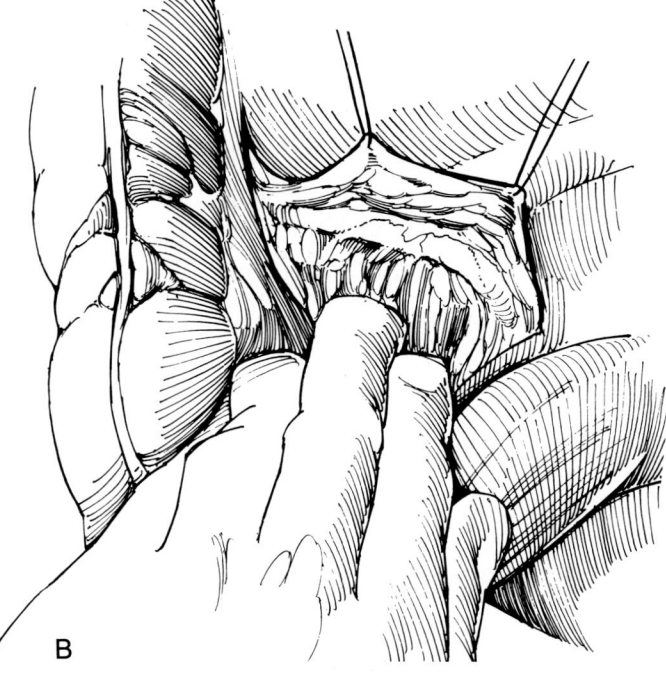

A

B

2 With the left thumb and forefinger, grasp the sigmoid colon at its junction with the rectum to elevate the tenia. Incise the peritoneal coat and muscularis for 5 to 6 cm with a #15 blade scalpel until the white submucosa is expressed.

3 Separate the muscle from the submucosa with a curved mosquito clamp for at least 1 cm on either side of the incision to provide muscular flaps to cover the anastomosis.

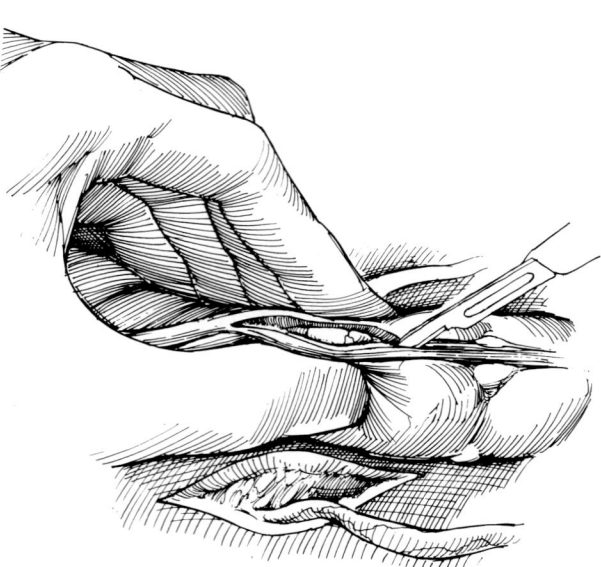

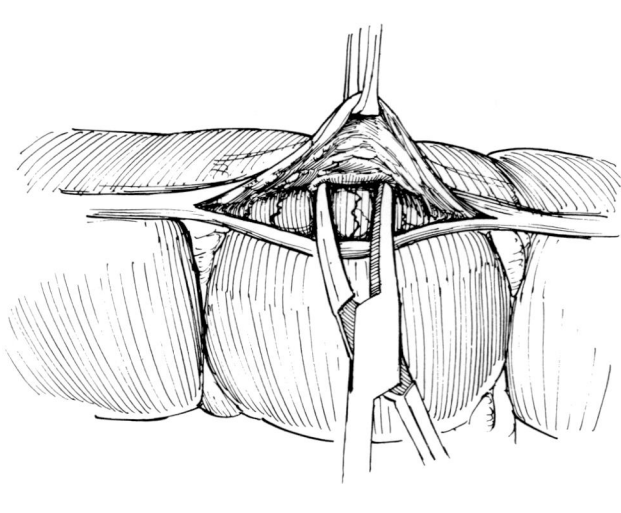

4 Tack the medial flap of the posterior peritoneum adjacent to the bowel incision on the right to the serosa with 4-0 or 5-0 synthetic absorbable sutures.

5 Hold up a bit of the submucosa in fine forceps, and excise the elevated tip to leave a 3-mm opening into the bowel. Mucus will exude; if not, insert the tip of a small clamp to be sure the bowel has been entered. The opening will enlarge surprisingly during the anastomostic procedure.

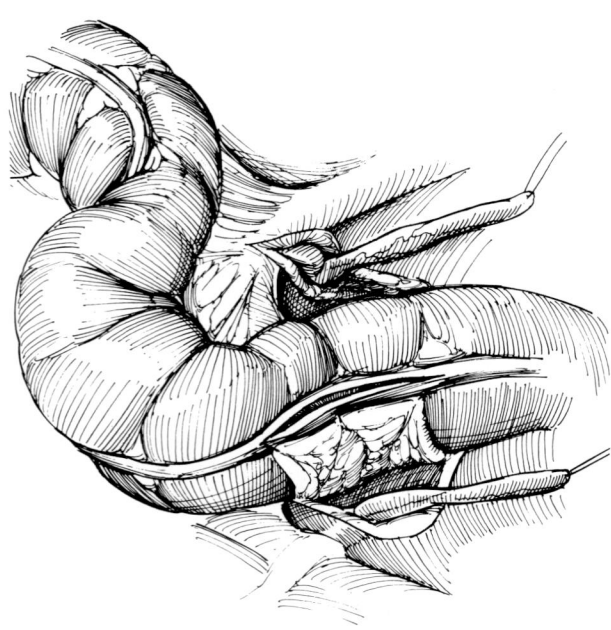

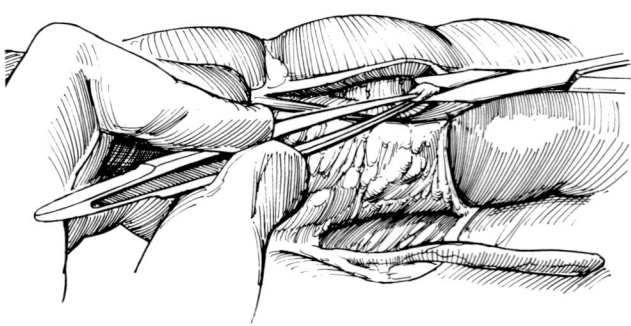

6 Trim the ureter to the proper length to avoid kinking. Spatulate it and replace the stay suture. Place a 4-0 or 5-0 synthetic absorbable suture through the mucosa and submucosa of the bowel from the outside in, then through the apex of the ureteral cut from the inside out. Place a second suture next to the first and tie both of them.

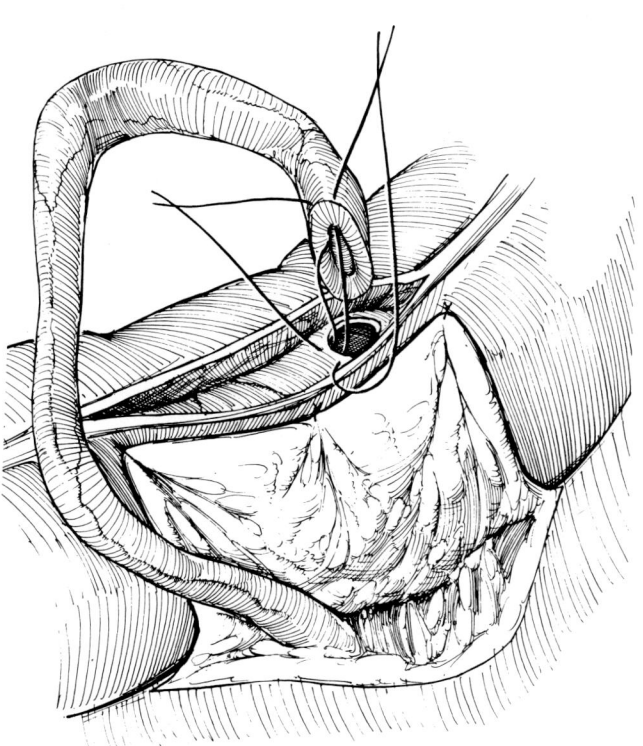

7 Run one suture down each side, locking a stitch occasionally, and tie them together at the tip.

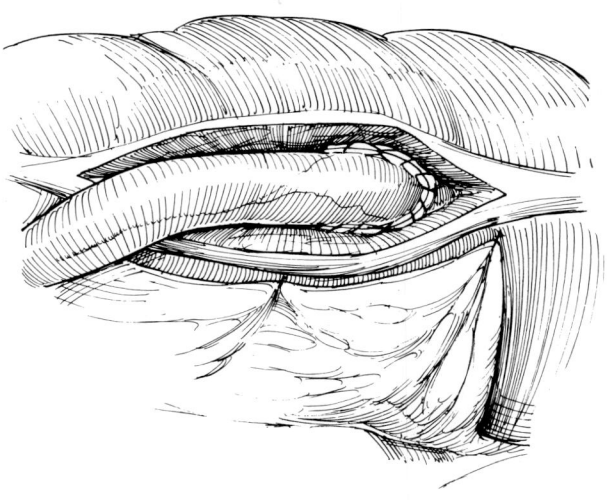

8 Approximate the seromuscular layer over the anastomosis with interrupted 4-0 or 5-0 synthetic absorbable sutures, taking care not to constrict the site of ureteral exit (leave the hiatus twice the diameter of the ureter). Bring the area of closure to the lateral flap of peritoneum, and suture it in place with 4-0 synthetic absorbable sutures.

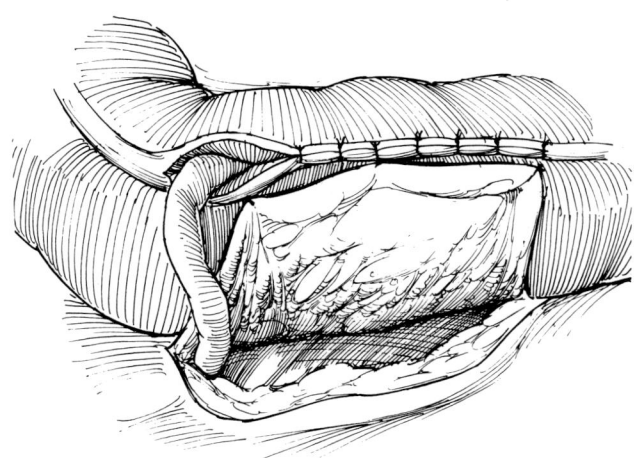

9 Repeat the procedure on the left side. Stents usually are not indicated. Close without drainage.

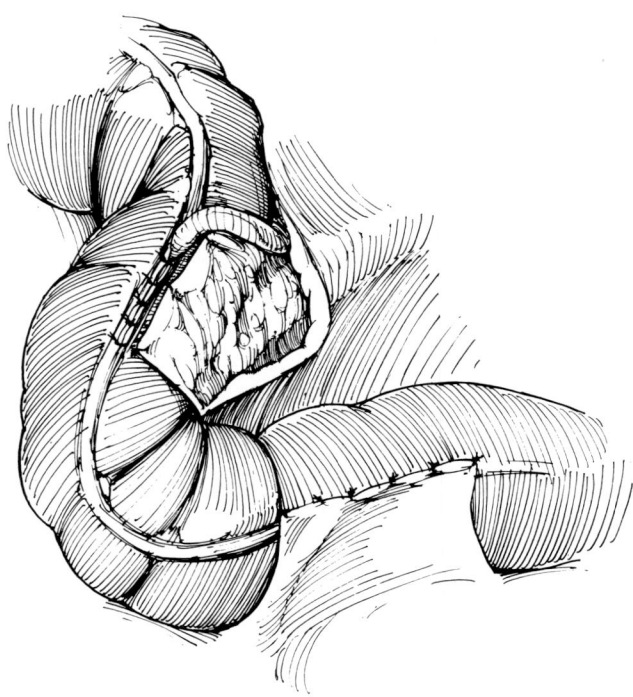

CLOSED TECHNIQUE FOR URETERAL IMPLANTATION
(KELALIS MODIFICATION)

10 **A,** At Step 5 of the Leadbetter technique, spatulate the ureter. Incise through the muscular coat of the colon for 1 or 2 cm—just enough to expose the submucosa. Pick it up in Adson forceps, and trim a very small button of mucosa and submucosa with fine scissors.

B, Anastomose the mucosa of the ureter to the mucosa at the opening in the bowel using interrupted 4-0 or 5-0 synthetic absorbable sutures in a watertight fashion. Incorporate the anastomosis into the bowel by placing a series of 4-0 nonabsorbable sutures over the ureter, starting the stitch laterally and exiting from the bowel wall approximately 1 cm from the tenia, then entering on the other side 1 cm from the tenia and exiting laterally. Tie the sutures successively from the distal end, making sure that the ureter is not constricted.

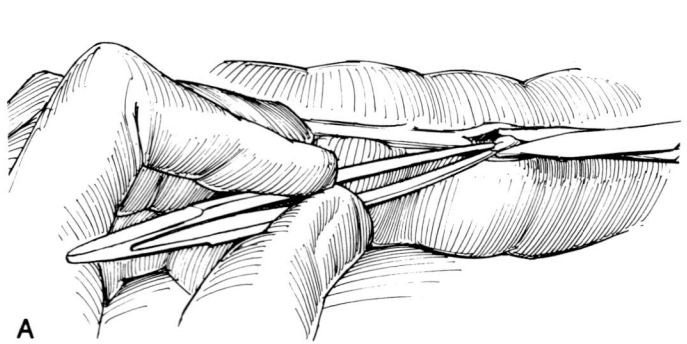

A

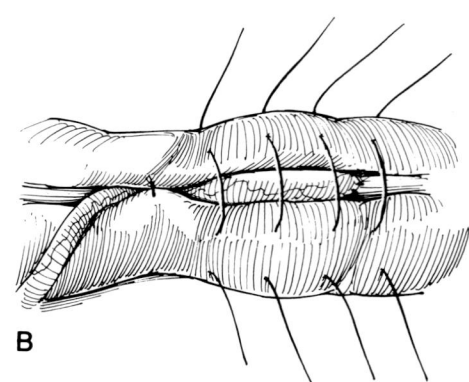

B

TRANSCOLONIC URETEROINTESTINAL ANASTOMOSIS
(GOODWIN)

11 **A,** *Incision:* Lower midline. **B,** Retract the sigmoid colon to the left, and incise the peritoneum over the right ureter, just below the crossing of the iliac vessels (where it is most easily identified); continue the incision to as low a point as possible.

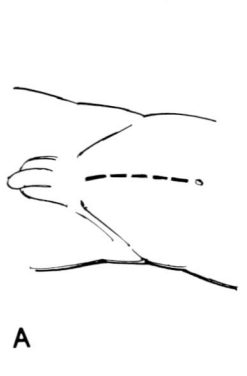

A

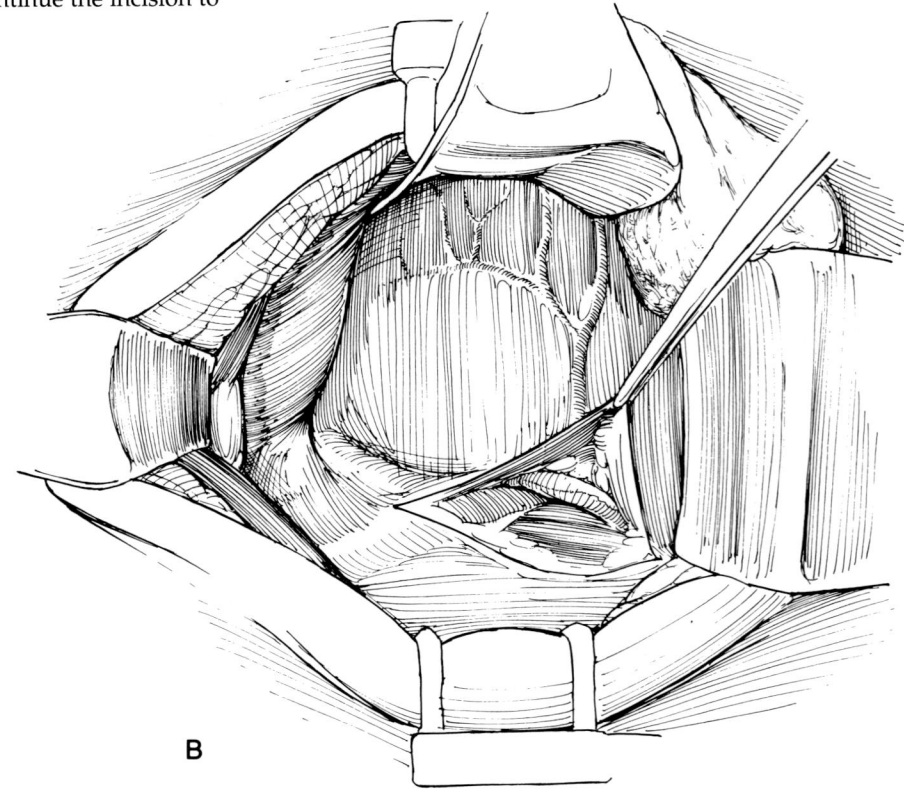

B

12 Free the right ureter sharply from the level of the sacral promontory, a distance of 10 to 12 cm toward the bladder, taking care to preserve the vessels in the adventitia. A small branch from the iliac artery is commonly encountered and should be left intact. Dissection of the ureter above its crossing of the iliac artery may jeopardize its circulation. Clamp the ureter distally with a right-angle clamp if it has not already been freed. Place a 4-0 silk stay suture just proximal to the clamp. Divide the ureter between, and ligate the stump with a 4-0 or 5-0 synthetic absorbable suture. Release the left ureter similarly.

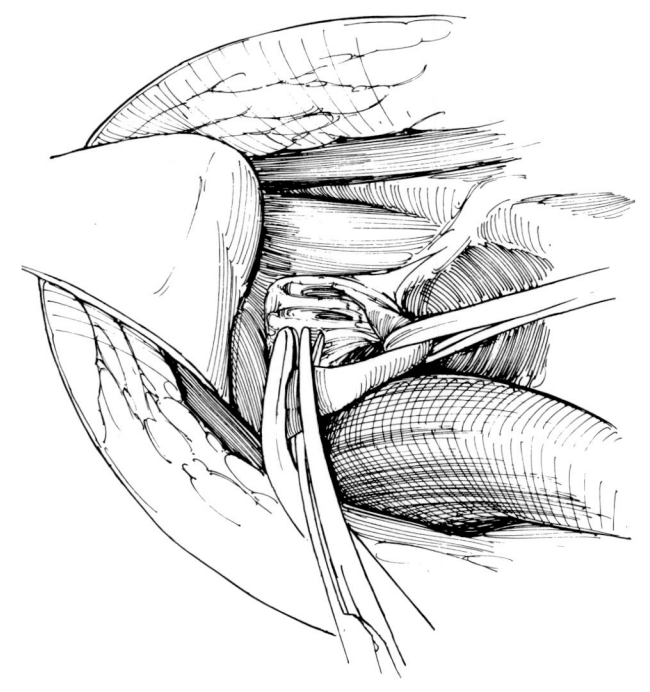

13 Grasp the rectosigmoid and deliver it out of the pelvis to permit positioning of the ureterocolic anastomosis as low as possible. Incise the bowel along the exposed tenia coli as low as feasible for 10 to 12 cm, cutting through the wall into the lumen. Stay sutures may be helpful.

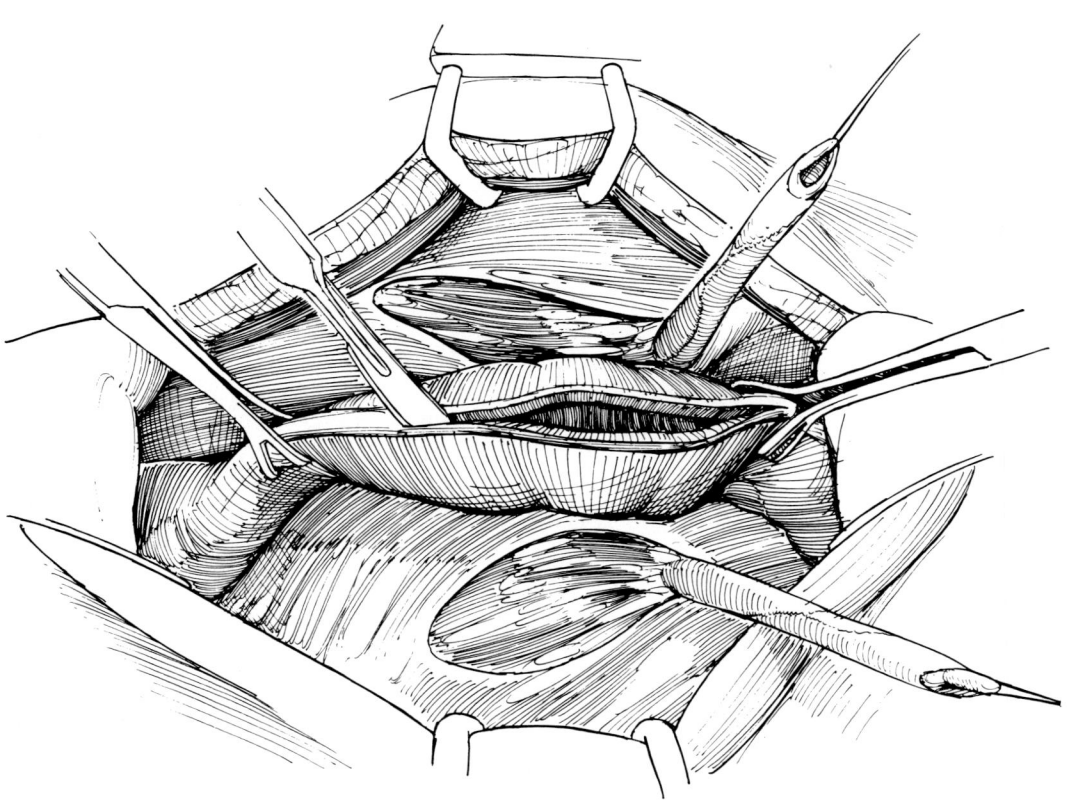

14 Insinuate the left index finger under the bowel, inserting it retroperitoneally through the defect used to expose the left ureter. Evert the posterior wall of the bowel through the colotomy. Place one or two stay sutures, and make a 1-cm transverse incision through the bowel mucosa and submucosa against the fingertip near the distal end of the exposed bowel wall. Alternatively, remove a button of mucosa and submucosa. Place a stay suture, and infiltrate the submucosa proximally with saline. Gently introduce a small curved clamp or iris scissors between the mucosal layer and the thin muscularis to make a tunnel 3 to 4 cm long, very similar to that made for ureteroneocystostomy. Alternatively, split the mucosa to lay the ureter in the trough and cover it.

Rotate the fine curved clamp so that the tip is directed posteriorly. Press it against the finger outside, and push it through the right lateral bowel wall into the retroperitoneal space. Avoid the vessels palpable in the mesentery. Spread the jaws of the clamp to make an adequate opening for the ureter in the muscularis. Pass the tip of the clamp retroperitoneally to the right, out through the peritoneal defect.

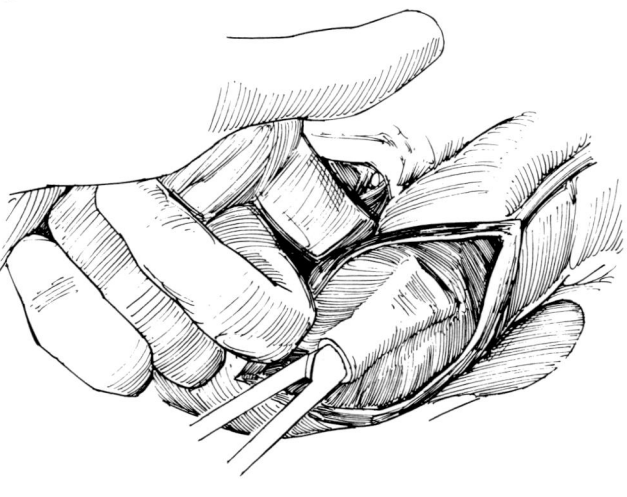

15 Grasp the stay suture on the right ureter, and draw the ureter into the bowel without tension. Repeat these maneuvers for the left ureter so that it will enter the bowel alongside the right one.

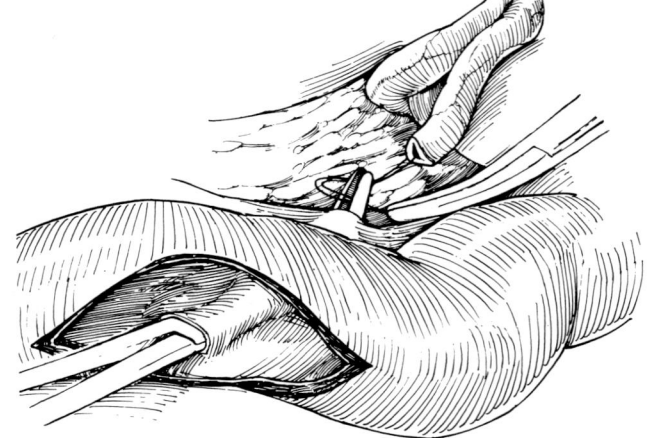

16 A, Trim excess ureteral length, and spatulate the ureters up to their point of entrance into the rectosigmoid while there is no traction on the stay suture. B, Suture the two ureters together along their medial edges for a distance of 2 cm, using several interrupted 4-0 synthetic absorbable sutures. Use the stay suture, not forceps, for manipulation.

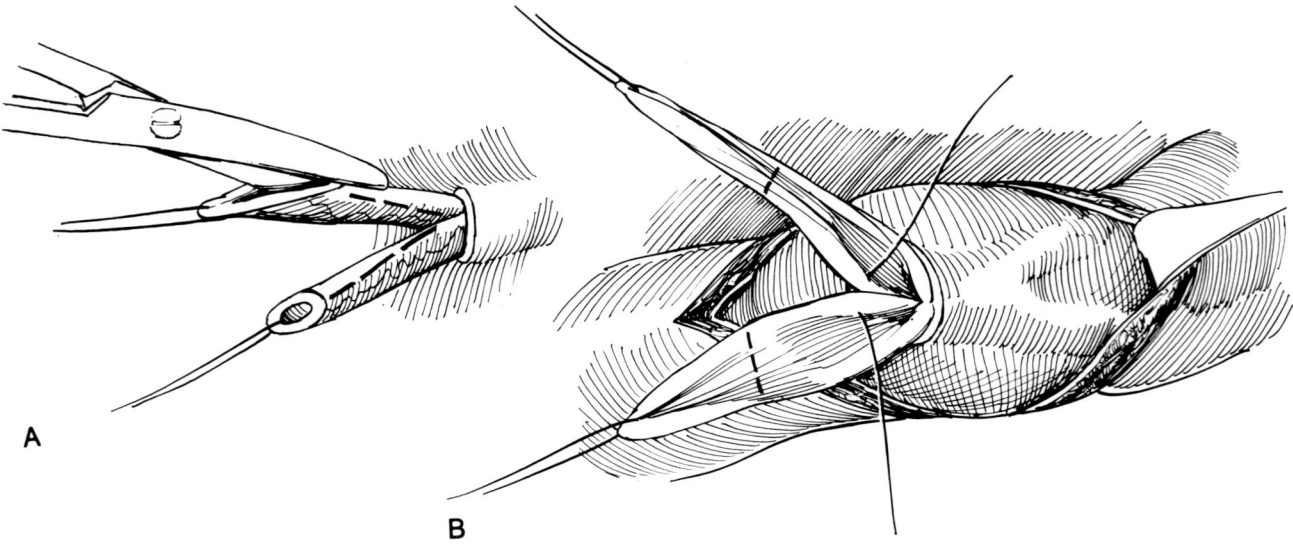

A

B

17 A, Continue the mucosa-to-mucosa anastomosis with interrupted sutures. Do not use forceps. B, Cross-sectional view.

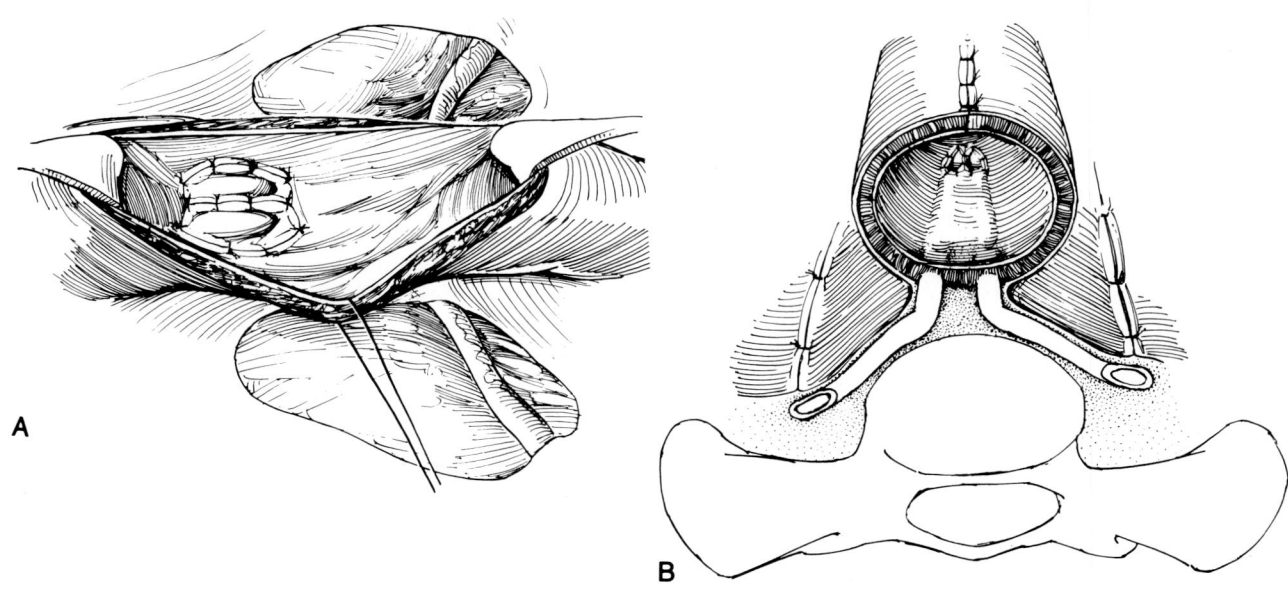

A

B

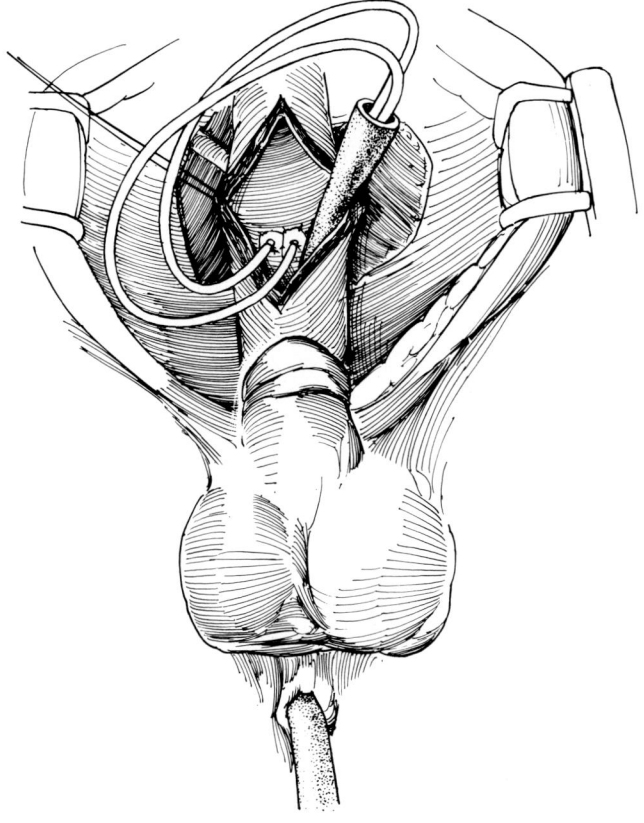

18 Stenting catheters (8 F infant feeding tubes, single-J catheters, double-J catheters or an open-ended stent) may be placed, cutting the distal end of the left one obliquely for identification. Suture each stent to the posterior wall of the bowel with a fine chromic catgut suture. If a rectal tube was not placed at the start of the procedure, pass one out the anus from above. Insert the stenting catheters into the upper flanged end to draw them out of the anus within the rectal tube.

19 Close the colotomy in two layers with continuous 4-0 chromic catgut sutures for the inner layer and interrupted 4-0 synthetic absorbable suture for the outer serosal and muscularis layers, and reapproximate the edges of the retroperitoneal openings. Insert a rectal tube from below. Alternatively, insert a large mushroom catheter into the rectum. Close the abdominal wound in layers.

At the end of the operation, suture the rectal tube to the anus, and tape the stents to the inside of the thigh with waterproof tape over tincture of benzoin (check them daily postoperatively). Perform a stentogram in 7 days; if the tract is intact, remove the stent. A contrast enema probably is not needed prior to removal of the rectal tube on the 10th day. Continue prophylactic antibiotics postoperatively for a month and watch for electrolyte disturbances.

MAINZ POUCH II (SIGMA RECTUM POUCH) (HOHENFELLNER)

The rectosigmoid colon may be detubularized to form a large pouch for urine storage.

20 Open the large bowel at the rectosigmoid junction along the tenia libera for 10 to 12 cm. Place two stay sutures approximately 4 cm apart at the site of the junction to create an inverted V. Anastomose the posterior wall with running 4-0 synthetic absorbable sutures for the seromuscular layer and 4-0 catgut for the mucosa. Implant the ureters from the free bowel margin if dilated (shown) or by the Goodwin technique if normal. Place ureteral stents.

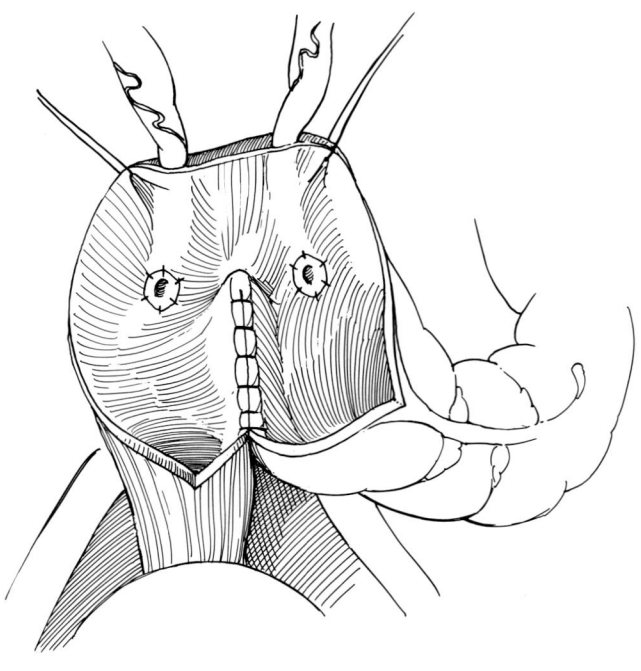

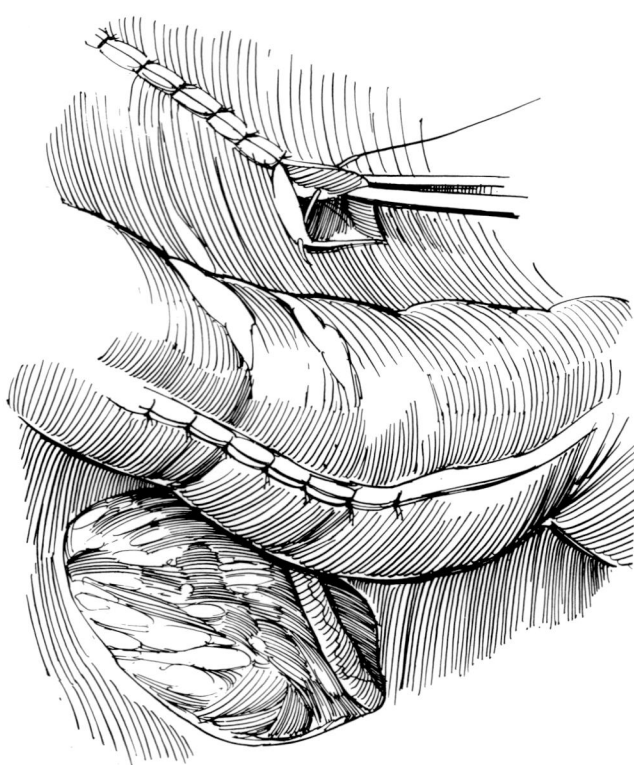

An *ileocecal ureterosigmoidostomy* (Rink and Retik, 1991) diverts the urine via the ileum into the sigmoid colon and may avoid carcinoma in the large bowel.

Isolate an ileocecal segment on the ileocolic vessels by detaching the ileal mesentery. The segment is composed of 12 cm of terminal ileum and enough cecum to contain an ileocecal intussusception. Grasp the ileum with Babcock clamps from within the cecum, and intussuscept it into the cecum. Hold it in place by the Hendren technique by dividing the ileal and cecal mucosa where they abut and suturing the margins with chromic catgut sutures to form a muscle-to-muscle connection. Anastomose the spatulated and combined ureters to the end of the ileum and make an end-to-side anastomosis of the cecum to the sigmoid colon.

21 Evaginate the "pig's ear" created by the posterior wall suture, and fix it to the fascia over the sacral promontory to stabilize the pouch. Insert a large rectal tube, and close the anterior wall in two layers.

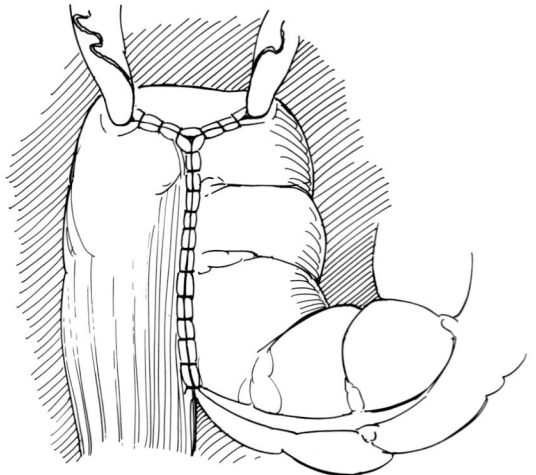

POSTOPERATIVE PROBLEMS

Oliguria and anuria most often are the result of inadequate intraoperative fluid replacement and hypotension. Try a challenge with furosemide (Lasix). Perform ultrasonography to detect hydronephrosis; if it is present, place percutaneous nephrostomies at once before anastomotic leakage occurs.

Leakage is heralded by fever and signs of peritonitis. Immediate reoperation is mandatory, although small leaks have been known to close spontaneously if the rectum is well drained. A *pelvic abscess* may develop after the first 5 to 10 days and requires drainage. Perform an ultrasound study (or a computed tomographic scan) to detect it.

Peritonitis, formerly a frequent complication and cause of death, now seldom occurs if the bowel is well prepared, suitable broad-spectrum antibiotics are given, and the anastomoses are extraperitonealized. *Incontinence,* especially at night, is common, even though many of the children had anal continence before diversion. When there are chronic urinary tract infections with *pyelonephritis,* the cause often is ureteral obstruction or reflux. Perform an enema with water-soluble contrast medium. Deterioration of the upper tracts is the result in a high proportion of patients. Early *obstruction at the ureteral anastomotic site* can be avoided by using a meticulous mucosa-to-mucosa technique, but late stenosis is frequent enough to require that intravenous urograms be made at least yearly so that reoperation can be done at the first evidence of upper tract obstruction or deterioration. Significant *hyperchloremic acidosis* usually is seen only in patients with existent or developing renal impairment. It may be prevented by a low-chloride diet with added sodium and potassium (as bicarbonate or citrate). Titrate the dose to keep the serum bicarbonate level nearly normal. Treat the decompensated patient with a rectal tube, fluids, and additional sodium and potassium bicarbonate. Frequent evacuation and retention of a rectal tube at night may reduce reabsorption and also avoid the not-unusual nocturnal incontinence.

Adenocarcinoma may occur at the site of anastomosis after an average interval of 25 years, with an incidence of 5 percent. The stools should be screened every 3 months, and colonoscopy is done yearly starting at the fifth anniversary. Should the ureterosigmoidostomy be converted to a ureteroileostomy or to cutaneous diversion, be sure to excise the terminal ureter and an adjacent cuff of colon to reduce later development of adenocarcinoma at the anastomotic site of the cutaneous diversion.

Commentary by R. Lawrence Kroovand

Intractable incontinence and upper tract deterioration unresponsive to nonoperative management remain the most common indications for permanent urinary diversion in childhood. Other indications include exstrophy of the bladder, lower urinary tract malignancy, and failed urinary tract reconstruction. Permanent urinary diversion should not be considered until all other forms of management have failed. Permanent urinary diversion may be either cutaneous (end-cutaneous ureterostomy; transureterocutaneous ureterostomy; or ileal, gastric, or sigmoid conduit) or internal (ureterosigmoidostomy). Vesicostomy, which can be a permanent form of diversion, is most appropriately used only for temporary cutaneous diversion in childhood.

Ureterosigmoidostomy is an internal urinary diversion that offers an alternative to cutaneous diversion whenever there are normal upper tracts bilaterally, normal renal function, and an intact anal sphincter. Some surgeons prefer this procedure to a cutaneous diversion because it allows for urinary control and also avoids external evidence of urinary diversion. Children with neurogenic disease generally do not have an intact anal sphincter and, therefore, are not candidates for ureterosigmoidostomy. The procedure has been used predominantly in children with epispadias and exstrophy. However, because these children may have an incomplete anal sphincter continence, they should be carefully evaluated preoperatively before ureterosigmoidostomy. Children with sarcomas of the prostate, bladder, or vagina who require urinary diversion may be considered for ureterosigmoidostomy, provided the rectum has not been irradiated.

A "two-stage" ureterosigmoidostomy has been advocated. In the first stage, a nonrefluxing sigmoid conduit is constructed. This permits evaluation of conduit function and anal sphincter tone at a later age, when assessment is more accurate. Once anal continence is documented, the conduit can be anastomosed to the intact sigmoid colon, establishing a continent internal urinary diversion. Preoperative evaluation should include an intravenous pyelogram (IVP) or isotope renogram and renal function studies. Anal continence may be tested preoperatively by use of a watery porridge enema. The ureters should be normal. A bowel preparation (both mechanical and antibacterial) is mandatory. Appropriately administered, polyethylene glycol–electrolyte solution (GoLYTELY) provides an excellent mechanical bowel preparation in children. Intravenous fluids should be administered during any pediatric bowel preparation to prevent dehydration and electrolyte imbalances.

The operative techniques described by Hinman are appropriate and require no comment. Although some surgeons prefer that the site of ureterocolonic anastomosis be as far distal on the rectosigmoid as possible, implantation higher on the sigmoid allows for conversion to a sigmoid conduit without refashioning the ureterocolonic anastomoses, should the ureterosigmoidostomy fail (note subsequent cautions).

Early complications of ureterosigmoidostomy include anastomotic urinary leakage, ureteroenteric anastomotic obstruction, and acute pyelonephritis. Long-term complications include hydronephrosis, chronic pyelonephritis, calculus formation, anal incontinence, and hyperchloremic metabolic acidosis with hypokalemia because of selective chloride reabsorption in the bowel and the exchange of potassium for hydrogen ions in the renal tubules. A degree of hypokalemia and acidosis is detectable in as many as 70 percent of those with ureterosigmoidostomy; however, this tends to be mild and asymptomatic unless there is coexisting renal damage; without treatment, growth retardation can occur. Sodium bicarbonate or sodium citrate and more frequent evacuation of urine may be adequate to correct the metabolic disorder. I prefer long-term prophylaxis with a potassium ion elixir to maintain normal metabolic balance and to prevent total-body potassium depletion, which can be present even with a normal serum potassium level. Even in those children with good anal sphincter function, some degree of anal urinary incontinence can occur, especially at night. Many may develop rectal irritability (proctitis) and perianal excoriation.

There are increasing reports of polypoid changes and colonic carcinoma at the site of ureterosigmoid anastomosis seen as early as 6, and as late as 31, years after the diversion, indicating a need for careful and continuing long-term follow-up. Because of these long-term problems, many authors question whether ureterosigmoidostomy ever should be done in children. To minimize psychologic disturbances from external diversion during childhood, I still find ureterosigmoidostomy useful for selected exstrophy patients. For the failed ureterosigmoidostomy or in adult life, the colon may be divided, and if the level of the ureteral implants permits, a segment containing the ureters is brought to the skin to create a sigmoid conduit. When converting an existing ureterosigmoid internal urinary diversion to a cutaneous diversion, to reduce the risk for malignant degeneration, it may be prudent to excise the ureterosigmoid anastomoses and create a new ureteroenteric anastomosis at a different site in the sigmoid colon. Any child with a urinary diversion of any type requires lifelong follow-up. A limited IVP 4 to 6 weeks after surgery rules out silent urinary obstruction. Upper tract surveillance is repeated yearly for 2 to 3 years and at least once every 2 years thereafter. For prolonged postoperative follow-up, the substitution of radionuclide scans and ultrasonography reduces radiation exposure. If renal function is abnormal, renal function studies and electrolyte levels are assessed several times a year. At each visit, the rectum is catheterized for residual urine, and a sample is obtained for urinalysis and culture and sensitivity. Many children will have asymptomatic acteriuria after ureterosigmoidostomy. This usually is well tolerated in the absence of reflux. Symptomatic urinary infections are treated appropriately. Long-term antibacterial prophylaxis may be indicated in some children Any perineal excoriation should be managed vigorously, a project best shared with an enterostomal therapist.

For ureterosigmoidostomy, periodic renal function studies and electrolyte determinations define the adequacy of timed "voidings" and the need for medication to correct any metabolic imbalance. Yearly proctoscopic examinations starting 5 to 10 years postoperatively are advisable to permit early detection of malignant changes at the site of ureterosigmoid anastomosis. An air pyelogram, hydronephrosis, renal parenchymal loss, or calculi are indications to convert ureterosigmoidostomy to cutaneous diversion, along with correction of the underlying pathologic condition. Although there are no consistent recommendations for the management of the defunctionalized bladder, reports of late development of malignancy in the defunctionalized bladder indicate a need for a protocol to follow these bladders systematically, including studies such as periodic bladder irrigations for cytologic study and cystography and endoscopy.

PART V

BLADDER AUGMENTATION

CHAPTER 88

Introduction to Bladder Augmentation
URETHRAL AND URETEROVESICAL JUNCTIONS PRESENT

If the urethra is intact, augmentation is indicated for the small-capacity, poorly compliant bladder, whether the problems are from intrinsic disease of the detrusor or neurologic overactivity, or they are secondary to spinal cord disorders or instability. This procedure is a necessary adjunct to functional rehabilitation of the exstrophic bladder. The upper urinary tract must be protected by antireflux mechanisms that are constructed from intussuscepted bowel segments forming a flap-valve in the intestinal wall or by tunnel implantation of the ureters.

Recently, the dilated, tortuous megaureter has been used to enlarge the bladder (Churchill, 1993), with the advatage of being free of mucus and absorption, and it is readily available in these cases. The ipsilateral kidney is removed after the pelvis and its blood supply are preserved, and the ureter dissected from the retroperitoneal with its segmental blood supply, especially the gonadal vessels, is preserved. The connection at the ureterovesical junction also is preserved. The ureter is opened on its lateral border, doubled on itself, and applied as a patch.

Except for interstitial cystitis, the bladder does not need to be excised during augmentation to permit good function. Excision complicates the procedure by requiring ureteral reimplantation. Attached bowel segments do act as diverticula when the communication with the bladder is restricted but not if the bladder is bivalved and the segment is detubularized. If the ureterovesical junction is obstructive or allows reflux, reimplantation into the bladder is preferable to a ureterointestinal anastomosis.

Important Points. Take a segment that is long enough to ensure adequate capacity but not so long as to jeopardize nutrition and foster electrolyte absorption. In certain cases (*eg*, irradiated bowel, cloa-cal exstrophy, or chronic renal failure, and in boys in whom excess mucus could obstruct the sphincter) use of the stomach may be preferable.

Evaluation before cystoplasty includes studies of renal function to ensure at least a minimum of reserve (*ie*, creatinine clearance greater than 40 ml/min and a serum creatinine level less than 2.5 mg/dl, unless the augmentation is preparatory to renal transplantation). Urine culture provides the basis for preoperative antibiotic therapy. In patients with interstitial cystitis, obtain a cytologic study to help rule out carcinoma *in situ*. Intravenous urography and renal scans define upper tract abnormalities, and a voiding cystogram can show gross distortions of the bladder, detect reflux, and ascertain whether urine is held at the bladder neck. An existing conduit also should be evaluated radiographically, and retrograde ureterograms should be made of the ureteral stumps, because these structures may prove useful in the repair.

The urethra and bladder neck should be visualized endoscopically under anesthesia to be certain that continence mechanisms are intact and that intermittent catheterization will be feasible, if required. Maximum vesical capacity can be determined at the same time. For patients with small bladder capacities even under anesthesia, insert a tube into the bladder percutaneously at this time, remembering that the peritoneum extends well inferiorly when the bladder is contracted, and cycle the bladder to see if the capacity will increase and if the continence mechanism is adequate. Alternatively, when intermittent catheterization is the goal, the bladder can be cycled using intermittent filling though a urethral catheter. Having the child do this will reveal the degree of motivation at the same time.

Urodynamic testing can document reflex activity, compliance, and sensation, with and without pharmacologic agents, and can determine the efficiency of voiding.

After augmentation, voiding dysfunction is inevitable. Resection of the bladder alters not only the sensation of filling but also the ability to open the bladder neck. Substitution of bowel for detrusor replaces the normal sustained detrusor contraction with involuntary and unsustained contractions characteristic of bowel. The result is poorly coordinated voiding, often with resultant residual urine with infection, stone formation, nocturnal incontinence, and, if the pressures are elevated, upper tract damage. Thus, not only must the capacity and compliance be increased by the procedure, but a balance must be established between urethral resistance and voiding pressure by altering sphincteric mechanisms or resorting to intermittent catheterization.

Formed from the terminal ileum, cecum, and ascending colon, four types of augmentation currently are in use: (1) ileocystoplasty, using a folded patch of ileum; (2) intact or detubularized colocystoplasty; (3) intact or detubularized cecocystoplasty; and (4) ileocecocystoplasty, using opened ileum to supplement the cecal pouch.

Artificial sphincters can be applied after bladder augmentation or substitution, usually necessitated by night-time incontinence. If some bladder remains, the cuff is placed about the trigone; if not, the cuff must be placed around the urethra or around the emergent segment of bowel, where it appears to be well tolerated if a wide cuff is used. It is important that the reservoir be compliant and store urine at low pressure. However, extra fluid must be added to the appliance reservoir at the time of insertion, because the bowel wall will shrink. The cuff must not be obstructive, and no other causes of outlet resistance should remain. However, if incomplete emptying persists, the child may have to resort to intermittent catheterization.

UNDIVERSION

Obtain serum creatinine levels and differential function by renal scan. Study the conduit function and bacterial content. Perform a voiding cystogram and cystometrogram of the native bladder. Perform cystoscopy and panendoscopy. Insert a suprapubic catheter if bladder cycling is to be done. For a neurogenic bladder, because it will be augmented, cycling is not necessary. The day following the initial studies, check the maximum bladder capacity by instillation through the suprapubic tube, and teach the patient intermittent catheterization. From these procedures, the need for bladder neck surgery and bladder augmentation can be estimated.

Three classes of patients are candidates for undiversion. In the first category are patients with sufficient ureteral length to require only cutaneous ureterostomy coupled with transureteroureterostomy. In the second are those without adequate length of the ureters so that a new ileal segment must be interposed. This may be supplemented by a bladder flap and augmentation with bowel, if needed. The third consists of patients with neurogenic bladders requiring excision and subtotal augmentation or substitution. Each case requires some imagination and inventiveness on the part of the surgeon.

Bladder neck reconstruction, insertion of an artificial sphincter, or construction of a continent stoma are options for the patient with sphincteric incontinence. Young, single adults most often desire undiversion. Even those patients with very poor renal function may benefit, because renal transplantation may be done later into a continent bladder.

PROBLEMS AFTER AUGMENTATION PROCEDURES

The most difficult problem to cope with is selecting the patient for the reconstruction procedure to avoid later problems. A child with marginal renal function and unsuitable bladder, ureters, or sphincters can have such problems. Most important is the capability of the child (and family) to want and care for a new system, especially the child's willingness to maintain a program of intermittent catheterization, if that should prove necessary.

Ureteral leakage becomes a problem if the ureter turns out to be too short for tension-free anastomosis. Preoperative estimation of length is important, and various techniques can be used intraoperatively to compensate (*eg*, psoas hitch, bladder flap repair, transureteroureterostomy, or as a last resort, interposed ileum). *Reflux* may arise from too short a tunnel after direct anastomosis or from failure of the constructed intestinal valve. *Stricture* at the site of ureterointestinal anastomosis may not appear for years.

Bladder dysfunction postoperatively leads to upper tract damage and incontinence. In a bladder with poor compliance, dysfunction can be avoided by augmentation with adequate bowel. In a patient with dyssynergia, pharmacologic manipulation and retraining may avoid complications.

Urinary infection is not a problem if the system is free of obstruction and empties satisfactorily. However, bacteriuria is common, and long-term antibacterial suppression usually is required.

Declining renal function results from any of the complications previously mentioned. Increased fluid intake will be needed postoperatively to compensate for fluid extraction from the bowel. Transient renal failure is not uncommon; in fact, a temporary rise in creatinine levels may be anticipated. Close follow-up, with regular determination of the serum creatinine level, is necessary. The reconstruction itself usually is not responsible for renal failure; rather, it is the progression of the underlying renal disease.

Wound infection with abscess formation is more common after colonic than after ileal operations. *Enteric fistulas* result from insertion of a tube through the bowel wall. Placement of a sump drain in the retropubic space and avoidance of nonabsorbable sutures and clips help. *Pelvic hematoma* is unlikely if good drainage is provided.

Inefficient evacuation of the bladder is the most common complication of cystoplasty, because peristaltic contraction is unsustained during voiding and works against outlet resistance. *Obstruction* present before cystoplasty must be detected urodynamically and corrected. Persistent outflow obstruction can be detected by determination of residual urine by catheterization or ultrasonography. Its site is determined by voiding cystography with or without pressure-flow studies. Resolution may require endoscopic incision of the bladder neck. Overdilatation of the urethra may help achieve balance in the female.

Incontinence can be a trying problem. Placement of a segment still capable of mass contraction will result in incontinence, which is why detubularized segments should be used. Too small a segment will fill too fast to its maximum capacity, at which point spontaneous contractions are stimulated. Opening the segment increases the capacity and reduces the incontinence. In spite of a normal outlet and good functional capacity, nocturnal wetting still may be a problem because of the relaxation of the sphincters. Diphenoxylate hydrochloride (Lomotil) decreases bowel contractility and increases capacity but has little effect on enuresis. Timed voiding every 4 hours and intermittent catheterization may be resorted to. If all these measures fail, consider surgically supplementing the augmentation. For the relaxed outlet, ephedrine and phenylpropanolamine may correct the problem. Otherwise, some form of continence procedure may be required.

For obstruction of the plicated ileocecal valve, try prolonged nephrostomy drainage, and revise if necessary. *Reflux* can occur when the ureters are im-

planted in the ileum and the ileocecal valve is incompetent. *Stenosis* of the vesicoenteric anastomosis results in a functional diverticulum with accompanying infection and vesical irritability.

Mucus secretion is a problem, usually greatest in the immediate postoperative period, because mucus production decreases with time if the bladder empties. The pouch must be irrigated completely and vigorously every 6 hours postoperatively, and the urinary flow must be monitored carefully, lest the segment overfill and the anastomoses become disrupted.

Renal function remains stable if the system drains effectively and the underlying renal lesion does not progress. For a patient with severely impaired renal function, in whom reabsorption may tip the balance, augmentation may be considered a preliminary step to renal transplantation.

Electrolyte imbalance, with increase in chloride and hydrogen ions, can affect the bone buffers and lead to stone formation. *Small bowel obstruction* from adhesions may require intubation or operation. Prolonged ileus can be a problem. *Neoplasms* can occur, even in augmentation with ileum.

The sites for postoperative problems and their remedies are outlined in Table 88–1, but the necessity for diligent lifetime follow-up must be reiterated.

Table 88–1. Complications With Corrective Options

Location	Complication	Corrective Options
Ureter	Stricture or loss	Ureteroureterostomy
		Mobilization of kidney
		Psoas hitch; bladder flap
		Ileal ureter
	Dilation	Tailoring
Ureterovesical junction	Stricture	Reimplantation
	Reflux	Reimplantation
		Ileal nipple
		Others
Detrusor	Reduced compliance	Pharmacology
		Neural manipulation
		Hydrodistention
		Augmentation
		Vesicostomy
	Increased compliance	Intermittent catheterization
Outlet	Contracture	Dilation
		YV-plasty
	Incompetence	Vesical neck repair
		Sling with intermittent catheterization
		Artificial sphincter
		Closure of neck
	Dyssynergia	Sphincterotomy
		Intermittent catheterization

CHAPTER 89
Ileocystoplasty
(GOODWIN)

Evaluate the child's general status and renal function. Determine vesical residual urine and capacity, detrusor compliance, and urethral function to select the appropriate procedure and to determine whether an increase in outlet resistance by bladder neck reconstruction or a reduction in outlet resistance is needed. Obtain an intravenous urogram and voiding cystourethrogram or loopogram to assess bladder size and ureteral length and configuration. A radionuclide scan helps define upper tract function. Cycle the bladder to increase its capacity. Preoperatively, consider the feasibility of intermittent catheterization. Is the urethra patent and accessible? Teach the patient how to perform self-catheterization. Espe-

cially consider the motivation of the patient for reconstruction, which must be strong to warrant operation. If capacity is limited or the outlet relaxed, warn the patient of the possibility of incontinence.

The ureters may be left in the bladder or may be reimplanted into the bowel via tunnels, with or without transureteroureterostomy. Implantation of the dilated ureter into the intussuscepted ileum is least desirable. In general, tunnels are preferable to nipples. Reimplant into the bladder whenever possible, although not at the expense of using ischemic ureter or reimplanting under tension.

Instruments: Provide an autosuture set with TA-55–4.8, TA-55–3.5, and EEA staplers.

1 **A,** *Position:* Supine. *Incision:* Make a lower midline transperitoneal incision (page 263), standing on the left side of the patient. Check the mobility and mesenteric length of the terminal ileum. The bladder may be opened at this time (proceed to Step 4), or the bowel may be prepared first.

B, Choose a 20- to 25-cm loop of ileum, leaving the last 10 to 15 cm of terminal ileum in place, as for an ileal conduit (page 373). Mark the ends and the center with stay sutures. Draw the center of the loop over the dome of the bladder to be sure it will reach the anterior part of the proposed vesical anastomosis. Divide the ileum between Kocher clamps. The mesentery, which should be well vascularized, needs to be divided for a shorter distance than for ureteroileostomy. Reapproximate the ileum. Irrigate the loop with saline solution until clear, then with 1 percent neomycin solution (kept away from the peritoneum), and finally with air. Divide the ileal segment along its antimesenteric border with straight Mayo scissors or with the cutting current. Alternatively, before opening the bowel, shape it into a loop and suture the adjacent serosal surfaces together with a running 4-0 chromic catgut suture.

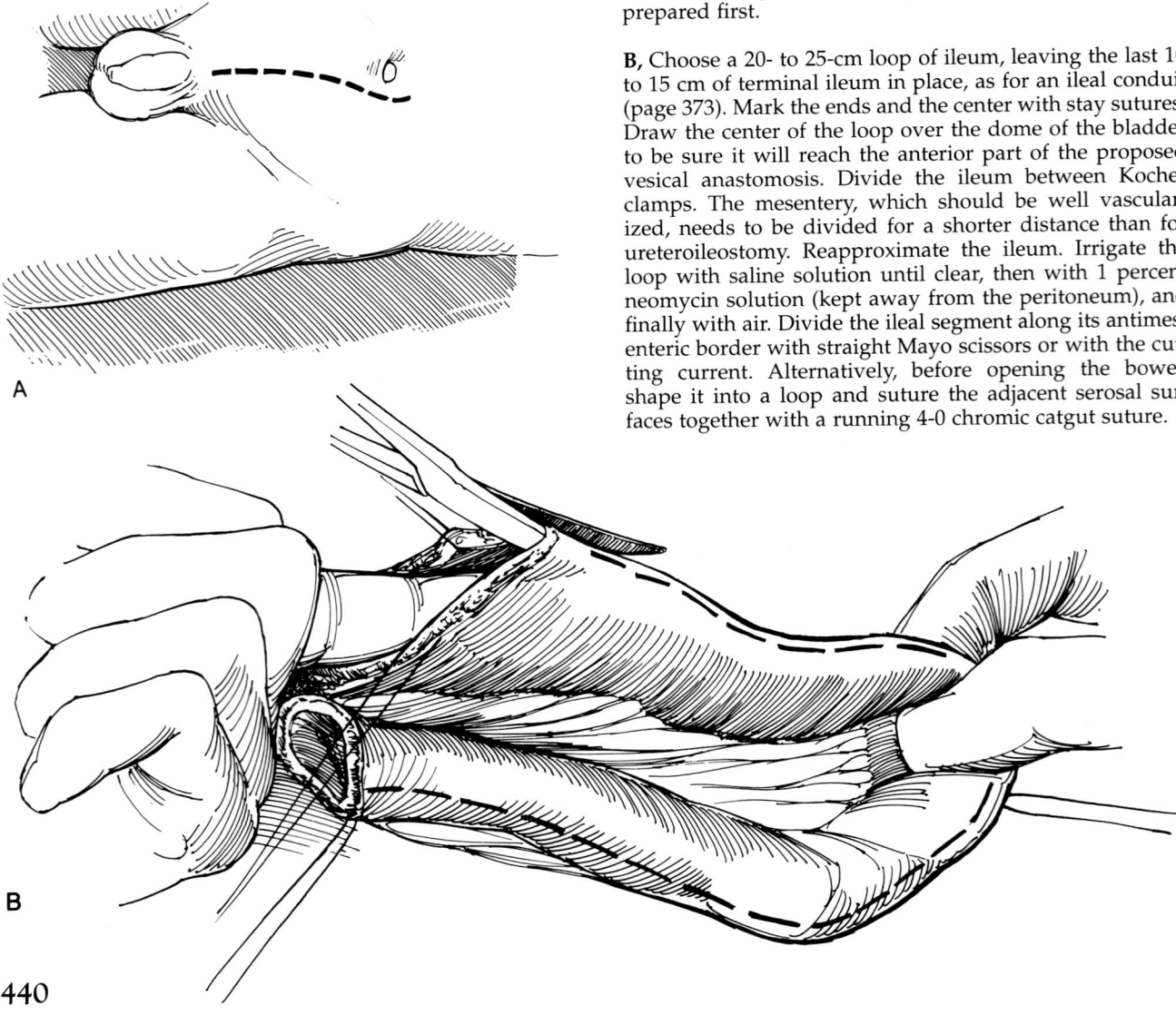

A

B

2 Suture the adjacent mucosal edges with a continuous 3-0 chromic catgut suture. Use an atraumatic tapered needle through all layers of the bowel. Tie the suture once on the outside to prevent bunching of the suture line.

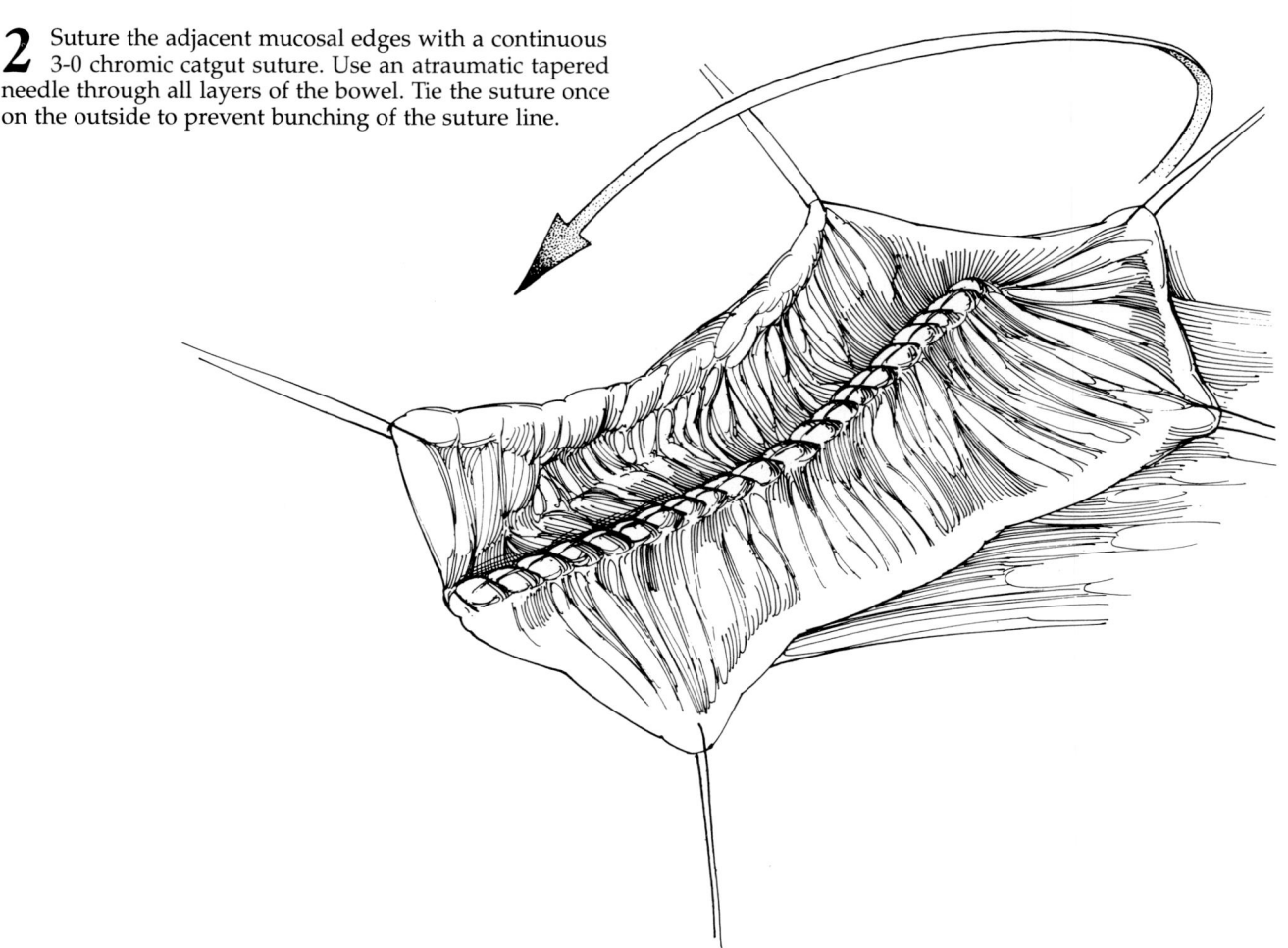

3 Fold the open end of the segment over on itself and suture it along each margin to form a cup. If a larger opening is desired for the anastomosis to the bladder, do not suture the edges together for their entire length. Watch for interference with the blood supply.

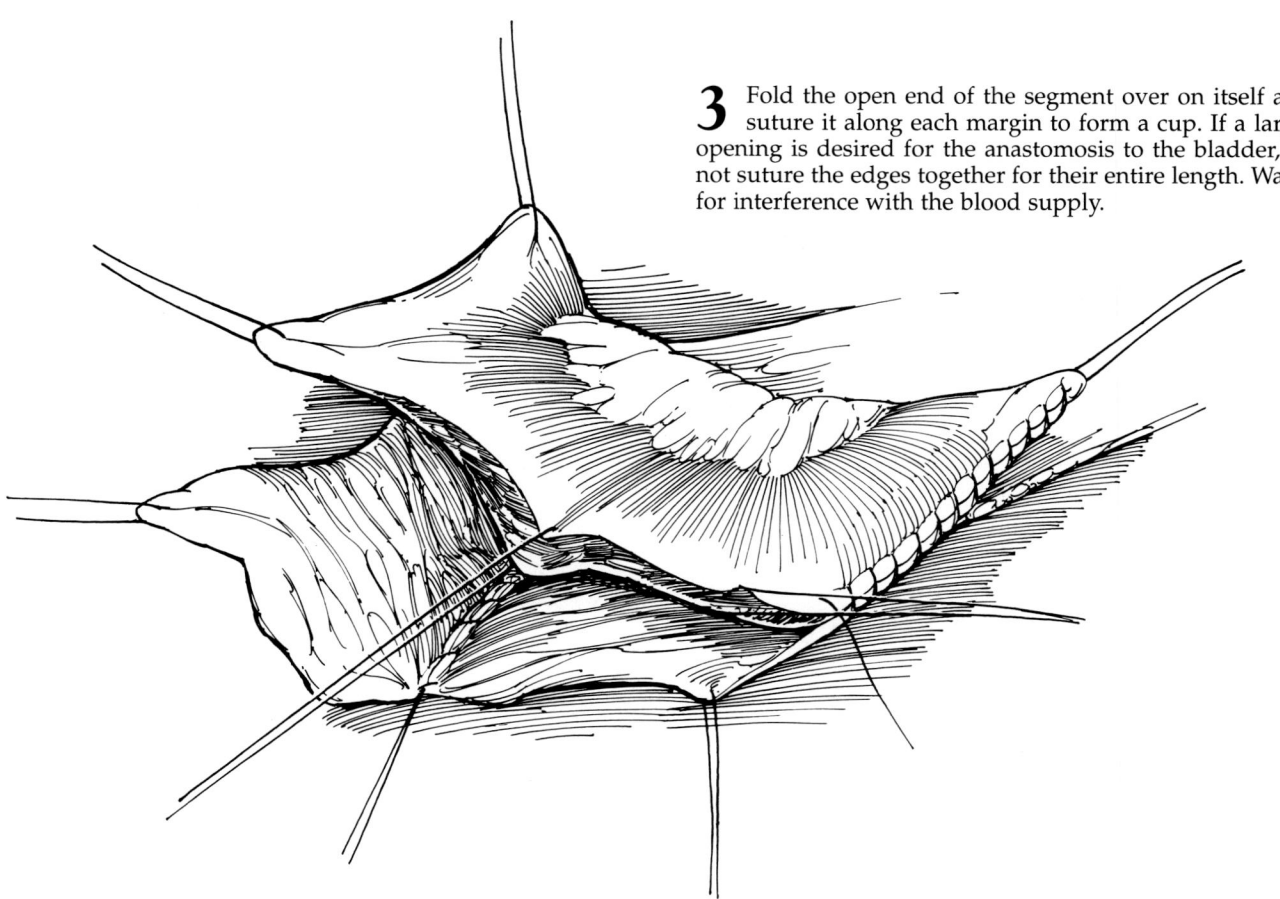

4 Grasp the bladder at the apex adjacent to the peritoneal reflection. Sharply divide the lateral peritoneal attachments as far as the superior vesical pedicle. Free the bladder anteriorly and elevate it into the wound. Open the bladder sagittally as far posteriorly as possible, using the cutting current and ligating large vessels with 4-0 catgut. Although a coronal incision is an alternative, a sagittal incision will suffice even for very small bladders. Insert infant feeding tube catheters to identify the ureters and place a Malecot cystostomy tube away from the suture line. The tube should be inserted through the wall of the bladder, but if the bladder is very small, it may be placed through the new augmentation as shown in the figure.

Place the posterior rim of the ileal cup adjacent to the posterior apex of the bladder incision and, starting posteriorly, run a 3-0 chromic catgut suture through all layers up each side to form a watertight closure. Tie the sutures several times during insertion to prevent gathering and take extra care where the suture lines meet. Reinforcement with 2-0 chromic catgut sutures may be helpful, especially posteriorly where tension can exist. An alternative method: before folding the superior end of the segment on itself, start anastomosing the inferior end to the bladder, and continue the suture to the midway point of the bladder incision. Now fold the doubled ileum over and start suturing from the midline anteriorly around each side. Continue the suture to approximate the ileal edges to form the "clam" in place.

A YV-plasty at the vesical neck should be considered only when intermittent catheterization is not planned. An artificial sphincter may now be applied; the chance of contamination is minimal because ileal contents are sterile.

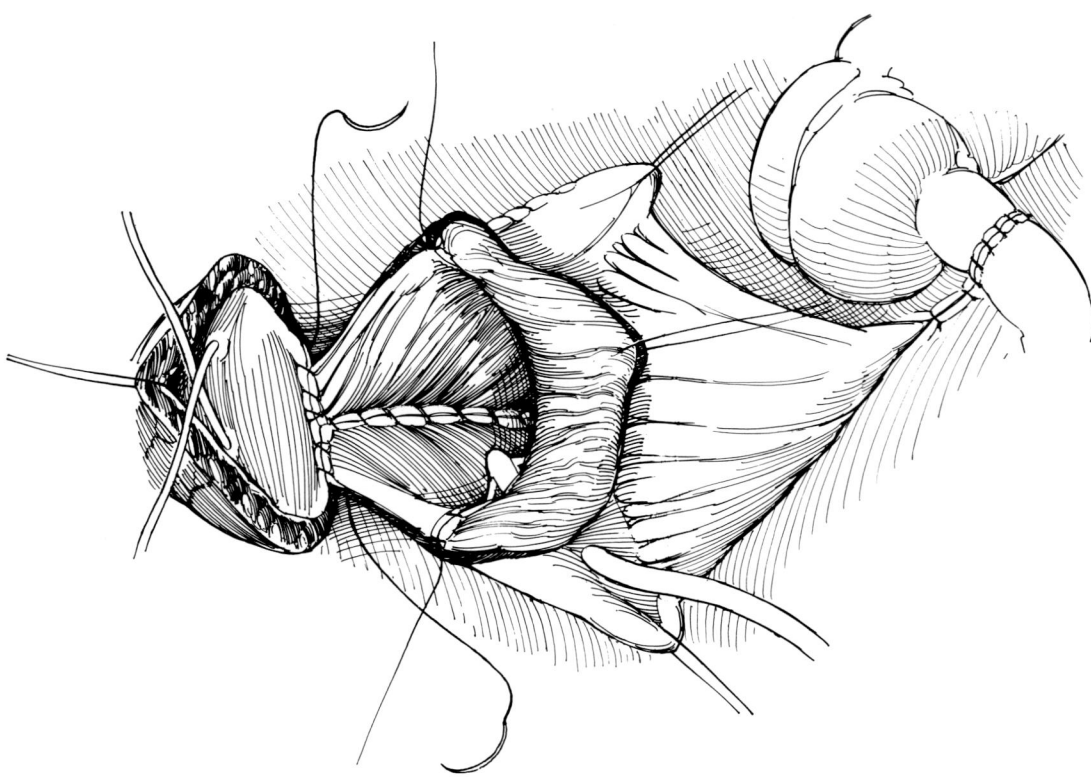

5 Remove the ureteral catheters and close the mesentery. If the peritoneum is especially redundant, incise it and wrap it around the mesentery of the augmentation to retroperitonealize the isolated bowel segment. Fix the mesentery of the segment to the posterior peritoneum to prevent an internal hernia. Free the omentum from the transverse colon and tack it posteriorly first and then wrap it around the repair to cover the suture lines. Test the augmentation by filling it with saline and reinforce it at the site of leaks. Place one (or two, if the anastomosis is tenuous) Jackson-Pratt drain for suction. Insert a silicone balloon catheter into the bladder through the urethra for extra security during the immediate postoperative period. Close the wound in layers around the drains.

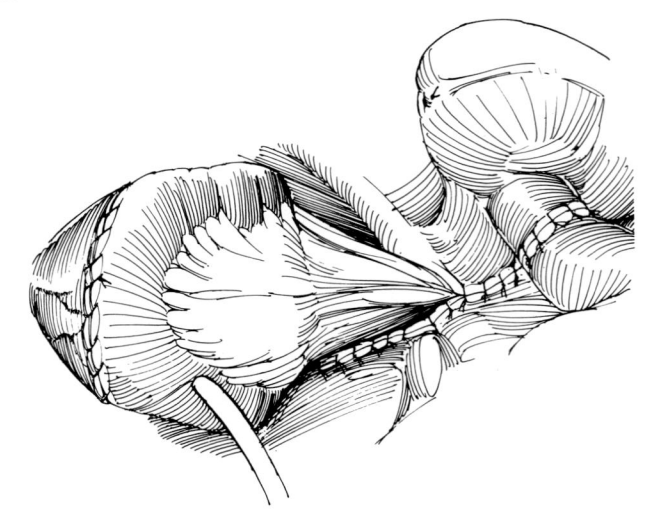

CONVERSION OF ILEAL CONDUIT (HANNA)

To provide a continent pouch, open the ileal conduit to be used as a patch. Reimplant the ureters by a nonrefluxing technique into this patch. Take a new ileal segment and form an intussuscepted nipple in its distal third. Open the remainder and apply the patch to it. For extra capacity, fold the opened loop on itself twice, suture the edges, and then fold the entire plate into a cup.

HEMI-KOCK PROCEDURE

6 Follow steps of Ileocystoplasty (pages 440–442). Resect a loop of ileum 5 cm long, and open the distal 30 cm on the antimesenteric border.

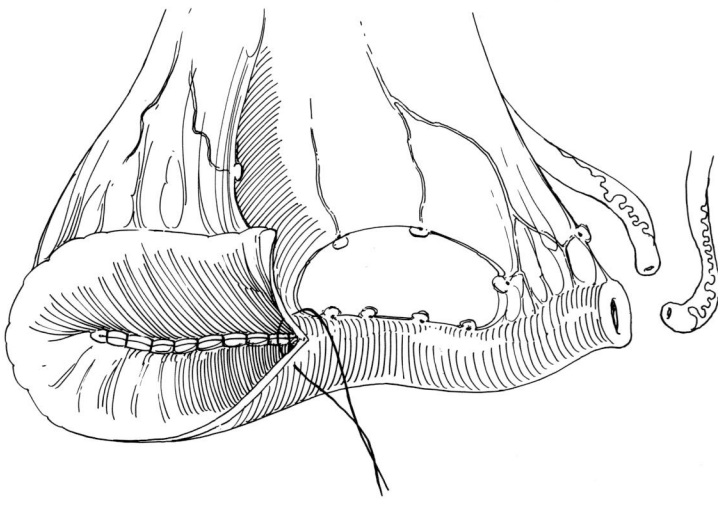

7 Fold the opened flap on itself to form a patch. Clear the mesentery from half of the more proximal segment, and intussuscept the ileum to form a nipple. Incise the full thickness of the outer wall of the nipple, denude the adjacent muscle in the pouch, and suture the two surfaces together with 3-0 synthetic absorbable sutures. Anastomose the cup to the remainder of the bladder and implant the ureters in the end of the proximal ileum with stents. Suture the pouch to the levator ani muscles on both sides. Insert a balloon catheter through the conduit and secure it and the stents to the skin. Postoperatively, monitor drainage from the ureteral catheter every 6 hours. If it declines, irrigate the catheters. After 2 weeks, do a cystogram at minimal pressure (15 to 20 cm H_2O). If leakage is seen, leave both catheters in place another week and repeat the study.

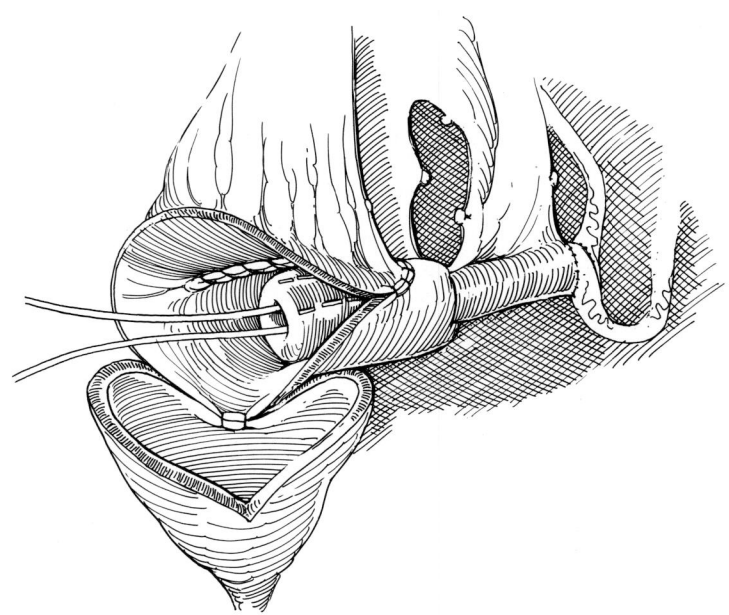

Postoperative Care

Maintain nasogastric suction until good-quality bowel sounds are heard. Have the system irrigated with normal saline three times a day to clear the mucus. The broad-spectrum antibiotics may be stopped after 5 days and the drains removed when drainage ceases. Before discharge, teach the child how to irrigate the bladder daily. Make a cystogram through the cystostomy tube in 2 weeks to ascertain the integrity of the anastomoses. Clamp the tube; if the child can either void or perform intermittent catheterization, remove it. Even if the child voids, he or she should check the bladder once a day for a couple of weeks for residual urine.

Commentary by Edmond T. Gonzales, Jr.

The use of bowel to refunctionalize the urinary tract has become increasingly popular with the introduction of clean intermittent catheterization and improved antirefluxing techniques for ureteral implantation into bowel. By combining these principles with the large-volume, low-pressure reservoir that can be constructed with an intestinal segment, either used to augment the bladder or as an entirely free-standing urinary reservoir, the progressive

deterioration of renal function seen with the ileal conduit can be avoided. The more recent introduction of new continent stomas, using appendix, ureters, tapered bowel, or bowel nipples, has allowed the development of innovative continent reservoirs. The days when an appliance was necessary any time urinary diversion was considered are long gone.

However, the use of bowel in these situations demands a dedicated commitment on the part of the surgeon to achieve optimal results. Meticulous technique is required to preserve blood supply to the intestinal segment and to maintain integrity of all suture lines. Continent catheterizable channels must be thoughtfully positioned to avoid problems with catheterization postoperatively. Mucus production does seem to decrease but never goes away entirely and will require constant management with a regular irrigation program. Calculi in the pouch seem to be another long-term problem. Finally, the risk of spontaneous rupture has added a new dimension of concern for the patients. Whether there is an increased risk of carcinogenesis remains controversial but bears special consideration.

Despite all of these issues, vesical augmentation and the development of continent stomas have improved the quality of life for countless patients with vesical dysfunction who present with incontinence and/or progressive renal parenchymal damage.

CHAPTER 90

Colocystoplasty and Sigmoidocystoplasty

(MITCHELL)

1 *Position:* The patient is placed supine. In girls, prepare and drape the perineum so that a catheter can be inserted aseptically. Instruments and preliminaries are the same as those for ileocystoplasty.

Incision: Stand on the patient's left side. Make a lower midline transperitoneal incision (page 263), from the symphysis to just above the umbilicus. Alternatively, if you are confident that an ileal or sigmoid patch can be used, make a transverse skin incision combined with a vertical midline incision in the fascia, a more-cosmetic but more-limiting approach. Pack the small intestine into the upper abdomen. Because there is a possibility that the appendix will be needed as a cutaneous conduit, do not perform an appendectomy.

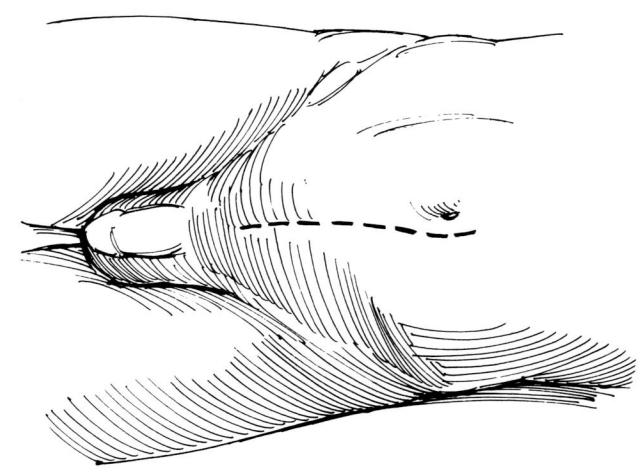

2 Study the colonic vasculature for the distribution of the sigmoid artery from the inferior mesenteric artery, and select a length of sigmoid colon of at least 15 cm, preferably 20 cm or more, which is mobile and has a very broad mesentery. Be sure to take enough bowel.

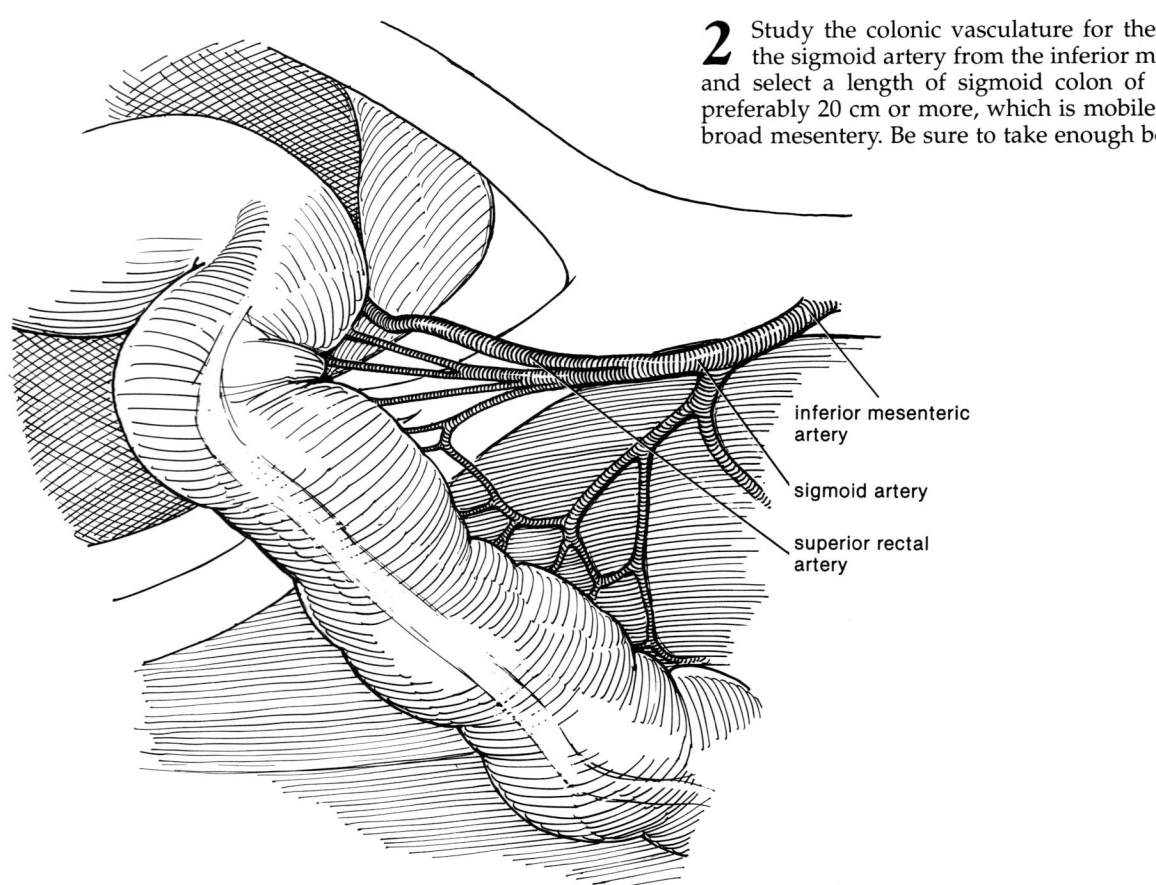

inferior mesenteric artery

sigmoid artery

superior rectal artery

444

3 Separate the loop of sigmoid colon from the retroperitoneum with scissors along the white line of Toldt. Mark the selected length with a silk stay suture. Pull the loop down to be sure the bowel can be reanastomosed without tension. Divide the mesentery, but not as deeply as for a sigmoid conduit (page 393). Divide the bowel between two pairs of Kocher clamps, and fulgurate the exposed mucosa.

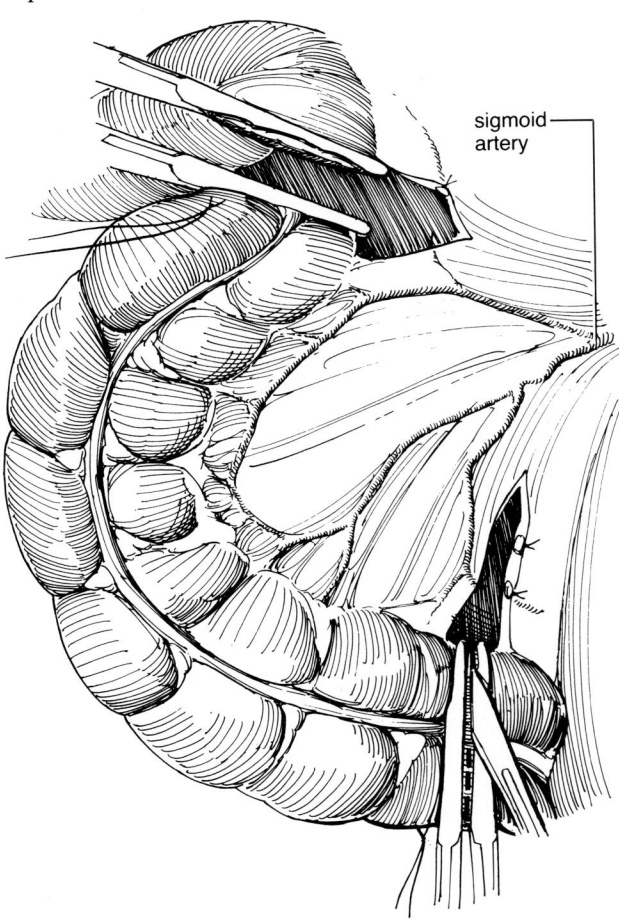

4 Reanastomose the colon in two layers with staples (page 33) or sutures after making sure the colon is anterior to the isolated segment. Place noncrushing intestinal clamps (Doyen) 2 cm proximal to each Kocher clamp; remove the Kocher clamps. Insert a posterior row of six or eight interrupted inverting horizontal mattress sutures of 4-0 silk.

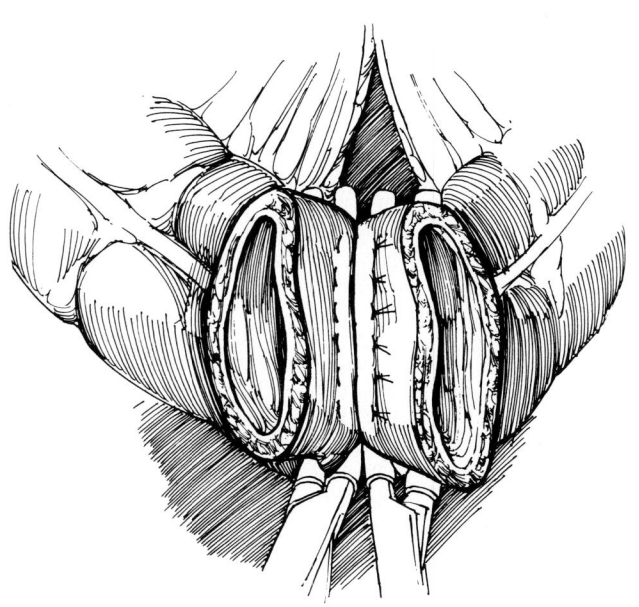

6 Tie the suture in continuity near each corner to prevent pursestringing. Construct the corners carefully, using one suture at a time, going from mucosa to serosa on one side and serosa to mucosa on the other (half-Connell suture). Tie another incontinuity knot at each corner anteriorly. Continue with an inverting suture from each end, going in and out on one side and in and out on the other (Connell suture). Tie the sutures in the midline. Remove the Doyen clamps. As an alternative to the running 4-0 polypropylene sutures, place a layer of inverting interrupted 4-0 silk sutures. Use of interrupted sutures in the inner layer prevents possible pursestringing with resultant narrowing at the anastomosis.

5 Start one double-armed or two single-armed 4-0 polypropylene sutures in the center posteriorly. Run the sutures in opposite directions. Take 3 mm of tissue in each bite, and keep the stitches close together.

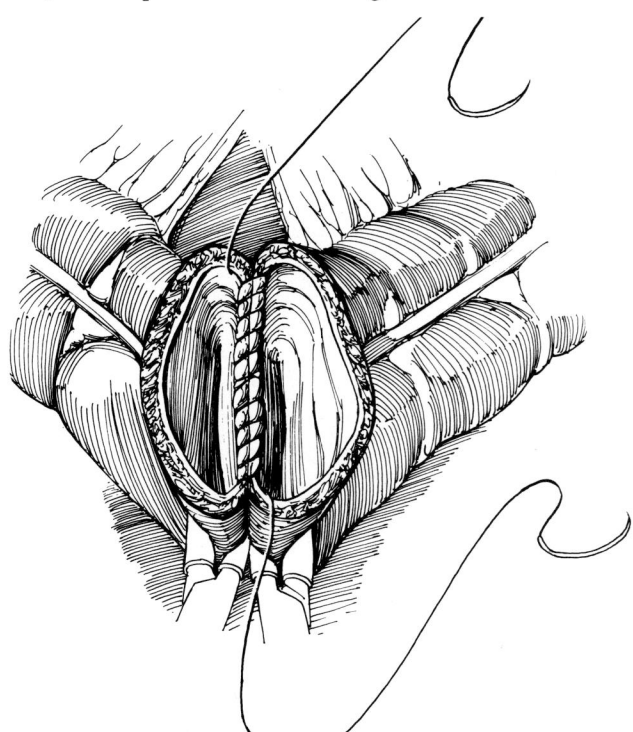

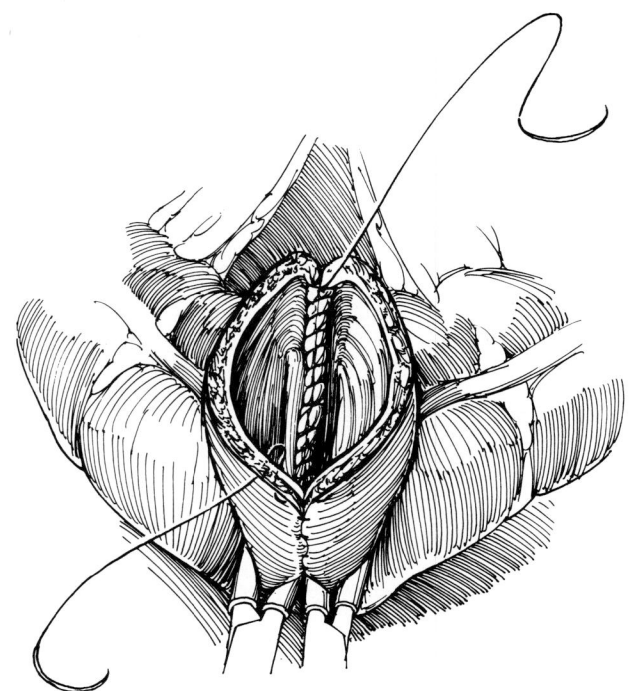

7 Place an anterior layer of interrupted inverting sutures of 3-0 or 4-0 silk through the serosa and superficial muscularis.

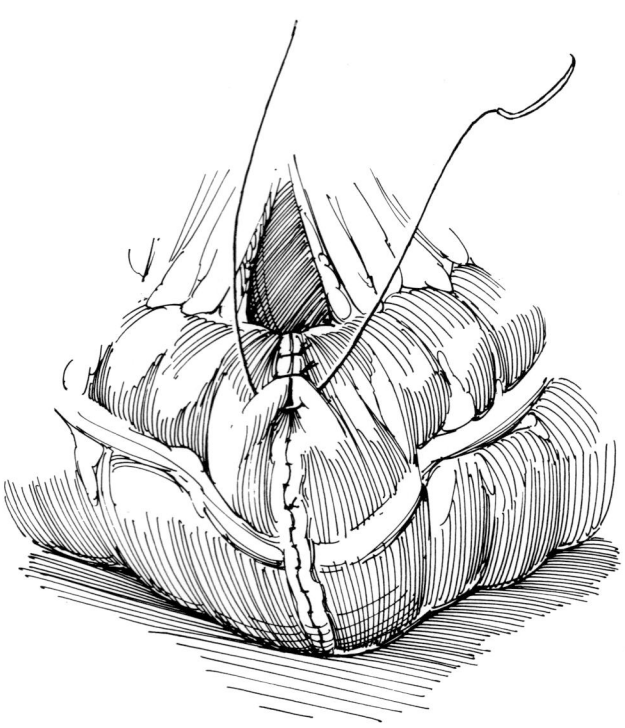

8 Close the mesocolon with a running 4-0 chromic catgut suture.

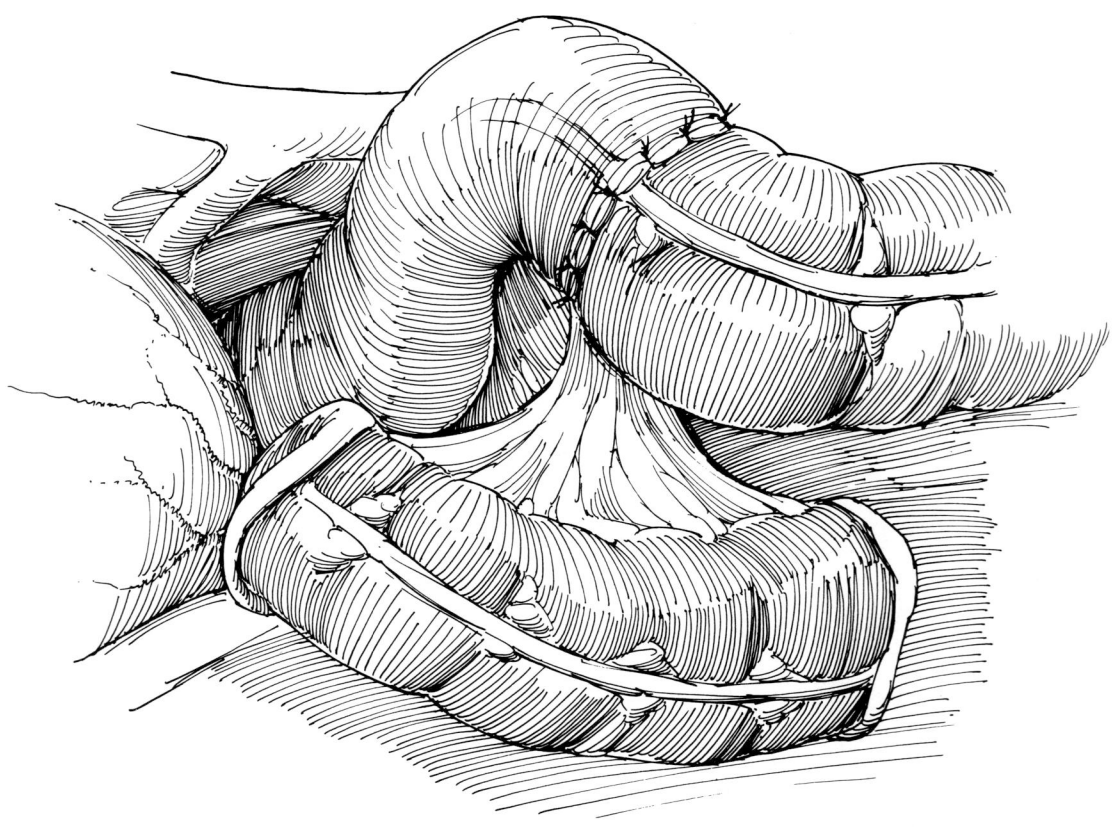

9 **A,** Place stay sutures at the mesenteric and antimesenteric borders of the proximal end of the segment. With the Kocher clamp still on the end of the segment, place a running inverting 3-0 chromic catgut suture to invert the mucosal edge.

B, Remove the bowel clamp and pull the suture tight, as the assistant helps invert the edge; run the suture back to its origin and tie it. Place a second simple running 3-0 nonabsorbable suture over this closure to ensure watertightness. Repeat the process at the distal end.

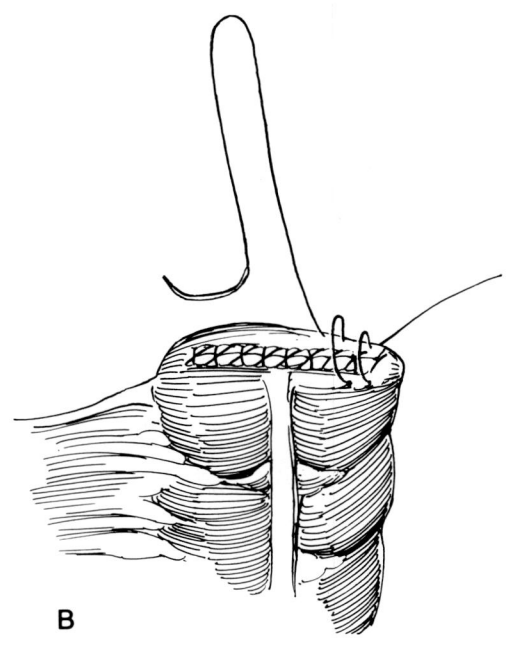

B

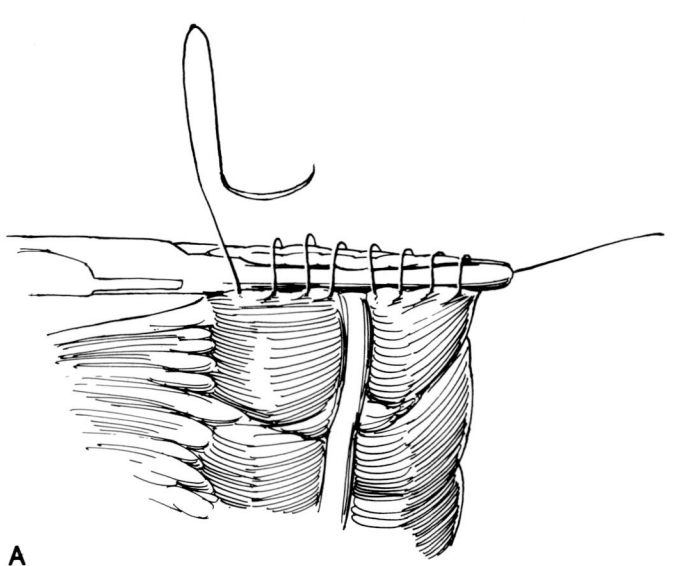

A

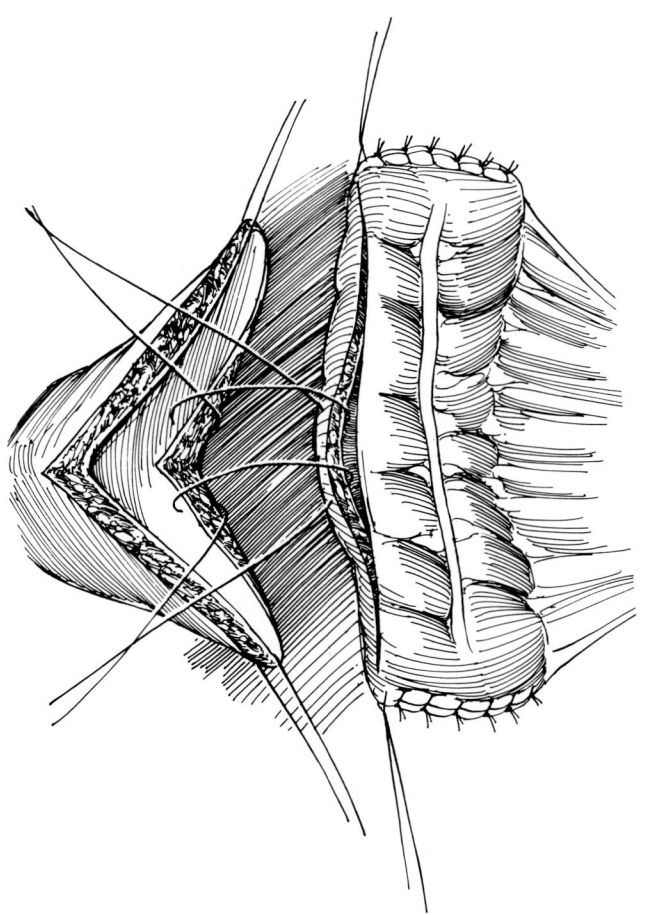

10 Open the segment along the antimesenteric border to within 1 cm of the suture line at each end. Isolate the segment with laparotomy pads, and carefully cleanse it with 0.25 percent neomycin-soaked sponges. The sigmoid cap is now ready for placement on the bladder. If possible, dissect the peritoneum from the dome and posterior wall of the bladder.

If this cannot be done, incise the peritoneum vertically over the fundus of the bladder to expose the anterior and posterior aspects. Open the bladder between stay sutures in a sagittal plane approaching the trigone posteriorly and the bladder neck anteriorly. The bladder opening should equal the length of the segment when it is stretched out by its stay sutures. If the bladder wall is totally resected, as for interstitial cystitis, insert ureteral catheters for guidance. In other cases, such as neurogenic bladder dysfunction, it usually is not necessary to resect bladder tissue. The bladder incision, however, must be extensive enough to prevent development of a diverticulum or an hourglass-type bladder. The ideal configuration after application of the cap is spheric. A transverse orientation, shown here, may fit better, but a sagittal orientation, shown in Figure 11, may be preferable, because by orienting the bowel sagittally, tension does not develop on the mesentery with bladder filling; in fact, it may become more relaxed.

Begin the anastomosis in the midline posteriorly, running a 3-0 chromic catgut locked suture posteriorly, including all layers of bladder and bowel.

11 Run this suture to the apex of the lateral wall or what used to be the dome of the bladder on each side. Do the same for the contralateral side. Place a second running 3-0 synthetic absorbable suture over this suture line to ensure a watertight inverted closure. If the bladder is very small, first suture the sigmoid cap to the bladder in the sagittal plane posteriorly and anteriorly, and then close the bowel on each side as the lateral walls of the new bladder. The bladder may contract with time, leaving a rim at the bladder neck. Place a 12 F or larger single-lumen plastic catheter in the urethra, and secure it with a 2-0 silk suture tied to its tip and brought through the bladder wall. Place a Malecot catheter (except in children with possible latex allergy, for whom a plastic catheter should be used) in one quadrant of the bladder, to be brought through the body wall later; avoid bringing tubes through the wall of the bowel. The size of the Malecot catheter depends on the patient's size. For smaller children, 18 F is the smallest that is acceptable; 22 to 24 F catheters are ideal, because the smaller sizes more easily become plugged with mucus in the postoperative period. Fasten the tube at the bladder wall with a 3-0 plain catgut suture.

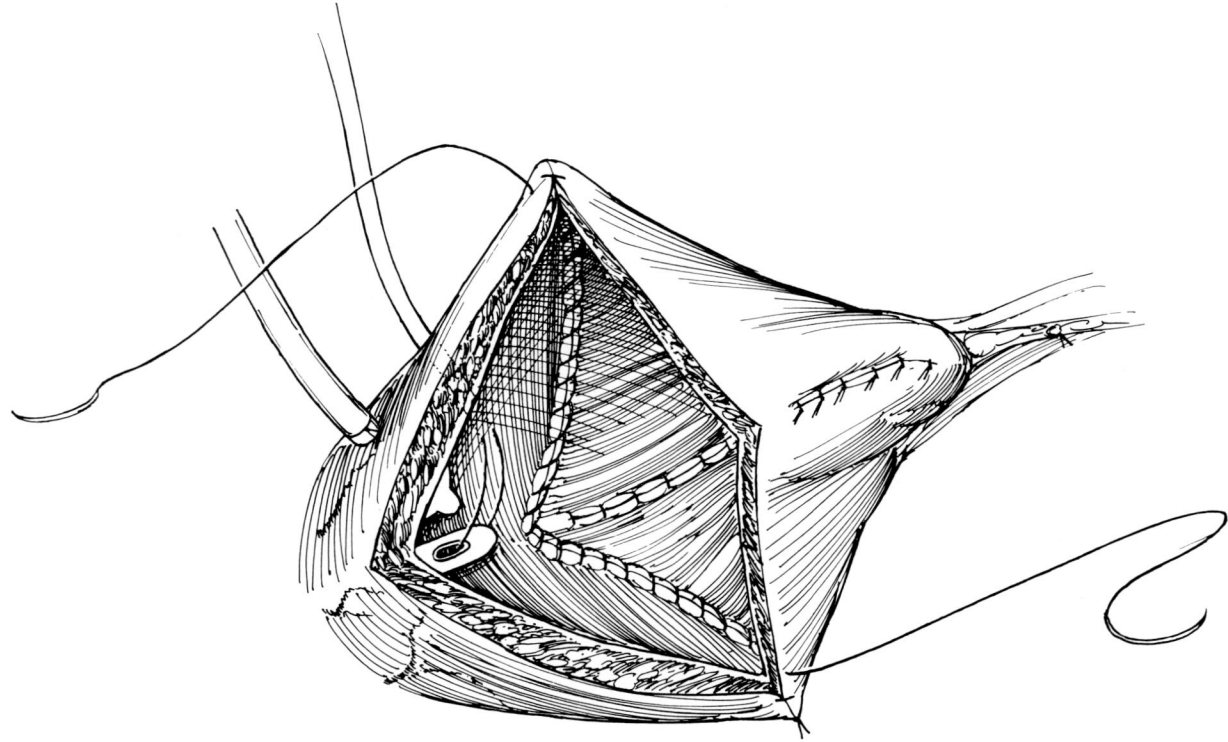

12 Close the anterior suture line in the same way as the posterior closure, except in reverse order, beginning in front and proceeding around both sides. Bring the cystostomy catheter through a stab wound in the body wall, and suture it to the skin. Bring the silk suture from the urethral catheter through the abdominal wall with a straight needle, and secure it to a button or cotton pledget. Place a Penrose drain (of 1/4 in or 1/2 in, depending on patient size) in the prevesical space, and bring it out through a separate stab wound. Patients with ventriculoperitoneal shunts are not drained. It may be wise to insert a silicone balloon catheter transurethrally to doubly protect from mucous accumulation. Close the wound in layers, and stitch the Penrose drain to the skin.

At first, irrigate the cystostomy at least three times a day with normal (or 3 N) saline to prevent mucous obstruction. Perform a cystogram in 1 week, and remove the urethral catheter if the anastomoses are intact. After 1 or 2 more weeks, clamp the suprapubic tube and start the patient on self-catheterization. If you personally know that this program is being carried out in a satisfactory manner, remove the suprapubic tube after another 1 or 2 weeks, but have the child continue irrigating at the times of catheterization to remove mucus. At first the bladder will be small. Anticholinergic agents and frequent catheterization are required. For the long term, have the child use a good-sized catheter (12 F or larger), because mucus will plug a smaller catheter and lead to subtle retention. Even if the child voids, he or she should check for residual urine at intervals.

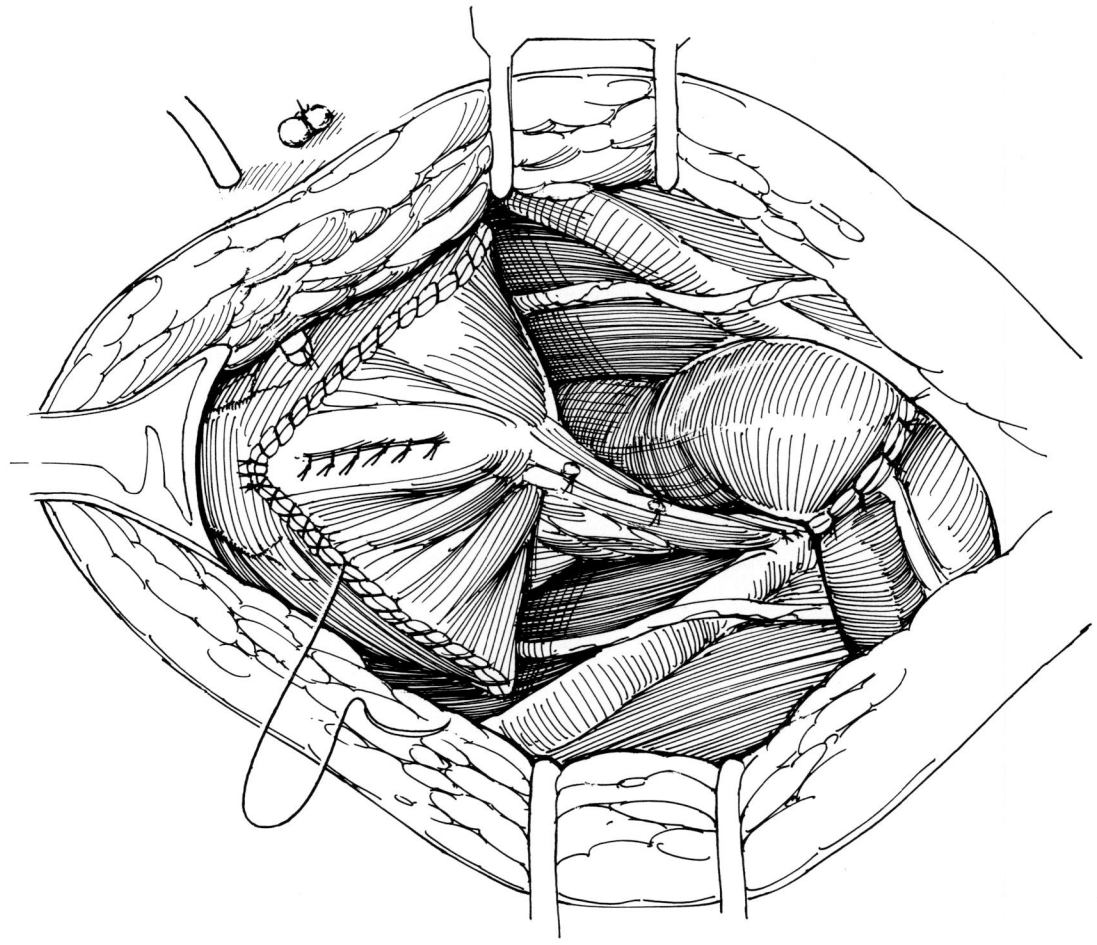

SIGMOIDOCYSTOPLASTY
(R. GONZALES)

The sigmoid is an alternative to the ascending colon used for a colocystoplasty, although it is more prone to mucous formation.

13 **A,** Select a 25-cm segment from the lower portion of the sigmoid colon, and check it for mobility. Incise the mesosigmoid and resect the segment. Reanastomose the colon (page 33). Irrigate the loop, and open it on its antimesenteric border, leaving the proximal few centimeters intact to receive the ureters. Form the bowel into an S shape, and suture the two sets of adjacent edges with running polyglactin sutures. Open the bladder widely in the sagittal plane. **B,** Anastomose the segment to the bladder with a running suture beginning posteriorly, tying the knots on the outside. Place a Malecot catheter (use a plastic catheter in children with myelomeningocele), and continue the suture line up the anterior wall.

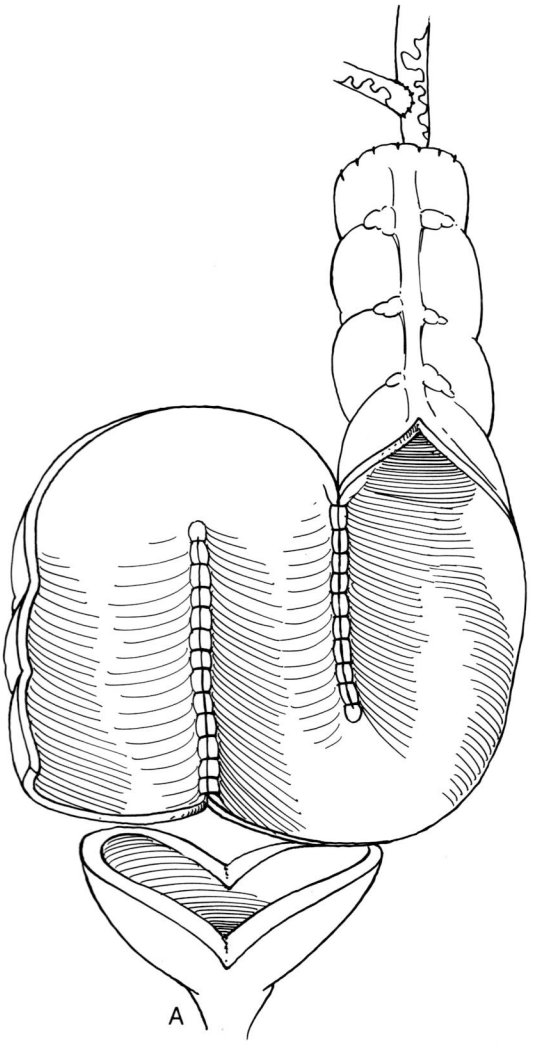

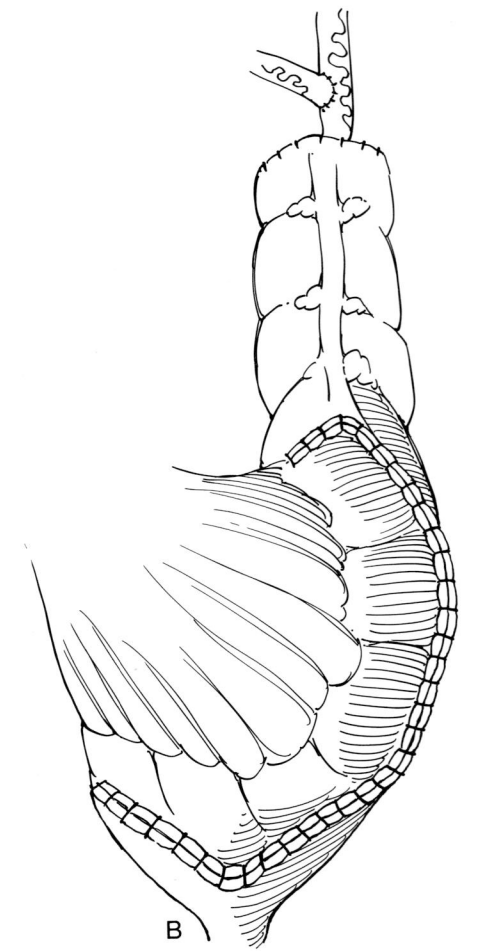

A

B

POSTOPERATIVE PROBLEMS

Mucus is formed profusely at first, but after 3 to 4 weeks, its secretion subsides to manageable proportions.

Colicky pain suggests *intestinal obstruction;* a silent abdomen suggests *ileus. Adhesions* may cause intestinal obstruction soon after the operation, and other causes may be an anastomotic stoma that is too narrow or herniation through an unclosed defect in the mesentery. Take lateral or upright films of the abdomen, and look for gas-fluid levels proximally and for empty bowel distally.

Leakage from the bowel anastomosis can occur occasionally, caused by ischemia from resection of too much mesentery. Place a long nasogastric tube, provide hyperalimentation, and continue suction drainage. For persistence after 10 to 14 days, reoperate. *Ischemia and necrosis* of the segment, seen as a dusky stoma during closing, come from tension on the mesentery, hematoma, or inadvertent ligation of a major vessel. The bowel will remain intact for 1 or 2 weeks, but intervention is needed if recovery has not occurred by that time. Perform endoscopy on the segment to see how much is involved; if it is only the terminal few centimeters, enough ileum may be pulled out to make a new stoma. Otherwise, another segment of ileum must be attached, or a new loop must be created. *Deficiency of vitamin B_{12}* occurs with use of the ileocecal region for augmentation. A supplement must be given yearly.

Commentary by Michael E. Mitchell

We have been pleased with this form of cystoplasty as a mechanism to increase bladder volume and compliance. The same basic technique may be used for large and small bowel, and with minor alterations, for the stomach as well. The advantage of closing the ends of the bowel and the sagittal orientation is that no tension develops on the mesentery with bladder filling. If anything, the mesentery becomes more relaxed as the bladder is pushed higher in the pelvis. It usually is necessary to fold the bowel back on itself at least once and sometimes twice to make a larger patch. In some circumstances, a transverse orientation of the sigmoid seems to fit better and works equally well. When I have made mistakes with this technique, it has been in the direction of not taking enough bowel. Always take a little more than you think you will need; 15 cm is minimal. Do not cut the segment to fit the bladder. In cases where the bladder is very small, it often is necessary to suture the sigmoid cap to the bladder posteriorly and anteriorly and then to suture bowel to bowel on each side to form the lateral walls of the new bladder. It usually is the case that the original bladder shrinks further with time to form just a rim of tissue at the bladder neck.

There is a natural tendency to be timid in the sagittal incision of the bladder. This is an important maneuver, because if the incision is not generous enough, the cystoplasty segment becomes nothing more than a diverticulum, and the anticipated dynamic advantages of the cystoplasty may not be realized. In the same sense, the antimesenteric incision in the bowel, converting the segment from a tube to a patch, is very important. In our review of 129 cystoplasty cases, the patients who had problems were those in whom the bladder was augmented with bowel in its tubular configuration. Of the patch-cystoplasty patients, fewer than 10 percent had problems with what we considered to be peristaltic contractions; most of these were believed to have segments that were too short.

We use only resorbable suture material on tissue that either conducts or stores urine (*eg,* renal pelvis, ureter, bladder, and bladder neck). Nonresorbable material, such as silk and staples, even if used on the outside, ultimately seems to be a potential nidus for stone formation and should be avoided if possible.

Because of the initial flood of mucus, we always leave two drainage tubes. The urethral catheter is removed at approximately 1 week after a cystogram has demonstrated that there are no leaks in the bladder. The patient usually is discharged with suprapubic drainage, which is continued for an additional 1 to 2 weeks. At that point, the suprapubic tube is clamped, and intermittent clean catheterization (ICC) is initiated. The suprapubic tube is not removed until the patient proves, beyond a shadow of a doubt, that ICC can be done effectively and regularly. The suprapubic tube usually is removed 1 or 2 weeks after the initiation of ICC. To control mucous production, which sometimes is quite significant initially, we irrigate the bladder three times a day with normal, and sometimes 3 N, saline solution. Usually after several months, irrigation can be reduced to once a day or, sometimes, only as needed. All patients are maintained on ICC until they prove, again beyond a shadow of a doubt, that they can completely empty with voiding. Some patients catheterize once or twice a day "just to be safe." Those patients who must do long-term ICC usually do best with a catheter size of 12 F or larger. Smaller catheters can lead to mucous plugs and unsuspected retention.

Finally, it sometimes takes considerable time (months) for even the augmented bladder to stretch after surgery. I do not hesitate to use anticholinergic agents during this period. Patients also are sometimes distressed to find that ICC needs to be performed quite frequently, at least as often as every 2 or 3 hours initially. This requirement usually is temporary and will change gradually but requires support from a caring physician.

Commentary by Barry A. Kogan

I rarely use colocystoplasty at this time. Although it has a predictable and ample blood supply and is easily mobilized into position, the sigmoid produces large amounts of mucus and tends to have significant contractions.

From a technical standpoint, I would make several suggestions. I generally use a transverse skin incision and fascial incision, because I believe this is a stronger incision in the early postoperative period. I do not close the ends of the bowel segment to be used for the augmentation, because I use the bowel more as a flat plate than as a tube. Usually, it fits nicely this way, but occasionally, it is necessary to close bowel to bowel in some places if the bladder is very contracted.

Most children requiring this procedure have neurogenic bladder dysfunction, and many of these have a latex allergy. Therefore, we avoid Malecot catheters and use a large silicone balloon catheter as a suprapubic catheter.

I generally do not worry about a two-layer closure, but I do check the anastomosis to make sure it is watertight and then try to mobilize the omentum to cover the dome and suture lines, in an effort to prevent or limit spontaneous ruptures.

CHAPTER 91

Cecocystoplasty

Study the child urodynamically before planning cecocystoplasty. This procedure is not suitable for a child with a relaxed bladder neck, because contractions of the bowel may open the neck and cause incontinence. If ileocecal cystoplasty is planned, inject the enema at relatively high pressure to check on the competence of the ileocecal valve. Prepare the bowel. If the conversion is from ureterosigmoidostomy, place a rectal tube.

1 *Position:* Place the child supine. *Instruments:* The same as those for ileocystoplasty; add a TA-40 or TA-50 stapler. *Incision:* Make a lower midline, transperitoneal incision (page 263). Stand on the left side of the table for most of the operation, although initial mobilization of the ascending colon may be more easily undertaken from the right. Examine the peritoneal contents, and pack the intestinal contents superiorly. Direct the operating light behind the bowel to study the ileocecal blood supply to select an appropriate segment.

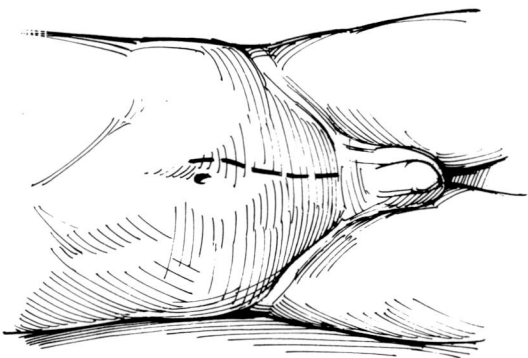

2 Mobilize the ascending colon with scissors from the right gutter along the white line of Toldt to the level of the hepatic flexure, and free the terminal ileum and cecum from their peritoneal attachments over the sacral promontory. Continue the peritoneal dissection medially to the ligament of Treitz, and separate the right colon and small bowel from the retroperitoneal surface.

Identify the ileocolic and right colic arteries, and divide the mesentery between them, almost to the origin of the

right colic artery. The stump of the ascending colon is dependent on the ileocolic artery coming from the superior mesenteric artery. Be careful not to cut the marginal vessel to the distal colon when dividing the short proximal stem of the right colic artery. If the mesenteric pedicle is unusually short, or if the pelvis is very deep, divide one or two additional perpendicular mesocolic vessels to obtain more freedom for the ascending colon. The segment will depend on the ileocolic artery for its blood supply.

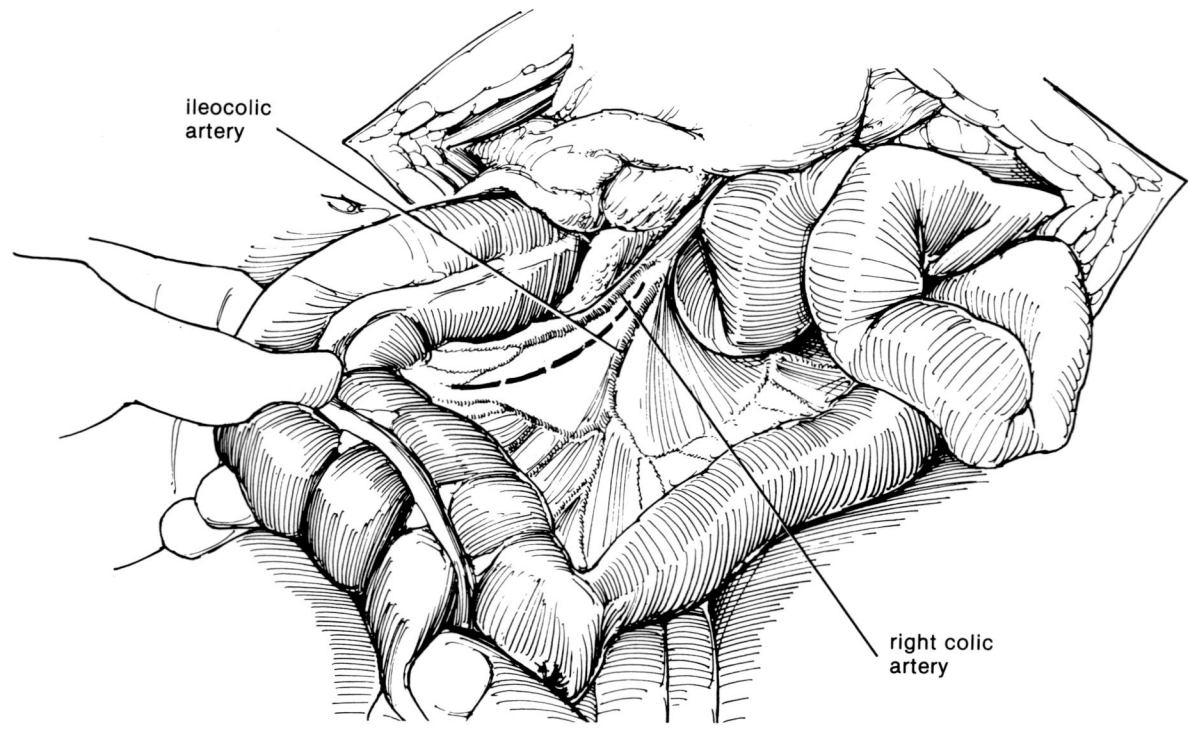

ileocolic artery

right colic artery

3 Divide the colon as close to the right colic artery as possible, either between Kocher clamps or with the GIA surgical stapler. Examine the mesentery to the cecum and terminal ileum to determine how much ileum must be taken to provide a very adequate pedicle for the cecum, which usually is 15 to 20 cm long. Place a stay suture, and divide the mesentery on the other side of the ileocolic artery. Divide the ileum between Kocher clamps or use the GIA stapler.

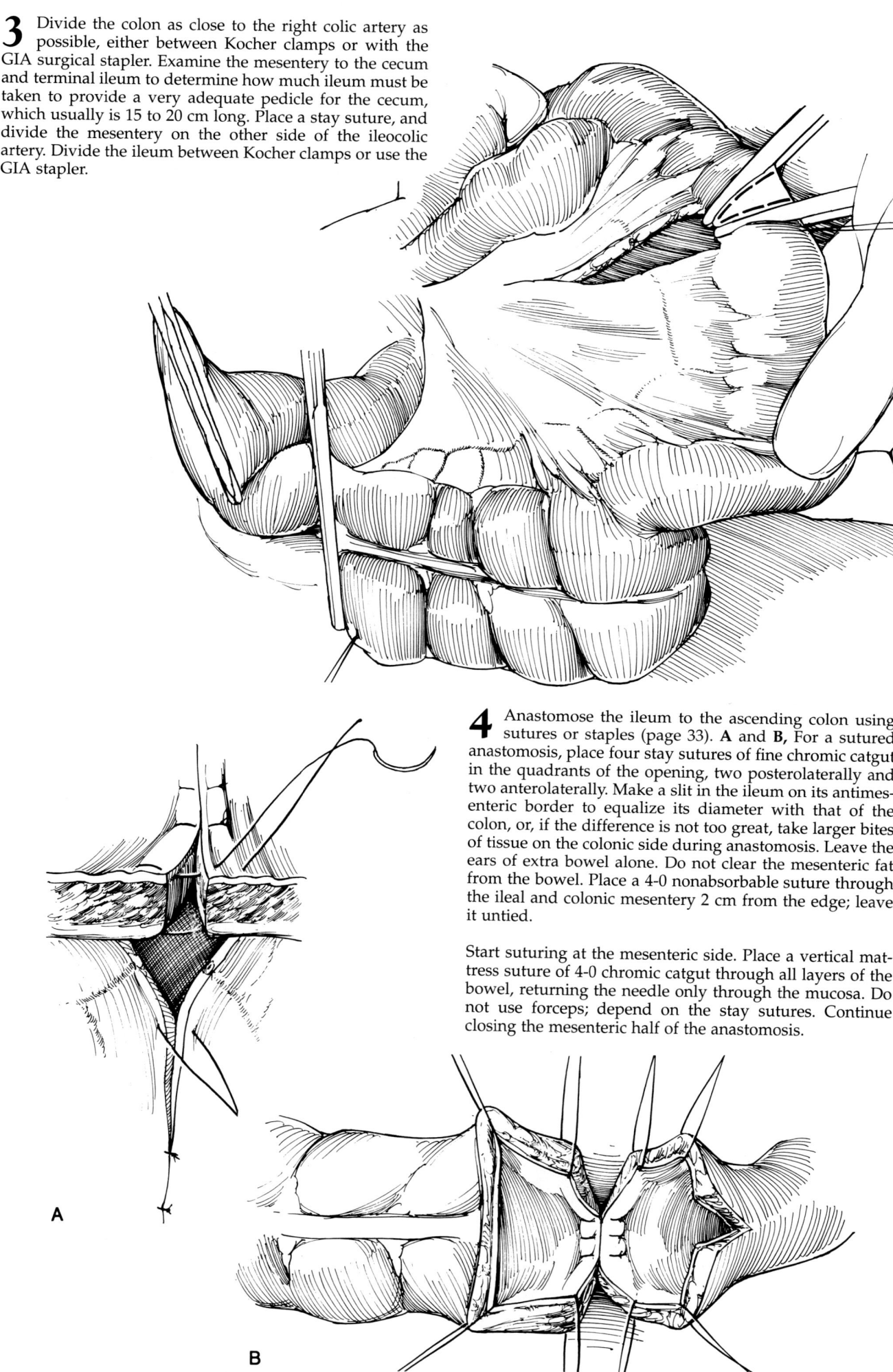

4 Anastomose the ileum to the ascending colon using sutures or staples (page 33). **A** and **B,** For a sutured anastomosis, place four stay sutures of fine chromic catgut in the quadrants of the opening, two posterolaterally and two anterolaterally. Make a slit in the ileum on its antimesenteric border to equalize its diameter with that of the colon, or, if the difference is not too great, take larger bites of tissue on the colonic side during anastomosis. Leave the ears of extra bowel alone. Do not clear the mesenteric fat from the bowel. Place a 4-0 nonabsorbable suture through the ileal and colonic mesentery 2 cm from the edge; leave it untied.

Start suturing at the mesenteric side. Place a vertical mattress suture of 4-0 chromic catgut through all layers of the bowel, returning the needle only through the mucosa. Do not use forceps; depend on the stay sutures. Continue closing the mesenteric half of the anastomosis.

A

B

5 For the anterior half of the anastomosis, place interrupted sutures of 4-0 chromic catgut through all layers except the mucosa; this will bring the mucosa in apposition inside the lumen. Cut each suture short.

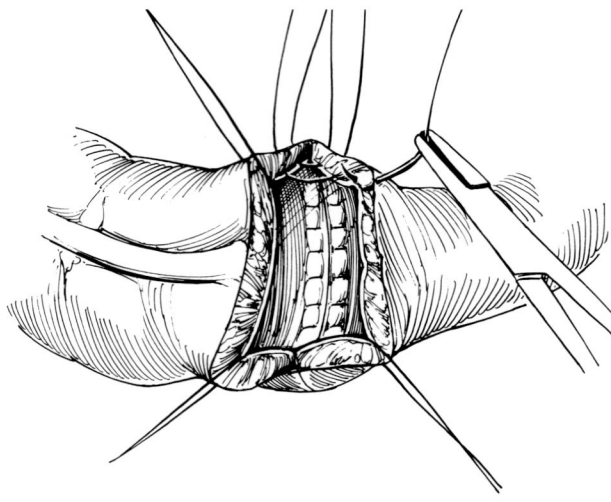

6 Place a seromuscular layer of 4-0 nonabsorbable sutures as a second layer anteriorly; it may be carried well laterally, using the original mesenteric suture to rotate the bowel. Complete the closure of the mesenteric defect. Alternatively, do a side-to-side anastomosis using GIA and TA-40 or TA-50 staplers (page 34). The omentum should be draped over the anastomosis and tucked into the fornices of the pelvis to keep the bowel from touching the raw surfaces.

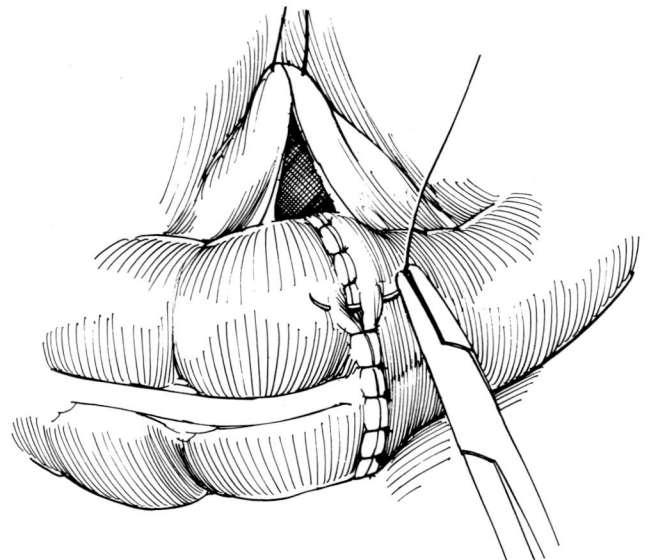

7 Make a small window in the posterior peritoneum, and pass the segment through it into the right gutter. Tack the mesentery that remains inside the peritoneal cavity to the posterior peritoneal surface to prevent an internal hernia. Close the margins of the window around the pedicle. Rotate the segment 180 degrees counterclockwise. Palpate for arterial pulsations in the mesentery to assess the viability of the intestinal segment.

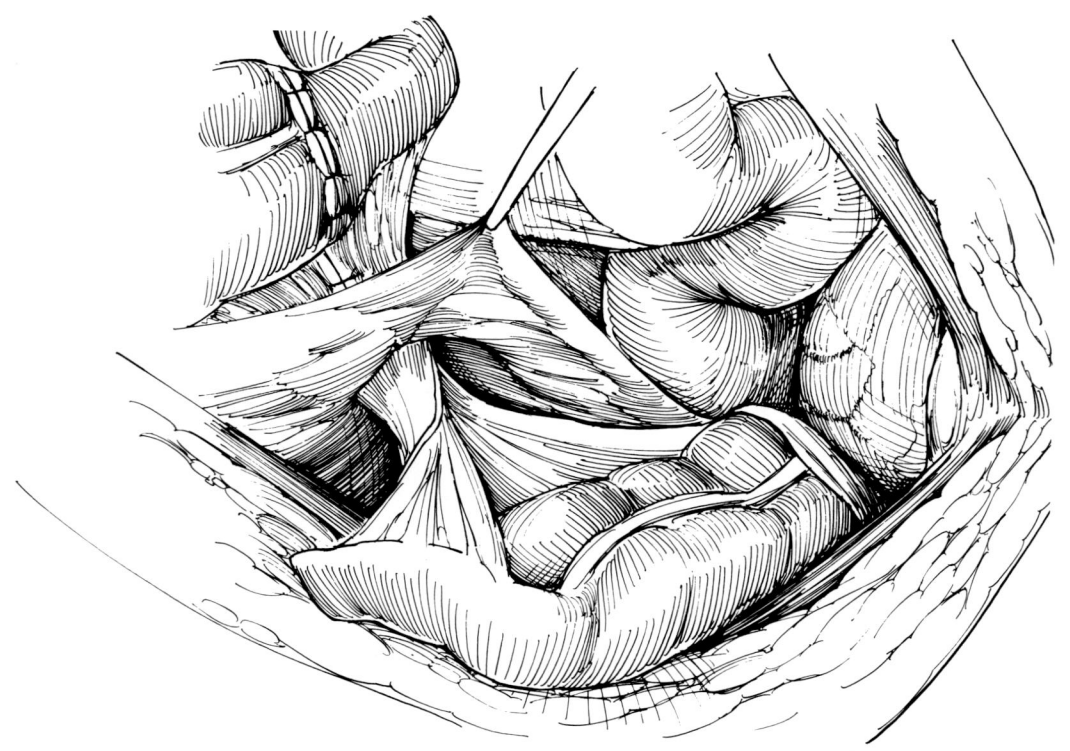

8 **A,** Discard the terminal ileum by dividing its blood supply close to the bowel wall and by dividing it 2 cm from the cecum. **B,** Close the stump with a full-thickness running suture of 2-0 chromic catgut. **C,** Invert the stump into the cecum with a layer of 3-0 synthetic absorbable sutures. Take care not to let the needle enter the cecum.

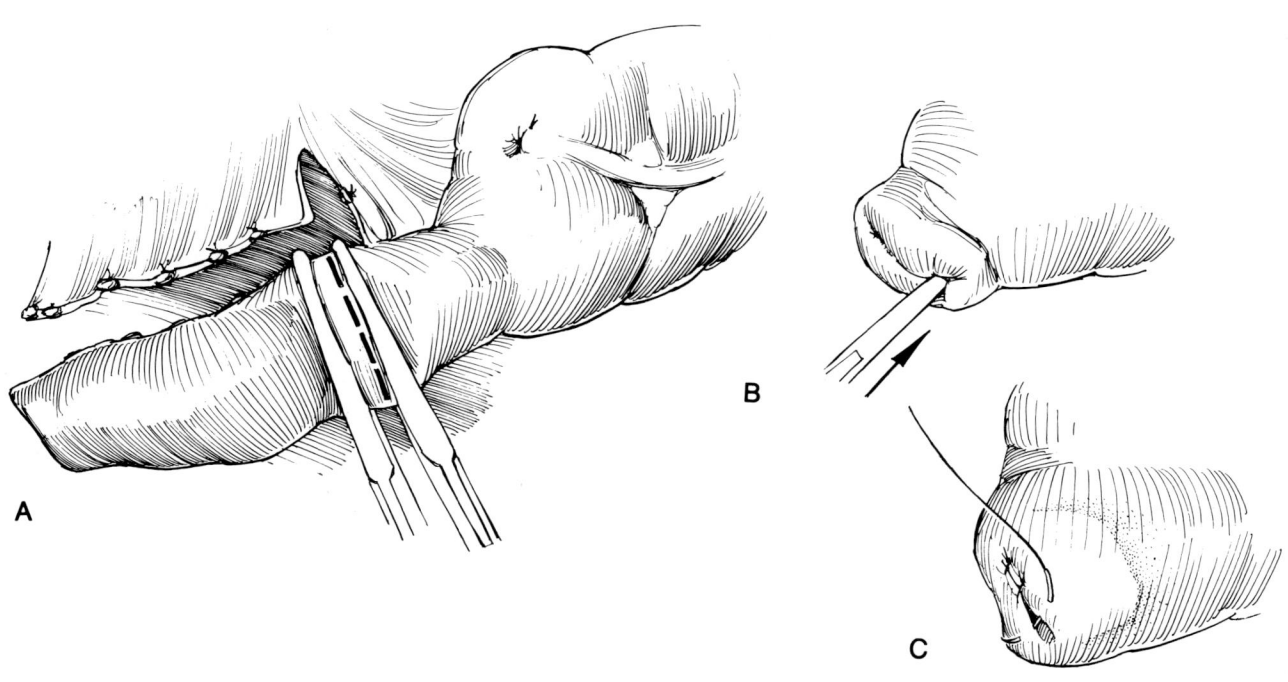

9 **A–C,** An alternative and preferable method to detubularize the segment is to open both ileum and cecum on the anterior surface. Fold the ileum over to fill the cecal defect. This enlarged pouch now can be anastomosed to the bladder. The terminal ileum is useful for ureteral anastomosis when most of the bladder has been resected or when the ureters are short from previous surgery.

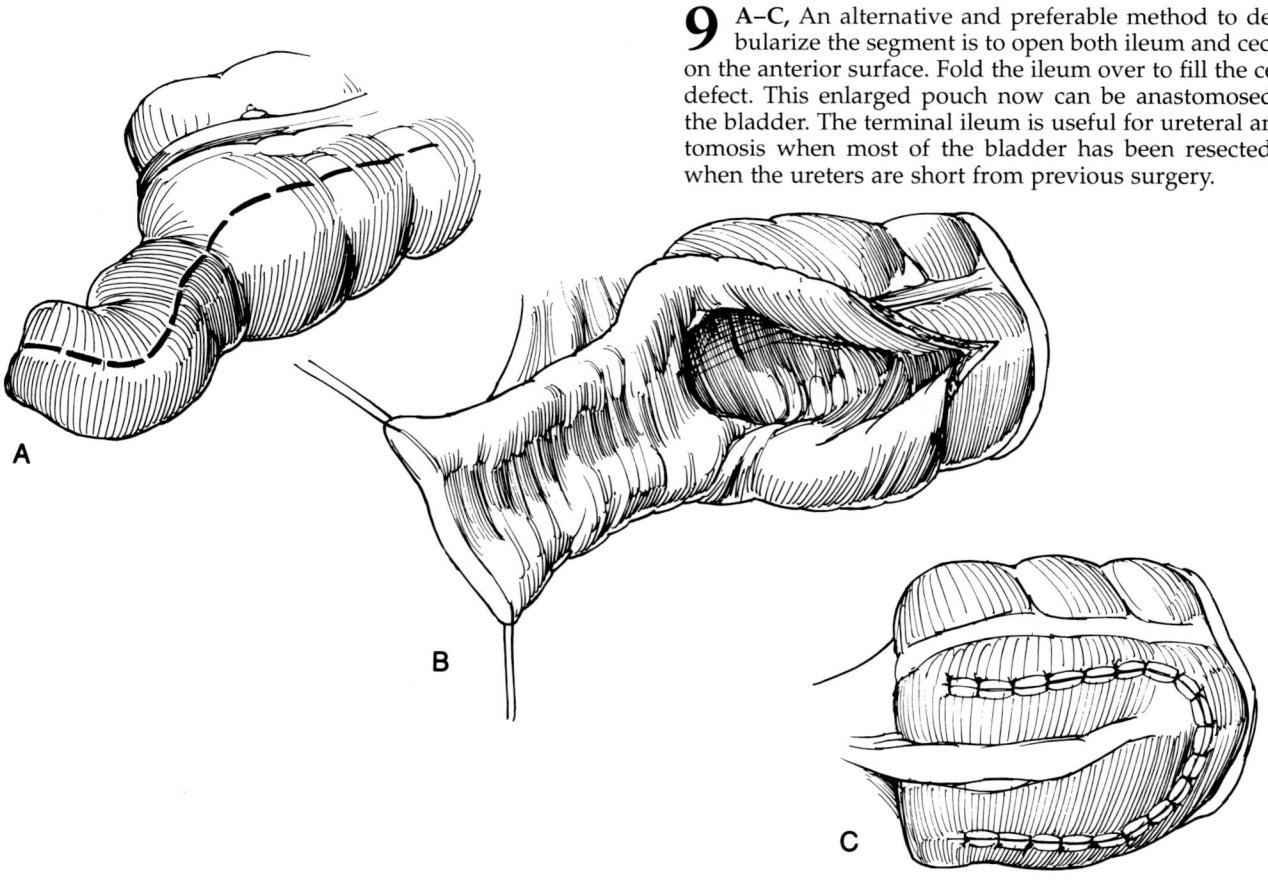

10 Bisect the peritoneum over the bladder.

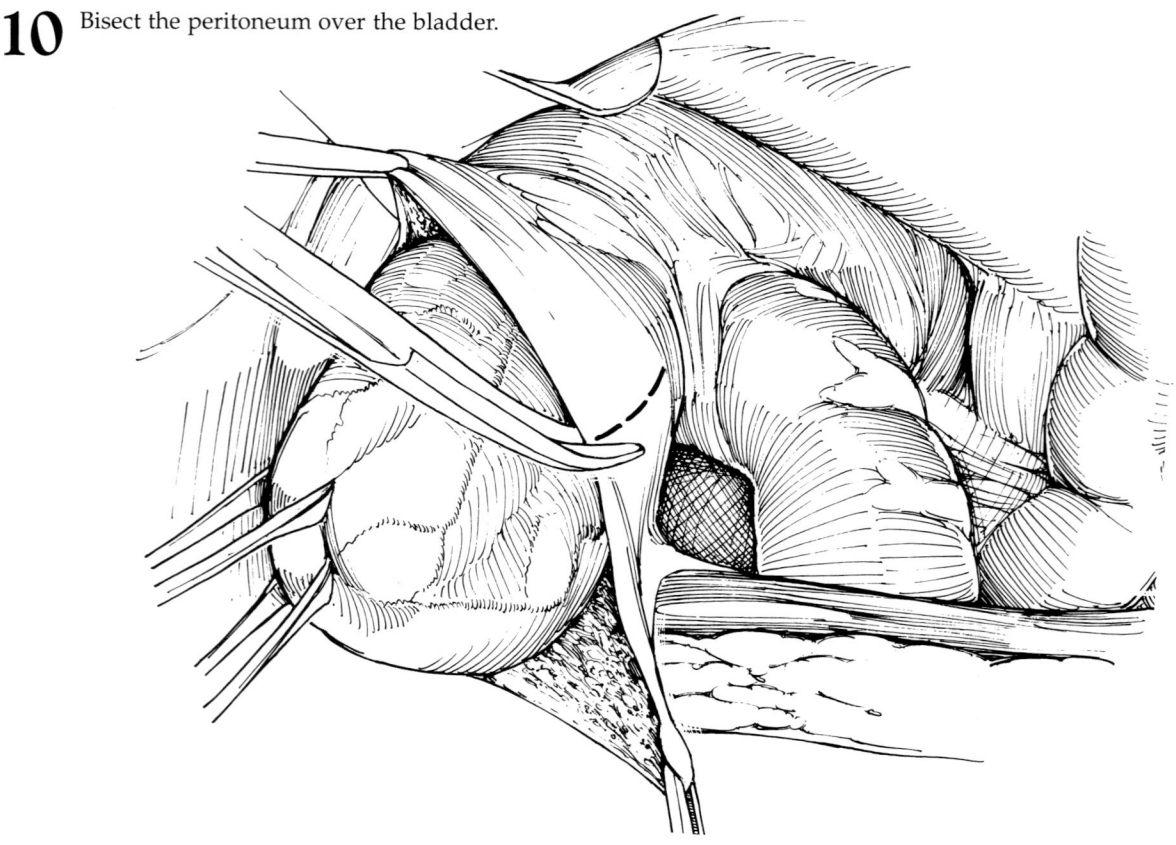

11 Incise the bladder in a sagittal plane from the trigone to the deep anterior wall, a distance at least equal to the stretched diameter of the cecal lumen, and place four stay sutures. Be sure to place a catheter in each ureter for identification. Trim the crushed edges of the cecum, caused by the Kocher clamp or stapler, and flush the bowel with 1 percent neomycin-bacitracin solution.

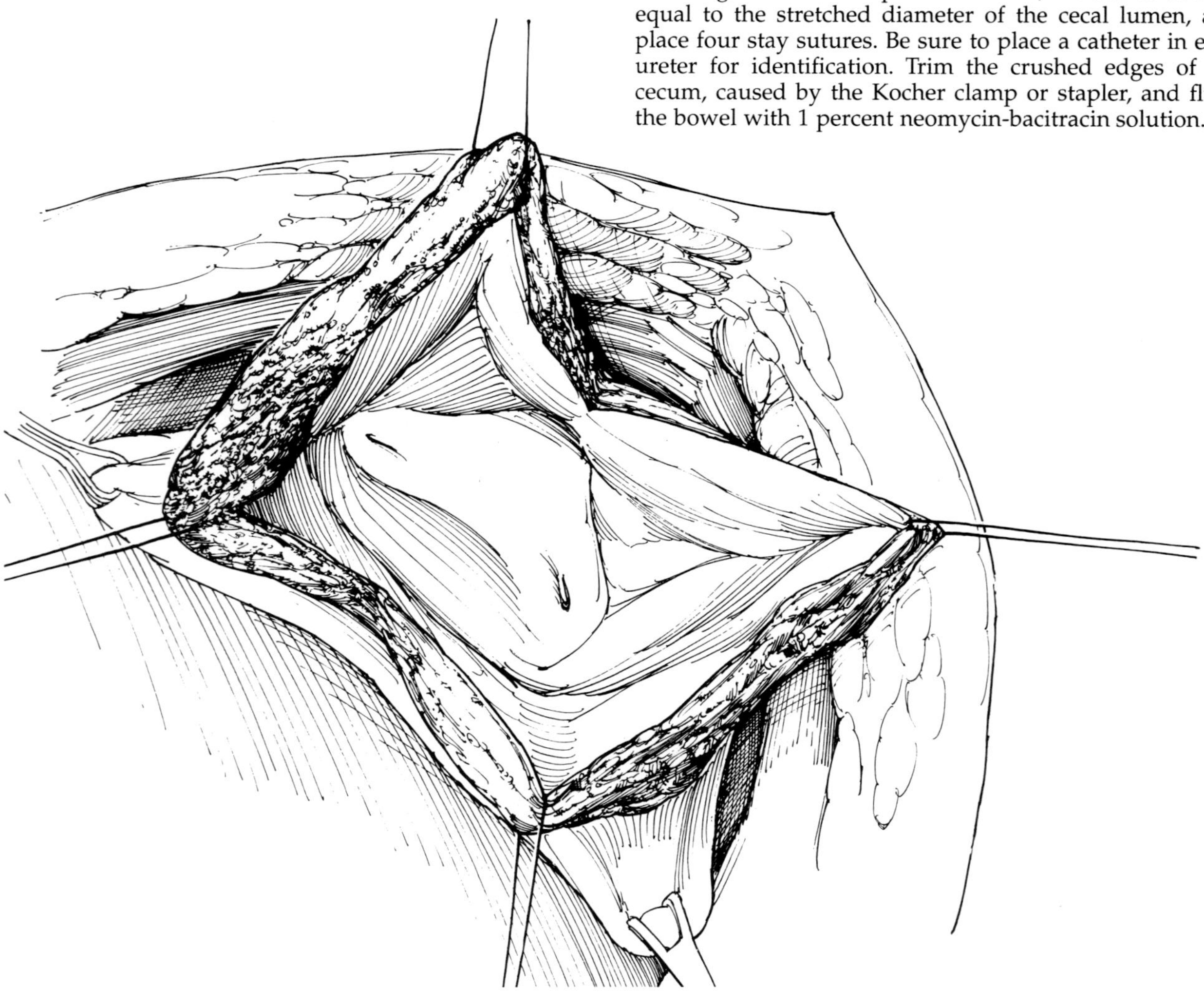

12 Stretch the cecal opening to fit the bladder defect. If necessary, increase its circumference by making two short, lateral incisions in it. Run a good-sized Malecot catheter through a stab wound in the anterolateral surface of the bladder, because mucus will be obstructive. If the remaining bladder is too small, bring the cystostomy tube out the dome of the reservoir. Start two sutures of 3-0 chromic catgut posteriorly, including the mucosa and submucosa of the colon and the urothelium of the bladder.

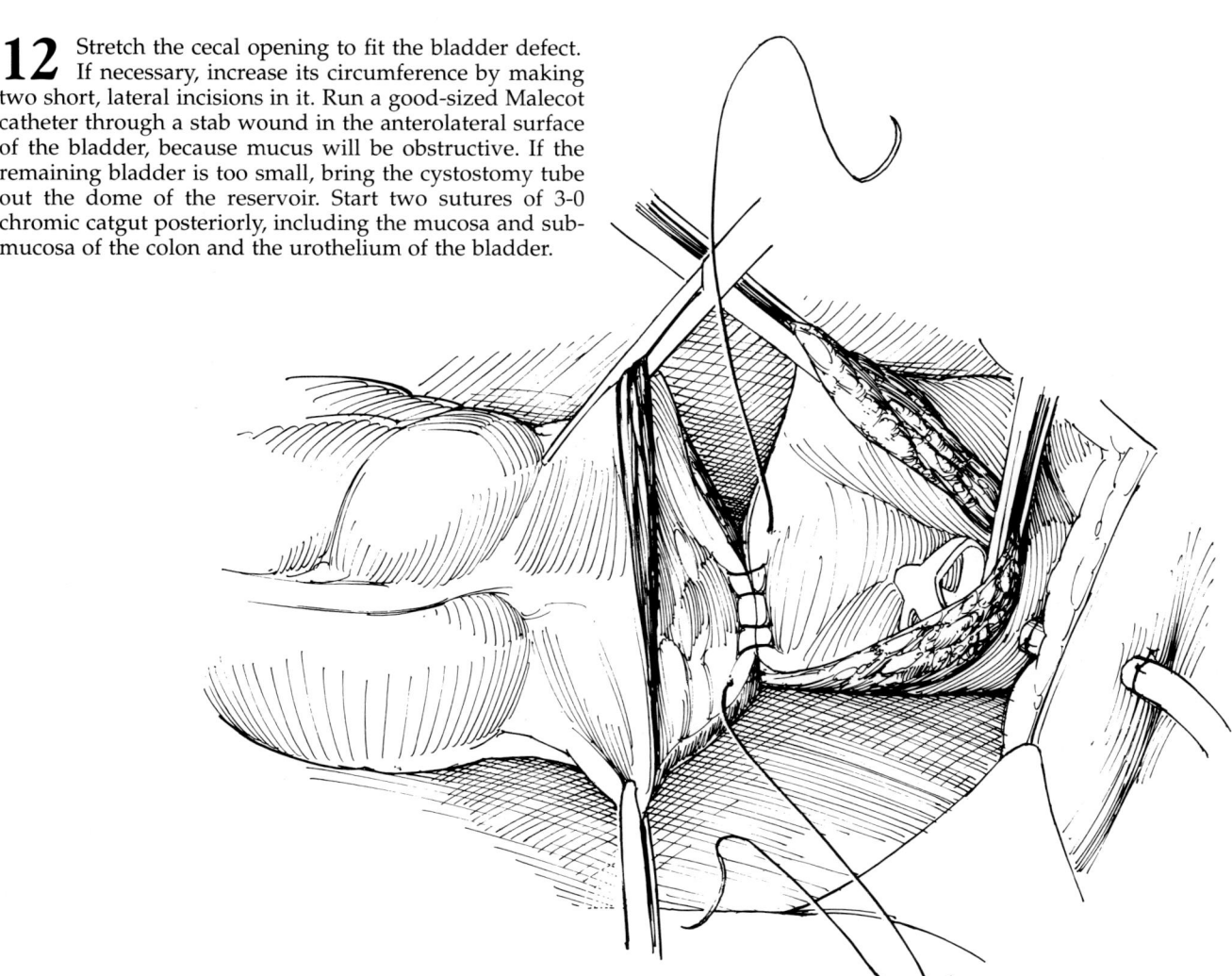

13 Run the sutures up each side and tie them anteriorly. Place a second seromuscular layer of 2-0 chromic catgut sutures. Alternatively, place four quadrant sutures, and run a full-thickness suture from each quadrant, taking care to keep the knots outside and the mucosa inverted. Avoid pursestringing. In a girl, suspend the vagina on the round ligaments, and tack it to the lateral pelvic wall to keep the bowel segment out of the cul-de-sac, where it could become obstructed. Suspend the new augmented bladder in either the right or left fossa or the midline, by suturing it to the posterior body wall. Having the suprapubic tube exit through the dome of the bowel helps hold it in place so that it will not fall into the cul-de-

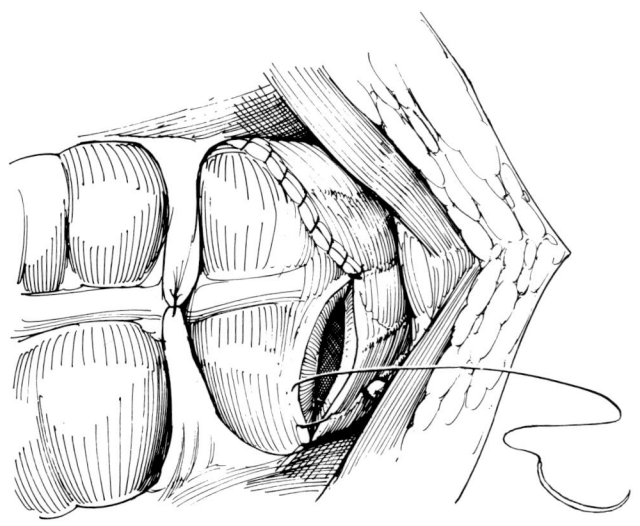

sac. Consider at this point the alternative of insertion of an artificial sphincter if the outlet is incontinent and the reservoir capacity and compliance are expected to be adequate, with a pressure consistently below 35 cm H_2O, the ureteral pressure. This is not an option if the bladder neck has been subjected to a prior operation.

Lavage the pelvis copiously with normal saline. Place a Penrose or Jackson-Pratt drain to the area. Close the peritoneum and body wall in layers, bringing the cystostomy tube through a stab wound and sewing it to the skin with braided silk. If the ureters have been anastomosed, bring the stents through stab wounds in the bladder and body wall. Because of the copious production of mucus, in addition to the cystostomy tube, insert an adequate silicone balloon catheter (or a straight catheter held by a suprapubic rein) transurethrally, and tape it to the leg.

Postoperatively, monitor the child closely; considerable fluid loss will have occurred during the procedure, and instability of fluid-electrolyte balance is to be expected. Wait 5 to 7 days before resuming oral feeding. Stop broad-spectrum antibiotics after 24 hours to reduce the chance of superinfection. Irrigate the cystostomy tube frequently to prevent plugging by mucus. Remove the drains 2 days after drainage stops, but continue irrigation three times a day. Remove the cystostomy tube on the 14th day, after making a cystourethrogram to detect leakage and to ascertain that the child can void. If the anastomosis is intact, remove the urethral catheter 2 days later. In 2 months, obtain an intravenous urogram and cystogram and determine the serum creatinine level. For a discussion of postoperative problems, see "Ileocystoplasty," Chapter 89.

Commentary by Rudolf Hohenfellner

Between 1983 and 1992, the detubularized ileocoecal segment was chosen for bladder augmentation and substitution in 21 children and continent urinary diversion in 46 children. Additionally, undiversion was carried out in 17 children. The indication for substitution in children is rare. (It is needed in more or less exotic cases and in girls with neurogenic bladder.) The following points should be kept in mind when cecocystoplasty is performed:

1. Perform subtotal resection of the bladder when just a cuff is left for the anastomosis (one-layer-deep anchor sutures). Stay close to the bladder to avoid a lesion of the ganglion pelvicum in the nonneurogenic case for postoperative residual free voiding.

2. Exact measurements of 12-cm of cecum and two pieces of 12-cm ileum are important (Hinman's capacity formula) for an adequate 450 ml reservoir. A suture running through all layers with 4-0 Maxon suture material (with a straight needle) for anastomosis is safe, watertight, and fast.

3. Dilated-wall, thickened fibrotic ureters and previously operated or irradiated ureters (for rhabdomyosarcoma) are implanted via a short tunnel (butterfly). Reflux is less dangerous than obstruction. (If reimplantation becomes necessary, it is carried out by a right flank incision, where pouch and ureters can easily be identified.)

4. The ileocoecal valve is preserved in case the augmentation fails and conversion into continent urinary diversion becomes necessary to construct the ileal nipple.

5. For bowel anastomosis, reconstruction of the ileocoecal valve using the fish-mouth technique is promising. The advantages are prolonged ileal transit time and less stool frequency—especially in neurogenic disorders and patients with short bowel, as well as in the irradiated group. The main disadvantage is prolongation of the operation time by 20 to 30 minutes.

6. Because of the risk of residual urine, the pouchostomy is left in place, sometimes for several weeks, until adaptation of the new bladder to the intact outlet mechanism is completed (detected by residual urine of less than 50 cm and decreased mucous production). The bladder is emptied every 3 hours to train pelvic floor relaxation and abdominal pressure.

7. If the negative base excess is less than -2.5, it is corrected immediately by sodium bicarbonate or potassium bicarbonate.

8. Because secondary malignancy is an important risk and increases over time, pouchoscopy is carried out once a year by using a scope with a magnification lens system (biopsy if certain areas are questionable). Adenocarcinoma or squamous cell carcinoma may be detected either at the implantation site of the ureter or where the bladder cuff is connected to the bowel. Among our own three cases, there was one case in which a carcinoma was detected 18 years after augmentation using sigmoid colon, one case of a carcinoma 20 years after ileal augmentation, and one case of a carcinoma 10 years after clean intermittent catheterization.

9. Following these observations, we *do not believe in afferent ileal nipples,* because they make it impossible to inspect the ureter bowel anastomosis for malignancy.

10. Results of bladder closure and subsequent bladder augmentation using the Young-Dees technique in patients with bladder exstrophy were disappointing. Conversion became necessary in five of eight cases (the same was shown in Ransley's series [1988]). For primary continent diversion as well as undiversion and conversion (Bricker or colon conduits) into continent reservoirs, it is important that the child is not mentally retarded because of the risk of overdistention and spontaneous rupture.

By the incorporation of the continence mechanism (efferent segment) *into* the reservoir, genuine continence is produced. In contrast, the narrowed efferent Indiana ileal segment, as well as the Hoffmann modified narrowed efferent ileal segment (combined with the Mainz pouch), guarantees continence only up to the leak-point pressure (3 to 4 hours) when the patient has to self-catheterize; otherwise the patient gets wet. Whenever possible, the appendix embedded in the tenia is the method of choice. The same is true for the ileocecal ileal nipple, although the technique is more sophisticated. However, the Manangadze procedure, which uses tapered ileum embedded in the tenia, is promising.

ANTIREFLUX ILEOCECOCYSTOPLASTY

Check for the presence of an adequate urethral continence mechanism. Serum creatinine level should not be higher than 2.2 mg/dl. Proceed as for augmentation cecocystoplasty Steps 1 to 8, thereby preserving 15 cm of the terminal ileal segment for use as an antireflux valve. Divide the ureters close to the bladder after inserting a stay suture in each. Ligate the ureteral stumps with 3-0 chromic catgut sutures. Dissect a tunnel bluntly retroperitoneally, and bring the left ureter to the right side.

14 **A–C,** The ileocolic valve should have been evaluated by a preoperative contrast enema to assess its competency. If reflux was noted at relatively low pressures, a more-secure nipple-type antireflux procedure should be planned. If the ileocecal valve was found to be competent, insert three layers of interrupted seromuscular sutures of 4-0 silk to invert 3 to 4 cm of the terminal ileum into the cecum.

Test for obstruction from the supplemented valve by inserting an 18-gauge needle into the ileum and filling it with saline with a three-way stopcock and syringe, using a length of clear intravenous tubing on the stopcock for a manometer. Test the competence of the ileocecal valve by transcecal instillation of saline.

15 As an alternative to supplementation of the valve, prepare a 6- to 8-cm window in the ileal mesentery, as for the intussusception described on page 407 for the Kock pouch. Draw the ileum through the ileocecal valve with Allis forceps.

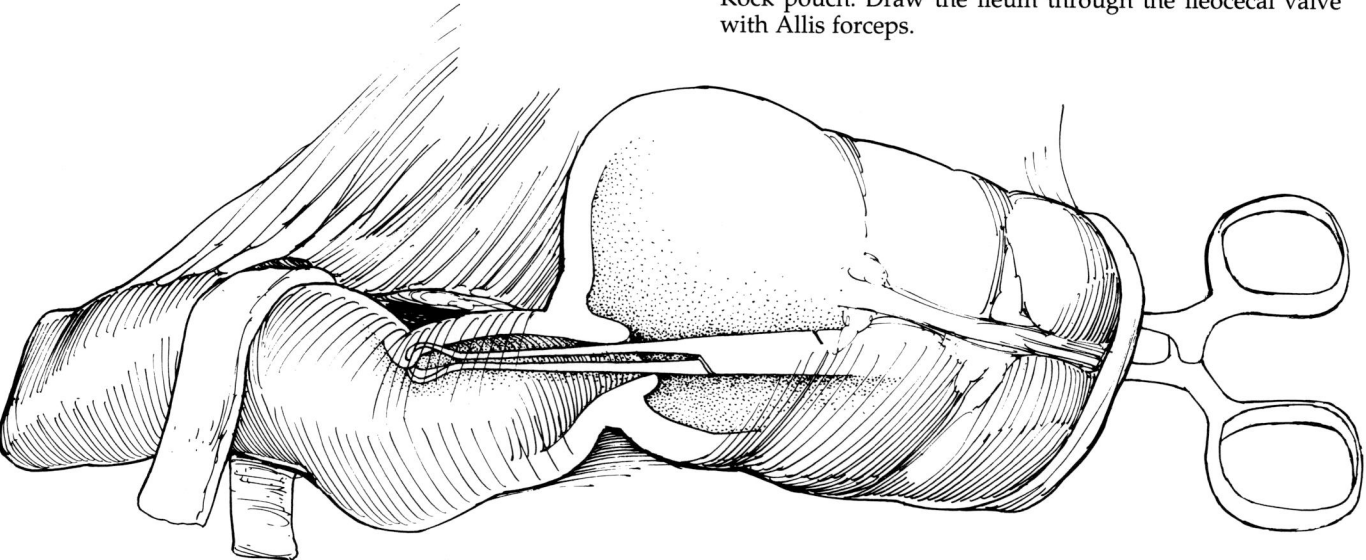

16 Fasten the ileum to the cecum with the aid of a strip of polyglycolic acid mesh and sutures.

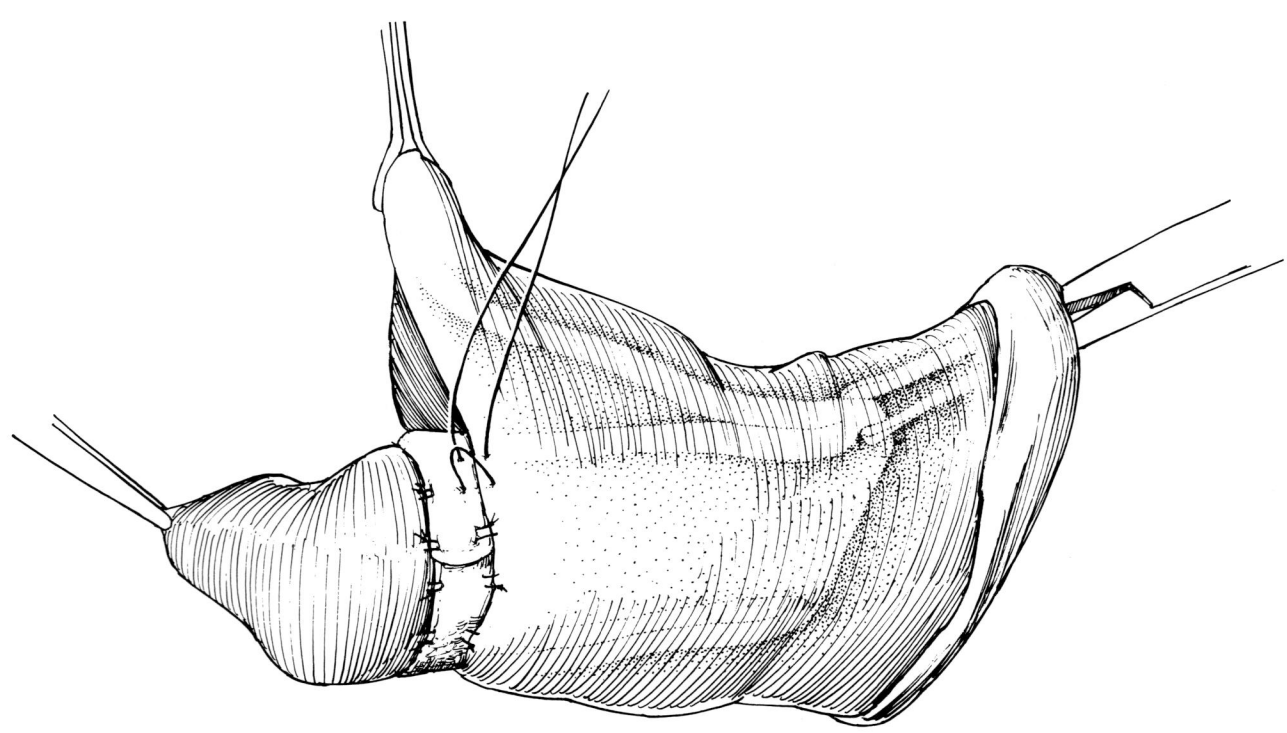

17 An alternative method that may be simpler and as effective that avoids devascularizing the bowel is to turn the cecum back to expose the nipple. Fix the nipple to the cecal wall by incising the wall of the nipple through the muscularis and the cecal wall into the muscularis, for a distance of 4 cm. Approximate the two raw surfaces with a row of 3-0 polydioxanone sutures applied to the serosa and muscularis. Supplement this with some nonabsorbable sutures around the site of entrance of the ileum.

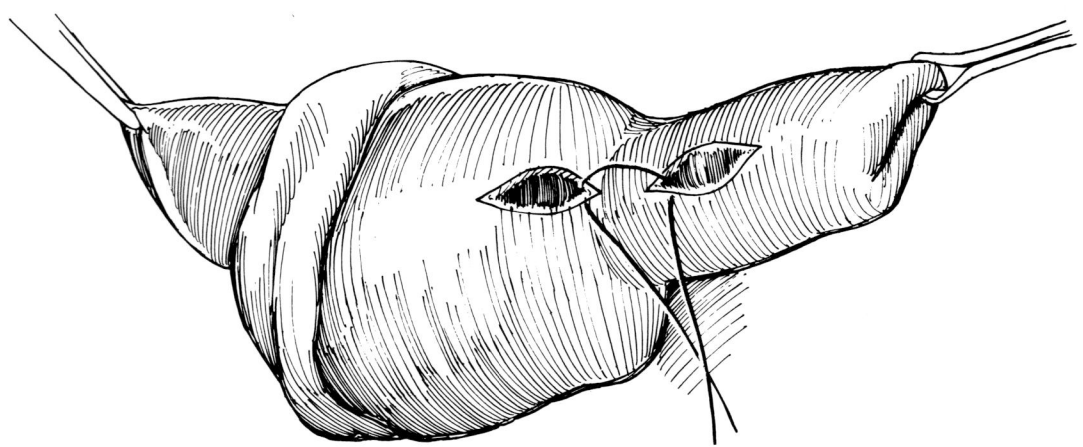

18 Bisect the peritoneum over the bladder or leave it in place to help make the closure more secure. Halve the bladder from just proximal to the bladder neck anteriorly to the midtrigonal area posteriorly. If reflux or hydronephrosis is present, resect the trigone as well and reimplant the ureters.

Place two silicone single-J tubes through the body wall and the anterior bladder wall preparatory to stenting the ureteroileal anastomoses. Place a Malecot catheter through a stab wound in the anterolateral surface of the bladder to enable clearance of potentially obstructive mucus. Select a convenient site along the ileal segment for insertion of the ureters. Excess ileum will be resected later. Proceed with ureteral implantation, as described for ileal conduit (pages 381–385). Mobilize the ureters down to the trigone, and free the left one carefully as far as the kidney, so that it may be pulled through retroperitoneally below the duodenum. Spatulate the right distal ureter and anastomosis to the right side of the ileum. Make a deeper spatulating incision in the left ureter, and use it to close the proximal end of ileum. During construction of each anastomosis, after the proximal suture is placed, hold a stent on a long clamp, and insert it up the cecum and through the intussusception into the ileum. Alternatively, it may be easier to pass an extra feeding tube down through the intussusception and out the cecum and tie the stent to it to guide it through the ileocecal valve; then cut the tie, pull the stent back to the level of the anastomotic site, and advance it up the ureter. Pass the stents out through the bladder wall, or the colic tenia if the bladder has been subtotally resected, and fix them to the skin with silk sutures.

Trim excess ileal length by dividing and ligating the vessels in the mesentery and by dividing the bowel beyond a Kocher clamp. Close the ileum in one layer with 4-0 silk pull-off sutures, as described on page 375. Tack it to the dome of the cecum unless it already was fixed, as previously described. An alternative method is to resect the ileum and turn in the stump, as depicted in Figure 8. Connect the ureters to the cecum with an antireflux technique (pages 427–433). When the ureters have been destroyed and ureteral substitution is required, start with a longer length of terminal ileum to be able to anastomose the upper ureter or pelvis to it.

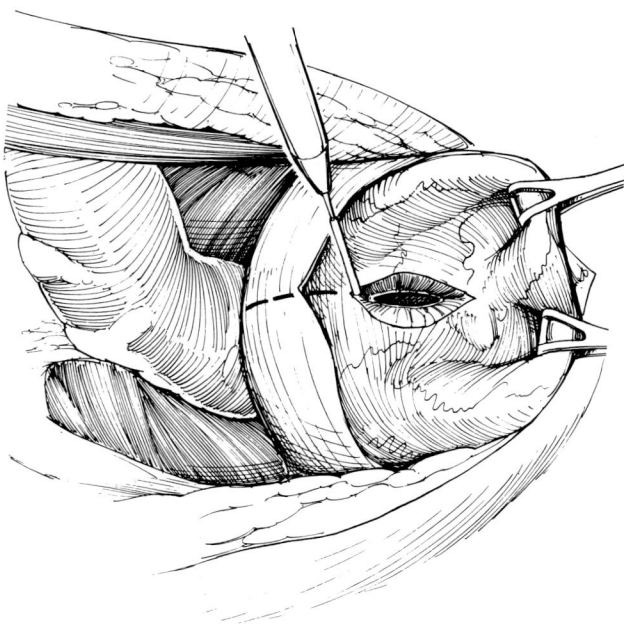

19 Trim the crushed edges of the cecum caused by the Kocher clamp or stapler. Adjust the size of the cecal opening to fit that made in the bladder by slitting the antimesenteric border. Suture the ascending colon to the bladder opening after rotating it counterclockwise 180 degrees, so that the mesenteric margin of the bowel fits into the interureteric ridge in the midline posteriorly. Start two sutures of 3-0 chromic catgut posteriorly to include the mucosa and submucosa of the mesenteric edge of the colon and the urothelium of the bladder. Run them up each side, and tie them anteriorly. A second seromuscular layer of 2-0 chromic catgut may be placed. Alternatively, use the technique described for colocystoplasty (pages 447–449). Place Penrose drains to the area for adequate drainage. Close the peritoneum and body wall in layers. Bring the cystostomy tube and stents through stab wounds, and sew them to the skin with braided silk. Insert a 5-ml silicone balloon catheter of suitable size through the urethra. Attach the stents and catheters to drainage.

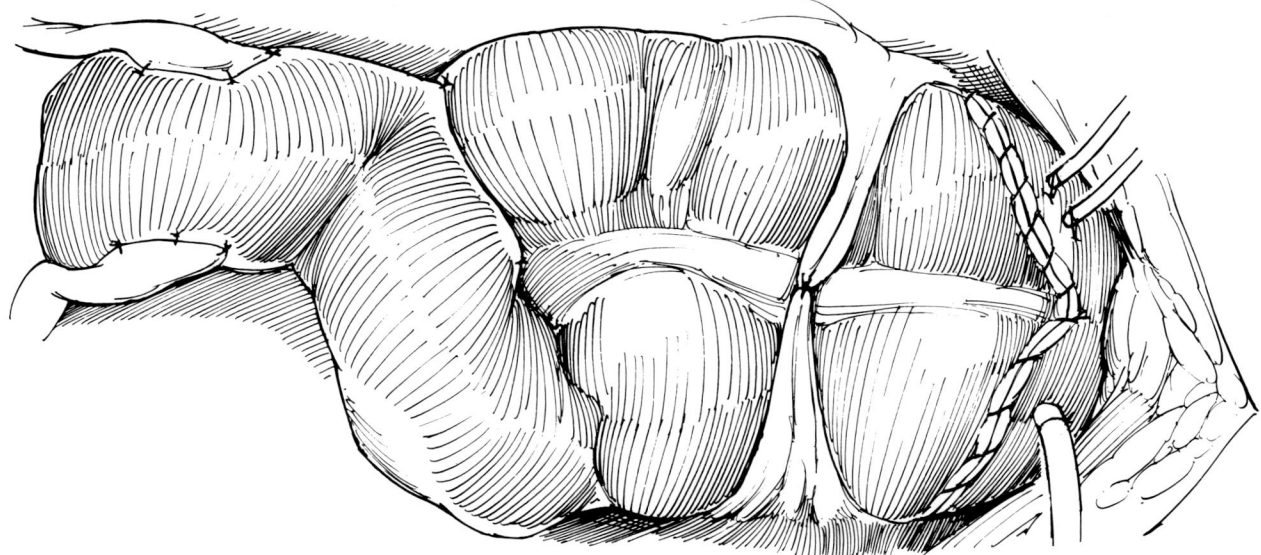

POSTOPERATIVE RESPONSIBILITIES

Adjust fluid and electrolyte levels assiduously. Irrigate the bladder through the cystostomy tube three times a day to evacuate mucus. Withdraw the drains after the drainage declines. Remove the ureteral catheters on the 10th postoperative day, and the cystostomy tube on the 14th day after obtaining a gravity cystogram. Finally, take out the urethral catheter after testing for voiding.

Commentary by Helen Parkhouse

Cecocystoplasty has few indications in pediatric practice. The long-term risk of neoplasia is potentially greater than for ileum or stomach, and mucous production is more difficult to deal with in children because of the small size of catheters used for intermittent self-catheterization. The most common indication for bladder augmentation in children is the neuropathic bladder. Because many children with neuropathic bladder also have renal impairment with metabolic acidosis, the use of bowel for augmentation may cause further metabolic problems. For this reason, gastrocystoplasty is preferred for children with renal failure, although the long-term results are unknown.

Cecocystoplasty certainly should be considered in children with coexisting congenital or acquired abnormalities (*eg*, short-gut syndrome) that preclude the use of small bowel or stomach.

CHAPTER 92

Ileocecocystoplasty

(MAINZ)

Bisect or trim the bladder wall, as described preparatory to bowel anastomosis (Chapter 91).

Follow the technique for ileocecal bladder substitution (Mainz) (page 263), but make the total length of the ileal segments only 20 to 30 cm by omitting the 25- to 30-cm tail.

1 **A,** *Orientation and incision:* Midline lower abdominal (page 413). **B,** Anastomose the bowel segments to each other, as described for bladder substitution (page

413). Test to see if the mesentery is long enough to allow the bowel plate to reach the resected edge of the bladder. **C,** If not, rotate the plate 180 degrees counterclockwise. Place a single row of through-and-through interrupted 3-0 synthetic sutures to connect the lower edge of the bowel plate to the bladder posteriorly. Anastomose the ureters into either the ascending colon or the inverted cecum, depending on the rotation. Insert two 90-cm J-stents or 5 F or 8 F infant feeding tubes into the ureters. Place stay sutures to stretch the tenia on each side of the proposed tunnel.

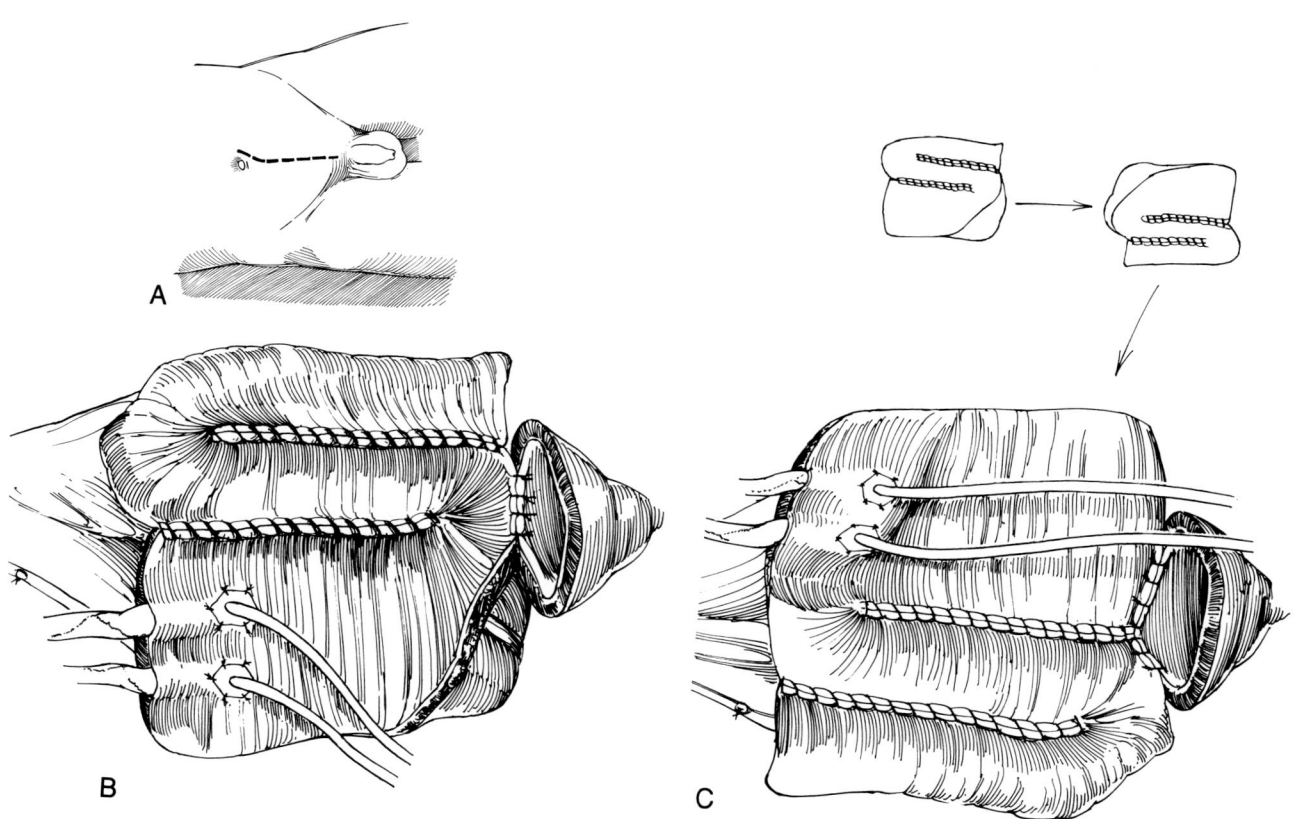

2 Place a 16 F Malecot catheter in the bladder through a stab wound, and bring the ureteral stents through separate stab wounds. Complete the anastomosis of the bowel and bladder anteriorly by a single row of through-and-through interrupted 3-0 synthetic absorbable sutures. Close the anterior wall of the pouch with a through-and-through running 4-0 synthetic absorbable suture. Take care to close only the mucosa at the site of ureteral entry. Insert a 22 F silicone balloon catheter transurethrally, and drain the area of bladder and ureteral anastomosis with two drains placed on gravity (not suction) drainage. Although watertight closure of the pouch is not essential, major leaks should be closed with additional sutures. Suture the cystostomy tube and stents to the skin. Repeatedly culture the ureteral urine. Remove the stents one at a time in 10 days and the balloon catheter at 2 to 3 weeks. Remove the cystostomy catheter after a cystogram shows no extravasation and spontaneous voiding occurs with less than 50 ml residual urine.

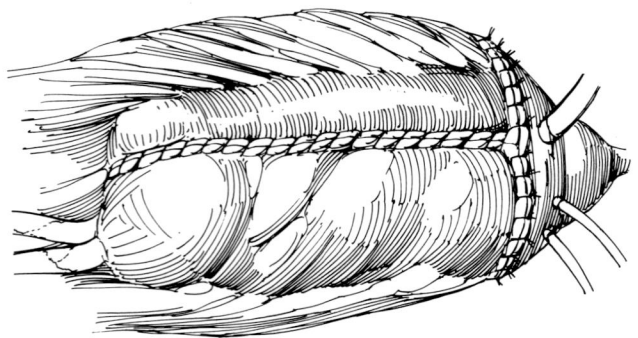

POSTOPERATIVE PROBLEMS

The problems associated with other forms of augmentation with bowel (page 450) may occur.

ILEOCECAL SPHINCTER PLICATION TECHNIQUE
(NISSAN-ZINMAN)

3 Insert a 30 F catheter in the isolated ileocecal segment retrogradely through the ileocecal valve. Intussuscept the ileum into the cecum, and fix it with three or four 3-0 nonabsorbable sutures.

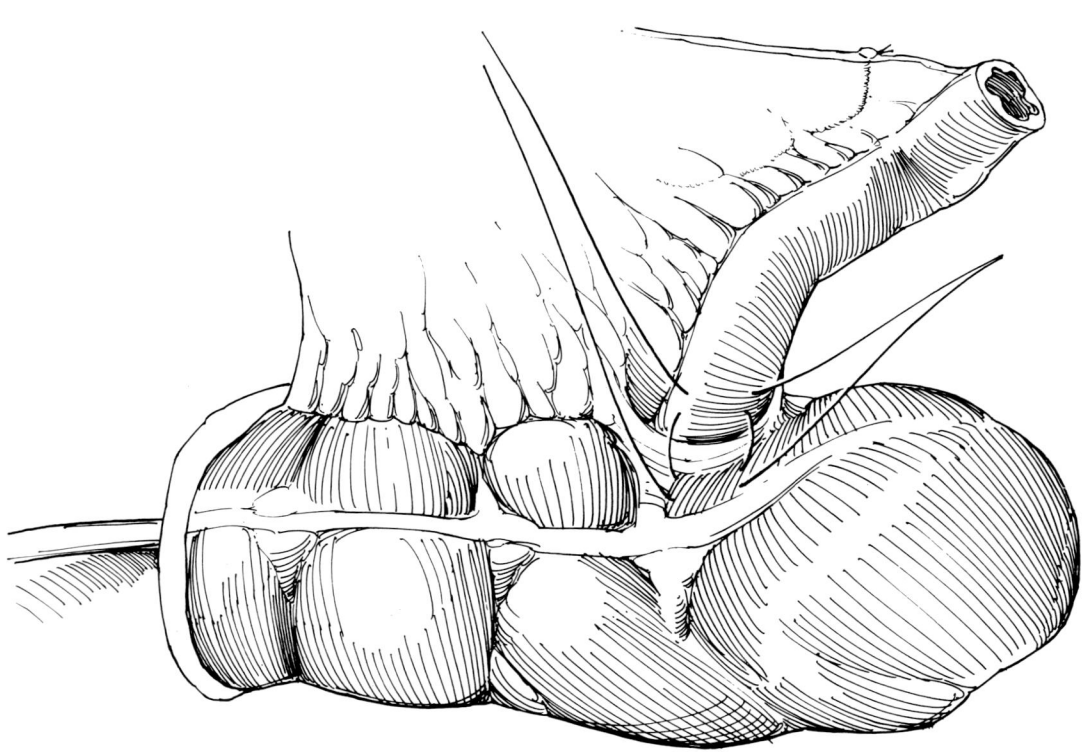

4 Wrap the redundant cecum around 6 to 8 cm of terminal ileum to enclose two thirds of ileal circumference. Fasten the ileum in place with a row of four or five 3-0 nonabsorbable sutures. Test the effectiveness of the valve by gravity instillation of saline tinted with methylene blue. The valve can be reinforced with another row of sutures if it leaks.

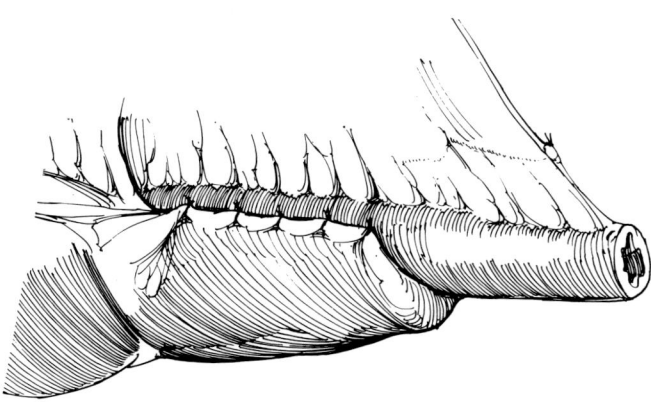

INTERNAL FIXATION TECHNIQUE (HENDREN-KING)

5 Clear the mesentery from the terminal ileum for 8 cm. Open the cecum along the anterior tenia. Incise the serosa of the ileum on the antimesenteric border.

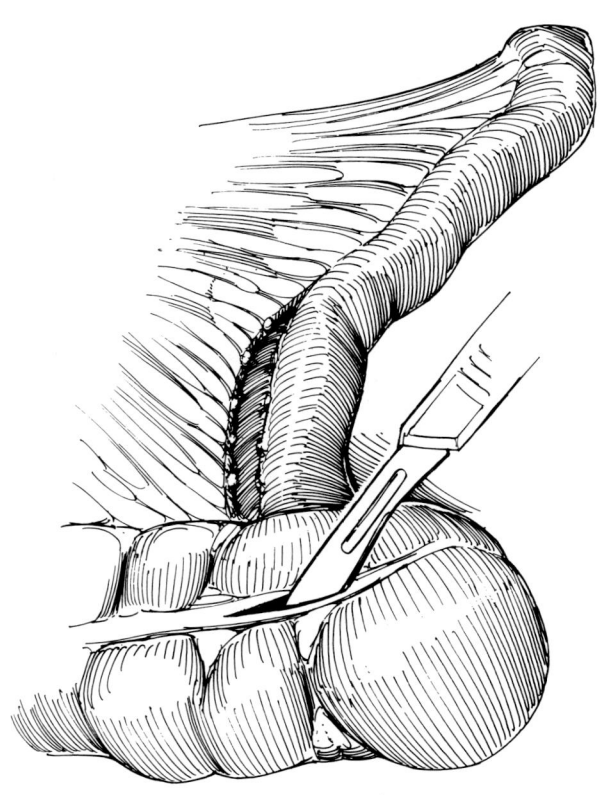

6 Draw 8 cm of the ileum into the cecum for a 4-cm nipple. Incise the full thickness of the posterior wall of the ileal nipple with electrocautery for 3 cm. Similarly incise the facing cecal mucosa into the muscularis. Suture the apices of these incisions together with a 3-0 synthetic absorbable suture.

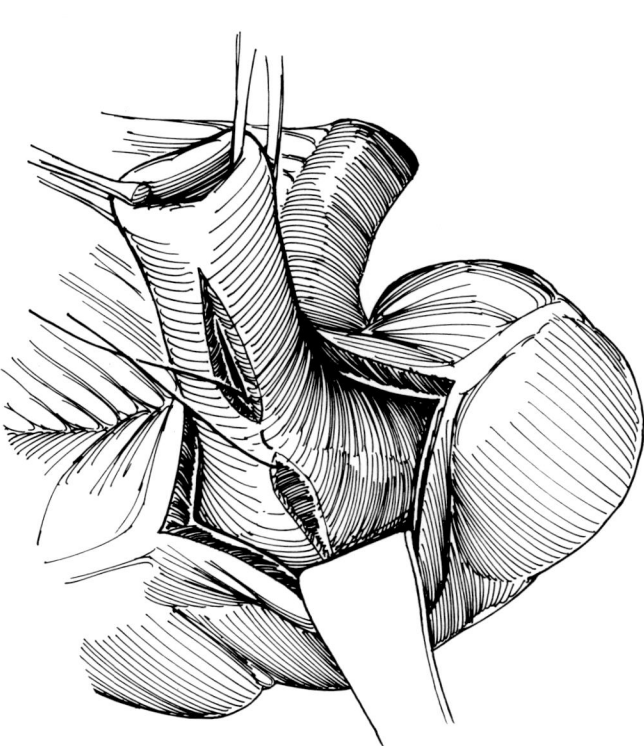

7 Proceed down each side of the defects with interrupted sutures.

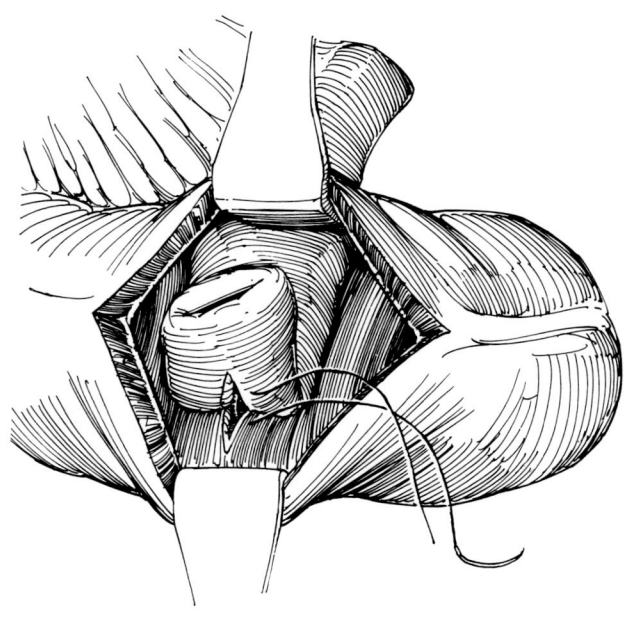

8 Close the cecotomy, and tack the ileum to the cecum with 3-0 nonabsorbable adventitial sutures at the site of entry.

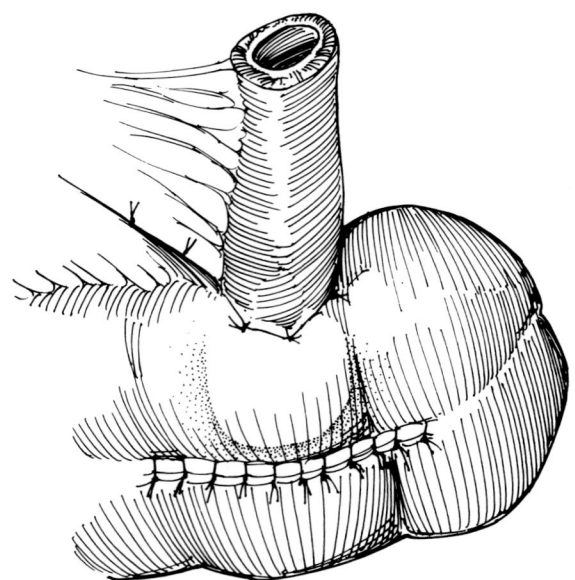

9 With either method, anastomose the conjoined spatulated ureters to the ileum with interrupted fine absorbable sutures. Alternatively, anastomose the right ureter to the side of the ileum and the widely spatulated left ureter to the open end of the ileum. Stent the ureters with infant feeding tubes or single-J catheters led through the remains of the bladder wall or through the anterior tenia. Place a tube in the bladder to remain 3 weeks.

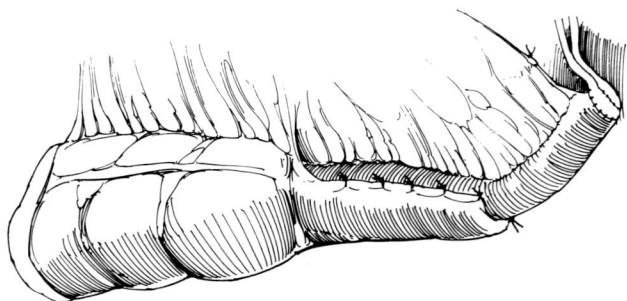

Commentary by Lowell R. King

The stabilized intussuscepted ileal nipple has proved to be reliable in preventing reflux in a patient undergoing bladder substitution with a detubularized ileocecal segment or an ileal cup. When the ureters are dilated from reflux or obstruction, it is our experience that good drainage can be reliably predicted when the ureters are implanted into the ileum above the type of stabilized intussusception illustrated here. In more than 60 cases we have performed, obstruction has not occurred. Reflux was present in three cases in the immediate postoperative period but persisted in only one patient, who required revision because of disintussusception of the nipple. In that particular case, loss of the nipple was caused by high intravesical pressures before muscle-to-muscle bonding of ileal nipple muscle to the cecal wall had a chance to occur. Perhaps most important, emergent reflux has not occurred with follow-up observation as long as 9 years, and we are becoming optimistic that the muscle-to-muscle bonding, together with the lateral attachment of the nipple against the bowel wall, will prevent disintussusception for the long term.

CHAPTER 93

Gastrocystoplasty
(MITCHELL)

Place the child on a liquid diet for 48 hours, and give magnesium citrate 24 hours before operation. The child may be admitted the day of surgery. Attempt to sterilize the urine.

1 Insert a nasogastric tube. The child will have been covered by preventive antibiotics.

Incision: Midline transperitoneal from xiphoid to pubis (page 83). Expose the bladder through the lower part of the incision, and open it sagittally in the midline ("bivalve"). The incision should extend from the bladder neck anteriorly to the trigone posteriorly. Control bleeding by electrocautery. Insert infant feeding tubes of suitable size into each ureter. Preparing the bladder first reduces acid spillage from the stomach, but in myelomeningocele patients with shunts, it may be better to open the bladder after the gastric patch has been prepared to avoid prolonged drainage of urine into the abdominal cavity. Place an artificial sphincter at this point, if indicated.

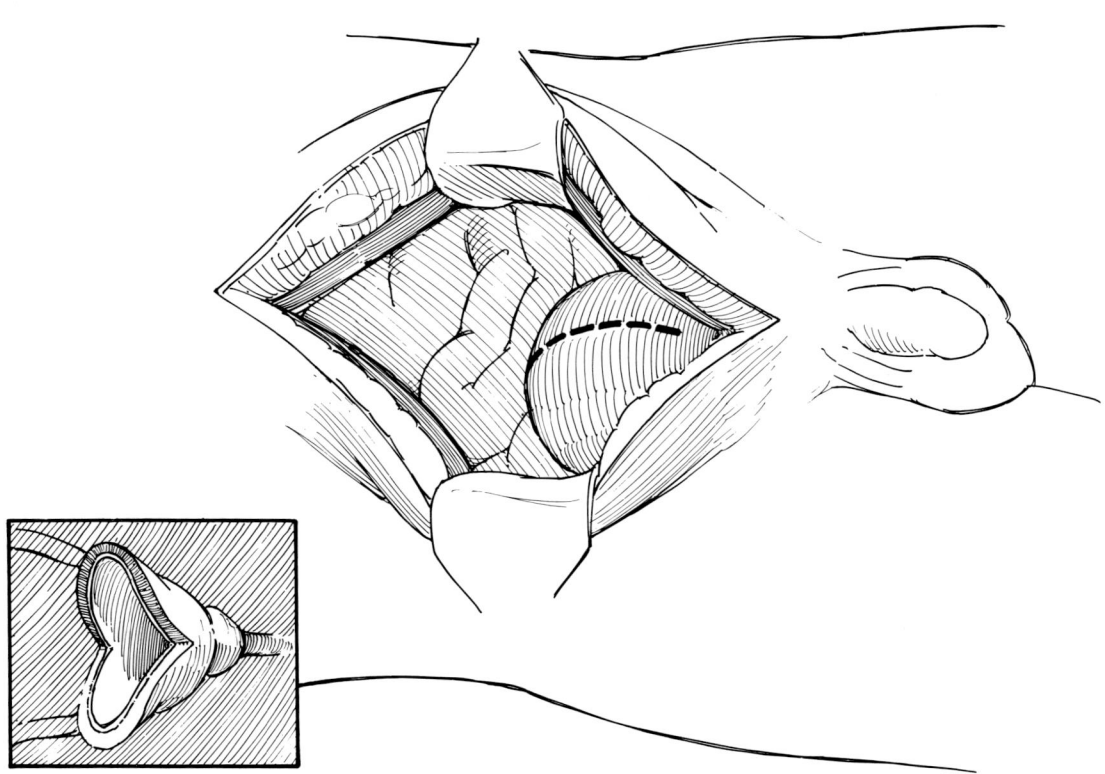

2 Extend the incision cephalad, and open the peritoneum. Reimplant the ureters, and prepare the bladder neck area for sphincter or sling, if indicated.

Right-sided pedicle: Draw the stomach into the wound with large Babcock clamps. Examine the right and left gastroepiploic arteries over the greater curvature of the stomach. The left gastroepiploic artery arises from terminal branching of the splenic artery. The right gastroepiploic artery is a branch of the gastroduodenal artery. Together they form the gastroepiploic arterial arch. The left gastroepiploic artery is found not infrequently to merge into the greater curvature or to taper to a small caliber, whereas the caliber of the right is more constant. For this reason, the right vessel usually is used to supply the flap.

Free the omentum from the transverse colon by dividing its relatively thin avascular connection. Incise the greater omentum 1 or 2 cm distal to the gastroepiploic artery on the right side with the electrocautery while clamping and tying the larger vessels (page 272). Leave the vessels intact on the left, so that the omentum may descend with the patch.

Select as large a wedge as possible—one that encompasses at least a third of the stomach. Because the right gastroepiploic artery will be the base, tend to make the wedge toward the left side of the stomach to have as long a pedicle as possible. Outline the proposed wedge with a marking pen after grasping the edges of the greater curvature with Babcock clamps and putting traction on them. The length of each arm of the wedge should approximately equal the width of the patch and should approach, but not reach, the lesser curvature. Divide the short arteries to the stomach starting at the right side of the proposed wedge and working to the right. Do this by passing a Providence clamp through the omentum on each side of the first short artery, to the right of the right arm of the wedge; elevate the artery, and draw a 4-0 synthetic absorbable suture under the artery. Tie the suture. Clamp and divide the artery close to the stomach, then ligate the end of the vessel in the clamp. Avoid traction on the gastroepiploic vessel to prevent arterial spasm. This technique also avoids retraction of the proximal (omental) end that could quickly produce a potentially harmful interstitial hematoma. Continue with the remaining branches, avoiding mass ligation and contact with the gastroepiploic arterial arch itself, to reach the gastroduodenal origin of the arch. Because an undivided branch could be torn easily when the flap is pulled into place, preserve a 5- to 7-cm band of omental vessels intact to protect the pedicle from avulsion. On the left side of the patch, the omentum is left attached to the pedicle so that it subsequently may be used to cover the repair.

Inspect the right gastroepiploic artery to be sure it has good pulsations before clamping and dividing the left gastroepiploic artery on the other side of the wedge. Spasm may be prevented by applying papaverine hydrochloride solution to it.

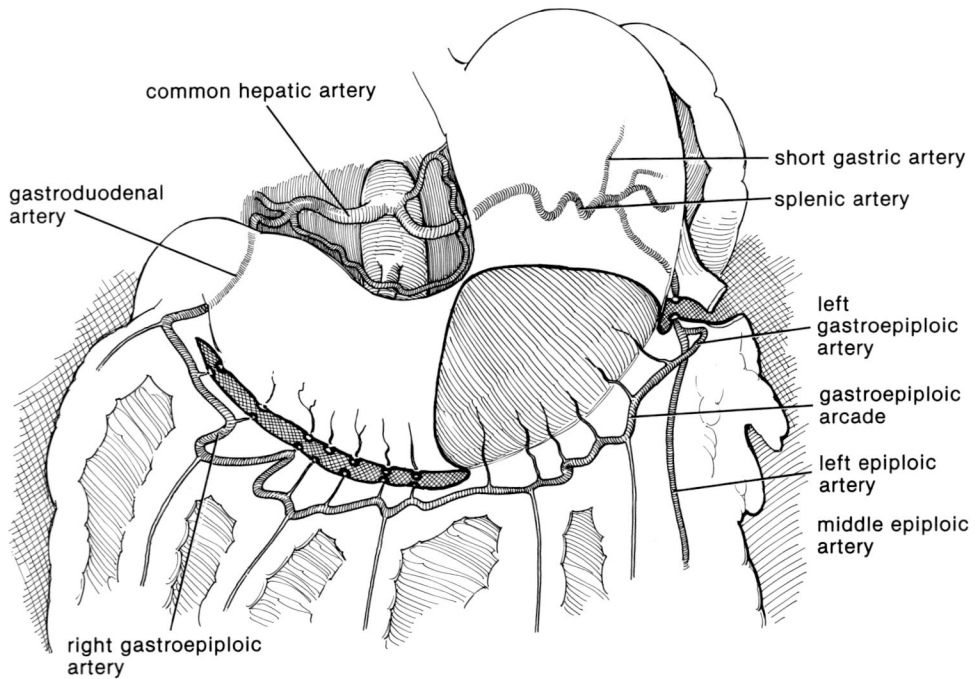

3 Place parallel bowel clamps on either side of the gastric wedge. Ligate the branches off the gastric vessels of the lesser curvature near the apex of the wedge to prevent significant bleeding. Pack the area with laparotomy tapes to minimize spillage. Excise the wedge, taking care not to injure the vascular pedicle. Place the wedge in a moist laparotomy tape for protection.

Alternatively (shown here), insert the 70- to 90-mm gastrointestinal anastomosis stapler (GIA-90) twice, and resect the wedge. Be careful not to damage the vascular pedicle when the instrument is placed at the right side of the

wedge. Place a moist laparotomy tape around the wedge before placing it in the pelvis; similarly protect the pedicle itself. If the stomach has a saccular shape, instead of taking a wedge, staple off the bottom with the GIA-90 stapler. Alternatively, by excising and not stapling, time is saved by avoiding cutting out the staples, but blood is lost during reconstitution of the stomach.

Make the pedicle as long as possible by dissection near the gastroduodenal junction. If greater length is needed, divide a few more vessels distally on the patch.

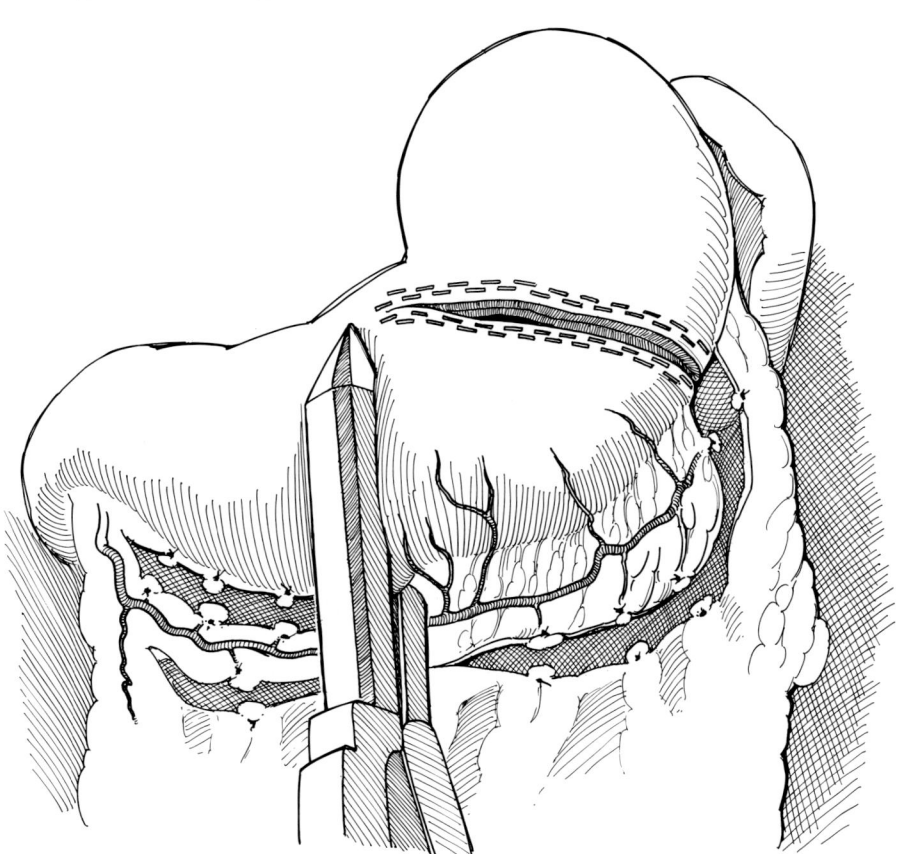

4 *Left-sided pedicle:* The short arteries are divided starting at the left side of the proposed wedge and continued to just distal to the origin of the left gastroepiploic artery, near its origin from the splenic artery.

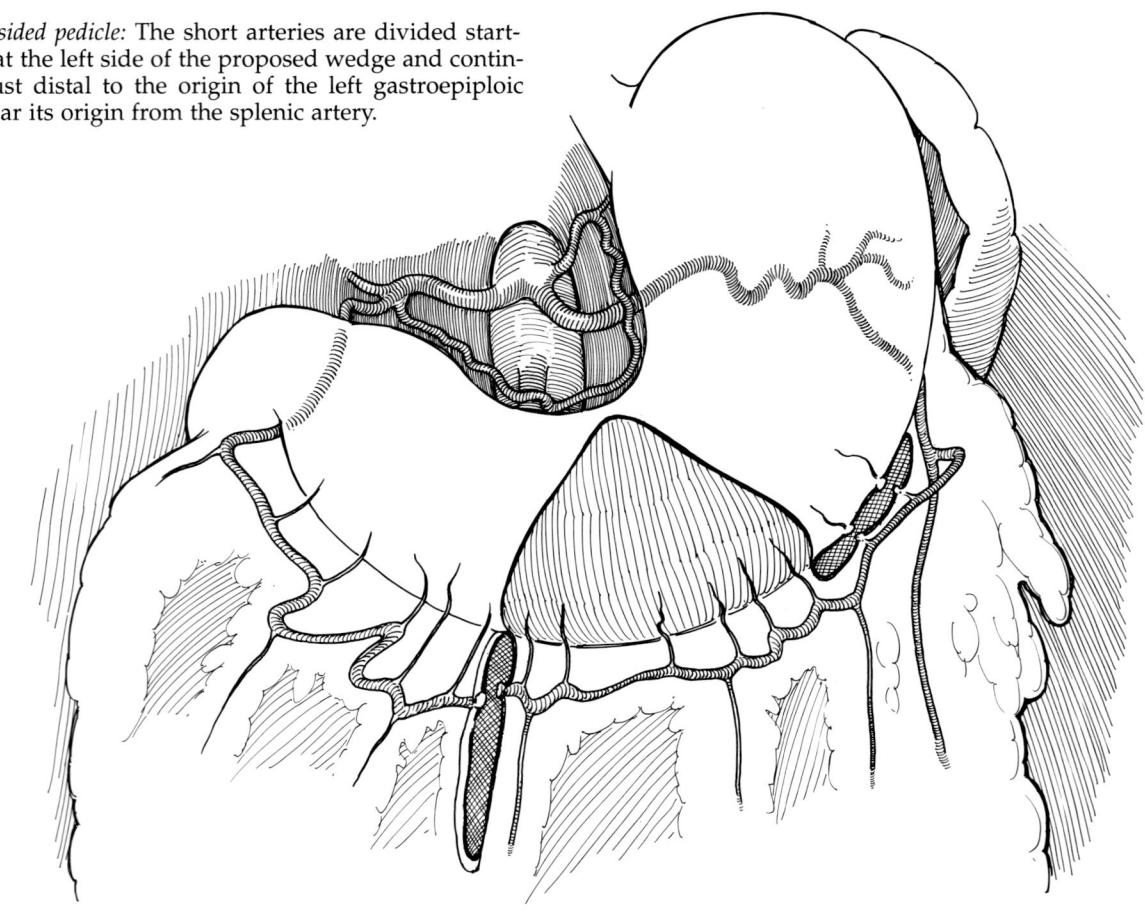

5 To close the stomach, place a posterior seromuscular row of interrupted 3-0 silk sutures, tie them, and then remove the staples, at least those on the anterior wall suture line. Place an inner through-and-through layer of running locked stitches with 3-0 synthetic absorbable sutures. Move the nasogastric tube into the antrum just proximal to the suture line.

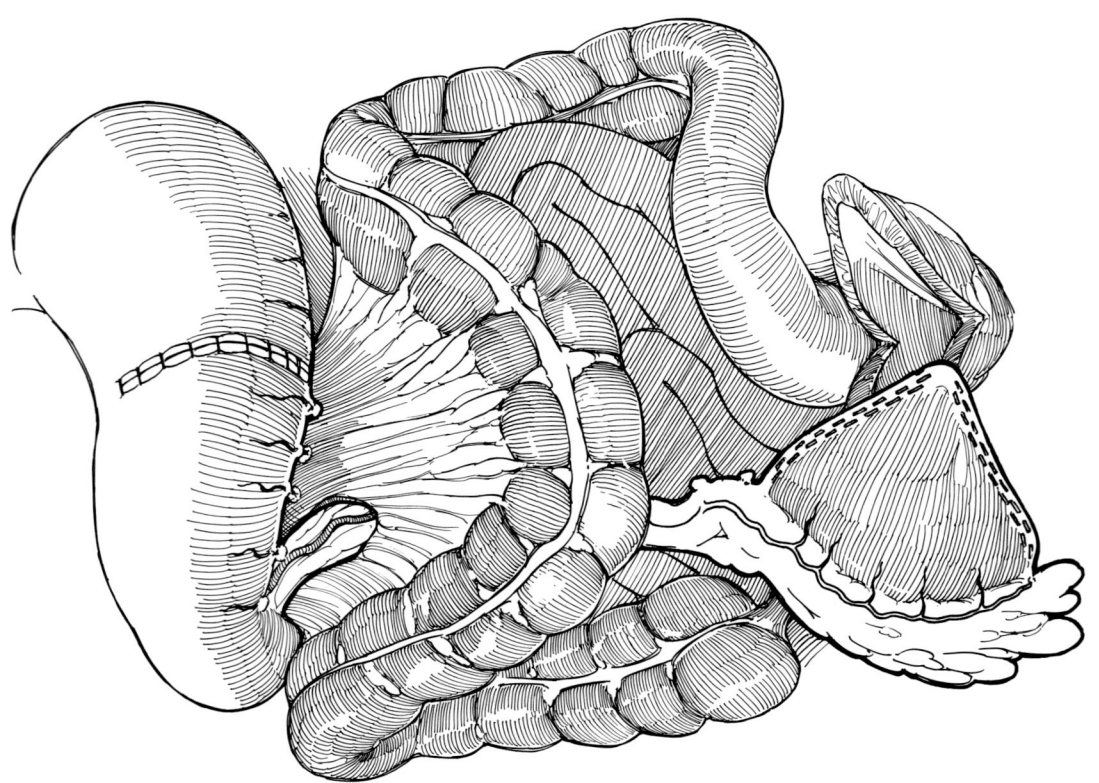

6 Pass the flap on its pedicle under the transverse meso-colon along the root of the small intestine and through the mesentery of the small intestine (arrow). Alternatively, elevate the right colon, and place the entire pedicle beneath its mesentery, siting it in the retroperitoneum. Avoid rotating the mesentery. Should the flap not reach the bladder, free more of the vessels connecting the artery to the duodenum. Recheck the pulsation in the artery in the pedicle.

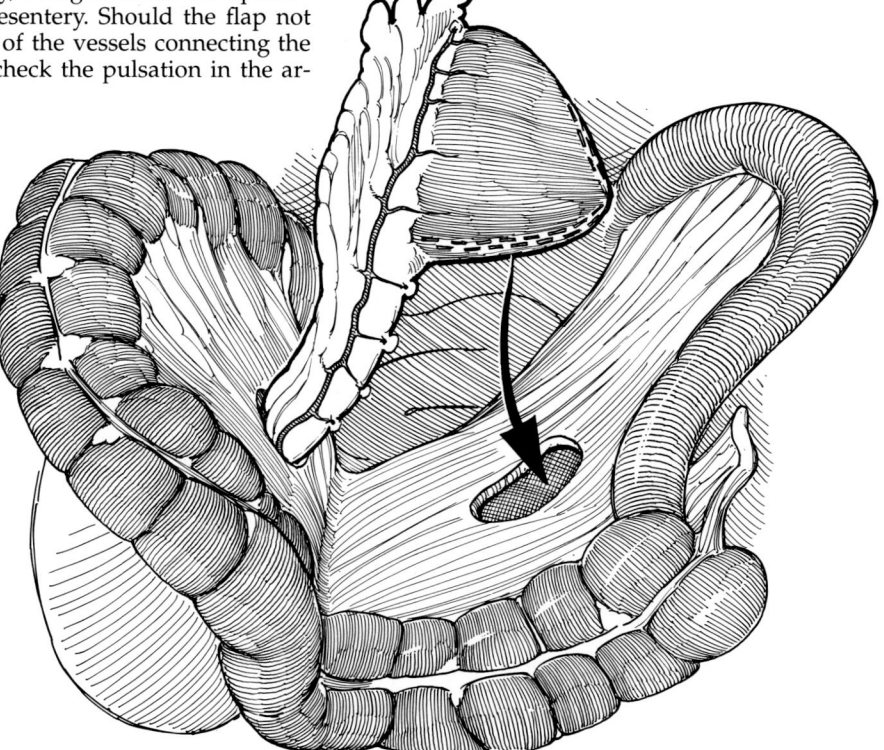

7 The former ventral side of the stomach flap will now lie anteriorly, and its apex will be fastened to the vesical neck, while the apex of the former dorsal surface extends to the trigone.

Remove all of the staples. Run full-thickness locked 3-0 chromic catgut sutures from the trigone up each arm to the dome from inside the bladder, and reinforce the suture lines with a second layer of seromuscular 3-0 synthetic absorbable sutures, placed from the outside.

Place a Malecot catheter of a caliber adequate to handle mucus (at least 16 F) through the bladder wall (or through the patch, if necessary). Remove the ureteral catheters unless surgery has been performed on the ureteral orifices.

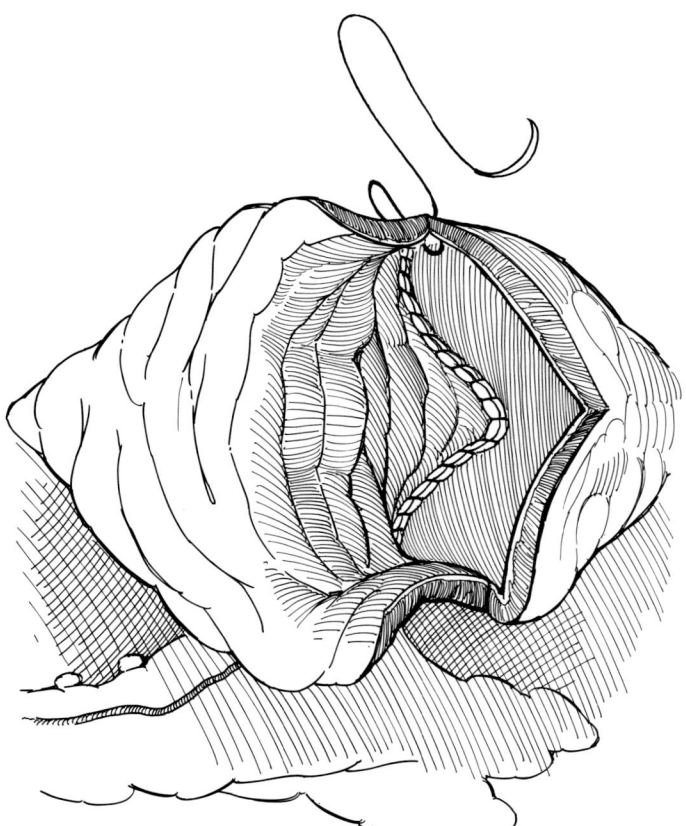

8 Insert a urethral catheter for added safety during the postoperative period, and fix it transvesically on the anterior abdominal wall with a stitch through its tip tied over a bolster.

Close the anterior portion with similar sutures (a running locked 3-0 chromic catgut suture from the inside and a running 3-0 synthetic absorbable suture from the outside). Test the suture line by filling the bladder; place additional sutures if needed. This also is a chance to see if filling disturbs the blood supply to the pedicle. Inspect the gastroepiploic artery in the pedicle again. Fix the pedicle to the posterior peritoneum along the root of the small bowel, or close the opened peritoneum over it with a running 3-0 chromic catgut suture. Place the left side of the omentum over the small bowel (and, if long enough, the anterior suture line), and use the portion from the left side that is attached to the patch to cover the posterior anastomosis. Drains are not necessary. Again, distend the bladder for a final check.

Maintain nasogastric suction until the child passes gas, then start easily digestible liquid feedings. Check the suture lines with a cystogram. Discharge the child after 1 week with the suprapubic catheter in place, and give suppressive antibiotics. Have the child return 1 or 2 weeks later to have the tube clamped, so that either intermittent catheterization or voiding may begin. If that goes well, remove the tube 1 week later. Check the results in 2 or 3 months by ultrasound and cystogram.

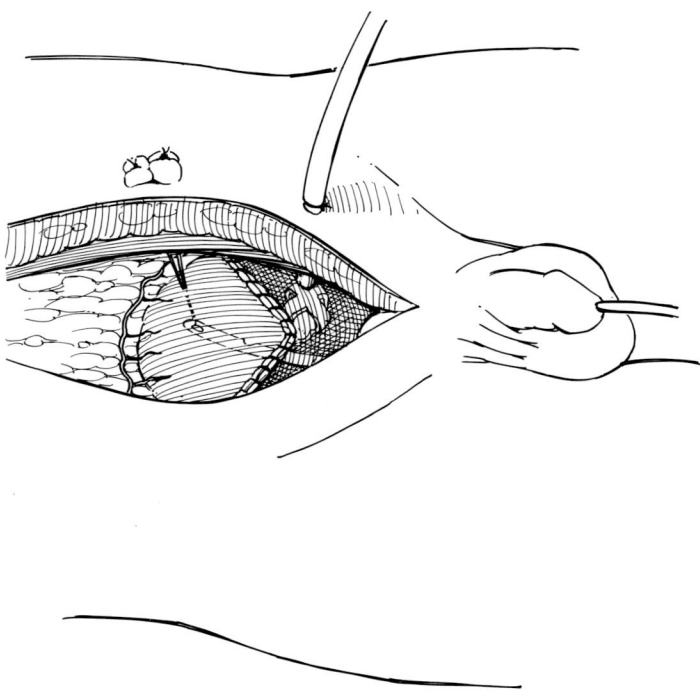

POSTOPERATIVE PROBLEMS

Penile burning from hyperacid urine is treated with an H_2 receptor antagonist, such as cimetidine. Giving the child an antacid tablet after meals clears the penile burning quickly. Urinary pH levels should be checked regularly. *Asymptomatic infections* do not need treatment. *Electrolyte imbalance* will be detected by monthly determinations for the first 6 months. It may become severe if the child has an episode of vomiting or diarrhea with resultant salt loss; if this occurs, salt replacement is mandatory.

Commentary by Richard C. Rink

Use of the gastric segment for bladder augmentation has allowed lower urinary tract reconstruction in many children who previously were not candidates. It has been particularly useful in the child with a paucity of bowel, such as the patient with cloacal exstrophy, or in one requiring reconstruction following pelvic irradiation, when the bowel is compromised. The other major indication for the use of stomach has been renal insufficiency with acidosis. The gastric segment will act as a chloride pump with net chloride and hydrogen ion transport into the urine to prevent further acidosis. In comparison with bowel segments, the use of gastric segments has lessened symptomatic lower urinary infections in our series. However, this may be offset by hematuria and dysuria.

Preoperatively, it is important to rule out any history of stomach abnormalities, such as ulcer disease or gastric emptying abnormalities. A severe salt-wasting nephropathy should be identified preoperatively. Children having this disorder are poor candidates because gastrocystoplasty may worsen the fluid and electrolyte abnormalities.

I would suggest caution using stomach for reconstruction in the child with normal sensation, because hematuria and dysuria have been seen in one third of our patients. This may lead to significant perineal pain in those with normal sensation and, at times, may be quite difficult to resolve. The gastric wedge taken for augmentation generally is smaller than for the gastric reservoir. Initially, we were somewhat conservative in the amount of stomach used, and this has been reflected in marginal urodynamic studies in some of the early patients in our series. I would be certain that at least one third of the stomach is used for augmentation to ensure that the most compliant, largest-capacity reservoir can be obtained. We have not seen problems with the native stomach postoperatively, because we have been taking larger segments. The use of the stapler to excise the wedge may prevent some gastric spillage and blood loss, but this is offset by wasting stomach tissue during excision of the staple lines. I excise the wedge between bowel clamps. It is helpful to ligate the branches of the gastric artery to the patch near the apex of the wedge to prevent blood loss. It also is helpful to back the bowel clamp off the stomach wall and run the inner layer on the back wall of the stomach closure first, because this acts as a hemostatic closure and prevents inverting a large portion of the stomach wall.

The pedicle must be secured to the posterior peritoneum to prevent its injury and to avoid an area for bowel herniation. We generally tack the omentum along the pedicle to the posterior peritoneum as it runs along the root of the small bowel. Alternatively, the entire right colon can be elevated and the pedicle placed in the retroperitoneum behind the bowel and its mesentery. We had four bowel obstructions in our initial 41 patients, and at least one involved the gastric pedicle. The wedge generally is rotated and anastomosed to the bivalved bladder, as described in the preceding technique. However, we have, at times, rotated this only 90 degrees to achieve a better "fit." This results in the gastroepiploic artery on the wedge running in an anteroposterior fashion on the bladder, rather than in its usual transverse lie. If there is tension on the pedicle when the artery reaches the bladder, length can be gained by two methods. More vessels from the gastroepiploic artery to the stomach and duodenum can be divided, or the initial short artery from the gastroepiploic artery to the wedge itself can be divided. The richly vascular plexus keeps this portion of the wedge perfused.

I do not leave ureteral stents, because urine will help buffer any early acid production. However, double drainage by urethral and suprapubic tubes is important during the initial healing phase. A Penrose drain is left in all patients, although in those with ventriculoperitoneal shunts, it is removed early.

Postoperatively, the child is placed on H_2 blockade and is maintained on this treatment for the 1st month. Although mucous production is reduced with stomach versus other intestinal segments, we still irrigate the bladder free of mucus every 8 hours in the hospital, and the parents are instructed to do this twice a day after discharge. Early on, "coffee-ground" urine may be present, which is concerning to the uninitiated. This will pass. When the child returns in 2 weeks, the suprapubic tube is clamped, and intermittent catheterization or spontaneous voiding is started. The catheter is removed only when it is established that the family or child can reliably catheterize, or that the child can spontaneously void to completion. Initially, catheterization may be necessary as frequently as every 2 hours, with awakening once at night to empty. The bladder would adequately stretch during the next 2 weeks to allow catheterizations every 4 hours during waking hours and avoidance of nocturnal catheterization.

With any associated viral illness resulting in vomiting, electrolyte levels must be checked to determine whether treatment of significant hypochloremic alkalosis is needed.

Commentary by Michael E. Mitchell

There are two foci of potential vascular obstruction in the pedicle of the gastric flap. One is at the gastric antrum, where angulation can occur if the right gastroepiploic artery is used as the pedicle. To avoid this, free the gastroepiploic vessels, so that there is no possible tethering by short vessels to the gastric antrum. Always check this area after the gastric flap is brought into the pelvis. The second focus is the distal end of the gastroepiploic artery where it enters the flap. It may be necessary to divide one or two of the most proximal short vessels to the flap to prevent angulation. This will not jeopardize the blood supply to this portion of the flap and will protect the blood supply to the entire flap. Vascular spasm rarely is observed during the completion of the posterior suture line of the bladder anastomosis. Watch for change in color of the gastric mucosa. Purple color or paleness is a sign of vascular compromise. Immediately check the proximal and distal ends of the pedicle, and apply papaverine to the entire length. Spasm occurs approximately 10 percent of the time but never should result in loss of the flap.

Remove the staples from the wedge-shaped flap just before suturing it to the bladder. (The wedge flap is opened along posterior staple line and anastomosed to the posterior bladder; then, the anterior staples are removed, and anterior anastomosis is completed.) This prevents needless blood loss and spillage of gastric juices. At the conclusion of the anastomosis of the gastric flap to the stomach, *all* staples should be removed from the flap.

The suprapubic tube usually is brought through the native bladder. However, if it is necessary to bring it through the flap, tissue adjacent to the tube should be sutured to the anterior abdominal wall, similar to a gastrostomy. This prevents needless intraperitoneal leakage with removal of the suprapubic tube.

Nasogastric suction needs to be used only 2 to 3 days postoperatively. Patients can leave the hospital 5 to 7 days after gastrocystoplasty. The suprapubic tube is removed only after complete bladder emptying (by voiding, catheterization, or other methods) has been proved. If ureteral reimplants into the flap portion of the augmented bladder are required, the posterior aspect of the suture line is completed, and the reimplants are performed with the standard tunnel technique. If the appendiceal Mitrofanoff technique is to be considered, it can be performed after the anterior closure and in the manner described by Barry *et al.* (1976) for reimplantation of the transplant ureter into the bladder. A direct-catheterizable channel from the umbilicus through the appendix-catheterizable channel to the bladder is thereby constructed.

Hematuria and/or dysuria are seen in 36 percent of patients with gastrocystoplasty. Five percent will have significant symptoms, and approximately 20 percent will require periodic treatment. The critical factor in these patients is serum gastrin levels. If the serum gastrin level is persistently elevated, consideration may have to be given to alternative means of augmentation. The presence of hematuria and dysuria without gastrin elevation usually is treated with H_2 blockers and, occasionally, with alkaline irrigation of the bladder.

PART VI

BLADDER SUBSTITUTION

CHAPTER 94

Introduction to Bladder Substitution
URETHRA PRESENT

Bladder replacement may be needed in a child with exstrophy when the bladder is taken to construct a continent urethra. In general, bowel substitution is a good alternative to diversion, although nocturnal incontinence can be expected in a number of cases.

Two general types of substitution currently are in use, one formed from opened ileum (Camey), the other from some rearrangement of the cecum and terminal ileum (Mainz, LeBag, Indiana).

The amount of bowel used should be small enough so that a capacity of 500 to 600 ml is not exceeded, because reservoirs larger than that promote excessive electrolyte absorption and use excessive lengths of bowel with resultant diarhhea. However, the new bladder must be large enough to keep the pressure low, because children tend to void at normal intervals but will void by abdominal straining and must arise at night to keep dry.

CHAPTER 95

Ileal Bladder Substitution

Prepare the bowel. Give prophylactic antibiotics perioperatively.

Incision. Make a midline incision (page 83). Expose the urethra.

U-SHAPED ILEAL BLADDER

(CAMEY)

Select a 35- to 40-cm loop of terminal ileum, the midportion of which will reach the urethra without tension. If this is not possible, use another method of substitution. After being sure the mesentery is long enough, divide the ileum at the ends of the segment and reestablish continuity (page 375).

1 Make a 1.5-cm incision in the antimesenteric border of the segment at its center or slightly to the right. Anastomose the ileum to the urethra using angle sutures through the ileum from inside out and posterior sutures from outside in. Push the openings together while gradually tightening the sutures. Tie the posterior sutures, but do not cut them until all sutures are tied. Hold the lateral sutures in clamps.

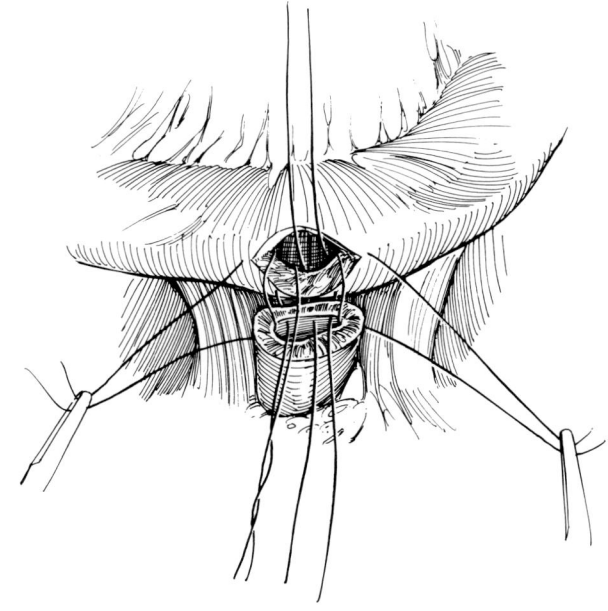

2 **A,** To construct a ureteroileostomy, incise one end of the loop on its antimesenteric border for 4 cm. Starting 1.5 cm from the end, divide the mucosa on the posterior wall longitudinally for 3 or 3.5 cm to expose the muscularis. Insinuate a curved clamp through the wall at the proximal end of the furrow from inside to outside to make a tunnel large enough for the ureter to pass through loosely. **B,** Pull 3 cm of ureter into the lumen, and secure it to the serosa outside with three 4-0 synthetic absorbable

sutures. **C,** Cut the ureter obliquely, and fix the tip to the mucosa and muscularis at the distal end of the furrow with three 3-0 synthetic absorbable sutures. Complete the anastomosis with lateral mucosal sutures. Avoid angulating the ureter where it enters the ileum—that could lead to ureteral obstruction. Leave the ureter lying superficial to the ileum. Repeat the procedure at the other end of the loop.

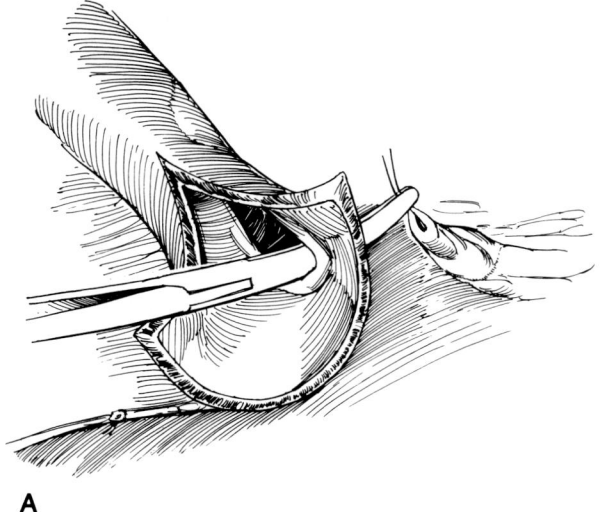

A

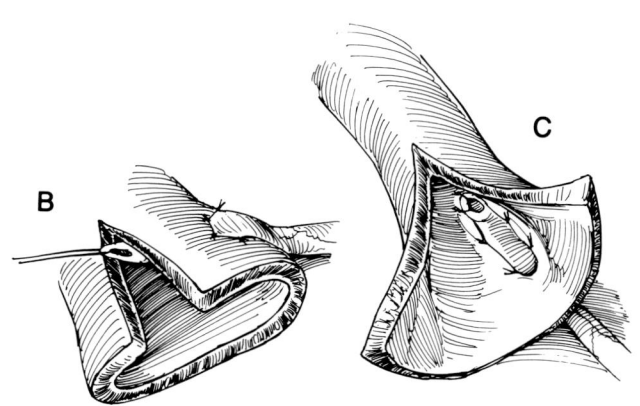

3 Cut extra holes in the end of a length of 8 F silicone tubing, and insert it up each ureter into the renal pelvis. Tack the stents to the ileal mucosa with a 4-0 plain catgut suture 1 cm below the site of exit from the ureters. Pass the other end of each stenting tube with a curved clamp out through the ileourethral anastomosis, then down the urethra. Insert a 20 F silicone catheter with extra holes into the urethra and up the right ileal limb. Rotate it so that the most-proximal hole faces to the left just above the anastomotic site. Suture the three catheters by two sutures each to the frenum.

Alternatively, bring the ureteral catheters through the ileal wall distal to the ureteral implantation and then through the abdominal wall, in which case, the ileal wall must be fixed to the retroperitoneum with two sutures surrounding the exit of the stents.

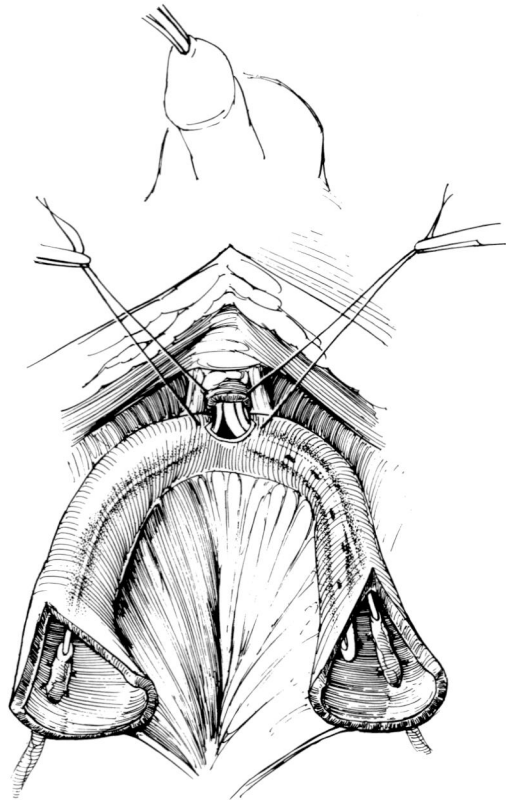

4 Complete the ileourethral anastomosis with four 3-0 synthetic absorbable sutures. Tie these sutures and the two lateral ones. Close the ends of the loops with continuous 2-0 synthetic absorbable sutures after trimming the acute angles created by the initial incision. Test for watertightness by filling the loop through the urethral catheter. Suspend the ends of the segment above the iliac vessels by fixing them to the lateral pelvic walls with 3-0 synthetic absorbable sutures. Close the defect in the mesentery, and bring the omentum down to cover the loop. Place three suction drains—one behind each limb of the ileal loop to exit anteriorly, and a third to lie behind the symphysis.

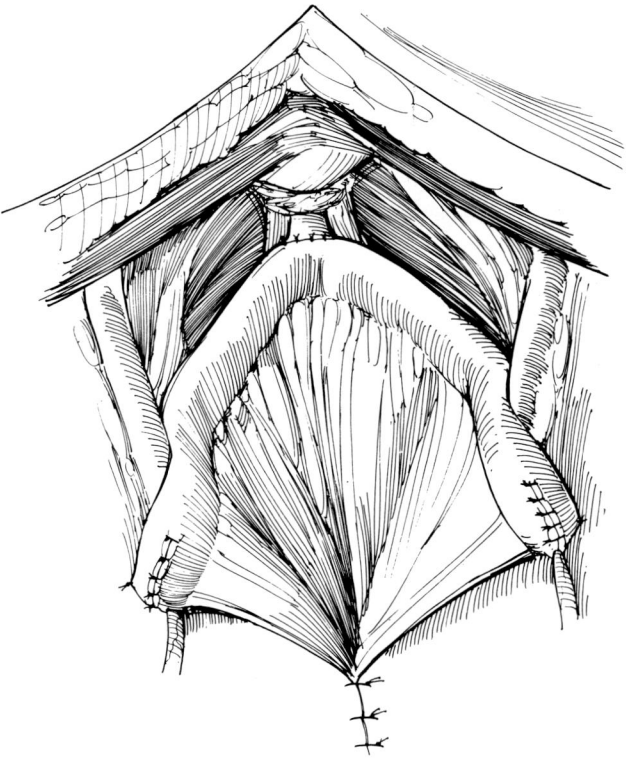

DETUBULARIZED U-SHAPED ILEAL BLADDER

(CAMEY)

5 Anastomose the ileum to the urethra 10 cm closer to the right end than to the left. Completely open the ileum on the antimesenteric border, and proceed with Steps 3 and 4, as previously described, anastomosing the ureters and inserting the catheters.

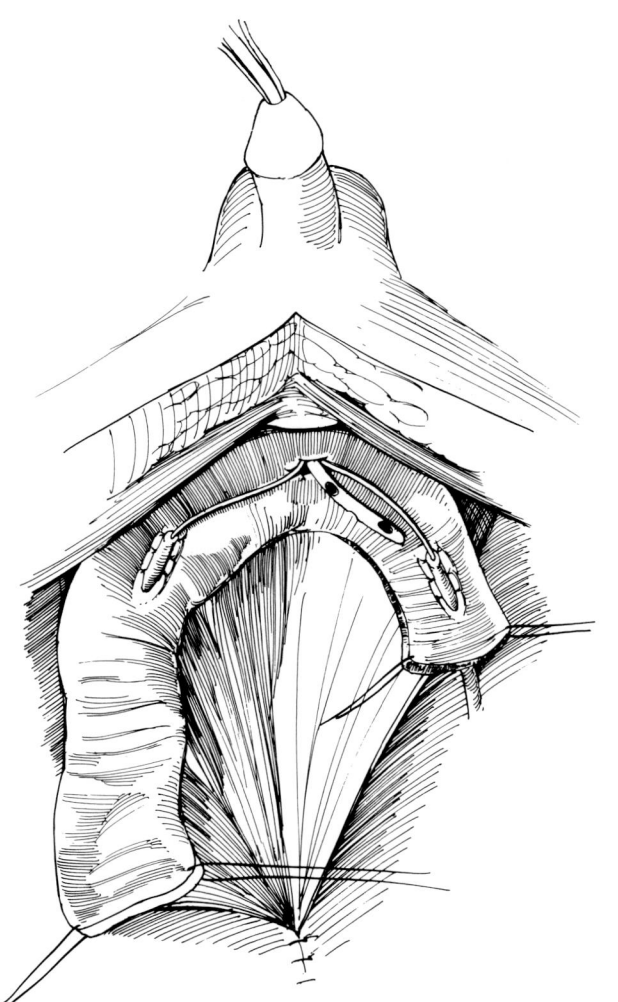

6 Fold the longer end of the ileal segment over to cover the shorter end, and join them, first along the upper margin, and then along the lower one, with running 2-0 synthetic absorbable sutures. Close the wound, bringing the drains through stab wounds. Tape and stitch the three catheters to the penis.

Postoperatively, irrigate the ileal bladder through the catheter four or five times every 3 hours with 30 ml of saline to evacuate the mucus. Maintain prolonged parenteral nutrition, even after passage of gas. Remove the drainage tubes as soon as the volume decreases, no later than the 12th day. At the same time, remove the ureteral catheters, but obtain a urine culture and a cystogram. If leakage occurs, let the ureteral stents remain for another week. Remove the urethral catheter 2 days later.

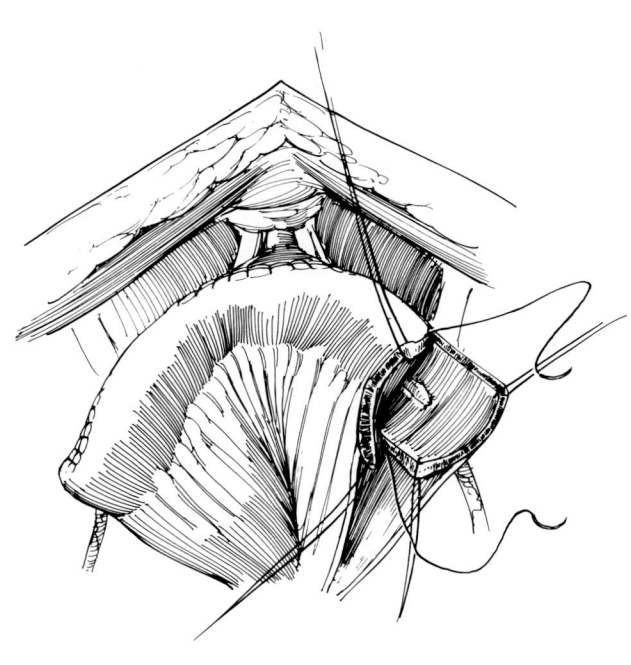

POSTOPERATIVE PROBLEMS

Obstruction at the ureteroileal junctions from edema may cause flank pain, low-grade fever, and decreased renal function, which may be due in part to ileal stasis and resorption and drug toxicity. *Small bowel obstruction* is uncommon, but prolonged ileus can be a problem. *Lymphoceles* may form and require laparoscopic drainage because of pressure on the new bladder.

Ileourethral fistulas may respond to prolonged catheter drainage, but a few require surgical correction.

Wound infection and pelvic abscesses may require surgical drainage. *Bacteremia, septicemia, and septic shock* usually are associated with displacement of catheters, for which percutaneous nephrostomy may be required. *Incontinence* is more likely if the neurovascular bundles are not preserved during cystectomy, but it is a special problem if the bowel is hyperactive.

Commentary by R. Bruce Filmer

Preservation of as much healthy membranous urethra as possible results in improved continence. To achieve this, sharp transection of the urethra at the apex of the prostate, without the use of a right-angle clamp, is recommended.

Because of the thicker muscular wall of the ileum, there is a greater chance of obstruction occurring at the antireflux ureteroileal anastomosis. Therefore, an adequate hiatus for the ureter must be made through the muscular wall of the ileum.

The 8 F ileal stent can be brought out through the ileal wall approximately 8 cm below the site of reimplantation and then through the abdominal wall. To avoid possible leakage out of the stent, the ileal wall at the site of exit of the stent should be fixed to the retroperitoneal tissues.

The detubularized form of the Camey procedure has a lesser incidence of urinary incontinence. However, even detubularized bowel segments can generate high-intraluminal-pressure contractions at times, which can be reduced with oxybutynin.

As with any form of intestinal bladder substitution or augmentation, mucous retention can be a problem initially. Mitchell has described the use of irrigations with 3 N saline as a better way to break down the mucus so that it can be irrigated more easily from the bladder substitution.

The insertion of a 20 F silicone catheter into a child's urethra might be impossible; for this reason, it may be necessary to pass a 20 F silicone catheter into the Camey procedure through the anterior abdominal wall. To avoid adhesions occurring at the ileourethral anastomosis, it is recommended that a Foley catheter be placed through the urethra into the bladder substitutions for at least 2 weeks.

ILEAL NEOBLADDER

(HAUTMANN)

An alternative method of increasing the volume for a given length of ileum is to open the cecum and part of the ascending colon, along with the equivalent of three segments of ileum. The four "elements" are arranged in a W shape, and the three adjoining edges are sutured together to form a flat plate, which is then folded on itself to form a large chamber. This neobladder is anastomosed to the urethra, and the ureters are implanted into the ileal plate. A similar technique may be used for augmentation of the bladder.

KOCK POUCH BLADDER SUBSTITUTION

An alternative to the Camey technique is to form a hemi-Kock augmentation (page 443) with an ileal nipple. Fold the free end on itself to cover the ventral surface. Suture it closed semitransversely. Push the corners of the pouch down between the leaves of the mesentery, bringing the posterior aspect of the reservoir anteriorly. Anastomose the base of the pouch to the urethra, and connect the ureters to the proximal end of the ileum.

CHAPTER 96

Ileocecal Bladder Substitution

(MAINZ TECHNIQUE)

1 Proceed as described for cecoileal reservoir (page 412), but make the ileal portion 20 to 25 cm shorter and omit formation of the nipple (Steps 5 to 9). Before closing the anterior wall of the pouch, make a buttonhole incision in the lowest part of the cecum or ascending colon, depending on the position after the rotation, and place a single row of five or six through-and-through 4-0 interrupted synthetic absorbable sutures to connect the bowel opening to the membranous urethra. Intraluminal sutures also may be inserted.

2 Intubate the ureters with J stents, and bring them out through the wall of the pouch and through the skin, rather than through the urethra. Place a silicone balloon catheter in the bladder through the urethra and place a cystostomy tube. Close the anterior wall of the pouch.

Remove the stents one at a time in 10 days, after culturing the urine from each kidney. At 3 weeks, obtain a cystogram. Clamp the cystostomy tube at the time the urethral catheter is removed, but leave it 2 more weeks for security. Other pouches (Indiana, LeBag) can be similarly anastomosed to the urethra.

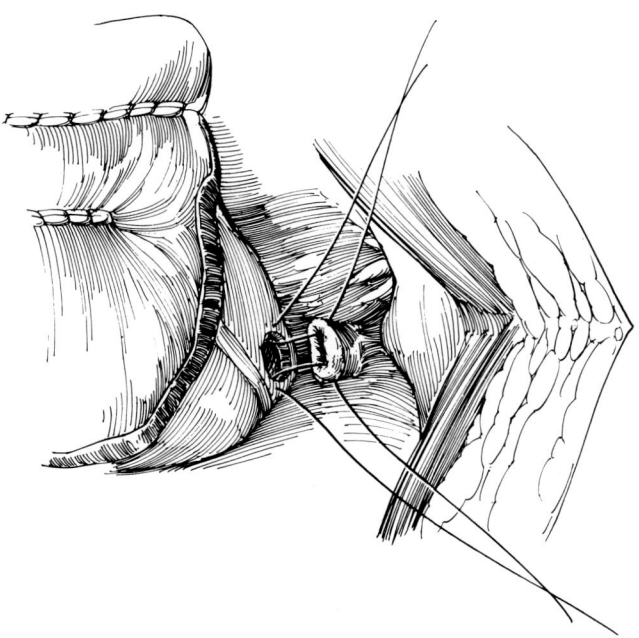

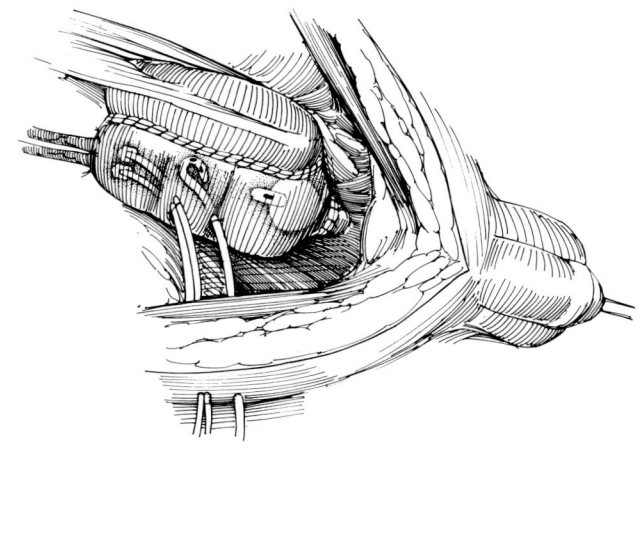

POSTOPERATIVE PROBLEMS

Complications with bladder substitutions are similar to those with a cecoileal reservoir. *Leakage* from the urethral anastomosis will subside with more prolonged catheter drainage. In addition, *incontinence* may result from improper selection of a child with sphincteric incompetence. *Strictures* at the anastomotic site usually can be managed by simple dilatation.

Commentary by R. Bruce Filmer

Because this procedure produces a low-pressure bladder reservoir, complete absence of ureteric reflux following the operation is less important.

The problem of mucous formation following this operation is managed in a fashion similar to that of the Camey procedure.

If the patients are unable to urinate on their own following removal of the catheters, intermittent catheterization is instituted. At that time, it may be necessary to continue to irrigate the bladder substitution with saline solution for a number of months to break down the mucus.

It is important not to hurry to remove the urine drainage tubes following an operation of this nature. Stepwise removal of the drainage tubes, as outlined in the text, is highly recommended.

CHAPTER 97

Gastric Bladder Substitution

1 Harvest the stomach as described for gastrocysto-plasty (page 467). Instead of forming an anastomosis to the bladder, remove the staples and suture the apex of the posterior wedge to the urethra. Partially tubularizing the flap may aid in making the anastomosis. Make 2-cm oblique tunnels in the plane under the gastric mucosa, and draw the ureters through them. Place a deep suture at the apex of each spatulated ureter, and suture the edges of the ureter to the gastric mucosa.

2 Insert a Malecot catheter into the reservoir. Close the edges of the flap, and complete suturing the apex of the pouch to the urethra with interrupted 3-0 chromic catgut sutures. Suture the wall of the stomach to the abdominal wall as for a gastrostomy to protect the exit site of the catheter.

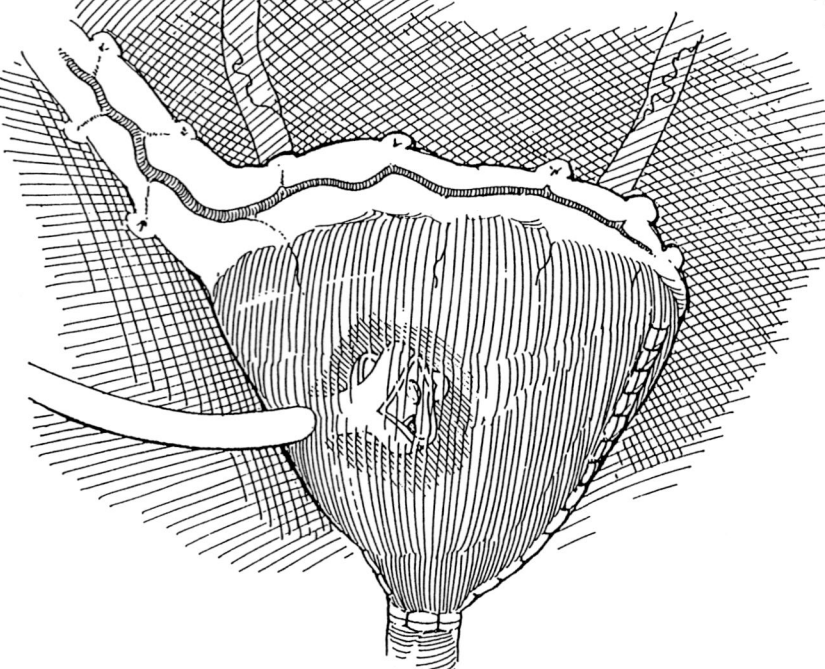

GASTRIC NEOURETHRA

If a urethra is needed because of loss of the native one, construct a new urethra from a portion of the stomach.

3 **A,** Mark and cut a strip 2 cm wide from one arm of the flap. Form it into a tube over a 10 F catheter. **B,** Slightly intussuscept the base into the reservoir to promote urethral resistance. Anastomose the distal end to the remains of the urethra.

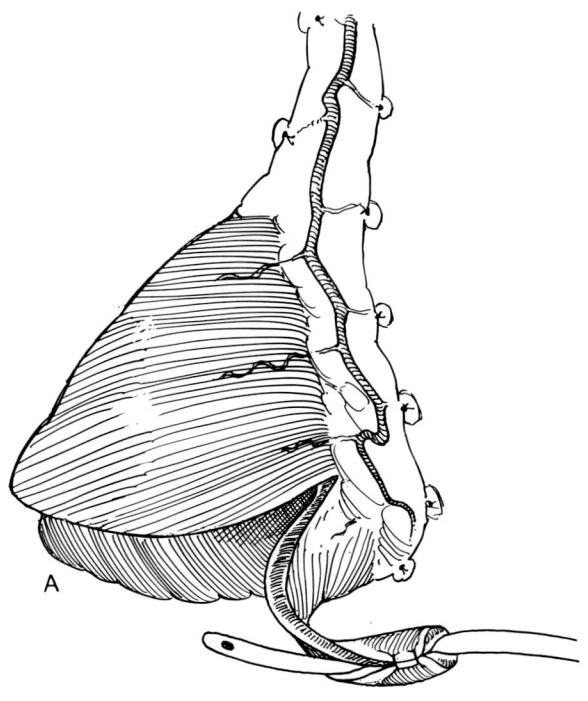

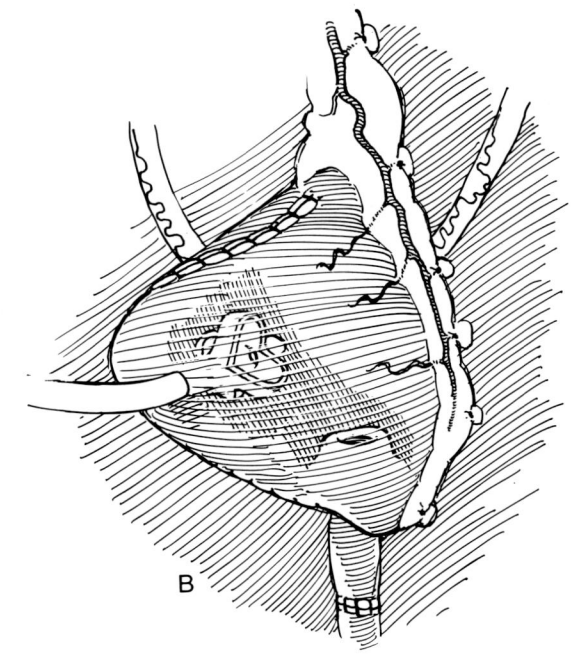

Commentary by Michael E. Mitchell

Gastric reservoir has proved to be a valuable addition to the surgical reconstruction in patients with complex problems, including those with classic exstrophy, cloacal exstrophy, some with severe cloaca malformations, and some who have had extensive radiation therapy for pelvic tumor. A short segment of small intestine may be added to the reservoir to balance salt loss by adding a resorptive surface and increasing the volume of the reservoir without significantly reducing the length of the intestine. The ureters are easily tunneled into the wall of the gastric reservoir to prevent reflux. The nature of gastric tissue also provides several options for continence mechanisms. The appendix, ureter, or even tapered small bowel may be tunneled successfully into the gastric reservoir to construct a continent catheterizable channel. Furthermore, as illustrated in this chapter, it is possible to construct a tube from the gastric reservoir to form a catheterizable channel. A nipple is constructed in a manner similar to that of a Janeway continent gastrostomy. The presence of hematuria and dysuria is not a problem in the continent reservoir patients; however, the possibility for salt loss should be considered, particularly in the patient with short-bowel syndrome.

Regarding technique, I find it easiest to position the new reservoir prior to reimplantation of the ureters. Therefore, it usually is easiest to anastomose the tip of the flap to the urethra before reimplanting the ureters. It is helpful to nipple the tip of the ureters to prevent stenosis. The suprapubic tube should be positioned so that the gastric bladder wall can be sutured to the abdominal wall, like a gastrostomy, to prevent leakage after removal of the tube. If it is necessary to create a catheterizable channel from stomach, great care must be taken to make a nipple at the base, to ensure continence, and that the channel is straight, to ensure ease of catheterization.

Mucus usually is not a problem after surgery, but initially, the bladder should be irrigated at least daily. Because of acid production by the gastric mucosa, patients should be receiving H_2 blockers initially. Omeprazole probably is *contraindicated* in this group, because it has greatest effect on stomach mucosa locally and therefore increases serum gastrin, which will selectively increase acid production of the gastric bladder, resulting in dysuria and hematuria.

SECTION 7
Testis

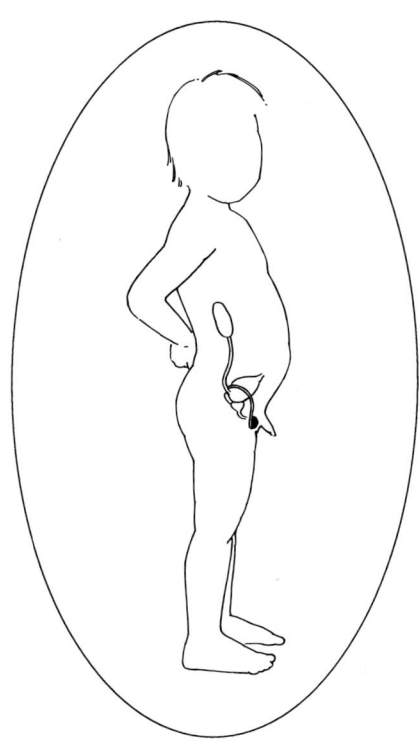

PART I

TESTIS RECONSTRUCTION

CHAPTER 98

Testis Biopsy and Inguinal Orchiopexy

TESTIS BIOPSY

Testis biopsy is usually reserved for adolescents and adults and performed under local anesthesia; however, for children, consider arranging for general anesthesia.

1 Stand to the left. Infiltrate the cord with 1 percent lidocaine when the youth is cooperative and has been sedated. To avoid puncturing the vas, do not inject near it.

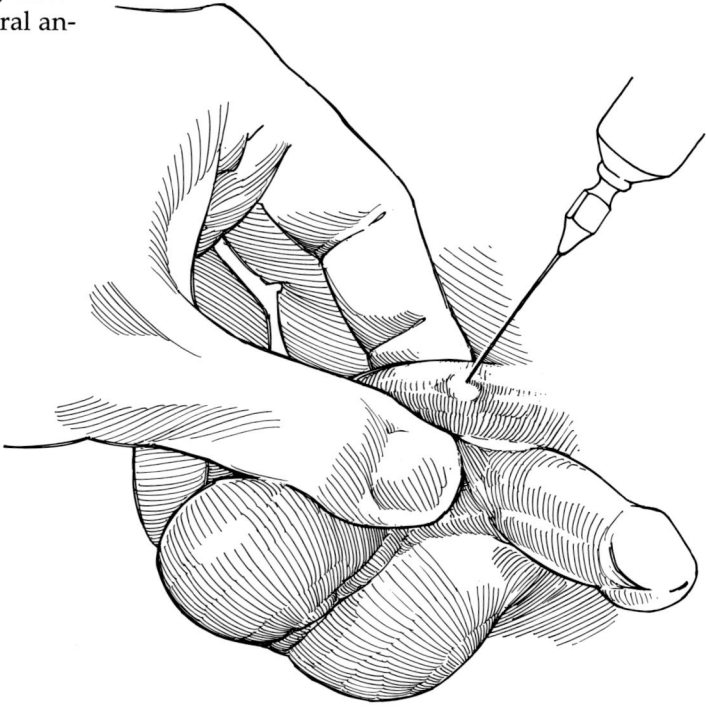

2 A, Grasp the testis in the left hand, and press it against the scrotal skin. Infiltrate the skin and dartos layer with 1 percent lidocaine without epinephrine. Do not inject the tunica albuginea. Incise transversely through the skin, dartos, and tunica vaginalis; these layers will retract as the scrotum is squeezed.

Incise the tunica albuginea transversely, the direction taken by the underlying small vessels. Do it sharply and quickly with a #15 blade for a distance of 5 or 6 mm to allow extrusion of a bead-sized portion of the testicular tubules.

B, Excise the extruded tubules with *the belly* of small curved scissors, and pass the biopsy specimen on the scissors directly into Bouin's solution (*not* formalin). Do not relax the grip on the scrotum.

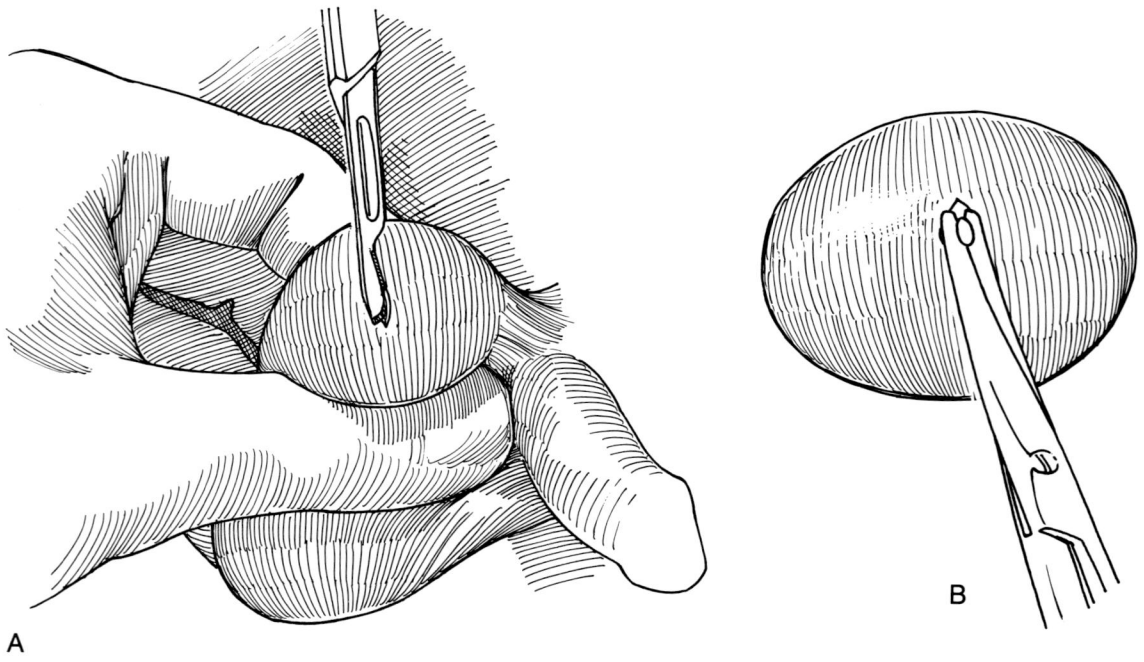

A

B

3 Close the tunica albuginea with two sutures of 4-0 plain catgut swaged on a needle. Observe for hemostasis; add more sutures it necessary. Release the grasp on the scrotum.

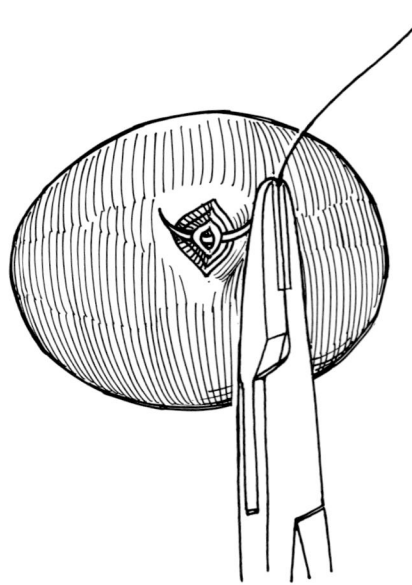

4 Approximate the skin, together with the dartos layer, with several stitches of 4-0 plain catgut. Repeat the procedure on the other side if indicated. Apply a nonadherent dressing and a large padded scrotal suspensory. In children, simply apply collodion to the incision.

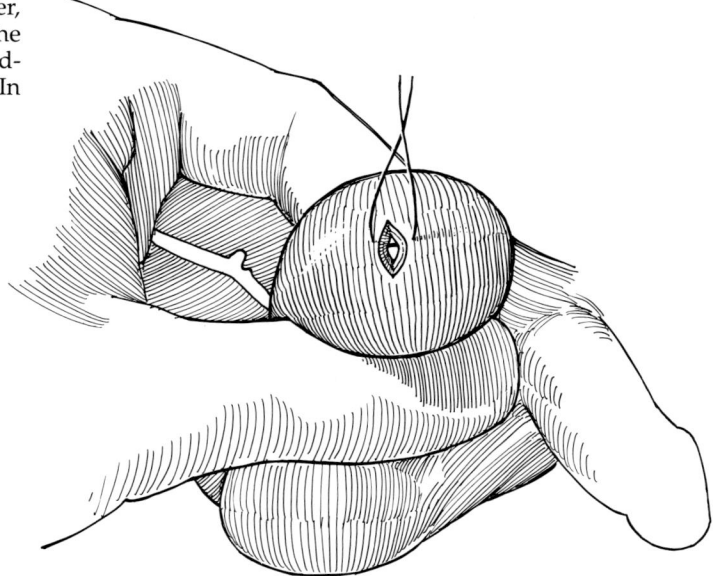

POSTOPERATIVE PROBLEMS

A *hematocele* can appear if the tunica albuginea is not closed over a subtunical vessel.

Commentary by Kenneth I. Glassberg

I anesthetize all children. In grasping the testis before making the incision, be sure that the epididymis lies posteriorly. When taking the biopsy specimen from the extruded tubules, use the belly of the scissors to lift it off into the Bouin's solution. Fulgurate the edge of the tunica vaginalis before closing to ensure hemostasis.

INGUINAL ORCHIOPEXY

Despite advances in endocrine management, after the presence of retractile testes has been ruled out and perhaps hormonal therapy has been tried, orchiopexy is still the most effective treatment for cryptorchidism. Because many studies have shown that damage to the germ cells begins very early, at least before the end of the 2nd year, treatment for true cryptorchidism must be done before such irreversible changes occur. Operations on infants require magnification and special technique, especially if the testis lies high, and require judgment that the testis is worth the effort of salvage. Furthermore, the need for a technique other than standard orchiopexy must be recognized before the testis is dissected from its bed and the option for long-loop vas orchiopexy is lost.

The surgical techniques gained by the use of the loupe and operating room microscope have fostered delicate handling and exact coaptation of tissues and the use of fine sutures, both important for pediatric urologic applications, such as hypospadias repair and orchiopexy.

The inguinal region in infants differs somewhat from that in adults, and these differences are important for surgery at this age. The superficial fascia is much thicker, resembling the aponeurosis of the external oblique, which, in turn, is relatively thin with delicate medial and lateral crura. The inguinal canal runs more transversely, and the cremaster is well developed with fibers that blend with those of the internal oblique. Before the child reaches 2 years of age, the bladder extends well into the abdomen and can be injured during medial exposure of the spermatic cord.

If the testis is not palpable, perform a laparoscopy and consider an abdominal approach (page 507) or be prepared for the Fowler-Stephens orchiopexy (page 496), staged orchiopexy (page 500), or microvascular orchiopexy (page 503).

Determine the serum testosterone level at 6 weeks of age. If it is low, consider early endocrine therapy. Before 2 years of age, consider a trial of luteinizing hormone–releasing hormone or human chorionic gonadotropin. In unilateral cases, if descent has not occurred by age 2, perform an orchiopexy. Include abdominal exploration if the testis is not apparent, and rule out anorchia. For bilateral cases, repair both sides at the same operation unless the testes are very high; repairing one side at a time is then wiser. Obtain consent from the parents for orchiectomy in case the testis proves to be not worth salvaging, and have a prosthesis of suitable size available.

Instruments: Provide a three-power loupe or an operating microscope plus a biopsy tray, a genitourinary fine set, a plastic set, fine Allis clamps, extra mosquito clamps, handheld bipolar electrocautery with needle tip, two small DeBakey forceps, and a ¼-in vessel loop.

5 *Position:* The child is supine with the knees bent, with the soles of the feet approximated to separate the upper legs. Prep and drape widely, in case abdominal exploration is required. *Incision:* Make a 3.5- to 4.5-cm semitransverse incision in the natural skin fold, from the edge of the rectus muscle to a point medial to the anterior superior iliac spine. Consider making it somewhat higher if the testis is not palpable. Divide and ligate the superficial circumflex iliac and superficial inferior epigastric vessels. Divide Camper's and Scarpa's fascias and expose the external oblique fascia laterally, as far as the inguinal ligament, as well as inferiorly to reveal the external ring. Place fine curved clamps on the edges of the superficial fascia to maintain exposure. Take care not to injure a testis lying in the superficial inguinal pouch. Push the protruding processus vaginalis down to define the external ring.

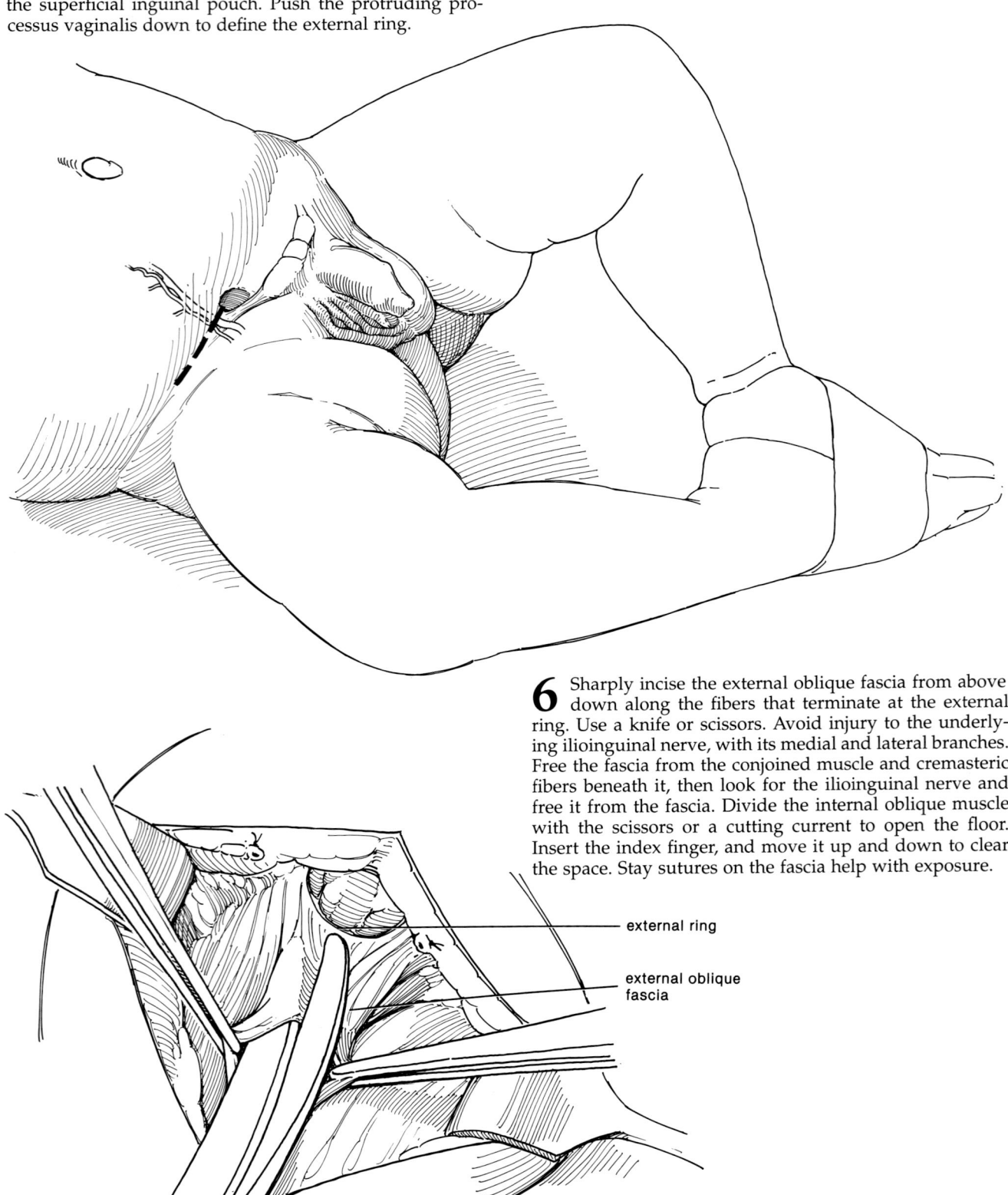

6 Sharply incise the external oblique fascia from above down along the fibers that terminate at the external ring. Use a knife or scissors. Avoid injury to the underlying ilioinguinal nerve, with its medial and lateral branches. Free the fascia from the conjoined muscle and cremasteric fibers beneath it, then look for the ilioinguinal nerve and free it from the fascia. Divide the internal oblique muscle with the scissors or a cutting current to open the floor. Insert the index finger, and move it up and down to clear the space. Stay sutures on the fascia help with exposure.

external ring

external oblique fascia

7 Identify the testis within the tunica vaginalis. In infants, use loupes, and work with inverted forceps, so that hands do not obstruct vision (page 14). Open the tunic before doing any dissection of the cremaster or around the cord. Do not mobilize the tunica vaginalis until you are sure you do not need the distal collateral blood supply for a Fowler-Stephens orchiopexy. Put traction on the testis, and check to be sure the artery is going to be long enough. If it is not and there is a looping vas, decide to do a long-loop vas orchiopexy (page 496).

With the aid of an assistant, pick up the overlying cremasteric fibers on either side with fine smooth forceps, and sharply and bluntly peel them down and off close to the tunic to be able to locate the communicating processus.

external inguinal ring

external oblique and aponeurosis

internal oblique muscle

right testis

cremasteric fibers

8 Open the tunica vaginalis anteriorly, and incise it proximally to the base of the cord. Remove the appendix testis and appendix epididymis, and fulgurate the bases superficially.

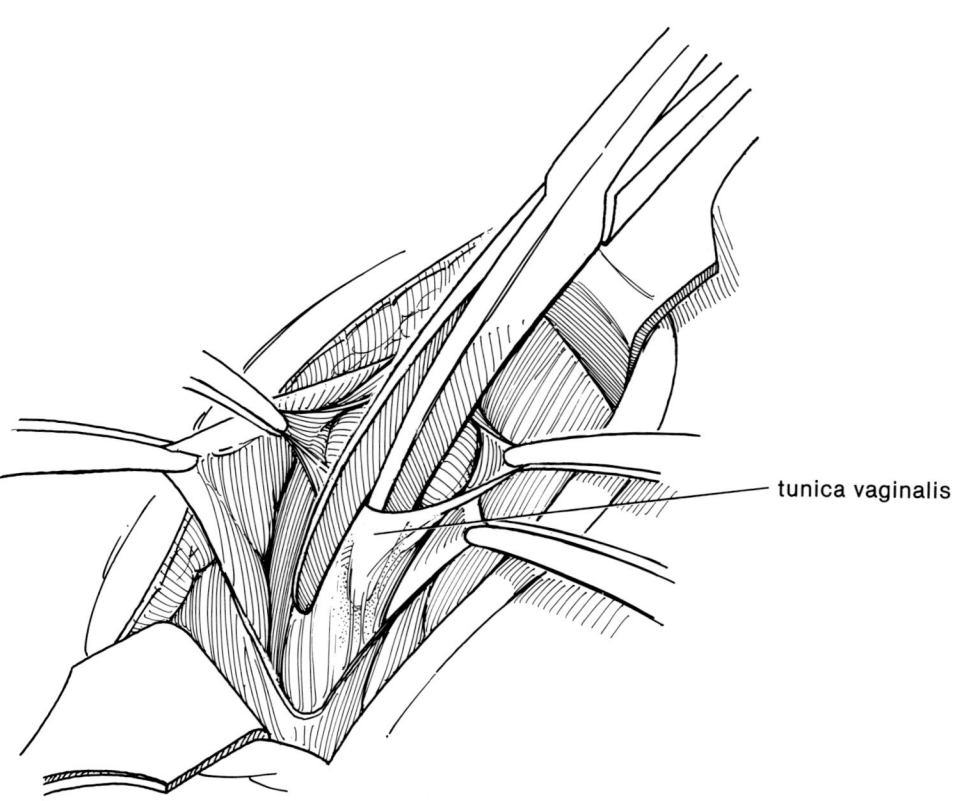

tunica vaginalis

9 Once it is apparent that the cord will become long enough, grasp the edges of the tunica vaginalis near the internal ring with fine forceps, and insinuate fine scissors or a small straight hemostat between the peritoneal lining of the hernia canal and the vessels and vas. The tunica vaginalis may appear to surround the cord. It is easiest to separate it from the vessels and vas just below the internal ring, dissecting from both the medial and lateral sides. Injection of saline in this plane may help the separation. Divide the free edges of the sac as the separation progresses. Divide the posterior and lateral connections of the internal spermatic (transversalis) fascia.

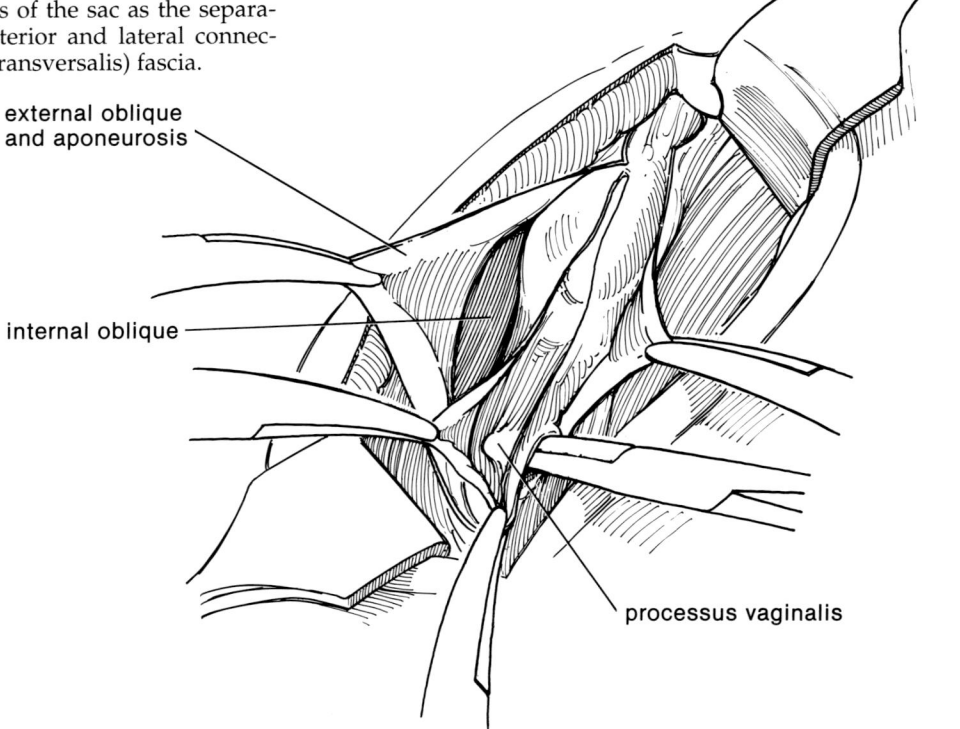

external oblique and aponeurosis

internal oblique

processus vaginalis

10 Complete the division of the sac, place mosquito clamps on its edges, and close the peritoneal opening with a 4-0 silk pursestring suture. With the usual small hernia sac, suture ligation is enough. It may be preferable to postpone this step; if you do it now, the subsequent retraction to expose the retroperitoneal dissection frequently will tear out the closure, so close it after this upward mobilization has been completed. If the peritoneum tears, oversew the opening into the peritoneal cavity with a fine continuous suture.

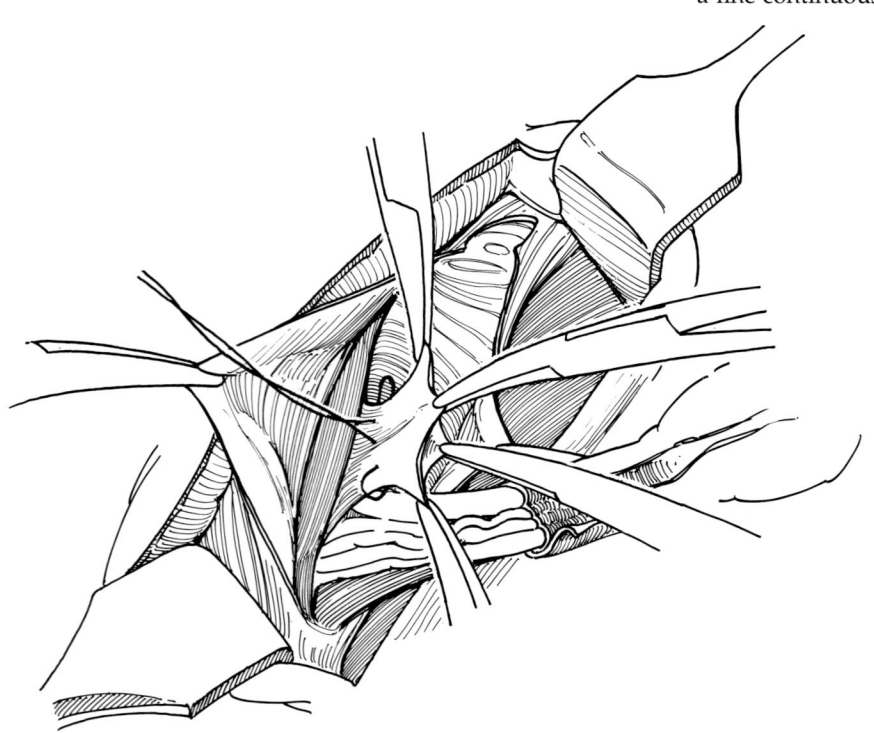

11 Trim excess tunic and cremasteric fibers from the cord distally, if it is necessary to lengthen it. Take care not to cut the deranged cord or splayed-out epididymis. Alternatively, do not open the entire tunic; rather, close the proximal end loosely to prevent dislodgment of the testis outside the sac. *Caution:* Avoid using the electrocautery unless the testis is well grounded; otherwise, the current will run up the relatively narrow cord and destroy it. Inspect the testis for size and anomalies. Gauge the length of the cord by pulling the testis over the symphysis. If it is too short, meticulously free the remainder of the tunica vaginalis and cremasteric fibers from it.

12 Locate and divide the inferior epigastric artery and vein(s) separately, and open the associated transversalis fascial layer. Usually, upward retraction provides adequate exposure of the cord after the transversalis fascia is divided, but, if necessary, open the internal ring by dividing the internal oblique muscles and more of the lateral spermatic fascia. Free the cord well retroperitoneally, using a peanut dissector to mobilize it medially, up toward the kidney, if necessary. Testes in the superficial inguinal pouch need minimal dissection of the cord. Dissect among the vessels, vas, and cord structures as little as possible, particularly in infants, to avoid atrophy. Perform a biopsy of the testis by taking a thin wedge near the upper pole opposite the epididymis and putting it at once without manipulation in Bouin's solution. Close the defect with one or two fine sutures.

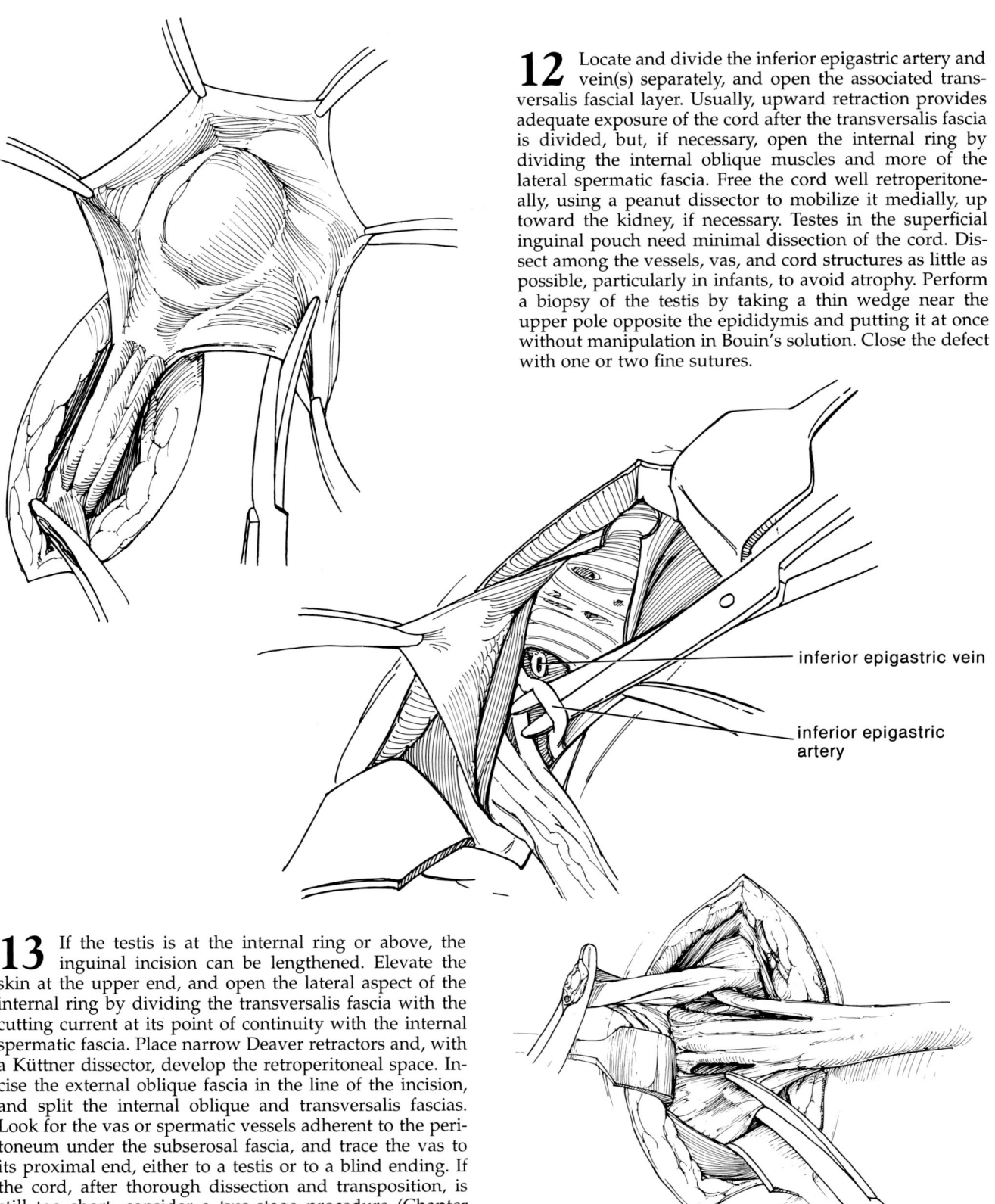

inferior epigastric vein

inferior epigastric artery

13 If the testis is at the internal ring or above, the inguinal incision can be lengthened. Elevate the skin at the upper end, and open the lateral aspect of the internal ring by dividing the transversalis fascia with the cutting current at its point of continuity with the internal spermatic fascia. Place narrow Deaver retractors and, with a Küttner dissector, develop the retroperitoneal space. Incise the external oblique fascia in the line of the incision, and split the internal oblique and transversalis fascias. Look for the vas or spermatic vessels adherent to the peritoneum under the subserosal fascia, and trace the vas to its proximal end, either to a testis or to a blind ending. If the cord, after thorough dissection and transposition, is still too short, consider a two-stage procedure (Chapter 100) or a microvascular orchiopexy (Chapter 101). A long-loop vas orchiopexy is no longer an option. If orchiectomy is done, consider insertion of a suitably sized prosthesis, which can be changed for a larger one at puberty. At this time, the safety of silicone prostheses has been questioned,

but because there are no better alternatives, advising the parents of the minimal risk and obtaining informed consent is a reasonable course to follow. Close the neck of the scrotum behind the prosthesis.

14 **A,** Pass the index finger along the usual course of descent of the testis into the scrotum until it reaches the "third inguinal ring" formed by the nondescent of the dartos fascia. Make a 2-cm incision with the scalpel through the scrotal skin, leaving the third inguinal ring intact. **B,** Develop a pocket for the testis from below by freeing the skin from the dartos fascia bluntly with the back of the knife or with scissors for 1 to 2 cm. **C,** Make a small opening in the dartos fascia tensioned over the finger, and grasp the edges with small Allis clamps.

B

A

C

dartos
fascia

tip of finger

15 Draw the testis out through the scrotum by passing a clamp from below against the index finger and grasping the edge of the tunica albuginea. Take care not to rotate the cord.

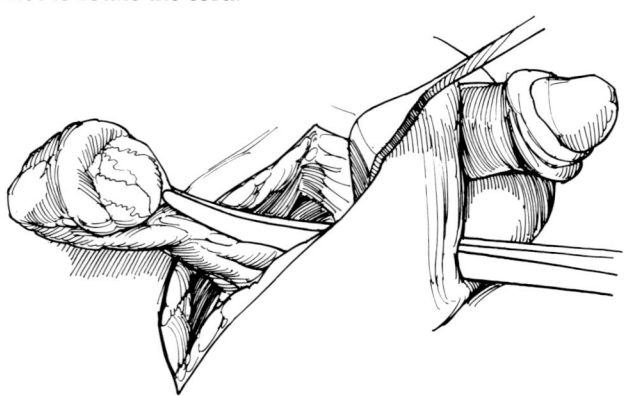

16 **A,** Close the dartos fascia behind the testis with a 4-0 synthetic absorbable suture at each end, catching a little of the tunic in the bite. **B,** Tuck the testis in the subcutaneous pouch, close the skin with 5-0 plain catgut subcutaneous interrupted sutures, and seal with collodion.

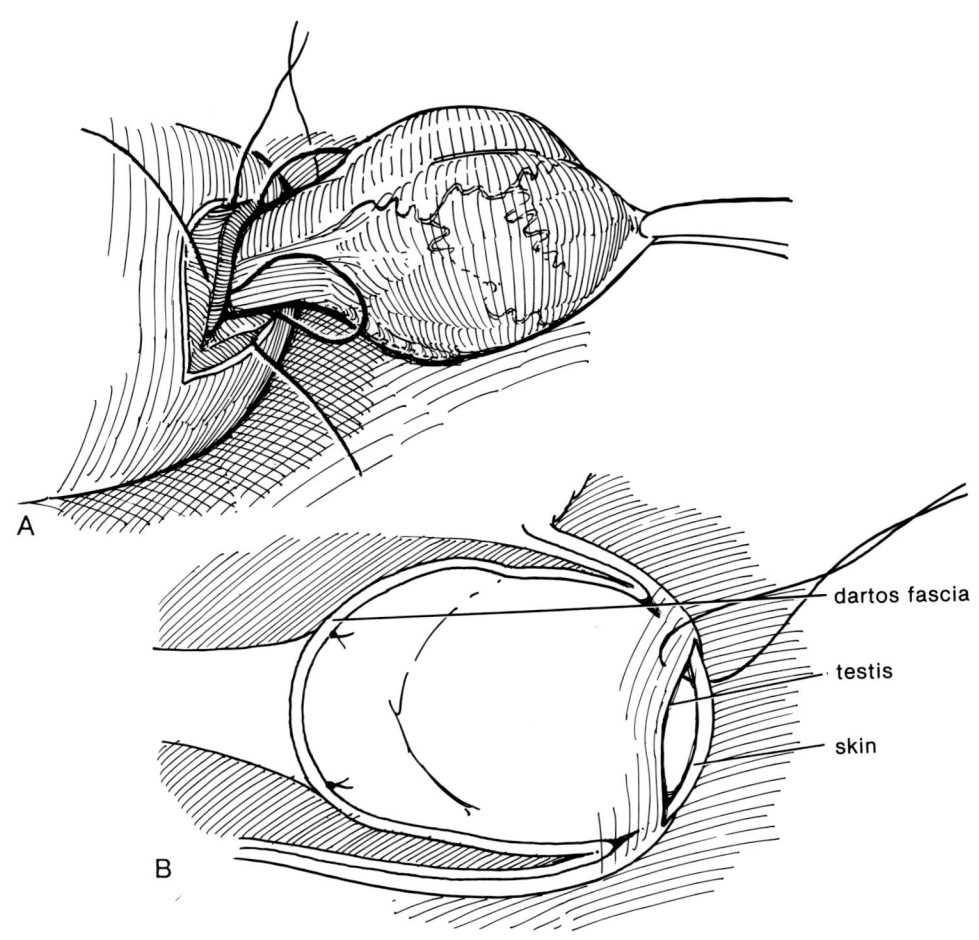

A

B

dartos fascia

testis

skin

17 Reapproximate the transversalis fascia over the cord, displacing the internal ring downward.

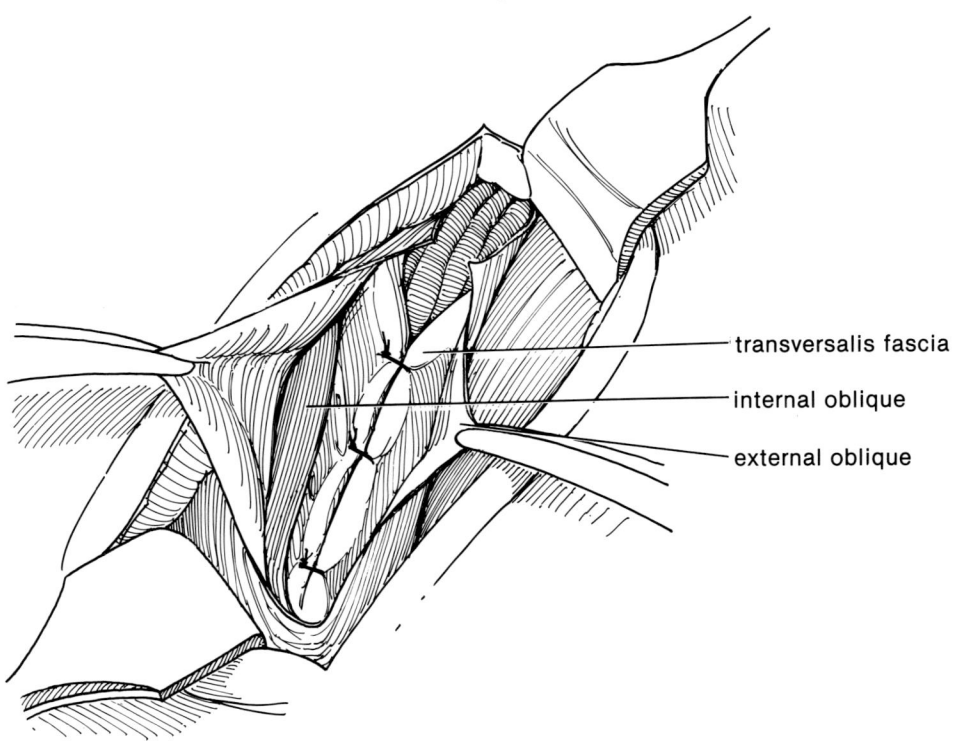

transversalis fascia

internal oblique

external oblique

18 Suture the internal oblique muscle to the shelving edge of the inguinal ligament over the cord with 3-0 to 4-0 synthetic absorbable sutures.

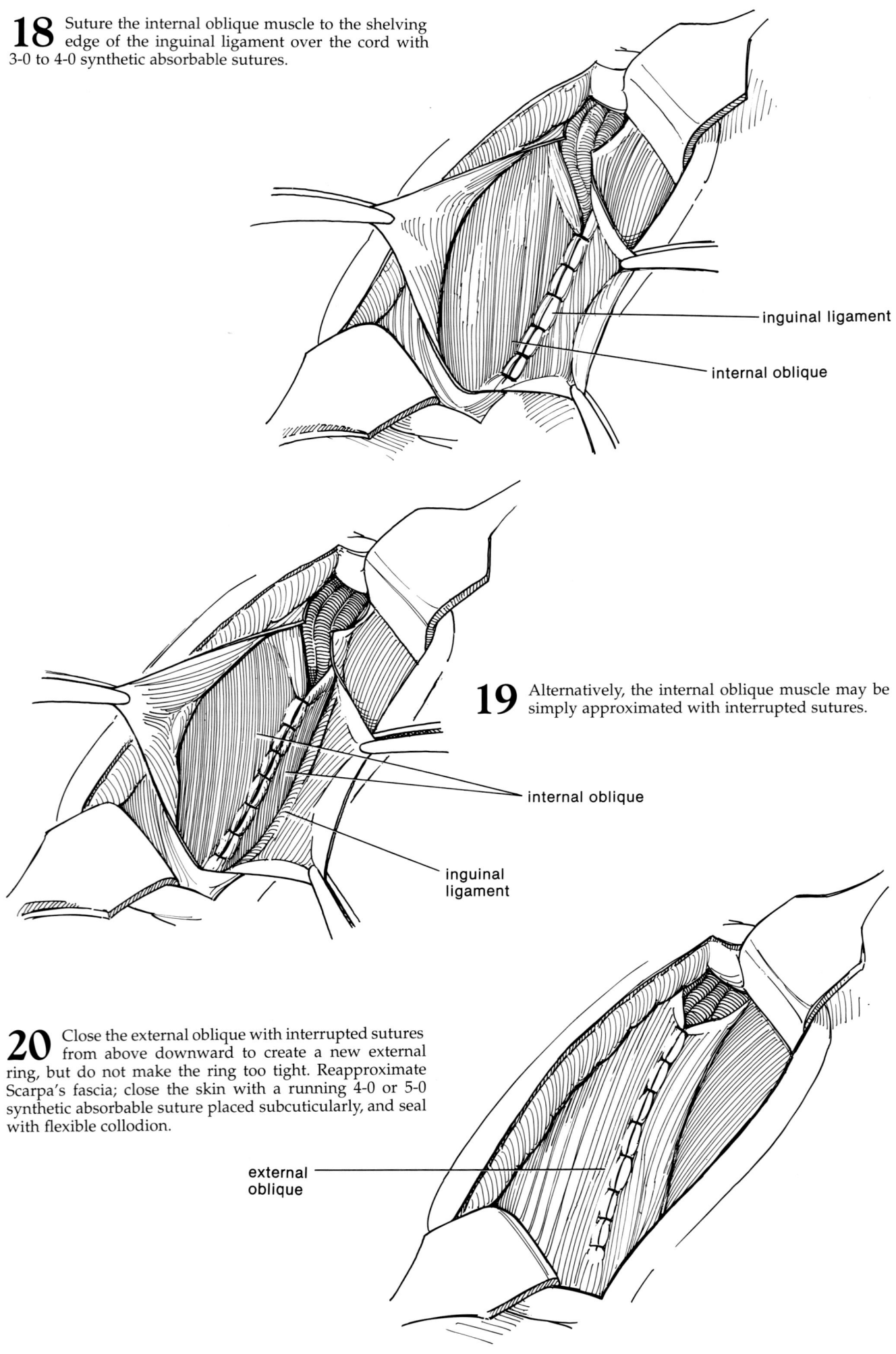

inguinal ligament

internal oblique

19 Alternatively, the internal oblique muscle may be simply approximated with interrupted sutures.

internal oblique

inguinal ligament

20 Close the external oblique with interrupted sutures from above downward to create a new external ring, but do not make the ring too tight. Reapproximate Scarpa's fascia; close the skin with a running 4-0 or 5-0 synthetic absorbable suture placed subcuticularly, and seal with flexible collodion.

external oblique

POSTOPERATIVE PROBLEMS

Inadequate testis position has an incidence as high as 10 percent as the result of incomplete retroperitoneal dissection. It usually can be corrected in a second operation. *Retraction* of the testis after operation occurs in a small percentage of cases.

Apparent atrophy is related to the preoperative size of the testis relative to age, but the most feared complication is *devascularization of the testis* during dissection of the cord, a complication that must be avoided by the use of loupes or microscope, fine instruments, and sequential dissection. Ischemia also can be produced by rubber-band traction. Orchiectomy for a small testis may be indicated later if there is a fear of cancer, and a prosthesis may be inserted.

Accidental division of the vas is possible. Immediate or postpubertal microvascular repair will correct the problem. The complication occurs more frequently in a nonpalpable case. *Epididymo-orchitis* can occur and is treated with antibiotics. *Postoperative scrotal swelling,* however, usually indicates edema rather than hematoma or infection. Progressive scrotal enlargement suggests uncontrolled bleeding and warrants exploration. Needle aspiration seldom is diagnostic and, if the swelling is due to bowel herniating through the peritoneal defect, may be harmful.

A *hydrocele* may form later from excess remnants of the tunica vaginalis. If it is small, it can be ignored; if large, it will require trans-scrotal repair (page 528). *Testicular extrusion* from ischemia of the scrotal skin is uncommon but may result if the area has been electrocoagulated or if rubber-band traction has been used, an unnecessary and potentially harmful practice, because it also can cause testicular atrophy. *Bladder injury* has been reported from ligation of the hernia sac that includes a portion of the bladder.

Commentary by John R. Woodard

I was told by one of his former residents that Dr. Robert E. Gross, the renowned pediatric surgeon and former Surgeon-in-Chief at the Boston Children's Hospital, considered orchiopexy to be his favorite operation. It is easy for me to see why this might have been a true story. As is beautifully described and illustrated by the author and illustrator, the procedure is an anatomically precise sequence of maneuvers that, when applied to properly selected patients, almost always leads to a successful result.

That is, the orchiopexy operation as it is described here should produce a scrotal testis in almost every young boy having an easily palpable testis at the start. In boys having a nonpalpable testis, we routinely perform laparoscopic examination, and for the truly intra-abdominal testis, would be prepared to select a technique other than this standard inguinal orchiopexy.

Precision is the key to success in orchiopexy. Each of the tissues and anatomic structures labeled in these diagrams should be easily identifiable in each case. In my experience, there are three important maneuvers that serve to add length to the cord and prevent subsequent testicular retraction: (1) complete transection of the cremaster muscle fibers, (2) good separation of the cord structures from the peritoneum just above the the internal ring as one accomplishes high ligation of the hernia sac, and (3) incision or division of all the lateral spermatic fascia to allow medial advancement of the cord. All patients undergoing orchiopexy require all three of these maneuvers. Further retroperitoneal dissection or transection of the inferior epigastric vessels adds only small amounts of additional cord length and only occasionally is necessary. Also, dissection of the fascia (and collaterals) between the testicular vessels and the vas deferens rarely is necessary and should be avoided in most cases.

A caudal block at the beginning or end of the procedure allows the child to awaken without pain and appears to minimize postoperative nausea and vomiting. We employ this in most cases.

INSERTION OF TESTICULAR PROSTHESIS

Be certain that the patients understand the possible complications from silicone prostheses.

Make a transverse inguinal or an oblique inguinoscrotal incision. Place two incisions if implantation is to be bilateral. With the index finger, stretch the scrotal sac vigorously, taking care not to tear it. Carefully select the correct size of prosthesis for the size of the child; it can be replaced with a larger size later. Most hospitals require that a prosthesis be discarded if it has been put in the wound and not used. Invert the scrotum into the incision, and suture the tab on a gel-filled prosthesis to the inverted scrotal wall with a 3-0 synthetic absorbable suture. Place a pursestring suture to close the scrotal neck, taking care not to pierce the capsule with the needle. In practice, it probably is unnecessary to either suture the tab (just trim it off) or place the pursestring.

Complications

Infection will require removal of the prosthesis. *Necrosis* of the stretched skin over the prosthesis can occur and should be prevented by placement of a smaller prosthesis. *Scrotal hematoma* formation is rare.

CHAPTER 99

Long-Loop Vas Orchiopexy

APPROACHES TO THE IMPALPABLE TESTIS

Unilateral Cases. Approach the testis through a standard transverse skin-crease incision; extend the incision superiorly through the internal ring if necessary to gain added retroperitoneal or transperitoneal exposure.

Bilateral Cases. Make bilateral skin-crease lower quadrant incisions, and explore each groin. Usually, extensive retroperitoneal dissection through these incisions will allow the testis to be placed in the scrotum. If the testes are not found, complete the middle of the incision and open the peritoneum, essential for adequate visualization of the internal spermatic vessels and of the cord if a long-loop orchiopexy is planned.

Commentary by Stanley J. Kogan

Exposure for Bilateral Impalpable Testes. I believe that the procedure described is the most concise and accurate way to accomplish exposure for bilateral impalpable testes. I explore both groins first through a transverse lower skin incision and then continue my surgery through each inguinal canal, opening them further for transperitoneal exposure, if necessary. Many impalpable testes will be found in this manner. If neither testis is encountered after opening the inguinal canal, I believe it is important to obtain good transperitoneal exposure immediately, because the Fowler-Stephens orchiopexy is much more safely done in this manner. I go transperitoneally, either by entering vertically through the midline fascia or by transecting both recti and connecting both inguinal canal incisions horizontally. I individualize the choice of entrance in each case ("surgical judgment") and do not have really good criteria that can be written down definitively.

ORCHIOPEXY WITH VASCULAR DIVISION

(FOWLER-STEPHENS)

Orchiopexy with vascular division is for the testis with a vascular cord too short to allow placement in the scrotum. It uses the secondary vascular loop accompanying the congenitally long vas. The main trunk and the internal spermatic artery anastomose with the vasal artery near the lower pole of the testis and close to the hilum. From this junction, a single artery bypasses the hilum, penetrates the tunica albuginea at the lower pole of the testis, and usually

divides into two branches in the tunica vasculosa. In the technique described, the internal spermatic vessels are divided, and the blood supply of the testis is then reliant on the vasal vessels and some small branches that track across the loop to join with twigs arising from the internal spermatic vessels.

The testis that is detected at the external ring or in the inguinal canal with a long-loop vas emerging from the external ring is ideally suited for this operation. A testis situated higher in the abdomen with the usual short vas is better suited for other orchiopexy techniques.

A first stage for vessel ligation is needed only if the testis or the loop of the vas deferens cannot be located by clinical examination. Through a short abdominal incision, the spermatic vessels and testis are identified, and the vessels are ligated as high as possible. Ligation may be more readily done by laparoscopic techniques (see page 513), which not only can determine the presence and location of the testis and the presence and course of the vas deferens but also allows clipping of the spermatic vessels.

1 Make an incision in the inguinal crease. Identify the special anatomic circumstances applicable to the use of this technique. Plan ahead; do not mobilize the posterior wall of the hernia sac proximal to the testis and epididymis or disturb the floor of the inguinal canal or the epigastric vessels. Expose the processus vaginalis as for a standard orchiopexy. Dilate the internal inguinal ring or, if necessary for greater retroperitoneal exposure, incise the internal oblique muscle. Three-power loupes can be helpful. Do not dissect behind the processus or the hernia sac.

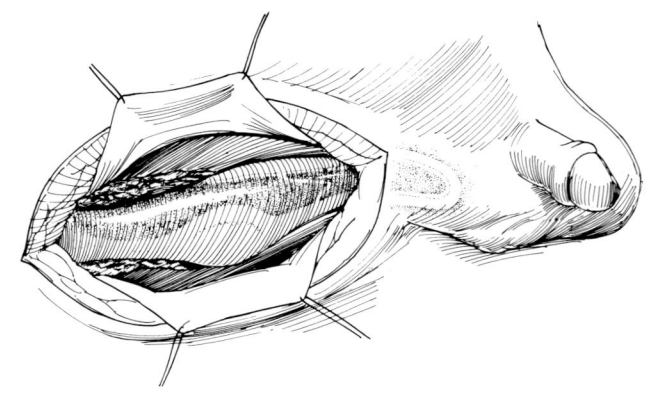

2 Open the hernia sac, identify the epididymis, and note the course of the vas with its several vascular arcades looping down the posteromedial wall of the sac below the testis. Place a traction suture superficially in the testis capsule; traction will determine if the testis has a long mesentery and can be brought into the scrotum by standard methods or a short one that requires division of the spermatic vessels. Dissect the sac well up inside the internal ring to the point where the vas turns medially, at the same time allowing the peritoneum lying more distally to remain attached medially and posteriorly to the vas. Inject saline under the peritoneum, then transect the processus, and close it with a 4-0 nonabsorbable pursestring suture.

Carefully separate the testicular vessels from the vessel to the vas and its accompanying vessels where they converge on the internal inguinal ring.

If the spermatic artery was not clipped at a first stage, test the collateral circulation by placing a small bulldog clamp high on the vascular pedicle, well above the testis; make a 3-mm longitudinal incision in the testis between the faintly visible vessels of the tunica albuginea, and watch for brisk bleeding. If bleeding persists for 5 minutes, collateral circulation is adequate. In the meantime, transilluminate the cord structures. First, identify the vascular anastomotic arcades between the vas and the spermatic vessels alongside the testis and epididymis, best seen through the back wall of the hernia sac, a view enhanced by the presence of venae comitantes. These arcades contribute to the blood supply, so divide only the arcade (or arcades) necessary to enable the loop of the vas to be straightened out and the

testis to be placed in the scrotum without tension. Before dividing a major arcade, gently compress the vessel and note whether bleeding from the tunica is impeded. Continued bleeding indicates that it is safe to divide the arcade, whereas arrest indicates a nonexpendable vessel.

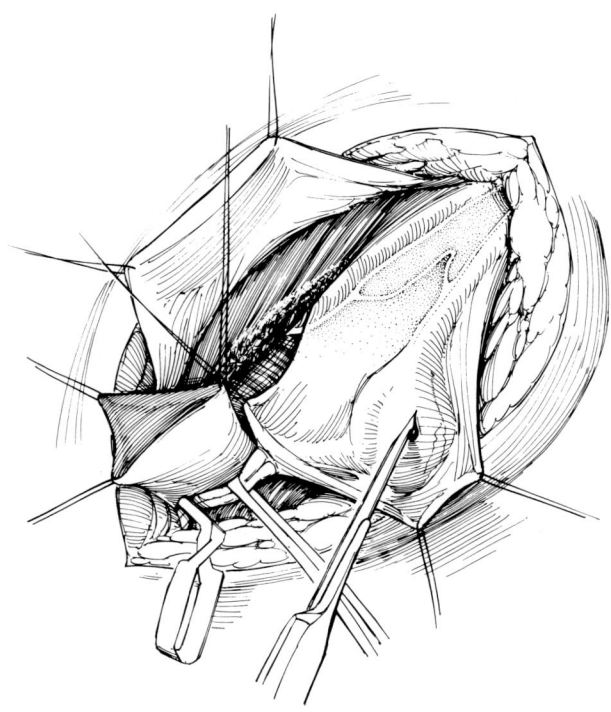

3 Close the tunica with a single fine atraumatic suture. Clamp and divide the pedicle above the bulldog clamp, and ligate it doubly. Grasp the areolar tissue adjacent to the artery, and temporarily release the bulldog clamp. Free, bright bleeding from the distal cut end indicates adequate collateral circulation to the testis. Ligate this end of the artery.

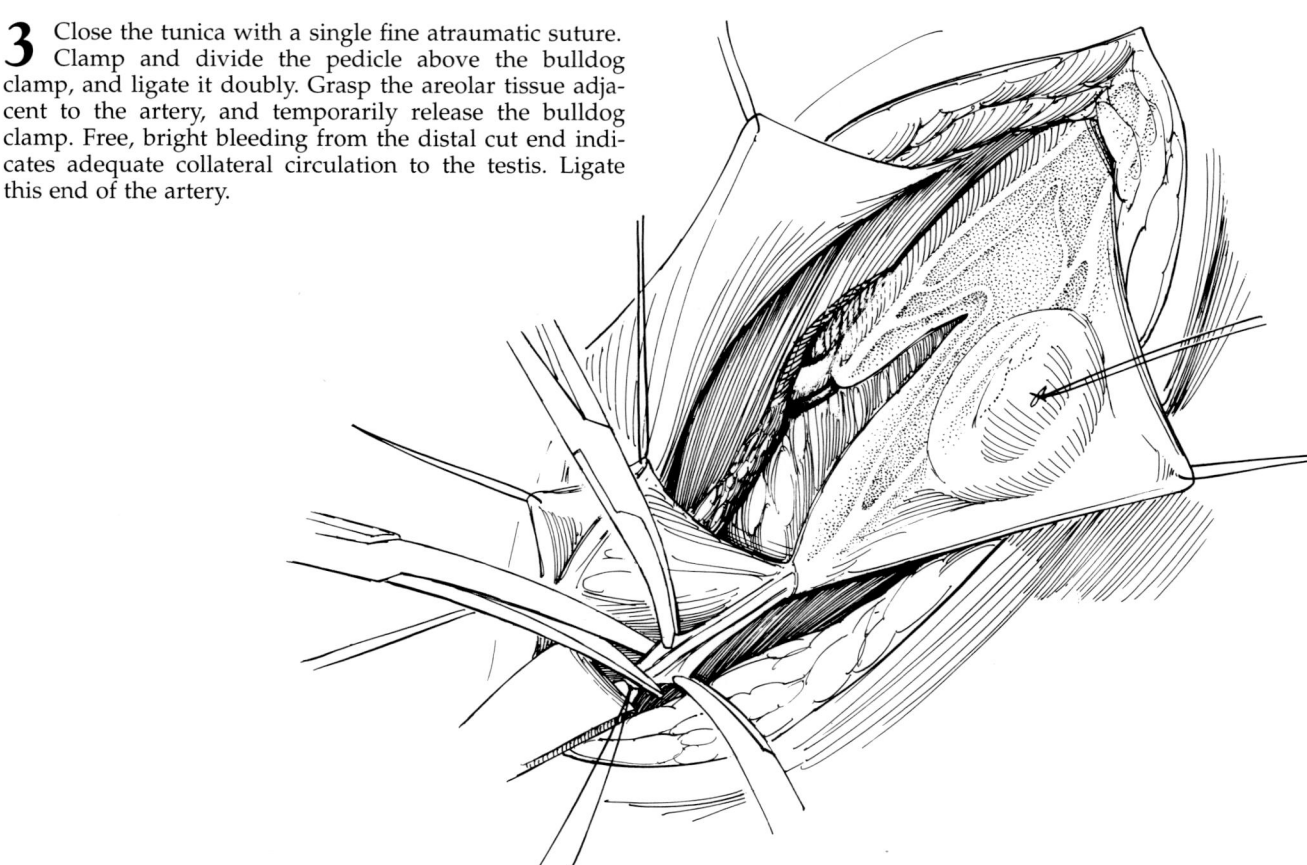

4 Turn the testis caudally into the scrotum. Continue as for a standard orchiopexy.

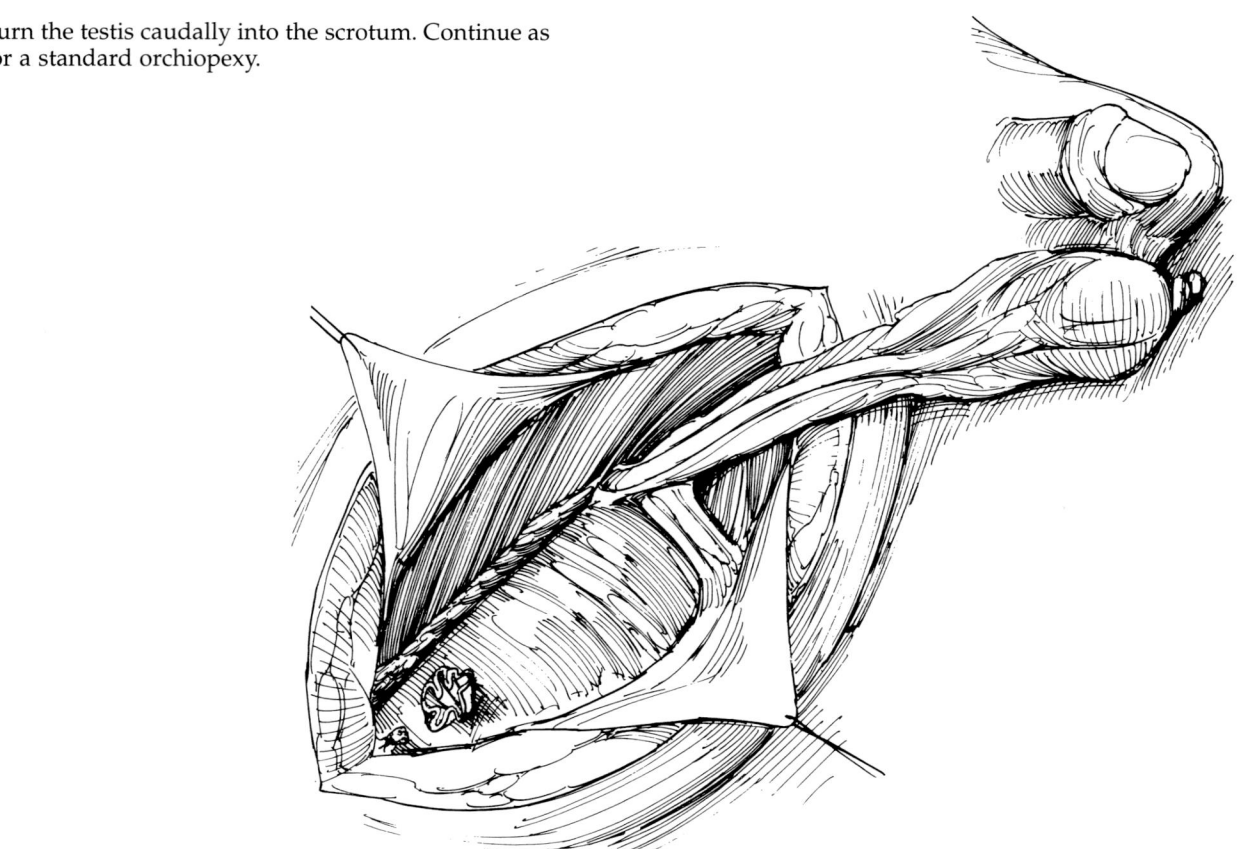

Postoperative Problems

Testicular atrophy is the major complication. This may be caused by failure to incorporate an adequate strip of peritoneum medially to, and accompanying, the vas with loss of collaterals, by injuring the vasal artery, or by ligation of the spermatic vessels too close to the testis so that the arcades cannot function. The irregular pattern of the blood supply contributes to the problem. Injury to the vas or the testis also is possible.

Commentary by F. Douglas Stephens

The testicular artery is the small trunk that is formed by the junction of the internal spermatic and vasal arteries. It forms near the hilum of the testis but does not divide and radiate from the hilum in the parenchyma in the manner of the renal vessels. Instead, it tracks under the lower pole in the tunica vasculosa beneath the tunica albuginea. It usually divides into two branches that course over the summit toward the upper pole, giving off end-artery twigs that dip into the septal compartments. Sometimes these two main branches can be identified because of the accompanying venae comitantes visible through the tunica albuginea. To avoid infarction of septal compartments when performing the bleeding test, incise into the vasculosa layer by a longitudinal incision of the albuginea only toward the upper pole and between the main branches, and use very fine atraumatic sutures to approximate the cut edges of the tunica albuginea, thus arresting the bleeding without incurring further infarctions.

This technique of orchiopexy is not recommended if the spermatic cord and vas deferens have been dissected or

skeletonized in a failed attempt to bring down the testis into the scrotum. Hence, on recognition of the long-loop vas, conduct the operation in the stages outlined herein.

If bleeding stops almost immediately after the bleeding test incision is made, the anastomosis between the internal spermatic vessels and the artery of the vas is inadequate. Microvascular anastomoses of the inferior epigastric to the internal spermatic vessels should be considered as the means by which the viability of the testis can be maintained after division of the internal spermatic vessels.

The anatomy of the blood vessels both outside and inside the tunica albuginea governs the steps in the operation that entail the division of the internal spermatic vessels.

Blood Vessels Outside the Tunica Albuginea. The testicular artery anastomoses by one or several terminal branches, with the vasal artery near the lower pole of the testis and close to the hilum. A single artery arises from the junction of these vessels, bypasses the hilum, and penetrates the tunica albuginea at the lower pole of the testis.

Blood Vessels Inside the Tunica Albuginea. Immediately beneath the tunica, the testicular artery commonly divides into two separate branches that course longitudinally toward the upper pole, giving off end arteries, which dip into and supply the tubules in the individual septa of the testis. Sometimes the vessel remains single, and sometimes the two branches at first run close together. These vessels are accompanied by veins that can be seen, if carefully scrutinized, as blue streaks under the tunica.

Precautions to Preserve the Blood Supply to the Testis. Transect the internal spermatic vascular bundle cranial to the internal ring of the inguinal canal and higher than the point of deviation of the vas deferens. In this way, the main testicular artery is divided before giving off delicate anastomosing connections to the vasal vessels. One or more of these cross-connections, which are best seen through the back wall of the hernia sac, may need to be divided under vision to free and turn down the testis from the descending limb of the loop of the vas and its main vessels. Venae comitantes enhance the visibility of these small channels.

Incise the tunica for the bleeding test longitudinally and toward the upper pole. Select a site for the incision between the main visible vessels in the tunica vasculosa or an area of nonvisible vascularity. Meticulous positioning and suturing curtail the extent of infarction that follows an incision in the tunica vasculosa that inadvertently divides a main trunk and its septal-end arteries.

Division of the testicular vessels and orchiopexy can also be applied to abdominal testes of patients with the triad (prune belly) syndrome. In these patients, however, the vas deferens is sometimes atretic in some part of its course; hence, the bleeding test would indicate a lack of supply to the testis from the artery of the vas.

Commentary by David T. Mininberg

Long-loop vas orchiopexy is an essential part of the armamentarium of the pediatric urologist that has facilitated successful orchiopexy for the high inguinal or abdominal testis. The key to success with this procedure is early recognition of the need to employ it. These testes often are impalpable. Diagnostic laparoscopy can be helpful in these cases to locate the testis and perform either laparoscopic orchiopexy, the first stage of a Fowler-Stephens procedure, by clipping the spermatic vessels or an inguinal orchiopexy if the testis is intracanalicular. (These procedures are well described elsewhere in the text.)

The key to a successful Fowler-Stephens operation is taking a broad tongue of attached peritoneum along with the testis and the vas down to the scrotum. This pedicled flap provides essential collateral circulation to the testis. The flap is raised by careful dissection of the hernia sac on its anterior aspect, avoiding the posterior wall. The resultant peritoneal defect is closed in standard fashion. Additional length without tension can be obtained by opening the transversalis fascia up to the epigastric vessels. A space can be developed readily under the vessels so that the testis and its vessels can be tunneled under the epigastric vessels. This avoids forcing the testis to climb over the vessels and also improves the angle of the passage down the inguinal canal. The benefits of this maneuver are enhanced by dissections along the vas down toward the pelvis. This allows even greater change in the angle of passage. The main pitfall of the Fowler-Stephens operation is late recognition of the need to perform it. If the testis and vas have been freed from all the contiguous structures, it will not be possible to carry it out successfully. Another potential pitfall is overestimating the potential value of the particular testis. There are testes that are so atrophic that they are best removed. The need for removal occasionally can be difficult to judge, but the small testis found in the long term may be from misjudgment at the start rather than from an operation that placed too much tension on the vascular pedicle.

CHAPTER 100

Two-Stage Orchiopexy

Ascertain the position or absence of the testis preoperatively. Apply strict aseptic precautions, because insertion of a silicone sheath is anticipated.

FIRST STAGE

Perform a standard orchiopexy, using all the methods described for lengthening the cord, including ligating the inferior epigastric vessels or resorting to the long-loop vas technique. Resort to the two-stage procedure for the inguinal testis that had not reached the bottom of the scrotum despite all maneuvers in the first stage.

1 **A,** *Incision:* Make a skin-crease incision. **B,** If after thorough mobilization, the testis still does not reach the scrotum, fix it to the pubic tubercle with 3-0 nonabsorbable sutures, or, if possible, place it in a high dartos pouch. The blood supply can be jeopardized by inserting a suture on a Keith needle in the tunica albuginea and bringing it through the scrotum to attach it to rubber-band traction.

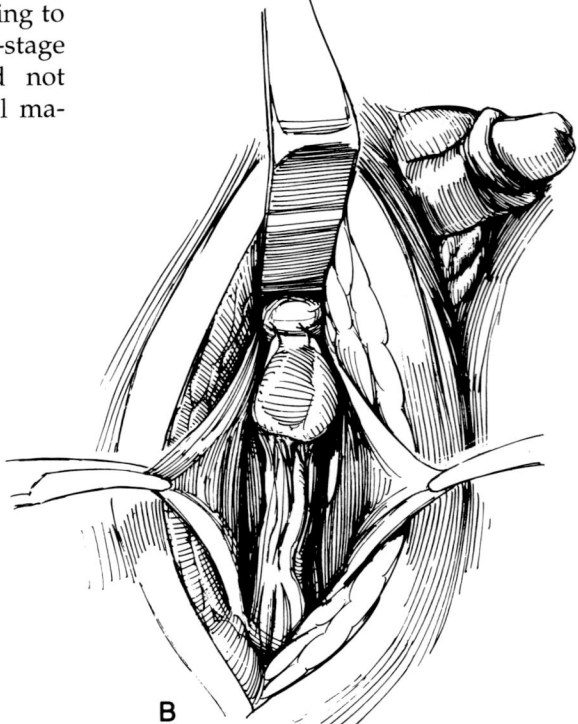

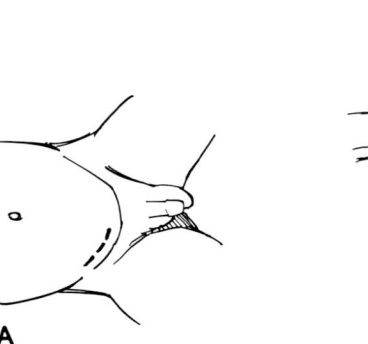

A

B

2 **A** and **B,** A silicone sheath placed around the cord (Corkery, 1975) can facilitate the second stage but will cause greater capillary oozing and more fibrosis. Cut a rectangle from a sheet of Silastic that is 0.007 in thick, long enough to reach from the internal ring to the tubercle, and wide enough to encircle the testis. Cut a narrow V-shaped notch at each end. **C,** Place the notched sheath around the testis and cord, and trim the sides to fit. First, close the tube around the testicular fixation sutures at the pubic tubercle with a 3-0 nonabsorbable suture. Continue along the edges with a running 3-0 nonabsorbable suture. Close the external oblique fascia with similar sutures for later identification.

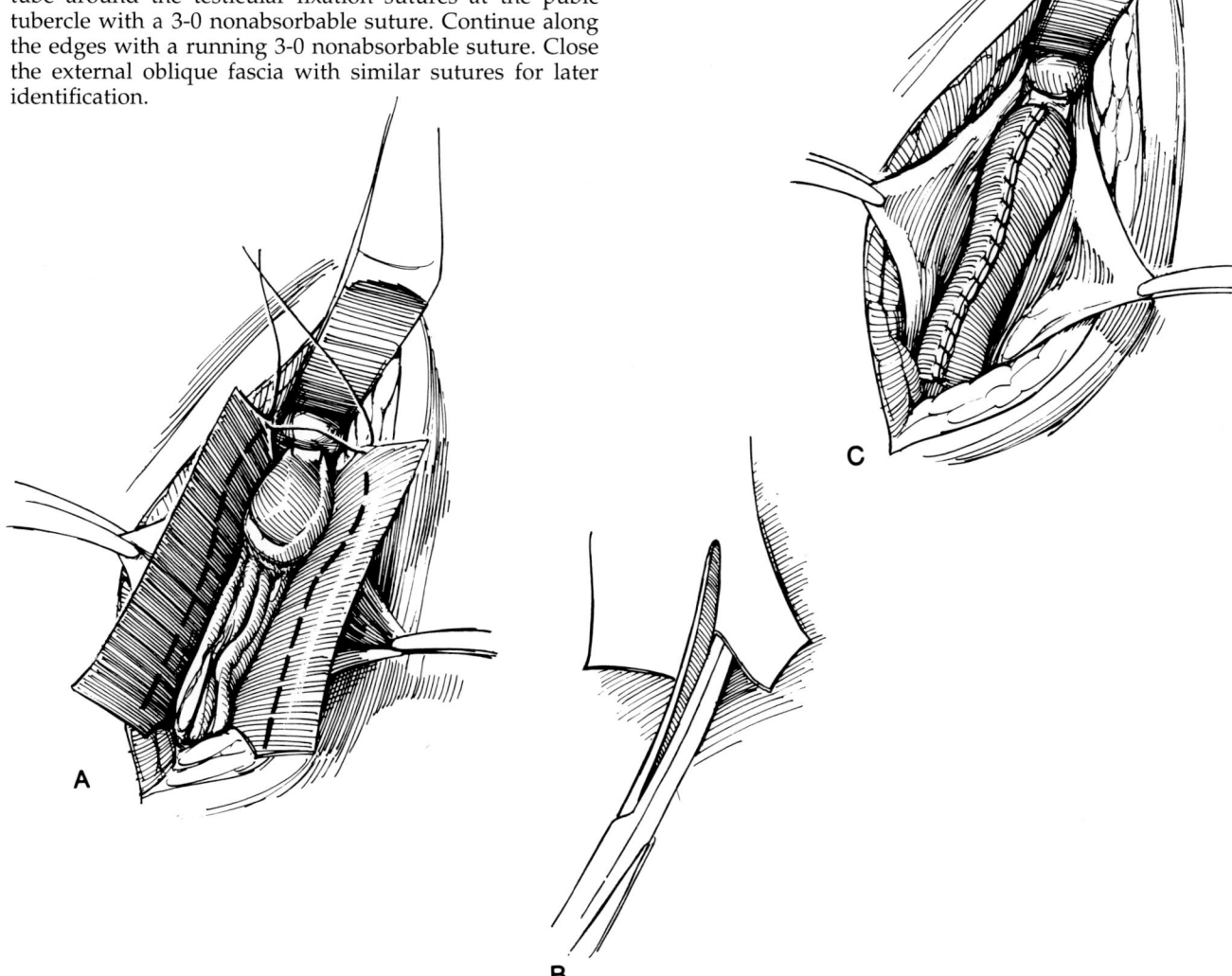

SECOND STAGE

At least 1 year later (sooner in infants) open the external oblique fascia identified by the nonabsorbable sutures. If a sheath has been inserted, dissect it out with its contents, separate the testis from the pubic tubercle, and slip the Silastic sheet out after cutting its sutures. Whether a sheath has been placed or not, dissect the testis and cord carefully using a loupe—this dissection can be tedious. Free adhesions proximally by opening the internal ring. Continue dissection in the retroperitoneal space, where it will proceed more easily. Adequate length usually is obtained. Scrotal placement and fixation are completed in the usual way.

POSTOPERATIVE PROBLEMS

Infection may require early removal of the sheath.

Commentary by John R. Woodard

The problem with two-stage orchiopexy is that it requires a second stage; that carries an increased risk for injury to the ilioinguinal nerve and the vas deferens. Because the optimal interval between stages is probably 1 year, the technique also results in a significant delay in achieving a scrotal environment for the testis. In my experience, this procedure is used when I have embarked on a routine inguinal orchiopexy and employed all of the usual maneuvers without gaining enough cord length to achieve a scrotal testis. Having gotten to that point in the operation, a Fowler-Stephens procedure probably would result in atrophy, so a two-stage orchiopexy is a better option. I have not used Silastic wraps, although those who do find them useful and satisfactory. My reticence has been due partly to the belief that the second-stage dissection, as tedious and difficult as it sometimes is, facilitates the gaining of additional length. Of course, the potential for infection of the Silastic sheath is a concern as well.

I find it useful to start the dissection during the second stage slightly lateral to the original procedure to allow accurate identification of tissue planes peripheral to the original scar. Beyond that, the second stage involves slow and meticulous dissection of the cord structures and testis with mobilization to the same extent as in the first stage.

Commentary by Stephen C. Shapiro

I have resorted to the two-stage procedure only occasionally among the more than 500 orchiopexies done in the past decade. The reason for this is that I believe it is important to make a decision concerning whether or not to perform a two-stage orchiopexy *before using* all the methods described for lengthening the spermatic cord, rather than after. Some of the testicles subjected to a two-stage orchiopexy, as described in the text, would be treated better with "orchiopexy-on-vas." This is particularly true if a long-loop vas is present; a patient with this type of testis is an ideal candidate for this procedure (the Fowler-Stephens orchiopexy). Accordingly, the testis and spermatic cord can be mobilized without ligating the hernia sac and without skeletonizing the spermatic cord structures. If it is apparent that the testicle will not reach into the scrotum, a decision can be made at that point to perform an orchiopexy-on-vas or a two-stage maneuver.

Certain truisms also apply. It is unlikely that an intra-abdominal testis will reach the scrotum without ligation of the spermatic vessels, even with a two-stage orchiopexy, except perhaps in an infant with prune belly syndrome. The two-stage orchiopexy, therefore, is best applied to the inguinal testis that will just not reach the bottom of the scrotum after thorough dissection. Most testes beyond the external ring can be brought into the scrotum in one stage. If after having mobilized the inguinal testis, ligating the hernia sac, and releasing the lateral spermatic ligaments, it becomes apparent that the testis will not sit comfortably in the scrotum, I have chosen simply to bring it into the lowest comfortable location, which usually is the upper scrotum. Scrotal fixation is then performed by the dartos pouch technique, and no attention is paid to retraction of the scrotum. I would advise against using a traction suture, because this could result in vascular compromise of the testis. It sometimes is surprising how low a testis eventually will lie in the scrotum after maximal mobilization despite retraction of the scrotum and obviously inadequate length. It is important either to ligate the inferior epigastric vessels or to bring the testis under them to shorten its course to the scrotum. If the testis is in an unsatisfactory position 6 to 12 months after the initial surgery, a second-stage operation can be undertaken.

I have not used the silicone sheath around the spermatic cord, because my initial experience with it resulted in infection and loss of a testicle. Instead, at the second stage, I simply mobilize the testicle again. The procedure is facilitated by 3.5 × magnification. I believe that it pays to wait longer than 1 year in an older child before undertaking this second-stage orchiopexy; however, 6 months or 1 year may be adequate in an infant. Because all intra-abdominal testes or high inguinal testes have been subjected to orchiopexy-on-vas, the two-stage maneuver has been successful in my hands in the several instances in which it has been employed.

CHAPTER 101

Microvascular Orchiopexy

Instruments: Provide a complete microvascular set-up with an operating room microscope, three-power loupes, and 10-0 or 11-0 nylon sutures on BV-6 or ST-7 needles.

1 *Position:* Place the child on a table extension to provide space for the surgeon's knees. *Incision:* Make a generous inguinal incision in the skin crease that extends well laterally to permit abdominal access (page 270).

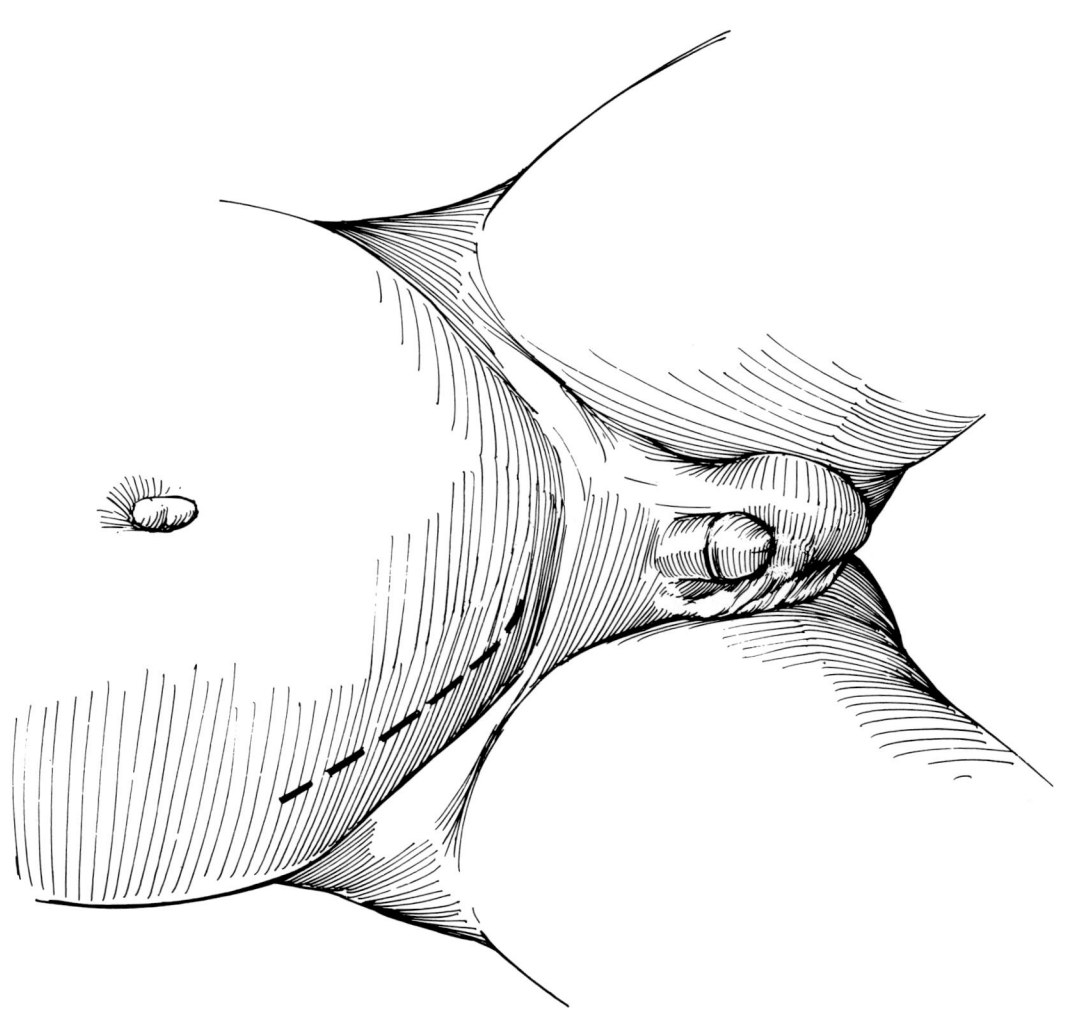

2 Open the inguinal canal, and identify the gubernaculum and the processus vaginalis. Open the peritoneum at the internal ring. Locate the testis, and place a traction suture. Expose the spermatic vessels. Move the testis into the retroperitoneal space, and carefully dissect the peritoneum off the vascular pedicle. Close the peritoneum. Using loupes for the dissection, bluntly dissect retroperitoneally, following the vessels to near their communication with the vena cava or renal vein and aorta. Ensure that the dissection of the vessels extends beyond the confluence of the pampiniform plexus to form a single vein. Preserve the vasal vessels in a large patch of peritoneum as the vas is freed into the pelvis. If the vas is too short, pass the testis under the lateral umbilical ligament (obliterated umbilical artery).

Expose the inferior epigastric artery and vein(s) by dissection through the internal oblique aponeurosis and the transversus abdominis, and hold them in a vessel loop. Ligate the side branches as far from the main vessel as possible, because one of them may be of suitable size to be used for the anastomosis. Ligate and divide the artery and vein high beneath the rectus muscle, placing a noncrushing microvascular clamp on the proximal end. Apply heparin solution (10 U/ml) to the cut ends. Ligate or fulgurate their muscular branches with bipolar diathermy.

Prepare a dartos pouch. Ligate the spermatic vessels. Divide them distal to the ligature, and look for backbleeding. Place the testis in the dartos pouch (pages 492–493). Close the peritoneal defect and the anterior part of the peritoneal cavity.

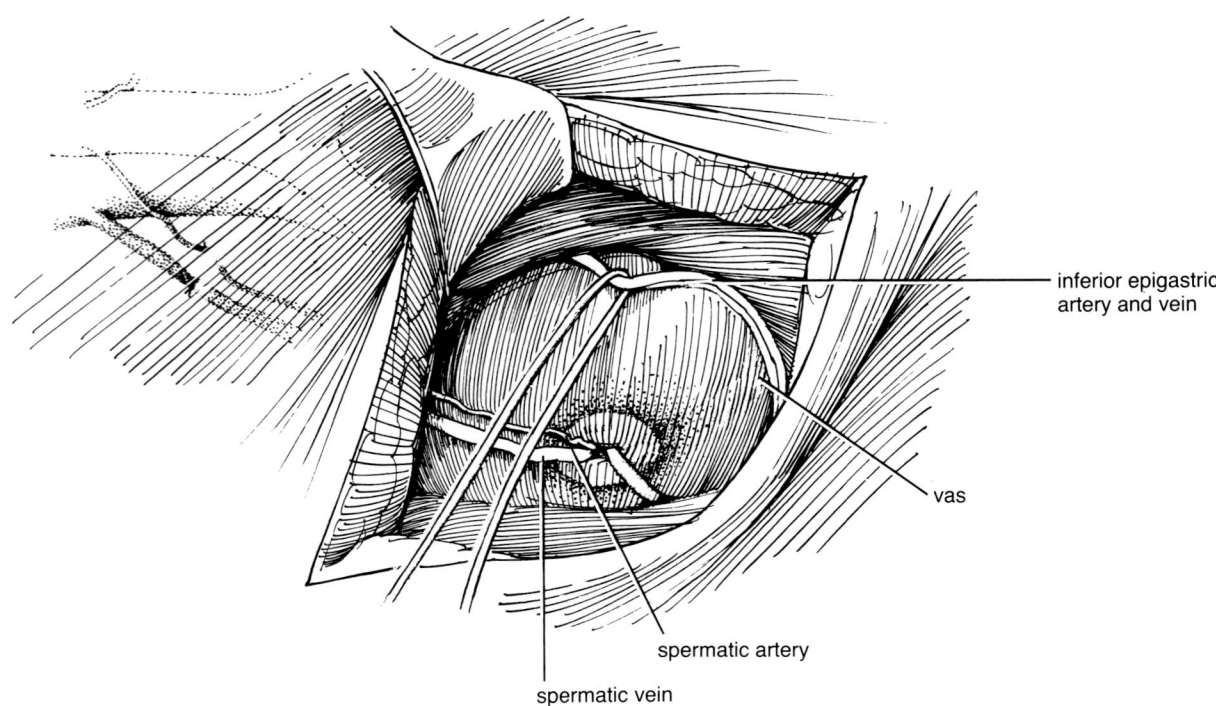

inferior epigastric
artery and vein

vas

spermatic artery

spermatic vein

3 **A,** Bring the spermatic and epigastric arteries into the microscopic field, and place them in a microvascular clamp. Perform vascular anastomosis with 10-0 or 11-0 nylon, commencing with a venous anastomosis. Expect a considerable disparity in size between the arteries. An oblique or a spatulated anastomosis may compensate for the difference. Ischemia time should be kept as short as possible. **B,** Observe the anastomosis for at least 20 minutes to be sure occlusion will not occur. If it does, resect and redo the anastomosis. Before closing, incise the testis and look for fresh bleeding. Fix the testis in the scrotum, and close the inguinal wound carefully to avoid obstructing the vessels.

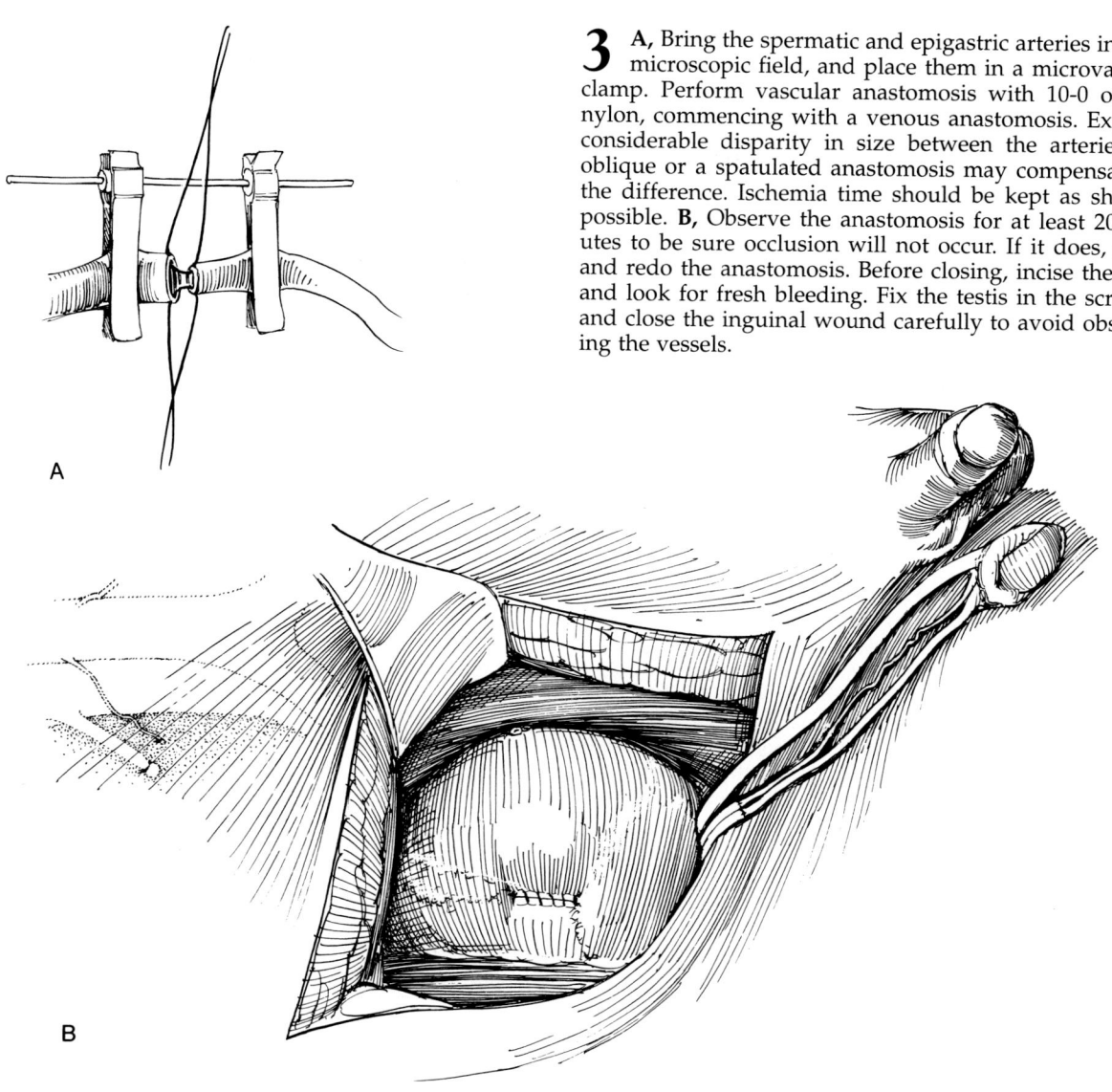

A

B

Commentary by A. Bianchi

The majority of palpable testes can be brought to the scrotum without tension by a minimally invasive "trans-scrotal orchidopexy." For the more difficult testis, the addition of a conventional inguinal approach may provide further vessel length. The reliability of microvascular anastomosis for vessels smaller than 1 mm in diameter has removed the problem of the short vascular pedicle, so that the high inguinal and intra-abdominal testis now can be safely transferred to the scrotum with a full blood supply. Concern regarding testicular vessel size in the infant under 2 years of age is unfounded. Indeed, the genitalia and the testicular vascular pedicle are particularly well developed, possibly consequent to the heavy hormonal stimulation during the pregnancy. Recent experimental work in rats has demonstrated the absolute importance of a full blood supply and, particularly, sufficient venous drainage from the testis, in preserving spermatogenesis. It is therefore no longer logical, and is indeed self-defeating, to advocate techniques that rely on the vasal and other collaterals, following division of the main vascular pedicle, because the severe chronic ischemic injury to spermatogenic tissue or testicular venous congestion, or both, renders any surviving testis virtually sterile.

The child with an impalpable testis first should have a laparoscopy to locate and assess the testis, its vessels, and the vas. The child and parents are then counseled regarding the indications for microvascular orchiopexy. Only one testis should be transferred at any one session. There are no special anesthetic requirements, except those that are routine for a safe 3-hour procedure. No anticoagulant or other adjuvant therapy is necessary. However, cut vessel ends are constantly washed with a heparin-saline solution (10 U/ml) during the anastomoses. An operating room microscope is essential and should preferably be equipped with a foot pedal control for focus, zoom, and X-Y coupling.

The child is placed supine on a heating blanket on the operating table, and the bladder is emptied by manual suprapubic compression. The surgeon and assistant position themselves comfortably, and the microscope is adjusted for position and focus. A laterally extended skin-crease groin incision is deepened through the fibers of the external oblique to identify the gubernacular structures and the processus vaginalis. The ilioinguinal nerve is displaced sideways and the processus vaginalis followed backward to the internal inguinal ring, where the inferior epigastric vessels are easily located. Care should be taken to avoid injury to a long-loop vas. The peritoneum is opened, and the testis is delivered out of the abdomen. The peritoneum is closed, and further careful blunt dissection of vessels and vas occurs extraperitoneally. Vessel dissection is taken high, toward the origin of the artery and beyond the confluence of the pampiniform plexus, to form a single testicular vein. One or two venous communications passing to the perinephric tissues are divided with sufficient length for additional venous anastomoses, if required. Vasal dissection is undertaken with due care to preserve the vasal collaterals. In the event of a short vas, additional length may be obtained by passing the testis beneath the obliterated umbilical artery. The testis with intact vas and vascular pedicle is then placed to one side. The inferior epigastric artery and its two venae comitantes are followed high beneath the rectus abdominis, dividing all muscular branches, to provide a long donor pedicle and a better arterial diameter match to the much smaller testicular artery. The inferior epigastric vessels are clamped proximally with graded microvascular clamps and then divided. Under magnification with the operating microscope, the artery and the larger vein are carefully cleared of adventitia. The vessel ends are cleanly cut back in circular or spatulate fashion to undamaged intima. A wide circular (venous) anastomosis and a long wide oblique (arterial) anastomosis are planned. The remaining inferior epigastric vein is preserved for a possible additional venous anastomosis or for vein donation, should a reverse interposition step-down graft be required for the difficult arterial anastomosis because of a marked mismatch in vessel diameter.

The testicular vessels are ligated high and divided. The testis is transferred through a prepared track to exit through a scrotal incision. Cooling with ice packs may be used but is not essential. Testicular perfusion definitively is contraindicated, for fear of intimal damage. The testicular artery and vein are prepared under magnification with the operating microscope and the ends cut to match the inferior epigastric vessels. The testicular vein, at a diameter of 1.4 mm, is a reasonable match to the inferior epigastric vein, at 0.8 to 1 mm. However, there is a marked mismatch in the arterial wall thickness and the luminal diameter between the testicular artery, at 0.5 to 0.8 mm, and the inferior epigastric artery, at 1 to 1.2 mm. In the event of more than one testicular artery, the diameter may be further reduced to approximately 0.3 mm. Only one arterial anastomosis is required, and the interposition of a reversed venous step-down graft is helpful in these circumstances.

One arterial anastomosis and one venous anastomosis usually are required. Interrupted sutures of 10-0 monofilament nylon on a 3.75-mm, 75-μm needle (Ethilon W2870, or similar suture) are used to accurately appose the intimal surfaces. Vessel ends are washed constantly with a heparin-saline solution (10 U/ml). The venous anastomosis is completed first, and the microvascular clamps are removed to relieve any venous congestion from an inadequate venous collateral circulation. On completion of the arterial anastomosis, the testis becomes revascularized.

Anastomotic patency lasting longer than 20 minutes usually is associated with a good long-term outcome. Vessel thrombosis will occur within 5 minutes and is an indication of an imperfect anastomosis, for which the only management is resection and reanastomosis. A testicular biopsy is taken. Incision of the tunica albuginea will show active arterial bleeding from a pink testis of normal appearance. The testis is placed in a subdartos pouch in the ipsilateral scrotum. All wounds are closed in layers (including subcuticular skin closure) with absorbable materials. No postoperative monitoring is necessary, or indeed possible, in the young infant. The child is mobilized and allowed home within 24 to 36 hours. Successful microvascular orchiopexy is associated with an uncomplicated postoperative course and an expectation of a scrotal testis of normal consistency and mobility thereafter.

At the Royal Manchester Children's Hospital between 1981 and 1992, 49 testes in 41 boys between 2 and 15 years of age were transferred to the scrotum by microvascular techniques. Eight children had a bilateral transfer, and 31 had a unilateral orchiopexy, some for a single residual testis after loss of the contralateral organ. There has been no mortality and virtually no morbidity. A total of 45 testes are present in the scrotum, providing excellent cosmesis and "genital normality." The psychologic relief for the child, and particularly for the parents, has been noticeable. Indeed, those with bilateral intra-abdominal testes insisted on the same procedure for the opposite side. No patients would accept orchiectomy as an option, even in full knowledge of potential malignancy in later life. Four testes have atrophied, either because of anastomotic failure or inherent abnormality. A few more than 50 percent of testes have shown varying numbers of spermatogonia, the remainder showing Sertoli cells only. There was no instance of *in situ* neoplasia. Most children in the series underwent the operation in the younger age group and still have not reached puberty. All testes in pubertal and postpubertal children have demonstrated good hormonal output and have grown to approximately 75 percent of expected volume for age. Postpubertal children are counseled regarding the malignancy risk and are taught the self-examination technique. Perhaps the most important indication for orchiopexy is the correction of an obvious genital anomaly. The provision of "normal genitalia" has a definite impact on the development of a normal psyche in the growing child and provides major relief for the parents. Enhanced spermatogenesis and reduced morbidity (torsion, hernia, and possibly malignancy) are also of major relevance.

Experience has shown that microvascular orchiopexy is a reliable and safe procedure. It is a further option in the successful transfer of the high inguinal and intra-abdominal testis to the scrotum. Whereas the child's age and the vessel diameter are no barrier, the skill of the surgeon most certainly requires laboratory and clinical development, if consistently high success rates are to be achieved. Techniques relying on vasal collaterals are associated with high atrophy rates and induce virtual sterility in surviving testes. Currently, there can be little reason for testicular transfer to the scrotum on anything less than a full blood supply.

Although microvascular orchiopexy is now a proven technique, its value in the management of the high testis on a short vascular pedicle requires long-term evaluation with reference to the development of the patient's psyche, his fertility, and the incidence of malignancy.

CHAPTER 102

Orchiopexy for Abdominal Testis

The nonpalpable testis usually is approached by starting with an inguinal incision and extending it as the findings warrant (discussed on page 496). However, laparoscopic inspection will show whether the vessels end blindly and the testis is absent, whether the cord structure end in the inguinal canal is attached to, at most, a markedly hypoplastic testis, or whether the testis is present intra-abdominally and can be approached directly without exploration. A high testis that has been localized laparoscopically can be exposed directly through a midline abdominal incision, or if shown to be hypoplastic, it may be excised by the laparoscopic technique.

EXTENDED INGUINAL APPROACH

With the expectation that the testis is relatively low, start with a standard orchiopexy incision, but do not extend the opening in the internal oblique muscle into the external ring. Expose the internal ring, and pull on the processus vaginalis at its point of exit to bring the intra-abdominal testis into view. Open the anterior surface of the hernia sac, and look for a long, looping vas deferens or an attenuated epididymis with a testis attached. A blind-ending vas and epididymis can be found in the inguinal canal, detached from the testes and outside the hernia sac.

If the testis is not discovered, open the external oblique muscle, retract the internal oblique muscle at the medial edge of the internal ring, and open the peritoneum. Look for the vas behind the bladder near the obliterated hypogastric vessels, and trace it along with the spermatic vessels to their end, often in a nubbin that denotes anorchia. The vas should be resected for pathologic examination. If a testis is found, place a fine traction suture in the tunica albuginea at the lower pole, and pull on it to assess vessel length. If it appears that enough length could be gained by high dissection of the vessels, proceed accordingly with a traditional orchiopexy. If traction shows that the vessels are too short, proceed to a long-loop vas orchiopexy (page 496). Alternatively, if dissection has progressed and release proves inadequate, fix the testis to the pubic tubercle, perhaps cover the cord with a Silastic sheath, and return for a second-stage orchiopexy (page 501).

An absent testis is confirmed by the presence of blind-ending vas and spermatic vessels. Finding only a blind-ending vas requires further abdominal exploration.

ABDOMINAL APPROACH

1 **A,** Make a midline incision in the lower abdomen from pubis to umbilicus. **B,** Separate the rectus and underlying areolar tissue. Open the peritoneum and pack the intestine aside. The testis often will be found lying intraperitoneally, usually behind the bladder and often on a short mesentery.

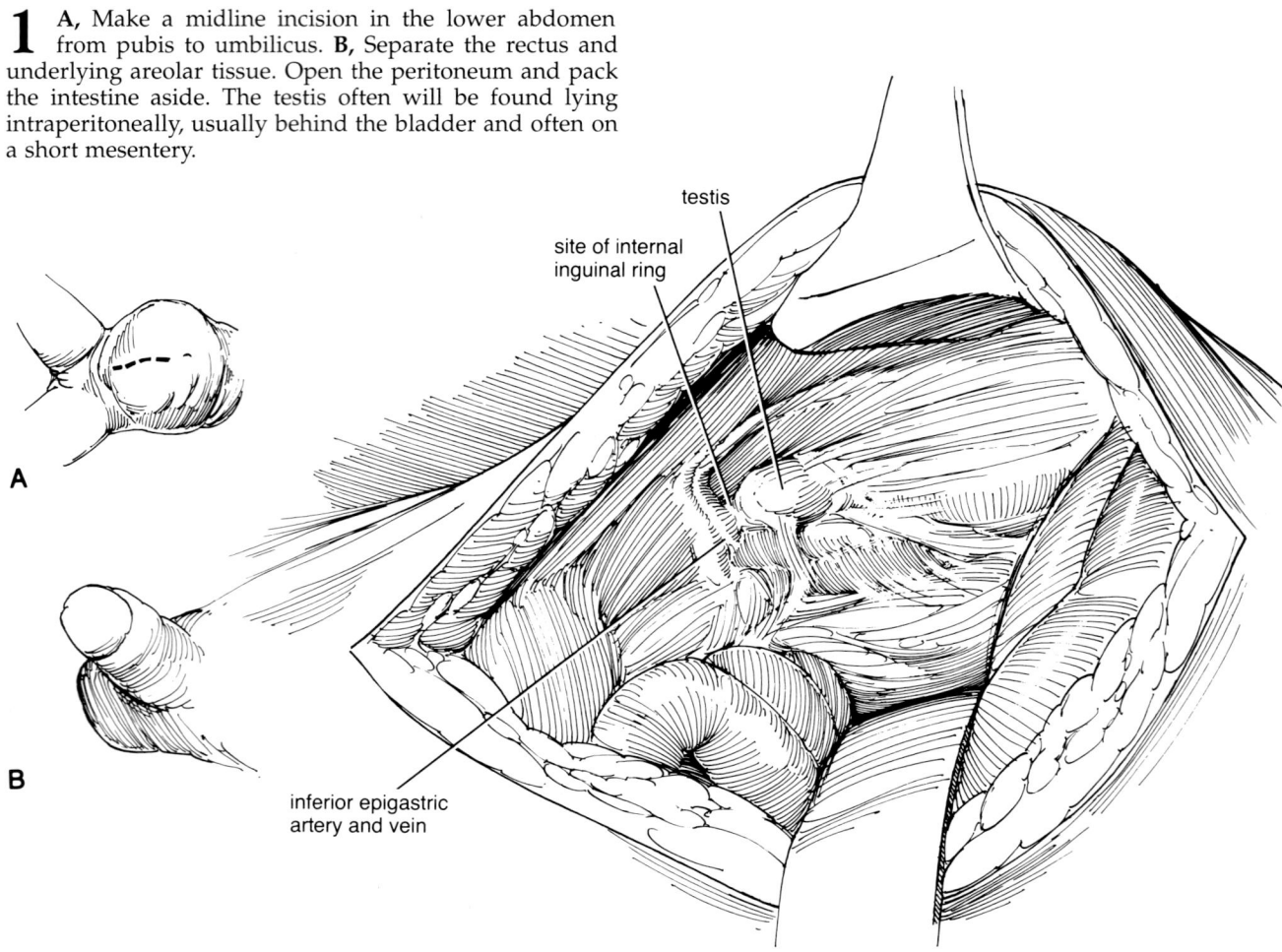

2 Incise the peritoneum obliquely, leaving a strip of peritoneum, and sharply free the vessels from the retroperitoneal tissue under direct vision.

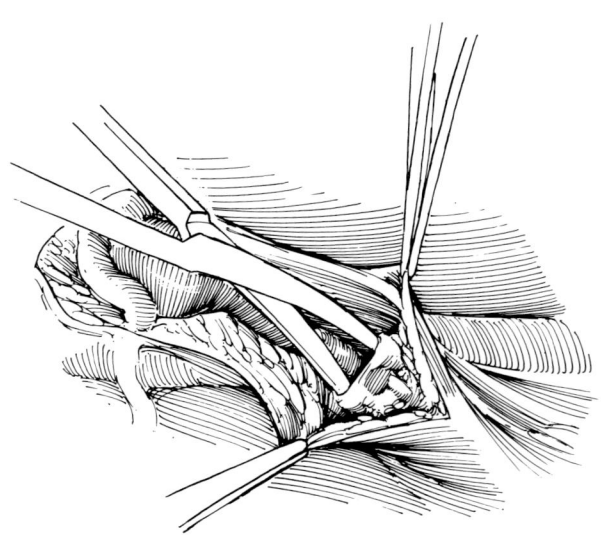

3 Similarly, sharply free the vas behind the bladder, leaving 1 cm of peritoneum on either side (not shown) until sufficient length is achieved to place the testis in the scrotum. Invert the scrotum through the external ring, as is done in palpating for a hernia, and place a curved clamp against the fingertip from above. In boys with prune belly syndrome, the ring will be relatively large. Push the clamp through the transversalis fascia and the conjoined tendon as the finger is withdrawn, then dilate the canal and scrotum with the clamp and finger as necessary to form a passage for the testis. Incise the scrotum over the finger.

Place a suture in the tissue adjacent to the testis that will be used to lead it through the canal to the bottom of the scrotum. Fix the testis in a dartos pouch by incising the scrotal skin and developing a pocket between the skin and dartos by blunt dissection. Make a small nick in the dartos, and introduce a curved clamp into the inguinal canal to grasp the suture to bring the testis into the scrotum with a little traction. Anchor the testis by closing the dartos behind it with two fine nonabsorbable sutures.

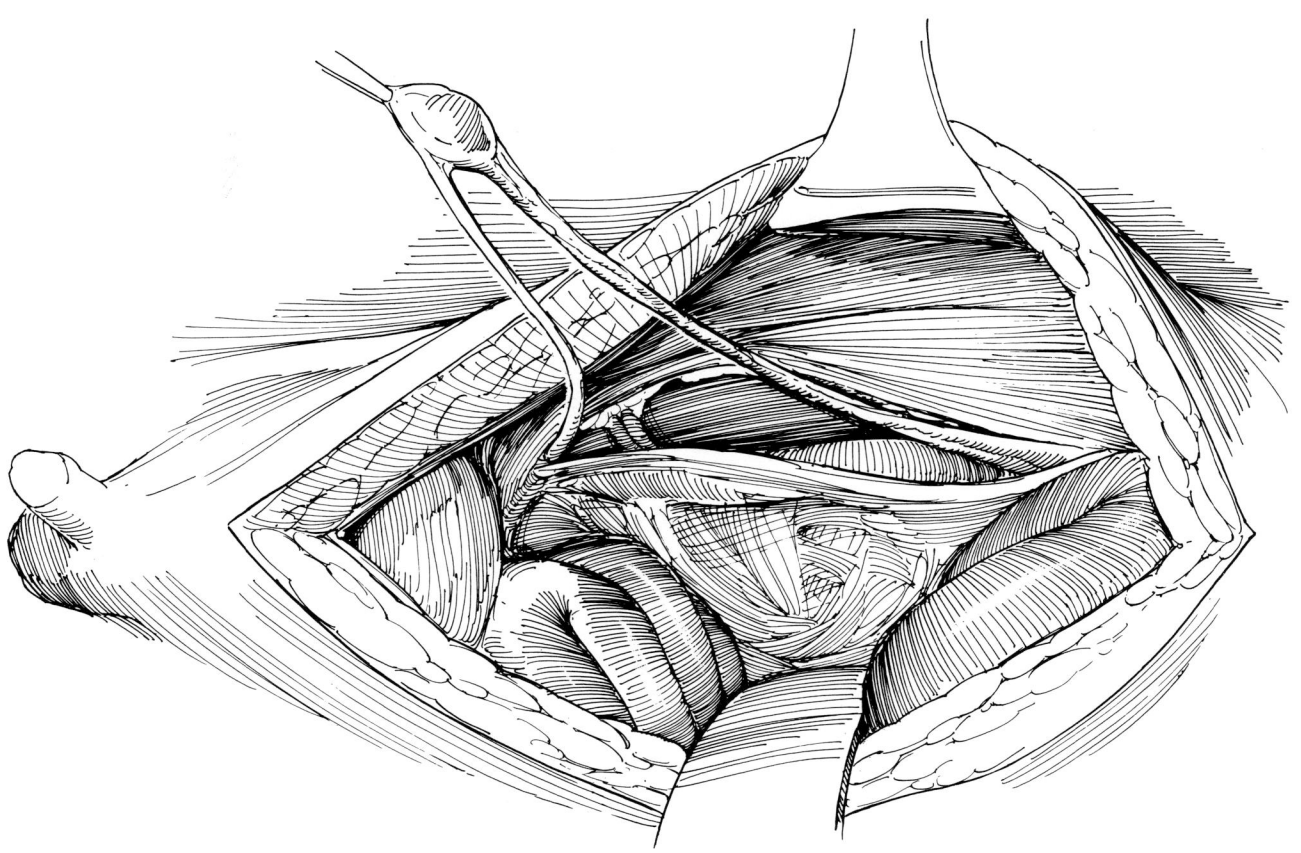

EXTRAPERITONEAL APPROACH

4 Make a lower abdominal midline incision from pubis to umbilicus. Separate the rectus muscles, and bluntly reflect the peritoneal envelope medially. Look first in the internal inguinal ring to pick up the cord structures. If found, bluntly free them along with the testis from the canal, bring them into the retroperitoneum, and divide the gubernaculum. The inferior epigastric vessels may prevent this maneuver; if they do, divide and ligate them. The internal ring may be too tight; divide it posteriorly and repair it later.

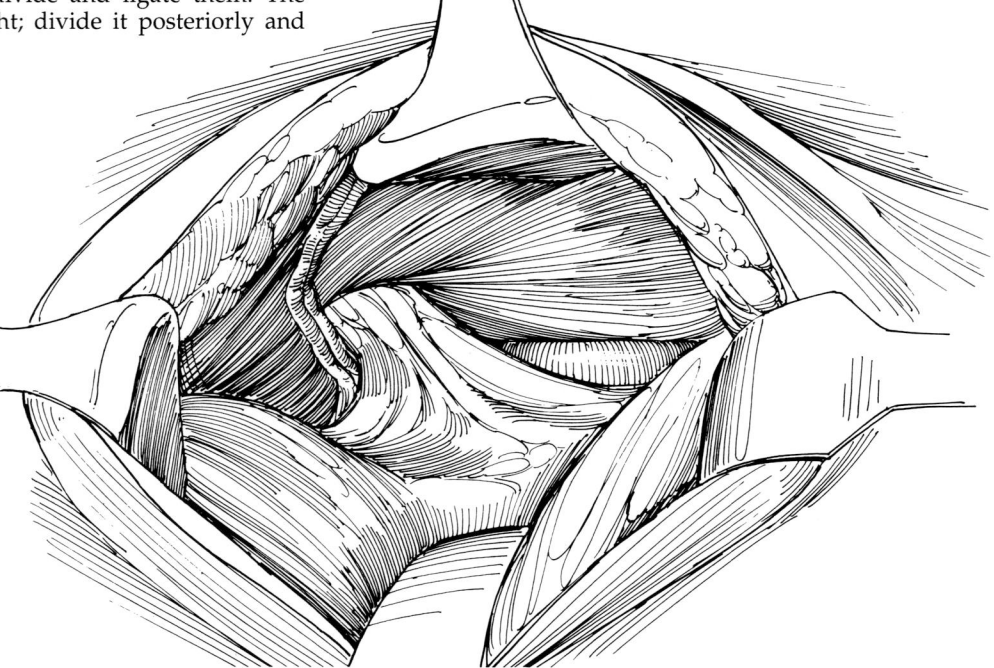

5 If the testis is not found about the internal ring, examine the posterior surface of the peritoneum, within which the testis is attached. Start by locating the vas deferens behind the bladder, and follow it into the canal to the testis, which will be concealed because it is intraperitoneal. The blind-ending vas and epididymis may be appreciably separated from the testis. If the vas ends blindly or in a rudimentary epididymis, identify the spermatic vessels and follow them. If they also terminate blindly, the diagnosis is an absent testis. If the testis is found retroperitoneally, incise the peritoneum around it, and close the peritoneal defect with a running 4-0 synthetic absorbable suture. A pedicled flap of peritoneum, inferior to the testis, can be left attached to the testis and placed in the scrotum with it (not shown). This flap can supplement the blood supply and is necessary if a Fowler-Stephens orchiopexy is done. Encircle the testis with a small Penrose drain for traction, bluntly and sharply free the vas down to the area of the prostate, and free the vascular bundle up to the level of the kidney.

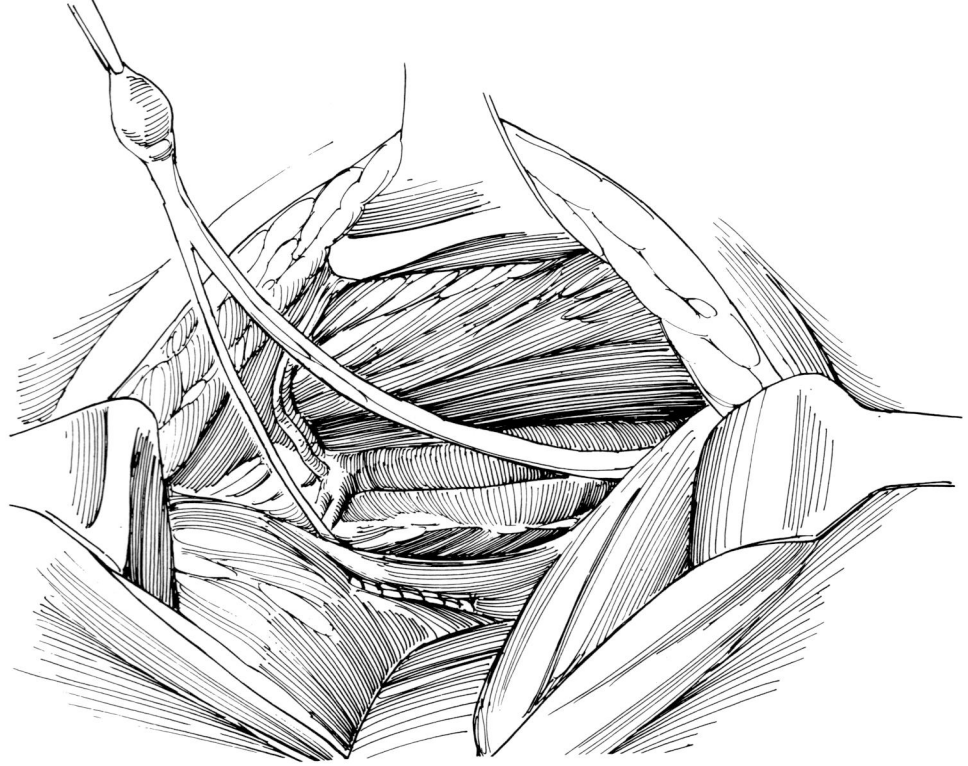

6 Make an adequate opening through the transversalis fascia and the tendinous end of the rectus muscle immediately superior to the pubis above the ipsilateral side of the scrotum. Create a scrotal pouch bluntly, and install the testis in the scrotum over the dartos, as described on pages 492–493, taking care not to twist the cord. Close the abdominal wall without drainage.

An alternative approach is through a muscle-splitting incision in a lower quadrant (page 267). Bring the testis medial to the inguinal canal to provide a direct route for the vessels. This incision will not provide enough exposure for high intra-abdominal testes.

For laparoscopic orchiopexy, see Chapter 103.

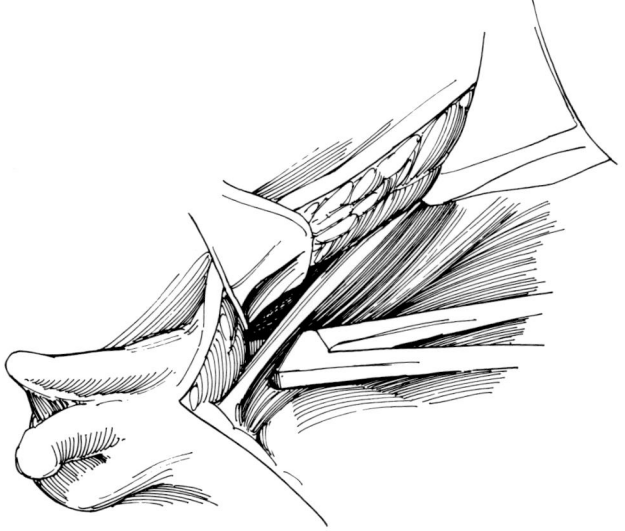

Commentary by David T. Mininberg

The description, with the illustrations, is an excellent guide to successful treatment of a nonpalpable testis. We personally favor the extended inguinal incision over the transperitoneal approach, because we believe this approach precludes the risk of future adhesions. In our experience, the blind-ending vas and epididymis often are found in the inguinal canal separated by a significant distance from the testis. Caution should be used in dissecting the cord until the testis is found and mobilized. If, in fact, the Fowler-Stephens orchiopexy should be necessary, we favor taking a generous tongue of peritoneum attached to the testis. This peritoneal flap will function as a pedicled flap with an additional potential blood supply to the testis. This maneuver allows the whole unit—testis and epididymis—to be placed in the scrotum.

We also favor scrotal placement by the dartos pouch technique.

Commentary by William J. Cromie

Extended Inguinal Approach. Start with a standard orchiopexy incision, open the external oblique from the external ring superiorly, and retract the internal oblique muscle medially. This will expose the internal ring, a small amount of preperitoneal fat, and the parietal peritoneum, extending to the processus vaginalis as it exits the intra-abdominal cavity. Often, the testis can be visualized directly at this point. The anterior surface of the processus can be incised and the sac explored for a long-loop vas deferens or an attenuated epididymis with the testis attached.

In most cases, no testis is found and, on opening the processus vaginalis at the internal ring, a blind-ending vas and testicular artery confirm the absence of the testis and make a diagnosis of monorchia. In some cases, the vessels and vas are not immediately apparent, and an exploration of the pelvis near the obliterated hypogastric vessels allows identification of the vas, which is then traced superiorly and laterally to its junction with the spermatic vessels near the area of the internal ring. The absence of the testis in either circumstance confirms the diagnosis of monorchia. In most cases, the vas should be resected for pathologic examination, and hemosiderin pigment frequently can be found within the distal tissues, confirming an *in utero* torsion.

If this exploration reveals the presence of an intra-abdominal testis, a traction suture is placed through the midportion of the tunica albuginea of the testis, avoiding significant polar blood supply to the testicle. Traction is placed on the vessels and, if it appears there is enough cord length for a traditional orchiopexy, the process vaginalis is resected, the cord skeletonized, and the testis placed within a subcutaneous dartos pouch in the appropriate hemiscrotum.

If the vessels appear too short and the boy has a long-looping vas, a Fowler test should be carried out to confirm collateral vasculature. This is followed by a Fowler-Stevens orchiopexy (page 496). On rare occasions, when a decision has been made to do a traditional orchiopexy and inadequate length is obtained, the testis can be affixed to the pubic tubercle, and the cord can be covered with a Silastic sheath to return for a second-stage orchiopexy in 6 to 8 months (page 500). It is important to note that the absent testis can be confirmed *only* by an intra-abdominal exploration. Although the testis is retroperitoneal embryologically, it is an intraperitoneal structure anatomically.

Abdominal Approach. It is important to note that abdominal adhesions may result from an abdominal approach. Using a classic Pfannenstiel incision in the inguinal crease, a transverse skin incision is employed exposing the rectus. Subcutaneous dissection is carried out to the umbilicus, and the rectus sheath and muscle are separated in the midline along with the underlying areolar tissue. The peritoneum is opened, and the intestine is packed superiorly. The testes usually are found lying intraperitoneally, posterolateral to the bladder, with a short mesentery covered by peritoneum.

The peritoneum is incised over the vas, leaving a wide strip of vascularized peritoneum to retain the vasal blood supply. The testicular artery is traced superiorly and ligated as close to the aorta as possible, leaving a large vascular network near the testis.

Sharp dissection of the vas is carried out, creating a pyramidal base that widens as the vas becomes closer to the seminal vesicles. This allows mobilization of the vas from the surrounding tissues to attain sufficient length, while at the same time retaining adequate collateral vasculature. Once appropriate cord length is achieved, the testis is brought into the scrotum, as described in the text. If there appears to be some slight traction, the tension suture in the testis can be brought through the skin inferior to the pouch incision and tied over a Silastic button. In most cases, there is adequate length to obviate this step.

Extraperitoneal Approach. I would recommend a transverse incision in the inguinal skin crease with a traditional Marshall-Marchetti exposure of the peritoneum, because it is cosmetically more acceptable and gives the same accessibility anatomically.

General Commentary. The surgical approach to the nonpalpable testis should be a planned and structured exercise. In bilateral nonpalpable testes, I believe laparoscopy is justified diagnostically and, in some cases, therapeutically in the form of a staged laparoscopic orchiopexy in highly selective patients, such as those with prune belly syndrome. I believe that laparoscopy is of equivocal value in the unilateral nonpalpable testis, because more than 75 percent of these patients have the vessels and vas entering the internal ring, making them accessible by an inguinal exploration. Most nonpalpable, intra-abdominal testes can be approached through a transverse inguinal incision in the skin crease. Careful exploration of the inguinal canal often will yield atretic vessels and a vas ending blindly but with a small nubbin of epididymis. It is important to confirm the confluence of the vas and the testicular artery at the internal ring to avoid missing a high intra-abdominal testis with a detached epididymis. Extension of the incision of the internal oblique aids in abdominal exposure, with minimal effort. High ligation of the testicular artery and provision of a wide pedicle of vascularized peritoneum over the vas are critical to attaining adequate vasculature to the testis. Bringing the testis directly transperitoneally through the external ring superior to the pectinate line also minimizes the dissection necessary for scrotal placement. Most of all, it is important at the outset to make a clear decision of the necessity of a Fowler-Stevens procedure, because any attempt to salvage a traditional orchiopexy using the Fowler-Stevens technique is perilous for the testis. I believe the abdominal approach should be reserved for unique occasions, often coupled with other surgical procedures, such as vesicostomy closure in prune belly syndrome. Because of the nature of this procedure, I have been loath to do bilateral simultaneous Fowler-Stevens orchiopexies on patients other than those with prune belly syndrome and a long-looping vas.

CHAPTER 103

Laparoscopic Methods for Impalpable Testis

TECHNIQUE OF LAPAROSCOPY

The performance of laparoscopy is somewhat different in children than in adults, because the distance between the anterior abdominal wall and the great vessels is smaller and the organs are closer, although the shorter instruments under development will help. In infants, where the distance is very small, first making a small paraumbilical incision allows the insufflating needle to be passed by direct observation. If the Veress needle is used, less pressure is required because of the less-resistant fascia of the child. One new trocar has coarse threads and can be screwed into the abdomen through a small infraumbilical peritoneal incision. Less gas will be needed to fill the small peritoneal cavity; it can be added at a slower rate. However, loss of pressure is greater in children, requiring operating at higher pressures than in adults (18 to 20 mm Hg). Transillumination of abdominal wall is easy in children, a fact that aids in the placement of trocars to avoid vessels in the abdominal wall. Anatomic details are more clearly seen in children because of the small amount of preperitoneal fat. This fact also reduces the chance for preperitoneal insufflation during insertion, but because the peritoneum is more loosely attached, it is more susceptible to emphysema. Also, the weak adherence to the abdominal wall makes the introduction of large cannulas difficult; an instrument introduced through a smaller port may be required to assist the entry of the larger-sized port.

Because children swallow air, it is important to decompress the stomach with a nasogastric tube; leave it in place for extensive procedures, because a distended stomach pushes the omentum into the field.

Caution the family that although the operation will be done through three small incisions, it still is a surgical procedure because hemorrhage and bowel injury can be serious complications. Moreover, warn that it may not be possible to complete the procedure; an open operation may be necessary after all.

If adhesions are anticipated, prepare the bowel by both mechanical and antibiotic means. Give a broad-spectrum antibiotic parenterally preoperatively and postoperatively. Whether blood should be matched depends on the type of procedure and the risk of vascular injury. It is wise to have a standby table with instruments for laparotomy ready in case of complications.

Use general anesthesia in children; the irritation of the diaphragm by carbon dioxide is painful, and any motion by the child is hazardous. Moreover, muscle relaxation is important because of the small intraperitoneal space with a greater liability for injury to intra-abdominal structures. Placement of an endotracheal tube is recommended to ensure absence of movement and to allow mechanical assistance to respiration as the intra-abdominal pressure rises. Be aware that hypercarbia from absorbed carbon dioxide (CO_2) may be a problem during long procedures. Prep and drape the child as for laparotomy, but leave the scrotum exposed.

INSERTION OF TROCARS

1 Place the child supine. Empty the bladder with a catheter, and leave the catheter indwelling. Determine by percussion that the stomach is empty; if in doubt, place a nasogastric tube, because a full stomach depresses the omentum into the route of the trocars. For orchiopexy and other pelvic procedures, insert a rolled towel under the lower back to create lordosis, and tip the table into a 10-degree Trendelenburg position to allow the intestine to drop out of the pelvis. Shift to a 30-degree Trendelenburg position for placement of the initial port. It can be helpful after the ports are inserted to tilt the table laterally 30 degrees to raise the involved testis above the intestine. Prep the entire abdomen, in case laparotomy is required. Test all equipment before starting.

For *insertion of Veress needle*, palpate the sacral promontory and aorta. Make a curved incision with a #15 blade in the inferior crease of the umbilicus that penetrates the linea alba where the body wall is thinnest. In infants younger than 1 year of age, it may be preferable to insert the needle above the umbilicus to avoid the yet-undescended bladder. The Veress needle has two parts: a sharp beveled sheath to pass through the body wall and a blunt obturator that springs forward to fend off the intestine. Check its mechanism and patency. Start the flow of CO_2 to ascertain resistance to flow and pressure. Press the needle firmly through the incision; you can feel it go through the linea alba and then through the peritoneum. The direction of pressure must be toward the hollow of the sacrum.

Check the position of the needle by aspirating with a syringe; there should be no return of blood or bowel contents. Check the position again by instilling 10 ml of the heparinized saline irrigating solution to find that it may be easily injected but not aspirated. (Aspiration would indicate preperitoneal placement.) It should be possible to swing the tip of the needle through 360 degrees. Check intraperitoneal pressure to be sure it is less than 7 mm Hg and shows shifts with respiration. Begin insufflation with CO_2 at a rate of approximately 1 L/min until the pressure, in a fully relaxed child, reaches 15 to 20 mm Hg, then quickly withdraw the needle. Realize that some anesthetists do not immediately achieve relaxation.

For *insertion of sheath and trocar* (site 1), incise the fascia of the linea alba with a #11 blade and place towel clips on either side to elevate the anterior abdominal wall. Insert the 11-mm sheath (a 5-mm port is large enough for infants) with its contained sharp pyramidal trocar, keeping the index finger extended to prevent it from going too deep. Point the trocar at the sacral promontory while pressing on the upper abdomen, and insert it into the abdominal cavity. When gas is heard escaping, quickly remove the trocar inside the sheath to let the valve in the sheath close the channel. Connect the CO_2 tube, and set the flow control to maintain a pressure of 15 mm Hg above baseline.

For *insertion of telescope*, insert a 5- or 10-mm laparoscope, and attach a full-beam video camera to the eyepiece to monitor the area on the video screen placed at the foot of the table. First, check to be certain no abdominal structures were injured during needle insertion. Systematically inspect the peritoneal cavity as for diagnostic laparoscopy.

For *insertion of working ports*, turn the lens to bring the anterior abdominal wall above the bladder in view, and while illuminating the abdominal wall from within, insert two 5-mm working ports, one at each McBurney's point (sites 2 and 3). Place them at the umbilical level in infants to have enough working distance. Avoid traversing the inferior epigastric vessels, which can be seen by transillumination.

Precautions: To avoid injury to abdominal structures, be sure to visualize the position of all instruments, and do not leave them unattended.

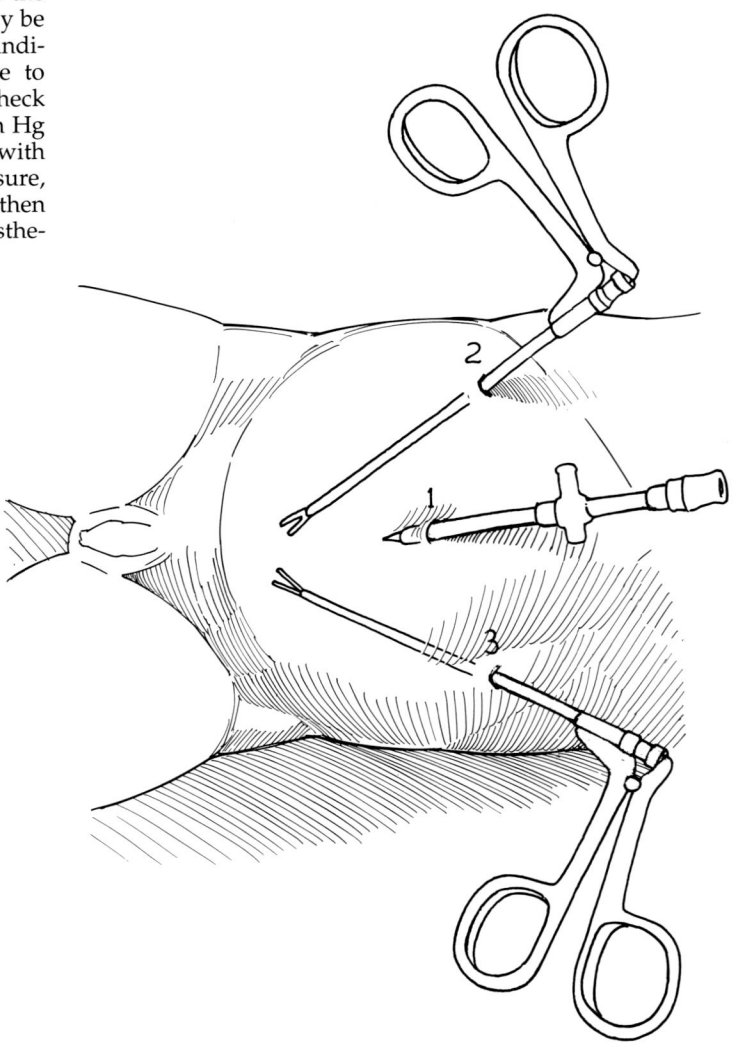

DIAGNOSTIC LAPAROSCOPY

2 For the impalpable testis, examination of the retroperitoneal area and internal ring is indicated before definitive surgery.

Place the primary access port (site 1), and inspect the abdomen. Because the preperitoneal fat is minimal, the structures of the pelvis are readily seen. In all cases, orient yourself by locating the medial umbilical ligaments (obliterated umbilical arteries), lying laterally and running from the hypogastric arteries to the umbilicus, and by finding the median umbilical ligament (urachal remnant), which is seen continuing from the bladder to the umbilicus. *Normal side:* Identify the spermatic vessels as they run into the external inguinal ring. Pull on the testis in the scrotum to bring the vas and vessels into prominence. If the pelvic structures are not well visualized, check on the CO_2 insufflator. *Impalpable side:* Five findings are possible:

1. The spermatic cord is seen passing through the internal inguinal ring, indicating a testis or remnant in the groin area. Press on the external ring to see if the testis can be pushed back into the abdomen. If it responds, either a standard orchiopexy or a laparoscopic orchiopexy is feasible. If standard orchiopexy is elected, it will be facilitated by laparoscopic mobilization of the spermatic vessels to the level of the kidney.

2. The testis is seen just above the internal ring, but a short patent processus is present. Here too, either type of orchiopexy can be done.

3. No testis is seen, but the cord structures disappear in the canal. Use the grasper to pull on these structures to identify the position of a testicular remnant in the groin. If there is a question about this, an inguinal exploration may be indicated.

4. The testis with adnexae is seen but lies well above the internal ring. This testis is best managed by staged Fowler-Stephens orchiopexy, with preliminary laparoscopic clipping or coagulation of the spermatic vessels.

5. No testis is seen. Look for blind-ending spermatic vessels as proof of testicular absence (vanishing testis). Even if a blind-ending vas is found at the internal ring, the entire retroperitoneum to the lower pole of the kidney must be examined, even if that means reflecting the colon by freeing its lateral attachments.

If an atrophic or dysmorphic testis is found, remove it either laparoscopically or transperitoneally through a 3- to 4-cm muscle-splitting incision in the lower quadrant.

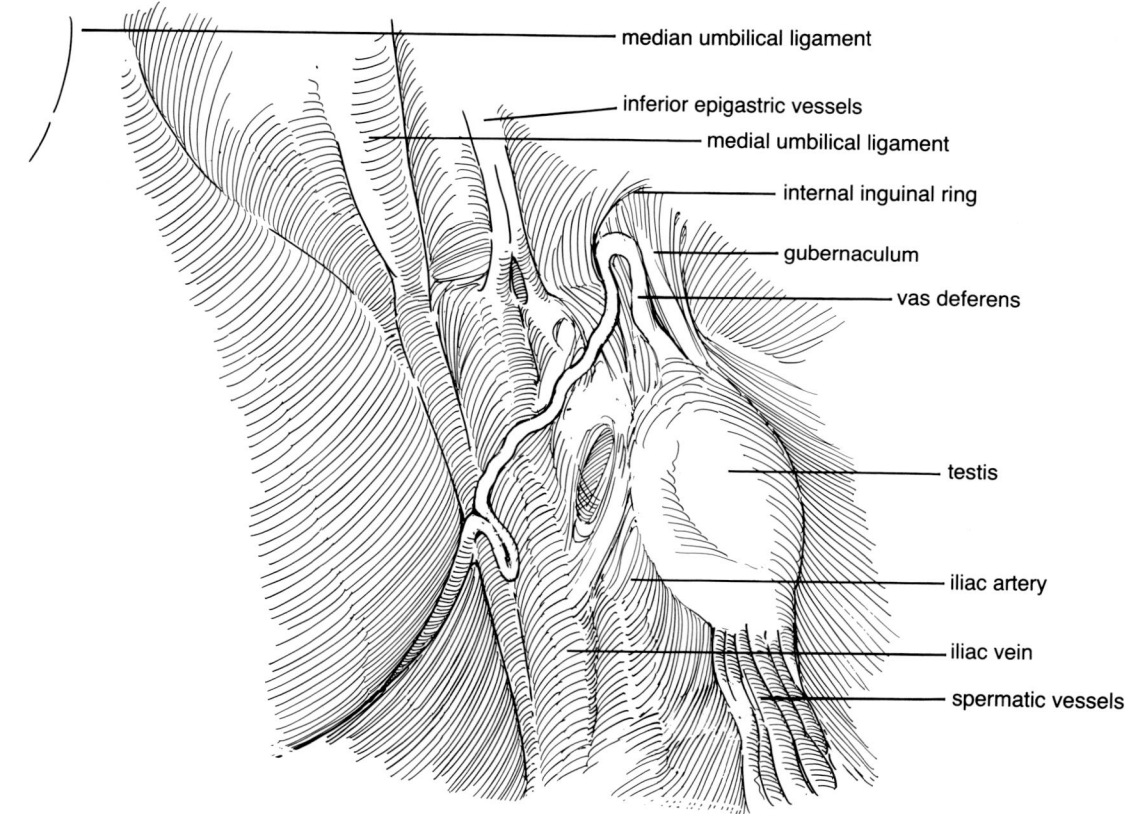

median umbilical ligament
inferior epigastric vessels
medial umbilical ligament
internal inguinal ring
gubernaculum
vas deferens
testis
iliac artery
iliac vein
spermatic vessels

FIRST-STAGE FOWLER-STEPHENS OPERATION: LAPAROSCOPIC VESSEL LIGATION (BLOOM)

This stage is needed only if the testis or the loop of the vas deferens cannot be located by clinical examination. Diagnostic laparoscopy can determine the presence and location of the testis and the presence and length of the vas deferens.

After placement of the telescope and one access port, inspect the testis and cord. Traction on the testis will help decide whether it will be necessary to clip the spermatic vessels (short vessels), to proceed at once with standard open orchiopexy, or to proceed with laparoscopic orchiopexy. Insert an electrode, and elevate and fulgurate the vessels with unipolar or bipolar current. Alternatively, if a large port has been inserted, pass a loaded Hulka clip applier through the sheath, and clip the spermatic vessels as high as possible. A second clip may be needed. Remove the instrument sheath, evacuate the CO_2 to a level of 6 cm, and ensure that the area has been inspected for venous bleeding. Remove the visualizing port. Close the fascial openings with 4-0 synthetic absorbable sutures, and close the skin with subcuticular sutures. Proceed with the second stage in 3 to 6 months.

SECOND-STAGE FOWLER-STEPHENS OPERATION: LAPAROSCOPIC ORCHIOPEXY

Perform the procedure on a come-and-go basis. Place the child supine.

For orchiopexy and other pelvic procedures, insert a rolled towel under the lower back to create lordosis, and tip the table into a 10-degree Trendelenburg position to allow the intestine to drop out of the pelvis. Shift to a 30-degree Trendelenburg position for placement of the initial port. It can be helpful after the ports are inserted to tilt the table laterally 30 degrees to raise the involved testis above the bowels.

3 Stand on the side opposite that of the abnormal testis, with your assistant across from you. Inspect the pelvic peritoneal cavity with a 30-degree lens. Locate the median umbilical ligament (urachal remnant) and the sigmoid colon. Look for the internal inguinal ring with its crescentic medial margin, first on the normal side and then on the other side. The spermatic vessels can be identified by having an assistant pull on the testis; the vas deferens will be seen adjacent to it. Move the colon medially for access to the spermatic vessels proximally. (Formal mobilization is not needed, because incision of the peritoneum results in its medial displacement.) Incise the peritoneum, starting around the internal ring distal to the gubernaculum and bordering the testis laterally (long dashed line). Take a generous triangular flap of peritoneum that extends laterally 1 cm from the spermatic vessels, ventrally 1 cm from the vas deferens from the internal ring into the pelvis, and medially along the vessels from the site of fulguration toward the pelvic vas to provide a large peritoneal covering that encompasses the vas deferens and the collateral blood supply. Bluntly mobilize the spermatic vessels to the site of fulguration, and free the vas deferens. During the dissection, watch out for the ureter, which runs over and lies medial to the iliac vessels.

Make a short incision in the peritoneum (short dashed line) between the bladder and the medial umbilical ligament, just lateral to the median umbilical ligament, at the site of the new inguinal canal.

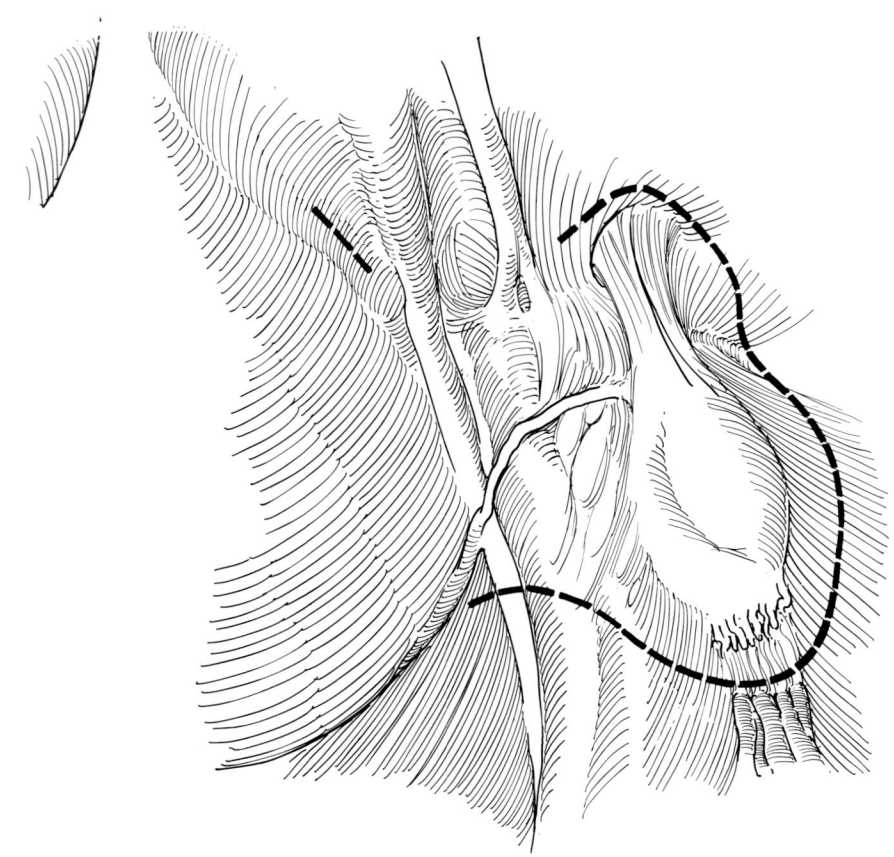

4 Free the testis from its bed, and start dissection of the gubernaculum as far distally as possible to preserve all collateral vessels. Raise the testis on the flap of peritoneum. Leave a broad isthmus of peritoneum on the vas.

If a hernia sac is present, free the peritoneum, but make an inguinal incision and proceed with a standard orchiopexy with repair of the hernia. In children, this is preferrable to laparoscopic repair with its residual clips.

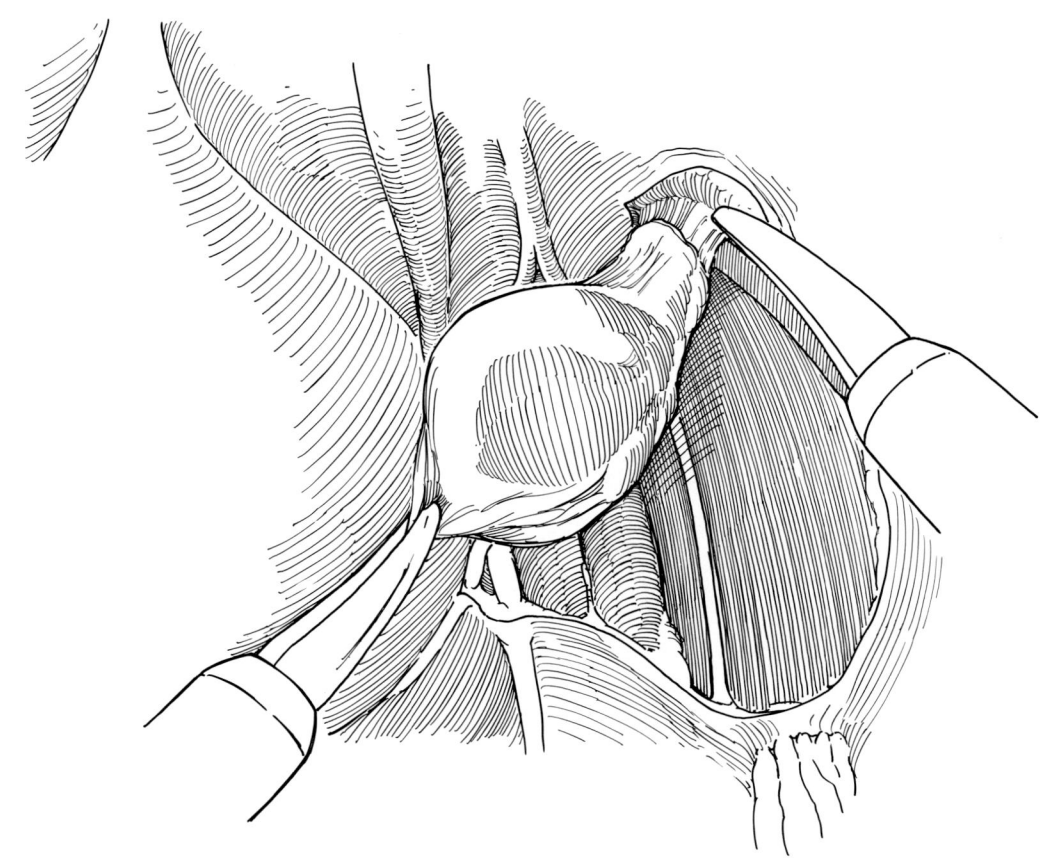

5 Make a 2-cm incision in the scrotum. Form a new inguinal canal medial to the medial umbilical ligament by passing a clamp from above through the peritoneal incision (short dashed line in Figure 3) along the ventral surface of the symphysis and out through the scrotal incision. Lead a clamp or cannula from below, grasp the testis, and draw it into the scrotum (through the cannula, if one is used). Place some traction on the testis, and divide any remaining retroperitoneal attachments from above. Fix the testis beneath the dartos with fine synthetic absorbable sutures (pages 492–493). Close the scrotal wound with a subcuticular synthetic absorbable suture. Replace the parietal peritoneum over the area of the patent processus vaginalis. Inspect the vas and associated structures for torsion and the operative area for bleeding. Aspirate most of the CO_2 to reduce peritoneal irritation and remove, in order, the instrument sheaths; finally, withdraw the visualizing port after inspection for bleeding is done at a pressure of 6 mm Hg. Close the fascial openings with 4-0 synthetic absorbable sutures, and close the skin with subcuticular sutures.

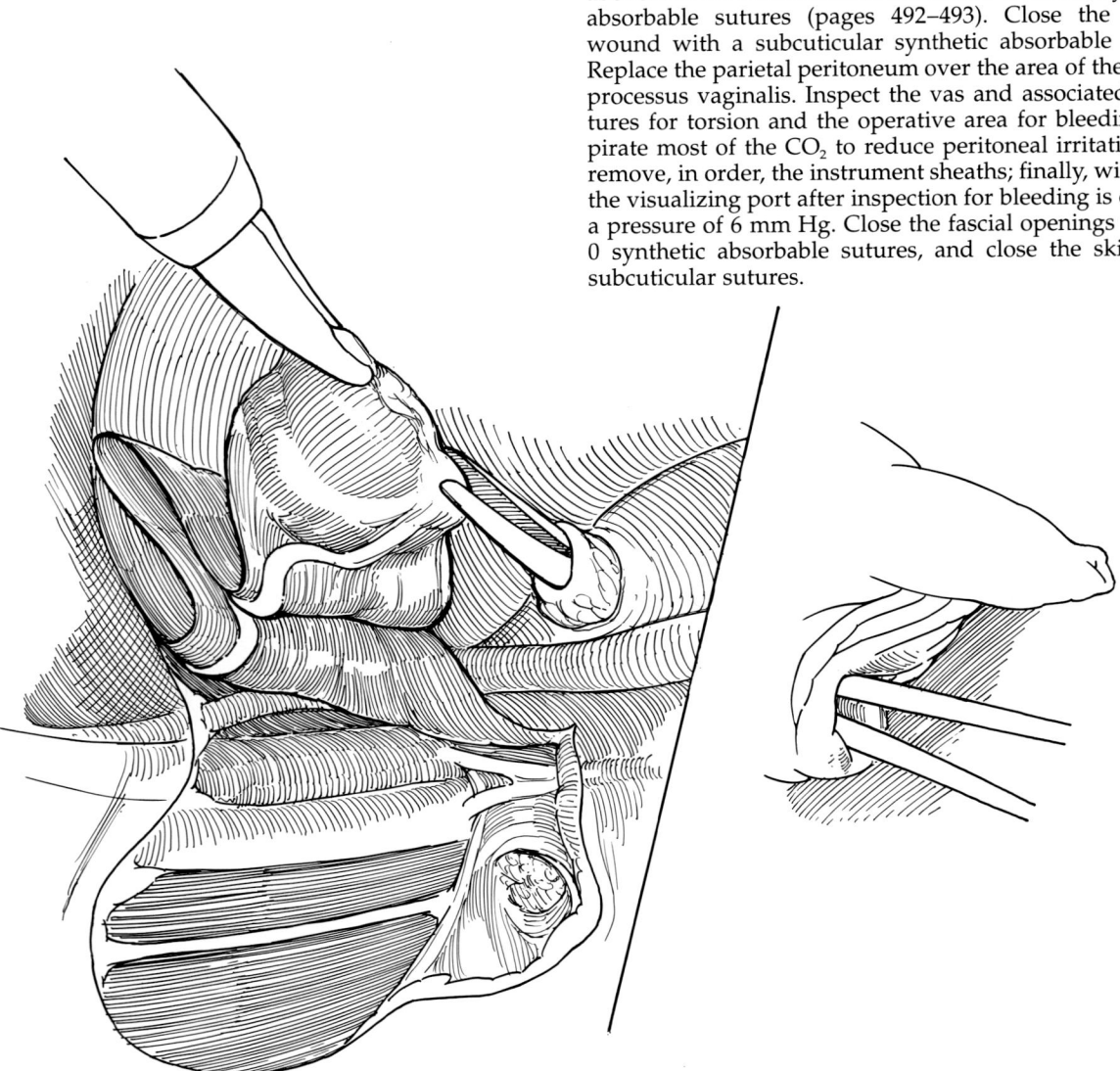

Problems With Laparoscopy

Most complications occur during initial trocar insertion or during insufflation. *Preperitoneal emphysema* makes identification of landmarks difficult. Emphysema of the omentum causes it to obstruct the view. *Puncture of a viscus* with the Veress needle is not harmful, so long as it is not connected to the CO_2 supply. Too high an insufflation pressure causes *tension pneumoperitoneum*, a phenomenon that might be missed in obese patients. *Puncture of the abdominal aorta* or other major vessels results in a spurt of blood. Leave the sheath in place for tamponade and as a guide to the site of injury, but proceed with emergency laparotomy. *Injury to the inferior epigastric vessels* by the sheath is recognized by blood dripping into the pelvis. The route the vessels pass through may be cauterized through the laparoscope, or the incision may be enlarged and the vessels transfixed

above and below the puncture site. For bowel injury from the trocar or sheath, open the abdomen, and repair the bowel. Resection of a bowel segment or fecal diversion seldom is needed. *Bladder puncture* is managed laparoscopically or by suture through a small suprapubic incision. *Ureteral injury*, especially from using electrocoagulation, requires stenting.

Postoperative bleeding is rare if the site of operation and the trocar sites have been closely inspected at low pressure at the end of the procedure. *Dehiscence* through the large port or incisional hernias might occur if the fascia is not closed. Suspect *bowel injury* if nausea, vomiting, and ileus occur. Institute nasogastric suction and explore if improvement does not follow.

Commentary by William J. Cromie

My comments are as follows: insufflation with CO_2 makes the anatomy of the pelvis and inguinal canal easy to discern. It is important to identify the landmarks of the internal ring and the junction of the vas and testicular artery with the testis. The wider the pedicle of peritoneum, the less is the likelihood of bleeding and injury to the collateral vessels. It is easiest to clip the testicular arteries more proximally, because there are fewer collateral vessels. This may require a little more superior peritoneal dissection, but it is worth the effort. It is difficult to discern when one has attained a sufficient cord length for scrotal placement. We have found that retracting the testis to the contralateral external ring is a fairly good way to judge adequate length. Once the testis has been placed successfully in the scrotum, we like to decompress the abdomen and examine the site of surgical dissection because insufflation tamponades venous bleeding and decompression allows identification of possible bleeding sites.

Commentary by Guy A. Bogaert

The high accuracy of laparoscopy makes it the diagnostic procedure of choice for impalpable testes. Advantages are its rapidity (approximately 15 minutes) and low morbidity. Additionally, one can begin a therapeutic procedure from the diagnostic laparoscopy: one or two accessory ports are enough for all procedures. In my experience, ports larger than 5 F are almost never necessary. If I find the testicle in the groin and decide to perform a classic open orchiopexy, I mobilize the testicular vessels laparoscopically up to the kidney to avoid tension on them after the testis is brought into the scrotum. If the vessels still seem too short, I suggest making a new "inguinal canal" laparoscopically and bringing the testis straight into the scrotum with the Prentiss maneuver. This is much easier and faster through the laparoscope, and the length gained is impressive. When you are ready to pull the testis into the scrotum through the new inguinal canal, after you insert a small clamp from the scrotum, let your assistant push against the symphysis to keep the CO_2 in the abdomen. After you have pulled the testis into the subdartos pouch, there will be no more leakage. Before ending the procedure, I make sure there is no hernia at the internal ring. If so, I recommend repairing it with an open procedure instead of placing foreign material in the defect and stapling the edges of peritoneum—not an attractive option in children.

I have found that in the second stage of the Fowler-Stephens orchiopexy, one can see the dilated collateral vessels around the vas deferens more clearly through the laparoscope. The magnification and the angle of dissection allow a more precise dissection around the delicate vasculature and the vas. Laparoscopy should improve the success rate of this procedure.

To remove a testis laparoscopically, I recommend placing it in a sterile condom or endoscopic bag before removal to avoid spillage of cells that might ultimately become malignant.

CHAPTER 104

Inguinal Hernia Repair

Inguinal hernias are indirect in infants and children, with rare exceptions, and are caused by a persistent processus vaginalis.

1 *Position:* Supine in frog-legged position. *Incision:* Stretch the skin, and make a 2- to 3-cm transverse incision in the prominent fold above the external ring. Carry it through Camper's and Scarpa's fascias, directly onto the external oblique aponeurosis. Identify the external ring by following the spermatic cord proximally until the vessels and vas can no longer be felt. A loupe may be helpful, especially in infants.

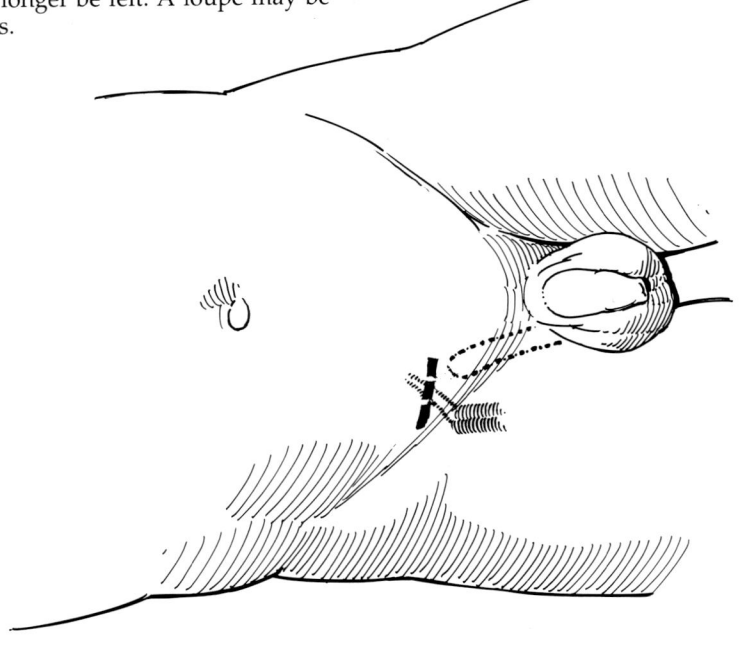

2 Grasp the subcutaneous fat on one side of the incision as your assistant grasps the other side, and separate the fat from Scarpa's fascia with fine scissors. Coagulate or ligate vessels encountered here. (In infants, Scarpa's fascia is relatively dense and may be mistaken for the aponeurosis of the external oblique.)

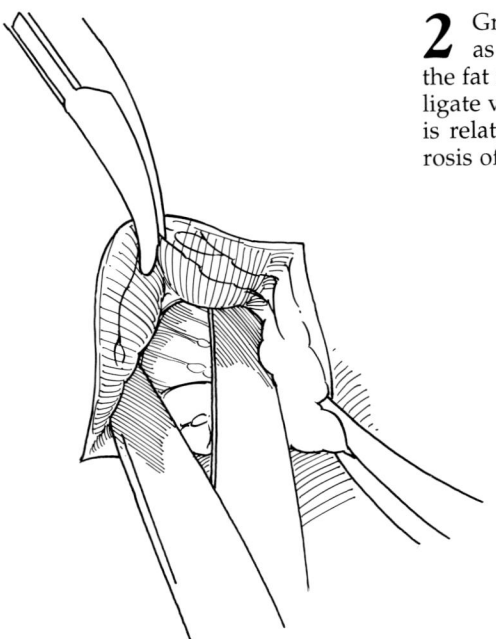

3 Lift Scarpa's fascia with fine forceps, and divide it in the line of the incision. Separate the fatty layer beneath Scarpa's fascia with scissors to expose the loose tissue over the external oblique aponeurosis. Have your assistant retract the upper and lower corners of the incision and expose the external ring (external oblique aponeurosis and external spermatic fascia) by dissection with the scissors.

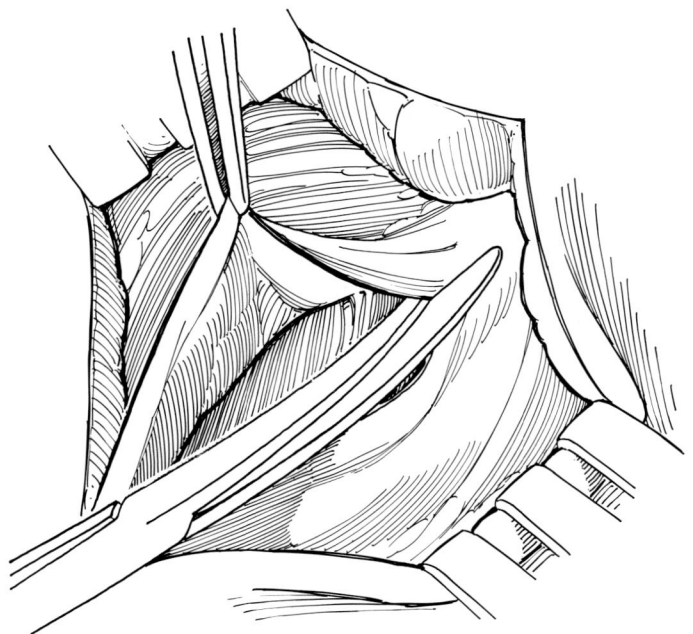

4 Elevate the edge of the external ring with scissors to avoid the ilioinguinal nerve, and divide the external oblique aponeurosis in the direction of its fibers. Alternatively, open the aponeurosis starting above the external ring with a knife, or, in infants, merely make traction on the sac to achieve high ligation.

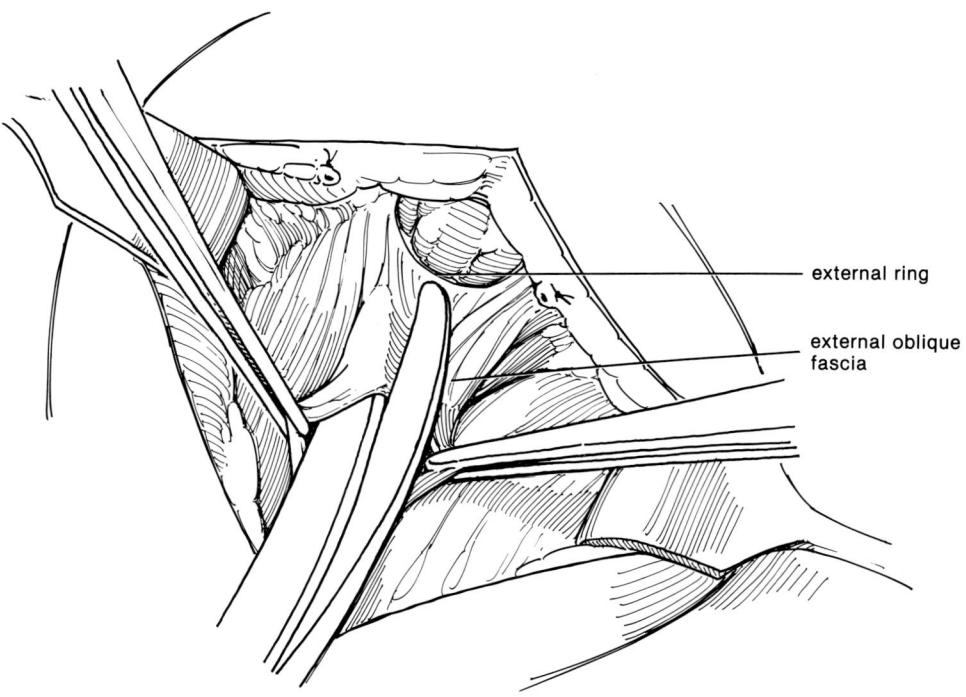

external ring

external oblique
fascia

5 Grasp one side of the cremaster as the assistant elevates the other, and incise it generously to reveal the internal spermatic fascia.

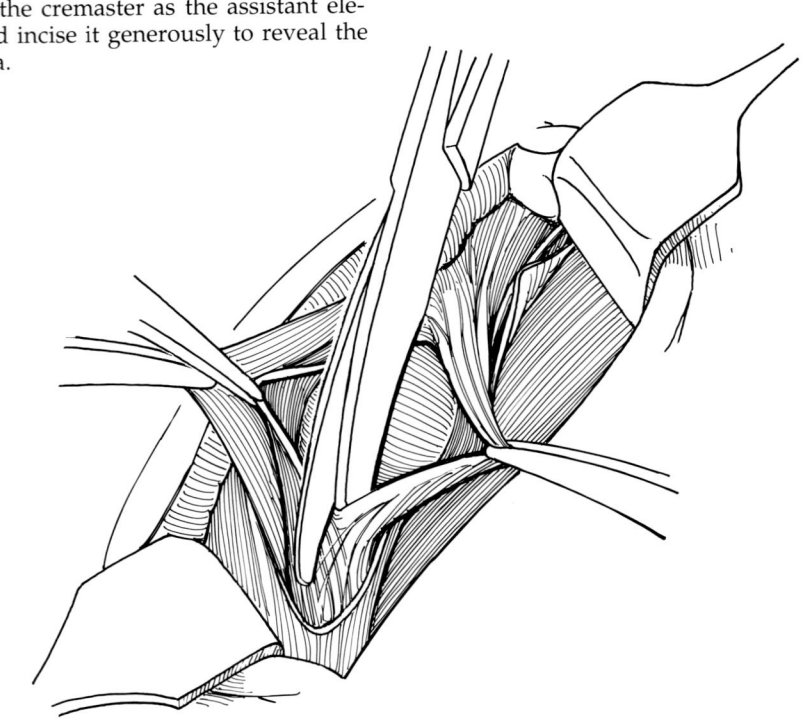

6 Similarly elevate the internal spermatic fascia with the hernia sac to expose the vas deferens and spermatic vessels lying laterally and posteriorly. Grasp the cord structures in a moist sponge, and free them from the sac for a short distance. It may help to open the sac to dissect it from the cord. Twist the sac and dissect proximally until the transversalis fascia is exposed or preperitoneal fat is seen.

At this point, it may be worthwhile to look for a contralateral occult hernia by instilling carbon dioxide at less than 20 cm H_2O into the peritoneal cavity through the opening in the hernia sac and palpate the contralateral groin.

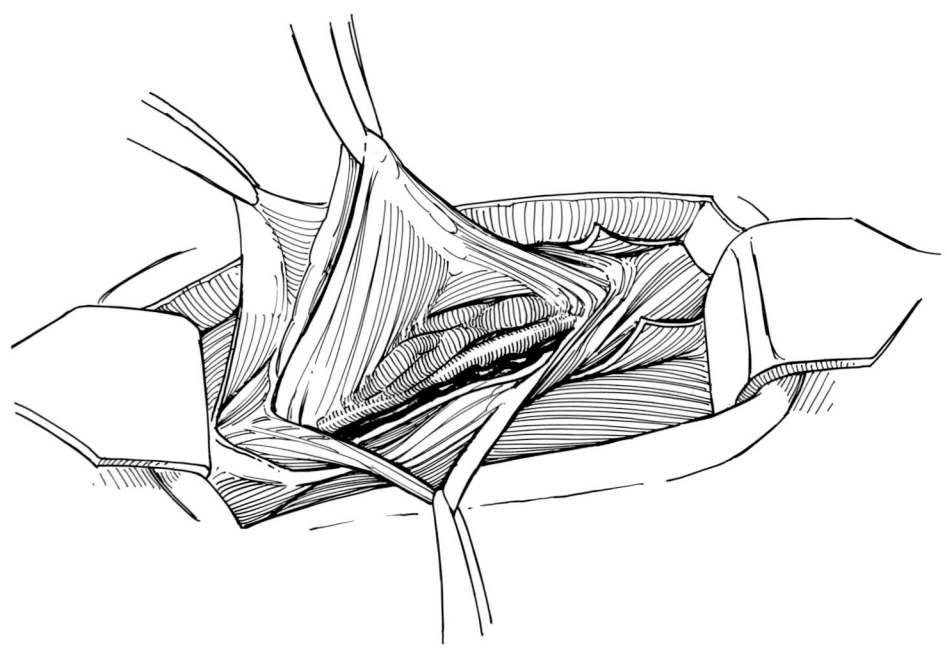

7 Suture-ligate the sac with a fine synthetic absorbable suture. Ligate the sac proximally with a tie. It is not necessary to trim the remainder of the sac unless you desire pathologic confirmation. Check the spermatic cord for injury. Approximate the external oblique aponeurosis with fine interrupted synthetic absorbable sutures, taking care not to encroach on the external ring, then join Scarpa's fascia with a few sutures. Close the skin with a fine running subcuticular absorbable suture. Consider local infiltration with a long-acting anesthetic solution.

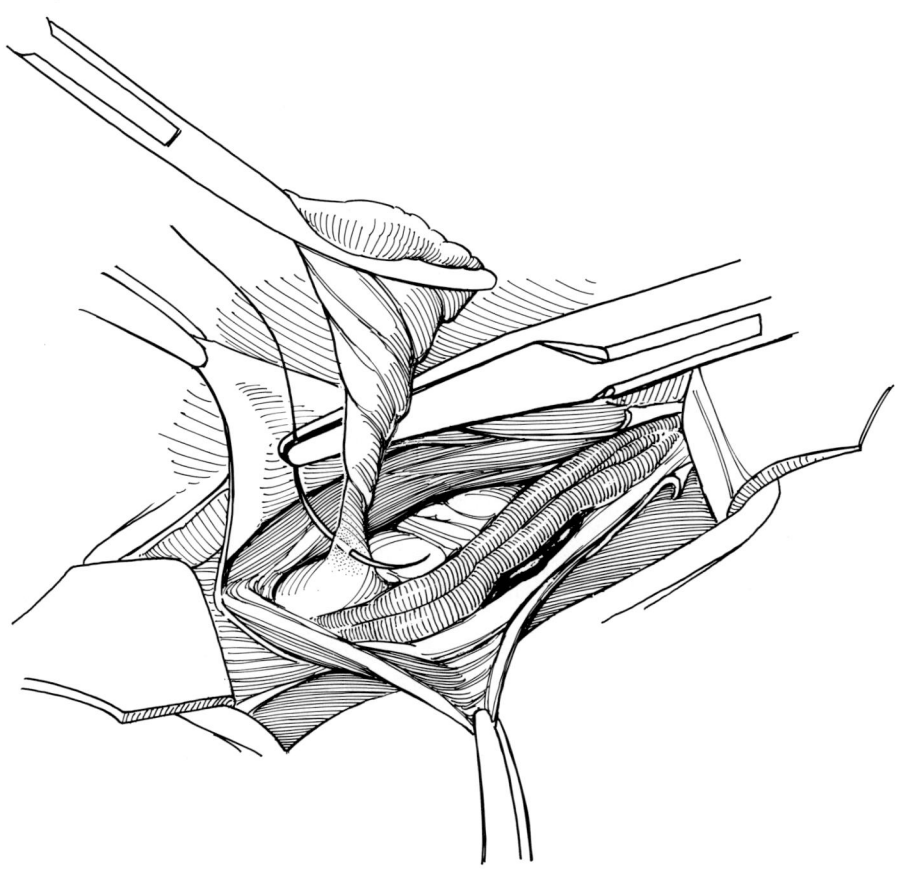

Commentary by Elliott Leiter

Adequate exposure with a transverse skin incision, converted to an oblique one at the level of the external oblique aponeurosis, is made possible by the extra skin mobility available in the pediatric patient. This gives an excellent cosmetic result, which translates into added parental satisfaction. In terms of surface anatomy, one can imagine the transverse incision to be located approximately midway between the external and internal rings. I try to keep the dissection of the subcutaneous fat to a minimum, and with practice, one can go right down to the external oblique aponeurosis with virtually no dissection at all. This reduces edema, transudate, and swelling and should result in better wound healing and a lower incidence of infection.

Freeing of the hernia sac from the spermatic vessels is easily accomplished when it is small and short but can be devilishly difficult with a wide, redundant sac that wraps itself almost circumferentially around the spermatic vessels. In these instances, I have found several tricks helpful.

First, do not start the dissection too far proximally. There, the sac usually is quite thin and diaphanous, and any tearing cephalad can make exposure for eventual peritoneal closure quite difficult. Second, dissect and divide the entire anterior and lateral surfaces of the sac by putting it on stretch between hemostats. Then, the final dissection off the spermatic vessels is usually short and can be accomplished with one of a variety of maneuvers, *eg*, scissors dissection, with or without saline injection, or careful incision of the sac over the vessels and then blunt and sharp elevation. In general, primarily for medicolegal reasons, I prefer to resect a small portion of the redundant hernia sac and send it to the pathologist for identification. For similar reasons, before closure I verify that the testis is still in the scrotum and has not retracted cephalad and so note it on the dictated operative report. The immediate postoperative period is made infinitely more comfortable for all concerned if a long-acting local anesthetic is injected subincisionly at the end of the procedure.

CHAPTER 105

Preperitoneal Indirect Inguinal Herniorrhaphy

1 *Incision:* Midline extraperitoneal or transverse lower abdominal. Retract the preperitoneal fat away from the anterior abdominal wall in the inferior part of the incision to gain an interior view of the inguinal area, and be able to identify the transversalis fascial sling (transverse arch) running anterior to the canal and the iliopubic tract lying behind. Expose the hernia sac as it extends between the peritoneum and the internal inguinal ring. Insinuate a finger under the neck of the sac, including the spermatic cord. Run a Penrose drain around the neck, and use blunt dissection to pull the whole hernia sac into the preperitoneal space.

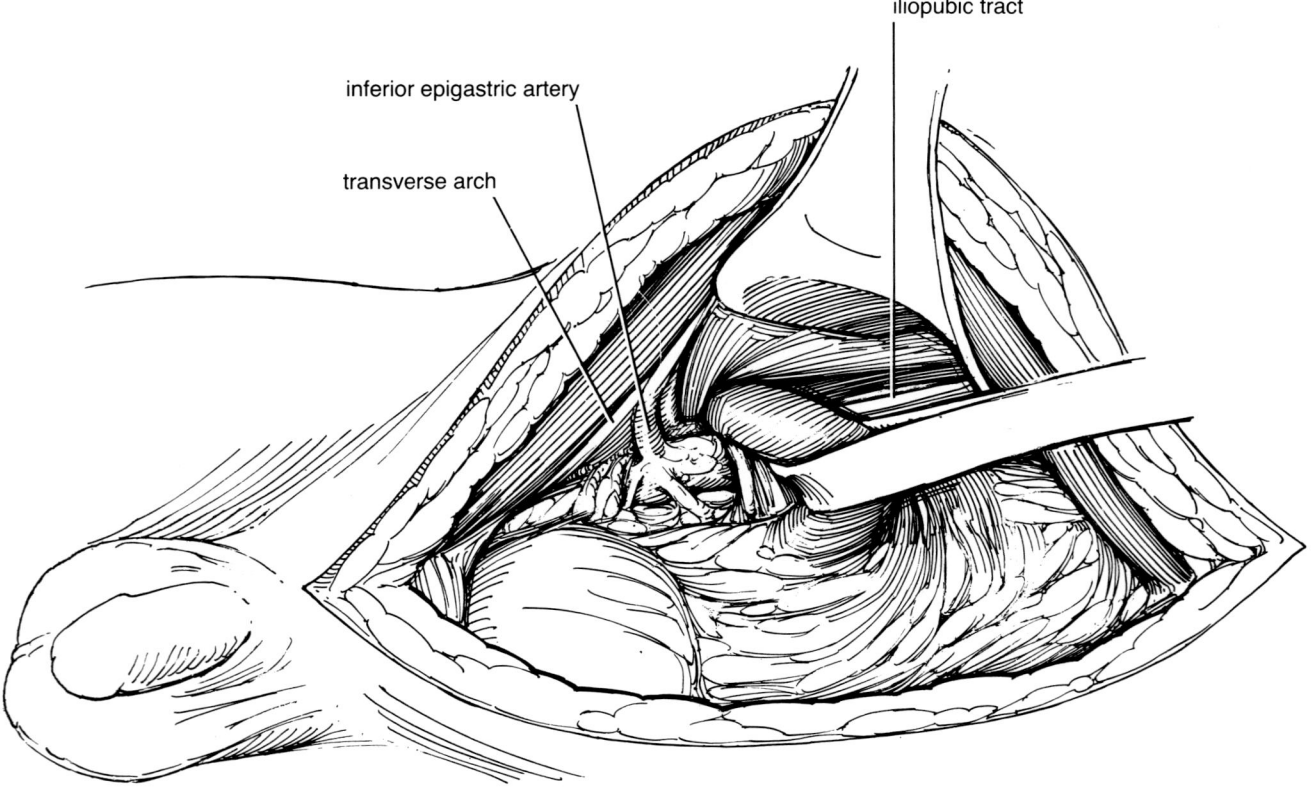

2 **A,** Separate the sac from the cord structures lying below it, and open it with scissors between clamps. **B,** Inserting a finger in the opened sac may facilitate freeing the two structures. If the sac extends distally, do not hesitate to divide it and leave that portion behind.

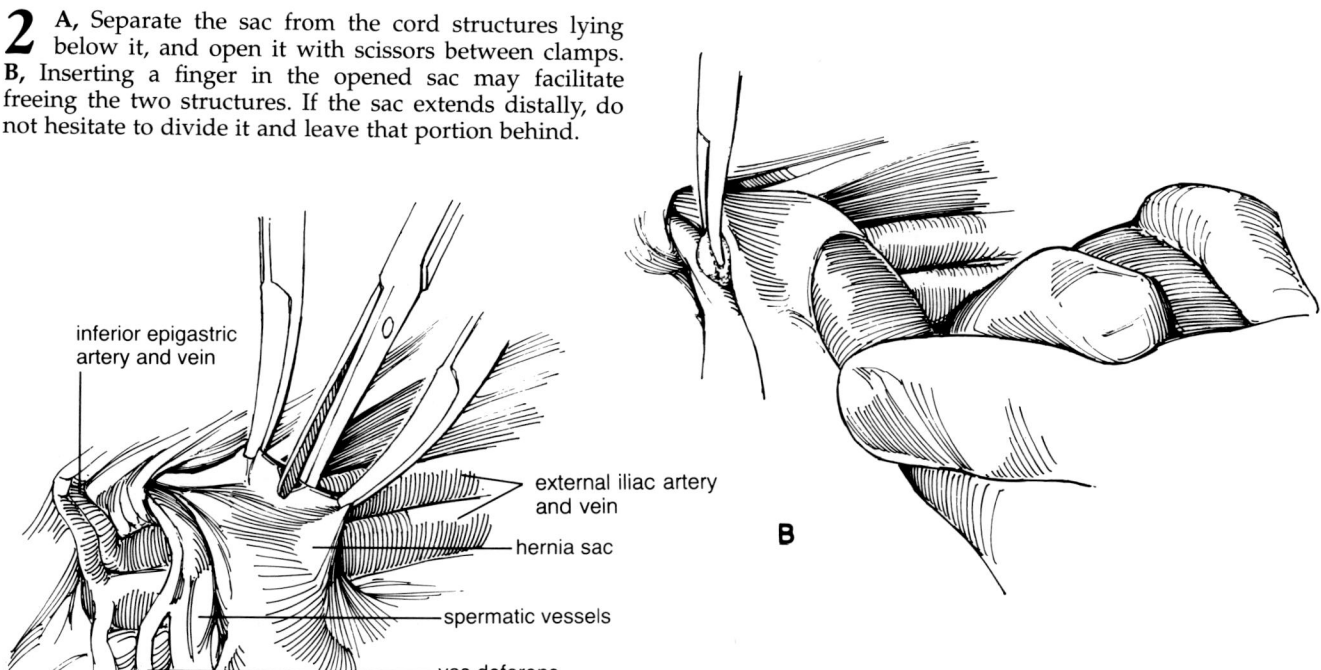

inferior epigastric
artery and vein

external iliac artery
and vein

hernia sac

spermatic vessels

vas deferens

A

B

3 Grasp the edges of the sac with clamps, and close the neck with a 4-0 silk pursestring suture. Trim any excess peritoneum.

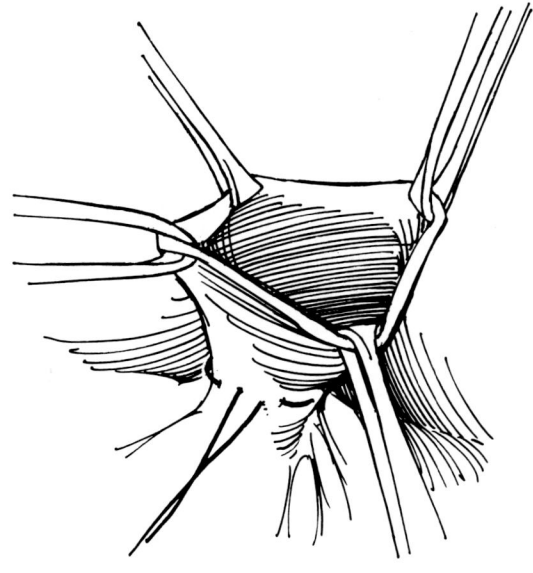

4 Place clamps on the edges of the internal ring, and retract the cord medially. Palpate both the iliopubic tract along the inferior margin of the ring and the iliac vessels lying posteromedially. They may be exposed by removing the overlying fat. If feasible, identify and preserve the deep inferior epigastric vessels just medial to the canal. Place two or three 4-0 polypropylene sutures in the iliopubic tract, pass them into the transversalis fascial sling medial to the cord, and tie them. Move the cord medially, and place several similar sutures in the tract and sling lateral to the cord. Close the wound appropriately.

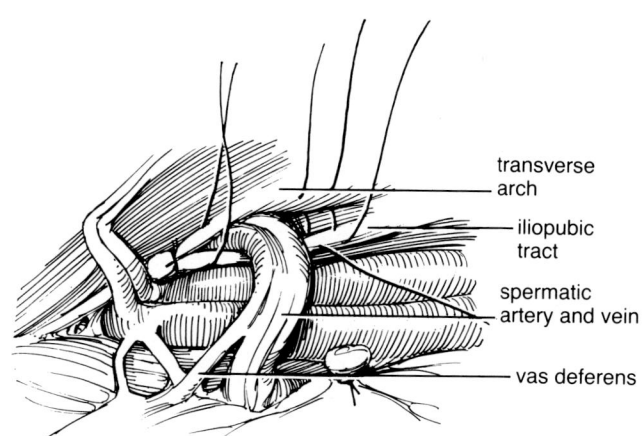

transverse
arch

iliopubic
tract

spermatic
artery and vein

vas deferens

Commentary by Elliott Leiter

My preference is to use a transverse suprapubic incision, primarily because it gives a much nicer final cosmetic result than does a vertical incision. Once again, the mobility of the skin in the pediatric patient allows adequate exposure for bilateral exploration and repair. I try not to grasp the sac with Allis clamps, because often they will tear the very fine tissue; I prefer to use hemostats for grasping and gentle traction. Otherwise, all the comments made earlier for inguinal hernia repair hold equally true for this approach.

CHAPTER 106

Reduction of Testicular Torsion

If an operating room is not immediately available, consider manual detorsion by rotation from within outward after a lidocaine cord block in adolescent boys, who will have intravaginal torsion. This maneuver is not suitable for newborns, in whom the torsion is extravaginal. Do not delay this emergency surgery. Warn the parents of possible loss of the testis.

1 *Position:* The boy is placed supine. Prep the entire genital area. In adolescents, block the cord with 1 percent lidocaine where it courses over the symphysis (page 57). In younger children, provide general anesthesia, aspirating the stomach if necessary. *Incision:* Grasp the scrotum with the thumb and index finger, and press the testis forward. Make a short transverse incision through the scrotum; it may be edematous. Extend it down to the tunica vaginalis, which may appear darkened from contained bloody serum.

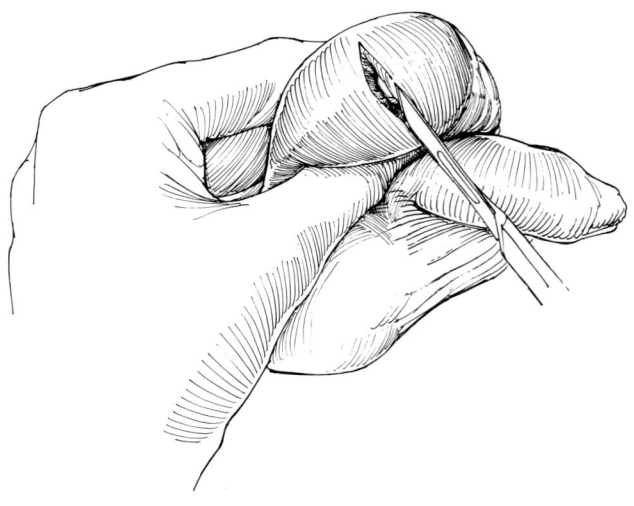

2 Open the tunica vaginalis, evacuate the accumulated hydrocele fluid, and extrude the testis. Observe its color after untwisting it. Wrap it in warm saline sponges; if it remains dark and the hydrocele fluid is sanguinous, consider excising it. Incise the tunica albuginea; if bleeding is not seen and if seminiferous tubules cannot be identified, remove the testis when the other one is normal to palpation and inspection. Replace it with a prosthesis, perhaps at a later time.

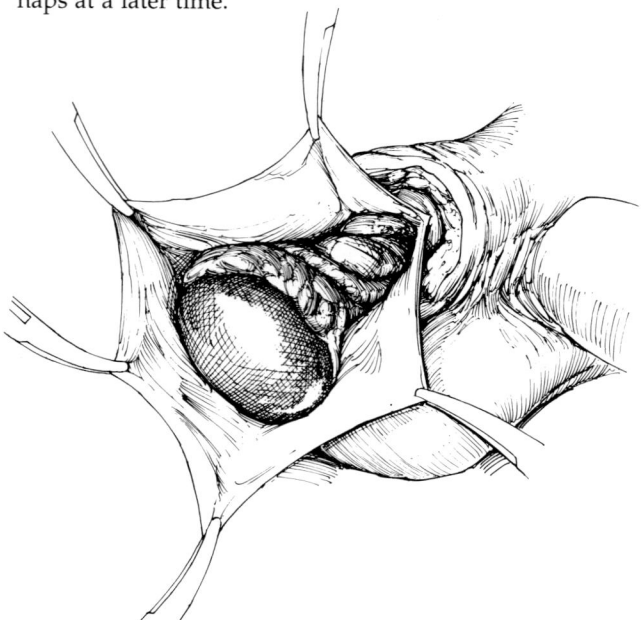

3 If the testis is not removed, trim the excess tunica vaginalis. Obtain hemostasis along the edge with thorough fulguration.

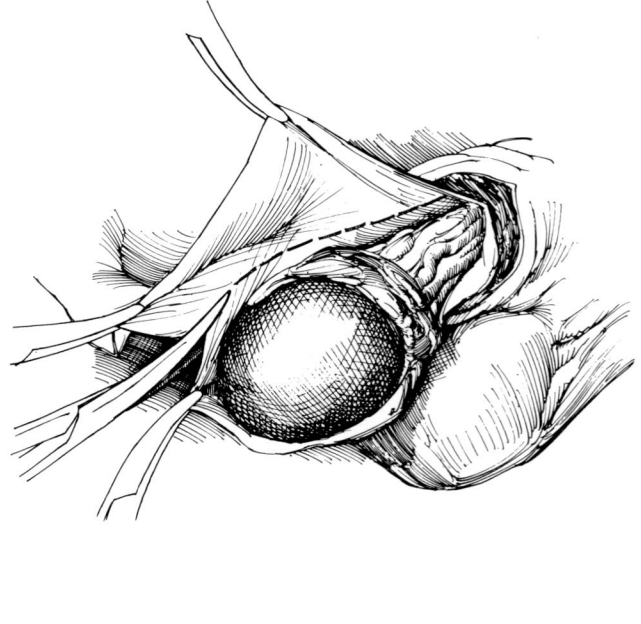

4 Place two or three interrupted 3-0 synthetic absorbable sutures in the cut edges of the tunica vaginalis to approximate the edges behind the testis, and obliterate the potential hydrocele sac.

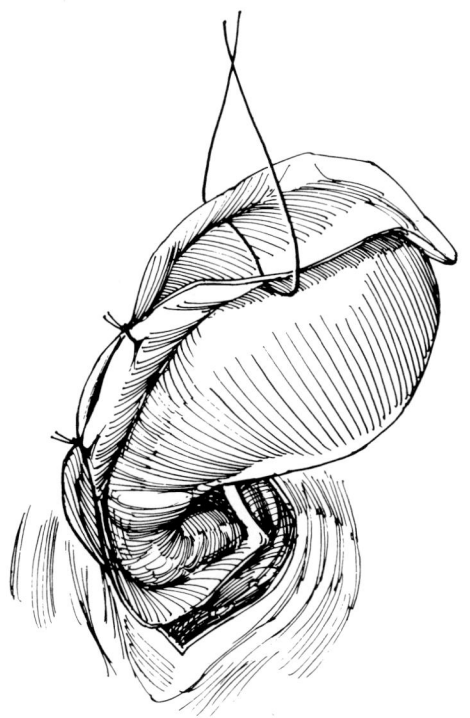

5 Invert the scrotal septum with a finger, and fix the tunica albuginea in three places, two laterally and one inferiorly, with interrupted mattress 3-0 synthetic absorbable or nonabsorbable sutures. Unless hemostasis is perfect, pass a clamp up through the bottom of the scrotum, incise over its tip, and draw a small Penrose drain out through the opening.

In all cases, open the contralateral sac and fix that testis in the same way. Close the dartos layer with figure-eight 3-0 synthetic absorbable sutures and the skin with a 4-0 or 5-0 synthetic absorbable subcuticular suture. Suture the drain in place. Place a dry dressing covered by a scrotal supporter.

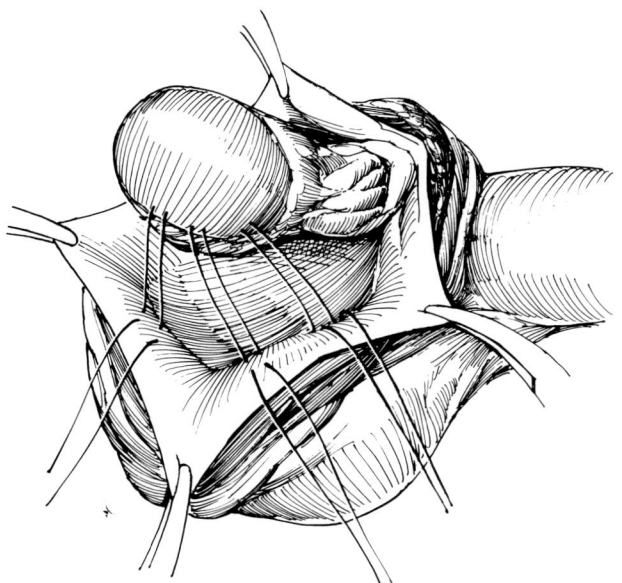

POSTOPERATIVE PROBLEMS

Hematoma is rare. *Retorsion* can occur; absorbable sutures may be a factor. *Fertility* could be affected if an ischemic testis is left in place.

Commentary by Kenneth I. Glassberg

In the neonate, a firm, hard, nontransilluminating mass in the scrotum in which one cannot delineate between the epididymis and testicle may represent a testicular torsion. This is especially true if there also are scrotal inflammatory changes. Most of these testes experience torsion prior to delivery, making early exploration unlikely to be successful in salvaging the testes. Because delayed contralateral torsion has been reported, the contralateral testis should be pexed as well. Also, one should be aware that a normal-appearing testicle on the contralateral side may only represent a testis that had experienced torsion even earlier than the testis in question. The normal-appearing testis may have been enlarged previously and now is passing through a stage in which it is of normal size prior to becoming a "nubbin" a few weeks later. Neonatal torsion, in general, is an extravaginal event.

Intravaginal torsion generally occurs between 12 and 18 years of age. The pain usually is sudden and sharp. The patient usually walks into the examining room in discomfort, limping, and has difficulty climbing onto the examination table. The scrotum usually is erythematous with varying degrees of swelling of the scrotal skin and its contents. The testicle is exquisitely tender, and it is difficult to differentiate the epidydidmis from the testis. Although colored Doppler ultrasound is proving with time to be a major factor in diagnosis and usually is more readily available than a nuclear medicine study, when the diagnosis is in doubt, an exploration should be done immediately—preferably within 6 hours on onset.

Because torsion is a vigorous event, fixing a salvageable testis and its contralateral mate with three nonabsorbable sutures is essential to prevent recurrent torsion.

There is concern that testicular torsion may be associated with a high incidence of infertility. Theories accounting for this incidence include an autoimmune phenomenon in which an autoimmune response is set up by detorsion against not only the involved testis but also its mate. Histologic findings suggest that these testes are abnormal even prior to torsion.

CHAPTER 107

Correction of Hydrocele

In a child, for a communicating hydrocele that persists longer than 24 months, plan a short transverse incision over the external ring to locate and divide the processus vaginalis, tying only the proximal end. For older boys with an acquired hydrocele, the Lord procedure is the best technique.

LORD PROCEDURE

Instruments: Provide at least eight small Allis forceps, a Wietlander retractor, and 4-0 synthetic absorbable and 4-0 chromic catgut sutures on half-circle needles.

1 If you are right-handed, stand on the boy's right side. Infiltrate the cord structures at the base of the scrotum with 1 percent lidocaine. Grasp the hydrocele in the left hand. Press it firmly to stretch the skin over the hydrocele, and compress the scrotal vessels. Make a 2-in incision between the visible blood vessels through the dartos muscle down *to* the surface of the tunica vaginalis. The initial incision includes the thin dartos layer and fine vessels, which may be fulgurated.

2 Pick up the full thickness of all the incised tissue with three or four Allis forceps on each side, each one catching the tissue immediately adjacent to the tunica vaginalis, the dartos layer, and the skin. By keeping the tissues under tension with the left hand, the Allis forceps can be placed to evert and compress the cut edge, thus controlling any bleeding and, most important, preventing dissection among the layers. At this point, separate the dartos layer from the tunica vaginalis to provide a pouch large enough to hold the testis after repair. Release the pressure on the scrotum.

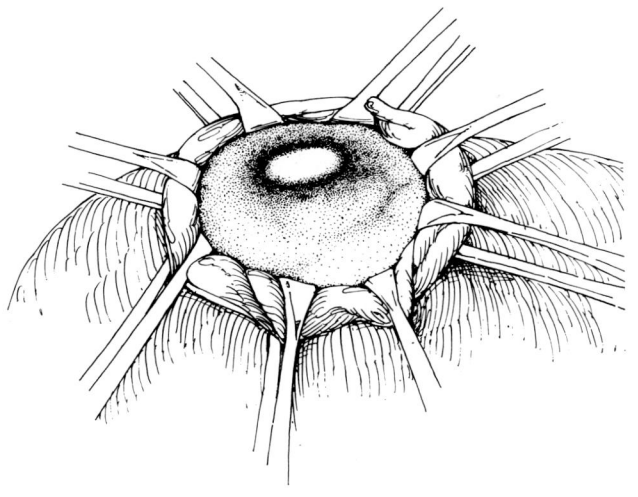

3 Hold the suction tip nearby, incise the tunica vaginalis, and evacuate the fluid. Expand the opening with scissors, and squeeze the testis out. Inspect and palpate it.

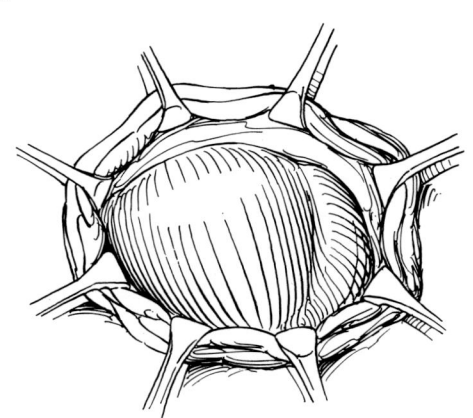

4 Lift the testis to stretch the tunica vaginalis. Plicate the peritoneal surface of the tunica vaginalis with 4-0 synthetic absorbable sutures. Do this by picking up the edge of the tunica with the needle and taking a small bite of the shiny surface held up by fine-toothed forceps every centimeter, until the junction with the testis is reached. Tie the suture.

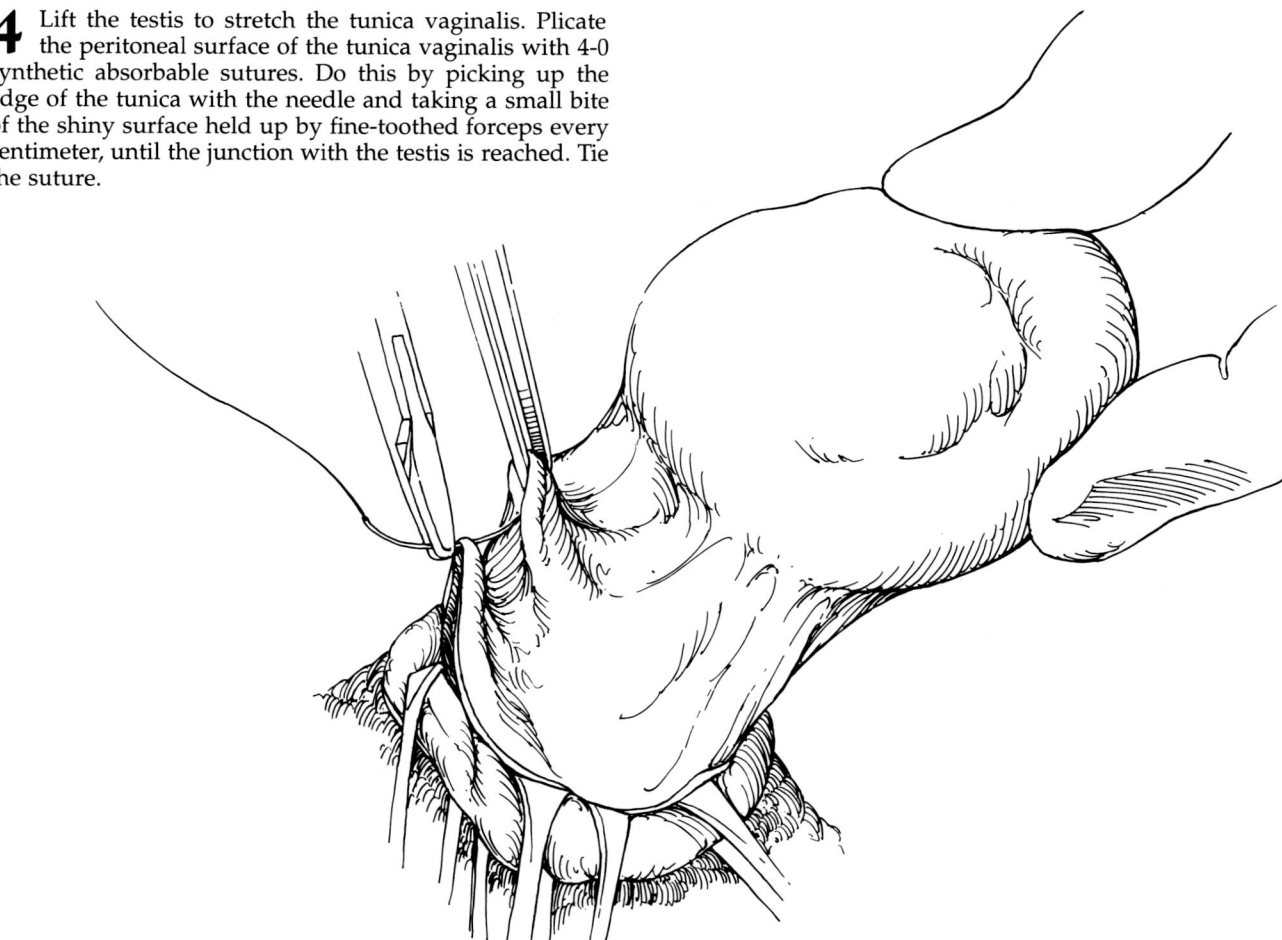

5 Repeat the suturing at intervals around the circumference of the testis, placing six to eight sutures in all. Replace the testis in the scrotum by squeezing it into the pocket beneath the dartos layer, with the aid of a flat, malleable retractor.

6 Remove the Allis forceps two at a time while rotating the next pair to allow placement of interrupted sutures of 3-0 chromic catgut that include full-thickness skin, dartos, and all the areolar tissue, thus obliterating any subcutaneous space. Traction on the ends of the wound with two towel clips may help with the eversion. Place a sheet of treated gauze and several 4 × 4 sponges over the wound, and apply a suspensory. Drainage is not necessary if the subcutaneous-fascial space was not violated.

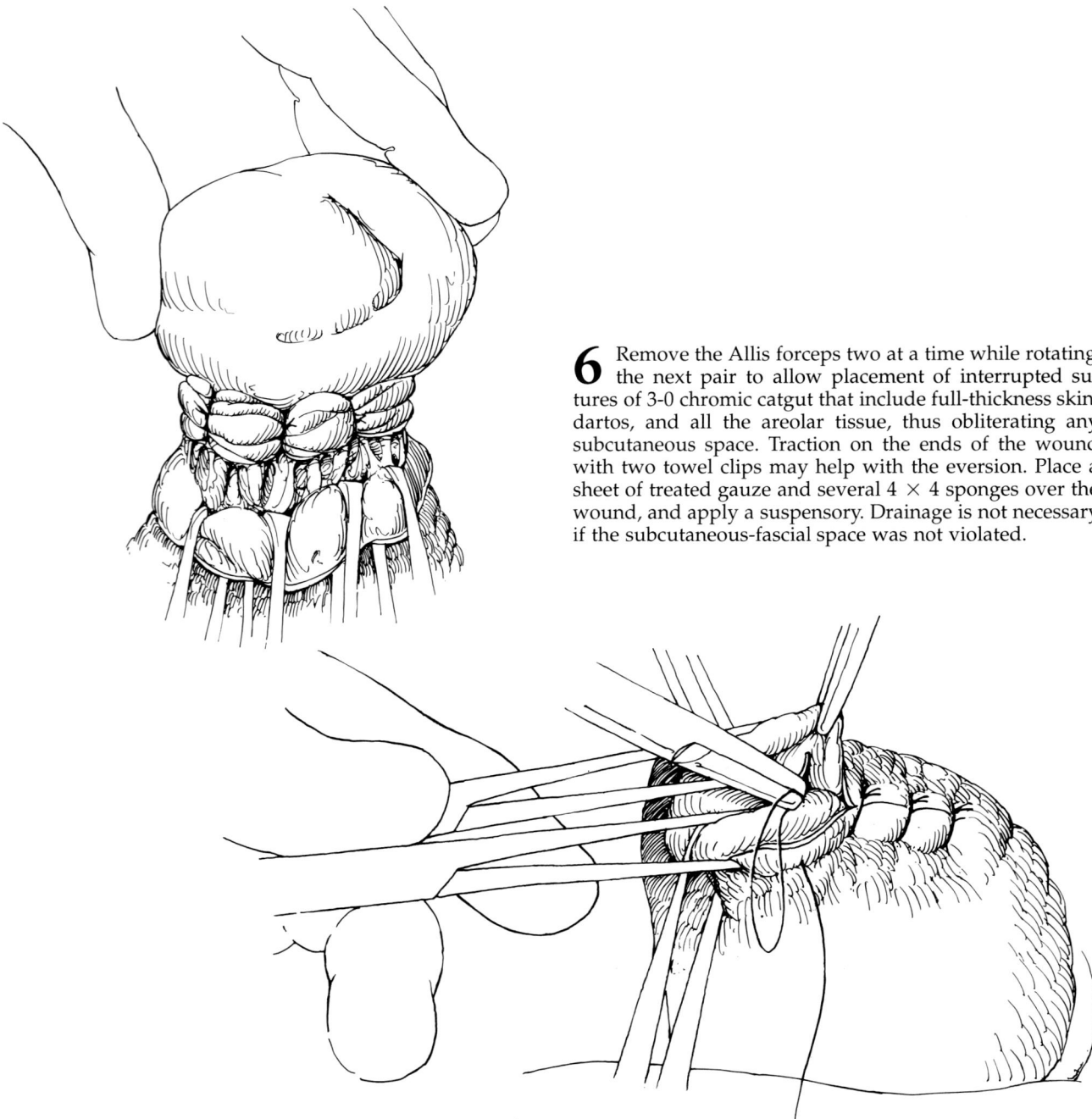

POSTOPERATIVE PROBLEMS

Hematoma formation is rare if the entire thickness of the scrotal wall is included first in the Allis forceps and then in the sutures at closure.

Recurrence of the hydrocele is likewise rare, because the operation leaves no dead space for a seroma around which the peritoneal lining can grow.

Commentary by Roelof J. Scholtmeijer

In children, virtually all hydroceles are communicating, and most infants with a scrotal swelling caused by a hy-

drocele will undergo spontaneous closure of the processus vaginalis with subsequent resolution of the hydrocele during the first 2 years of life. Hence, surgical repair usually is reserved for persistent swellings in boys 2 years of age or for a hydrocele that is very large or increasing in size. If a patent processus cannot be excluded, an inguinal approach should be performed. A Lord operation, done when a patent processus still exists, results in a high recurrence rate.

The important aspects of the Lord procedure are that this operation is less traumatic, easy to perform, and can be done under local anesthesia, especially in older boys. Plication of the peritoneal surface can be done more easily by placing the sutures first, after which they can be tied one by one. Closure of the scrotum with 3-0 plain catgut is safe and will ensure less irritation of the healing wound.

CHAPTER 108

Varicocele Ligation

Palpate the spermatic cord while the boy is erect and doing a Valsalva maneuver. A venogram may be useful in some cases. The Doppler stethoscope can help provide confirmation. Proceed to varicocelectomy if dilated veins are detected.

Position. Supine, with the head elevated 10 degrees.

Instruments. Provide a basic set; a headlamp; three-power loupes; Sims, Wietlander, and narrow Deaver retractors; vascular forceps; tenotomy scissors; and peanut dissectors.

ABDOMINAL APPROACH (PALOMO)

With this approach, adequate collateral will remain should the artery be compromised. It is more easily done on slender boys.

1 *Position:* Place the boy supine with a footplate to allow shifting to the reverse Trendelenburg position to fill the veins. Prep the scrotum. If the boy is old enough, use local anesthesia. *Incision:* Make a short semioblique incision through the skin and subcutaneous tissue over the site of the *internal* inguinal ring. Insert a Wietlander retractor.

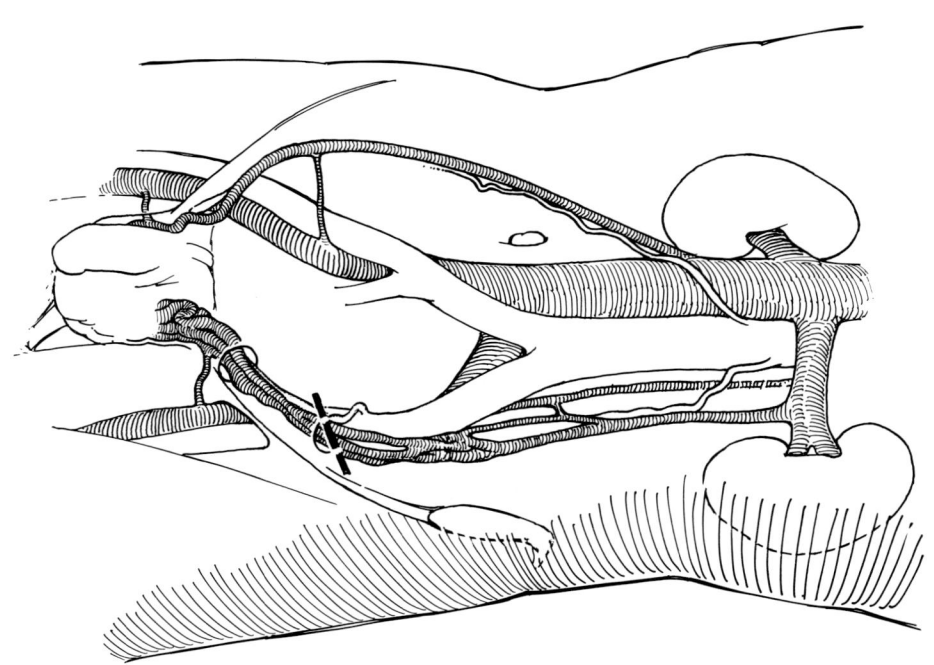

2 Incise the external oblique fascia in the direction of its fibers.

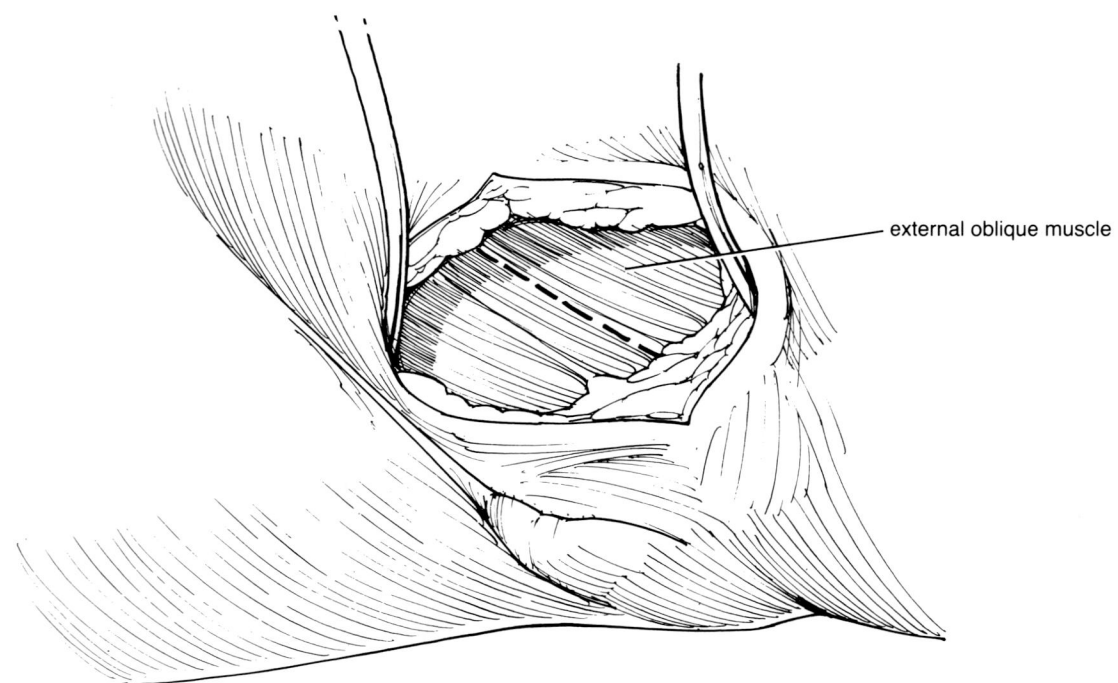

external oblique muscle

3 Separate the internal oblique muscle bluntly by inserting a curved clamp. Incise the transversus fascia.

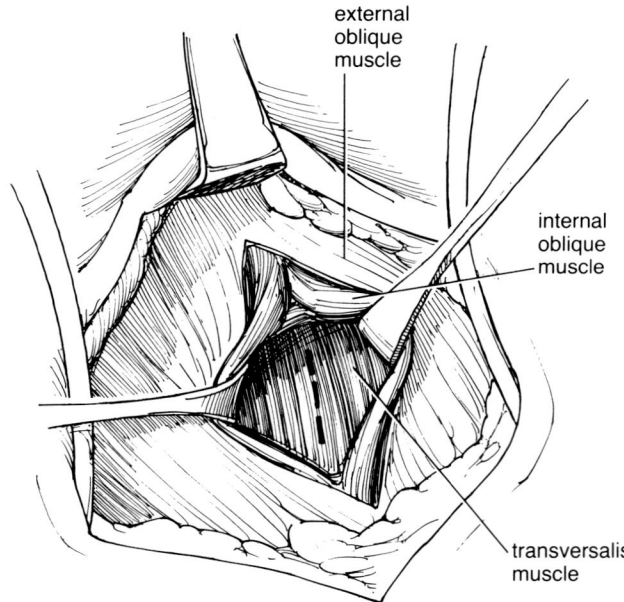

external
oblique
muscle

internal
oblique
muscle

transversalis
muscle

4 Enter the retroperitoneal space 3 to 5 cm above and medial to the inguinal ligament.

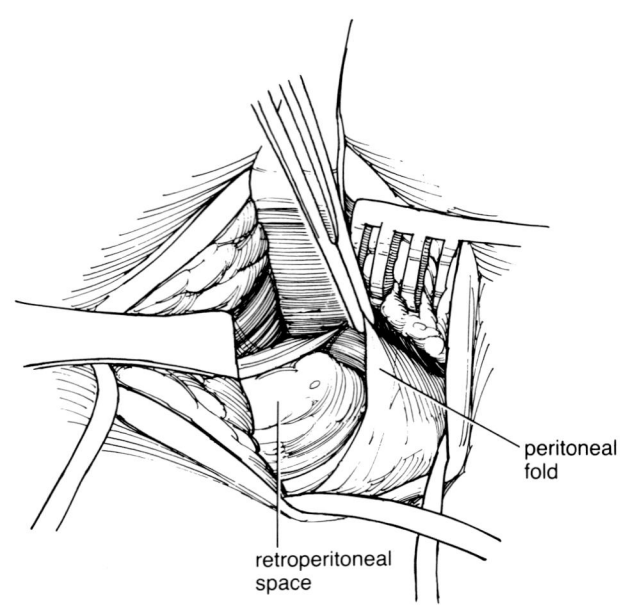

peritoneal
fold

retroperitoneal
space

5 Push the peritoneum medially with the peanut dissector, exposing the vessels as they rise to join the vas. Pulling on the testis at this point may be helpful in locating the vessels. A retractor placed medially could hide the spermatic veins on the posterior peritoneum.

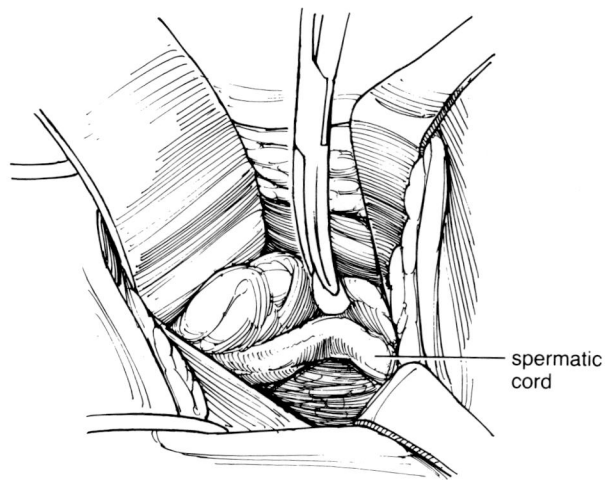

spermatic cord

6 Place a curved clamp or drain behind the vessels to elevate them into the wound. With loupe magnification, use sharp and blunt dissection to isolate all (usually three) of the flabby veins from the adjacent artery and lymphatic vessels. If the artery is not apparent, skeletonize the cord by bluntly stripping the spermatic fascia. Drip papaverine solution onto the cord to cause the artery to dilate and become visibly pulsatile. Inadvertent ligation rarely is harmful, because adequate circulation comes from vessels to the distal cord structures. The veins also may be made more obvious by dripping papaverine solution on the spermatic artery to increase the circulation to and from the testis. Placing the patient in the reverse Trendelenburg position may fill the veins and help identification. Perform intraoperative venography if identification of all collaterals is in doubt, especially in children. To do this, ligate the largest vein proximally. Tent it up, make a small nick, insert the plastic cannula of an 18-gauge needle, instill contrast medium distally, and expose a film. Ligate each vein with two silk ties and divide between. However, complete transection of all vessels at this level does not risk testicular viability, because the vasal and cremasteric vessels remain intact. Do not resect a segment, which would require unnecessary pathologic examination. Irrigate the wound, and close each layer of the body wall. Infiltrate the subcutaneous tissue with 0.25 percent mepivacaine for prolonged regional anesthesia. Place a subcuticular 4-0 synthetic absorbable suture to close the skin.

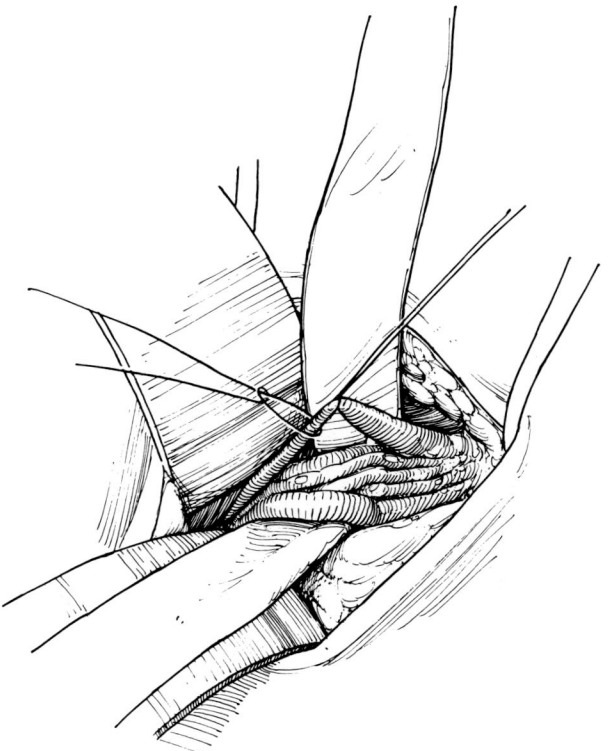

INGUINAL APPROACH
(IVANISSEVICH)

This approach allows management of the internal spermatic veins where they come off the cord structures at the level of the internal inguinal ring. It is easier, especially in the more obese patient, and requires less assistance.

7 *Position:* Place the boy supine. *Incision:* Make a 4-cm incision two fingerbreadths above the symphysis pubis in line with the lateral aspect of the scrotum beginning above the palpable external ring, extending obliquely along the course of the canal. Divide and ligate the superficial epigastric vessels that cross the lower end of the incision.

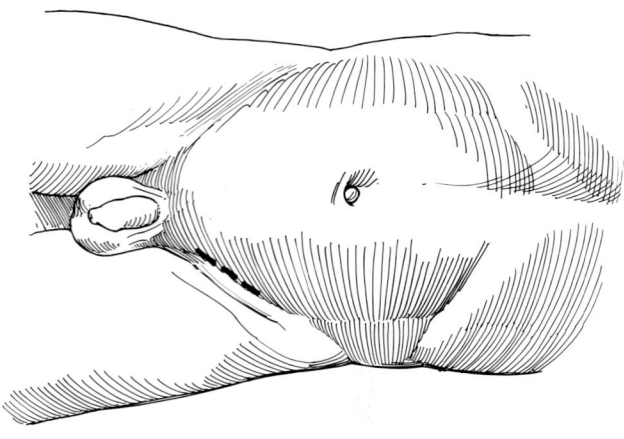

8 Divide Scarpa's fascia, and bluntly clear the connective tissue overlying the external oblique fascia and external ring. Insert a self-retaining retractor. Incise the fascia in the line of its fibers, beginning at the external ring and extending above the internal ring. Avoid the ilioinguinal nerve beneath. Pick the cord up between thumb and forefinger to palpate the vas and artery. Elevate the spermatic fascia with clamps to allow separation of the cord by blunt dissection.

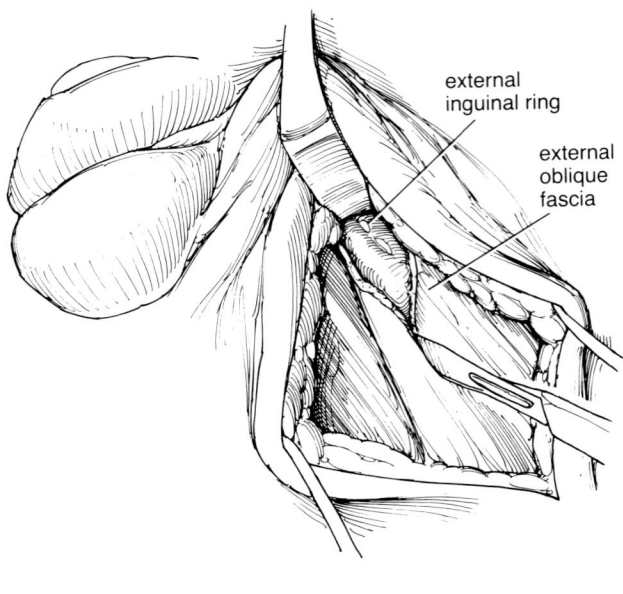

external
inguinal ring

external
oblique
fascia

9 Pass a curved clamp under the cord near the pubic tubercle and draw a Penrose drain or vessel loop through for traction to allow mobilization of the cord.

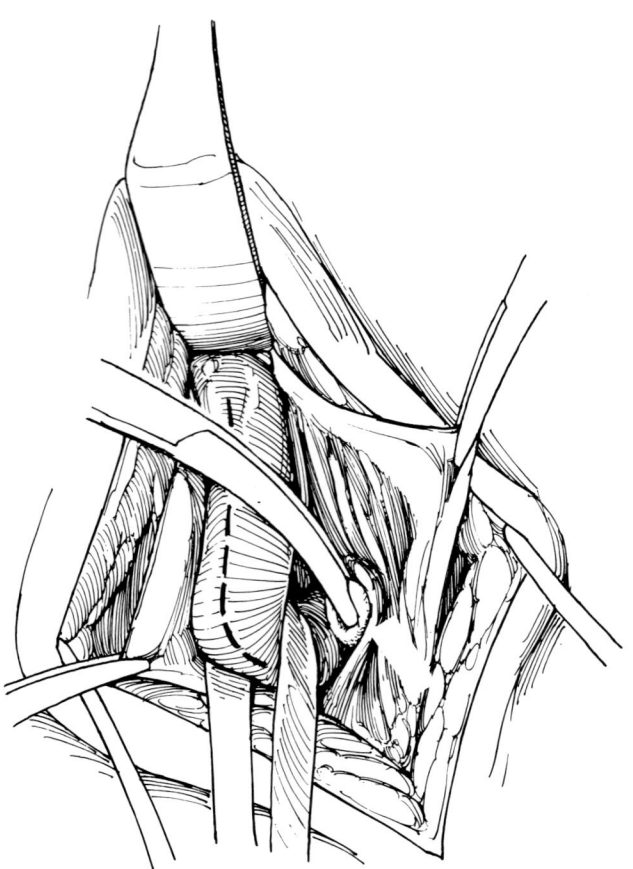

10 Hold the cord in the wound by fastening the ends of the drain to the drapes on each side. Open the cremasteric fascia. Sweep the underlying vas back out of the field. Aided by three-power loupes and microvascular forceps, dissect the spermatic fascia from each of the (usually) three branches of the spermatic vein from each other and from the more tortuous artery and the lymphatics for 2 to 3 cm in both directions. Papaverine dripped onto the cord will help visualize the artery and the veins. Look for and ligate the cremasteric vein that runs from the spermatic cord to the pudendal vein at the external ring.

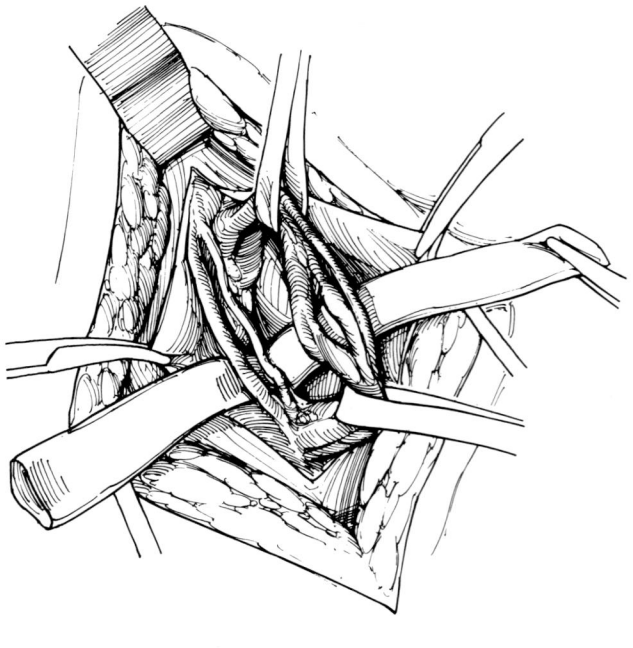

11 Doubly clamp each vein in succession, and ligate each end with 4-0 silk ties. Place the patient in the reverse Trendelenburg position to be sure no veins are overlooked. Remove the Penrose drain.

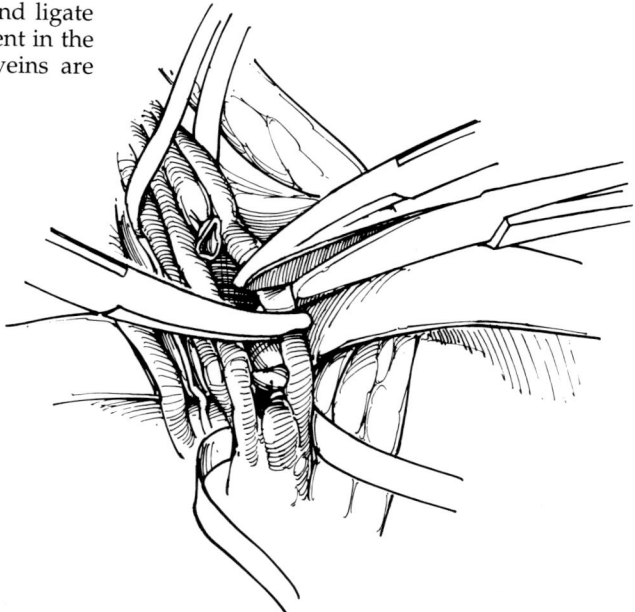

12 Close the external oblique fascia with interrupted 4-0 synthetic absorbable sutures, starting laterally and using the tied sutures for elevation of the edge. At the external ring, hold the cord down with a peanut dissector while placing the last stitch. Close Scarpa's fascia with a few fine sutures, and close the skin subcuticularly. Apply support for the scrotum.

Advise the boy to avoid activities that cause pain.

An alternative technique that ensures complete venous ligation (Goldstein et al., 1992) involves making a short inguinal incision in the skin and the external oblique fascia, encircling the cord, and drawing the testis out of the wound where the external spermatic veins can be readily identified and ligated, along with any other veins accompanying the gubernaculum. After the testis is returned to the scrotum, the cord itself is dissected under an operating microscope to ligate all the small veins except those with the vas deferens but spare the artery and adjacent lymphatics.

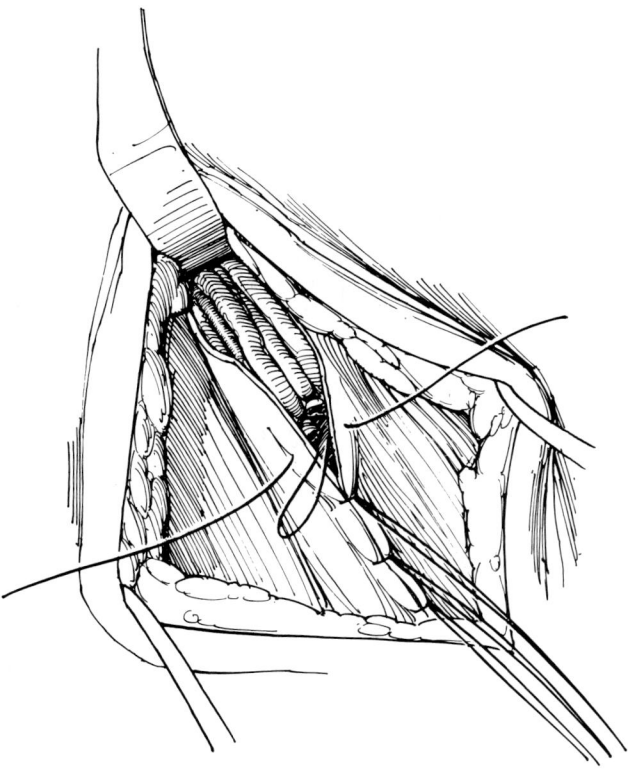

POSTOPERATIVE PROBLEMS

Damage to the artery can occur with subsequent testicular atrophy. It is less likely with the retroperitoneal approach. Injury to the vas deferens should be repaired immediately. *Recurrence* or persistence of the varicocele is not rare, resulting from missing a vein or because the varicocele was caused by actual venous obstruction from the so-called nutcracker phenomenon.

Commentary by A. Barry Belman

Varicoceles in adolescents occur at the onset of puberty and are present as frequently as in adults (15 percent). However, the indications for surgery differ, because in the adult population, infertility is the usual complaint. In adolescents, presentation usually follows a visit to the primary physician with the varicocele noted when the patient is examined upright. Rarely does the patient have any complaints referable to the findings, and generally, he is unaware of its presence despite the fact that these usually are quite large (Grade II-III or III). Indications for recommending surgical intervention are quite soft; however, the main objective remains finding a significant (more than 20 percent) variation in testicular size.

Testes may be measured using a standard orchidometer or sonographically (the latter adds cost to the evaluation that may not be justifiable). Hormonal levels are not affected by the presence of a varicocele. However, follicle-stimulating hormone and luteinizing hormone levels may rise higher than normal in response to gonadotropin-releasing hormone stimulation in men with varicoceles. This has been used diagnostically to substantiate an adverse affect from the abnormality. However, long-term results as to its significance have not been demonstrated.

Spermatic venous ligation is recommended on the presumption that fertility will be negatively influenced in the future by the varicocele. Growth of the testis in 80 percent of these boys postoperatively suggests that the varicocele was indeed detrimental. Unfortunately, no long-term controlled study exists comparing two groups of adolescents to determine if surgery is beneficial in this population.

CHAPTER 109

Laparoscopic Varicocele Ligation

The details for initiating laparoscopy are described in Chapter 103. Place an 11-mm video port just below the umbilicus, an 11-mm port in the suprapubic area, and a 5-mm port in the contralateral side midway between the umbilicus and the anterosuperior iliac spine. Stand on the right (the side opposite the varicocele), and manipulate the midline and left instruments. The assistant, holding the laparoscope, will view a mirror image of the procedure on the monitor at the foot of the table. Rotate the table to elevate the affected side, and initiate a 30-degree Trendelenburg position.

1 Identify the internal ring by following the vas deferens. Move the sigmoid colon medially; freeing it may be necessary. Compress the scrotum, and observe the filling of the spermatic veins. Try to identify the spermatic artery before manipulation of the vessels causes arterial spasm. Grasp the peritoneum approximately 5-cm proximal to the internal ring and slightly lateral to the spermatic vessels with grasping forceps passed through the midline port, and expose the vessels through a short T incision using laparoscopic scissors passed through the ipsilateral port. Using a straight grasping instrument in combination with the curved dissector, free the vessels from the retroperitoneal connective tissue and the psoas muscle.

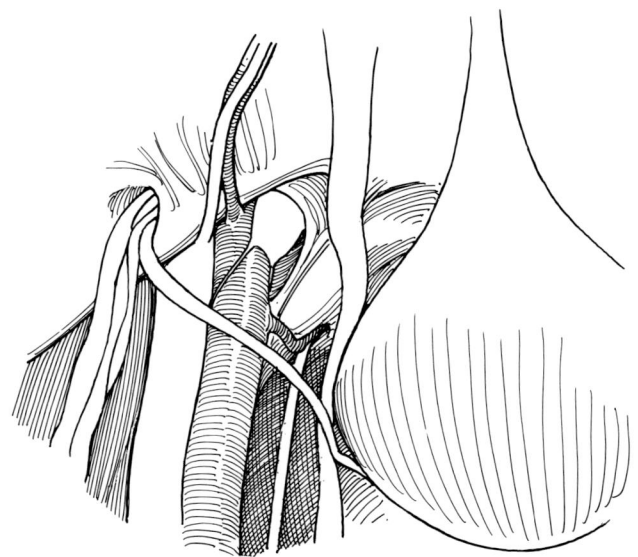

2 With two graspers, dissect the veins into multiple bundles while separating the spermatic artery from them. Traction on the testis helps identify the vessels. Avoid electrocoagulation near the delicate pedicle. Elevate the bundle, and push the spermatic artery out of the way with a dissector. Vasospasm may make identification difficult; it can be reduced by dripping papaverine or lidocaine through an aspirator-irrigator. Isolate the spermatic veins.

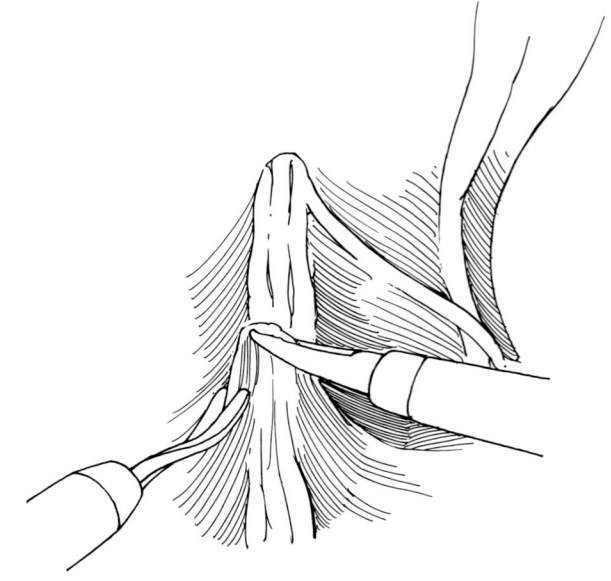

3 Place two 9-mm titanium endoclips proximally and two distally on each of the veins. Cut the veins between the paired clips with endoscissors. Smaller veins still may be present about the artery; tease them away, and clip them or fulgurate them with a fine electrosurgical probe or an Nd:YAG contact laser probe and divide them with scissors. Inspect the area to be sure of hemostasis, and check the result by again compressing the scrotum. Place the boy flat and in a reverse Trendelenburg position. Again look for any oozing, and aspirate any blood or irrigant that may have collected. Remove all but the one port, and open the valve to allow the carbon dioxide to issue from the abdomen. Place a single synthetic absorbable suture in the fascia below the umbilicus at the site of the 11-mm insertion site, and seal the skin incisions with sterile adhesive strips.

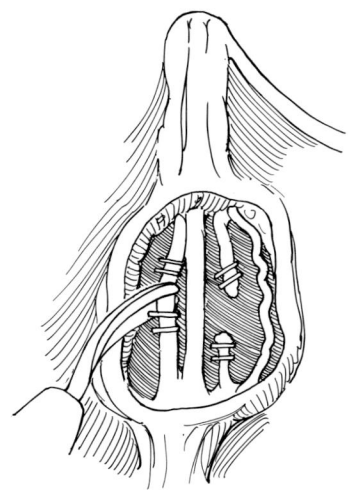

The large varicoceles of adolescents may resolve slowly postoperatively, and the pampiniform plexus may remain palpable.

Commentary by Stuart S. Howards

It is not clear at this time whether the advantage of laparoscopic varicocele ligation of decreased postoperative discomfort outweighs the increased cost and potential complications of this approach. Hopefully, with more experience, it will become evident whether the laparoscopic or open surgical approach is superior. It can be difficult to identify and preserve the testicular artery during a laparoscopic repair. Although every effort should be made to preserve the artery, there is considerable evidence that because of collateral circulation, it can be sacrificed at this level without causing any significant testicular damage.

Commentary by Howard N. Winfield

Over the past 3 years, laparoscopy has advanced from a diagnostic to a therapeutic surgical intervention in the field of urology. One of the initial procedures to be considered was laparoscopic varix ligation. This has been applied primarily for men with male factor infertility, but it also has been employed in the adolescent age group when testicular atrophy or pain is associated with a clinical varicocele.

The technique we use is similar to that described in this chapter, with a few modifications. To decrease the risk of bowel or vascular injury by the blind initial punctures with the Veress needle and 10/11-mm trocar-sheath unit, we now routinely use the "open laparoscopy" technique to place a Hasson cannula. Our working port arrangement consists of a 5-mm lateral port on the ipsilateral side and a 10/11-mm port on the contralateral side. A suprapubic port is not used, because we have found this to be quite painful for the patient.

Like Dr. Hinman, we also spend considerable time in dissecting the testicular artery(s) away from the veins. We have incorporated a 5-mm laparoscopic Doppler probe to aid in identifying the testicular artery, which usually is in the posteromedial aspect of the testicular bundle. The Nd:YAG contact laser probe aids to tease away and coagulate tiny testicular veins closely adherent to the artery. If the veins associated with the vas deferens or other collaterals are noted to be of significant size, these also are carefully transected.

All said and done, it is important that the urologic surgeon consider all other options available to the patient prior to surgery for correction of the varicocele. An inguinal or subinguinal incision under local anesthesia certainly is minimally invasive and may be safer for the patient. At this point, my approach has been to encourage the laparoscopic procedure in patients who have bilateral varices and/or have failed inguinal surgery. One certainly can make a good argument for the laparoscopic approach in children, because the small vas deferens should never enter into the operative field and be damaged, as may occur through the groin.

As long-term data are accumulated, it may be that the laparoscopic varix ligation is superior to other forms of therapy. Based on our first 50 patients who have undergone this procedure where follow-up is more than 12 months, the pregnancy rate is 34 percent and the recurrence rate only 2 percent. Furthermore, time to return to full activity is 3 to 5 days. A prospective, randomized study currently is underway comparing different therapeutic options for the management of the clinical varicocele.

PART II

TESTIS EXCISION

CHAPTER 110
Simple Orchiectomy

1 *Position:* Supine. *Anesthesia:* Use general anesthesia for children. Local anesthesia by infiltration of the cord (page 57) is effective and safe if the boy is old enough. Stand on the boy's right side, pull the testis down to relax the cremaster, and grasp the cord with the left hand, placing the thumb in front and the index finger behind the cord at the top of the scrotum. With the needle approaching the index finger, infiltrate the cord with 1 percent lidocaine solution without epinephrine through a 2.5-in, 25-gauge needle.

Grasp the testis with the fingers and thumb to tense the overlying skin. Make a transverse incision in the scrotum to avoid the scrotal vessels. A vertical incision in the scrotal raphe is suitable if bilateral excision is planned. Incise the dartos muscle and cremasteric layers onto the bluish tunica vaginalis. Control bleeding vessels with the electrocautery held in the other hand. Push the scrotal layers away with sponge dissection, and deliver the testis within the tunica vaginalis into the wound. Alternately, open the tunica vaginalis before delivering the testis.

2 Draw the testis down to expose the epididymis and cord. Bluntly dissect the spermatic vessels from the vas deferens. Divide and ligate the vas with 3-0 synthetic absorbable suture. In adolescents, clamp each group individually, and ligate them with the same type of suture. It may be wise to use a suture-ligature for the spermatic artery, because this vessel retracts after division, and loss of the ligature results in major (hidden) retroperitoneal bleeding. Should this occur, quickly extend the incision to expose the retroperitoneal space via the inguinal canal. In children, individual ligation is not necessary; the entire cord may be clamped, especially with torsion, and the cord suture-ligated. Before closing, electrocoagulate any bleeders in the dartos and subcutaneous tissue to avoid a distressing scrotal hematoma. Close the dartos layer with a running synthetic absorbable suture and bring the skin together with the subcutaneous tissue with interrupted 4-0 or 5-0 synthetic absorbable sutures or with a fine subcuticular running suture, with or without a Penrose drain pulled back into the scrotum. A fluff pressure dressing probably does not stop significant oozing.

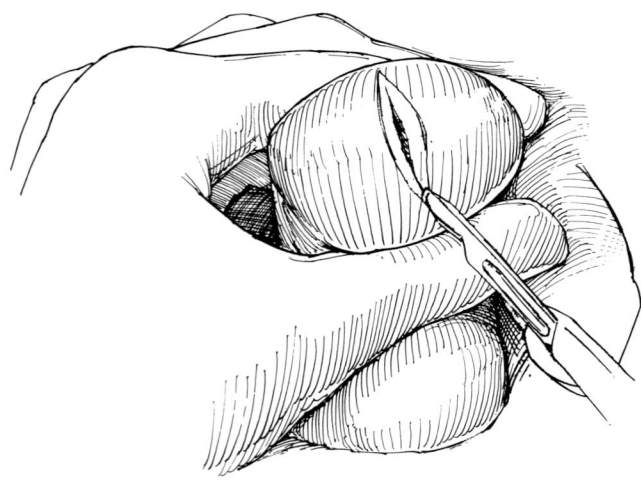

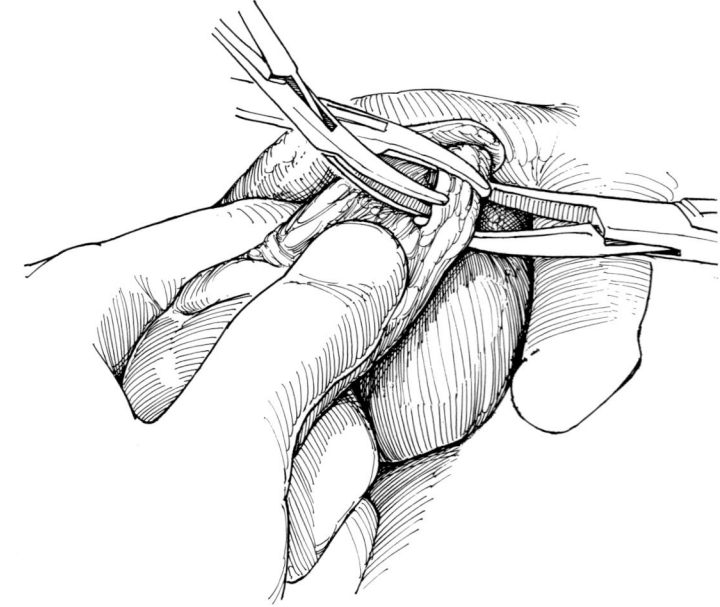

POSTOPERATIVE PROBLEMS

Continued oozing with formation of a *scrotal hematoma* is the most common complication and results from incomplete hemostasis in the several loose layers of the scrotum. Placement of a drain before closure avoids the hematoma but should not be necessary if good technique is followed. Drain a hematoma only if it becomes distressingly large or infected.

Commentary by H. Gil Rushton

Testicular torsion would be the primary indication for a "simple orchiectomy" in the pediatric population. One always should perform a contralateral simple orchidopexy in these cases. In this setting, one frequently encounters significant thickening of the scrotal wall and venous oozing as a result of scrotal edema and hyperemia.

Leaving an adequate stump of the spermatic vessels extending beyond the edge of the clamp will reduce the risk of bleeding associated with slippage of the ligature. I would only recommend spermatic cord block as the primary form of anesthesia in a postpubertal adolescent, because younger children generally are not cooperative enough to perform this procedure under local anesthesia.

CHAPTER 111

Laparoscopic Orchiectomy

Follow the technique and insert the sheaths as described on page 103. Place the child in a three-quarters torque position so he will not have to be moved. Through a small subumbilical incision, open the peritoneum (obviating the risk from the Veress needle), and insert a screw-in port (Surgiport).

1 Locate the small testis endoscopically, and incise the peritoneum over the upper pole to identify and fulgurate, or, if the port is large enough, clip the spermatic vessels. Dissect the testis from its bed along with a short length of vas deferens. Pull on the gubernaculum and fulgurate it. Clip the vas on the distal side. Usually the testis is small or atrophic, so it can be withdrawn through the sheath or removed after enlarging one of the accessory ports without the need for a bag. Alternatively, place the testis and adnexae in a specimen retrieval bag or a sterile condom, and draw the mouth of the bag to the sheath of the trocar at the anterior abdominal wall. Withdraw the sheath, clamp the bag, and draw the testis through the puncture site. Inspect the bed.

Alternatively, locate the testis endoscopically, make a small localized incision, and excise the testis with clamps, sutures, and scissors.

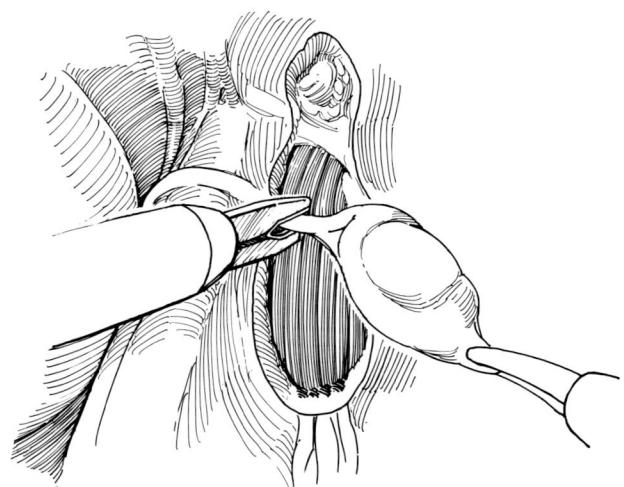

Commentary by H. Gil Rushton

The laparoscopic removal of the testis is indicated in the case of an atrophic or hypoplastic undescended intra-abdominal testis when orchiopexy is not considered more appropriate, particularly in the postpubertal adolescent. Other less-common indications would include the removal of abnormal premalignant gonads found in some intersex states, such as testicular feminization and mixed gonadal dysgenesis. If laparoscopic examination demonstrates that the testis has actually migrated into the inguinal canal, a small groin incision can be made to remove the testis.

CHAPTER 112

Radical Orchiectomy

Obtain serum markers for alpha-fetoprotein (AFP) and human chorionic gonadotropin (hCG-β). After radical orchiectomy, obtain a chest film, perform abdominal and thoracic computed tomography, and repeat measurement of serum markers. Stage the disease at that time. For boys with Stage I, IIa, or IIb seminomas and normal AFP levels, obtain radiation therapy postoperatively; for boys with bulky or disseminated seminoma or other germ cell tumors, treat according to stage.

1 Prep and drape the lower abdomen to include the genitalia. Incise the skin above and parallel to the inguinal ligament, as for inguinal hernia repair. Divide the subcutaneous fat, and ligate the several veins with 3-0 synthetic absorbable sutures as encountered.

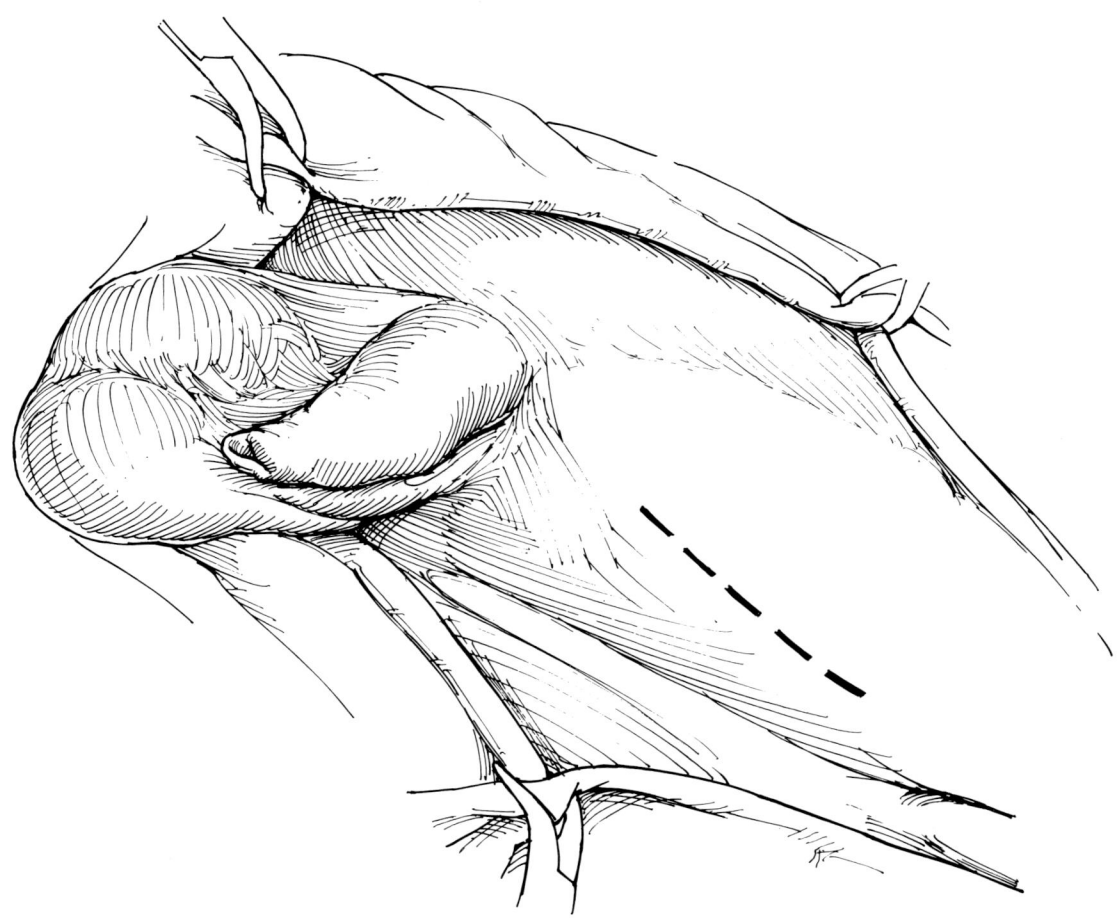

2 Identify the external ring, and incise the external oblique fascia sharply, taking care not to cut the ilioinguinal nerve lying just beneath it.

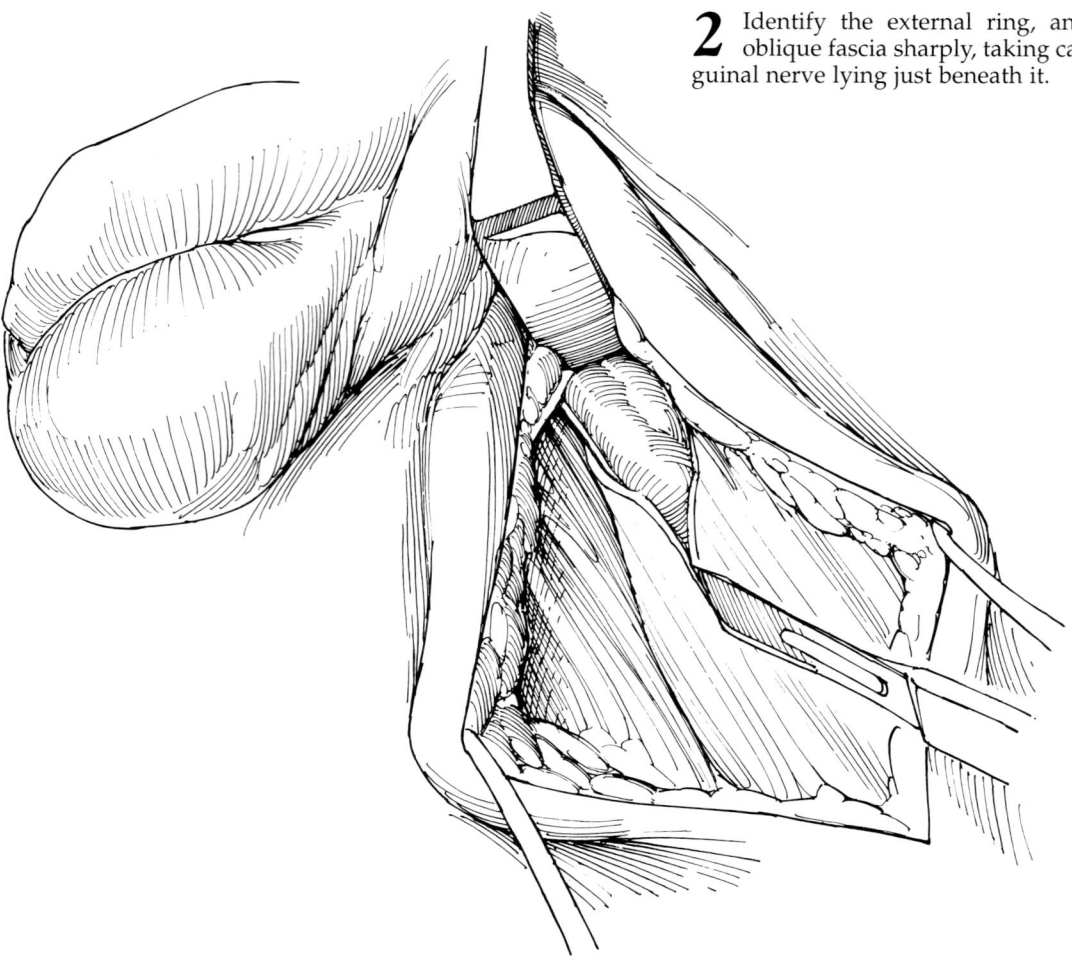

3 Grasp and elevate the lateral and medial edges of the external oblique fascia, and bluntly dissect the spermatic cord inferiorly to expose the pubic tubercle.

4 Repeat the dissection medially, elevating the medial fascial edge so that all of the cord structures, including the cremaster muscle, can be surrounded with a Penrose drain.

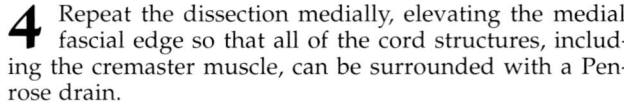

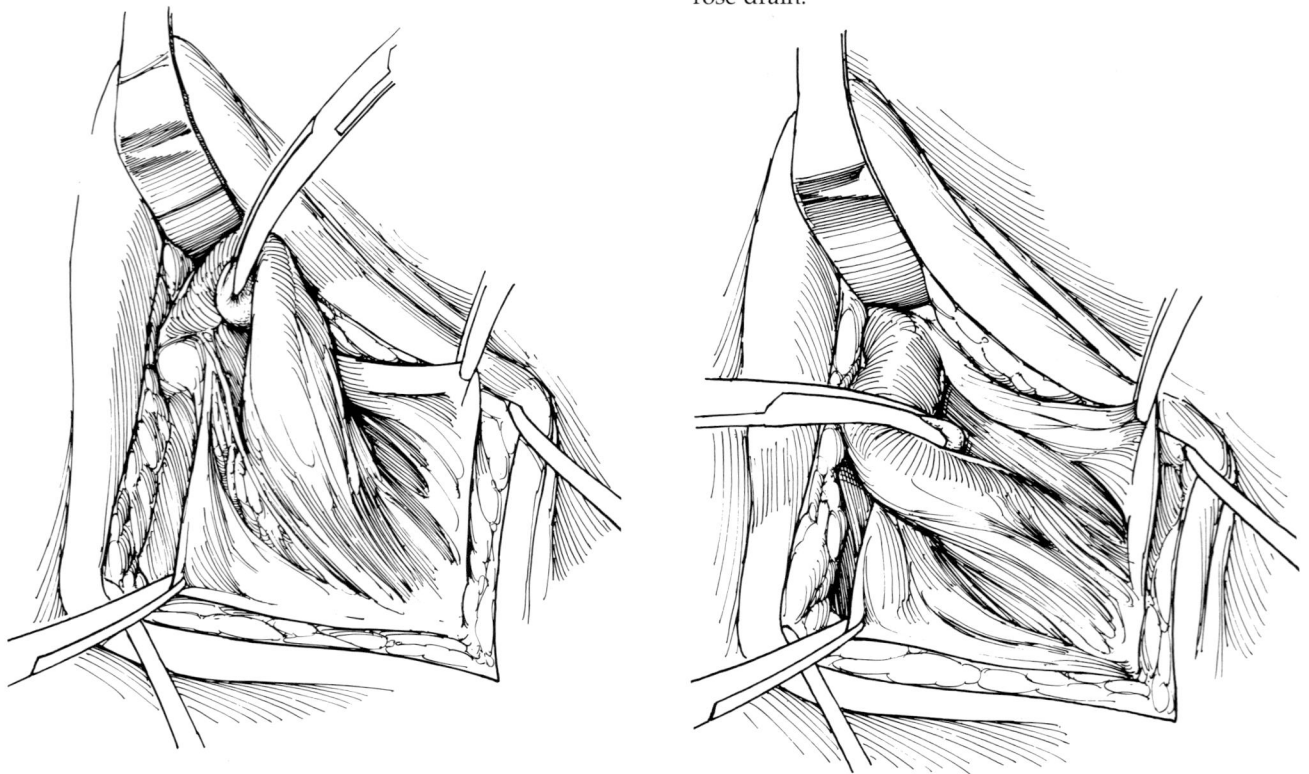

5 Lift the Penrose drain and free the cord to the internal ring. Watch for a perforating cremasteric vessel that must be tied. It is good technique to follow the vas medially to separate it from the vessels and to clamp and divide it between nonabsorbable ligatures.

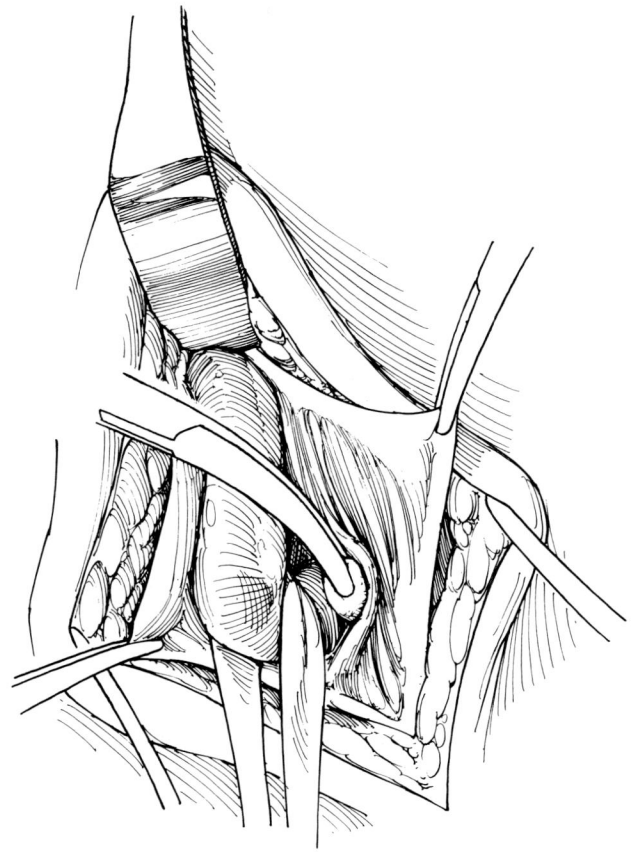

6 A and B, Pass a 14 F catheter, preferably latex, around the cord 1 in below the ring. Draw it up and clamp it as a tourniquet, or use a noncrushing clamp.

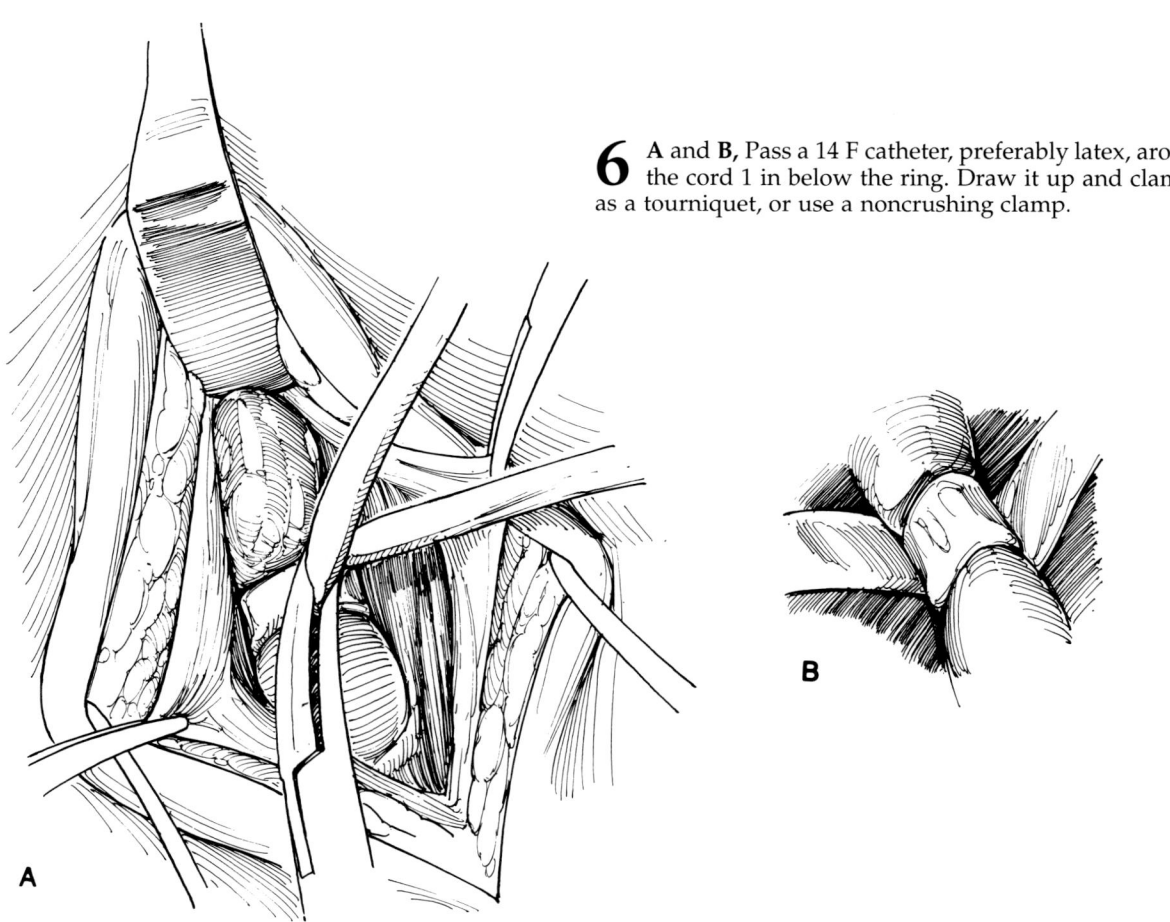

A

B

7 Stretch the neck of the scrotum and push the testicle upward. For large tumors, Scarpa's fascia may need further division, but avoid extension of the incision over the symphysis.

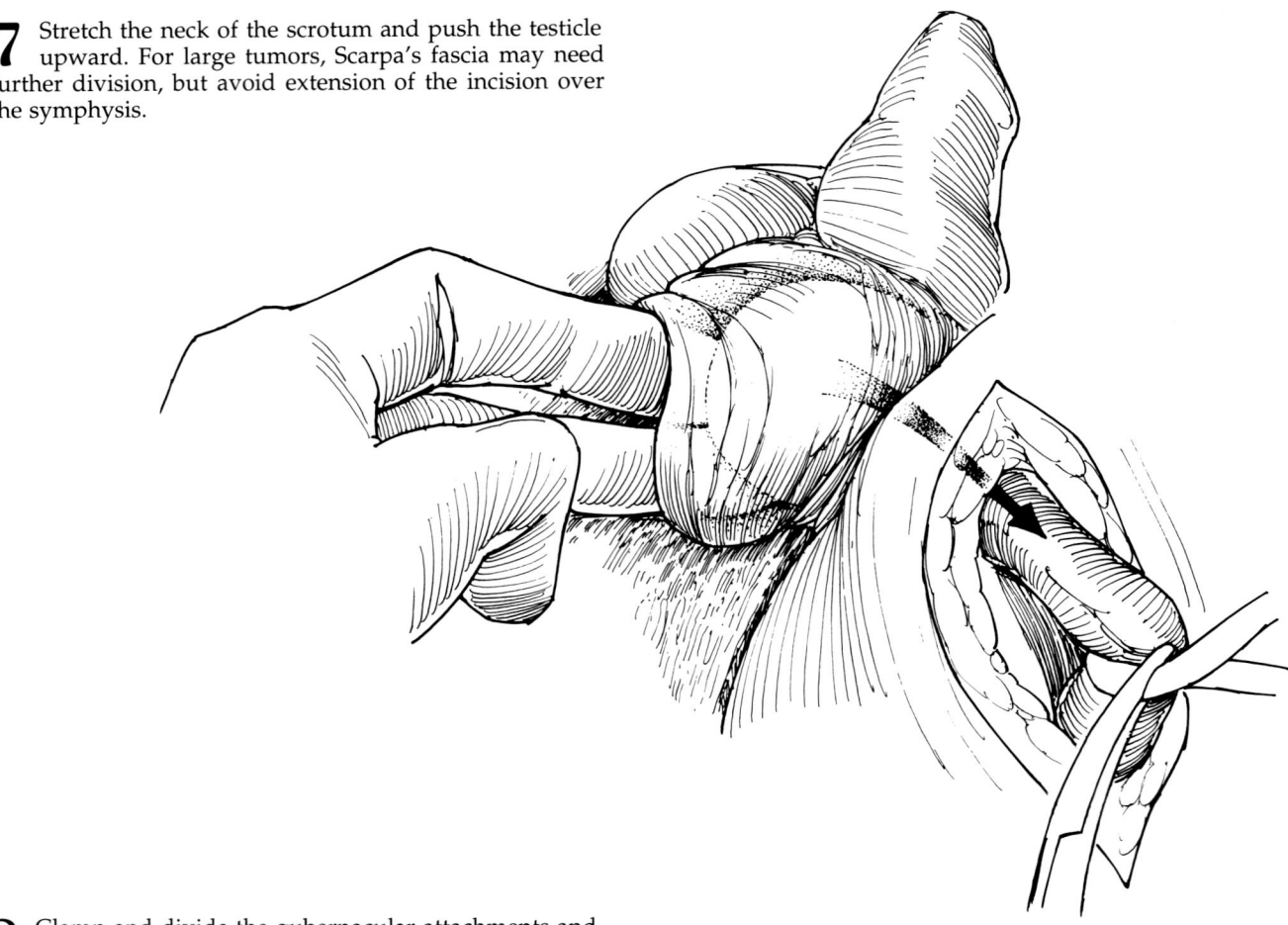

8 Clamp and divide the gubernacular attachments and ligate them.

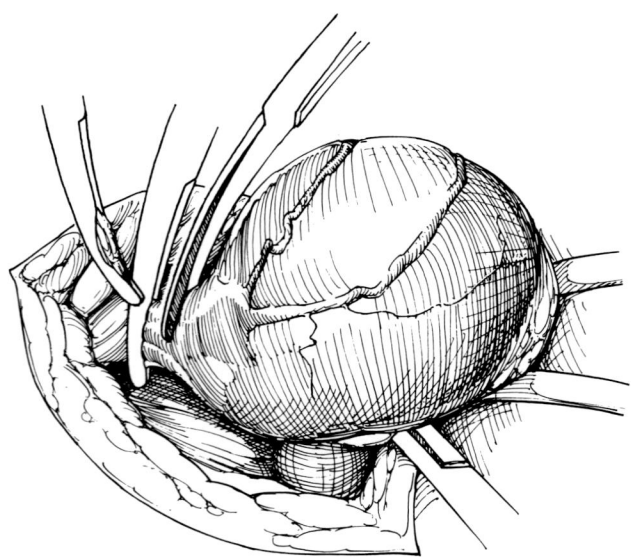

9 If at this point any there are any doubts about the diagnosis, place the testis on a sterile towel, where the tunica vaginalis may be opened and the testis inspected directly. Rarely will frozen section biopsy be necessary. However, it can be done without risk of spread if the testis is draped out of the field, and the surgeon changes towels, gloves, and instruments after removing the testis.

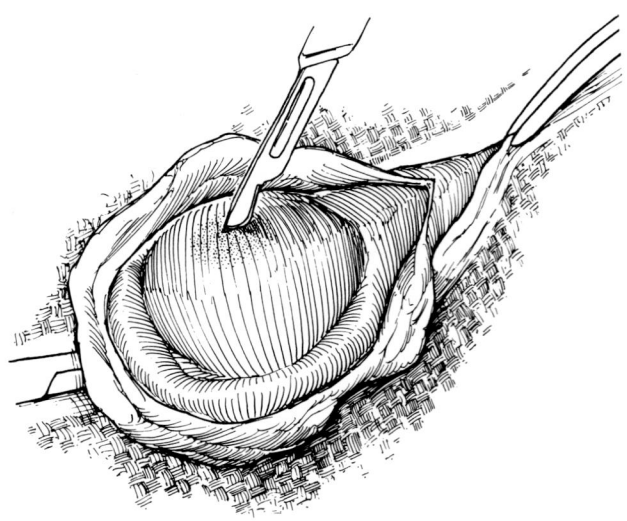

Open the internal oblique muscle at the internal ring for 2 or 3 cm, and dissect the vas and spermatic vessels as far as feasible through this incision.

10 Doubly clamp, divide, and doubly ligate the cord at the internal ring above the tourniquet, using 2-0 or 3-0 nonabsorbable sutures, preferably colored. Cut the ends of the sutures sufficiently long for later identification at node dissection. The cord should now lie retroperitoneally so that it can be reached readily during node dissection. Observe for hemostasis, and irrigate the wound. Should the ligatures slip, the cord will retract above the canal. Immediately open the external and internal oblique in the line of the incision, and grasp and religate the free end of the cord.

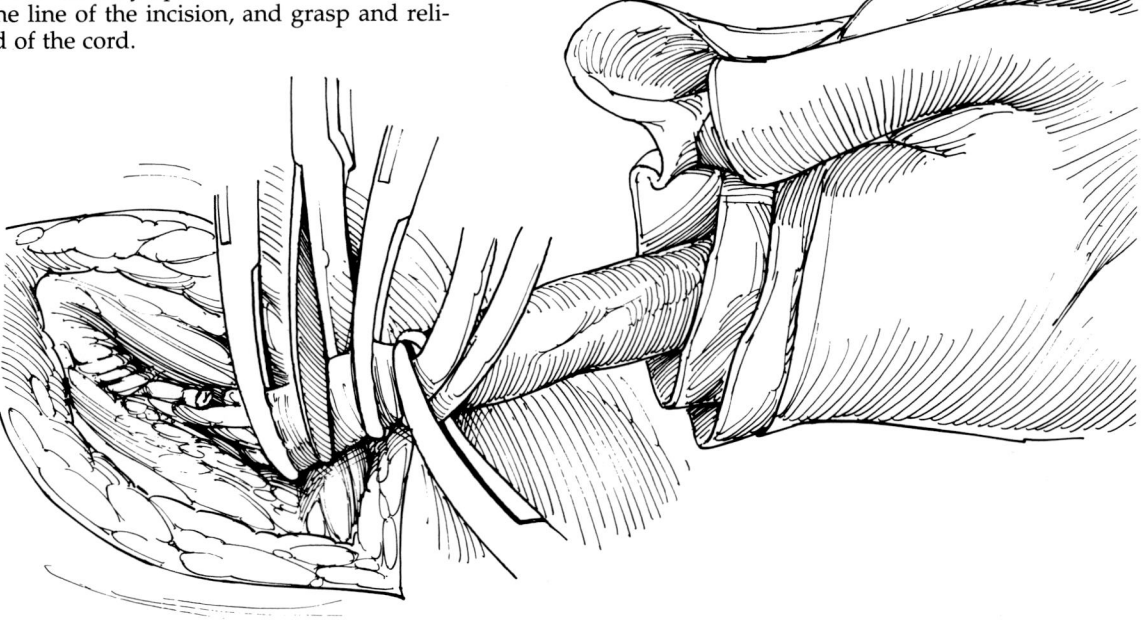

11 **A,** Suture the conjoined tendon to the shelving edge of the inguinal ligament. **B,** Imbricate the external oblique fascia with 3-0 synthetic absorbable sutures. Close the subcutaneous tissue with fine synthetic absorbable sutures, and run a 4-0 synthetic absorbable suture subcuticularly. Do not place drains. Use fluffs to compress the empty scrotum, or suture it to the lower abdomen over a gauze roll. Concomitant placement of a testicular prosthesis is not advisable; moreover, the patient usually prefers a scrotum free of all masses.

If an epidermoid cyst is suspected by palpation or sonography, expose the testis as described in Step 9. Obstruct the cord, open the tunica vaginalis on a towel, and excise the translucent cyst. Obtain a frozen section. If doubt still exists, clamp the cord and remove the testis.

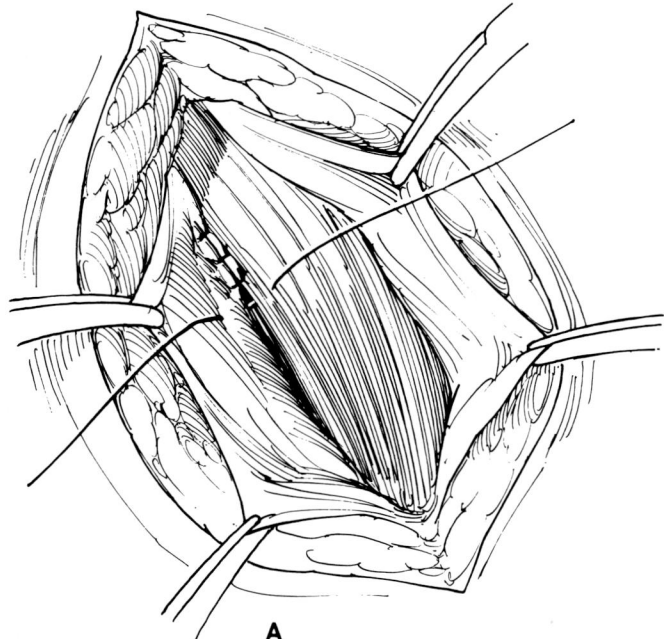

A

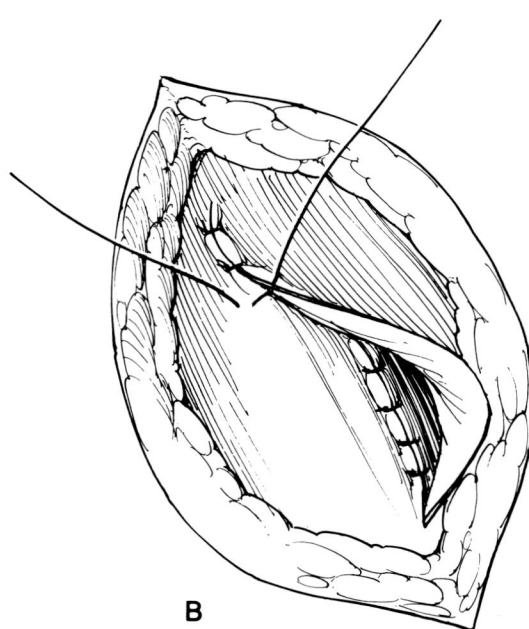

B

POSTOPERATIVE PROBLEMS

Hemorrhage can be a major complication from lack of separate control of vas and vessels and from improper ligation of the cord. An expanding hematoma or evidence of retroperitoneal bleeding warrants reopening and extending the inguinal incision to reach the retracted vessels.

Commentary by Randall G. Rowland

Sensitive serum markers (hCG-β and AFP) and scrotal ultrasound have greatly reduced the need to "explore" a testis for a mass that is within or adjacent to a testis. The diagnosis of testicular cancer is made with a high degree of certainty preoperatively in most of cases. The surgical techniques described in this chapter are widely accepted. Control of the gonadal vessels cannot be emphasized enough to prevent the development of a retroperitoneal hematoma. Also, as in any inguinal procedure, the surgeon must take great care to avoid entrapping the ilioinguinal nerve during closure of the wound.

CHAPTER 113

Retroperitoneal Lymph Node Dissection

For nonseminomatous tumors found on radical orchiectomy (page 541), proceed with staging as follows:

1. *Abdominal and pelvic computed tomographic (CT) scans:* If findings are negative or show only small involved nodes, proceed with staging retroperitoneal lymph node dissection (RPLND). For large nodes, give chemotherapy first.

2. *Whole lung tomograms:* If findings are positive (Stage III), give chemotherapy. Subsequently, do RPLND if CT scan findings show positive nodes; otherwise, watch the patient carefully. If the lungs are clear, proceed with RPLND.

3. *Nodal pathologic staging:* If node findings are negative (Stage I), watch the patient. If they are positive (Stage II), either watch the patient or give chemotherapy. As markers, use alpha-fetoprotein with a metabolic half-life of 5 days and hcg-β with a metabolic half-life of 30 minutes. For solid masses in the pelvis observed on sonography and urography, obtain a CT scan to delineate rhabdomyosarcoma, neuroblastoma, sacral teratoma, and lymphoma.

Evaluate the patient's respiratory status, especially if he has received bleomycin. Review the results of the intravenous urogram to establish the presence or absence of renal obstruction or any malfunction on the side of the nodal mass. Provide for monitoring with intra-arterial lines and Swan-Ganz catheters. Order adequate blood for replacement. Patients with large nodal masses need as many as 6 units, typed and cross-matched. Additional blood products should be available, as well as 1 to 2 L of 5 percent albumin.

Prepare the bowel. Hydrate intravenously the night before; give mannitol intraoperatively, but avoid furosemide after cisplatin therapy, gentamicin therapy, or both.

Explain the probability of dry ejaculation as the boy grows older and, in advanced cases, the possibility of removal of contiguous structures, including an excision of the aorta, vena cava, or ipsilateral kidney. Insert a balloon urinary catheter. Place a nasogastric tube intraoperatively.

A transabdominal approach is more quickly and easily performed. It facilitates bilateral dissection in the contralateral suprahilar and iliac areas, but for muscular children or for bulky nodes, the thoracoabdominal incision will give better exposure and less postoperative ileus.

Commentary by Randall G. Rowland

Improvements in staging studies have allowed more accurate preoperative assessment of patients with germ cell tumors, which, in turn, permits assignment to the appropriate treatment modality. Fortunately, the application of aggressive surgical and chemotherapeutic treatment has yielded very high cure rates in patients with this disease. As a result, efforts are now focused on reducing the severity or extent of treatment and reducing or eliminating its morbidity (such as infertility from loss of emission caused by sympathectomy during RPLND). Modifications of RPLNDs are nerve sparing in two ways. Modified or reduced templates of dissection spare the contralateral sympathetic chain, whereas prospective nerve-sparing techniques of dissection also spare the sympathetic nerves and their postganglionic branches that traverse the field of dissection. Preserving the tissue around the origin of the inferior mesenteric artery (IMA) and the bifurcation of the aorta is critical for preservation of emission, regardless of the site of the primary tumor.

When limited template or nerve-sparing dissection techniques are being used, the mesentery of the left colon is left intact from the area of the IMA caudally to the pelvis. The tissue along the inferior aorta and the left common iliac artery can be removed by elevating the IMA and its surrounding tissue or by mobilizing the left colon at its lateral border. This mobilization of the left colon allows good access to the area in question by a lateral approach.

The application of these limited templates and/or prospective nerve-sparing techniques must be tempered by the preoperative staging results and intraoperative findings. Templates must be extended in the presence of gross evidence of retroperitoneal metastasis to encompass all grossly enlarged nodes or masses to ensure a margin of safety. Prospective nerve-sparing techniques may have to be abandoned to ensure complete removal of potential tumor-bearing tissue in the presence of gross retroperitoneal masses.

Although RPLND is an extensive procedure with many potential major complications, the rate of occurrence of complications is low in the hands of experienced surgeons. Overall, patients tolerate these procedures well, which certainly is due, in part, to the age range of 18 to 25 years in which germ cell tumors are the most common.

SECTION 8

Penis and Urethra

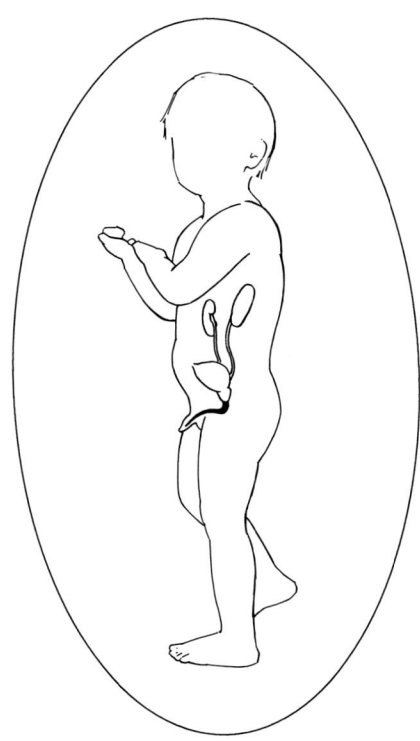

PART I

PENILE PLASTIC OPERATIONS

CHAPTER 114

Basic Instructions for Hypospadias Repair

OBJECTIVES OF HYPOSPADIAS REPAIR

The aims of repair are to completely relieve the chordee for unrestricted erection; to bring the urethra to the tip of the penis; to effect a solid stream with no splattering, splashing, or backflow on micturition; to render the external surface of the penis symmetric with no abnormal tissue tags or fistulas; and to allow the patient to assume normal sexual function. Remember that a one-stage procedure is best, but performing a staged procedure is better than being forced to redo the procedure. Success is directly related to the experience of the surgeon. For a successful result in hypospadias repair, the penile tissues must be handled with great care. Experience in mobilizing and rotating skin flaps is needed, as are the minutia involved in plastic surgical techniques. It is not enough to review pictures and follow descriptions; training in the techniques is essential. Knowledge of a few methods is not enough, because the one used must be the best for the individual situation of the boy.

AGE FOR OPERATION

Select a time between 6 and 18 months, within the psychologic window in the period of least damage to the infant's psyche. At this age, the infants do not remember, and they are also easiest to manage in diapers. Some pediatric urologists prefer a time between 6 and 9 months; others prefer to operate after 24 months, when the boy's penis is larger and he can be kept amused in the hospital. Parenteral testosterone may be administered to increase the size of the penis and especially the size and vascularity of the prepuce, should it be needed for proximal and perineal hypospadias repair.

The surgeon and nurse should give considerable support to the parents and their need to know what to expect.

OUTPATIENT REPAIR

An uncomplicated hypospadias operation can be done without hospital admission. Have the parents and child visit you sometime before the date of surgery for history and examination, as well as for instructions in feeding and preoperative care. Arrange an appointment for a complete blood count, urinalysis, and any other test suggested by the history. You or your nurse can explain the procedure, hand out suitable booklets for details, and obtain the most informed consent possible, given the difficulties of explaining procedures to parents and the need to adapt the operation to the tissues. Arrange for the anesthetists to evaluate the child, especially if any problems are anticipated. Separate preputial adhesions at this time, preferably 1 month before operation, to allow maturation of the inner face of the prepuce. The day before the procedure, have one of the outpatient staff call the parents to be sure everything is clear.

Ask that the patient and family arrive 2 hours before the time of the operation to complete the final details. Obtain consent if it was not done on the initial visit. Arrange for the parent and child to meet the anesthetist and surgical nurses outside the operating room. Premedicate the infant or child according to orders by the anesthetist.

Halothane is a good agent for induction, and isoflurane is good for maintenance. Monitor the patient with a precordial or esophageal stethoscope, a Doppler blood pressure recorder, and a rectal temperature probe. Add bupivacaine for regional block in genital operations, and consider its use as a caudal block for postoperative comfort.

It is good to have someone informing and reassuring the family as the operation progresses. At the end, place the child in the postanesthesia care unit for a short time before his return to the holding area and the parents. Discharge the child when he is fully awake and able to take fluids. Instruct the parents on the care of the indwelling catheter and be sure you or an associate are available around the clock for questions or emergencies and are able to have a bed available if it is needed. Make a telephone call to the parents the next day to check on progress.

PROPHYLACTIC ANTIBIOTICS

Prophylactic antibiotics are not essential, except for salvage repairs, although administration intraoperatively of a systemic antibiotic may be wise. If antibiotic coverage is needed, begin immediately and continue for 1 week postoperatively.

PREPARATION OF THE GENITALIA

Use povidone-iodine soap, but do not apply any substance like povidone-iodine solution that stains the skin and so could obscure its vascularization. If a skin graft in older boys is planned, do not shave the genitalia until you have identified a hairless area for grafts and flaps.

SELECTION OF THE OPERATIVE TECHNIQUE

Reclassify the degree of hypospadias *after* mentally correcting the chordee but before deciding on the particular technique you plan to use. The shape of the glans helps in the decision; the cone-shaped glans usually is accompanied by a fibrous urethral plate requiring division followed by a tubed transverse island flap (page 588), and a tunneled glansplasty, whereas with a flat glans, the plate usually is normal, so that it may be preserved for application of an onlay flap.

One-stage operations are preferable to two-stage operations not only for the avoidance of further surgery but also for the use of virginal skin. In any case, do not promise the patient or parents that only one stage is necessary.

The choices for repair are the meatal advancement and glanuloplasty (MAGPI), the Mathieu technique, the Hodgson XX technique, the mobilized inner face flap (Duckett, 1981), the external face flap (Standoli, 1982), one of the Hinderer perimeatal flaps, and free grafts of skin (Devine *et al.,* 1963) or bladder or buccal epithelium. With abundant dorsal vasculature, mobilization of the inner or outer face of the prepuce as a patch or tube (Duckett, 1981) is effective. Island flaps laid on as patches are increasing in popularity as the poorer vascularization of the Mathieu and flip-flap procedures is recognized.

Much depends on the position and characteristics of the meatus. The Allen-Spence procedure is suitable if the meatus is at the corona or just proximal to it.

The MAGPI technique also will correct this defect and achieve a better-appearing reconstruction. If the meatus on the glans is abnormal (*eg*, fish-mouth), a flap turned over from the shaft, as in the Mathieu or the flip-flap, will replace it. If the meatus is in midshaft without chordee—not a common situation—an onlay island flap without tubularization of its inner face or a perimeatal-based tube repair (Mustardé, 1965) will be needed. With mild distal chordee, a MAGPI may be possible, but a type of Mustardé procedure may be better.

With ventral deflection and some fibrous chordee, an onlay island flap may suffice. If the chordee is fibrous and extensive but the meatus lies on the distal portion of the shaft, a mobilized transverse island flap (Duckett, 1981) is most suitable. However, if the meatus is more proximal, a two-stage repair is advisable. Beware of penile rotation during the second stage of such a repair. Also, during a planned one-stage procedure, if the viability of the skin appears questionable, change to a two-stage procedure. A dorsal, relaxing incision (Browne, 1936) should be used rarely, if at all.

For secondary operations, if the prepuce is still available, an island flap may be applied. Otherwise, a free tube graft may be used, obtained from the residual prepuce on the shaft, or if that is not available, from the buccal mucosa or bladder epithelium or nongenital skin, in that order of desirability.

Remember that penile skin itself has a random blood supply, but the vessels in the dartos fascia that supply it run axially from the superficial external pudendal arteries, with one or the other side usually dominant, a fact that can be determined by transillumination. The dorsal surface of the corpora cavernosa has a meager blood supply; if a split-thickness graft is applied, it must be thin to encourage the entry of new vessels.

In all cases, try to provide an intermediate layer between the new urethra and the skin. One way is to remove the skin from one edge of the preputial or penile flap and bring the subcutaneous dartos layer across (Durham Smith, 1973). A flap of scrotal fat or a mobilized tunica vaginalis (Snow, 1989) can be used for the same purpose. Finally, success is more likely to be the result of the experience of the surgeon than the technique applied (Duckett, 1981).

PREOPERATIVE INVESTIGATIONS

Urologic investigation may be indicated in a boy with perineal hypospadias, severe chordee, bifid scrotum when other anomalies are possible, and in those with a history of infection or family history of urinary disease. Intersex investigations are indicated in those with perineal hypospadias with impalpable gonads.

INSTRUMENTS

Select instruments for delicate handling of tissues. A full list would include genitourinary fine and micro sets, fine Allis clamps, two pairs of Bishop-Harmon forceps, jeweler's forceps, sharp tenotomy scissors, iris scissors with the tips ground down, McPherson-Vannas scissors, blunt Castroviejo scissors, four small two-prong skin hooks, two small one-prong skin hooks, plastic scissors, a peanut dissector, and plastic needle holders. Also include the following: a three-power loupe or commercial magnifying visor; infant sounds; bougie à boule; fine lacrimal probes; grooved tunnel sounds if perineal urethrostomy is contemplated; 8, 10, and 12 F Robinson catheters; 5 F and 8 F infant feeding tubes; a pediatric stilet; a Dow Corning 8 F trocar cystocatheter (Cystocath); lubricant; rubber bands; a marking pen; a 23-gauge butterfly needle and syringe; microsponges; a #15 blade knife; #39, 64, and 69 Beaver blades and handle; Andrews and Frazier suction tips; and ophthalmic electrocautery. Have appropriate fine sutures at hand (synthetic absorbable suture, nonabsorbable suture, plain catgut, and chromic catgut).

NERVE BLOCK

Long-lasting bupivacaine (0.5 percent) mixed with quick-acting lidocaine (1 percent) in a volume of 3 to 4 ml, either infiltrated as a ring block at the base of each crus just below the symphysis or injected vertically in the midline deep to the notch of the symphysis through a 1½-inch 22-gauge needle (page 57), when placed at the beginning of the operation in the morning, will last well into the postoperative period in the afternoon and also reduce the amount of general anesthesia required. A caudal block is a good alternative or supplement.

ARTIFICIAL ERECTION

Place a rubber band or red rubber catheter at the base of the penis, secured with a hemostat. Introduce a butterfly needle through the glans into one corpus cavernosum. (Direct puncture of the cavernous body may cause a hematoma.) Distend the penis with normal saline solution (±10 ml). Avoid overdistention. The erection may be maintained during dissection of the chordee; repeat the erection to check after the chordee has been corrected.

SURGICAL TECHNIQUE

The tissue must be handled delicately if the operation is to succeed. The surgeon must know how to mobilize skin flaps while preserving all their vasculature and tissue viability. "Intern" with a pediatric urologist with a good referral practice so that you can see (and help with) these complex procedures. The diagrams of the operative steps can only be reminders.

Use magnification and pinpoint monopolar electrocautery for dissection. Handle the tissues with microhooks—never with forceps. Crushed tissue cannot heal primarily. Close tubes with precise suturing. Avoid strictures with adequate spatulation, ensuring good blood supply, and avoiding tension.

Use 1 × or 2 × loupes. Less suitable is a 175-mm microscope with the stand placed at the end of the table, although very small sutures (7-0 and 8-0) can be used at this magnification. Use microsurgical instruments and sutures; as confidence is gained, magnification becomes a boon.

For traction, insert a 4-0 silk or chromic catgut suture on a tapered needle vertically in the tip of the glans—not transversely on the dorsum, where it will leave two disturbing scars. Stretch a rubber band around the holding clamp, and fasten it to the drapes to maintain the position of the penis during ventral dissection. Press a finger under the shaft, and use skin hooks to immobilize the penis during this dissection. Clamp the traction suture to the drapes to avoid false rotation.

Close the edges of grafts with running, inverting locking sutures to prevent reefing. Do not close glans flaps too tightly over the new urethra; make these flaps very loose. Remember that the width of the graft in millimeters is equal to the French size. Place subcutaneous sutures where possible to take tension off the skin closure. Use blue-tinted saline injection into the urethra to test for leaks and fistulas.

The possibility of ischemia is reduced if the connective tissue layer underlying a flap is preserved and approximated and if the flaps are not made too long. Of course, suturing under tension impairs the blood supply. Fluorescein is not helpful; it shows inflow of blood but not outflow. Sometimes, the flap or adjacent skin can be salvaged by excising it, removing the subcutaneous tissue, and reapplying it as a full-thickness graft. Avoid lily gilding procedures; however, trimming skin tags is a worthwhile procedure. Opening intradermal suture tracts is done in the office under local anesthesia. For a circumcising incision, place it at the site of the original circumcision, even if that is well down the penile shaft, with the assurance that the blood supply will be coming from both sides. A ventral, vertical incision at the penoscrotal junction will contract and form a drawstring. Use a Z-incision instead. Topical irrigation during the procedure is done with a kanamycin-bacitracin solution, alternating with Normosol-R.

HEMOSTASIS

A solution of 1:100,000 epinephrine in 1 percent lidocaine may be injected through a 27.5-gauge, 1½-inch needle around the corona, meatus, and chordee area. Wait 7 minutes for it to act. This injection will make dissection less bloody, but if the operation is prolonged beyond 90 minutes, rebound vasodilation can be expected. Avoid electrocoagulation; if necessary, use a low-current monopolar unit. Once the skin flaps are applied, bleeding seems to stop, and a pressure dressing will complete the hemostasis.

During the operation, a tourniquet is not necessary for hemostasis. A gauze-covered finger held behind the penis over the dorsal artery provides hemostasis along with support. Some surgeons, however, use a rubber band around the base, releasing it every 20 minutes, even though considerable oozing occurs after release. For this reason, fulguration must be aggressive if it is used.

DISSECTION OF CHORDEE

The severity of chordee roughly parallels the degree of hypospadias. Thus, the majority of boys with the meatus at the corona will have at most a glanular tilt; however, 35 percent have significant chordee.

The major cause of chordee is adherence of the ventral skin to Buck's fascia and the tunica albuginea of the corpora. If chordee persists after skin release, it is caused by corporal disproportion and only can be corrected by a dorsal tuck. Experience teaches that all chordee must be corrected, and that the artificial erection is a boon in ensuring complete correction.

1 Circumcise the corona proximal to the meatus, and expose the tunica albuginea of the corpora cavernosa. Dissect proximally against the tunica under the skin and fibrous dartos causing the chordee while preserving the urethral plate. Use small, blunt-tipped curved scissors, cutting back and forth as you move proximally superficial to the urethral plate to whatever length the dysplasia dictates, even beyond the penoscrotal junction. If necessary, dissect well around the lateral aspects of the glans. Produce an artificial erection to clear any remaining fibrous tissue. If any chordee persists, consider making superficial transverse incisions in the tunica albuginea in the intercorporal groove, or consider incising the septum itself longitudinally and rotating the corpora by placing dorsal plicating sutures that bridge the neurovascular bundle. Be aware of the possibility of corporal disproportion, correctable by dorsal Nesbit-type tucks. The urethral plate must be transected usually only for very severe chordee without hypospadias, and the urethra completed with a tubed flap. Unwanted spontaneous erections will subside with sublingual nitroglycerine (which produces headaches) or by the injection of 0.2 ml of a 1:100,000 solution of epinephrine in normal saline into one corpus through a butterfly needle.

SUTURING

For the skin and subcutaneous tissues, absorbable sutures are best, because they do not require anesthesia for removal. Useful is 7-0 chromic catgut for the skin. (Colored ophthalmic sutures on a cutting needle are handy.) Catgut sutures are absorbed most rapidly but maintain their strength the longest when exposed to urine. Monocril sutures lubricated with glycerine may be substituted for catgut. Polyglycolic acid sutures are not as good as polyglactic sutures—they last too long and may promote fistulas. Place vertical mattress or subcuticular sutures in the skin if necessary to avoid overlapping or inverting the edges. For deep sutures, polydioxanone has the disadvantage that it loses strength most rapidly when exposed to urine, especially infected urine; polyglycolic sutures are better. Coat the suture with mineral oil to allow easier passage of synthetic sutures through the tissues. Tissue glues (Tisseel) may have a place in skin closure.

MUCOSAL GRAFTS

For the rare complicated case in which sufficient preputial skin is not available, bladder epithelium or buccal mucosa may be substituted. Harvesting the mucosa is straightforward, but the application of the graft may be more difficult than for skin. The technique is suitable for midurethral repair not extending to the tip and also for complete substitution if a 1-cm preputial skin tube is used for the terminal part to prevent weeping and stenosis that would require regular self-dilation for 3 or 4 months postoperatively. The bladder must be large enough to allow the harvest of adequate epithelium for a graft.

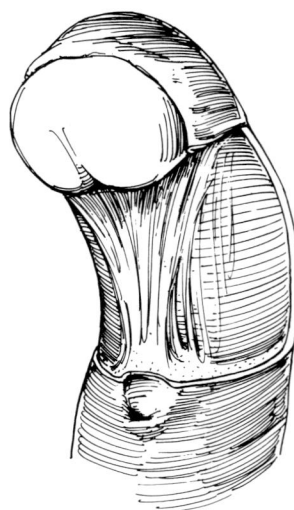

Bladder Epithelial Graft

2 **A,** Carry the correction of the hypospadias as far as possible before obtaining the graft. Insert a catheter or place a perineal urethrostomy. Distend the bladder with saline solution or air. Make a transverse lower abdominal incision (page 261) and retract the rectus muscles. Incise the exposed anterior surface of the bladder, just to the underlying epithelium. Peel the muscle from it with scissors and peanut dissectors to expose an area of suitable size for the graft.

B, Mark the outline of the graft with a skin-marking pen before the bladder is entered. Make the outline wide to allow for loss during suturing, usually 10 percent longer and 20 percent wider than needed, but realize that, in contrast with skin grafts, it will not shrink appreciably after placement. Place traction sutures at the four corners. Excise the graft with scissors along the marks. Obtain a 1 × 2 cm full-thickness graft from the prepuce, and clear it of subcutaneous tissue. Suture the two grafts together to form one long graft. Trim the epithelial portion of the graft to length. Proceed at once to roll the combined graft around a 12 to 14 F silicone tube stent, and suture it with an inverting, running, lock stitch of 7-0 synthetic absorbable suture. Be sure to have the scrub nurse keep the graft constantly moist.

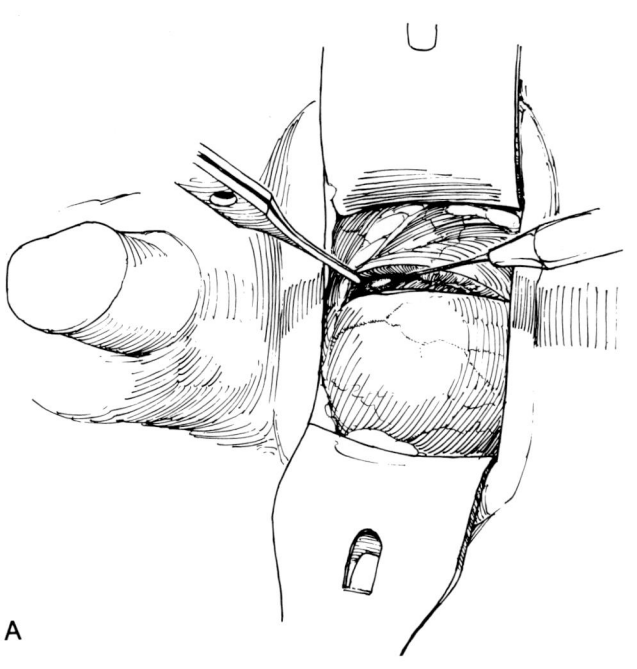

A

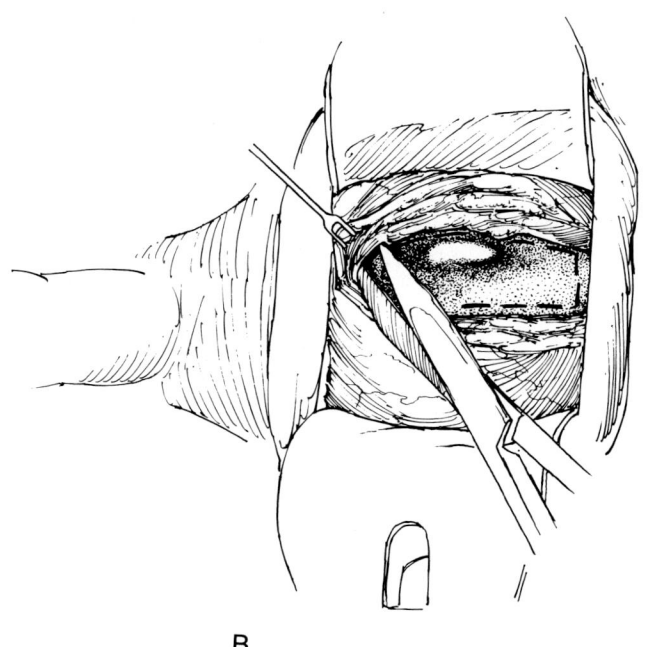

B

3 Insert a Malecot catheter in the bladder, and bring it out through a stab wound. Close the bladder in one layer; do not attempt mucosal approximation. Your assistant can be doing this at the same time that you apply the graft. Place a Penrose drain. Dress the penis and immobilize it with plastic foam. Do not remove the stent earlier than the 10th postoperative day, because the healing process takes considerably longer for this thin graft. Sponge the meatus with neosporin before the boy makes the first void. If voiding is then satisfactory, remove the cystostomy tube on the same day. In most cases, the parents will need to dilate the urethra at home with a tapered sound.

Complications include stenosis of all or part of the graft, diverticula, as well as proximal and distal strictures. Fistulas are uncommon, but protruding bladder epithelium has been a problem, which is reduced by stretching and trimming the graft at the meatus before suture.

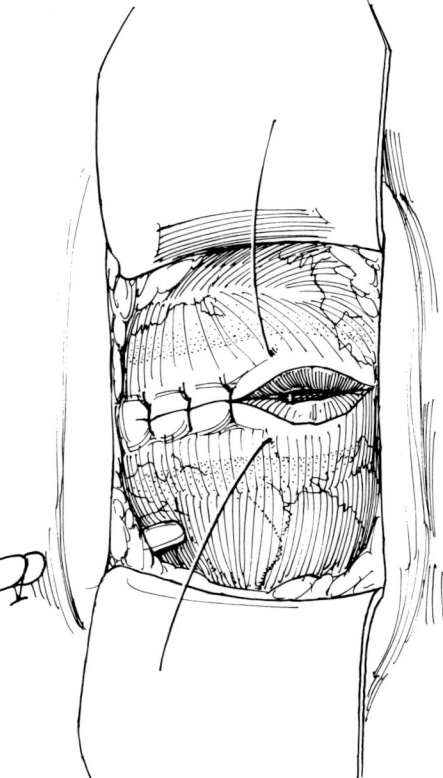

Buccal Mucosal Graft

4 The graft may be obtained from either the inner cheek or the inner surface of the upper or lower lip. Because the mouth cannot be sterilized, the graft will hold bacteria, but this has not been found to be clinically important. Intubate the child nasally during anesthesia and identify the parotid duct. Insert a mouth gag (Steinhauser mucosal retractor).

Injecting a mixture of 1 part epinephrine and 100,000 parts of 1 percent lidocaine beneath the mucosa may facilitate dissection and reduce bleeding. Sponge the surface and outline the graft with a marking pen. **A,** On the lip, mark a flap up to 4 cm long and 1.3 cm wide.

B, On the cheek it may be wider, extending from the parotid duct orifice to the inferior vestibular fold, but seldom is longer than 5 or 6 cm. Both cheeks may be used if a large graft is required. In any case, two strips may be sutured together side to side to make a wider graft or end to end to make a longer one. It is desirable to have the graft 10 percent larger than the urethral defect. Place four fine sutures at the corners of the graft to elevate the edges, so that the mucosa will not be traumatized with forceps. Incise the margins with a #15 blade. Dissect just beneath the submucosa to avoid obtaining too thick a graft, and watch out for the parotid duct in the cheek opposite the second molar tooth. The buccal neurovascular bundle lies in the buccinator muscle, and the facial nerve runs beneath it, so this layer should not be entered. Obtain hemostasis with pressure; bleeding postoperatively may be controlled by internal pressure and external ice packs. Trim any remaining fat from the cheek graft; this will foster quick imbibition. The lip graft is thicker and, consequently, stiffer. If the graft is too thick, try to remove some of the submucosa, although this may be difficult. A sticky protruding meatus is not created by buccal grafts, so a meatal skin patch is unnecessary.

The defect in the lip does not require closing; instead apply benzocaine (Orabase). The cheek wound may be closed with a running 5-0 chromic catgut suture. Regular mouthwashing with povidone-iodine solution renders infection a rare complication.

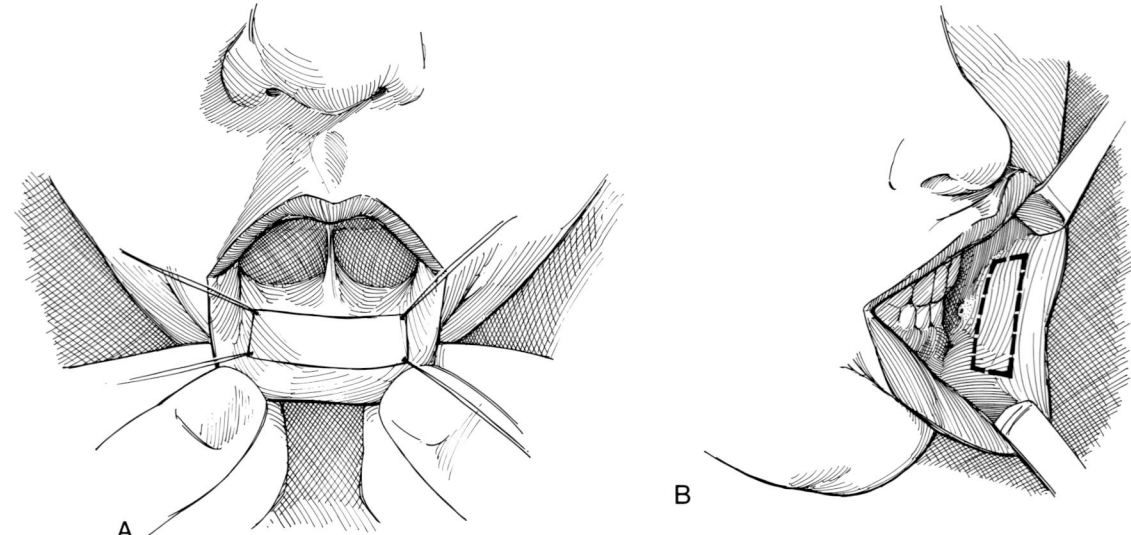

5 For urethral lengthening, spatulate the proximal end of the graft, insert the stent into the proximal urethra, and suture the graft to the urethra over a 12 or 14 F sound at a site that can be covered readily with subcutaneous tissue and skin. Use running 7-0 chromic catgut sutures. Tunnel the graft through the glans, or, preferably, split the glans to cover the graft with two flaps of vascularized tissue and skin. Be sure the channel is large enough. Suture the distal end to the glans. Secure the stent to the glans with a stitch. Cover the graft with previously mobilized penile skin. For forming a urethral tube, apply the graft to a catheter of suitable size, with the mucosa inside and the suture line dorsally. Run a 7-0 synthetic absorbable suture to approximate the edges, but do not go too close to the ends, because a spatulated anastomosis is desirable. Suture the proximal end to the spatulated urethral stump with interrupted fine sutures, and bring the distal end to the tip of the glans either by tunneling or by forming two flaps. Cover with local skin.

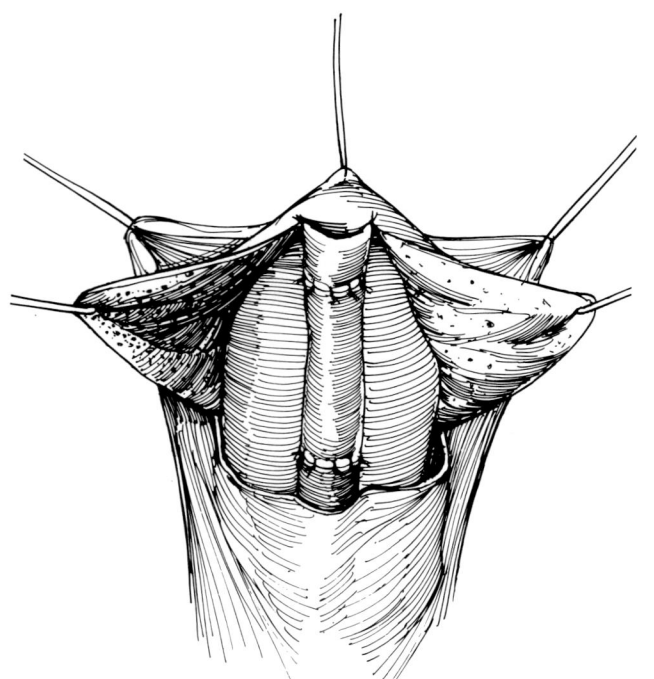

6 Test the repair before closure of the skin. Fill the bladder and press on the abdomen. Alternatively, instill dilute methylene blue into the meatus with a blunt-tipped syringe while compressing the urethra proximal to the repair.

A, Another testing technique is to introduce an 18-gauge angiocatheter into the tip of the suction tube at the level of the penoscrotal junction. Withdraw the suction tube and the trocar of the angiocatheter, leaving the plastic catheter in the lumen.

B, Attach a 20-ml syringe and inject saline to test the integrity of the repair. The addition of a little methylene blue to the saline helps detect tiny fistulas.

A diet of soft food and daily cleansing of the mouth with povidone-iodine solution are advised.

Complications include damage to the buccal neuro-vascular bundle by dissecting the buccinator (damage to the facial nerve that lies deep to the buccinator is highly unlikely). Bleeding is corrected by resuturing under cover of local anesthesia. For infection, usually in a hematoma, removal of the sutures will drain the area, and antibiotics will control the infection.

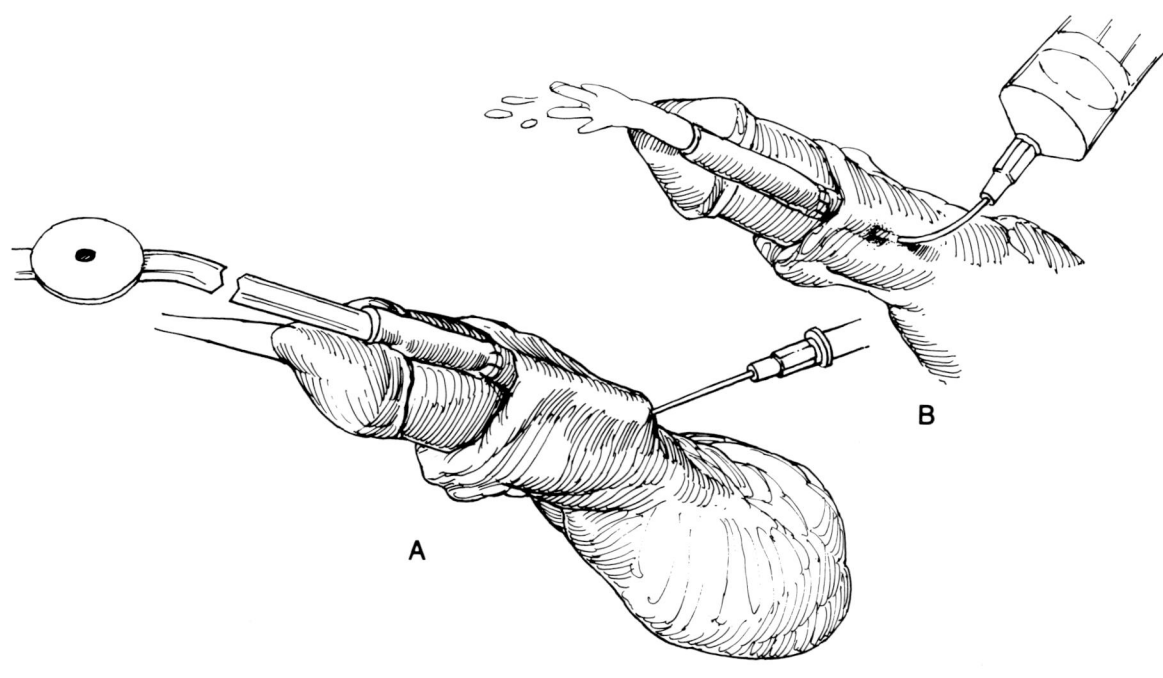

URINARY DIVERSION

Diversion of urine away from the suture lines always has been a problem, because tubes induce bladder spasms. Many techniques have been tried to minimize them. Whatever system is used in infants, collect urine in a double diaper. Young children will tolerate a tube that terminates in the bulbous urethra, but in older children, voiding becomes painful. A catheter ending in the bladder, especially one with a balloon, stimulates bladder spasms that force urine out around it.

Select the type of urinary drainage suitable to the site of repair, so that voiding will not occur during the early period. The simplest method, one that combines stenting with drainage, is to insert a fine silicone tube, such as 6 F neurosurgical shunt tubing (Firlit-Kluge) with its wandlike end, into the bladder through the urethra until it just starts to drain; trim it 3 cm from the meatus, and fasten the end to the glans in two places with nonabsorbable sutures. Leaving a long stay suture on the end to be taped to the abdomen is extra insurance against upward migration. Let the tube drip into the diaper. Inserting it only to the bulbous urethra maintains continence in older boys but causes pain on voiding.

7 **A,** As an alternative to diversion, make a tube from a length of Silastic tubing sufficient to reach from 1 cm above the repair to the meatus by cutting a longitudinal strip from it that removes a fourth of the tube's circumference (Mitchell and Kalb, 1986). Trim both ends obliquely.

B, Insert the tube with neurologic forceps, cut it flush, and suture it to the meatus with two fine nonabsorbable sutures. Test for patency by passing a 5 F or 8 F infant feeding tube through it. If necessary, this tube also can serve to drain the bladder. Alternatively, cut a Mentor stent into 5-in segments, sterilize one of them with gas, and use it as a stent. Do not be concerned if the child delays voiding for 24 hours. Remove the stent in 9 days.

A balloon catheter should never be used. It leads to infections and does not allow for a trial of voiding. The balloon usually rests on the trigone and produces excessive bladder spasm, whether it is used for perineal, urethral, or suprapubic drainage. Also, it has a small lumen, compared with a straight catheter, especially a plastic one. If used, allow it to drain between a double layer of diaper. Because the smaller tube tends to obstruct, suprapubic trocar cystostomy, although not as secure as open cystostomy, provides better drainage. For a trocar cystostomy, use an 8 F Cystocath, and allow it to drip in an outer diaper. Perineal urethrostomy (page 350) rarely is needed. Bladder spasms can disrupt a repair; give suppositories of methantheline bromide and opium, one third of one daily.

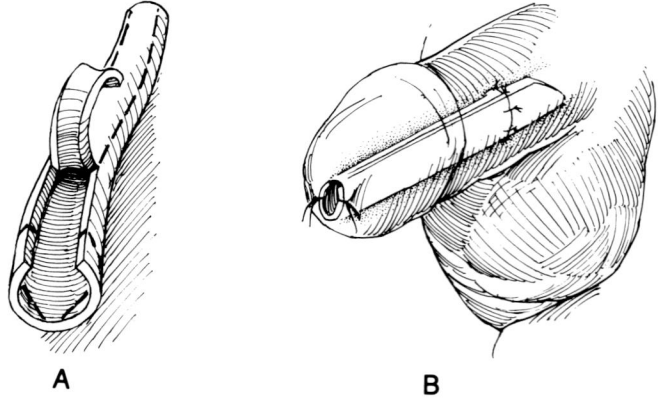

A   B

8 *Drains:* Use a drain only if hemostasis is unsatisfactory and a hematoma appears imminent. Make a suction drain from a butterfly needle with the adapter cut off and holes cut in that end (Devine). Insert the tubing subcutaneously, and place the butterfly needle into a sterilized vacuum blood collection tube.

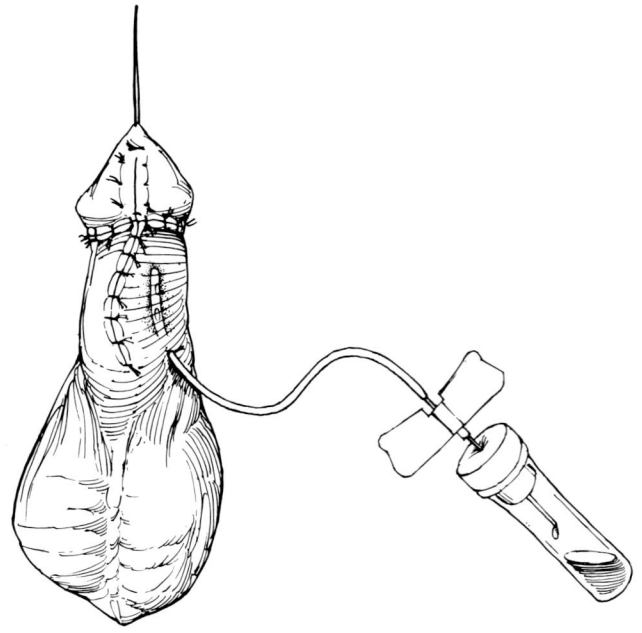

DRESSINGS

Apply a dressing to immobilize the area and prevent edema and hematoma. An improper dressing can cause the best operation to fail. Two types are in use: concealing and nonconcealing. In any case, mineral oil applied to the skin will reduce adherence of the dressing. Concealing dressings immobilize the area, provide some pressure, and are comfortable, but they prevent inspection. They may be partially or totally concealing, depending on the layers and the taping. Impregnated (Xeroform) gauze is covered with fluffs held in place with elastic adhesive (Elastoplast). One modification consists of covering the penis with a 4 × 8 in gauze sponge that does not encircle it completely, held in place by 2-in elastic adhesive tape splayed out dorsally to adhere to the pubic area, which is prepared with tincture of benzoin. Another popular modification uses an absorbent plastic film (Tegaderm or Op-Site) applied over Telfa gauze or tincture of benzoin. The glans can be left exposed for inspection, although this probably is not necessary. The dressing may be removed in 3 to 4 days. For a nonconcealing dressing for hospitalized boys, apply cotton padding over absorbent plastic film, and keep it wet with cold saline. Order a change of dressing three times a day. Edema is reduced, and the wound is readily inspected; however, more work is required.

POSTOPERATIVE CARE

Consider providing a caudal block with bupivacaine at the end of the operation. Give analgesics, such as acetaminophen, and antispasmodics, such as meperidine with promethazine (Demerol with Phenergan), atropine sulfate, or oxybutynin (Ditropan). Opium-belladonna suppositories cut in thirds longitudinally are effective. Trimethoprim (Septra) may be given for 3 days. In some cases, one may need to have the parents insert the nozzle tip of a small ophthalmic ointment tube into the meatus daily. Although one can calibrate the urethra with a small caliber sound or a bougie à boule in the office in 2 weeks (a painful procedure), a proper repair should maintain caliber without interference. See the child and remove the dressing in 3 to 7 days. The penis should be soaked in the bathtub daily thereafter. If the child is sent home with a stent in place, the instructions to the parents include its care and an appointment to return in 10 to 14 days for stent removal. If a suprapubic tube was necessary, remove it in 14 days. Check and observe the repair and observe the stream at 1, 2, 4, and 6 weeks, and then in 6 months, 1 year, 3 years, and 6 years.

Commentary by R. Lawrence Kroovand

The issue of whether residents should learn how to perform hypospadias repair is one that I have been wrestling with for a long time. I think that a lot of residents who have trained at a variety of programs over the past 5 to 10 years feel that they can perform practically any type of urologic procedure. As far as hypospadias repair is concerned, in many programs, the pediatric urologist may draw out the flaps and allow the resident to perform most or all of the dissection and to place most of the sutures. This practice clearly gives a resident a sense of having performed the hypospadias repair itself, when in reality, he or she probably does not understand many of the nuances involved in the surgical procedure. Thus, in a urology residency, I think it is appropriate for residents who are interested in going into pediatric urology or who are technically adept to perform parts of hypospadias repairs, but I do not think that they should be allowed to think that they have the judgment and experience necessary to perform these repairs on a regular basis.

POSTOPERATIVE PROBLEMS

It is probable that the result obtained from hypospadias repair is optimum if the surgeon, although he or she may have a limited repertoire, uses those techniques that are not only based on sound principles but are ones known from experience to be well done.

Bladder spasms not only cause a child to move about with pain but also cause urine to be forced through the repair. Stop antispasmodic drugs before removing the catheter. Do not reinsert the catheter should it fall out; if necessary, insert a cystostomy percutaneously.

Constipation may result from the antispasm regimen and lead to straining and urine leakage. It is important to give stool softeners and recommend a suitable diet.

Bleeding is not a common problem. If hemostasis has been incomplete, insertion of a miniature vacuum drain and application of a mild occlusive dressing will control the ooze. Be sure to remove any hematoma first, and do not apply the dressing too tightly.

Hemorrhage usually can be arrested by compression but may require reopening the wound.

Infection begins after injury to the tissues; therefore, be gentle during the operation. Preoperative genital scrubs, perhaps perioperative antibiotics, and washing with povidone-iodine solution in the operating room help. Tub baths may be used if the operated area appears inflamed.

Devitalization of skin flaps from ischemia may not result in failure if the underlying structures are well vascularized. Edema is inevitable but controlled by a pressure dressing. An *erection* in a postpubertal patient is a problem best controlled with amyl nitrite inhalants. Diethylstilbestrol is of no value.

Ischemia of skin flaps results from taking too small a flap and creating tension or from removing too much of its underlying support and blood supply. Look for blanching during suturing from excessive tension and an absence of bleeding from the cut edge, a situation that will lead to local necrosis. Take special care with the wings of the split glans—any separation of them creates a fistula. Treat a fistula acutely, as you would a wound separation. Use sterile adhesive strips; alternatively, one later can try breaking a piece of silver nitrate from a stick and applying it to the fistula to destroy the epithelium. If *wound separation* occurs on removal of the dressing, reapproximate the edges with sterile adhesive strips, although a later repair usually is necessary. Edema from rough handling of the tissues is the usual cause and, of course, could have been avoided.

Late complications are meatal retraction or stenosis, stricture, fistula formation, persistent chordee, stones or hair in the urethra, and formation of a diverticulum. Meatal stenosis can be corrected by advancing the urethral epithelium, if there is enough of it, or by splitting the terminal urethra ventrally, using the MAGPI technique. A persistent proximal stricture that does not respond to one dilation or to visual urethrotomy and a stent should be marsupialized and later repaired as a fistula, usually with an island flap. Small fistulas usually will close spontaneously. Wait 6 months, dissect them out, close them, and cover them with collodion in a come-and-go procedure. Look for distal narrowing in each case. For two-stage procedures, watch for penile rotation.

Commentary by Norman B. Hodgson

General Comments. The essence of hypospadias repair is adapting the available tissues to the needs of the child. This has been expressed in a seeming endless variety of ways in which there is a common thread: in most of the depictions and descriptions, the focus is in the cuticular layer. That has always limited the perception of the choices. From my perspective, the emphasis should be on the quality of the dartos and the attendant blood vessels. I know that is hard to depict, but it is the determining factor in outcome expectancy (a 1990s buzzword), and it defines the choice of operation (there now are approximately 220 different techniques).

Imagine the frustration of Ormond Culp with his watershed of cases. The tissues had been manipulated, large chromic sutures had been used with resultant scarring, the chordee was still there, there were holes around and about, the instrumentation was gross, and latex was the material for drainage. In his gentle, offbeat manner, he was able to dissuade the uninitiated from attacking the formidable. As consulting editor for the *Journal of Urology* in the 1960s, he was responsible for delaying the introduction of one-stage repairs until Bill Scott came to Milwaukee for a visit and was shown a group of children. The delay was for the best, because those were the formative years.

The learning curve of tissue management always will demand sufficient case material for growth. This dictates that not everyone will do these procedures; rather, one surgeon per million patients will tend to, and should, do them all.

Hypospadiac disability continues to occur but in sharply declining numbers. Thankfully, most of the repairs are done in some variation of a single-stage procedure. Most children are handled as outpatients or with brief hospitalizations. The overall cost of management has been sharply reduced. All in all, the management of the problem has

(thanks to our evangelists) become a success story in hands across the world. Still, the writings and subtle variations continue to surface. Tissue glues and other sealants are used by some surgeons. I am constantly amazed at the subtleties that God provides to guide the appropriate choice. The variations in the raphe, the redundancy of the dimples, the arching of the axial vessels, the density of the prepuce, the elasticity of the dartos and the skin, the configuration and size of the glans, the "in your face" fibrosis of chordee (here I am, take me, but do it right) all connive to challenge the intellect and hands of the operator. It must be frustrating to the uninitiated and uninterpretable to the disinterested.

Comments on One-Stage Hypospadias Repairs. Fortunately, knowledge regarding one-stage repairs is well disseminated so that the appropriate choices and nuances that seemed subtle now can achieve an appropriate focus. The concept that the child selects his own operation is quite true, because the combination of chordee and preputial distribution predicts the choices and eventual outcome. The quality of the tissue, as witnessed through the dartos, limits the choices and defines the character of the healing process.

I start with an incision tracing the raphe as it splits into its diversion to the preputial hood. I then carry it back toward the coronal margin, as suggested by Firlit, to provide for Firlit flaps, which may be swung onto the ventrum for covering. The tissues are valuable but not universally applicable, so they may or may not come into play in the final closure. This incision then allows mobilization of the shaft skin and visualization of the dysplastic bifurcated corpus spongiosum. At this juncture, an artificial erection demonstrates the components of the chordee. Does this involve glans tilt, fibrous dysplasia of the spongiosum, or, indeed, corporal disproportion? All of these can be elements in the presentation of curvature and disfigurement. Resolution of chordee proceeds.

Having accomplished that, the release of the glans wings can then guide the surgeon toward the repair.

The surgeon is obligated on the ventrum to remove thin cutis lateral of the midline and not join the urethral meatus to the tip of the glans. These tissues are dysplastic and will not serve the repair well. Their dartos is thin or nonexistent, and attempting to sew these will add only frustration. At this point, the best procedure for the child can be determined. The initial appraisal will rule in or out the glandular reconstruction procedure, such as the Arap or Zaontz, (notice that is an A-to-Z alphabetical order) for it has been described repeatedly by a number of different surgeons and is only occasionally (*ie*, rarely) of value. The child must present with just the right amount of tissue to allow the tubularization to proceed. The covering tissues ordinarily will have to come from elsewhere, and even with the tiny sutures now available may well experience impaired healing. These procedures are relatively straightforward in their presentation, but because of their simplicity, will be more commonly chosen than they should be.

Similarly, the Mathieu procedure demands an excellent dartos layer for covering of the suture line, and this is not as commonly present as one would hope. When it is sparse, supplemental denuded rotational flaps can be brought from either side but this might create problems in glans closure or bulk. Thus, the natural attention is directed toward the two-faced preputial flap. Its transposition to the ventrum depends on the vessel supply and distribution, which can be defined by transillumination. It can be developed on the ventrum with preputial extension with meatal continuity (Broadbent), by mobilized patches (Hinderer, Orandi), or from a fully mobilized flap on the dorsum. If a hinged flap is rotated at the ventrum by a transverse incision of the prepuce at the coronal margin (Hodgson IV, Asopa), the tissues fall to the ventrum, and the strip selected may come from the inner face, the verge, or the first part of the outer face. Choice is made according to the thickness of the tissue and the width of the strip needed. This can be isolated by incision or excision to provide the necessary dartos healing surface.

An axial incision can be made down into the prepuce to select a tangential flap, if the tissues so align (Hodgson XX). Lastly, its double pedicle creates ventral problems (ventral tissue abundance) that may be hard to resolve.

In my multiple writings, I chose a series of numbers to outline these choices, but they reflect mainly the options of the two-faced flap.

Suture choice will depend on the individual surgeon, and each have their proponents, but all of the suture is fine at 6-0, 7-0, and 8-0. Subcuticular inverted knots for skin closure with no sutures penetrating the skin are now in vogue.

Currently, I accomplish urinary diversion with a Kluge-Firlit tube, which is remarkably well tolerated by the bladder and less prone to produce bladder spasms. In our setting, urine continues to be collected in double diaper. The patient is an outpatient.

Buccal flaps seem to have an advantage over bladder epithelium or free skin grafts. On the other hand, preputial tissue continues to be the first choice.

A mobilized inner face flap (Duckett) is available for the longer defects but has been used less commonly in recent years.

There is an abundance of choices that follow these same principles, all going to the same end. Most young surgeons have these options in their armamentarium, so it will be fascinating to see which ones they ultimately select.

Commentary by E. Durham Smith

More than 300 operative techniques for the repair of hypospadias have been described, and any author clearly has a selection problem to be able to describe appropriate techniques in a short chapter. In this chapter, Dr. Hinman handles this well by not urging any particular technique—rather, he provides the essential points of surgical technique common to all repairs. Details of the construction of the neourethra are found in subsequent chapters.

Accordingly, this commentary focuses mainly on two areas: chordee correction and the selection of operative techniques appropriate to the clinical situation.

Chordee. The assessment of chordee and its total correction is far more important than the actual site of the urethral orifice, which changes after chordee is corrected, a point made in the text. Also stressed is that the major cause of chordee is adherency of ventral skin to underlying structures. The old concept that chordee was a central white fibrous band distal to the orifice defied experience, in that most of us could never find it! Two points should be stressed. First, the whole shaft of the penis should be exposed by a 38-degree circumferential cut of prepuce and penile skin, freeing all skin back to the base of the penis or beyond. This is because most of the chordee structures are *proximal* to the orifice, not distal to it. Second, the surgeon needs to deal with each element of the chordee in a progressive seriatim manner—free all skin first; in most cases, this is all that is required. Recheck for chordee by artificial

erection or simply by placing traction with the fingers on the *lateral* shaft of the penis. If there is still chordee, dissect fibrous tissue from the corporal tunica (a vascular exercise) or in the intercorporeal groove. If chordee persists, the urethra itself may require release from its distal site to a more proximal position. Finally, although not performed until a later step of the repair, the ventral deficiency of skin is made up by transference of dorsal preputial and penile skin to the ventral side.

The text suggests that in severe chordee without hypospadias, the urethra may need to be transected. Years ago, when the importance of skin tethering was not appreciated, transection was commonly performed. In recent years, I have not found this necessary on a single occasion, although it may be required in rare cases.

Selection of Technique. The inevitable argument of one-stage versus two-stage repairs continues. No one could argue that, given the right circumstances, the completion of a repair in one stage is preferable to submitting the child to two operations. However, the key to the debate is "the right circumstances." Unfortunately, an attitude has been fostered, especially in the United States, often with evangelistic zeal, that one-stage repair is sacrosanct and must be attempted at all times, whereas two-stage repair is reactionary, conservative, and out of context with modern surgical techniques. The result is a plethora of techniques of increasing complexity to "bridge the gap" in efforts to complete the repair in one stage, including long pedicle tubes, and free bladder and buccal mucosal grafts. These techniques are more difficult to perform and potentially carry more surgical hazards. They are dexterously performed with beautiful results in certain centers of excellence where the volume of cases is large and the surgeons have immense experience. But it is quite a different matter to advocate such repairs for the larger bulk of surgeons, who may see fewer than 15 patients with hypospadias a year. It is simply not possible to develop the necessary operative skills for such complex procedures on such a clinical volume. The bad results of such a policy are all too plain to see as one travels the world to many centers. A failed one-stage repair is not necessarily a minor complication but often a complex problem requiring a complete redo, perhaps in multiple stages.

For the surgeon of moderate or small experience, a technique is required that is simple in concept, easy of execution, and absolutely reliable in results. These objectives are achievable by certain types of two-stage repairs. Furthermore, the acceptance of the two-stage concept also simplifies the operative choices; in fact, the technique described by this commentator can, if necessary, be a "universal" operation, applicable to any clinical situation. Only one technique is required to be learned, and expertise thus can be maintained, even with a small clinical volume. Having to perform two relatively uncomplicated operations, each requiring less than 45 minutes in the operating room, is a small price to pay for a constantly predictable result, especially because one or both stages can be done on an outpatient basis. Compare this with the multiple hours of complex operation required to construct mucosal free grafts or pedicle tubes, the surgical hazards of blood supply to such tubes, the presence of an anastomosis, the complexity of instrumentation, and so forth, all in an effort to save one stage. For these reasons, one applauds the author's statement, "one-stage procedure is best, but a staged procedure is better than being forced to redo."

This is not to say that one-stage repairs should never be done. I do one-stage repairs; however, the guidelines of choice are not dictated by prejudice but by specific clinical features. One, as mentioned, is the experience of the surgeon. Another is the extent of the chordee, and a third, not mentioned in the text of this chapter, is the shape of the glans and depth of the central ventral groove. The significance of the latter is that a wide, splayed glans with a deep groove is an optimum precurser of a flip-flap repair, because it permits the closure of the glans tissue over the tube; conversely, a narrow cone-shaped glans with a shallow groove makes this difficult and is likely to result in a stricture.

I have no serious disagreement with the author's recommendations regarding selection of technique, except for the choice of pedicle island tubes for those with marked chordee. Pedicle tubes in Duckett's hands are superb, but in *principle,* transferred tubes (either on a pedicle or as free grafts) involve the complexity of an anastomosis, a more precarious blood supply than a Duplay tube constructed of penile and preputial skin already *in situ,* and no anastomosis, as in this commentator's technique.

Recommendations. My recommendations are simple:

1. An orifice in the coronal groove or more distal in the glans and minimal chordee—one-stage MAGPI repair.
2. An orifice on the distal shaft or coronal groove with skin-tethering chordee only, and a wide, splayed glans with a deep central groove—one-stage flip-flap repair.
3. A distal orifice with marked chordee and/or cone-shaped narrow glans, all with more proximal orifices either before or after release of chordee—two-stage Smith repair.

The literature does not support the Denis Browne repair or its modifications, scrotal repairs, pedicle tubes in nonexpert hands, and all free grafts. Free grafts have the highest rate of fistula formation and stricture of all repairs.

Hypospadias Disability. Comment is appropriate for the repair of hypospadias disability, *ie,* failed repairs with fistulas, residual chordee, strictures, deformed shape, skin shortage, and so forth. One supports the general concepts of the last paragraph in this chapter. In practice, I find it best to lay the whole repair open back to healthy urethra, and start with a two-stage repair again. It often is said that it may be impossible to construct a tube from existing penile and preputial skin, because previous repairs have created gross deficiency of these tissues. For that reason, intervening grafts, such as bladder mucosa, are recommended. In more than 500 repairs as of 1994 and many scores of cases since, including many people with hypospadias disability I have not once found such a skin deficiency that precluded a Duplay tube, nor has a free graft ever been necessary. There nearly always is some skin laterally or distally that can be mobilized and grafted to the glans as a first stage, but if it cannot, ventral skin always can be found by releasing skin from the dorsum, even to the extent of releasing the whole dorsal surface to the base of the penis. A large dorsal defect is easily closed by a Wolfe free skin graft from the inner thigh, which heals well on the penis. With ample skin now available on the ventral surface, a normal tube *in situ* can be constructed at a second stage. A free graft on the dorsal surface, unrelated to urine flow, is quite a different matter from a free graft within the urinary tract.

Commentator's Two-Stage Repair. The present text includes reference to an important part of this repair—namely, the overlap technique of denuded skin closed as an intermediate layer. With this technique, of 303 cases done before 1978, fistulas occurred in 2.3 percent, and of 200 cases since, the fistula rate was 1 percent (Smith, 1984). From 1984 until my retirement, many additional cases were performed with the same incidence of fistulas.

Other Comments. The recommended age for operation is supported (Smith, 1983), although I prefer the later second window at 2 to 3 years. Fundamental to age and more important that any particular recommended age is the amount of parental and house staff support. Given good parents, well-informed and unflappable, supported by a pediatric milieu in the hospital, the so-called "stress of hospitalization" is minimal at any age; however, the converse also is true.

For control of postoperative pain, we routinely use caudal injection and find it more effective than regional block. A fine-artery hemostat applied to the tip of the penis for stabilization of the penis actually is less traumatic than a suture; the latter often cuts out and leaves more sac than that from the hemostat.

I agree that a penile tourniquet is not necessary, but in the early stages of training the young surgeon, it is a help to be working in a bloodless field.

A Comment About Catheter Drainage. A per-urethral stent that does not reach the bladder is useful, as recommended, but I found some children have pain on voiding. We have standardized the use of a suprapubic stab cystostomy, which is easy to insert and almost never produces bladder spasms. It has no balloon, and it is easy to remove at the bedside. We prefer the Bonnano or Stamey catheter. Bladder spasms are lessened by (1) strapping the catheter firmly to the abdomen so that it cannot move in or out (childproof and nurseproof), (2) low-pressure suction, and (3) acidifying the urine with vitamin C. We do not use any catheter for the first stage of a two-stage repair but routinely use a stab cystostomy for the second stage or for a one-stage flip-flap reconstruction. Both stages can be done on an outpatient basis, certainly for the first stage, but for the second stage with the catheter in place, most parents prefer to leave the child in the hospital. We have not used perineal urethrostomy for more than 15 years.

The text has a long series of techniques for fistula repair. One cannot quarrel with this, except that it obscures the importance of three points: urethral mucosa must be closed separately as one layer, a wide overlap technique of skin closure (commentator's technique, as is used in the second stage of urethral reconstruction) for at least 1 cm proximal and distal to the fistula must be used, and checking for urethral stenosis must be done. I have not used the rather complicated technique described for a simple meatotomy.

REPAIR OF STRICTURES

Strictures and urethrocutaneous fistulas account for most of the late problems after hypospadias repair. Proximal strictures, usually at the site of the proximal anastomosis, should be dilated early. For those strictures not responding to dilation, try direct-vision internal urethrotomy. Excision and anastomosis seldom are applicable, but a patch graft or urethroplasty sometimes can be used. Placing a mesh graft after excising the scar and then returning to perform a Thiersch-Duplay repair may be a means of closing the defect without tension (Schreiter, 1984). As a last resort, a stricture can be exteriorized as a fistula and closed at a second stage.

9 **A,** *Meatotomy:* For secondary stenosis, make a circular incision around the stricture opening. Mobilize the distal end of the urethra for 1 cm. Trim the strictured area.

B, Make three stellate incisions through the thickness of the wall at angles of 60 degrees for 5 to 7 mm. Cut three V-shaped flaps at 60-degree angles on the surrounding skin, and elevate them.

C, Transpose the flaps, and suture the apex of each skin flap to the proximal end of the urethral incision; then suture the apex of the mucosal cut into the appropriate skin incision. Use 5-0 monofilament or chromic catgut sutures. Cover with impregnated gauze after placing a small silicone catheter. Collodion also may be used as a seal.

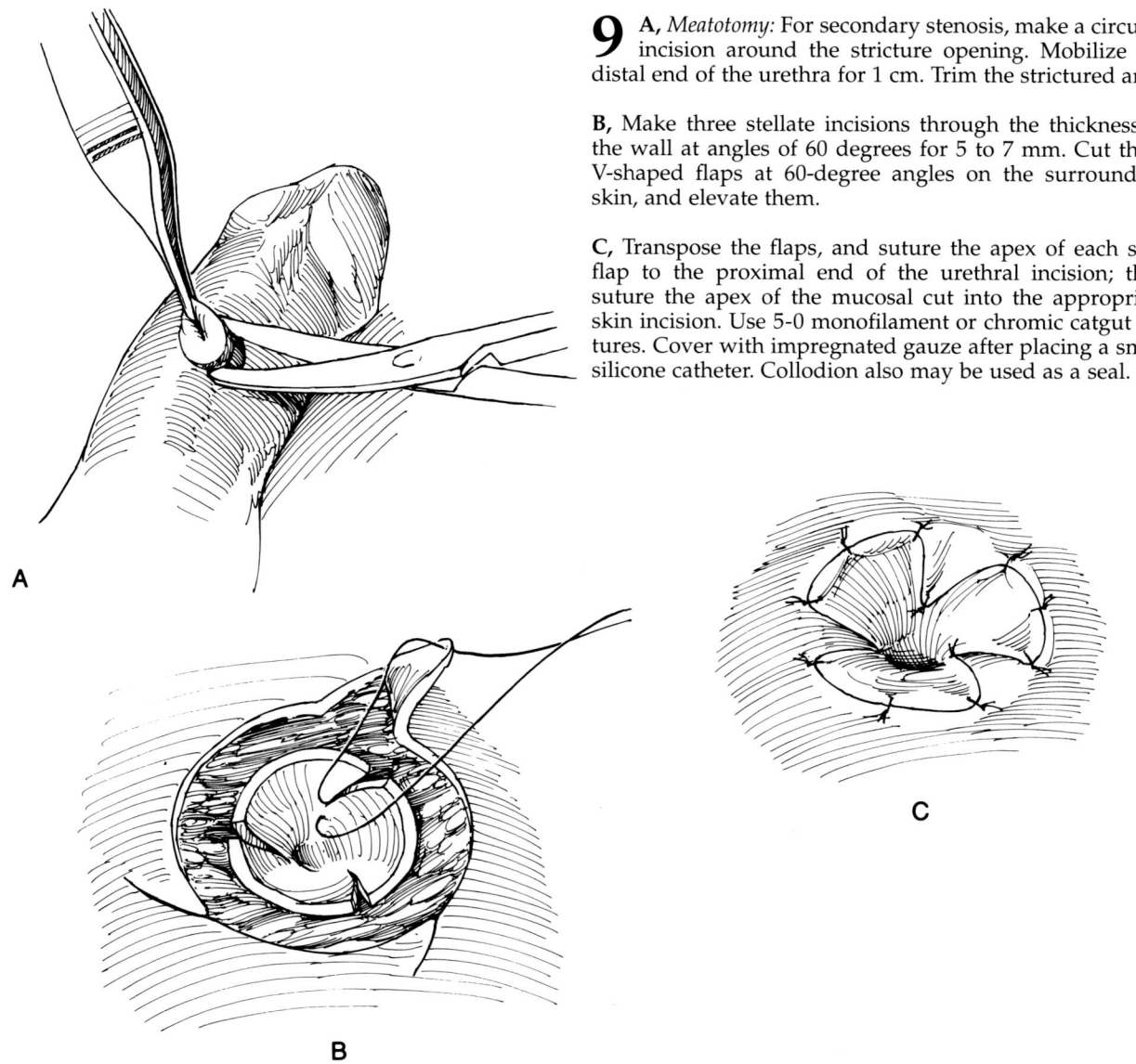

A

B

C

CLOSURE OF URETHROCUTANEOUS FISTULA

Fistulas may be the result of distal obstruction; check this first. They may be secondary to impaired vascular supply to the neourethra, use of nonabsorbable suture material in creating the neourethra, crossing suture lines, using poorly vascularized skin flaps to cover the neourethra, postoperative wound infection, or urinary extravasation. Because of these many factors, closure of a fistula is not always successful, and the success rate falls with the number of attempts. Large defects require a more extensive procedure like a Johanson second-stage urethroplasty. Before resorting to surgical repair, try to apply part of a silver nitrate stick to the opening. If that fails,

try trimming the epithelium from a small fistula, and invert it with a Michel clip, loosely applied.

For repair of larger fistulas, the principle is to avoid overlapping suture lines. Place a traction suture in the glans. Calibrate the urethra with bougie à boule to detect strictures distal to the fistula.

Compress the proximal urethra, and inject dilute methylene blue through a blunt adapter on a 10-ml syringe to inflate the urethra; this may detect more than one fistula, some being very small. Place a suitably sized silicone balloon catheter in the urethra. Insert a lacrimal probe through the fistula to determine its track.

Simple Advancement Flap Closure

10 **A** and **B,** Mark the proposed incision to encircle the fistula on one side and to extend widely beyond the circle laterally on the other side. Do not be afraid to make a large incision. For subcoronal fistulas, make a transverse incision; for those on the shaft, make a longitudinal incision. Also, mark a small flap to draw in the loosest and most normal skin.

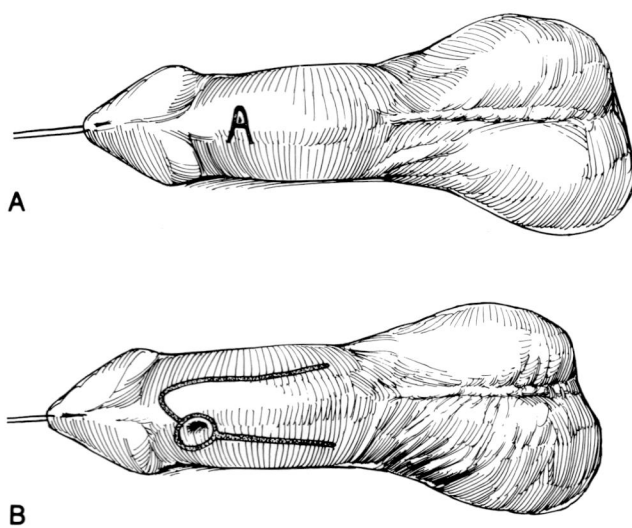

A

B

11 **A,** While wearing a loupe, elevate one skin edge with fine double-pronged skin hooks, and dissect widely with tenotomy scissors to free the skin down to the tract.

B, Continue this dissection around the fistula to its base. Use a needle electrode delicately on the bleeders.

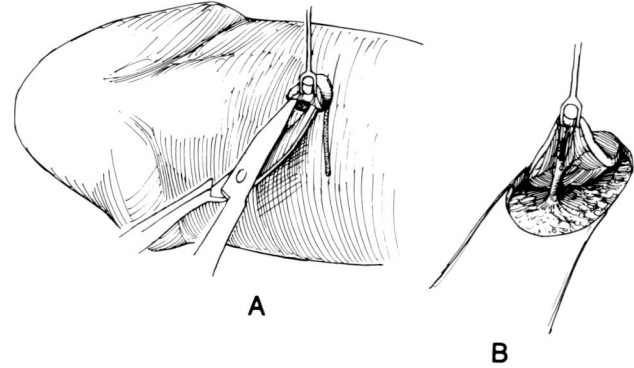

A

B

12 **A** and **B,** Divide the fistula 1 or 2 mm from the urethra, which is identified by the indwelling catheter. Run a 6-0 or 7-0 synthetic absorbable suture across the fistula or, if very small, place two or three interrupted sutures to invert the fistula into the urethra. Start and end the suture well away from the fistula.

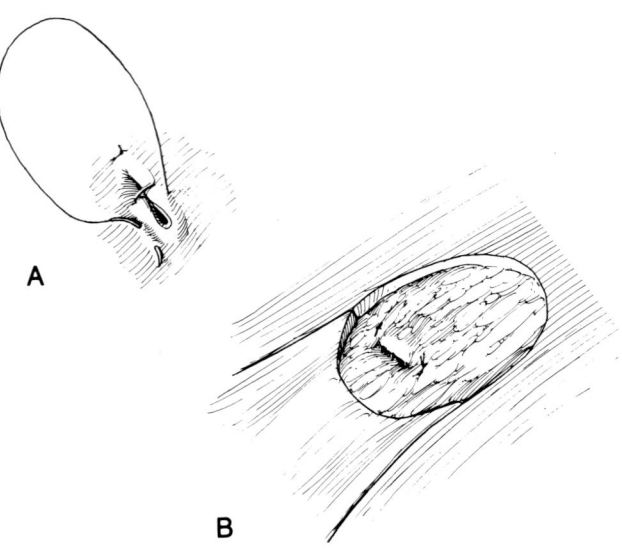

A

B

13 **A,** Incise and raise a generous skin flap. Advance and fasten it to the deep tissue at the far side of the defect with two subcutaneous 4-0 or 5-0 synthetic absorbable sutures. If at all possible, interpose subcutaneous tissue.

B, Close the skin edges with a 5-0 synthetic absorbable suture running subcuticularly around the perimeter. Remove the catheter. Apply a collodion dressing.

For more secure coverage, a rotation flap may be applied (page 44).

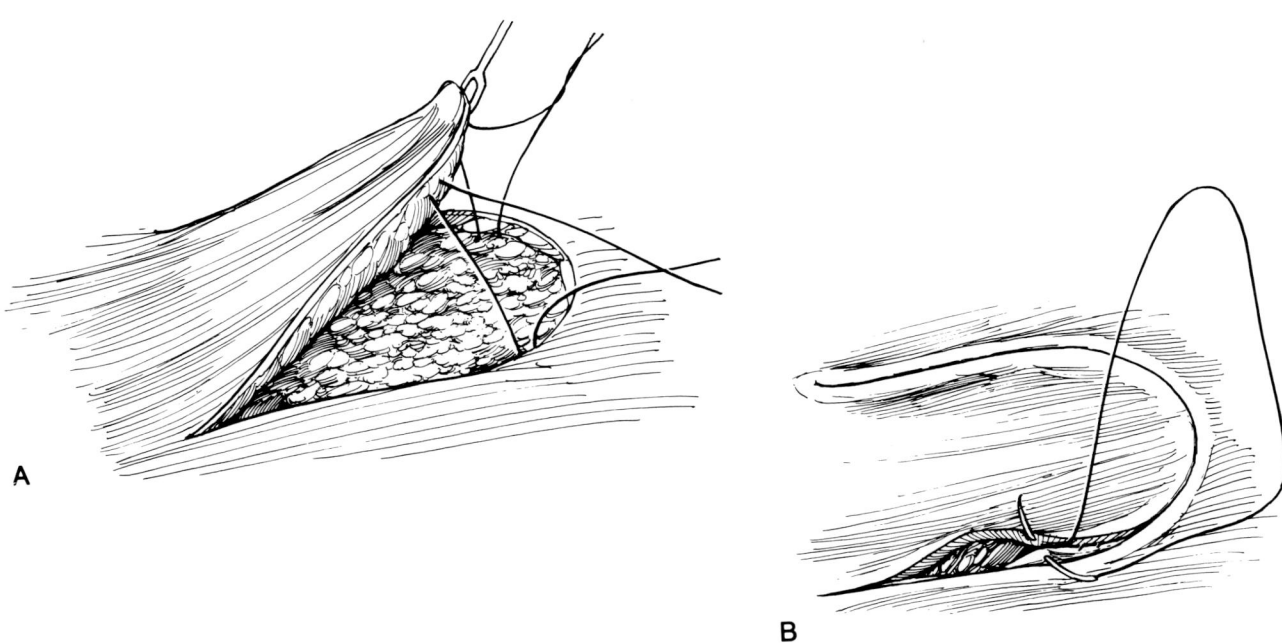

A

B

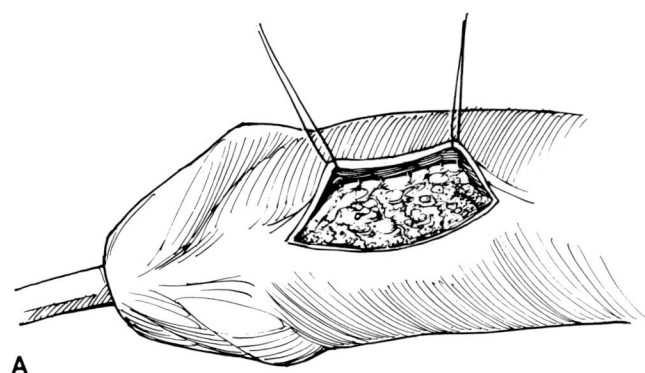

A

De-epithelialized Flap Closure
(Durham Smith)

14 **A,** Alternatively, use a de-epithelialized flap. Make a longer ventral incision, and undermine the flaps laterally, keeping close to the corpora to preserve blood supply. After closing the fistula transversely, remove the epithelium from the surface of one skin flap to create a dermal subcutaneous flap.

B, Suture the edge of this flap across the fistula to the base of the opposite flap. Suture the free skin edge to the line of de-epithelialization.

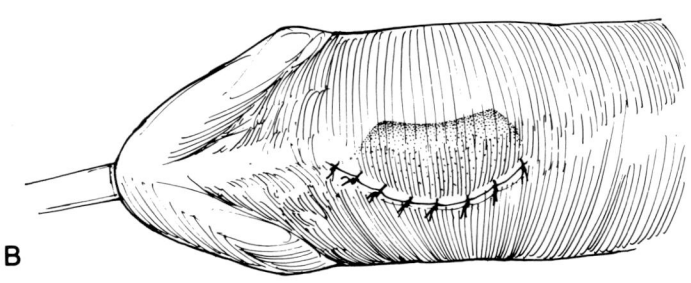

B

Repair of Coronal Fistula

15 **A,** To repair a fistula in the corona, excise the tract through a transverse incision. Free the lateral and proximal skin widely. **B,** Remove the epithelium from the margin of the glans distal to the fistula. Invert the fistula with fine interrupted sutures.

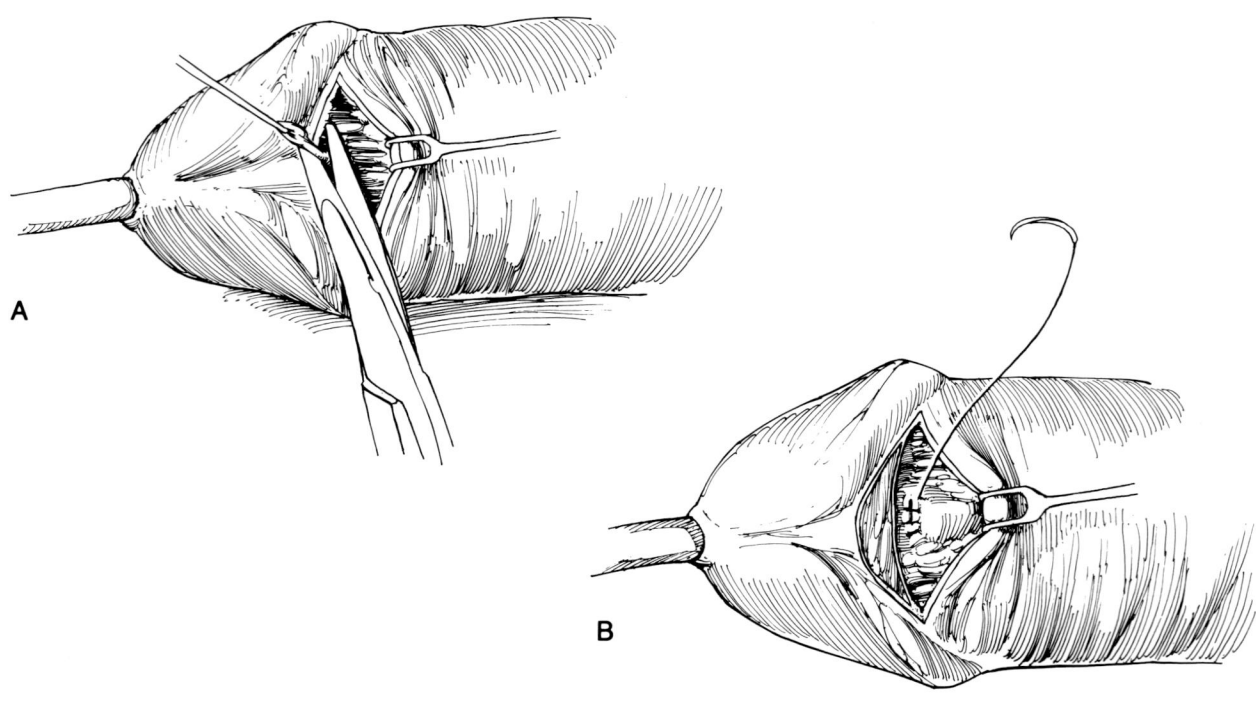

16 **A,** Place a row of 6–0 synthetic absorbable sutures to bring the subcutaneous tissue over the fistula onto the glans.

B, Suture the proximal skin edge to the edge of the denuded glans with 6-0 synthetic absorbable interrupted sutures. Apply a light dressing, and remove the catheter.

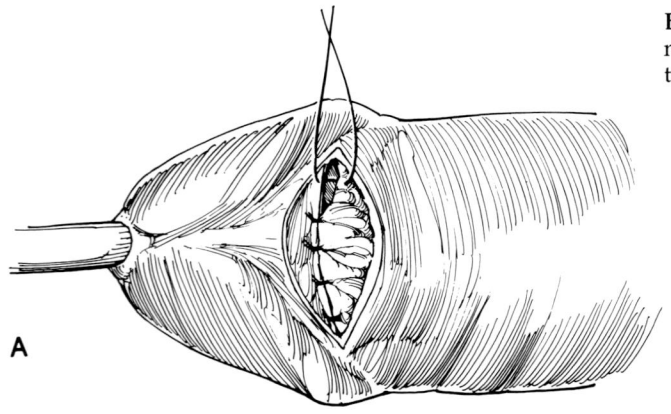

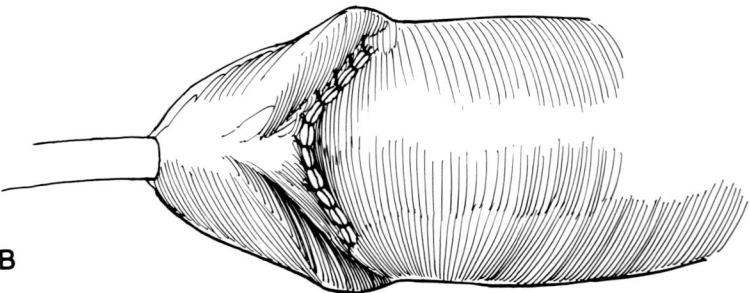

Repair of Scrotal and Perineal Fistulas

Place the child in a frog-legged position with the soles of the feet held in opposition with tape over the arches. Inject dilute methylene blue via the meatus. Press on the bulb to force the dye through one or more fistulas to identify them. Place a metal sound in the urethra.

17 **A,** Mark and incise an asymmetric ellipse of skin around the fistula. **B,** With traction on the skin edges, dissect the tract down to the sound and transect it.

18 **A,** Trim the fistula almost flush with the urethral wall. **B,** Invert the mucosal edge with a running 6-0 synthetic absorbable suture as a subcuticular inverting stitch, so that it will be flush with the urethral lining. **C,** Free enough subcutaneous tissue on one side to cover the defect without tension, and approximate it with 5-0 or 6-0 synthetic absorbable sutures. **D,** Close the skin with interrupted 6-0 synthetic absorbable sutures. Relieve tension, if present, with mattress sutures bolstered on beads. Place a 5-ml silicone balloon catheter into the bladder, if the urethral defect was large.

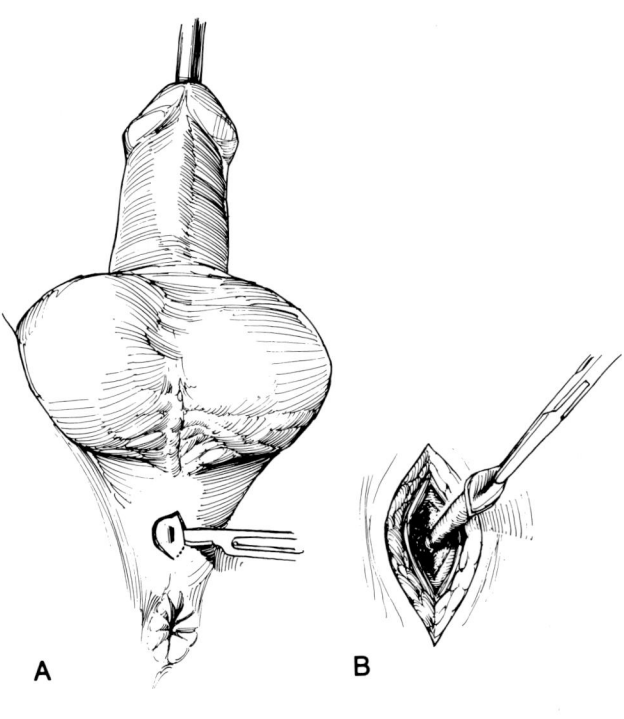

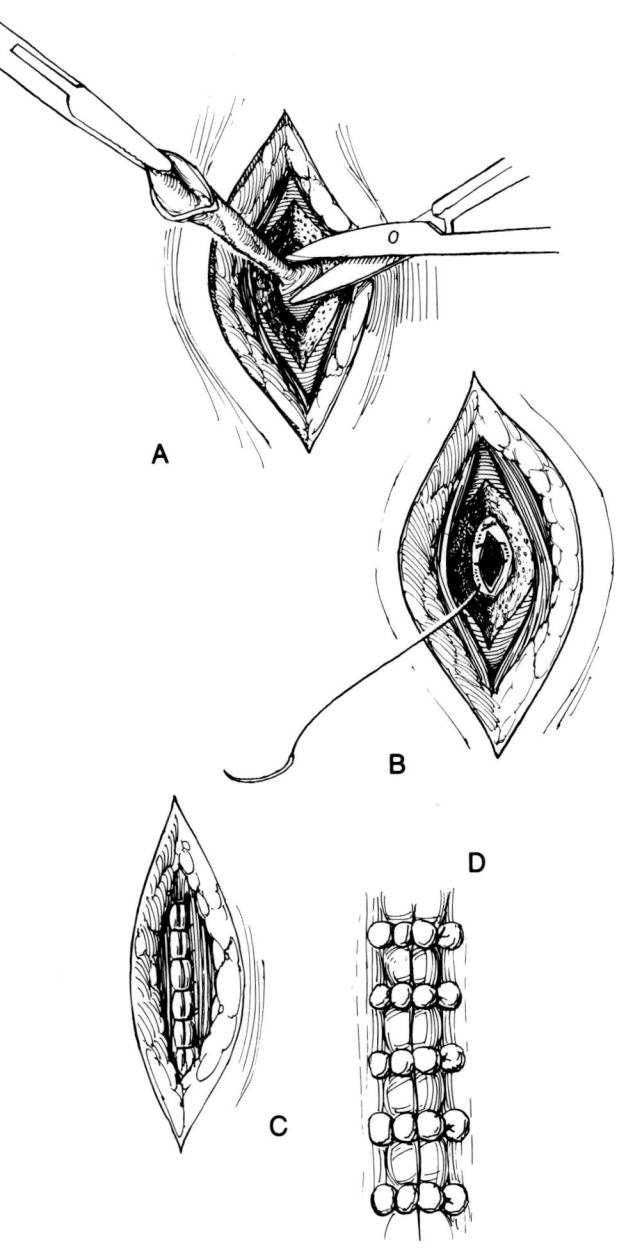

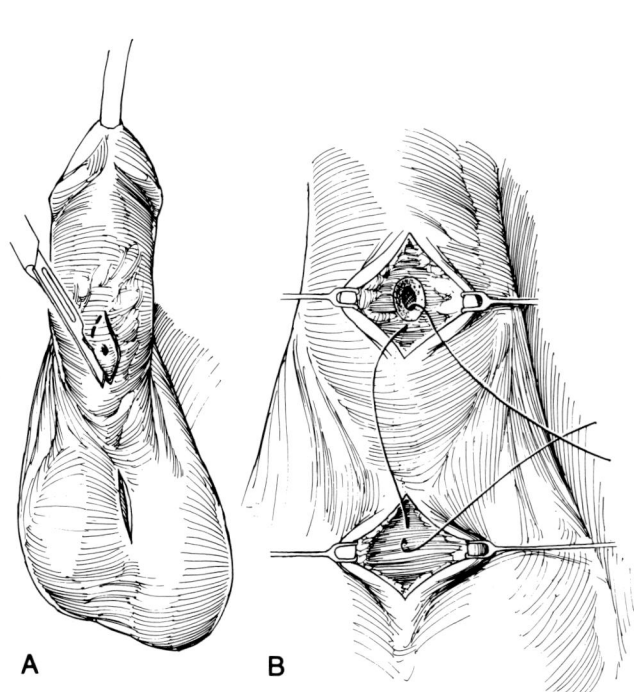

Repair of Severely Scarred Defects

19 **A,** Insert a 5-ml silicone balloon catheter of suitable size. Excise the scarred area generously. Make a vertical incision on the scrotum equidistant from the penoscrotal junction. **B,** Tack the urethral edge circumferentially to the dartos layer of the scrotum with interrupted 6-0 synthetic absorbable sutures. In an older child, insert a small Penrose drain to the area through a stab wound.

20 **A,** Close the skin edges with 3-0 chromic catgut. Remove the catheter in 2 weeks. **B,** Two or 3 months later, divide the scrotal skin asymmetrically and free the two flaps. Bring them together with subcutaneous 4-0 synthetic absorbable sutures. Close both skin defects with a subcuticular 5-0 synthetic absorbable suture.

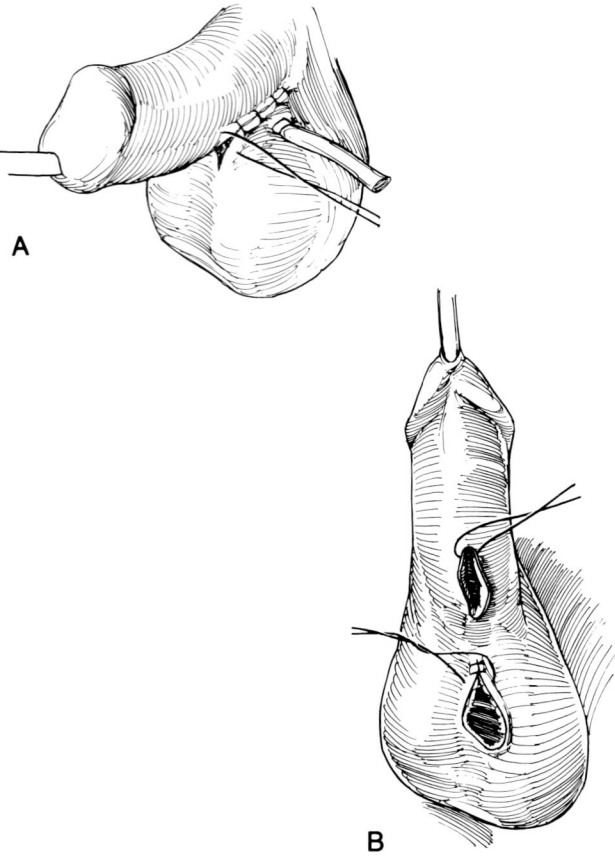

Commentary by A. Barry Belman

Urethrocutaneous Fistula. This is the most common complication of hypospadias repair. Some factors that may lead to urethrocutaneous fistula include distal obstruction, impaired vascular supply to the neourethra, use of non-absorbable suture material in creating the neourethra, crossing suture lines, poorly vascularized skin flaps to cover the neourethra, postoperative wound infection, and urinary extravasation. The incidence of this complication ranges from 4 to 56 percent.

Meticulous surgical technique and application of the fundamental rules of plastic surgery are mandatory in hypospadias operation, as well as in management of its most common complication.

However, closure of a urethrocutaneous fistula is no longer a major undertaking and usually can be accomplished rather easily and highly successfully as an outpatient procedure, without diversion or catheterization.

The principles are quite simple: (1) do not be afraid to free up enough normal tissue to get a good multiple-layered closure; (2) the fistula itself should be closed flush with the urethra, using a fine subcuticular inverting stitch with 6-0 or 7-0 suture; (3) the suture line can be completely covered by application of the de-epithelialized flap technique adapted from Dr. E. Durham Smith's (Durham Smith, 1973) two-stage hypospadias repair. Three full layers thus can be closed, including the final skin closure, over the actual fistula in most instances; (4) hemostasis must be excellent and can be best achieved using needletip electrocautery; and (5) most important, distal obstruction must *not* exist.

I use collodion as a skin dressing, which tends to seal the wound. As it dries, collodion contracts, compressing the skin edges. With the spectacular success being achieved these days with fistula closure, one really should have no concern about attempting a single-stage hypospadias repair in all but the most severe cases of perineal hypospadias with penoscrotal transposition.

In reviewing our experience, we conclude that repair of urethrocutaneous fistulas can be accomplished with a high degree of success. Although some small fistulas will close spontaneously in the early postoperative period, in our experience, the use of silver nitrate to cauterize the tract locally is of little help. Additionally, to achieve maximum success, we believe that 6 months probably should elapse between the previous procedure and any attempts at closure to allow resolution of induration and to reduce bleeding when performing the skin flap mobilization. The techniques are versatile and satisfactory in the more complex as well as in the simple cases. Our more recent experience substantiates that almost all but the most severe fistulas can be closed successfully as an outpatient procedure without the need for urinary diversion or urethral stenting, thus minimizing morbidity, hospitalization, and cost.

Excision of Diverticula

If the neourethra is made too wide, minimal meatal stenosis will cause it to distend, causing dripping of urine after voiding. Also, a leak from the inner suture line may create a pool that subsequently is re-epithelialzed as a diverticulum. Hair in the urethra from earlier techniques of repair usually is not a problem (other than requiring occasional trimming), unless it lies in a pool of urine in a urethral diverticulum, where it fosters the formation of stones. The treatment is correction of the diverticulum with depilation while the surface is exposed.

For repair, fill the diverticulum retrogradely to determine its dimensions. The simplest procedure is to make a longitudinal incision through skin and urethra, excise the excess urethral skin asymmetrically, and close the defect in three layers over a stent. For a more secure technique, if the ventral skin is free, deglove the penis before incising the diverticulum and urethra. Incise vertically over the urethra to form flaps for coverage of the repair. Resect the diverticulum. Insert a catheter or stent. Close the edges of the diverticulum meticulously with fine inverted interrupted synthetic absorbable sutures. Close the subcutaneous tissue with the vest-over-pants technique, and close the skin with a fine subcuticular suture. For repair of bulbar diverticula, see page 672.

Persistent Chordee

The neourethra must be freed from the corpora, and the chordee excised. Alternatively, tucks can be taken in the dorsum of the corpora cavernosa, or grafts can be placed. The loss in urethral length is made up with a Mustardé repair or a free graft of skin or bladder mucosa. Secondary scarring can be treated with Z-plasty (page 42).

21 Dorsal chordee may be corrected by making two parallel incisions on each side of the dorsal neurovascular bundle at the side of the curvature and approximating the lateral edge of each to the other with inverted nonabsorbable sutures (TAP procedure).

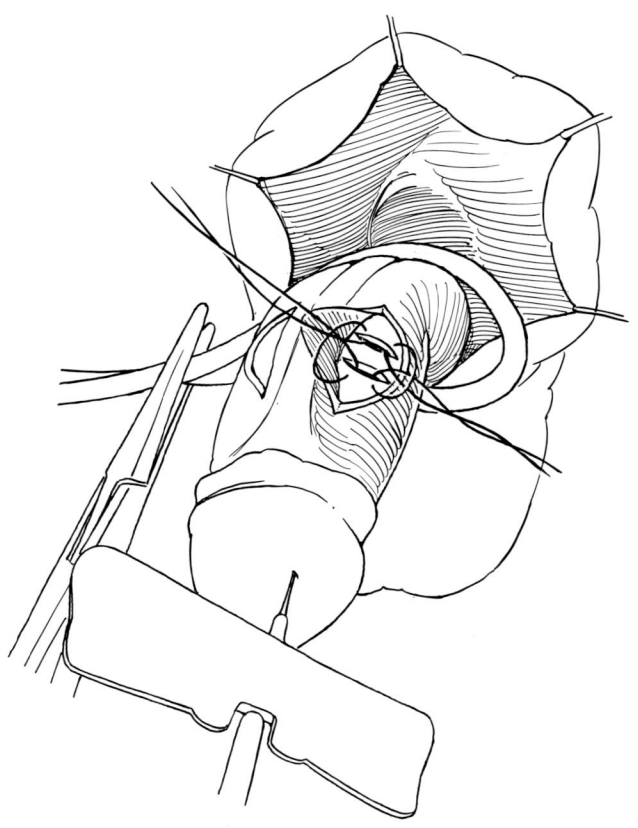

Congenital Curvature Without Hypospadias

Deglove the shaft, mobilize the urethra, and resect the fibrous chordee. Penile torsion can be corrected at the same time by reattaching the shaft skin in correct alignment. The excess preputial skin is split dorsally and brought around the shaft to cover the ventrum. A dermal graft may be necessary in a few cases. If mobilization is insufficient, bisect the urethra, and replace the deficiency with a tubed island flap. A good alternative is dorsal tucking although it may shorten the penis (page 633).

Complex Hypospadias Repair

For reoperation after multiple previous failures, observe the following five precepts: (1) obtain wide exposure; (2) excise all abnormal tissue remnants, including the old urethra; (3) look for and use the best-quality skin that is available, and plan for skin cover at the outset; (4) correct the chordee first and reconstruct the urethra; and (5) correct all the problems at one stage if possible. However, do not hesitate to revise any part that proves inadequate, resorting to a second stage. In difficult cases, it is best to first re-create the deformity without worrying too much about loss from taking it apart, and then set about repairing it. For example, incise the glans deeply to revise the meatus. Thin out the spongy tissue so that the glans is flat. Cover the raw undersurface, inserting a graft if necessary. Use subcuticular sutures. If placed continuously, those made of Prolene are easier to pull out than nylon. For the second stage, consider a tube graft tunneled under the skin cover placed at the first stage. Always use suprapubic diversion.

CHAPTER 115

Meatotomy

VENTRAL MEATOTOMY

1 *No-suture method for infants:* Instill 1 percent lidocaine through a 25-gauge needle passed through the meatus and directed at the frenulum.

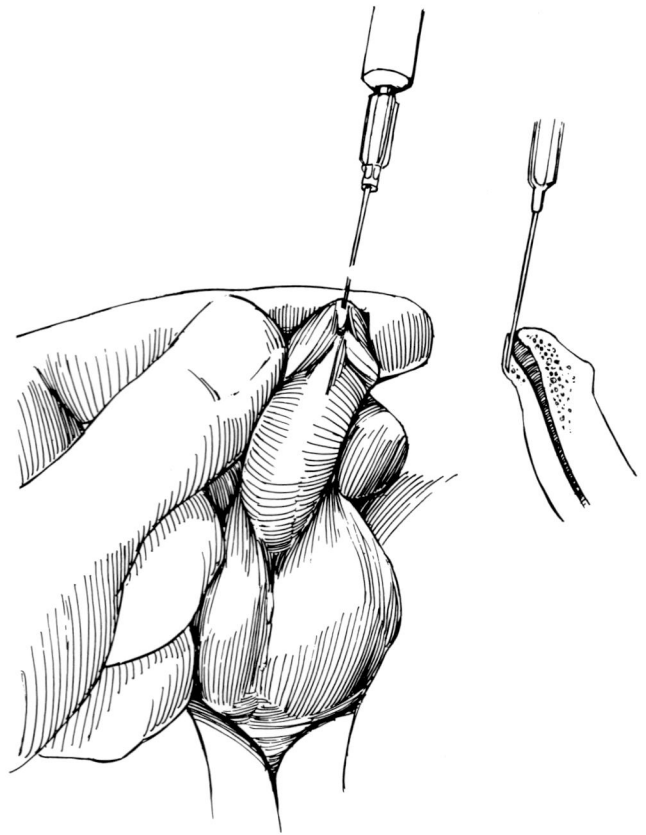

2 **A,** Clamp the ventral meatal lip with a fine clamp. Insert it deeply, because healing will reduce the depth of the cut. **B,** Divide the thinned tissue (now avascular) with scissors.

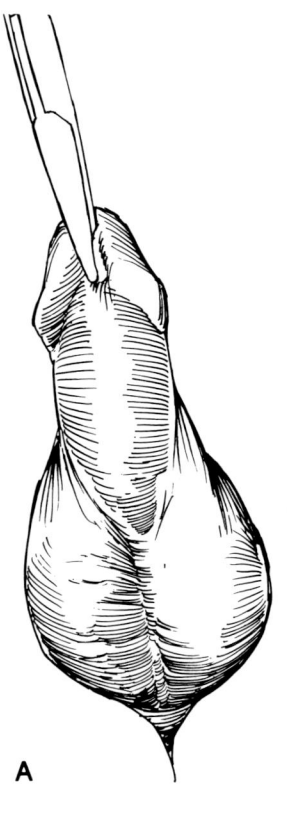

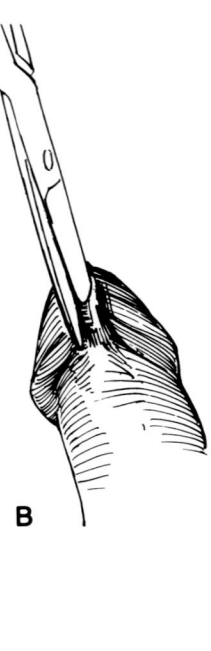

A

B

3 Apply petroleum jelly (Vaseline) or ophthalmic antibiotic ointment to the cut edges, and instruct the mother or father to do the same at home. The parent will need to use the tip of the ointment tube or an infant feeding tube three times a day at first to keep the edges from becoming resealed, and they should check the caliber for 3 months.

4 *Suture method for older boys:* **A,** Instill 1 percent lidocaine through a 25-gauge needle passed through the meatus and directed at the frenulum. Incise the ventrum with scissors, creating a V-shaped defect. Take care not to create hypospadias. Calibrate with an appropriately sized sound. **B,** Place up to five 3-0 or 4-0 plain catgut or synthetic absorbable sutures to approximate the edges of the V.

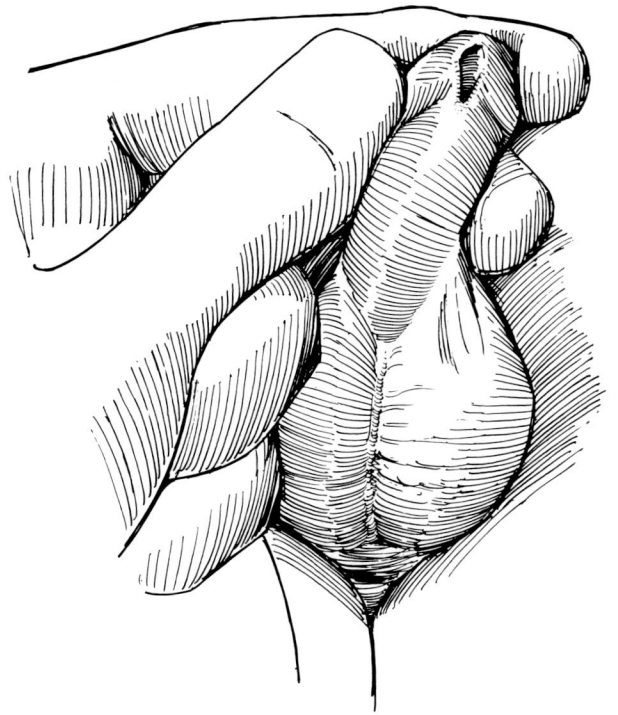

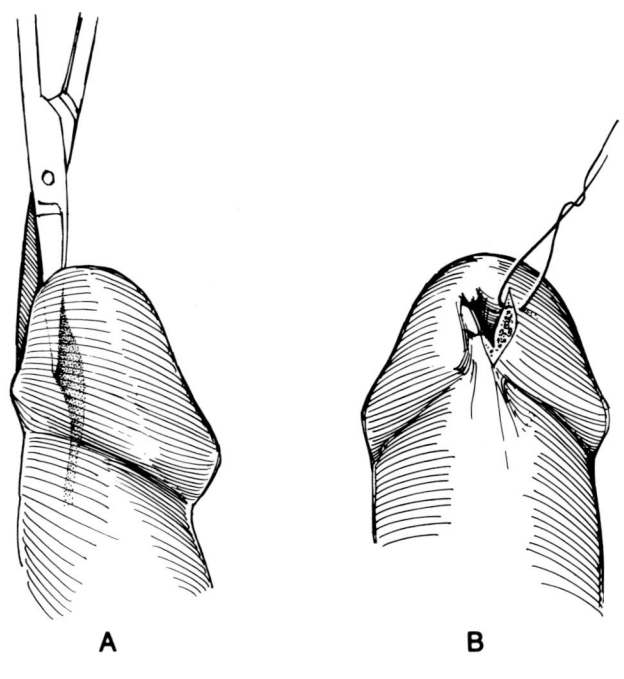

A   B

DORSAL MEATOTOMY FOR STRICTURE OF THE FOSSA NAVICULARIS

5 If the child has had previous urethral manipulation, it is useful prior to urethral instrumentation to insinuate a #15 (for children) or #10 (for adolescents) Bard-Parker knife blade into the meatus, cutting-edge up. Withdraw the knife, applying moderate upward pressure to incise the roof of the fossa navicularis and meatus. Repeat until a lubricated sound of appropriate size passes readily.

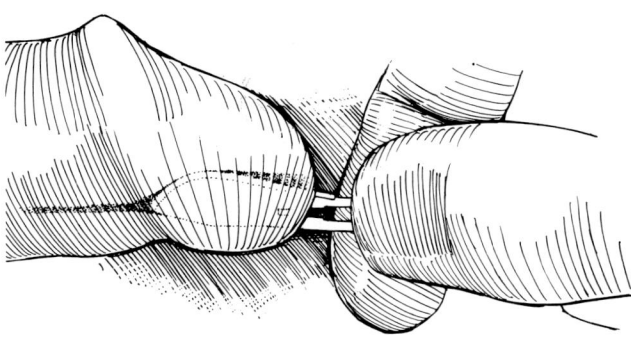

Commentary by David A. Bloom

Although meatal stenosis is a rather mundane problem for the surgeon, it is a matter of intense concern for the child and his family. Most cases, I believe, are the long-term result of inflammation of the exposed meatal lips. After circumcision, they may become periodically inflamed from rubbing against urine-soaked diapers. In the early part of the century, this reaction was called *ammoniacal meatitis.* The cycle of inflammation and healing with minute cicatrix formation ultimately can lead to meatal stenosis, which typically presents in circumcised boys after toilet training. In most instances, meatal stenosis is not a clinical problem. I think a legitimate problem exists when two of three conditions occur: (1) serious abnormality of the stream (severe angulation, spraying, diminished caliber), (2) stranguria, and (3) inability of the doctor to evert the meatal lips or pass a 5 F feeding tube.

Treatment requires two steps: first, meatotomy to restore the normal aperture; and second, a program of intermittent insertion of a catheter (every 2 weeks for 1 month, then monthly for 2 months) will maintain the opening during the healing period. This second step requires some degree of cooperation from the patient; our experience has taught us that if the meatotomy was traumatic, the calibration program will be difficult. For that reason, we do not hesitate to use a general anesthetic for those few boys with significant meatal stenosis; procedures on the genitalia of youngsters under local anesthesia are unhappy events for all participants.

CHAPTER 116

Coronal Repair

(SPENCE-ALLEN)

DISTAL HYPOSPADIAS WITH
SLIGHT CUTANEOUS CHORDEE

1 Place a traction suture in the glans. Divide the septum between the false dorsal and the true ventral urethras. Insert an 8 F infant feeding tube.

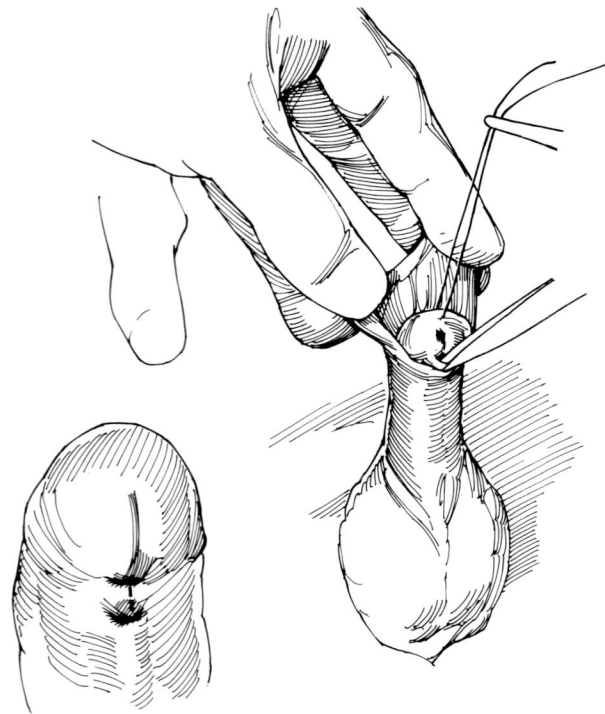

2 Choose a site on the dorsal hood just over the corona and make a transverse incision through the superficial layer of the prepuce. Expose the dorsal vessels, and separate them bluntly with a clamp to make an opening slightly smaller than the size of the glans.

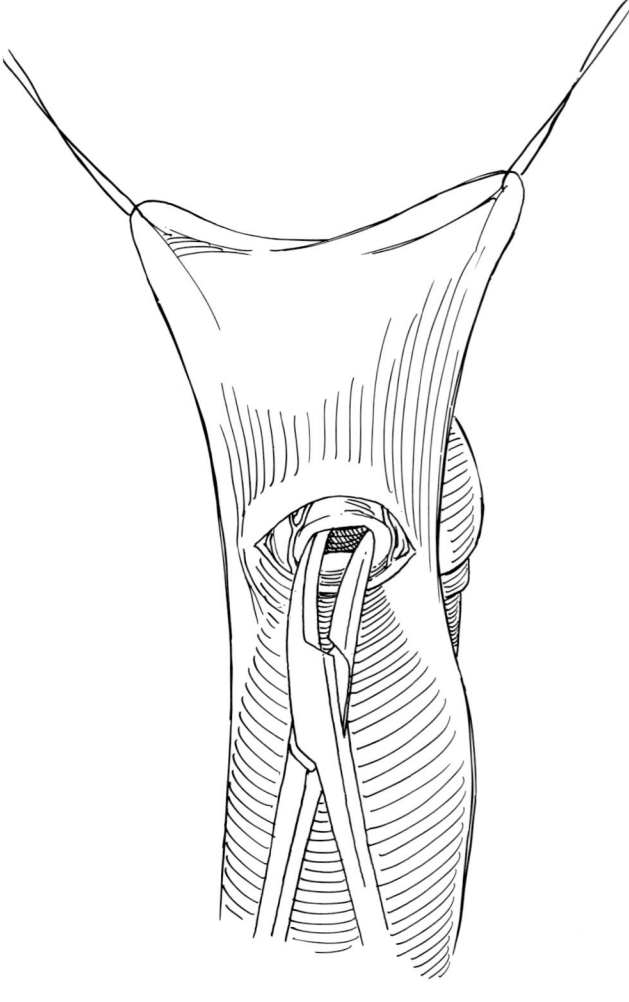

3 Mark and incise the skin 3 to 4 mm proximal to the glans, as done for circumcision, except make the incision on the ventrum run a few millimeters proximal to the meatus.

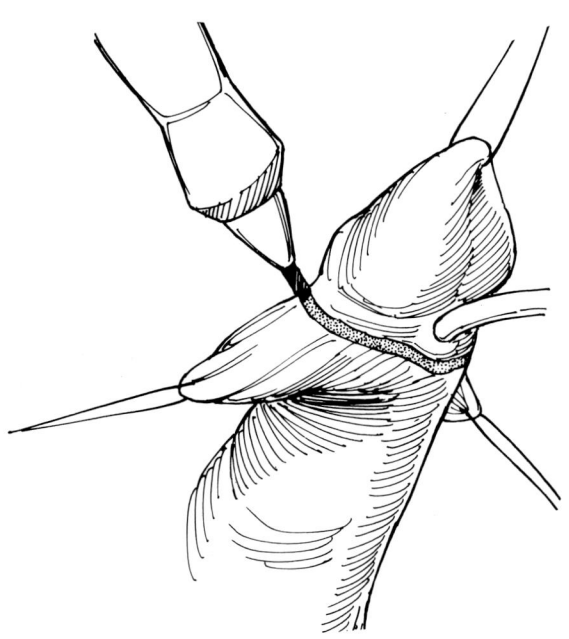

4 Dissect the skin from the shaft to release the chordee. Avoid contact with the thin urethra.

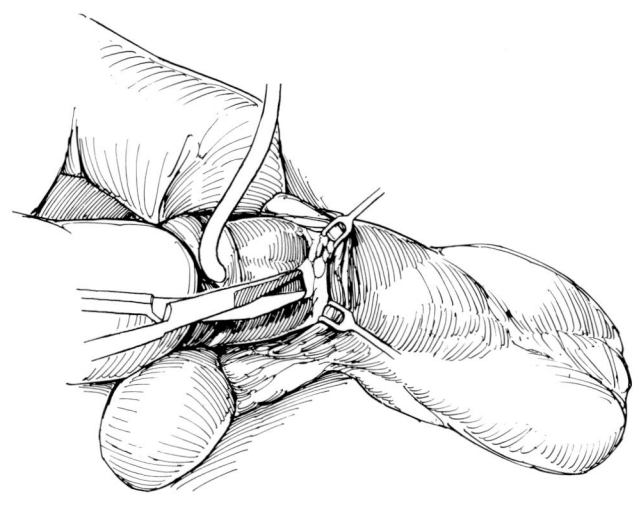

5 Open the dorsal hood and bring it to the ventrum by passing the glans through the buttonhole between the blood vessels.

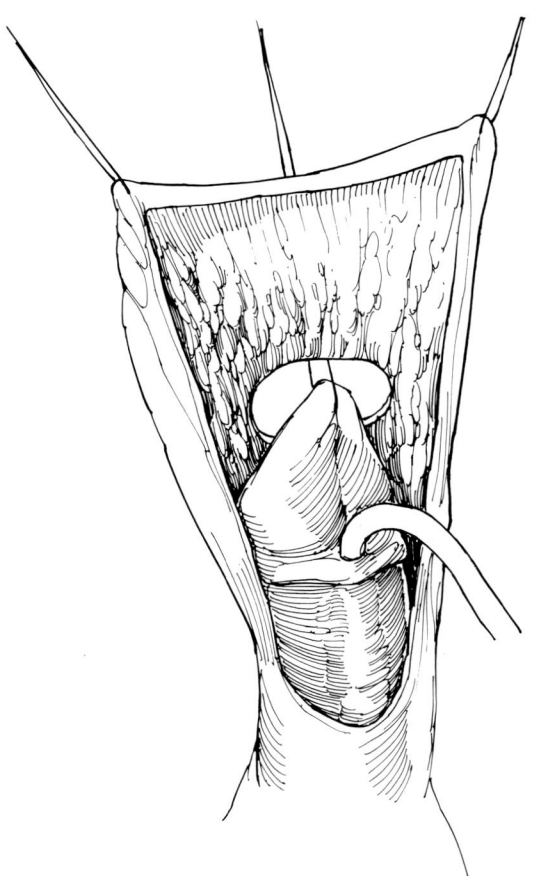

6 Suture the flap to the coronal skin and to the skin on the shaft with 5–0 chromic catgut. Trim the dog ears, but do so very carefully so as not to interfere with the blood supply to the flap.

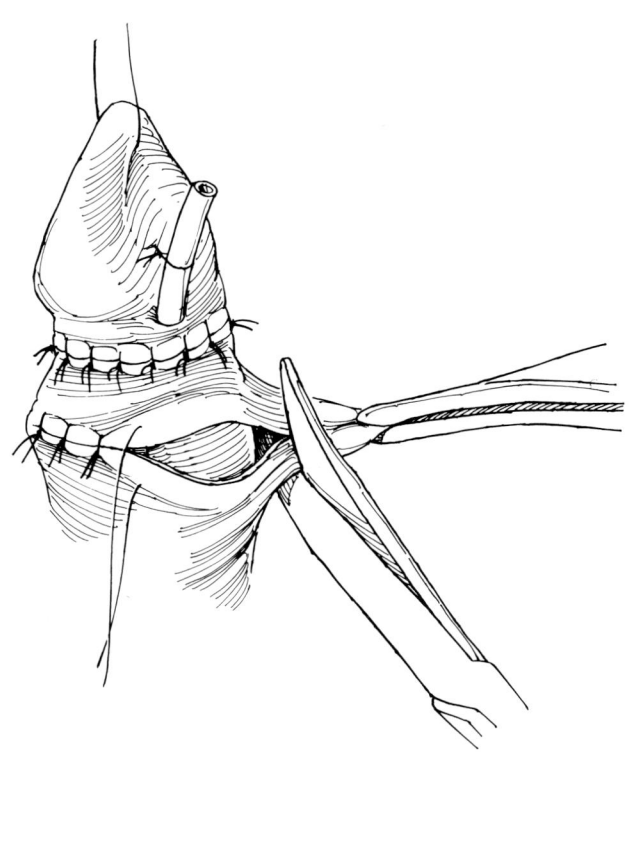

Commentary by Terry D. Allen

Prior to the development of this procedure, lesser degrees of hypospadias usually were treated in a formal way with staged operations, as were the more advanced forms of the anomaly at that time. Because this exposed the child to the complications associated with staged repairs, Dr. Spence was never happy with this approach. One day, in dealing with such a case, he carried his circumferential incision proximal to the urethral opening rather than distal to it as was the custom. With the confidence of youth, I was quick to point out that this would not relieve the chordee and thus could not be a satisfactory solution to the problem. The postoperative results proved me wrong and led me to investigate why it had worked. The result of this was the realization that the adherent skin was a major factor in the production of the chordee and that it was not necessary to free up the urethra in these minor cases to straighten the penis.

The advantage of the operation was that it was simple and essentially free of complications. It gave a nice cosmetic appearance when viewed from the dorsum of the penis, but it had the disadvantage that the meatus was not in the glans where it was expected to be. This was no cause for concern from a functional standpoint, but it failed to completely resolve the image problem in some patients, and occasionally we would see older boys and adolescents return to the office with a request to advance the urethra out onto the glans.

Today, there is little need for the procedure. Newer operations are available that offer a better cosmetic outcome in a single-stage outpatient procedure, and those doing most of the hypospadias repair today are skilled pediatric urologists with little interest in any compromise to the outcome for the sake of simplicity.

Commentary by Harry M. Spence

The operation that Dr. Allen and I devised well over 25 years ago took advantage of the Nesbit buttonhole and of the fact that the atretic corpus spongiosum and its overlying skin caused the chordee, as Don Smith had pointed out earlier. The procedure has stood the test of time and remains a simple way to correct a commonly occurring lesser deformity, which although minor in nature, not infrequently has psychologic implications in adulthood. The few times I have gotten into trouble have been when I stretched the indications where the meatus was located too far proximally. Here, the more elegant one-stage operations of Devine, Hodgson, or Duckett are in order. I learned from Ormond Culp that the blind-ending dorsal urethra of variable length is always present and is best demonstrated by probing with the blunt end of a milliner's needle. The thin veil-like septum can then be incised throughout its extent. Such division permits a forward, rather than a downward, trajectory of the stream without incising glanular tissue.

CHAPTER 117

Meatal Advancement and Glanuloplasty

MAGPI CORRECTION OF DISTAL HYPOSPADIAS WITHOUT CHORDEE (DUCKETT)

For the meatal advancement and glanuloplasty (MAGPI) procedure to be applicable, the meatus should be not more than 1 cm proximal to the glans, and the skin on the ventrum proximal to the meatus should be thick and mobile enough to be lifted off the urethra, so that it will move forward. If the parameatal skin is of poor quality, resort to an onlay repair. The principal goal of this operation is to provide good support for the glans, so that it will remain elevated with the meatus at the tip. For a widemouth, flat, fixed meatus that cannot be moved into the glanular groove, a Mathieu procedure (page 581) or an onlay island flap (page 588) is more appropriate.

This is an outpatient procedure performed under general anesthesia. Insert a vertical traction suture in the glans. Infiltrate the subcoronal area and glans groove with 1 percent lidocaine, containing epinephrine 1:100,000 to improve hemostasis. Blocking the dorsal penile nerves with 0.25 percent bupivacaine hydrochoride (page 57) will decrease the need for intraoperative anesthesia and will decrease pain postoperatively.

1 Incise the ventral skin proximal to the coronal sulcus and the meatus circumferentially.

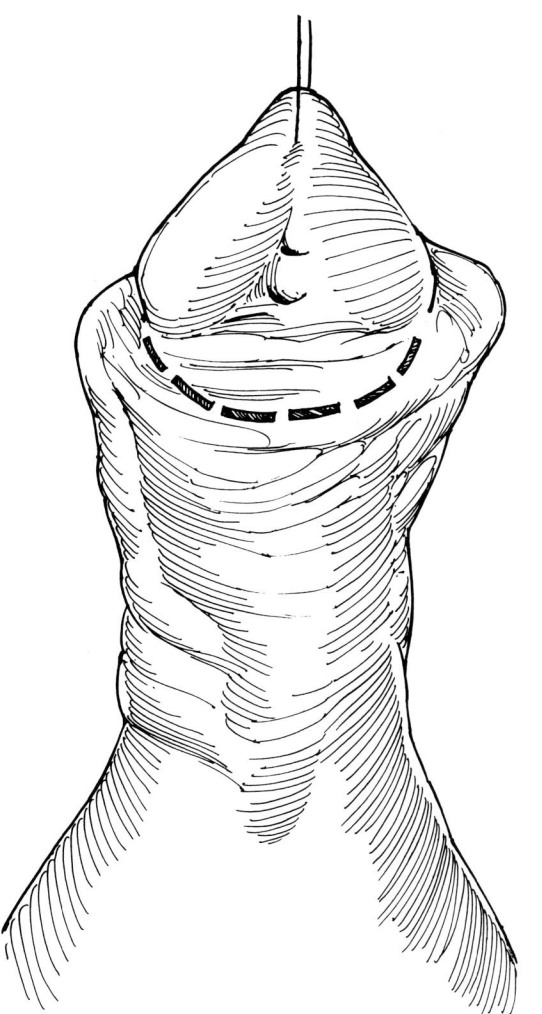

2 Mobilize the skin of the ventral shaft proximally as a sleeve, taking care not to injure the delicate urethral wall. Free the skin to the penoscrotal junction. Clear all tissue from the corpora causing tethering. Ascertain that the penis is straight with an artificial erection. Any residual curvature is probably caused by corporal disproportion and will be corrected by dorsal tucks.

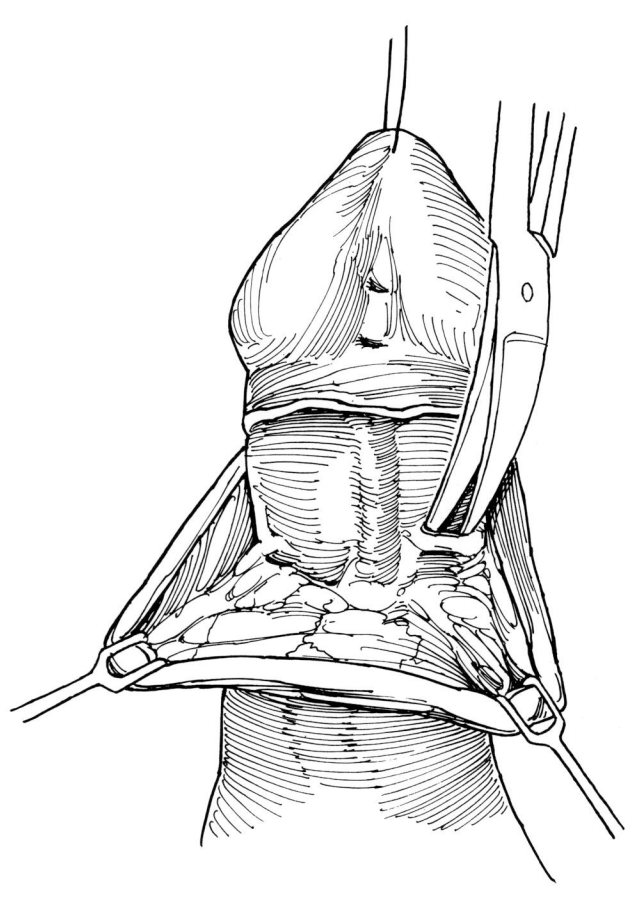

3 Starting inside the dorsal edge of the meatus, make a vertical incision to the distal end of the glanular groove. The vertical cut widens the dorsal meatal margin, even when meatal stenosis exists. Occasionally it may be desirable to excise a wedge if the bridge of tissue is prominent distal to the meatus.

4 **A** and **B,** Suture the edges of the meatal V to the groove in the glans with fine sutures as a Heineke-Mikulicz transverse closure to advance the meatus and flatten the groove.

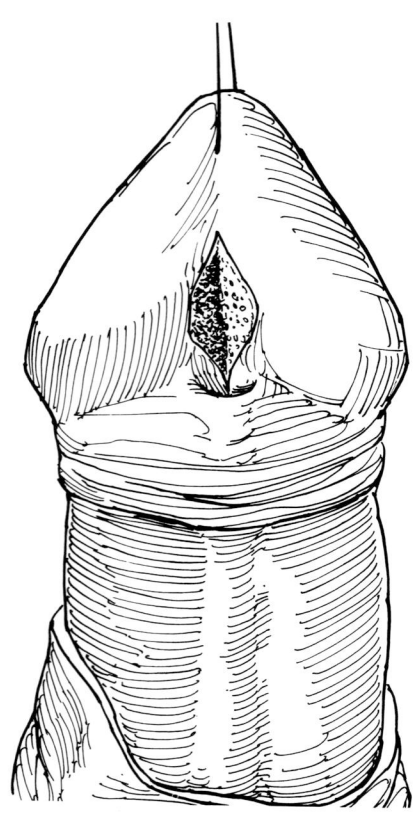

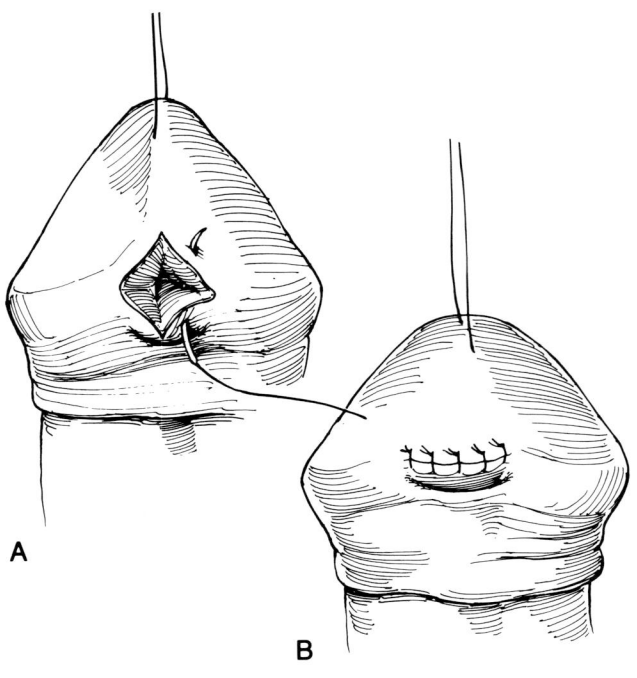

A

B

5 Lift the proximal edge of the meatus with a traction suture, pulling it toward the tip of the glans to form an inverted V as the glans wings are pulled together. Excise the glans tissue on the medial margins of these glans wings to provide support for the glans.

6 Approximate the deep glans tissue with one or two layers of 5–0 synthetic absorbable sutures. Close the glans epithelium with sutures of fine chromic catgut.

Correct any persistent ventral tilt of the glans by tacking the dorsal coronal edge of the glans to the dorsal tunica albuginea on either side with two fine nonabsorbable sutures. It is even better to make a dorsal vertical incision dorsally proximal to the glans and close it transversely (Heineke-Mikulicz). Avoid the midline structures.

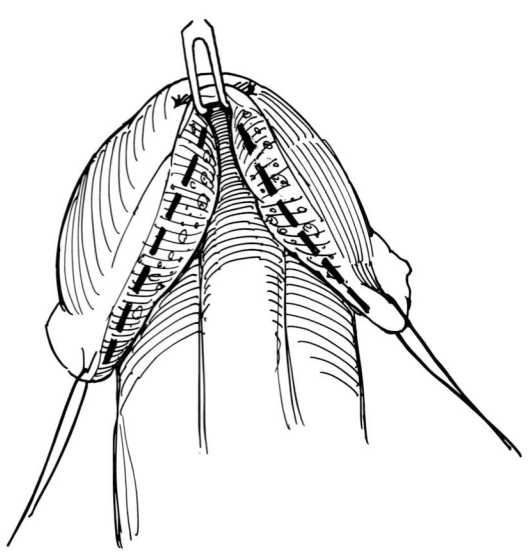

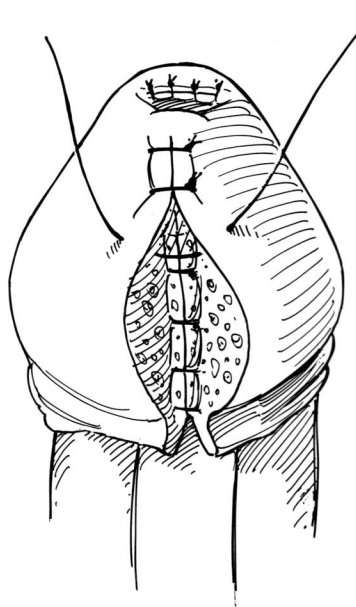

7 Align the median raphe and trim the excess preputial skin at a point proximal to the wrinkled portion. Suture the edges with 6–0 chromic catgut sutures or with fine subcuticular sutures. Trim the edges of the skin to improve appearance.

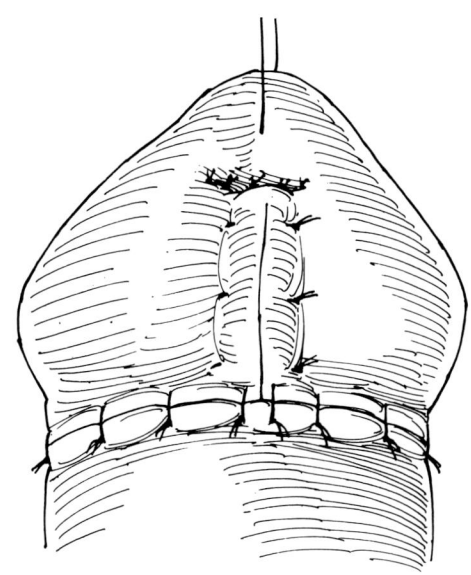

8 **A** and **B,** If the ventral skin is deficient, split the preputial skin dorsally. **C** and **D,** Bring the edges ventrally as Byars flaps. Trim the flaps to preserve symmetry.

It is not necessary to insert a catheter or stent.

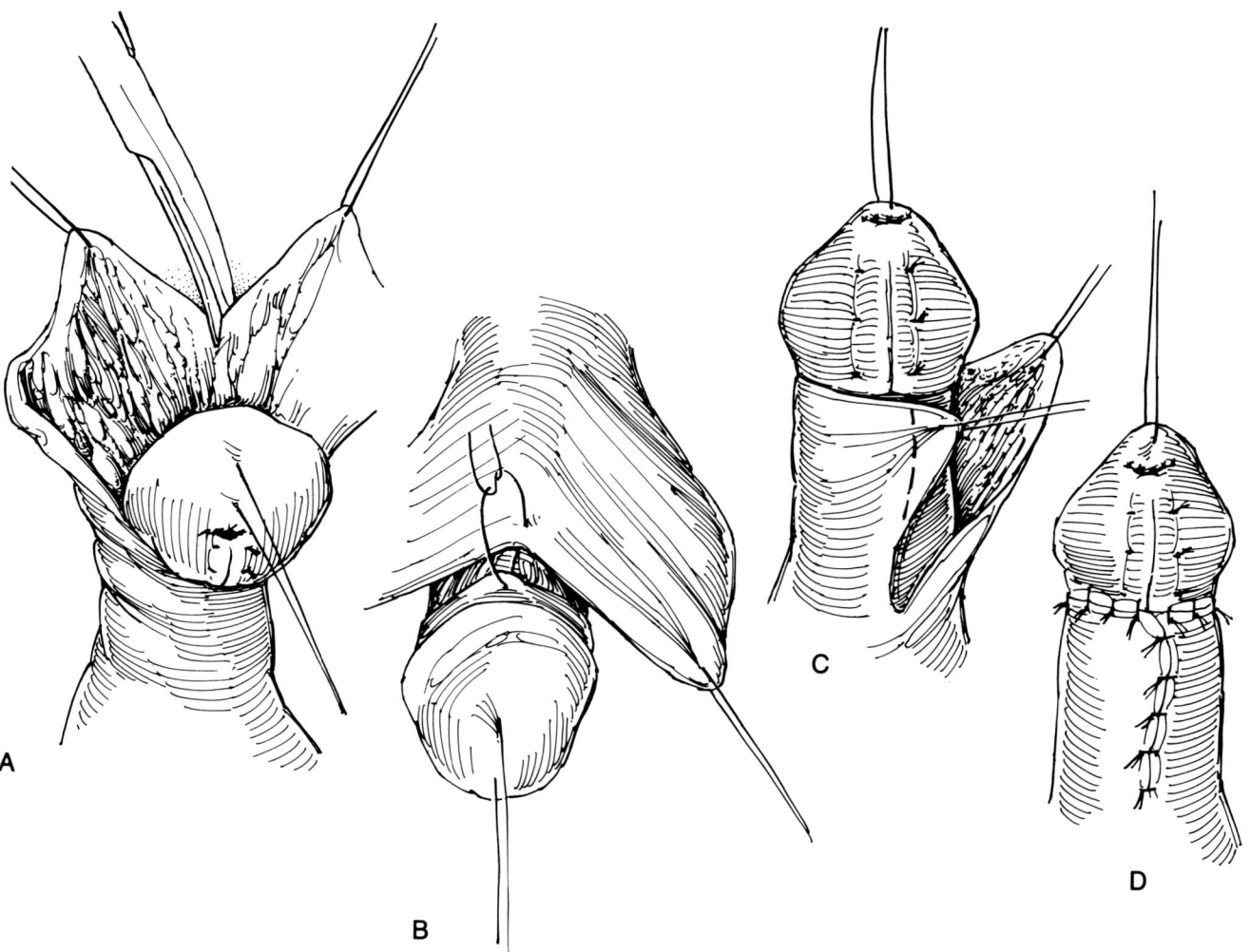

POSTOPERATIVE PROBLEMS

Meatal stenosis is the result of an inadequate meato-plasty. The dorsal vertical incision did not open the meatus widely and/or did not adequately deepen the urethral groove. *Meatal regression* results when the glans wings are not firmly coapted ventrally to provide support of the glans.

Commentary by John W. Duckett

The MAGPI procedure for hypospadias has been one of the more difficult techniques to describe and teach. Despite its simplicity, there is a gestalt about the concept that is difficult to describe in specific terms. Hypospadias comes in such variable configurations that specific indications for the MAGPI are difficult to enumerate. The main complication encountered by others using the MAGPI procedure has been glans breakdown and meatal retraction. It is most important to bring the glans wings together in the midline, excising excess skin on their medial edge and approximating two layers of deep glans with a superficial epithelial layer. This firm, conical reconfiguration of the glans will avoid meatal regression. It is important to excise these glans skin edges to approximate glans tissue primarily with the ventral meatal edge brought well forward.

An error is to try to extend the MAGPI where it is inappropriate. A fixed meatus without the typical bridge of tissue between meatus and glans is an inappropriate case to attempt a MAGPI.

Another error is failure to incise the dorsal meatal edge, leaving a meatal stenosis. It is important that the dorsal meatal edge be incised so that it can be closed transversely. No meatal stenosis should ever occur with a MAGPI.

When the technique was first published, we urged that one learn it by observing others who have mastered the technique. I still think this is an appropriate lesson, because it is difficult to depict its variability in an atlas.

A recent review of our MAGPI experience is cited in the references.

MODIFIED MAGPI REPAIR (ARAP)

An alternative procedure to the MAGPI, the Arap procedure advances the ventral aspect of the urethra and extends the operation to cases of more proximal hypospadias.

Advance the meatus as described for the MAGPI operation by a longitudinal incision in the glanular groove with transverse closure. Make a circumferential incision proximal to the corona and deglove the shaft.

9 **A,** Place traction sutures on the ventral skin on either side of the midline from 1 to 1.5 cm apart. Pull distally on these sutures to create two flaps.

B, Suture them together in the midline, thus forming a floor for the glanular urethra. Suture the deep tissue of the glans together in the midline, and approximate the epithelium of the glans. Close any ventral defect with Byars flaps or as a single pedicle flap; trim excess skin. Drainage tubes are not necessary.

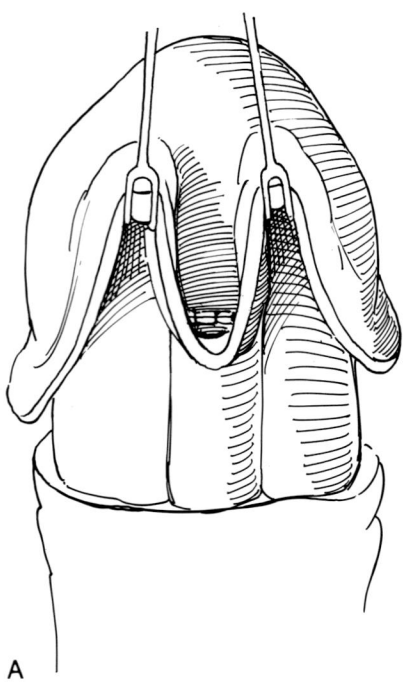

A

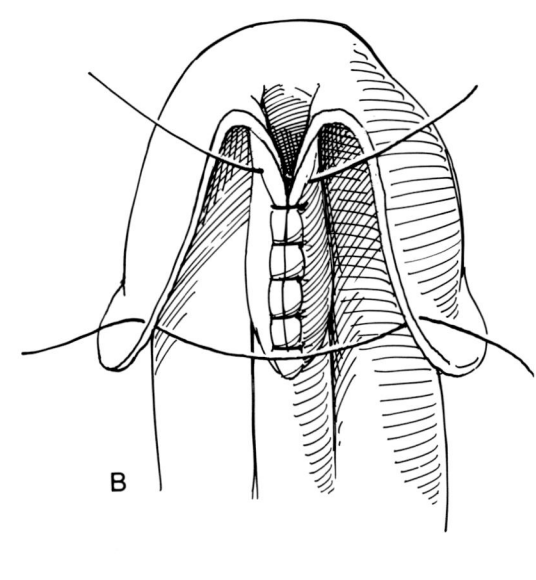

B

Commentary by Laurence S. Baskin

The Arap procedure is an ingenious variation of the MAGPI operation originally described in 1981 by John Duckett. This modified meatal advancement and glanuloplasty repair is designed for more distal hypospadias. Its success depends on the mobility of the distal urethra after release of the skin and dartos fascia. This concept also has been successfully used in the stretch MAGPI. As illustrated, a nice cosmetic and functional result can be obtained with the Arap procedure if the glansplasty provides adequate support to the new urethra.

In practice, however, patients with distal hypospadias tend not to have a dorsal lip of tissue in the glandular groove that lends itself to the classic Heineke-Mikulicz rearrangement that is performed in the MAGPI repair. These patients typically have a flat urethral plate that is more amenable to an onlay island flap, or if the distance is short, a Mathieu-style repair. Furthermore, in distal hypospadias, the ventral skin along the urethra often is quite thin, necessitating resection to healthy urethral spongiosum and leaving a gap too great for the Arap procedure to bridge.

The Arap procedure has its place in hypospadias surgery, the caveat being appropriate case selection.

PYRAMID PROCEDURE FOR REPAIR OF MEGAMEATUS-INTACT PREPUCE HYPOSPADIAS VARIANT (DUCKETT)

The large meatus is concealed beneath an intact prepuce, with a deep cleft forming the glanular groove. Techniques such as the MAGPI or Mathieu will not correct the large meatus. The Pyramid procedure exposes and excises the excess tissue in the terminal urethra and reconstitutes the meatus of proper size, while bringing it to the tip of the penis.

Place four traction sutures: one on the tip of the glans, one on each side of the meatal base, and one at its ventral margin. After infiltration with lidocaine-epinephrine to reduce bleeding, make a tennis-racquet incision near the glanular groove and around the meatus. Using iris scissors, mobilize the urethral cone (pyramid) proximally until it becomes normal in size. Develop glans wings on either side. Remove a wedge from the excess ventral urethral tissue, and approximate the edges with a continuous 7–0 synthetic absorbable suture to provide a normal caliber to the urethra. Bring the wings together with two layers of fine interrupted sutures, and place 7–0 interrupted chromic catgut mattress sutures in the skin. Test the urethral caliber with a 10 or 12 F bougie à boule; observe the quality of the stream by applying pressure over the bladder. Follow the repair with a circumcision if desired.

GLANS APPROXIMATION PROCEDURE (GAP) (ZAONTZ)

The Glans Approximation Procedure (GAP) is designed for the repair of glandular and coronal hypospadias in the presence of a wide and deep glanular groove with a noncompliant or fish-mouth meatus, utilizing the Thiersch-Duplay principle.

10 **A** and **B,** Incise the cleft in the glanular groove if it is present. Close the defect by slightly advancing the dorsal side of the meatus and suturing it with fine sutures to form a smooth urethral plate. Mark the glans wings in a thick U about the meatus with a marking pen, and excise a band of epithelium with tenotomy scissors, including the marked line. Approximate the urethral edges, first with a running suture of 7–0 chromic catgut placed subcuticularly, and then with interrupted imbricating stitches to the glans tissue. It is not necessary to form glans flaps. Reapproximate the skin of the glans with interrupted sutures.

For an improved cosmetic effect, form a mucosal collar (Firlit) by raising a V-shaped flap from the inner preputial lining on each side and bringing the flaps together in the midline.

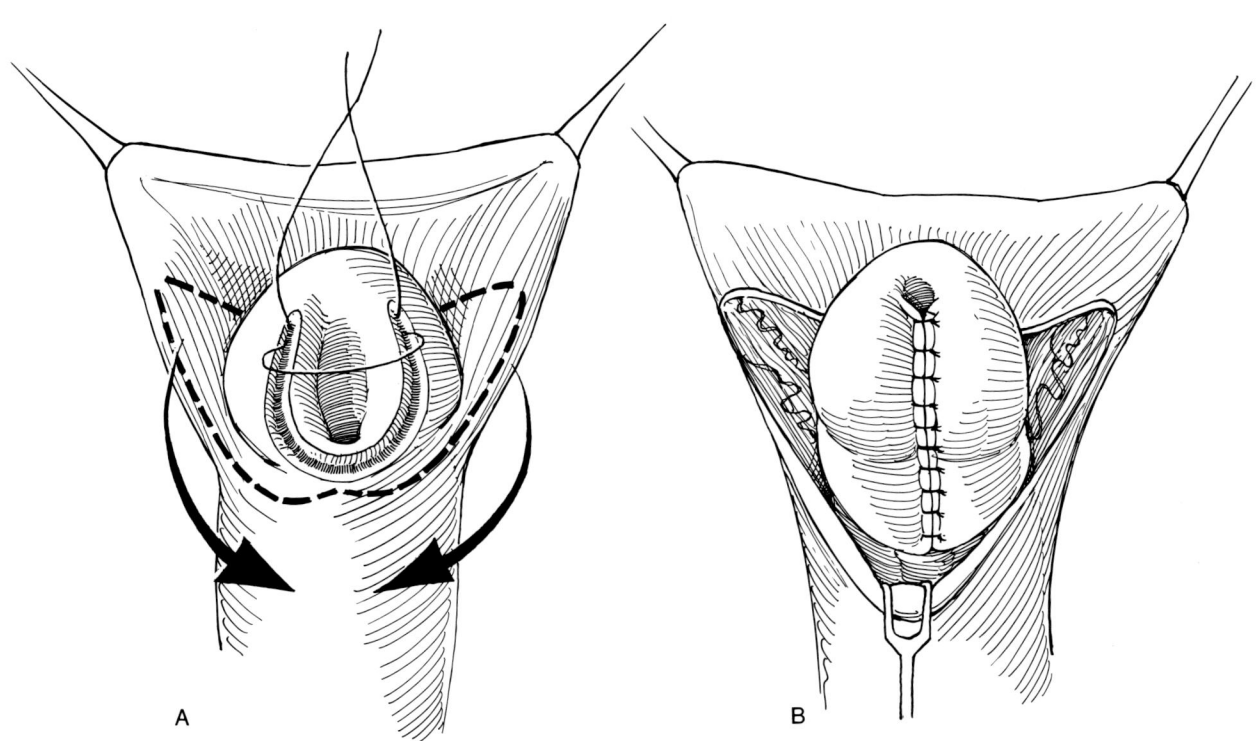

A   B

Commentary by Barry A. Kogan

There are innumerable published and unpublished hypospadias repairs. Were there not enough, there are any number of variations of them as well. These attest to the fact that no one repair is optimal; each has advantages and potential risks. Regarding distal hypospadias in particular, it is only in recent years that repairs have been consistently performed. In general, the lesion is not associated with major abnormalities of urinary or sexual function. Thus, the problem is primarily one of appearance and the related psychologic ramifications. Hence, in an era in which there were significant complications associated with repairs, it was quite reasonable not to operate on these minor lesions. Today, however, we have a number of approaches associated with minimal morbidity and a high success rate, so these lesions are commonly repaired.

The procedures used in most instances include the MAGPI or the Mathieu procedure. We have used these for outpatient repairs with a very high success rate and very few complications. For those patients with a deep glanular groove, however, we currently use the GAP, because the cosmetic results are unsurpassed. No dressing is required, and recently, we have not used a catheter to drain the bladder in children under 18 months of age.

We have performed this procedure in more than 25 patients, ranging in age from 6 months to 8 years. The cosmetic results have been outstanding, and there has been only one fistula, occurring early in the series in a child who was catheterized postoperatively and had numerous bladder spasms.

GLANULAR RECONSTRUCTION AND PREPUTIOPLASTY PROCEDURE (GRAP)
(GILPIN)

The Glanular Reconstruction and Preputioplasty (GRAP) procedure is a one-stage procedure suitable for outpatient surgery that leaves the penis, as the name suggests, with an uncircumcised appearance. It is not suitable when chordee is present.

Mark, incise, and raise the margins of skin and glanular epithelium on either side of the glans groove, forming a U around the meatus. Close the skin as a tube with 8–0 synthetic absorbable sutures. Test the suture line to be sure it is watertight. Place a catheter in the neourethra. Raise glans flaps, and close them over the neourethra with two layers of 7-0 synthetic absorbable sutures. Hold the prepuce up with two stay sutures placed far enough apart on the preputial hood that when they are approximated ventrally, the distal margin of the prepuce will form a preputial ring of adequate diameter to prevent phimosis. Make a Y extension from the original incision along the margin between the inner and outer preputial surfaces, almost to the stay sutures. Close the inner preputial edges vertically in two layers with 7-0 synthetic absorbable sutures to cover the neourethra. Confirm that the prepuce is fully retractable. This leaves a vertical defect on the ventrum that is closed as a Z-plasty to allow the prepuce to extend over the glans.

CHAPTER 118

Perimeatal-Based Flap Repair
(MATHIEU)

The Mathieu procedure is suitable for hypospadias with slight chordee. It uses the glanular urethral groove as the roof of the distal urethra and a meatal-based flap as the floor. It also preserves the prepuce. The Mustardé repair (page 583) is similar but tubularizes the meatal-based flap. If the perimeatal skin is very thin, consider a vascularized or free graft. The Horton-Devine "flip-flap" procedure is an obsolete operation, which has been given up even in Norfolk (Duckett).

DISTAL MEATUS WITH SIGNIFICANT CHORDEE

Create an artificial erection to evaluate chordee.

1 Insert a Prolene monofilament suture swaged on a fine tapered needle in the glans for traction. Mark lines of incision 0.6 to 0.8 cm apart for a glans flap on either side of the glanular groove. Continue the incisions for a proximal urethral flap. Infiltrate the subcutaneous tissue with 1:200,000 epinephrine in 1 percent lidocaine (optional), and incise along the marks. Incise the prepuce circumferentially 1 cm away from the glans.

2 Develop the lateral portions of the glans as wings. Raise the flap from the shaft, taking care to preserve its subcutaneous tissue with its blood supply. Fold it up over the distal urethra in the glans, and approximate it on either side with interrupted 5–0 synthetic absorbable sutures. Tack the subcutaneous tissue of the flap to the deep tissue of the glans. Test for a watertight suture line by instilling saline under pressure. Correct all leaks with additional sutures.

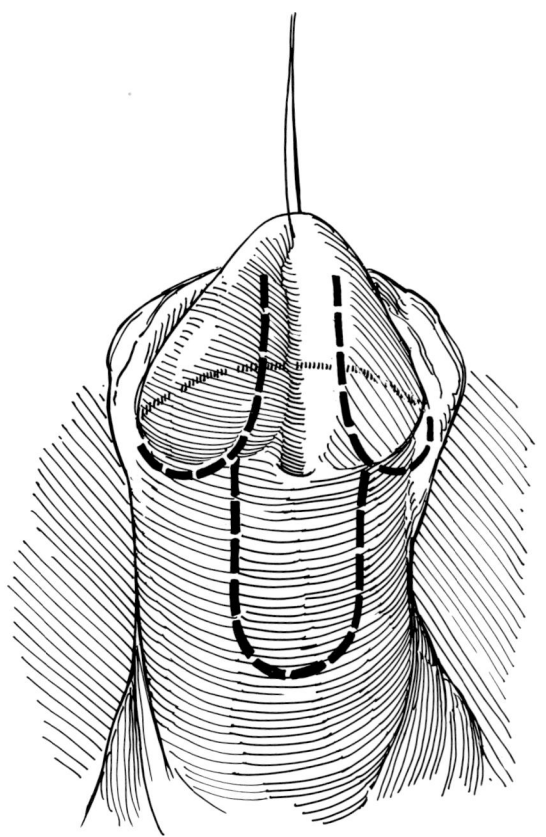

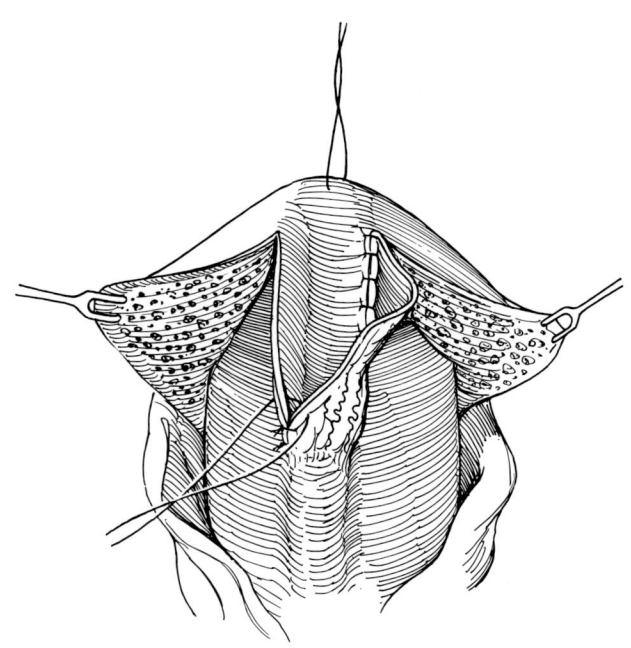

3 Approximate the glans flap with fine interrupted sutures (undermine the flaps to avoid tension). To prevent meatal stenosis, keep a large sound in the meatus while suturing.

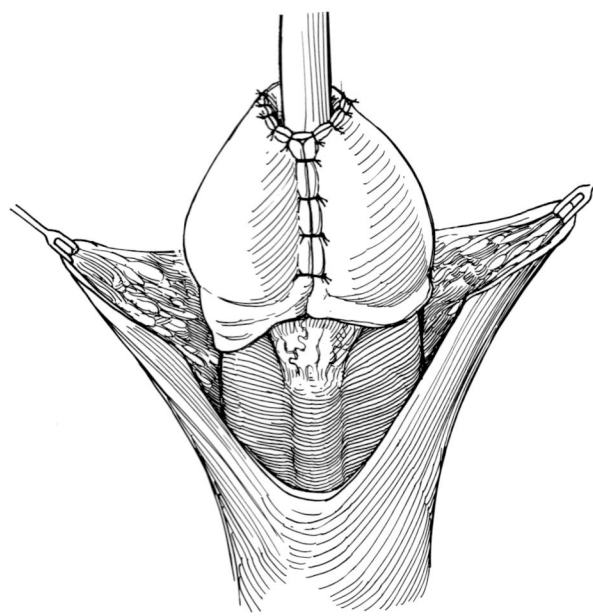

4 Draw the shaft skin around as Byars flaps. A portion of one of these flaps may be de-epithelialized and used to provide a layer to cover the repair. Close the circumcision defect. Trim excess skin, and close the ventral defect.

Finally, calibrate the urethra with a curved sound corresponding to the size of a normal urethra for the child's age. Pass an 8 F silicone catheter into the bladder, and tether it to the penis by the traction suture.

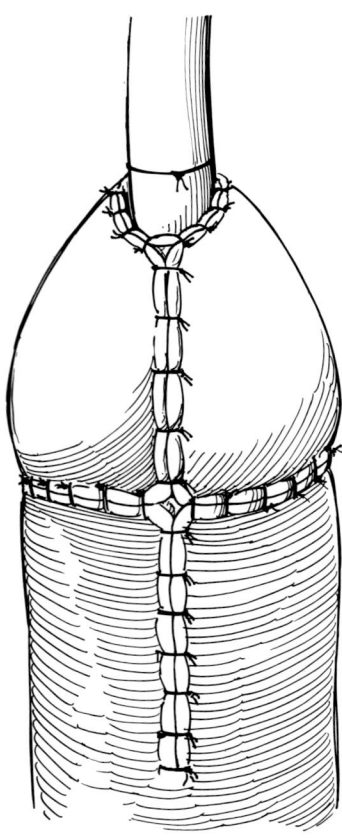

Commentary by Blackwell B. Evans, Sr.

Ideal candidates for the Mathieu procedure should have a straight penis, but glandular tilt and limited distal chordee may be corrected easily by a dorsal wedge resection of the corpora, as described by Nesbit. Great care should be exercised to protect the neurovascular bundle when performing the dorsal wedge resection. Additionally, distal chordee may be managed with this procedure by elevating the proximal portion of the glanular urethral groove and dissecting the base of the glans free from the corpora, as described by Horton and Devine in their flip-flop procedure. Unfortunately, if the glanular urethral groove is not of adequate length, the chordee may be re-created on closing the urethra.

As the meatal-based flap is developed, the base should be avoided during dissection, preserving the adventitial blood flow. The glanular urethral groove and the proximal urethral flap must have final dimensions that will provide an adequate distal urethra but at the same time not result in a patulous, flaccid pocket, a common complication of this procedure. It is especially important to invert the edges of the neourethra proximally to avoid dog ears, which will contribute to fistula formation. Many surgeons prefer to close the proximal urethral flap to the glanular urethral groove with fine interrupted sutures, but my personal choice is a running suture on each side, nearly to the neomeatus. The urethral closure is then completed with two or three fine interrupted 6–0 or 7–0 sutures, followed by a simple running closure of the adventitia, promoting a watertight closure, thus limiting fistula formation. If there is any question of closure strength, one or two single sutures may be placed along the course of the running closure. To permit accurate placement of individual sutures to control leaks, closure of the urethra should be tested by instillation of normal saline into the neomeatus prior to skin closure.

Optical loupes contribute to the precise placement of sutures during urethral closure and, for us, have reduced fistula formation.

The lateral flaps of the glans must be given sufficient elevation to provide approximation over the glanular urethra without tension. If approximated under tension, the tissue may necrose and result in a juxtaglanular meatus.

To cover the ventral closure with penile skin, the glans penis may be passed through a buttonhole in a dorsal hood, with typical tailoring and closure, as described by Nesbit. The foreskin may be split, as described by Byars, and passed ventrally to cover the neourethra, using the best-looking flap to cross the midline, or more appropriately, closed in a Z-plasty fashion. These closures sometimes require trimming of excess skin at a later date. A Nesbit hood or Byars flap closure avoids having the junction of four suture lines at the base of the glans, as diagrammed here. It is my experience that both glanular separation and fistula formation are more frequent when the four suture lines meet at the base of the glans penis. Skin closure is best accomplished with a 5–0 running suture and an occasional interrupted suture for security in the event that a portion of the running suture gives way. Care must be taken to avoid a drawstring effect in such a closure. My preference has been to first place a few interrupted subcutaneous stitches, which approximate the tissues with the tension on the subcutaneous tissue rather than on the skin itself. The skin edges are then approximated with a simple running suture of 4–0 or 5–0 suture material.

On completion of the procedure, the urethra should be calibrated according to the patient's age with a McCrea sound. An 8 F silicone catheter generally is adequate to drain the bladder for a brief time following the Mathieu procedure.

CHAPTER 119

Perimeatal-Based Tube Repair
(MUSTARDÉ)

For mild chordee that requires separation of the meatus from the coronal sulcus, perimeatal-based tube repair makes a tunnel in the glans rather than a V-flap and avoids splitting the glans. The technique is not suitable for repeat operations, because it requires good vascularization of the flap. By placing the single suture line dorsally against the corpora, the risk of fistula formation is reduced.

Insert a Prolene stay suture in the glans. Incise the meatus laterally if necessary.

1 Mark and incise a skin flap 1.5 to 2 cm wide (equivalent to 15 to 20 F) on the shaft proximal to the meatus that is long enough to reach the distal end of the glans. Excess skin can always be trimmed later.

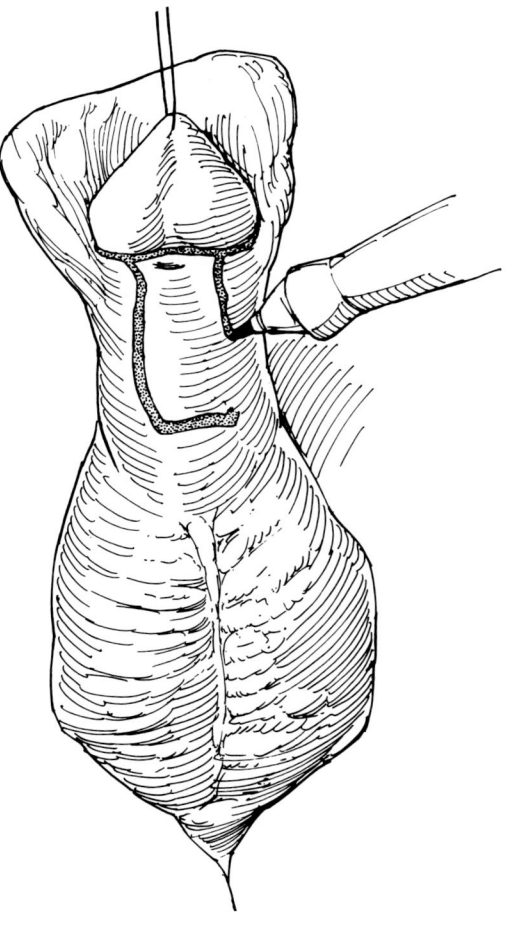

2 Incise the prepuce circumferentially at the corona. Direct the tips of the scissor to the midline, and develop a space as they are spread apart. Avoid cutting, but transect any fascial bands distal to the meatus producing tilt of the glans.

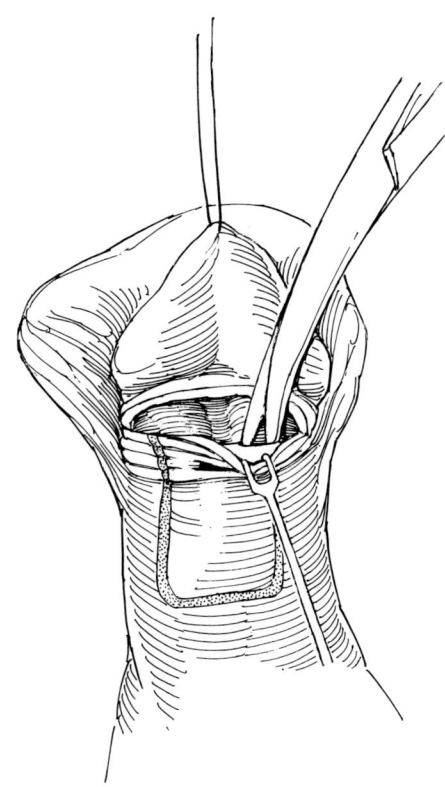

3 **A,** Tunnel through the glans by first directing fine tenotomy scissors to separate the undersurface of the glans from the underlying corpus on each side. Create a separate tunnel over each corporal tip, and divide the septum between them. Alternatively, if the glans is flat, open it widely to form two glans flaps.

B, Direct the scissors horizontally to reach the apex of the glans. Lift the glanular tissue with toothed forceps, and remove a generous divot of skin and glanular tissue. This opening must be tubular, not tapered. Use compression to stop the bleeding. Bring the scissors out through the tip, and spread the blades to make the tunnel wide enough to easily admit the double-thickness skin of the flap.

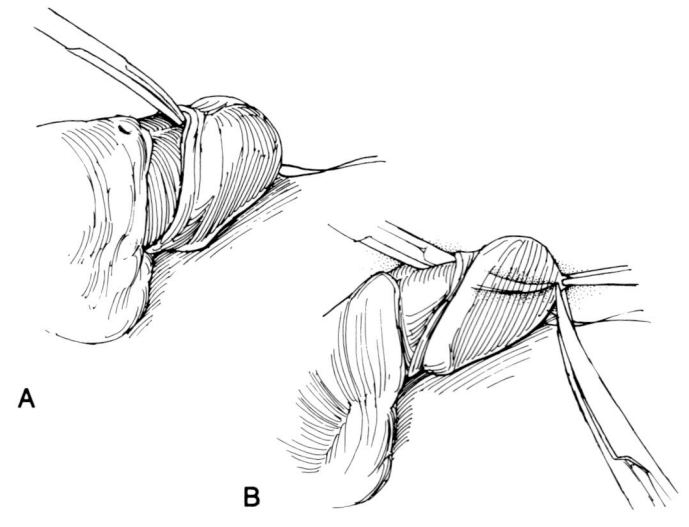

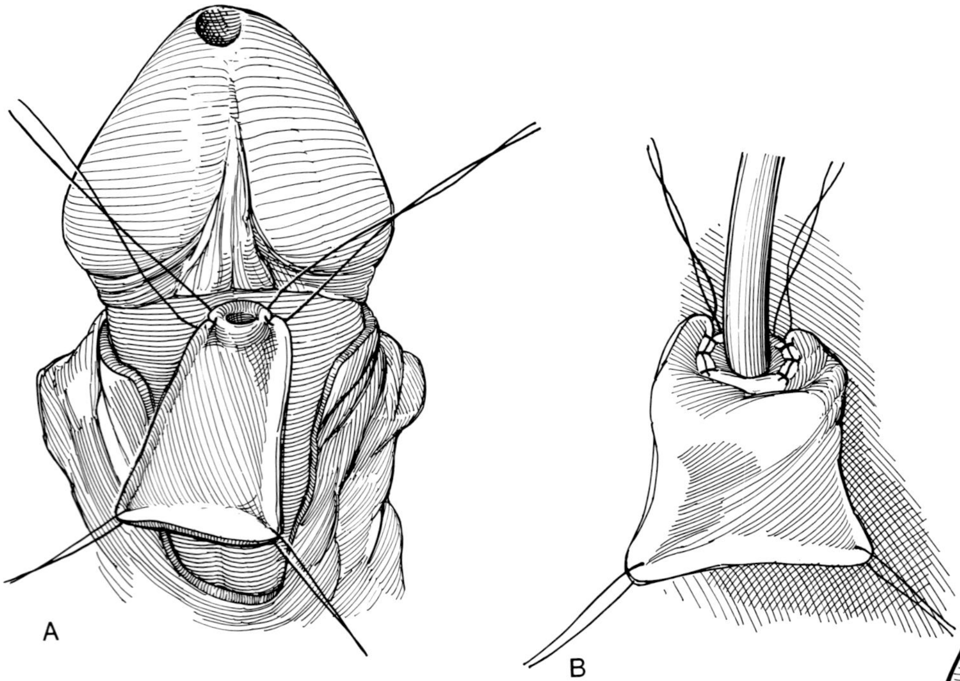

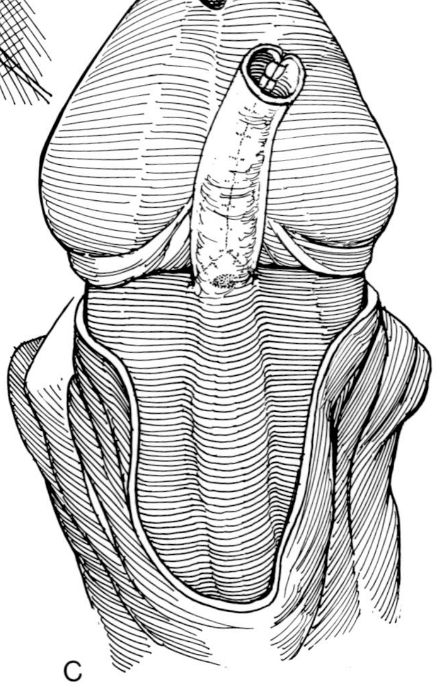

4 **A,** Recheck the outlined length of the flap to be sure it is still adequate. Incise the margins of the flap. Place stay sutures in the four corners, and free the flap from the corpora, leaving as much adventitial tissue on it as possible to preserve the blood supply. Free the lateral skin margins left on the shaft generously.

B, Carefully place one or two 6–0 or 7–0 synthetic absorbable sutures subcuticularly at the junction of the flap with its base. Start the tubularization over a catheter-stent.

C, Continue the closure with an interrupted inverting subcuticular suture of 6–0 or 7–0 Vicryl. Too much suturing will devitalize the edges of the flap; because the suture line will lie deep in the wound, free of pressure from the urinary stream, precise closure is not necessary.

5 Draw the skin tube and stent through the glanular tunnel. Suture the two peripheral corners together, and attach them to the dorsal end of the opening in the glans (stent not shown).

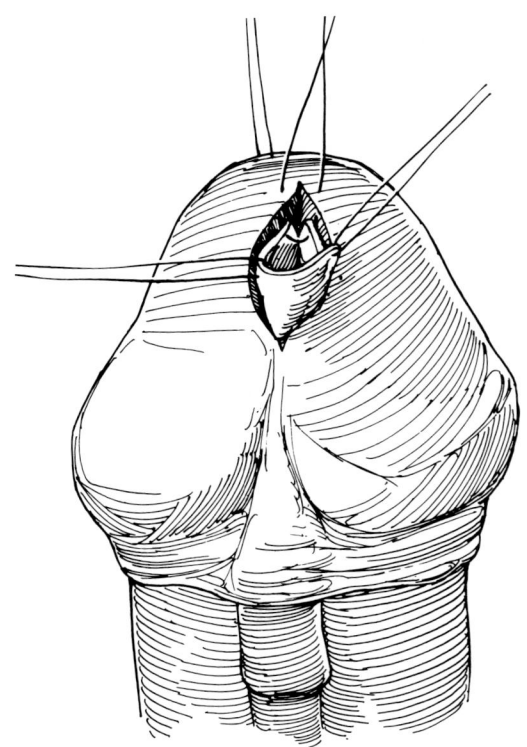

6 Trim the end of the flap to conform to the opening; cutting it obliquely makes the lumen larger. Suture its edges accurately to the glans with interrupted 6–0 synthetic absorbable sutures. Tuck any proximally projecting skin tags into the tunnel.

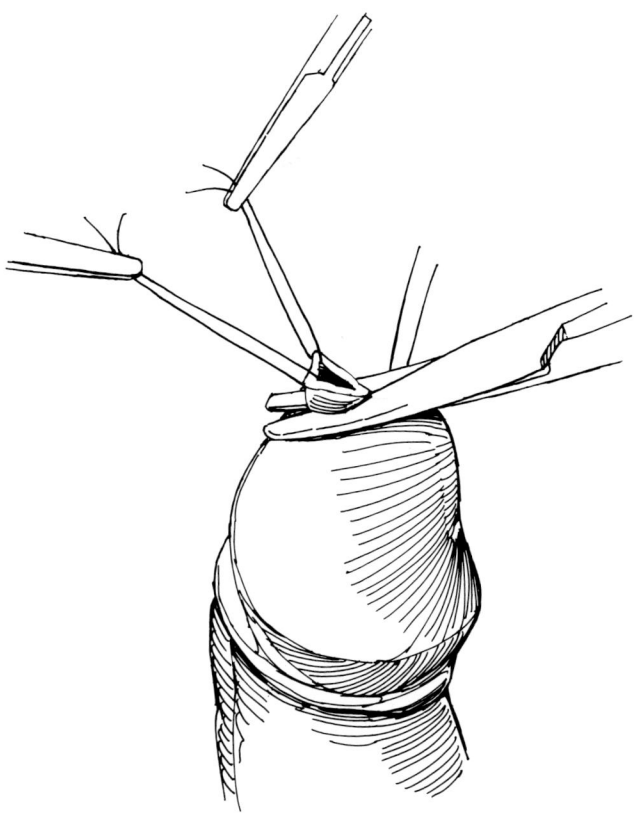

7 **A** and **B,** Open the prepuce by incising it vertically, and bring the wings around to cover the defect on the shaft. De-epithelialize the distal part of one flap, and pass it over the urethra into the tunnel to provide a second layer of coverage. Excise excess skin to achieve a good appearance, and approximate the wings so that the suture line lies in the midline.

C, Although not as good cosmetically, a buttonhole may be made in the prepuce to bring it over the glans. Insert a stent and fasten it to the glans with the stay suture. Loosely apply a Bioclusive dressing to remain until it loosens and can be taken off. If the "drippy tube" is used for diversion, remove it in 3 weeks.

For *diversion,* the drippy tube method (Winslow) (not shown) may be used. Fill the bladder through an 8 F infant feeding tube in the urethra. Place an 18-gauge spinal needle suprapubically, and pass a Prolene suture through it into the bladder; retrieve it transurethrally with an alligator forceps through a small panendoscope. Repeat the maneuver with a second suture. The sutures are now available for fastening to the end of a stenting catheter to be drawn into the bladder through the repair. The end is then cut off, so that drainage is free and no penile suture is needed to hold it.

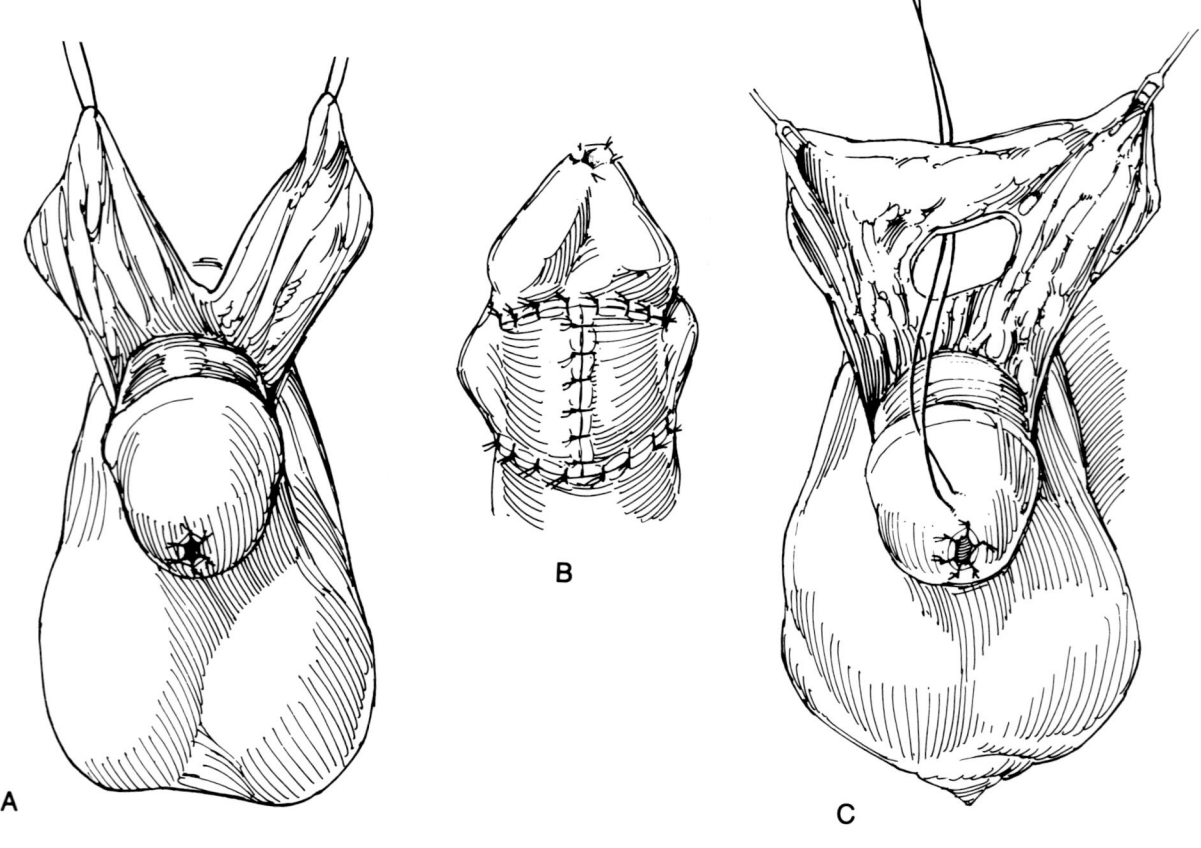

Commentary by Charles J. Devine, Jr.

The Mustardé operation would not be the routine procedure for distal hypospadias, especially when there is a significant amount of chordee. It is a useful technique to advance the urethral meatus to the tip of the penis, and if the vascularity of the skin is good, it can be applied when previous surgery has not brought the urethra as far distally as we and the patient think it should be. Some surgeons repairing hypospadias still believe that a subcoronal meatus is an excellent result.

The flap, when elevated, is a random flap; it has no major artery. During its mobilization, the scissors should be used to spread the tissues of the dartos fascia, preserving the delicate vessels within it. If there is bleeding, the vessel should be controlled with the bipolar cautery at a low-power setting. Heat generated will be confined to the tissue between the tips and will not be transmitted to other vessels within the pedicle. During creation of the tunnel through the glans, the tips of the scissors should be kept against the tunica of the corpora cavernosa, and again, most of the dissection should be accomplished by spreading the tips of the scissors rather than cutting away at this tissue. Buck's fascia inserts into the undersurface of the glans, and there are no large vessels in this space. When the tube is constructed, it is brought through the glans tunnel and secured to the epithelium of the glans. In the past, we used 6–0 chromic sutures for this and for closure of the skin. However, the new Ethicon "Monocryl" synthetic sutures are hydrolyzed in the process of absorption and leave no marks.

The dressing, the use of stents, and the techniques of urine diversion have evolved greatly within recent years. These simpler modalities have markedly shortened the hospital stay of these children. We have progressed from a suprapubic tube and a stent, past stents through which the patient voided after a feeding tube that was passed and left to divert the urine for a day or so had been removed, to the current technique—a "drippy tube" that my colleague, Dr. Boyd Winslow, has improved by securing it to a button on the abdomen. We perform a cystoscopy in all patients with hypospadias as the first step in the surgery, because we have occasionally found more-proximal urethral anomalies, *eg*, valves. Passage of sutures through a hollow needle passed into the bladder dome simplifies fixation of the tube, which is left in place for approximately 3 weeks. Lastly, we have not used a compression dressing for years. To cover the penis, a single wrap of Bioclusive dressing is applied loosely and stuck together on the dorsal side. This furnishes adequate pressure and, being clear, allows the status of the penile skin to be observed. The adhesive material will loosen in a week, and the dressing peels off easily. *Note:* Other wraps, such as Tegaderm or Op-Site, have a different consistency and have not been satisfactory for this purpose.

CHAPTER 120

Transverse Preputial Island Flap

ONLAY PREPUTIAL TRANSVERSE ISLAND FLAP
(DUCKETT)

When only minimal chordee persists after takedown of the ventral skin, use an onlay flap to preserve the urethral plate. The tubed transverse island flap is reserved for those with greater degrees of chordee that is not amenable to dorsal tucking.

1 Place a stay suture on a tapered needle in the glans. Infiltrate the ventral meatal area with 1 or 2 ml of epinephrine-lidocaine solution and wait 7 minutes. Using a magnifying loupe, mark and incise the coronal sulcus circumferentially 8 mm from the glans, and extend the incision as two parallel cuts 0.6 to 0.8 cm apart down the shaft and around the meatus as a U to release the tethering skin and dartos fascia, leaving the urethral plate intact. Mobilize the skin and superficial fascia from the proximal urethra with dissection around the lateral aspects of the shaft and distally into the glanular tissue. Do not dissect behind the plate. This may correct the chordee. Test by artificial erection. If chordee persists, plicate the dorsal tunica albuginea (Figure 4B).

2 Develop glans wings by extending parallel incisions onto the ventrum of the glans that continue out to the end of the glanular groove. Mobilize glans wings by dissecting in the plane between the glans and the tips of the corpora. If there is a lip in the glans groove, correct it with a longitudinal incision and transverse closure, as in the meatal advancement and glanuloplasty (MAGPI) technique (page 575). Take a wedge from the urethra proximal to the meatus to cut it back into well-developed spongy tissue, and trim any excess of thin urethral epithelium to provide a clean edge for suturing.

Place four traction sutures in the opened prepuce to fan out the ventral surface. Mark the skin for the flap and incise along the marks. Develop a plane well down to the base of the penis between the flap and the dorsal skin to form a substantial pedicle. Take great care not to devascularize the flap while raising it.

A smaller flap also may be obtained from the ventral skin of the shaft, as described under penile urethroplasty (page 688), using Byars flaps, as needed, for coverage.

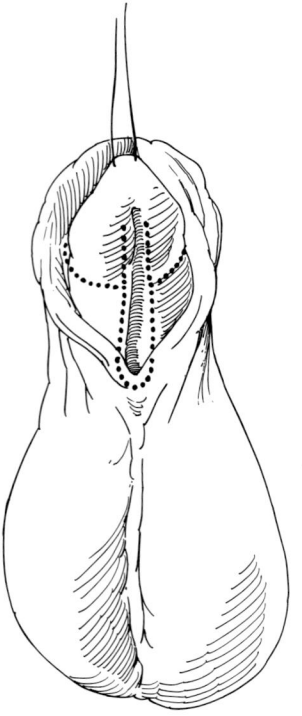

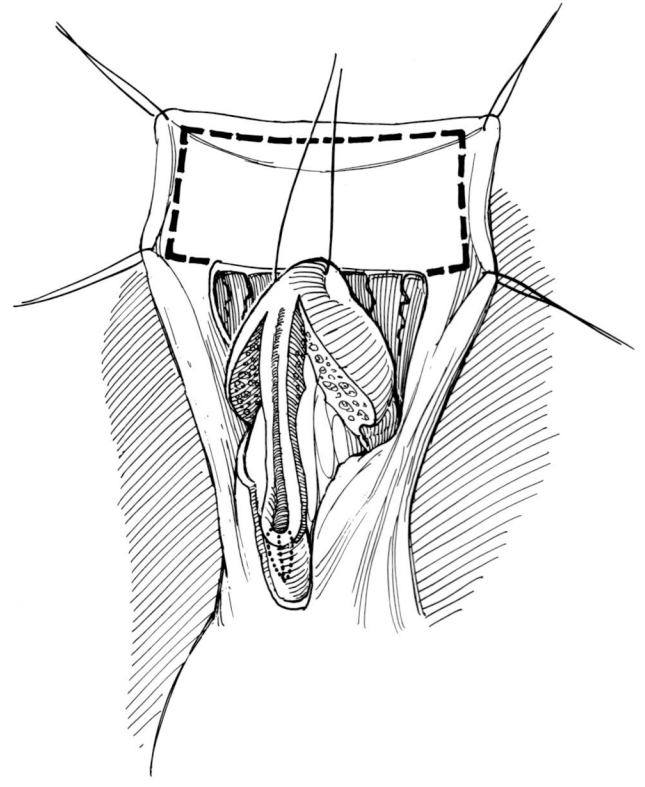

588

3 Rotate the flap ventrally. Trim the skin generously, because only a portion of it is needed to form a 12 to 14 F urethra in combination with the urethral plate. Discarding excess skin ensures adequate blood supply to the remaining strip. Alternatively, instead of resecting the redundant skin on right side of the flap, remove the epithelium from that portion not used for urethral coverage, and use the dermal layer for cover.

Suture the edge nearest the pedicle to the urethral plate starting at the tip, using a continuous 6–0 synthetic absorbable suture. Continue around the former meatus and up the shaft. Alternatively, if a de-epithelialized flap was developed, it now will lie on the left side of the repair. Turn it back for cover.

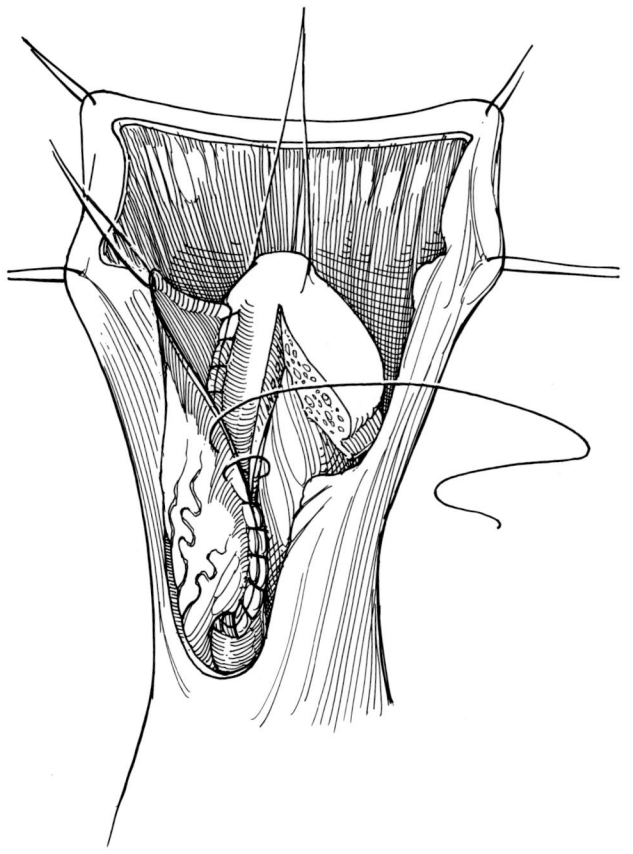

4 **A,** Suture the glans flaps together in the midline, and reapproximate the skin to cover the shaft. Insert a 6 F urethral stent into the bladder, to remain 7 to 10 days.

B, Preservation of the urethral plate may leave some chordee. Proceed with orthoplastic dorsal tucks by making two parallel incisions approximately 8 mm apart dorsally in the tunica albuginea on one side of the midline near the coronal sulcus. Bring the two incisions together with inverted nonabsorbable sutures that start from inside out at the proximal cut and outside in at the distal cut, thus drawing the two openings in apposition while ducking the intervening bridge. Repeat the procedure on the other side.

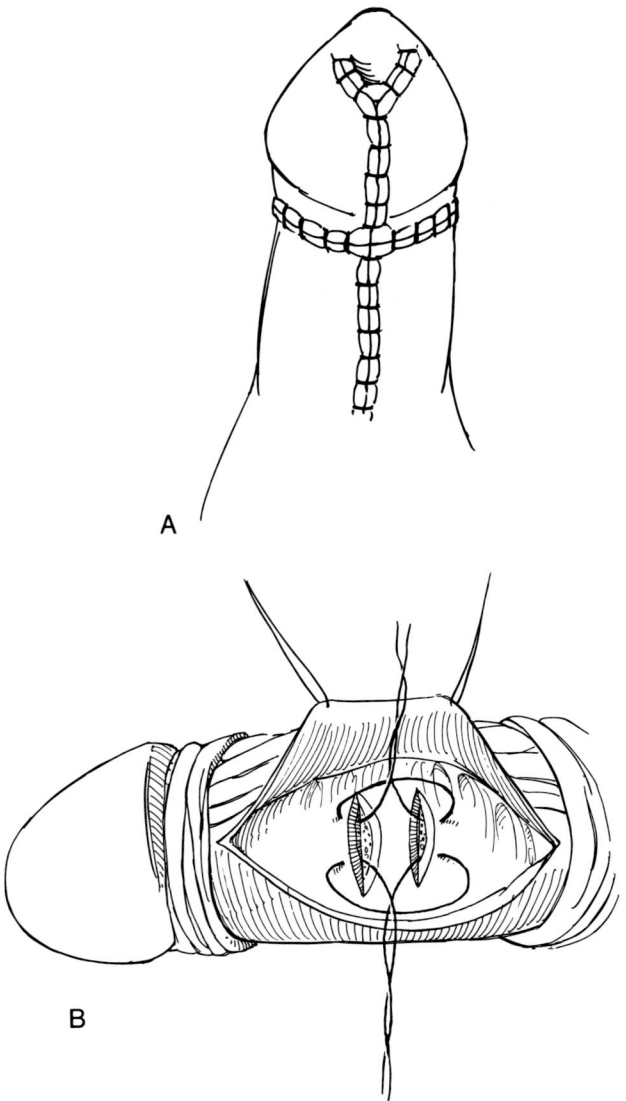

A

B

TUBED TRANSVERSE PREPUTIAL ISLAND FLAP
(DUCKETT)

If release of the urethral plate is required to correct the chordee, the missing portion may be replaced with a tube of preputial skin placed as an island flap.

5 Mark and incise the coronal sulcus circumferentially 8 mm from the glans, and extend the incision down the shaft and around the meatus as a U to release the tethering skin and dartos fascia, leaving intact a normal spongiosum supported by the urethral plate. Mobilize the skin and fascia from the proximal urethra with dissection around the lateral aspects of the shaft and distally into the glanular tissue. Test by artificial erection. If chordee is appreciable, proceed with a tube repair. If the urethral plate remains and there is no curvature on artificial erection, an onlay island flap is the preferred procedure.

Trim the meatus of poor-quality skin. Dissect the dorsal penile skin from Buck's fascia in the avascular plane.

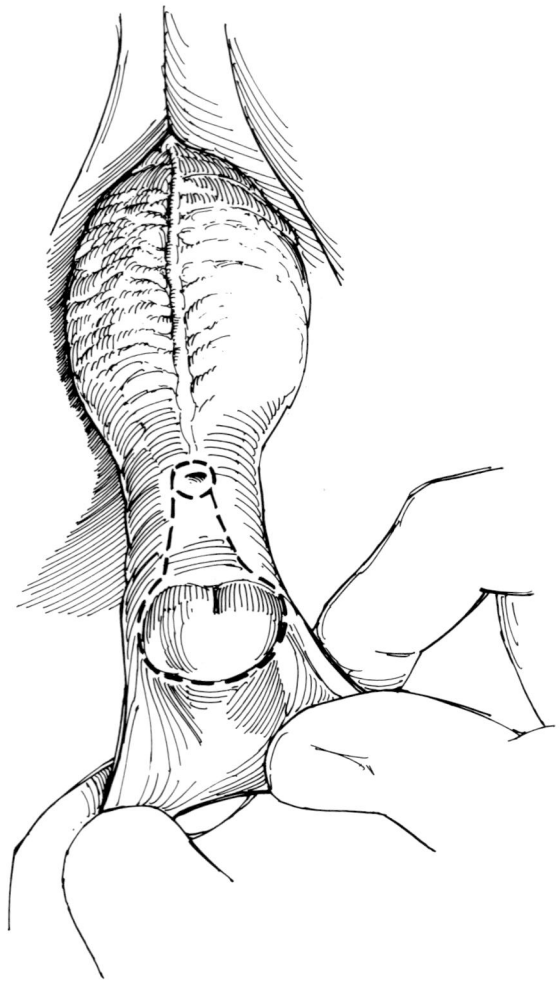

6 Place four fine traction sutures to fan out the ventral surface of the prepuce. Mark the skin for the neourethra to provide the needed length to bridge the gap and a width of 1.2 to 1.5 cm. Incise along the marks, just into the subcutaneous tissue.

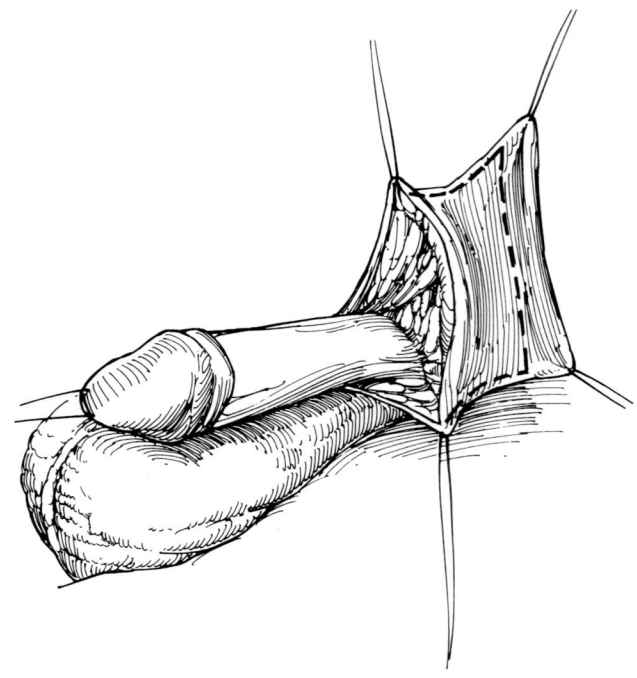

7 Develop a plane well down to the base of the penis between the flap and the outer prepuce to form a substantial pedicle. The vasculature of the pedicle usually is obvious, but take great care not to devascularize the flap.

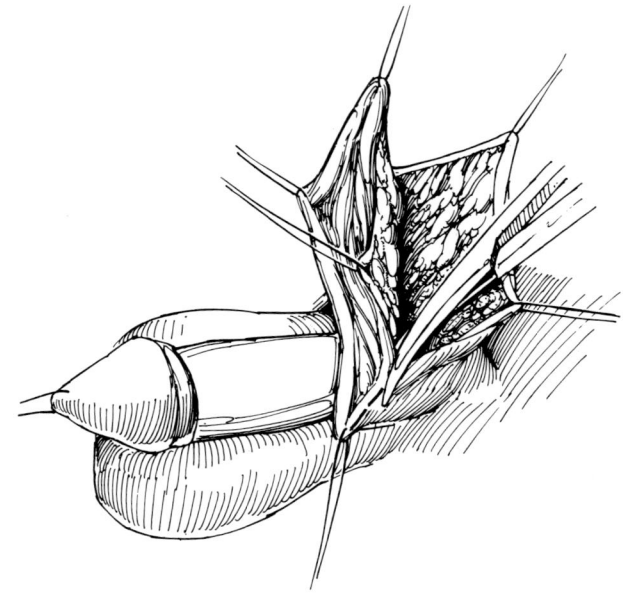

8 Roll the flap over an 8 F catheter, and approximate the edges with a running subcuticular 6–0 or 7–0 chromic catgut suture. Place interrupted sutures at the ends to allow trimming. Examine the ends of the flap for ischemia, and trim them appropriately. Test the caliber with a 12 F bougie à boule.

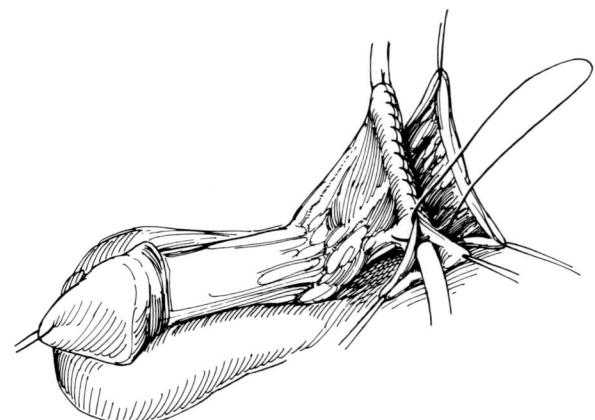

9 Rotate the graft around its base so that the right side of the flap is proximal. Avoid torsion by adequately freeing the base of the pedicle. Trim and spatulate the urethra, and suture the flap to it, so that the suture line of the flap lies against the corpora. Use 6–0 synthetic absorbable sutures placed with the knots outside in an interrupted manner. Fix the anastomotic area to the corpora with several sutures.

Insert plastic scissors flat against the corpora cavernosa in the plane between the cap of the glans and the corpora, and snip a path to the tip of the glans. Remove a large plug of glans (0.2 × 1.5 cm), and reach inside the meatus to excise excess glanular tissue to provide a wide channel, at least 18 F in caliber. Check the caliber with bougies à boule. If the tunnel is not adequate, split the glans and form glans flaps.

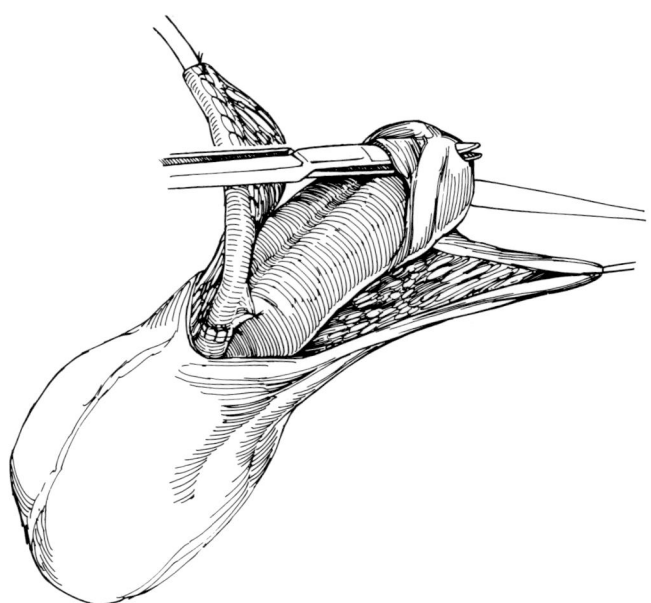

10 Pull the tubed flap through the glans channel, keeping the suture line against the corporal bodies. Pull it out to straighten it, so that no redundancy remains, then trim the excess length. Suture the tubed flap to the new meatus with interrupted 6–0 chromic catgut sutures. Fix the tube to the corpora along the shaft to prevent kinking of the anastomosis. Instill saline to check for leaks; place extra sutures as needed. Insert a 6 F Silastic tube as a stent, so that the end lies just within the bladder in infants. Cover the anastomosis with pedicle tissue, tacked in place to cover the whole repair, being careful not to interfere with its vascular supply.

Remember that if the flap looks devascularized, it can be defatted and converted into a graft.

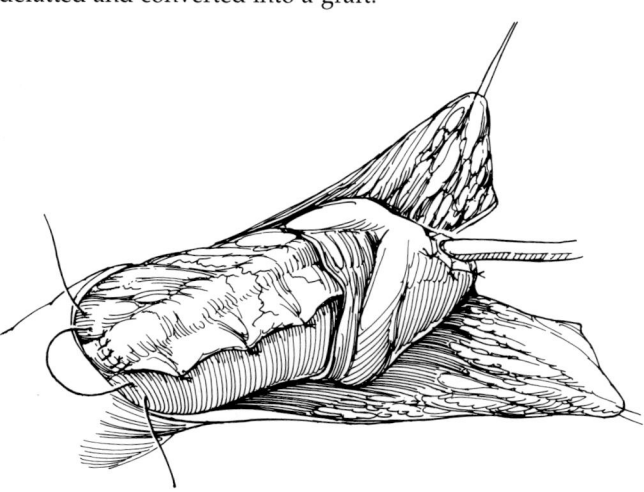

11 Divide the prepuce dorsally, and suture it ventrally with fine horizontal mattress chromic catgut sutures, excising the lateral triangles to fit. If insufficient skin is available, the skin may have to be incised on the dorsum. Check the position of the stent, suture it to the glans with a 5-0 Prolene suture, and cut it short, permitting urine to drip freely into the diaper. Test for leaks. Dress the penis with Tegaderm. Instruct the parents to keep the glans free of encrustations. Remove the stent in 7 to 10 days. Calibrate the repair with a straight 8 F sound in 3 weeks.

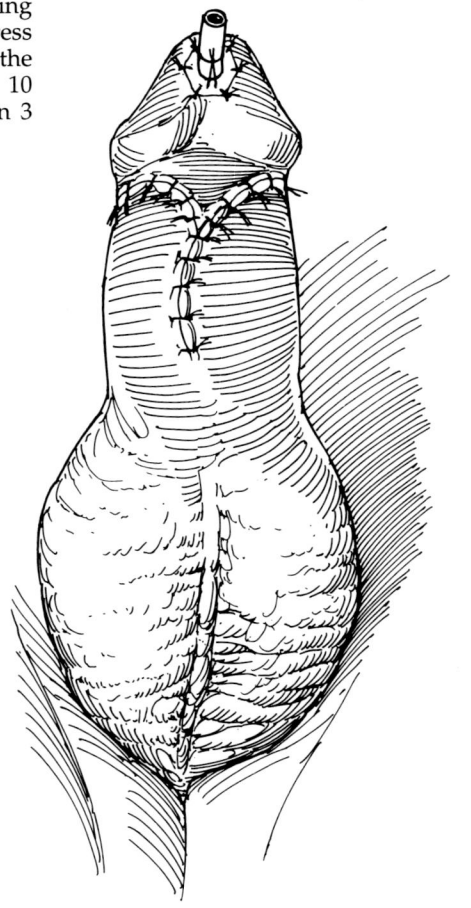

POSTOPERATIVE PROBLEMS

Fistulas are the most common problem. Unless they are very tiny, do not attempt closure for 6 months (pages 563–568). *Strictures* are not rare, usually consequent on kinking from overlap of two suture lines or from ischemia. Open repair usually is needed. *Meatal stenosis* may require meatoplasty (page 570). A very wide urethra, resembling a *diverticulum*, necessitates open excision of the extra skin. If chordee is present after repair, resort to dorsal tucks.

Commentary by John W. Duckett

This series of figures depicts the tubularized transverse preputial island flap, which is the classic technique that we have developed. In a recent review, we found it less frequently used today; an onlay island flap is favored. After the first skin incision, if the penis is straight, the urethral plate can be extended onto the glans, developing glanular wings. An onlay of transverse preputial tissue will form a floor for the urethra, and the glans is wrapped around this. One third of our procedures now use this maneuver, whereas only 10 percent use the tubularized flap. The remaining are either Magpi techniques or meatal-based procedures.

The most common error with this technique is making the glans channel too narrow, constricting the pedicle of the neourethra as it traverses the glans and causing ischemia and meatal stenosis. Great care must be taken in making a generous glans channel.

To avoid fistulization, it is important to test the repair by injecting saline to identify the gaps in the sutures, closing these to avoid leaks. It also is important not to make the tube too wide, because it will develop a diverticulum, even without meatal stenosis. This also is a problem with the onlay flap technique.

We use bougies à boule to calibrate the repair as we are operating to make sure it is appropriate for the penis size and the situation.

Our current dressing technique is to compress the penis onto the abdomen using a Telfa strip under a folded 4 × 4 gauze and medium-sized Tegaderm. (The 6 F urethral stent is now supplied by Kendall.)

Clearly, the most important elements for a successful hypospadias outcome are delicate tissue handling, familiarity with mobilizing skin flaps, and compulsive attention to detail characteristic of plastic surgical principles. It is worthwhile to apprentice oneself to a urologist who is doing these complex hypospadias reconstructions before being tempted to proceed, utilizing these diagrams and simplified steps. There is indeed a learning curve that can be most discouraging.

CHAPTER 121

Double-Faced Transverse Island Flap
(HODGSON XX-ASOPA)

This procedure uses pedicles from the superficial external pudendal system for both the flap that is tubularized and the one that provides cover.

1 **A,** Make a submeatal circumcising incision, and retract the edges of the prepuce. **B,** Encircle the meatus, and tack its dorsal wall to Buck's fascia at the corners. Free the glans wings from the corpora after incising a wedge in the ventrum of the glans and folding it between the edges of the wings. At this point, decide whether a transverse island flap, a free graft, or a perimeatal flap is suitable. The last may be satisfactory if a well-vascularized flap with an adequate attached dartos can be fashioned. Otherwise, choose one form of an island flap, the double-faced transverse island flap being the most anatomically sound.

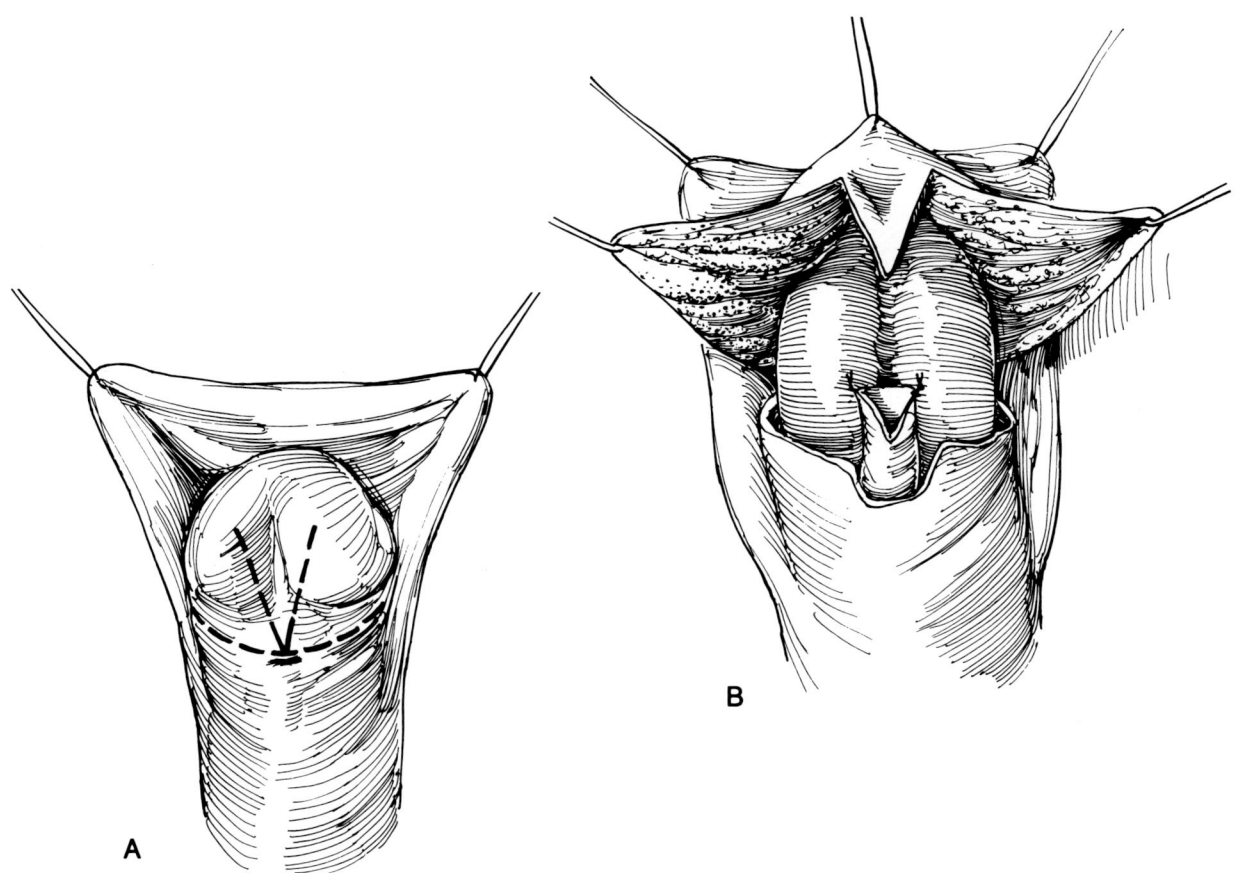

2 Incise the prepuce vertically to form asymmetric flaps. Mark and incise an island on the inner preputial fold of the smaller flap, and excise and discard it. Mark, incise, and partially mobilize a larger island on the larger flap, leaving the center of it attached to the flap in a transverse direction.

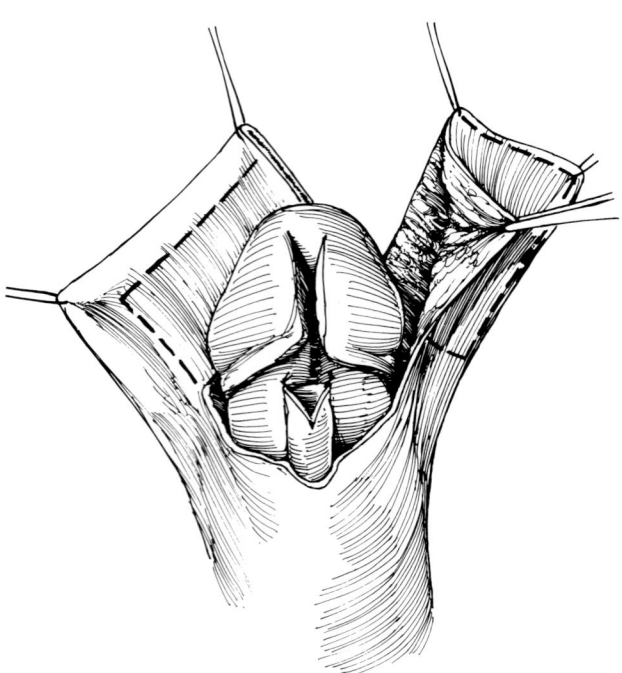

3 Roll the inner layer of the larger flap over a 12 F tube, and suture it with 5–0 synthetic absorbable sutures.

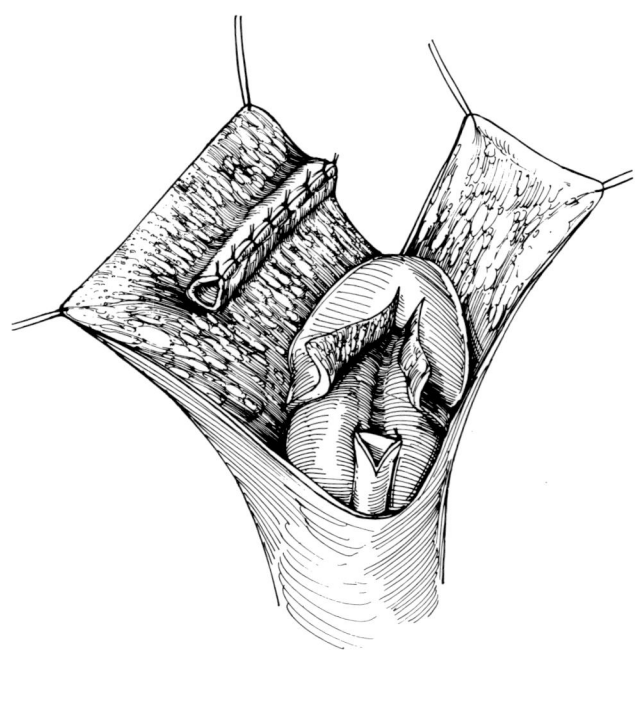

4 Rotate the tube, and suture it proximally to the spatulated urethra and distally to the V-flap at the meatus, using 6–0 or 7–0 chromic catgut sutures. The pedicle must be freed to the penopubic angle to prevent rotation of the penis after application of the flap. Mobilize a second layer composed of subcutaneous tissue and pedicle to cover the anastomoses.

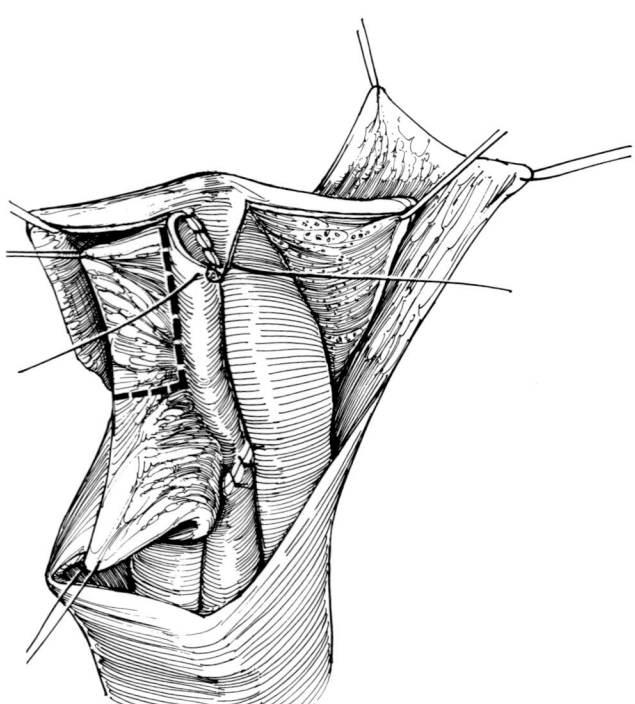

5 Bring the glans flaps over the new urethra. Trim the smaller preputial flap to fit. Draw the rest of the larger flap across to cover the repair. Insert a 6 F silicone tube into the bladder. Apply a Tegaderm dressing over tincture of benzoin.

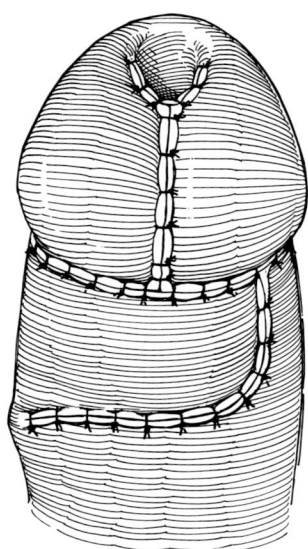

Commentary by Norman B. Hodgson

As can well be imagined, description of the variations on a two-faced flap have caused me considerable difficulty over the years. Time has shown that a glanular split is preferable to a V-flap in avoiding secondary meatal stenosis.

The many numbered flap techniques were chosen methods for depicting what, in reality, turned out to be a series of experiments. The initial goal was to complete the repair of hypospadias defects in a single operation and to achieve a cosmetically satisfactory or superior end result. As time has passed, the Hodgson II and III techniques have fallen into disuse. They were double-pedicle flaps to enhance the healing process, but they left a not-inconsiderable bundle of tissue on the ventrum and have since been replaced by more versatile techniques. The Hodgson III has little applicability for the longer defects because of the relative paucity of available skin in that area to accomplish the new urethra. In addition, the limitation of glanular advancement by the Denis Browne denudation has been replaced by various glans-split or glans-wing mobilization techniques, all of which have more nearly approximated a normal glans configuration. Although these procedures had some merit in the earlier phases of one-stage repairs, they too have been replaced by the current spectrum of procedures, such as the Hodgson XX or mobilized transverse island flap. (The appellation *Hodgson XX* was picked randomly, because I had difficulty conveying the earlier nuances, so each modification got a new number up to XIII, at which point a sudden jump was made to XX, for no other reason than it looked good.) The Hodgson XX has the merit of a nonmobilized tangential inner-face preputial flap rotated to the ventrum through a dorsal, cutaneous releasing incision, which protects the integrity of the superficial external pudendal vascular system. Actually, as is well known, the definition of that vessel system was not fully known until 1982, although Standoli, Duckett, Quartey, and Hinderer had each emphasized the ability to exploit and use those vessels when they had gained some character. The Hodgson XX would then be applied when the vessels were suspect or marginal in their transilluminated appearance. The main benefit of the Hodgson XX is in the rotated nonmobilized superficial external pudendal vascular system that allows ventral presentation of the inner face of the prepuce for urethral patching. The subtlety of that benefit escapes some reviewers, but its usefulness is real and its healing virtues are many. I really do not disown types II and III, but along

with the Model A Ford, the 1958 Ford Thunderbird, and the DC-3, they have a place not currently but historically.

The current environment stipulates minimal or no hospitalization with a home-care setting, free of discomfort with markedly diminished complications or healing defects. Much of the current success has been the result of new materials, such as 7–0 Vicryl or Dexon S sutures, or the occasional use of polydioxanone. The move has been away from chromic catgut because of tissue reactivity. Dissective processes are commonly done with magnification and pinpoint electrocautery. Tissues are handled with microhooks, all with directed emphasis to primary healing. The tubes are created with delicate suturing and are anastomosed over wide spatulations. Drainage of the neourethra is accomplished with fine (6 F) drain tubes, and dressings are commonly elastic membranes, such as Tegaderm. The recent addition of Telfa padding beneath the Tegaderm has enhanced the healing process.

Urinary diversion always has been a problem because of the complications of bladder spasms; a multiplicity of techniques has been called on to minimize them. Currently, my favorite and most successful drainage has been accomplished through the Figure-4 catheter (Bard), used as a cystostomy drain tube. The bladder spasms have been minimized, and the drainage is satisfactory. Urine ordinarily is collected in a double diaper. The surgery can be accomplished on an outpatient basis or with a 24-hour stay, and subsequent wound care is managed in an office setting. For severe hypospadias persisting after multiple repairs or a perineal defect underendowed with appropriate vascularized flaps, the leaning of the surgeon has been toward free grafts of bladder epithelium, which create their own set of problems, but have, on the whole, been rewarding.

We now have plenty of choices among the meatal advancement and glanuloplasty (MAGPI), Mathieu, Hodgson XX, mobilized inner face flap (Duckett), external face flap (Standoli), one of the Hinderer perimeatal flaps, and free grafts of skin (Horton-Devine) or bladder epithelium. If the dorsal vasculature is abundant and in no way suspect, the Duckett mobilization of those tissues (inner or outer face) as a patch or tube can succeed readily. Both John Duckett and I have found ourselves doing more and more patching and fewer and fewer Mathieu procedures, because the supporting tissue of the longer flip-flaps have become suspect.

CHAPTER 122

Tube Repair

(THIERSCH-DUPLAY)

Tube repair is applicable when previous procedures have failed, but it also may be used as a second stage after first-stage correction of chordee or when it had not been possible to complete the procedure in one stage.

1 Mark a V-incision on the glans, as for a perimeatal-based procedure. To form the urethral tube, mark two parallel lines on the ventrum spaced suitably for the age of the patient (*ie*, 1.5 cm apart in infants, 2.5 cm in children, or 3 cm in adults). Place these incisions more to one side, so that the urethral suture line at closure will not coincide with that of the skin. Incise along the marks. Begin with a knife, then proceed with blunt-tipped scissors to cut an edge in the skin at right angles to the surface. Mobilize the edges of the strip minimally (the figure exaggerates the dissection). Insert a small silicone tube into the bladder.

2 Form a glans flap and glans wings. Mobilize and incise the distal end of the ventral strip vertically in the midline to receive the V-shaped glans flap, and suture the flap in place with 6–0 chromic catgut sutures.

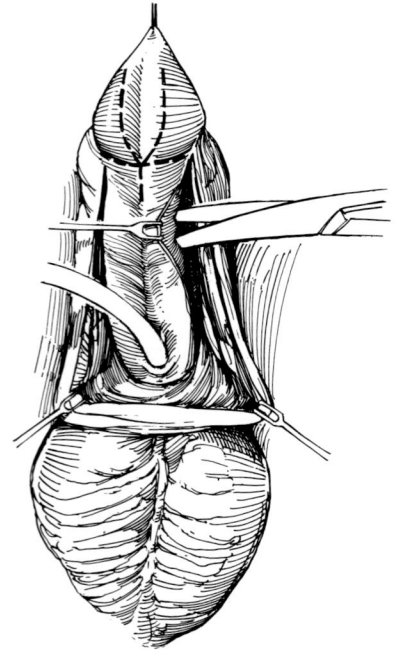

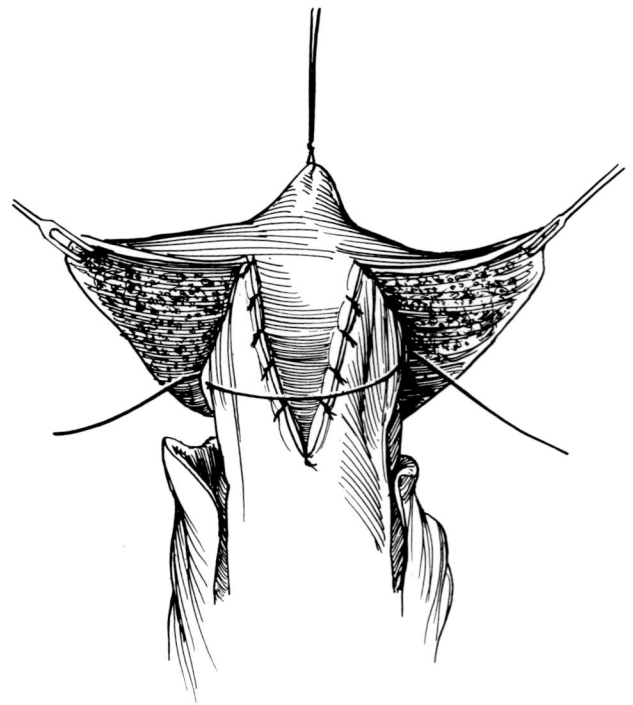

3 Elevate the edges of the strip with skin hooks, and tack them together in three or four places. The suture line will lie to one side. Run a 6–0 polydioxanone suture subcuticularly. Close the glans with a layer of synthetic absorbable deep sutures, adding fine interrupted sutures on the surface.

4 Make a Z-plasty if the skin is scarred and tight, or make a dorsal relaxing incision, which may be covered with a split-thickness graft. Place some subcutaneous sutures, and close the skin eccentrically with either a running subcuticular suture or interrupted sutures. Dress the penis appropriately. Remove the catheter in 10 days.

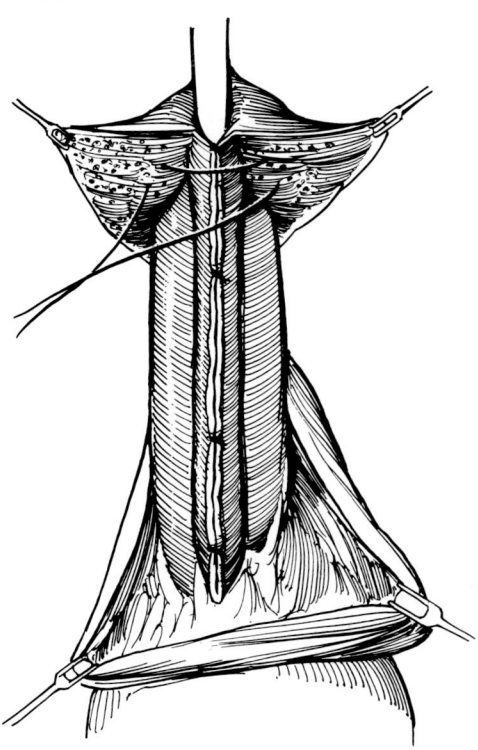

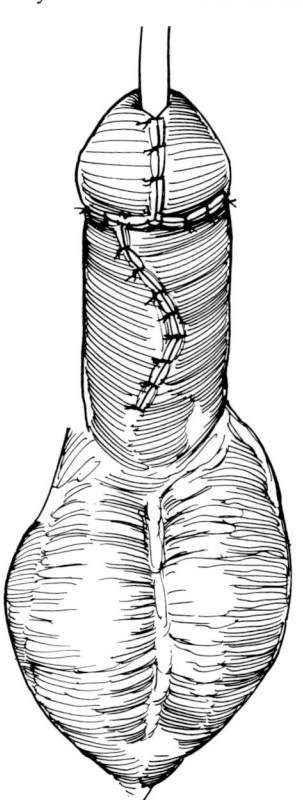

Commentary by George W. Kaplan

There are a number of technical nuances to this operation. In estimating the size of the neourethra, I have used the caliber of the native urethra (as determined with bougies à boule) and then added 2 mm as a "fudge factor." Hence, if the child's urethra calibrated as 14 F, I would outline a 16-mm strip. Additionally, I no longer bother to offset the suture lines, because I have found that the longer side often will not come across without mobilization, and I would prefer not to mobilize that strip. I usually divert the urine with a small silicone Foley catheter, although silicone tubing as a splint is perfectly acceptable.

I no longer use the type of glansplasty depicted in Figure 2; rather, I have employed a modification of the Barcat repair in which the distal portion of the strip (which usually is redundant) is mobilized, and after the urethroplasty is completed, the distal portion of the urethra is laid into a deep groove in the glans and sutured thereto. I usually use slightly finer suture material (usually 7–0 or 8–0 Vicryl), but 5–0 Vicryl is used to reapproximate the glans subcutaneously.

In the formation of the urethra in Figure 3, I prefer to use a complete resutured urethra. The curve of the U-incision that passes proximal to the native urethral meatus is relatively closely applied to the meatus (perhaps 2 mm from the ventral edge of the meatus). The entire epithelium is inverted into the lumen of the neourethra, and the suture line is continued out to the end as a subcuticular closure. The urethra is then tacked to the split in the glans dorsally, and after the glans is reapproximated, the neourethra is tacked to the glans circumferentially. I feel it important to bring some subcutaneous tissue over this closure to minimize fistula formation. This subcutaneous tissue can be obtained by using E. Durham Smith's technique (1973) of de-epithelializing one edge of the skin, provided there is sufficient skin to do so. If not, a flap of subcutaneous tissue can be rotated up from the scrotum to cover the urethral closure and then tacked over the closure with fine absorbable suture. I prefer to close the skin with interrupted sutures so that I can better tailor the closure. I really do prefer to avoid relaxing incisions. If, preoperatively, I recognized that a relaxing incision would be necessary, I probably would choose a free graft of bladder epithelium, which I would then tunnel under the tissue between the native urethral meatus and the corona. Often, I attempt to use a Z-plasty closure to avoid contraction of a midline scar. Lastly (based on our experimental observation of urethral wound healing), I tend to leave the catheter for only 7 days, because urethral re-epithelialization is complete by that time, and I feel that the foreign body beyond the time of urethral re-epithelialization acts as a nidus for urethritis rather than assisting in wound healing.

CHAPTER 123

Free Tube Graft and Partial Island Flap

FREE TUBE GRAFT
(HORTON-DEVINE)

1 **A,** Insert a cystostomy tube (page 346). Place a traction suture in the glans. Mark a V-shaped incision on the glans, and run it around the meatus. Infiltrate the area with 1 ml of 1:200,000 epinephrine solution in 0.5 percent lidocaine. Incise the coronal sulcus.

B, Elevate the wings of the glans with skin hooks and begin dissection of the ventral tissues that produce chordee. Continue freeing behind the meatus and urethra until the penis can be shown to be straight by artificial erection. Trim and discard the thinned tissue from the terminal urethra, and notch it on the ventral edge. Separate the glans from the corpora. Cut the glans flap (page 596), and excise the bulges of tissue at its base.

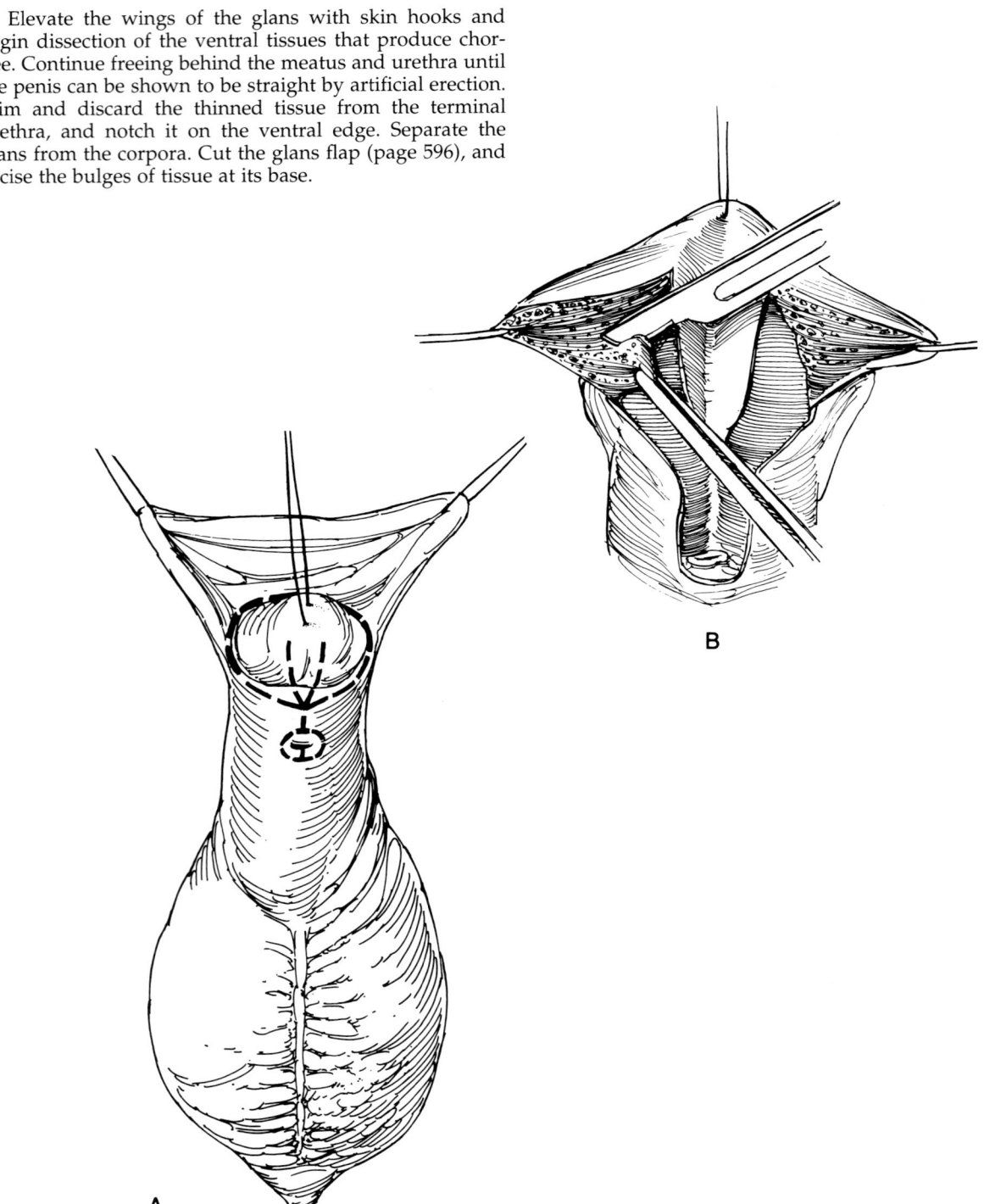

B

A

2 **A,** Unfold the dorsal prepuce, and place four stay sutures in it at least 1.4 cm apart and at a length that is 10 percent longer than that needed to replace the urethra, because 75 percent circumferential shrinkage of the graft is expected.

B, Cut the graft from the inner face of the prepuce, and defat it over the finger or on a board coated with double-surfaced dermatome tape.

C, Attach the full-thickness, fat-free graft, skin surface inside, to a suitably sized catheter at a site that will allow the end of the catheter to lie in the bladder. Use interrupted 5–0 or 6–0 synthetic absorbable sutures. Cut both ends of the graft obliquely, and insert one end of the catheter into the bladder.

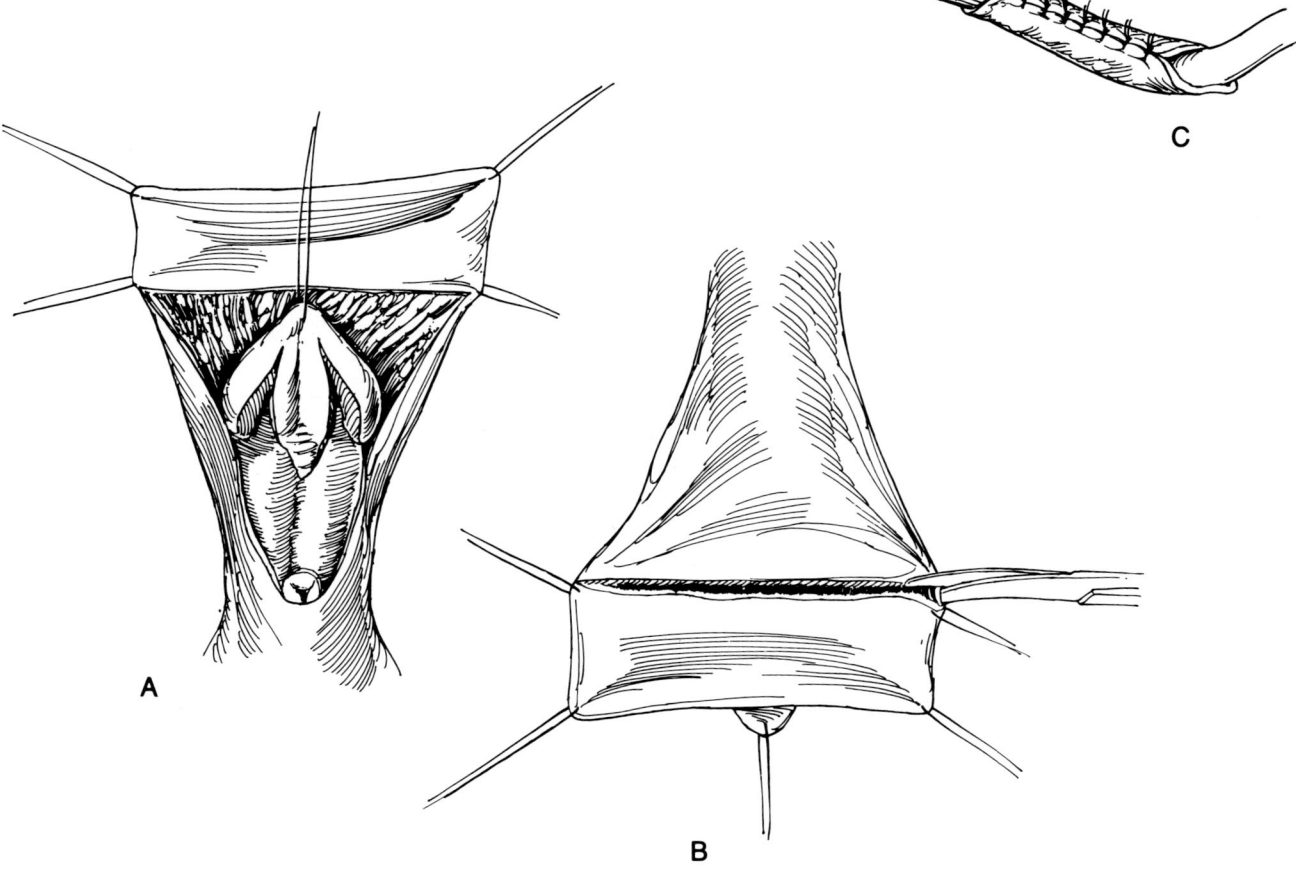

3 Suture the dorsal side of the proximal end of the graft to the spatulated end of the urethra with 5–0 synthetic absorbable sutures, and continue around to the ventrum. Place a suture from the tip of the glans flap through the apex of the oblique cut in the graft.

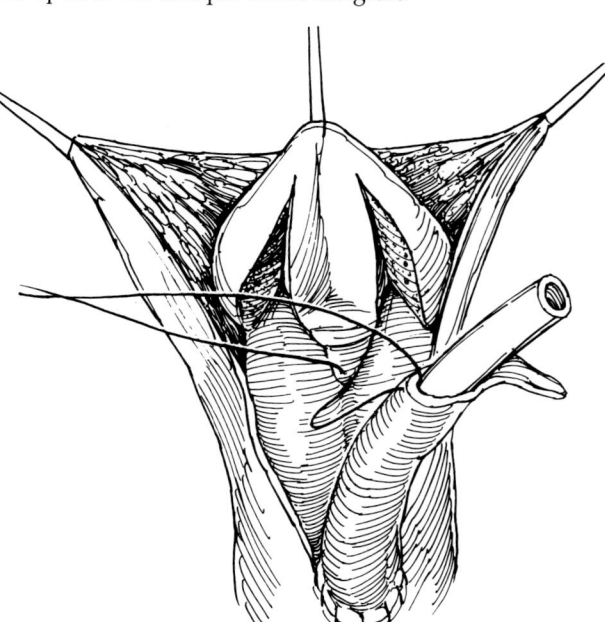

4 Complete the approximation of the flap and graft.

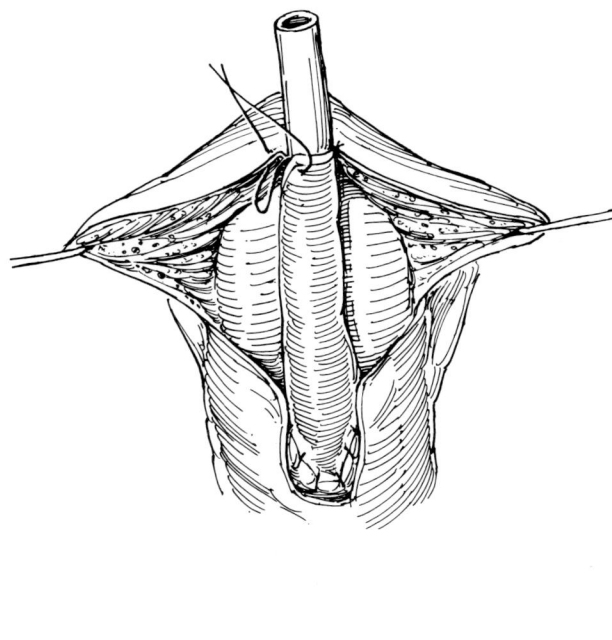

5 Close the glans flaps over the graft with three or four 5-0 synthetic absorbable sutures, and suture the graft to the edges of the glans at the new meatus with 5-0 chromic catgut sutures. If possible, bring in a layer of subcutaneous tissue to cover the proximal anastomosis.

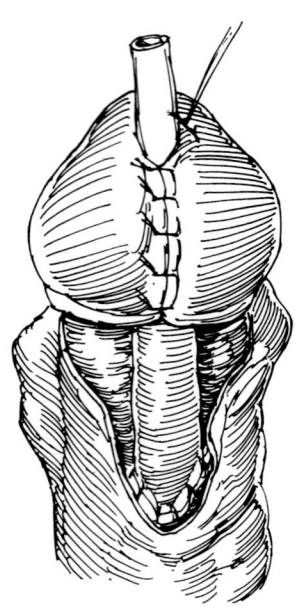

6 Split the remaining prepuce, and approximate it ventrally, trying to keep from superimposing suture lines. Suture the cut-off catheter to the meatus and leave it in place for 10 days.

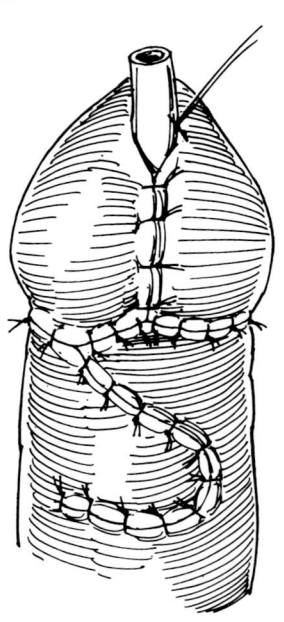

7 **A,** For longer, proximal defects, obtain coverage for a limited proximal tube from adjacent skin by incising the hairless skin around the proximal end to partially raise a flap. **B,** Close the proximal skin tube over a catheter first; then complete the closure of the skin.

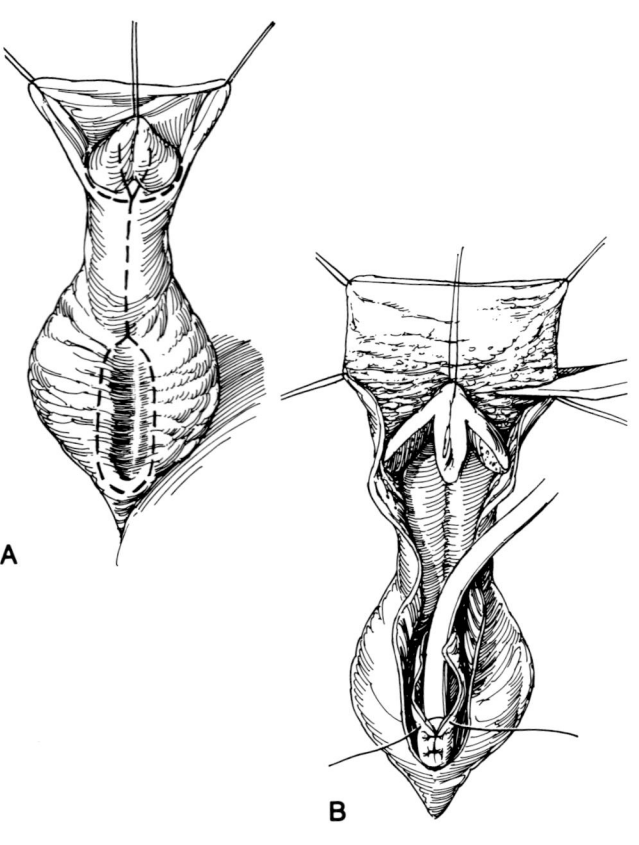

A

B

8 **A,** Harvest the graft and anastomose it to the end of the proximal skin tube. **B,** Close the glans, as described previously, and approximate the residual preputial flaps ventrally.

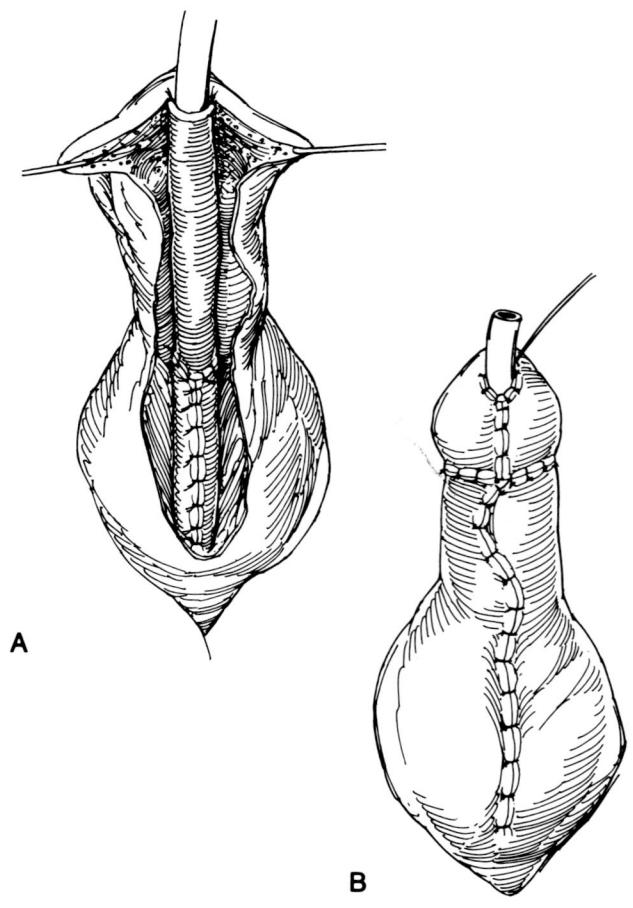

A

B

PARTIAL ISLAND FLAP
(KAPLAN)

9 **A** and **B,** Rather than apply a double-faced island flap (page 593), form such a flap, but dissect the inner preputial skin from its dartos pedicle, clear it of fat, and use it as a free tube graft. Cover the ventral defect by rotation of the remainder of the island flap, the outer layer of preputial skin, on its dartos pedicle.

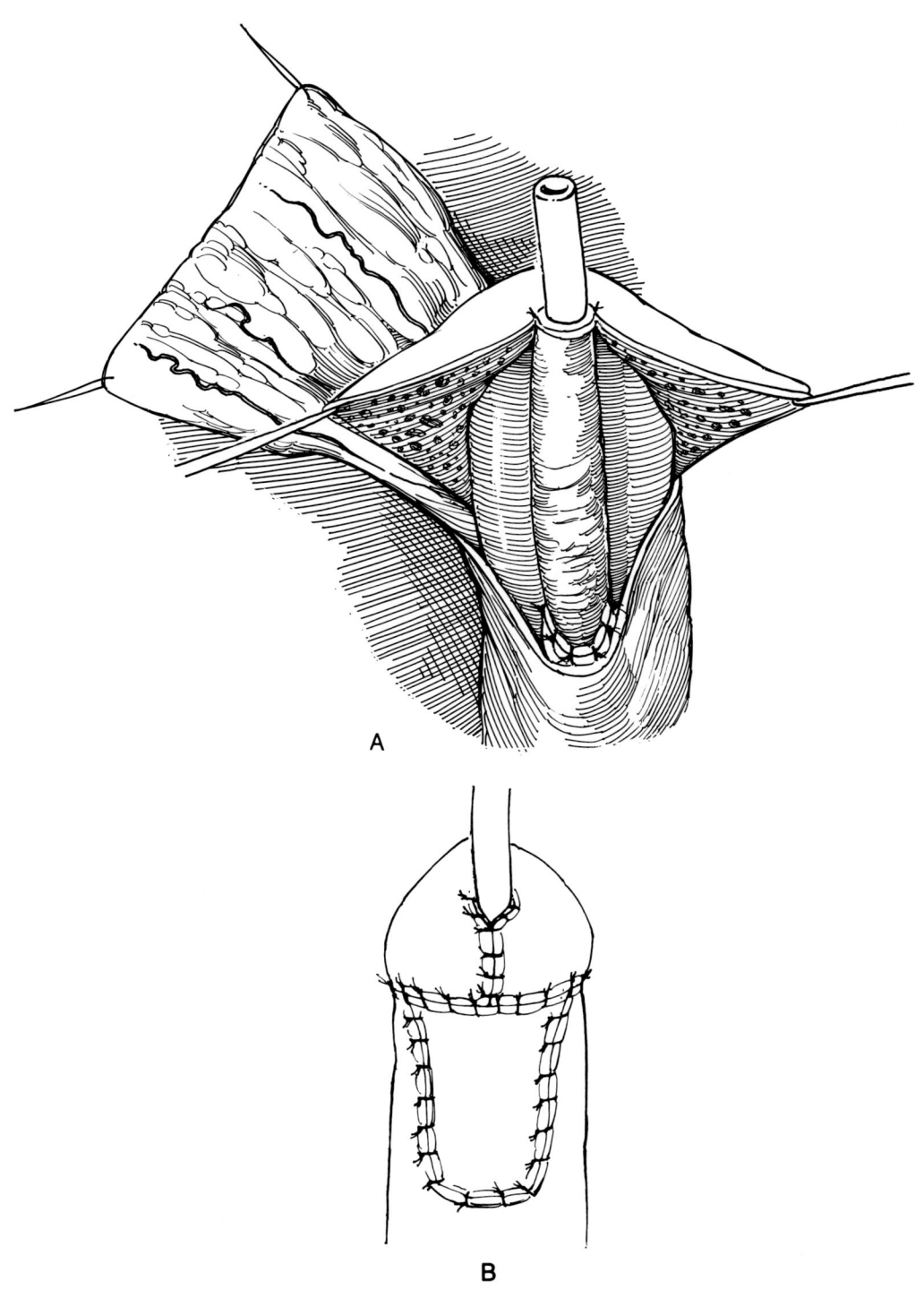

A

B

Commentary by Ahmed Shafik

The Important Aspect of the Operation. This procedure represents the modern trend in managing first- and second-degree hypospadias in a one-stage performance. The results are successful in more than 75 percent of the cases. The use of preputial skin is most suitable as a urethral graft because of its hairlessness and pliability. Other sites, such as the groin and medial aspect of the arm, are suitable donor areas only in circumcised males.

It is, however, to be noted that the vascularized preputial skin technique represents a natural progress of this technique with a much lower complication rate.

Tips, Short Cuts, and Alternatives. The measurement of the width of the graft should be equal to the circumference of a catheter with a diameter comparable to the proximal urethra. Still, it is preferable that the graft be stented over a catheter with a smaller diameter. This would allow easier manipulation of the graft and lessen the danger of too much pressure by the catheter on the suture line, which may predispose to dehiscence and fistula formation.

Sutures preferably are applied through the dermis of the graft and urethral submucosa. This makes the suture line slightly inverted to the inside. This tip allows better watertight healing of the suture line.

Although perineal urethrotomy may be an alternative to cystotomy as a method of urinary diversion, the latter has the advantage of allowing testing of the repair (usually after 1 week). If leakage occurred, the period of diversion could be prolonged.

Skin closure preferably is achieved by transverse mattress sutures, which allow eversion of the edges. The sutures should be loosely tied to allow for postoperative edema; otherwise, necrosis may develop at the suture line.

PART II

PENILE RECONSTRUCTION

CHAPTER 124

Microphallus

At 6 weeks of age, measure the penis and consult a table of normal sizes with standard deviations. Determine levels of luteinizing hormone, follicle-stimulating hormone (FSH), testosterone, and dihydrotestosterone, and testicular size and position. Normal testosterone and FSH levels usually indicate nonendocrine microphallus, only amenable to surgical improvement. Try a course of human chorionic gonadotropin (hCG) to detect those boys with mild hypogonadism.

Operation is indicated only for correction of the anomalous type of microphallus, not the endocrine type. A very small dysmorphic penis should be recognized at birth. Consider excising it and raising the child as a girl, because such a phallus is unlikely to reach a size adequate for the male role.

The type of operation will vary with the type of anomaly.

FIRST STAGE

1 Place a traction suture in the glans and an infant feeding tube in the urethra.

2 Make a circumferential incision at the junction of the prepuce with the subpubic skin. Develop a plane between the subcutaneous tissue and Buck's fascia, and dissect to the point of divergence of the corpora cavernosa.

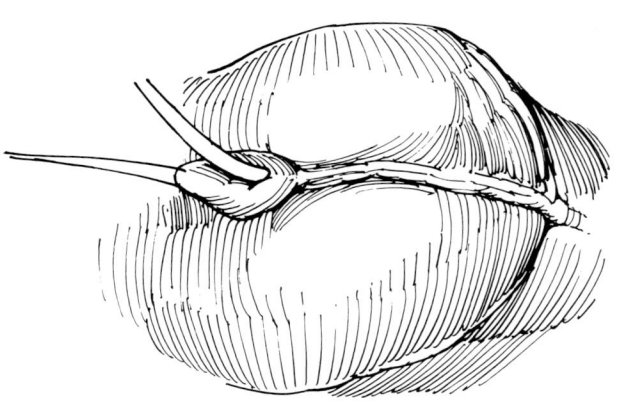

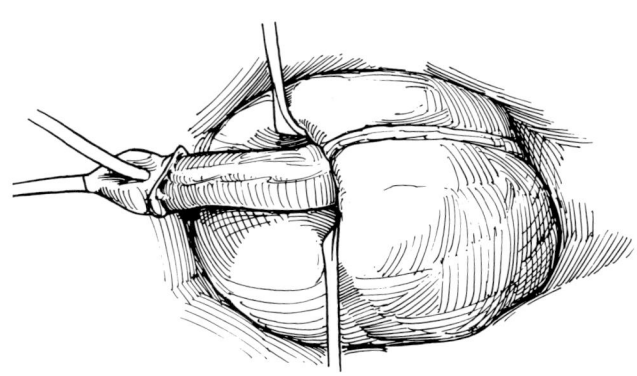

603

3 Incise the scrotum transversely at a distance from the base of the penis equal to the length of the shaft after dissection. Make a subcutaneous tunnel to connect the two incisions, and draw the penis through by the traction suture and catheter. Join the coronal margin to the scrotal skin edge, and close the basal incision with 5–0 chromic catgut.

SECOND STAGE

4 Insert a small catheter and stitch it to the glans. Make a U-incision in the scrotum, passing around the glans. The flap must be wider than the projected shaft diameter, because it also must enclose its own subcutaneous tissue. Free the flap, including the attached penile shaft.

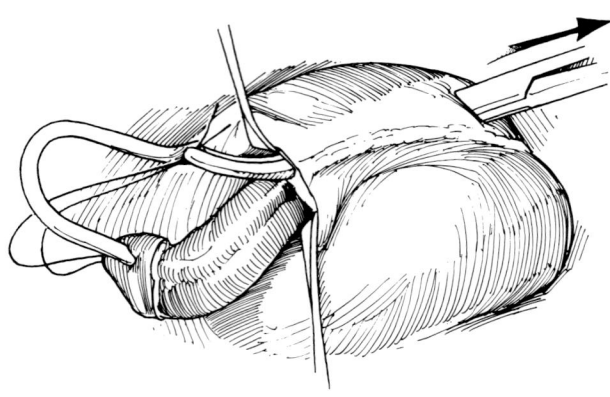

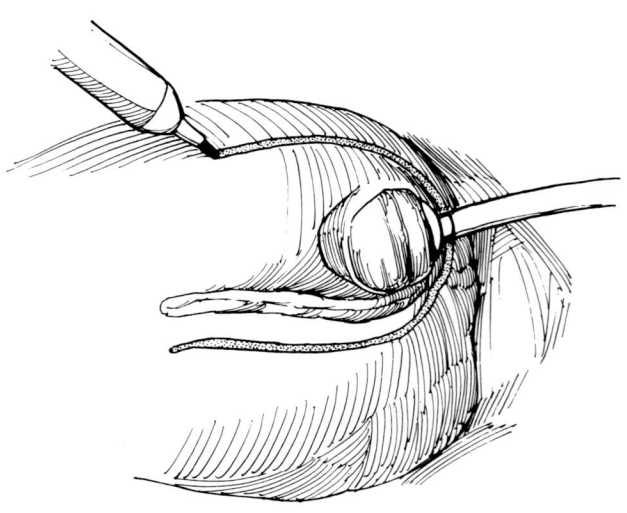

5 Close the scrotal defect with 5–0 chromic catgut sutures.

6 Approximate the edges of the flap with 5–0 chromic catgut sutures. If tension is suspected, place a series of 3–0 nonabsorbable sutures with beads and perforated lead shot instead. Dress as for hypospadias repair.

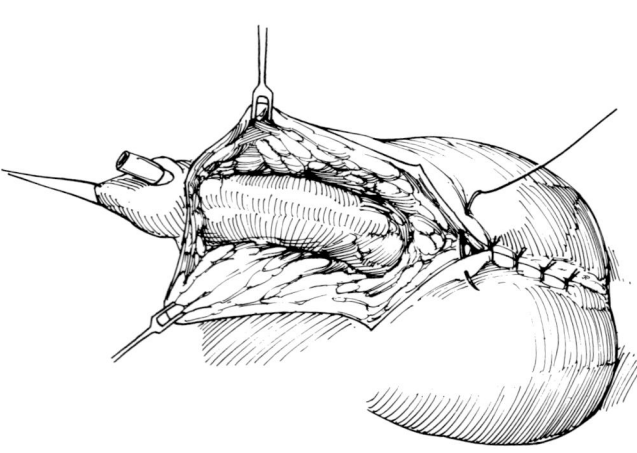

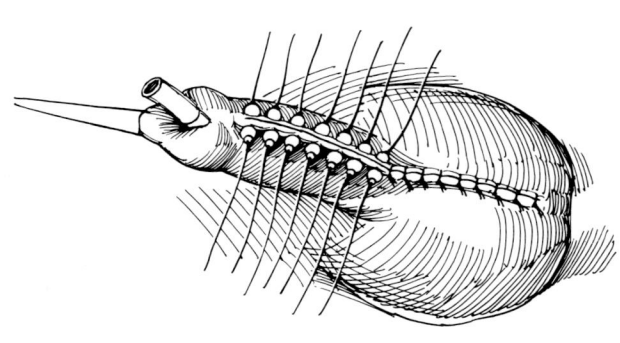

Commentary by Edmond T. Gonzales, Jr.

The newborn infant with a small penis demands a prompt and thorough endocrine evaluation. In most published series, hypogonadotropic hypogonadism has been the most common abnormality, at times associated with recognized syndromes such as Kallmann's, Prader-Willi, and others. A classic micropenis, which is a normally formed, small phallus with a glanular meatus, implies normally functioning testes that were stimulated during the first trimester of pregnancy by hCG but were quiescent during the remainder of the pregnancy because of deficient fetal gonadotropin. If micropenis is present in association with hypospadias, either inadequate secretion of testosterone by the testes (primary gonadal dysplasia, enzymatic abnormality) or incomplete utilization of testosterone by the end organ (androgen receptor deficiency, 5α-reductase deficiency) is more likely. Less-common causes of small penis are thought to represent primary abnormalities of the primitive genital tubercle.

The primary consideration in management involves an early decision regarding the sex of rearing. A micropenis with a normally formed urethra can be expected to respond to parenteral testosterone. It has been suggested that initiation of treatment during the 1st year of life will result in hyperplasia of the phallic tissues, whereas treatment later in life may result only in hypertrophy. Hyperplasia will provide more tissue for androgen stimulation and growth during adolescence, whether puberty is natural or induced. In most cases, penile growth is substantial with androgen therapy, and the penis will reach normal size in infancy. It is recommended that these children be followed throughout childhood and be given boosts of androgen stimulation if penile length measurements begin to fall off the standard growth curve.

Micropenis associated with a urethral anomaly may not respond as well to androgen therapy, because some of these cases represent primary end-organ failure. A careful psychosocial evaluation of the family must be included in the overall evaluation process. Once androgen therapy is begun, the family will identify the child in the male gender. If adequate growth does not occur, it may be best for the child if a change in the sex of rearing is considered. Such a role reversal will require understanding and emotional strength on the part of the parents. One technical consideration remains—an accurate estimate of penile length may be difficult to ascertain when severe chordee and anterior displacement of the scrotal tissues are present.

The small dysmorphic penis, in most cases, probably is best managed by excision and a change in the sex of rearing, if the child is seen in the newborn period. Although increased penile length can be obtained by extensive mobilization of the crura from the inferior ramus of the pubis and rearrangement of the shaft skin, normal phallic size is unlikely, and the patient probably will never function satisfactorily in the male role.

CHAPTER 125

Concealed and Webbed Penis

CONCEALED PENIS
(DEVINE)

Consider liposuction, at least initially, for the child with a large amount of prepubic fat.

1 **A** and **B,** Forcibly retract the prepuce, exposing the tight paraphimotic skin. **C,** Incise the paraphimosis vertically. **D,** It becomes almost a transverse incision after retraction.

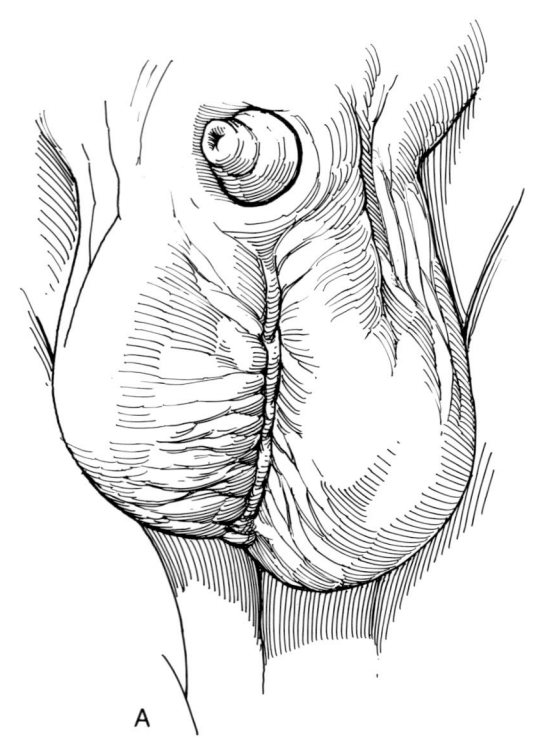

A

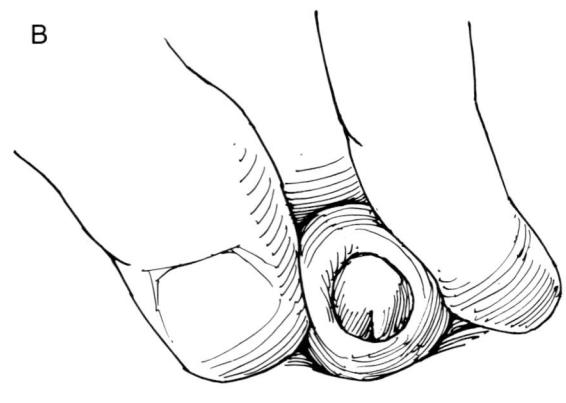

B

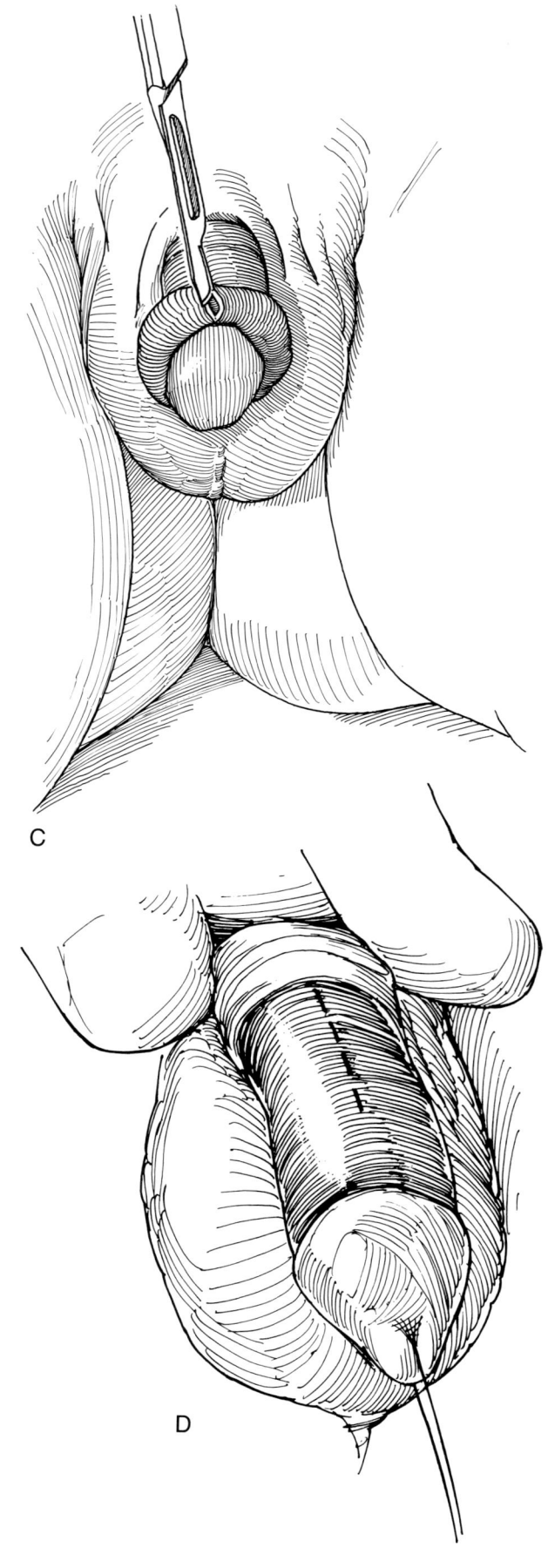

C

D

2 Locate and dissect the dysgenic bands of tissue from the dorsum of the penis, especially distally.

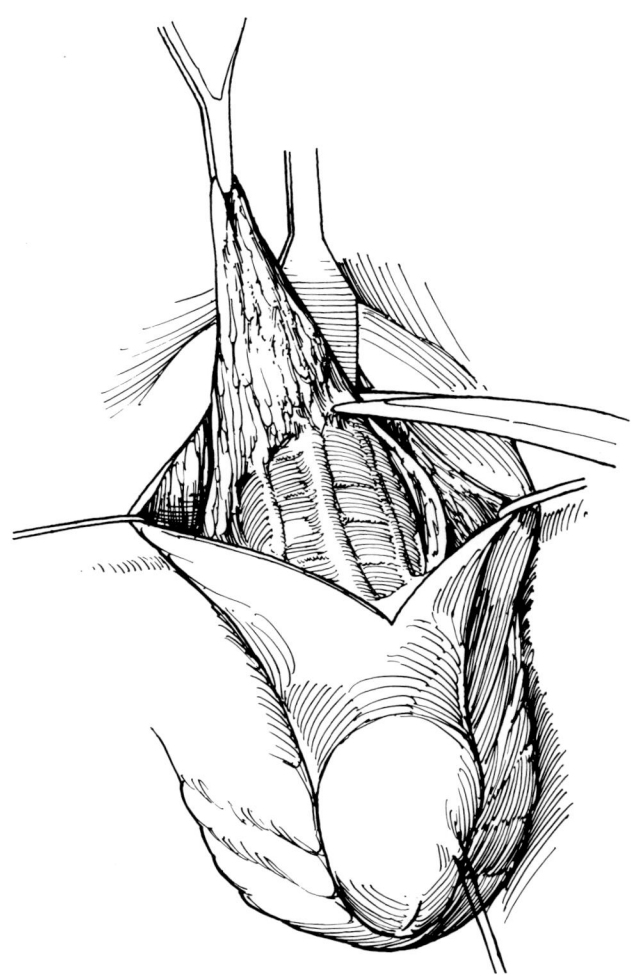

3 Pull the initial longitudinal dorsal incision transversely and extend it to divide the remaining skin circumferentially.

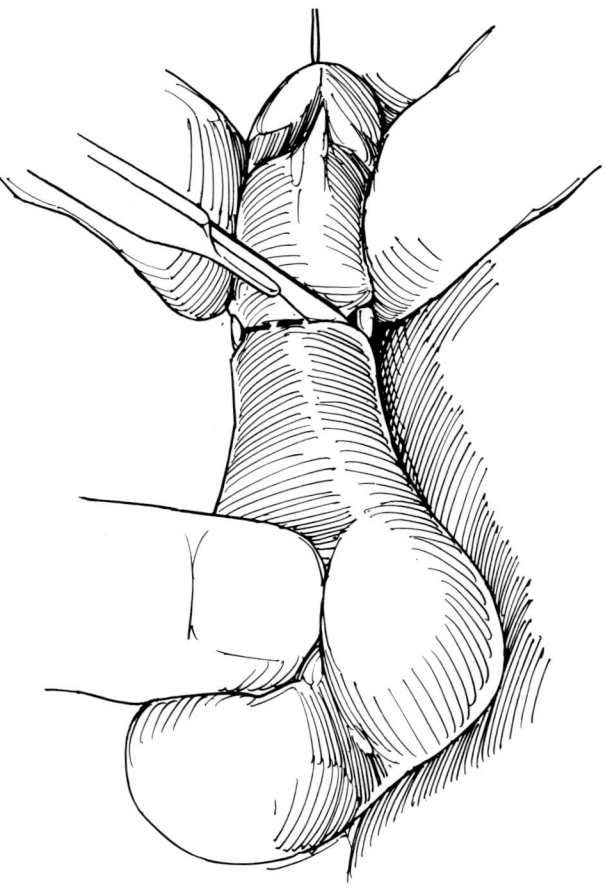

4 Remove any ventral bands. A large suprapubic fat pad may be excised if care is taken to isolate the spermatic cords while removing it. Anchor the skin of the lower abdomen to the fascia over the pubic area, and fasten the penile skin to the corpora at the base of the penis with nonabsorbable sutures.

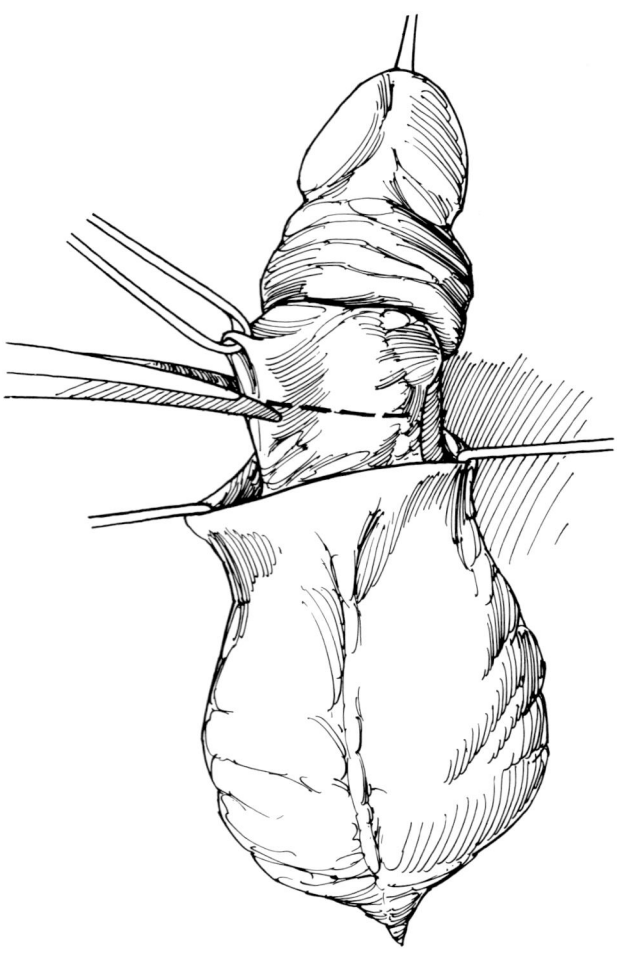

5 Approximate the skin edges transversely with interrupted 5–0 chromic catgut sutures.

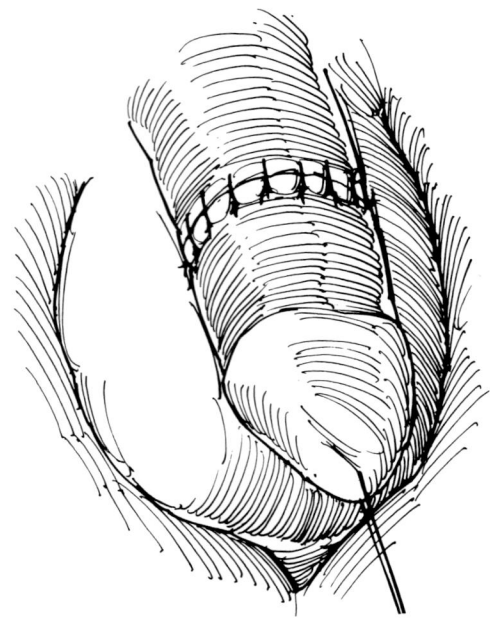

Commentary by Charles J. Devine, Jr.

Concealed penis is an entity that some pediatric urologists insist is a developmental stage that will resolve as the patient achieves puberty when the penis will make its appearance, to the great relief of all involved. These usually are the same physicians who insist that no male child should be circumcised unless circumcision is a tenet of religion. However, concealed, hidden, buried, or cryptic penis is a reality, and most newborn male Americans are still circumcised today. Unless concealment of the penis is recognized, this can be an anatomic, psychologic, and litigious disaster.

Concealed penis is caused by a developmental anomaly in which the dartos fascia has not developed into the normally elastic configuration that allows the skin to slide freely on the deep layers of the shaft but has become a very inelastic structure, restraining the extension of the penis and holding it beneath the symphysis. Here, the dartos fascia is continuous with Camper's and Scarpa's fascias of the abdomen, which normally are of limited elasticity. One identifies this condition by pulling on the glans penis and noting that although the shaft can protrude through the prepuce, it quickly contracts within it. Correction is not accomplished by trimming the prepuce to fit the penis but by cutting the inelastic fibers of the dartos fascia layer and allowing the penis to extend to fit the prepuce. Thus, release of the penile shaft may reveal sufficient length that all of the skin of the prepuce will be needed to cover the shaft, and none can be excised. As a consequence, when the condition is suspected, the initial incisions should be designed to allow development of such flaps.

Since the causes of this defect were recognized, we have treated 20 patients. Nine had no other anomalies of the penis except for concealment; two of these nine were adults. In the others, the penile concealment was associated with either epispadias or hypospadias.

We have found a normal penile shaft concealed beneath the surrounding tissues, held there by dysgenic bands of tissue in the dartos fascia layer. The insertion of these bands has varied from near the coronal margin to near the base of the penis, and the degree of concealment has been more severe with the more distal location of that insertion. In these more-severe cases, division and resection of these bands have not completely remedied the situation, and we have had to remove the suprapubic fat pad.

We recently treated a child who appeared to have just an exceptionally redundant prepuce with phimosis; however, the dysgenic bands and restrained penile shaft were easily palpable. Several other children must have had similar presentations, because they had been circumcised in an attempt to correct the problem. One of our patients had undergone four circumcisions. With release of the dysgenic bands, the penis emerged nicely, and fortunately, there was just enough skin to cover the penile shaft.

Distinct abnormal bands insert proximally into what appears to be Scarpa's fascia. They do not insert on the pubic or suspensory ligament nor does the suspensory ligament have to be divided to release the penis. Not all of our patients have had prominent suprapubic fat pads, but in those that did, we noted that a better immediate cosmetic result could be obtained by removing that fat. We normally isolate the spermatic cords to avoid injury to the structures in that area. We place fixation sutures of Prolene to anchor the skin of the lower abdomen to the pubic area and to anchor the penile skin to the corpora at the base of the penis.

We have tried to provide a good immediate cosmetic result. By the time these children have come to us, they and their parents have developed real concern as to whether they will grow up to be "real men." Some of our colleagues have suggested that reassurance is the best form of management, because they have seen similar patients in whom they felt that the situation would remedy itself at puberty; however, the two adult patients of ours attest to the fact that this is not always true. The latest of our patients had gone through some of the changes of puberty, and the fat pad had diminished. However, the bands remained, and some residual fat had to be removed. Furthermore, most of our parents and patients have already had reassurances before reaching us, and they have desired something further. Parents fear that their sons will suffer emotionally while awaiting midadolescence to see if nature will "take its course." We feel that boys become genitally aware long before passing through puberty, and we empathize with these concerns. We feel that our procedure offers a good cosmetic solution for these patients. We do not advocate its use for every boy whose penis looks small but rather for the boy whose penis is concealed, as we have discussed.

Commentary by Arnold H. Colodny

The standard operation for a concealed (buried) penis consists of making a circumcising incision, completely degloving the penis, and then attaching the skin to the base of the penis circumferentially, reestablishing the penoscrotal angle. This simple procedure often corrects the underlying defect that allows a penis to invaginate or intussuscept into the pubic fat pad. Excision of dysgenic bands or liposuction or excision of the pubic fat pad is rarely, if ever, necessary. There are some penises that seem to have a deficient suspensory ligament of the penis. If this defect is not recognized and corrected, one may get a recurrence.

If a concealed penis develops after a circumcision, it usually is because of a failure to excise enough of the mucosal (inner) surface of the foreskin. This allows the circumcising incision to heal in front of the glans of the penis, resulting in a buried penis. A corrective operative procedure, if necessary, is much easier if one waits at least 6 months following the circumcision.

I have used a new incision for the past 2½ years that allows easy access to the complete circumference of the penis and the underside of the symphysis pubis to recreate the suspensory ligament, if necessary.

We have utilized this incision in 16 patients. The first patient was one with a plexiform neurofibroma that surrounded the penile shaft and extended into the scrotum. There were eight patients who had a diagnosis of a concealed penis; these were all secondary cases or those where a deficient suspensory ligament was present. The other patients were complicated hypospadias patients. One patient had a diverticulum that involved the entire neourethra in the shaft of the penis and extended into his right hemiscrotum. This approach gives better exposure to all aspects of the penis than previously reported incisions. Exposure at the base of the penis is easily achieved. Retraction of or incision into the penile shaft skin is unnecessary.

Using a median raphe incision proximally does not interfere with the vascularity of the shaft skin or cut across any of the lymphatics and so does not result in lymphedema. No overlapping suture lines are present.

Patient discomfort following these 16 operations was minimal. Lymphedema was absent. Excellent functional cosmetic results were obtained. The only complication was a urethrocutaneous fistula after a bladder mucosal graft in a hypospadias cripple, which was closed easily.

WEBBED PENIS

6 **A,** Place a traction suture in the glans and a second one in the distal edge of the skin fold. Sharply divide the edge, keeping at a distance from the shaft to leave enough skin on the shaft for ventral closure. **B,** Approximate the ventral skin edges.

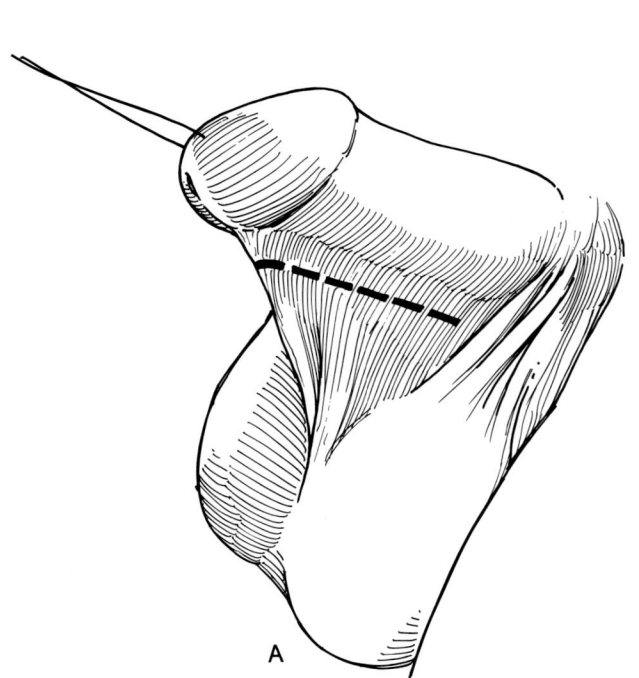

A

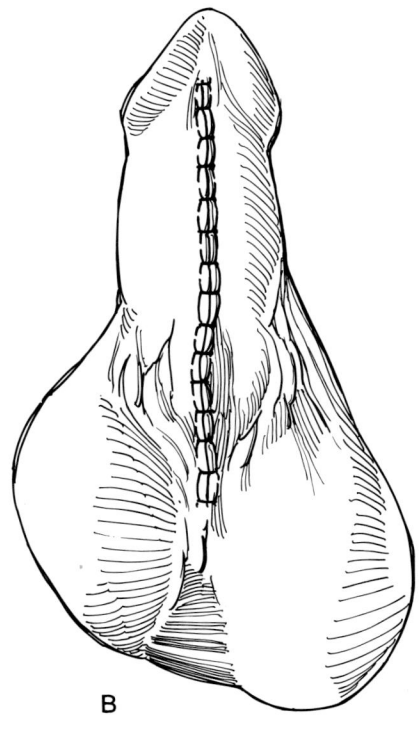

B

CHAPTER 126

Epispadias Repair

Consider the following four problems together: short urethra, short corpora cavernosa, chordee, and deficient skin. Be certain to make a more than adequate repair the first time; later attempts tend to fail.

PENILE EPISPADIAS

If the phallus is small, give testosterone enanthate ± 3 mg/kg intramuscularly or 25 mg monthly for 3 months (preferable to testosterone cream).

2 Using optical loupes, incise at the coronal sulcus. Free and open the prepuce dorsally.

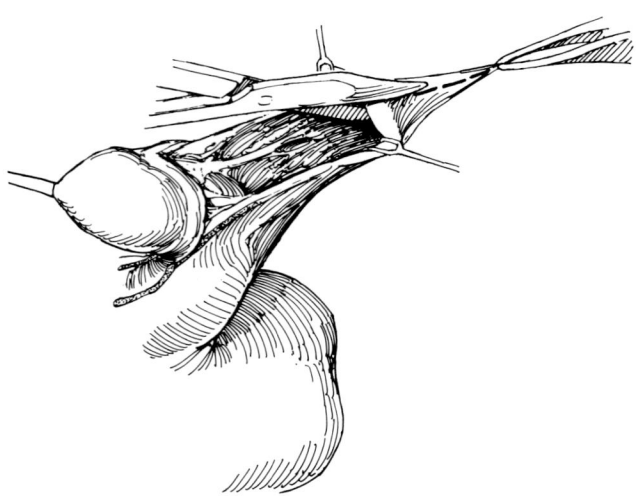

3 Place a small silicone balloon catheter, a length of silicone tubing, or a pediatric sound in the urethra. Incise and lift up the ventral skin flap. Sharply remove all the chordee. Take care not to injure the urethra, which lies superficially. Check for residual chordee by producing an artificial erection.

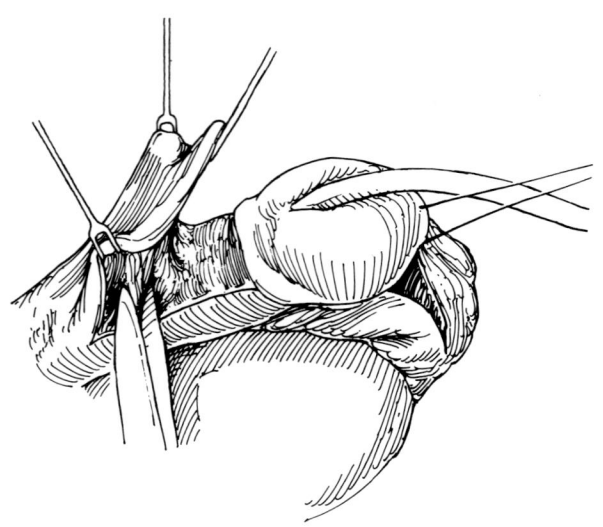

1 Mark a circumcision incision and two lines on the shaft approximately one fourth of the circumference apart.

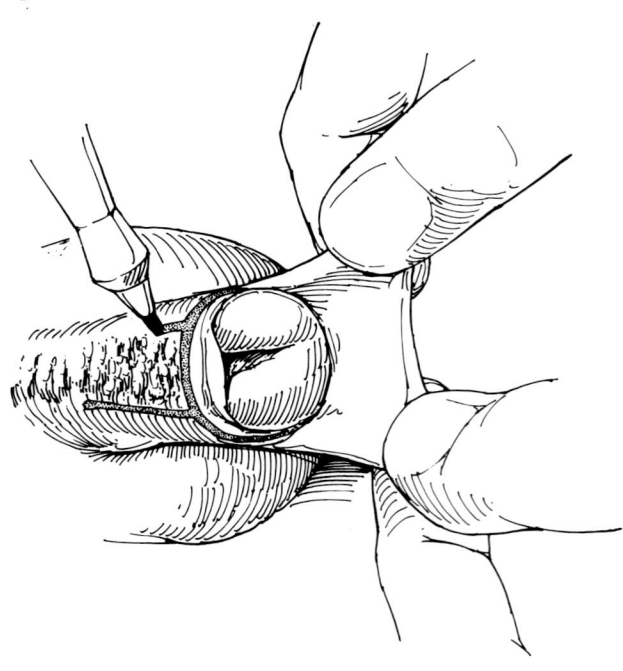

4 Mark and make two incisions in the glans, well separated to leave adequate mucosa to form a tube. Free the edges, so that they can be rolled to the midline and sutured with running 5–0 synthetic absorbable subcuticular sutures.

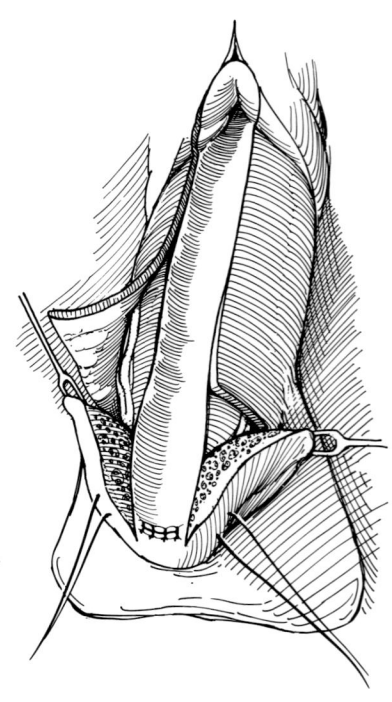

5 **A,** Place several 5–0 synthetic absorbable sutures to approximate the substance of the glans. **B,** Close the skin with a running subcuticular suture.

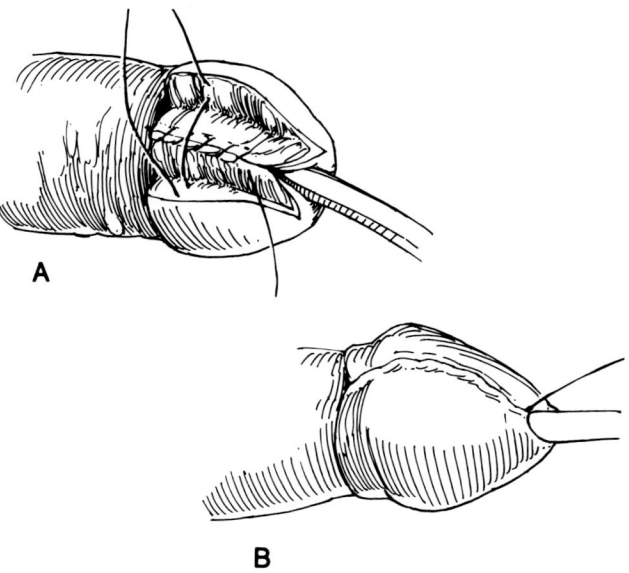

A

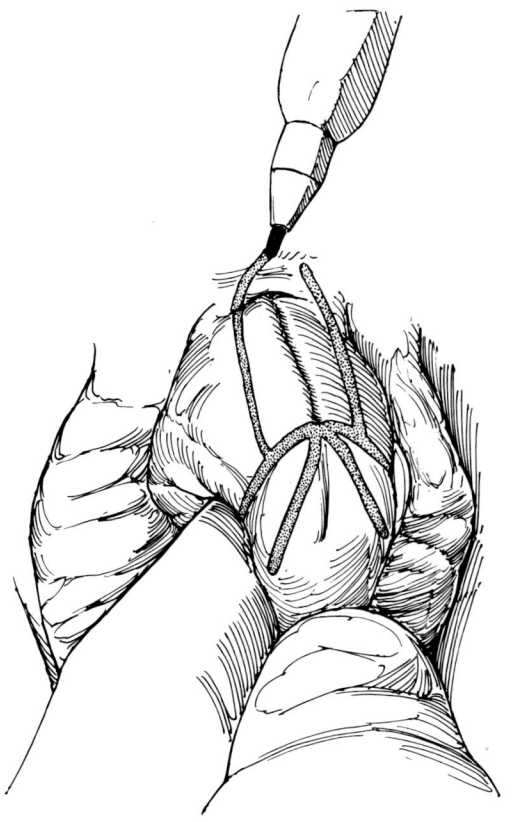

B

PENOPUBIC EPISPADIAS

Skin Graft Technique

7 Insert a perineal urethrostomy (page 350). Mark three incisions. One is U-shaped on the dorsum, encircling the meatus and terminating at the coronal sulcus. The second is a circumcising incision around the coronal sulcus. The third is a V in the glans to form the glans flap.

6 **A,** Split the prepuce. Fasten the apex of the V to the skin at the corona with a 5–0 chromic catgut suture. **B,** Swing the flaps around, and suture them together in the midline (or in a Z-fashion) on the dorsum. Trim excess skin from the dorsal flap, and suture the flap in place. Dress as for hypospadias repair. Leave the catheter or tube in place for 4 days.

For repair of epispadias with incontinence, see Chapter 62, "Reconstruction for Vesical Exstrophy."

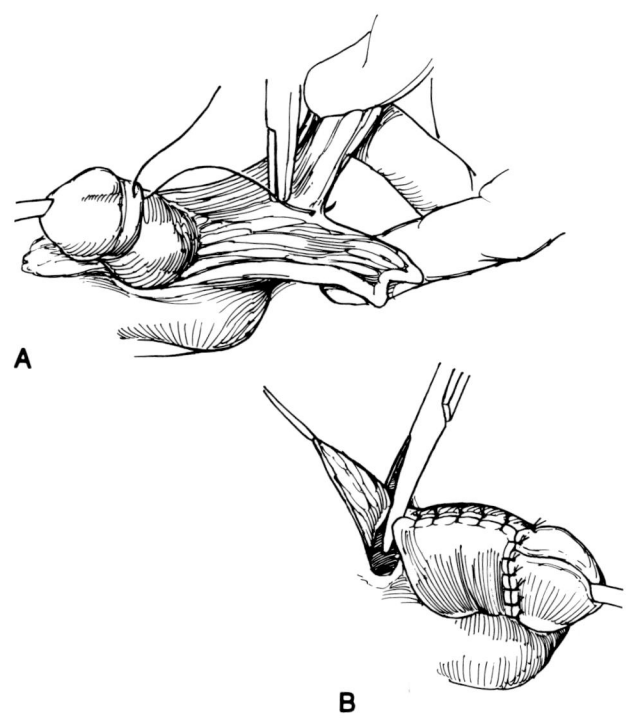

A

B

8 Incise the skin on the dorsum, and raise the urethral plate to be able to mobilize this dorsal skin and urethra back to the symphysis.

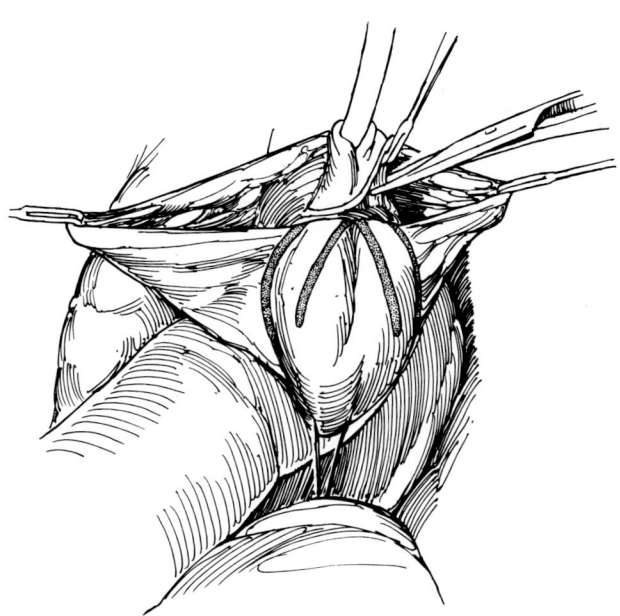

9 **A,** Clear dorsal fibrous bands to release the chordee, trimming directly down to the corpora cavernosa. Check for complete release by artificial erection. Two or three Z-plasties in Buck's fascia and the tunica albuginea can be done to gain greater length. **B,** Distally, the neuro-vascular bundles lie laterally, but as the symphysis is approached, they assume a more normal, central position.

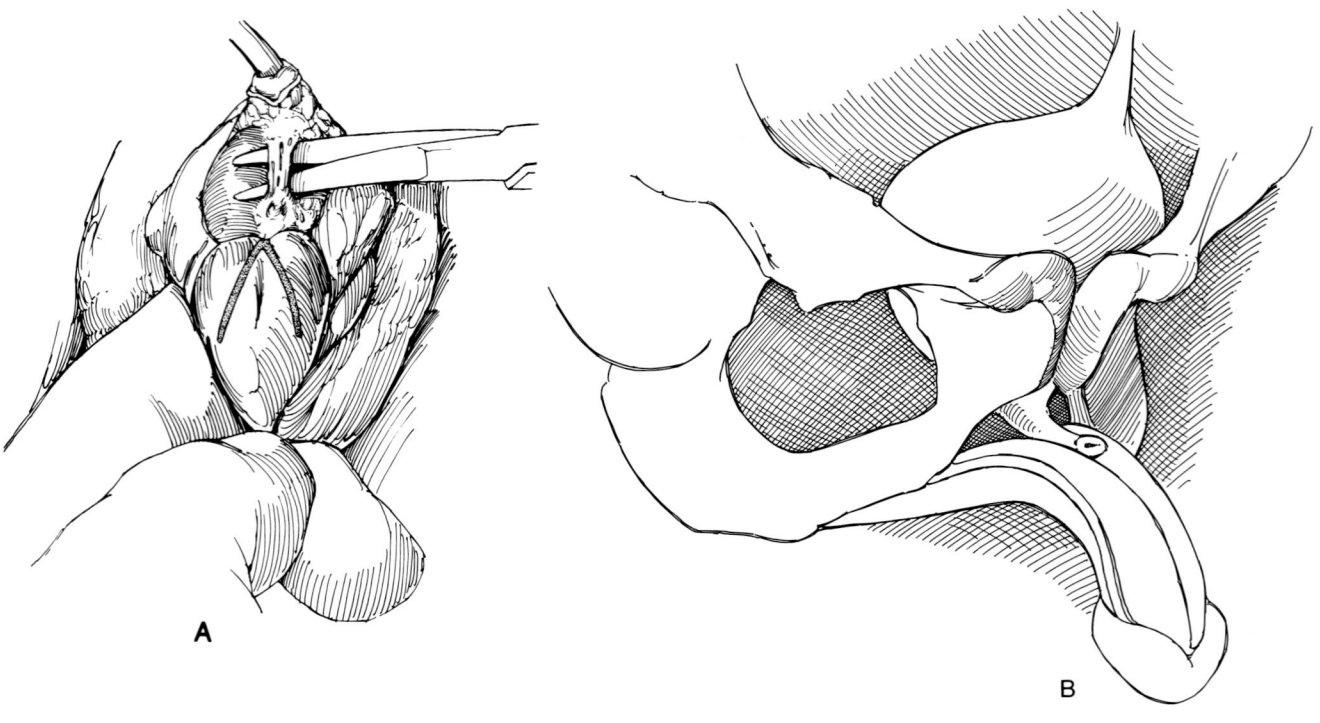

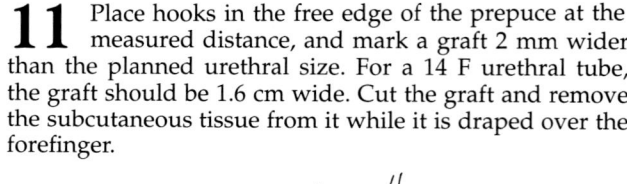

10 Make a circumcising incision. Unfold the prepuce, and denude the shaft laterally and ventrally. Measure the length on the dorsum from the stub of urethra to the end of the penis.

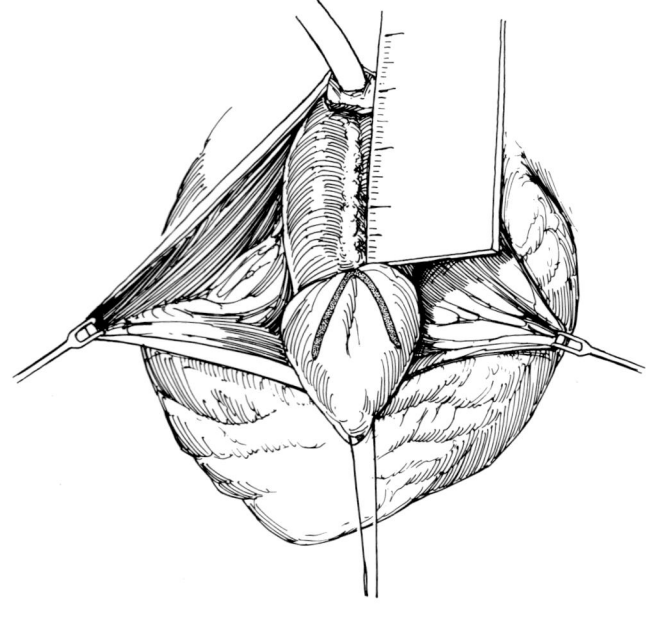

11 Place hooks in the free edge of the prepuce at the measured distance, and mark a graft 2 mm wider than the planned urethral size. For a 14 F urethral tube, the graft should be 1.6 cm wide. Cut the graft and remove the subcutaneous tissue from it while it is draped over the forefinger.

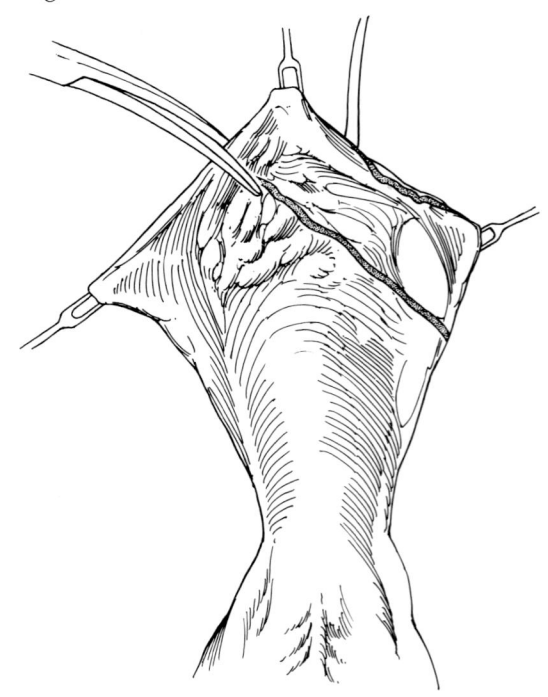

12 **A,** Place the graft skin side down onto an 8 F red rubber catheter or 9 F infant feeding tube approximately 8 cm from its tip. Place an interrupted 6–0 synthetic absorbable suture at each end, and hold the long ends against the catheter with clamps. **B,** Run one of these sutures to approximate and invert the edges. Close the last few millimeters of the intended distal end with interrupted sutures.

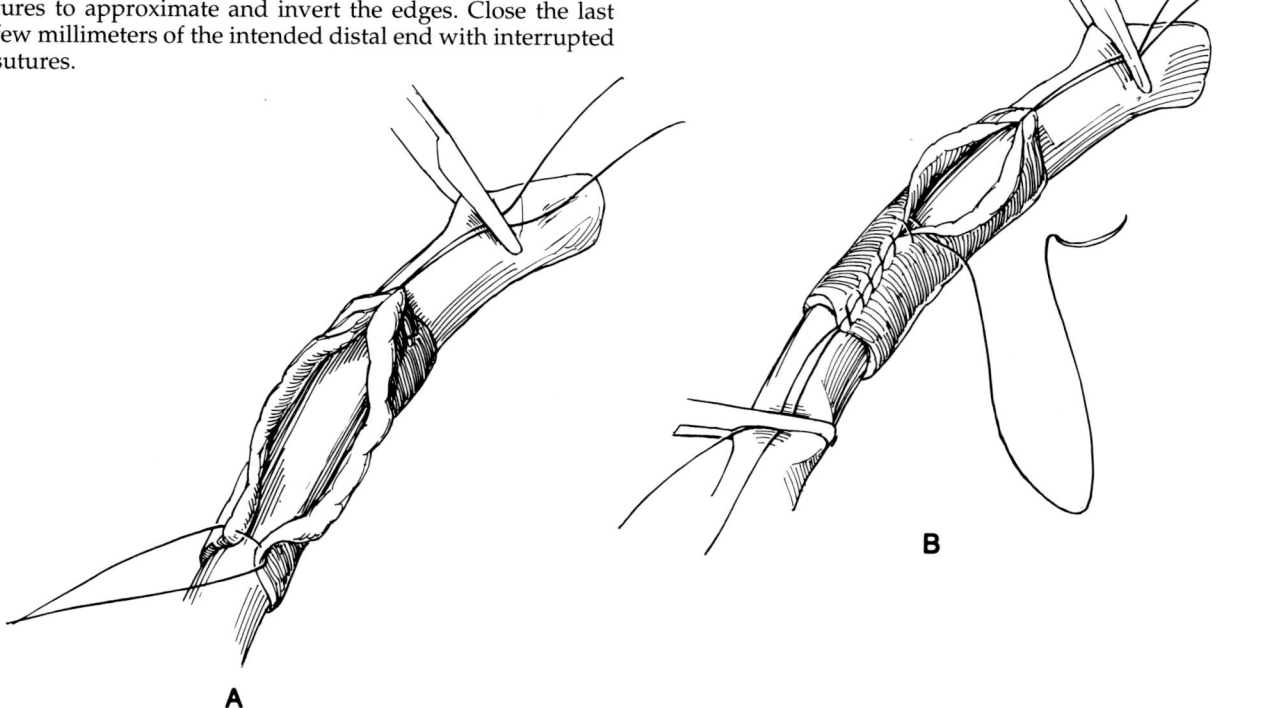

A

B

13 Form a short extension of the urethra by closing the edges of the original U-shaped incision on the dorsum. Notch the underside of the extension to spatulate the end.

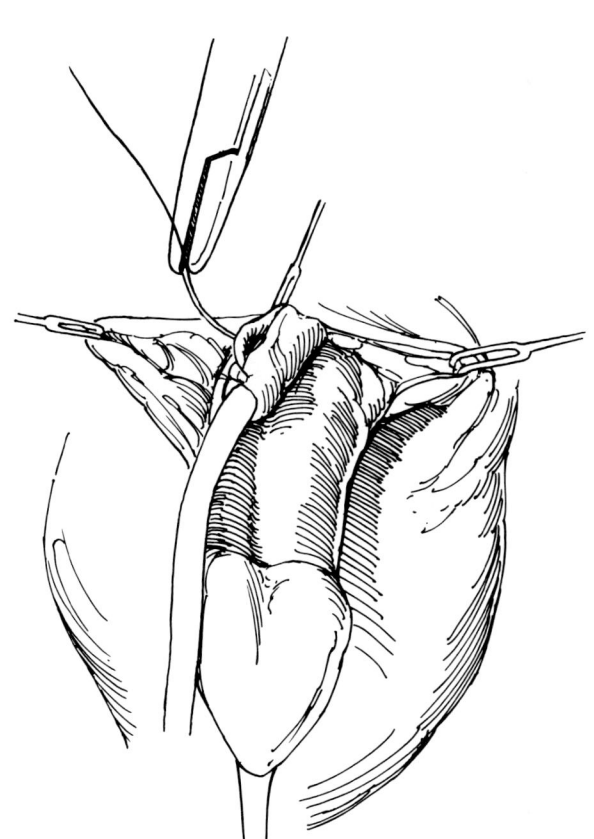

14 Incise the glans at the previously marked V.

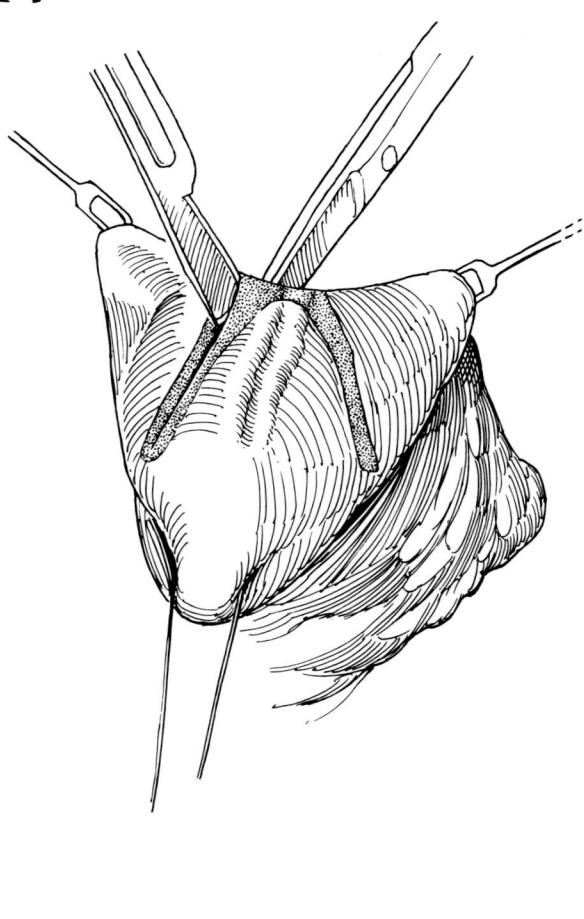

15 Undercut and trim the central wedge.

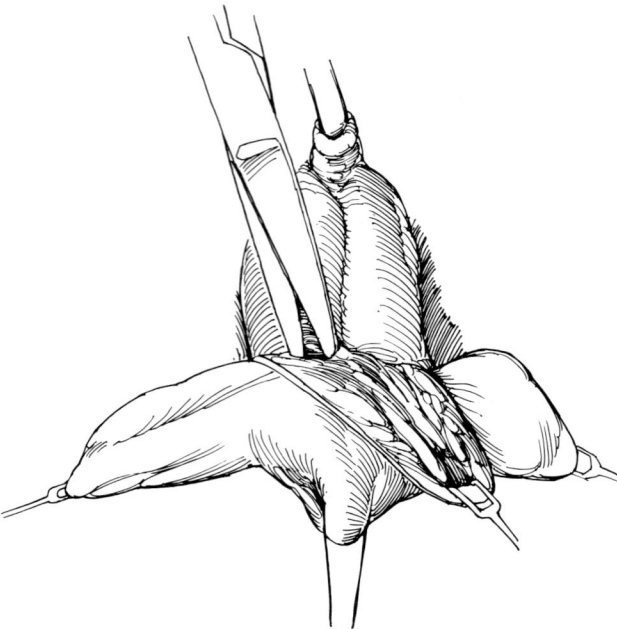

16 Tack the wedge to the corpora with 6–0 chromic catgut sutures. Insert the stent with the graft rotated, so that the sutures in the graft lie against the corpora. The tip of the stent should not reach the bladder. Anastomose the graft elliptically at its proximal end to the spatulated urethra.

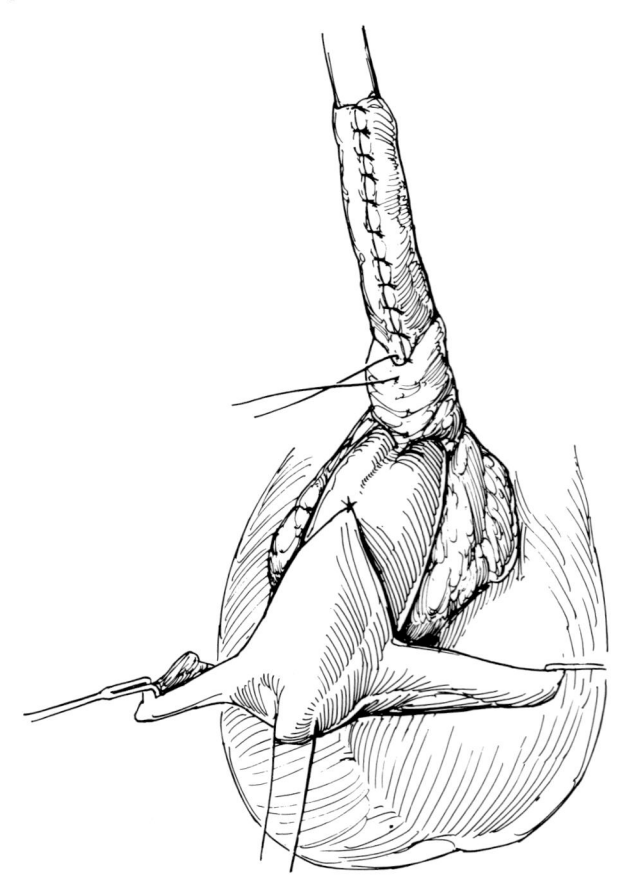

17 **A,** Incise a length of the interrupted suture line of the graft to receive the tongue of the glans flap. **B,** Suture it in place.

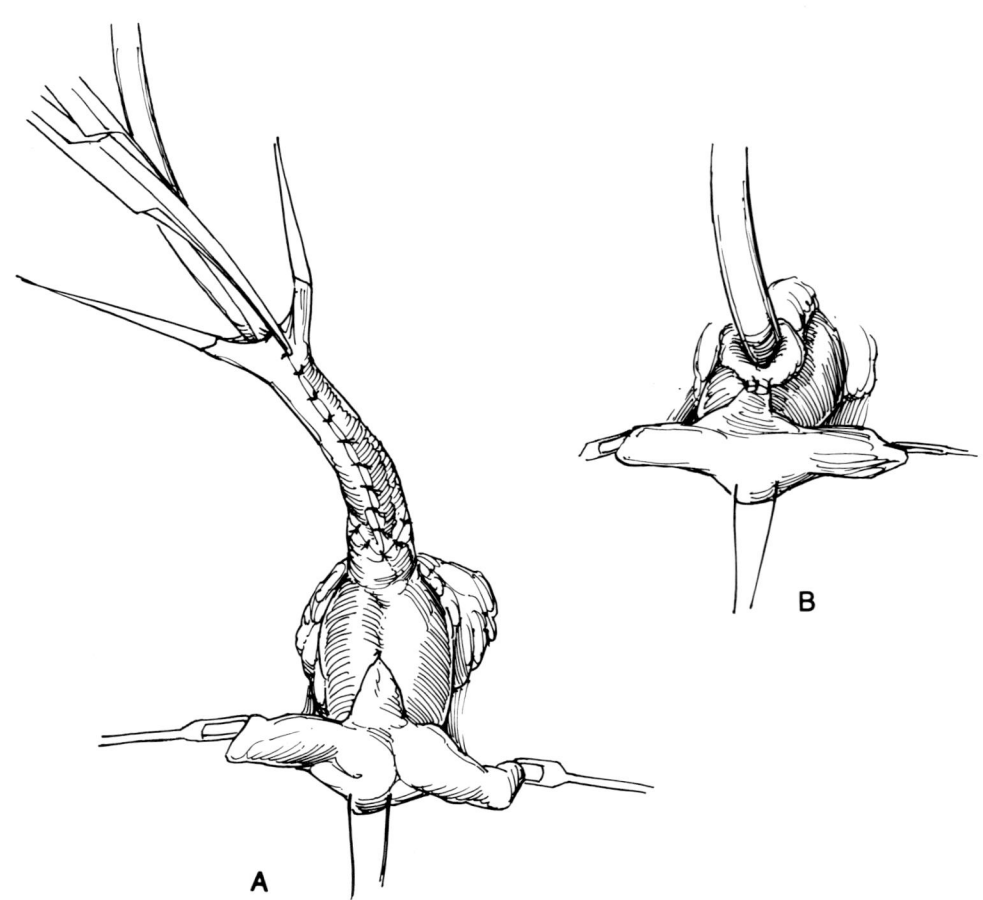

A

B

18 Bring the wings of the glans to the midline over the graft, and suture them to each other and to the graft to form a new meatus.

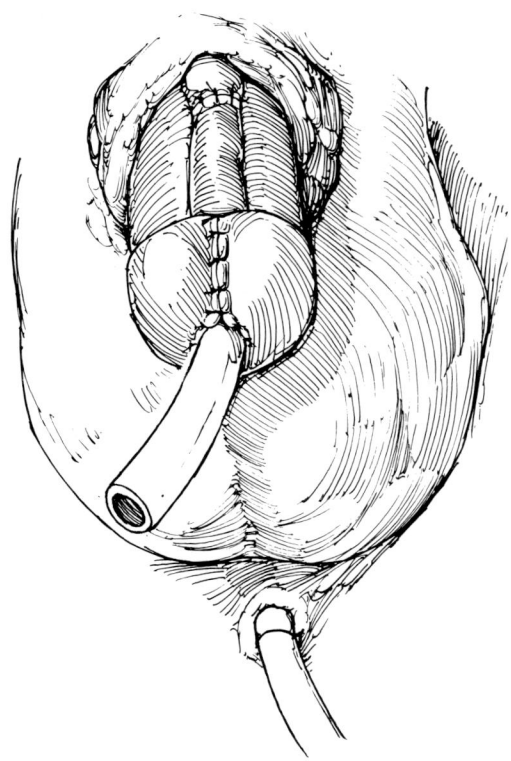

19 Approximate the preputial skin by rotating it over the dorsum. Trim and anchor the stent to the glans with heavy silk, to be left 7 days. Block the base of the penis with 2 ml of 2 percent lidocaine. Cover with a Tegaderm dressing. If recurrent chordee is feared, substitute a small silicone balloon catheter for the stent, or place a perineal urethrostomy. Place a heavy traction suture in the glans, and tie it over a bar in a bottomless Styrofoam cup. Maintain traction on the penis for a week or 10 days. If a perineal urethrostomy has been placed, remove it in 10 days. Keep the boy in bed. Antibiotics should be given to provide coverage. Culture the urine and change the drainage bags regularly. If insufficient penile length has been obtained, repeat the procedure in 6 months.

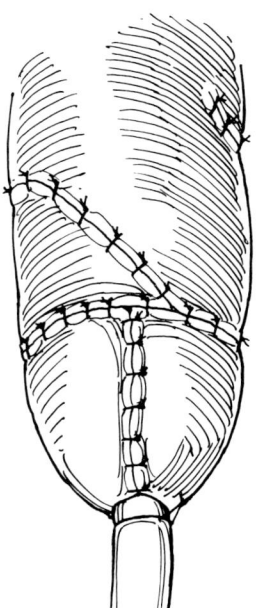

Dermal Patch Graft Release Technique

The dermal patch graft release technique has been resorted to for severe dorsal chordee that was not corrected by freeing the connective tissue over the dorsal corpora, as demonstrated by artificial erection.

20 Incise the corpora transversely on the dorsum, continuing well to the lateral borders. The neurovascular bundles will lie laterally and should be protected by dissection and by retraction in vessel loops.

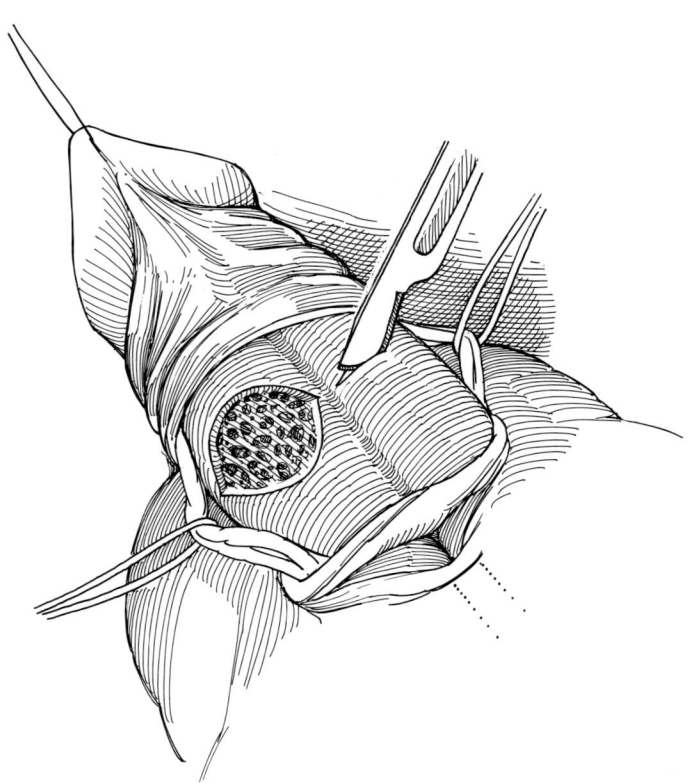

21 A, Mark two ellipses the length of each penile incision on the skin of the left lower abdominal quadrant. B, Sharply remove the epidermis and discard it. C, Excise the dermal patch and close the defect.

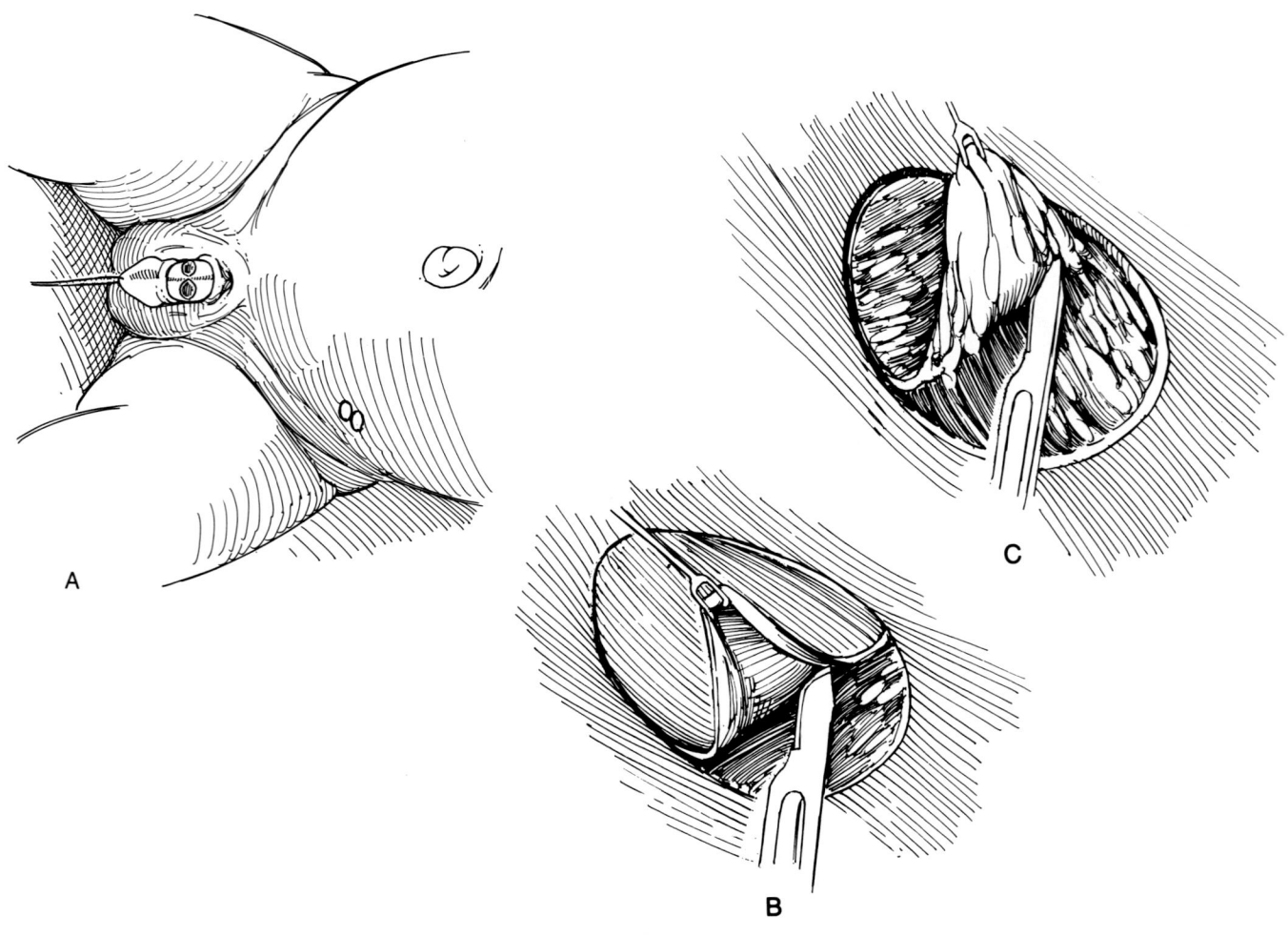

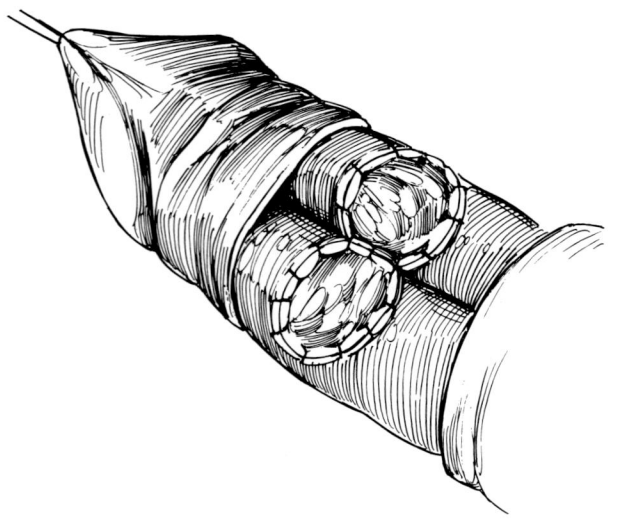

22 Insert the grafts in the defects, and fasten them in place with 4–0 synthetic absorbable sutures, with the knots inverted.

An alternative is to deglove the penis and form a ventral preputial island flap; bring it around dorsally, and place it either above or between the corporal bodies. At the same time, free the urethra from the corpora to allow it to retract, and detach the crura of the corporal bodies from the inferior pubic rami, taking care to avoid the branches of the pudendal vessels. Anastomose the tubularized flap to the urethral stump over a stent.

Urethral Translocation Technique
(Cantwell-Ransley)

Repair the epispadias at 14 to 18 months of age, unless there is a question about the bladder neck repair, in which case, delay the epispadias procedure.

23 Place two traction sutures in the glans. Mark two parallel incisions on the dorsum on either side of the urethral groove 1.8 cm apart for the length of the penis (long dashed line with pubic extension). Make a deep incision longitudinally in the urethral plate just proximal to the glans (short dashed line).

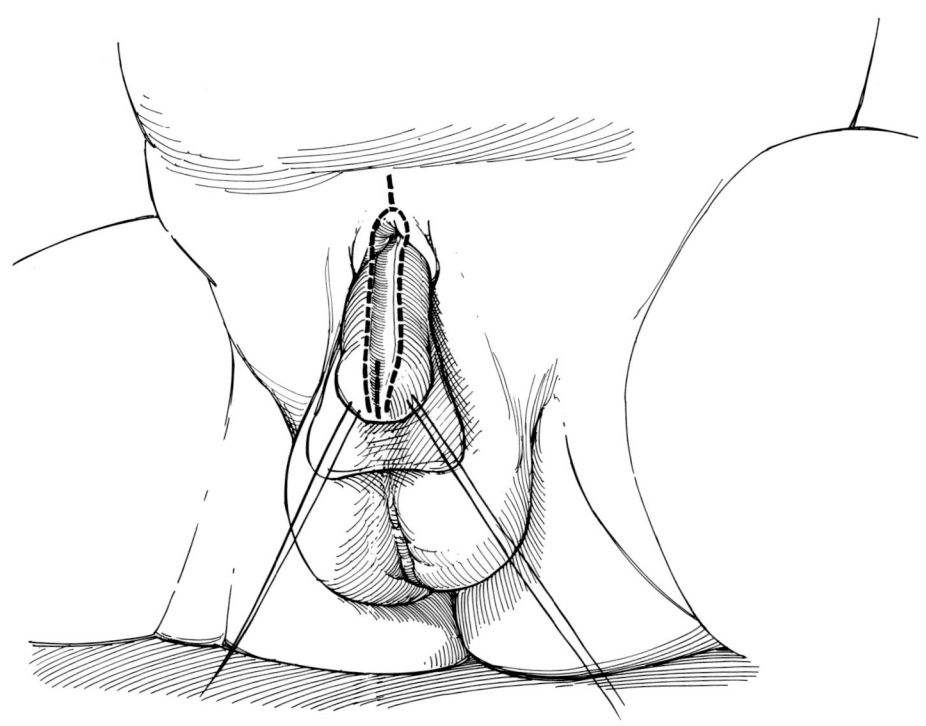

24 Close the incision in the urethral plate transversely to bring the plate to the penile tip by the IPGAM (reversed MAGPI) maneuver.

Excise triangular pieces of glans and form glans flaps. Dissect the skin of the shaft free throughout its length. Make a Z-incision at the base to release the split suspensory ligaments. Dissect the skin from the entire ventrum, being careful to preserve the proximal mesentery connecting the urethral plate to the base of the penis between the corpora.

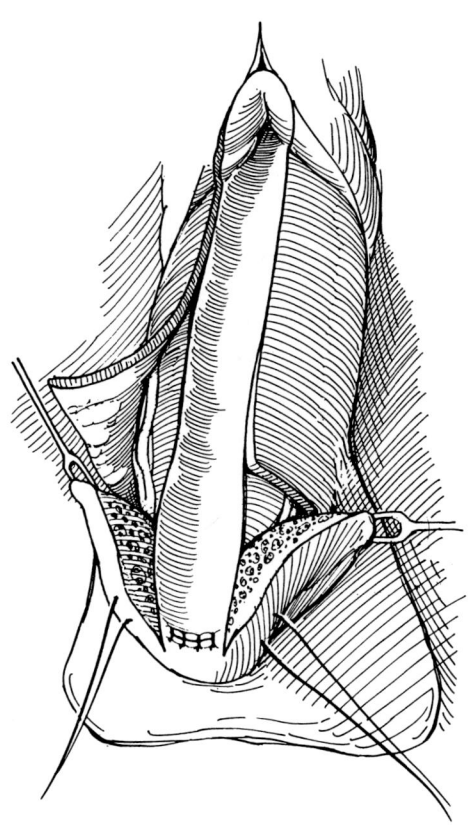

25 Expose Buck's fascia ventrally, and separate the corporal bodies in the midline. Hold each corpus with a vessel loop, and develop a plane between them and the urethral plate, both proximally and distally within the glans. At the same time, dissect the neurovascular bundles from beneath Buck's fascia over the corpora, and hold them in loops. Incise the tunica albuginea of each corpora transversely at midpoint (dashed lines).

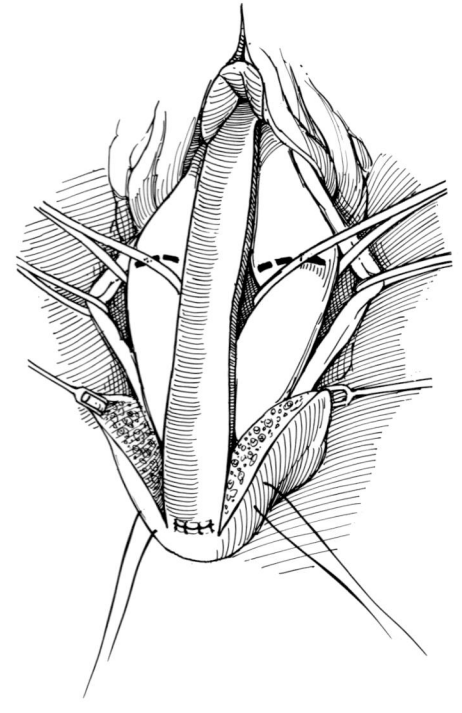

26 **A,** Close the urethral plate over an 8 F silicone stent with 6–0 synthetic slowly absorbable sutures. The transverse incisions in the corpora at midpoint are opened into diamond-shaped defects by traction on the penis. Suture the two diamond-shaped defects to each other, converting the original transverse incisions into a longitudinal closure.

B, Suture the corpora to each other over the new urethra with a running Connell stitch of 6–0 synthetic absorbable suture. Add more sutures between the corpora dorsally to further rotate them and move the urethra ventrally. This is especially important adjacent to the glans.

Outline and incise a flap on the inner surface of the prepuce.

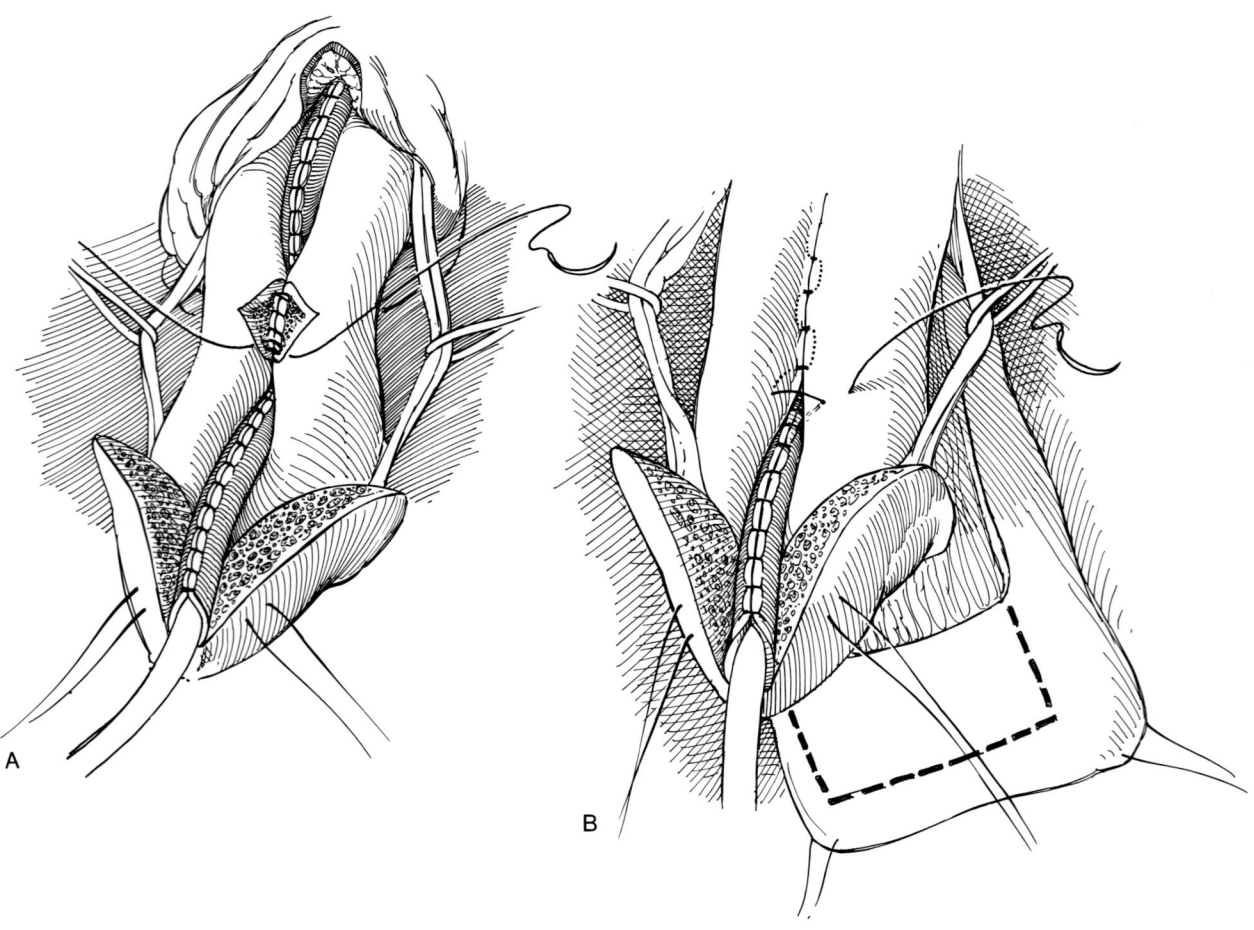

A   B

27 **A,** Approximate the glans flaps with subcuticular mattress sutures, and close the epithelium over them with fine interrupted sutures. Bring the preputial flap to the dorsum, and attach it to the skin as an island. Form flaps from the remainder of the prepuce and ventral skin to cover the rest of the penis. **B,** Alternatively, if there is sufficient ventral skin, bring it around and suture it dorsally.

Close the basal Z-incision with interrupted sutures. Tack the stent in place, and apply a Tegaderm dressing.

IPGAM (Inverted MAGPI) Procedure

28 **A,** Incise the distal margin of the glans vertically (see Figures 23 and 24). **B,** Close the incision transversely to form a deep groove and move the new meatus ventrally. Mark and make two parallel incision on the glans and a U-shaped incision on the pubic skin around the meatus.

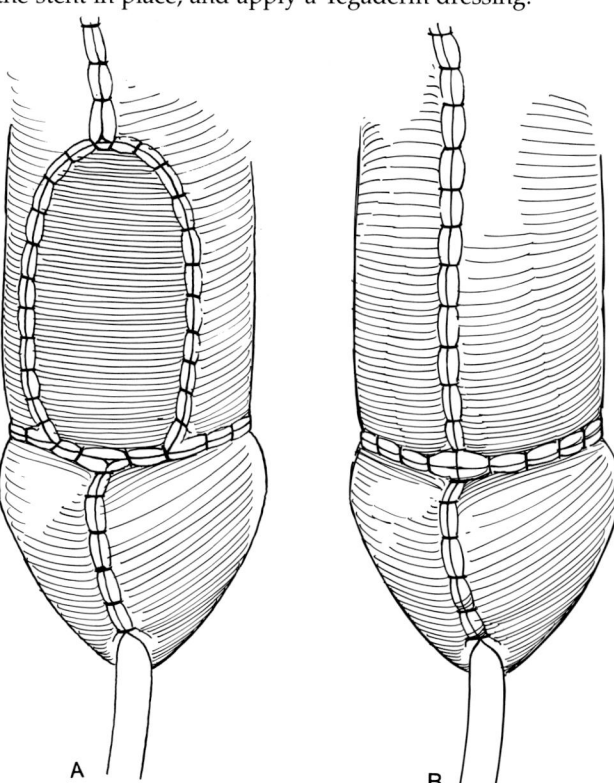

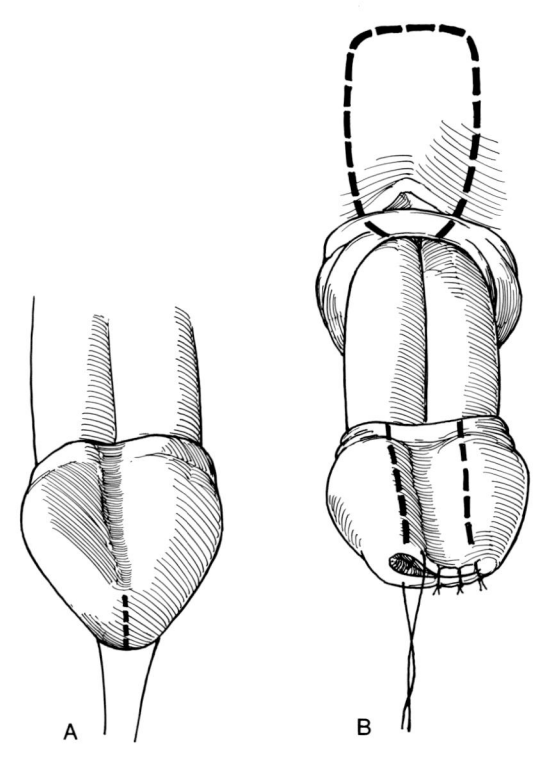

29 Mobilize the glanular urethra and tubularize it. Mobilize the upper flap, and close it ventrally into a tube. Form a flap from the skin above the meatus and tubularize it.

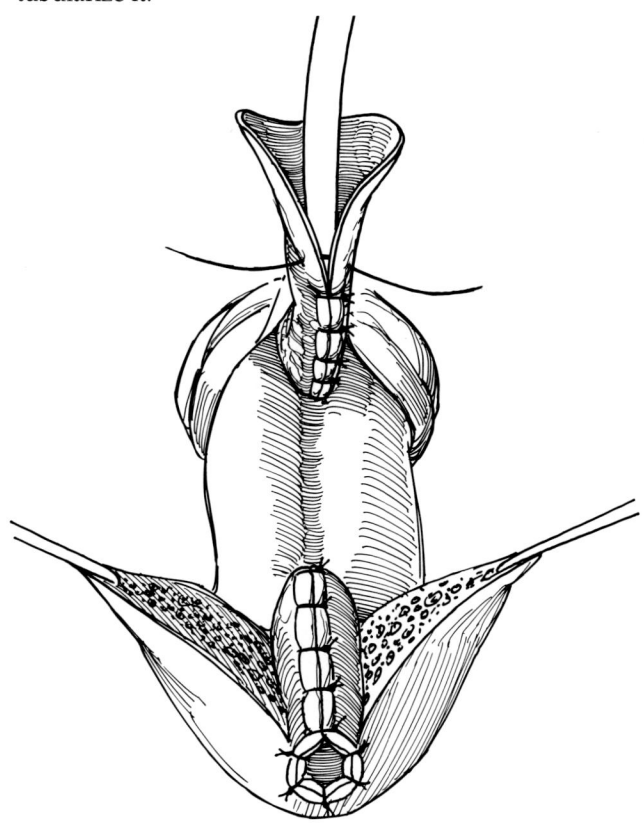

30 A, Anastomose the skin tube to the glanular urethral tube. Close the glans flaps. B, Split and approximate the ventral skin over the dorsum of the shaft.

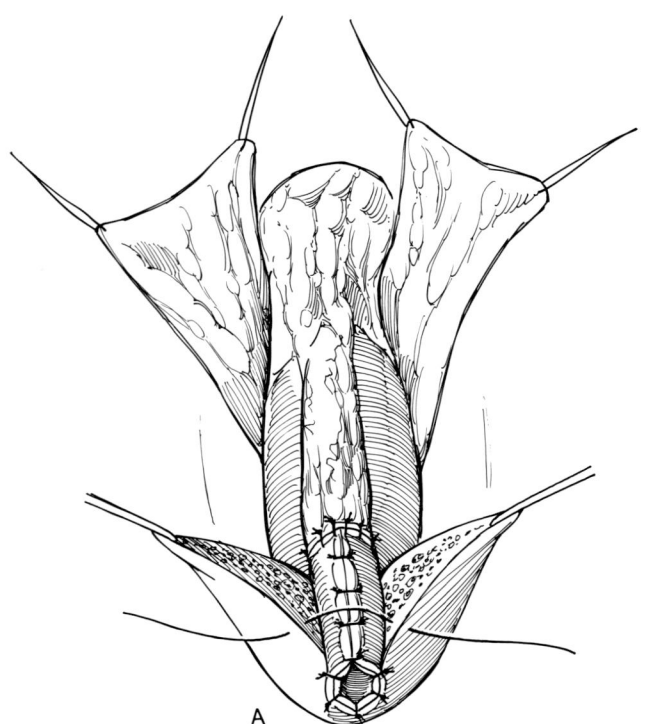

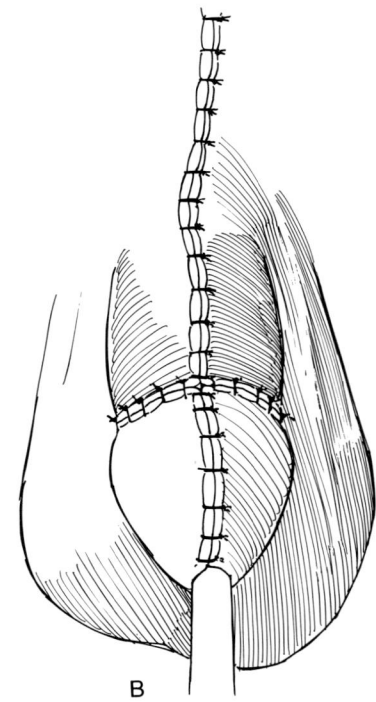

POSTOPERATIVE PROBLEMS

Fistulas are relatively common but are reduced by avoiding tension and preventing infection.

Commentary by Ricardo Gonzales

The important general points of the technique are: (1) use of optical magnification, (2) use of bipolar cautery, (3) use of fine monofilament absorbable suture material, and (4) atraumatic surgery with careful handling of tissues. Specific points include the identification and preservation of the dorsal neurovascular bundles, preservation of the urethral plate whenever possible, and the excision of small strips of glans lateral to the urethral plate to avoid leaving a cleft glans. In all cases, with the exception of the more distal glanular epispadias, I now use the Cantwell-Ransley technique. This operation is applicable to all cases of either isolated epispadias or those associated to bladder exstrophy. I begin by placing two traction sutures in the glans; then I perform the IPGAM procedure. In dissecting the circumference of the corpora, it is important not to injure the neurovascular bundles, but I do not necessarily dissect them and lift them off the corpora as originally described. Medially, during the dissection of the corpora, it is impor-

tant to preserve the tissue that joins the ventral aspect of the urethral plate to the ventral penile skin to maximize the vascularization of the urethra. In infancy, the age in which I prefer to correct this malformation, excellent straightening of the penis can be obtained by suturing the corpora as shown, without necessarily making corporal incisions and anastomosing the corpora together. This maneuver may be necessary in older children and adults and in redo cases. However, the proximal dissection of the corpora from the pubic rami is important in all cases. To tubularize the urethra, I prefer a 7–0 running extraepithelial polydioxanone suture (PDS) reinforced by a second layer of the same suture material. I also use 7–0 running PDS in the skin, with excellent cosmetic results. At the proximal end of the urethroplasty, avoid leaving a diverticulum that may make catheterization difficult. Remember that in cases of exstrophy, some of these children will need either temporary or permanent intermittent catheterization after the bladder neck reconstruction. In infants, I do all repairs with a 7 F Silastic stent with multiple perforations, with the proximal end just inside the bladder neck. The coverage of the dorsal skin defect is best obtained with an island flap of the ventral prepuce. Rotation of the penis by traction of the subcutaneous vascular pedicle must be avoided. The penis can be left without a dressing, but generally I prefer a double layer of Tegaderm.

CHAPTER 127

Circumcision

Circumcision, a procedure performed on an organ of great personal concern, must be done with precision. The newborn should be mature and in good health. Prep the penis with iodophor solution. Infiltrate the base of the penis with 1 ml of 1 or 2 percent plain lidocaine (Xylocaine) through a 26-gauge needle, even if, in older boys, general anesthesia is used. A tourniquet may be applied at the base for initial hemostasis.

DOUBLE-INCISION TECHNIQUE

1 **A,** Mark the site of the corona of the glans onto the unretracted prepuce with a marking pen.
B, On the ventrum opposite the frenulum, provide a V.

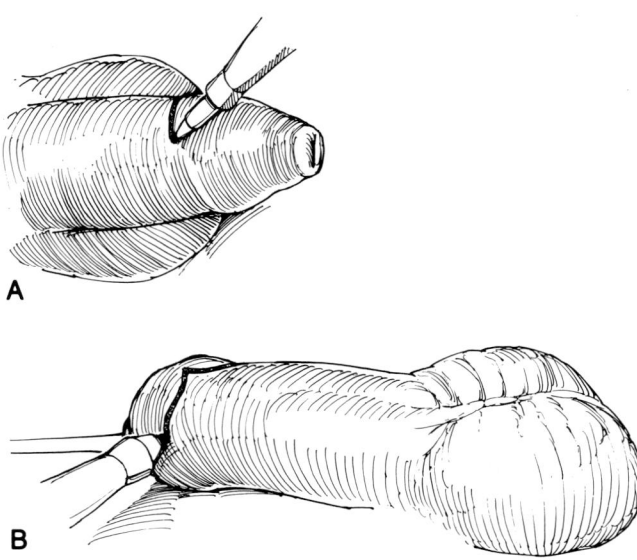

2 Retract the prepuce, freeing it completely from the glans using a mosquito clamp and traction from moist gauze held over the thumb and fingertips. Clear the lumps of smegma. Mark the second incision 0.5 to 1 cm proximal to the sulcus to leave enough membrane for suturing, going straight across the base of the frenulum. Identify the urethral meatus.

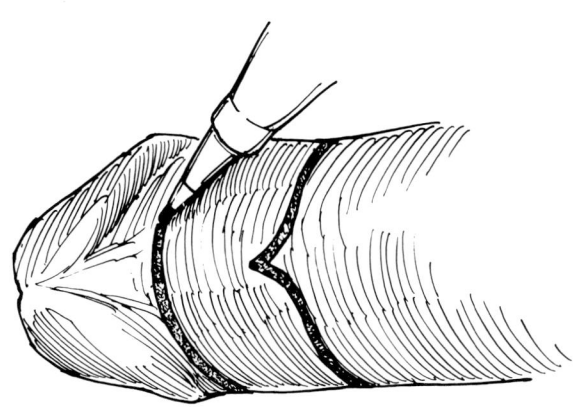

621

3 **A,** Incise along the marked lines proximally.
B, Also incise distally.

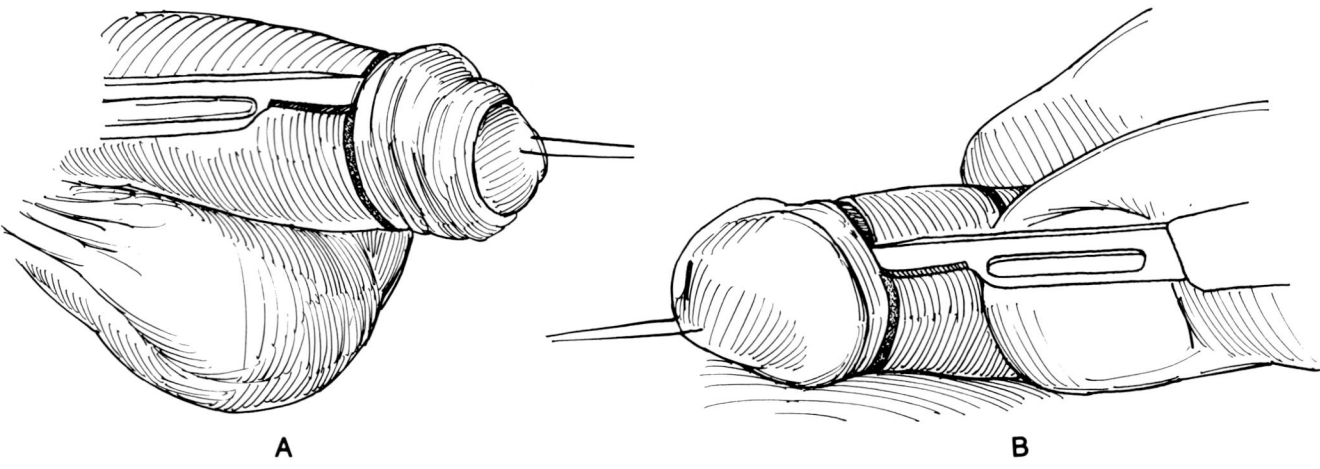

A

B

4 On the dorsum, divide the skin with scissors.

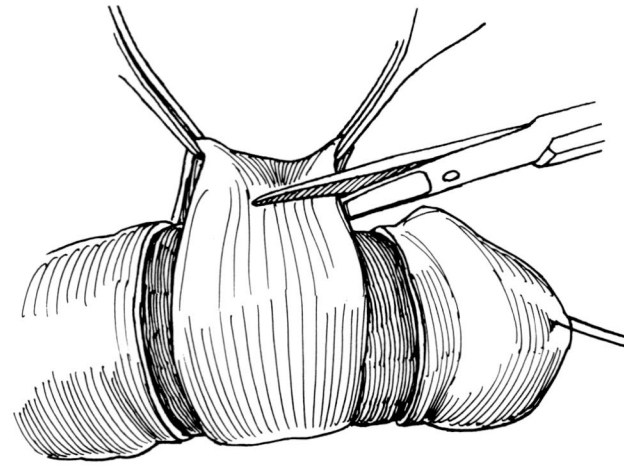

5 Elevate the edges and free the skin from the dartos layer. Fulgurate bleeders or tie them with 5-0 plain catgut. Inspect the frenular area, and secure and ligate the artery or arteries. Release the tourniquet, and complete the hemostasis with electrocautery.

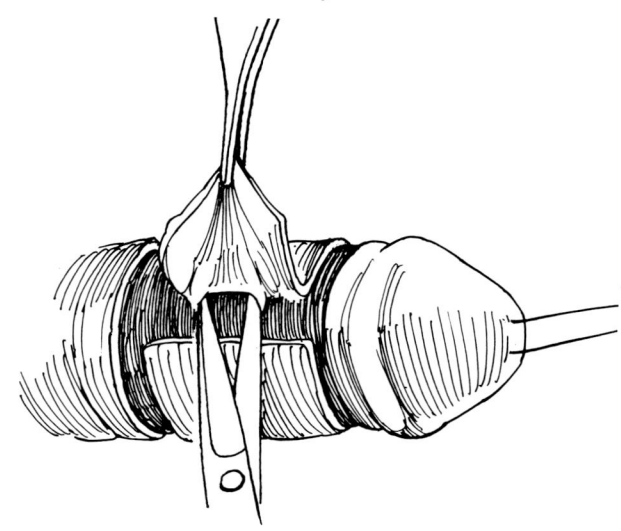

6 Place 4–0 plain catgut sutures through the skin of the shaft and corona in each of the four quadrants. Leave them long, holding them in mosquito clamps. Place two sutures between each pair, plus two more to approximate the V at the frenulum. End-on mattress sutures may be needed at the frenulum.

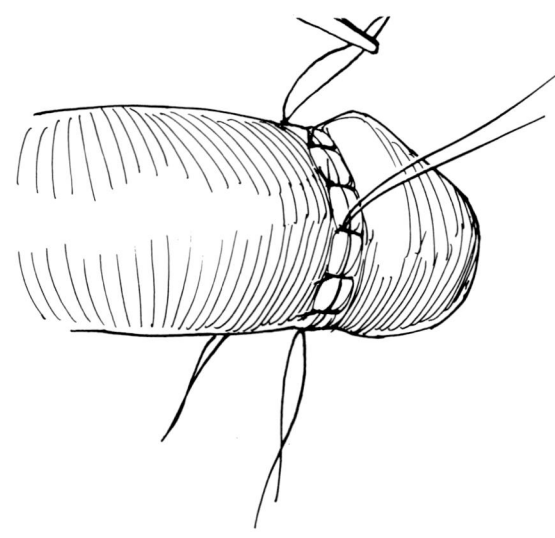

7 Take a strip of 1-in petroleum jelly (Vaseline) gauze in a clamp and coil it on itself by rotating it with the clamp like waving a flag; pull the free end to form a helical tube.

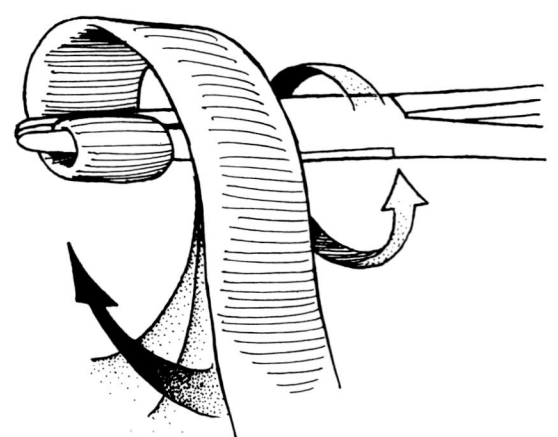

8 Tie the tube successively into the four quadrant sutures, loosely enough to avoid constriction should erection occur. Trim a 4 × 4 gauze to cover the tube, and secure it to the pubic region with plastic tape.

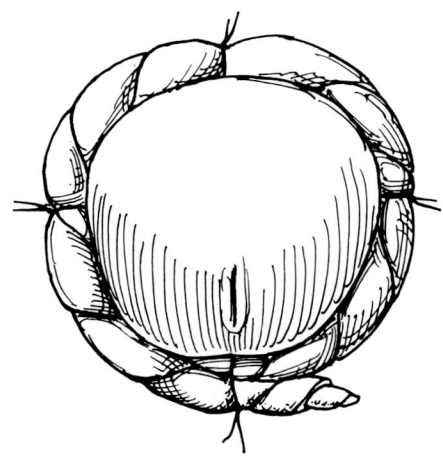

ALTERNATIVE TECHNIQUE
(FOR SMALL BOYS)

9 After anesthesia, mark the skin at the coronal level with the prepuce in place. Make a dorsal slit to the mark, and grasp the edges.

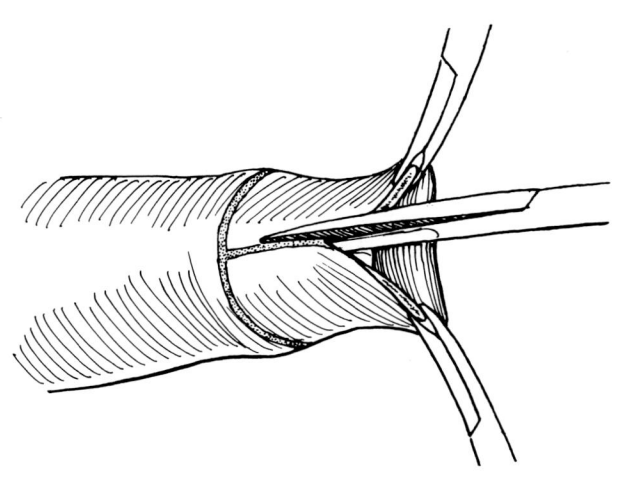

10 Divide both layers of the prepuce on the marked line.

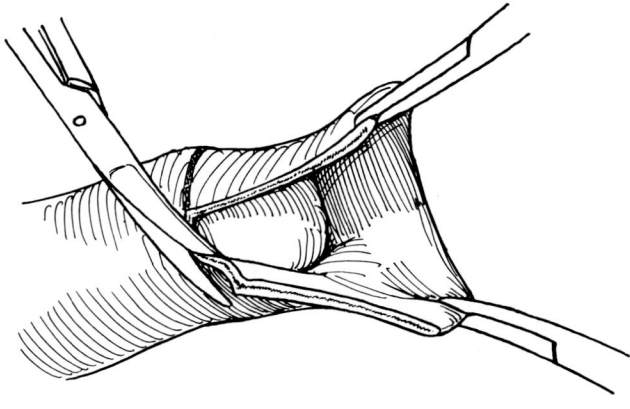

11 Provide a V at the frenulum. Reapproximate as described in Steps 6–8.

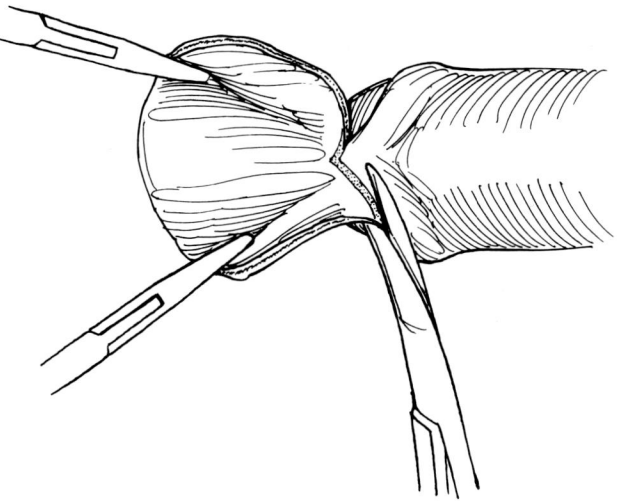

POSTOPERATIVE PROBLEMS

In the adolescent, *skin necrosis* may occur if epinephrine is used in the local anesthetic. Avoid electrocoagulation. If it is used, apply a saline-soaked sponge around the penis, and avoid holding the organ away from the body. Meatal stenosis should be treated at the time of circumcision (page 570). In infants, *bleeding and infection* occasionally are seen and are managed in the usual way. Severe infections with systemic spread are rare, but any infection should be treated adequately.

If *too much skin* is removed in one area, it may re-epithelialize. If removal is extensive, place a skin graft. When too much inner preputial membrane is left, while excess outer skin is removed, the penis becomes "buried." It can be released by circumcising the junction and covering the defect with the preputial tissue. If *too little skin* has been removed, phimosis may occur as the suture line contracts. A very redundant residual prepuce may require recircumcision. Skin bridges usually can be divided with small scissors without anesthesia.

Glanular necrosis (or even loss of the whole shaft) may result from contact of the cautery with a clamp. *Division of the glans* may occur while making a dorsal slit. *Chordee* can result from delayed healing of the ventrum. *Urethral injury* results from sutures hurriedly placed to stop bleeding. *Urinary retention* can occur later with secondary phimosis or immediately from a dressing that is too tight.

The worst complication results from *not recognizing hypospadias* before circumcision; the resultant loss of preputial skin makes hypospadias repair very difficult.

PLASTIBELL TECHNIQUE
(FOR INFANTS)

Wait for 24 hours after birth. Obtain informed consent. Before starting the procedure, read the printed instructions accompanying the Plastibell device. Identify the baby and restrain him adequately in papoose restraints. Be strict about aseptic technique. Prep and drape the penis.

For local anesthesia (page 57), which should be used, palpate the inferior border of the symphysis pubis with the index and middle fingers of one hand. With the other hand, inject 1.0 to 1.2 ml of 1 percent lidocaine *without* epinephrine from a 3-ml syringe, by inserting the needle at this point and directing it 0.25 to 0.5 cm toward the ten o'clock position, just under the symphysis pubis. Aspirate carefully to avoid accidental intravascular injection. Withdraw the needle, and repeat the injection in the two o'clock position. Inject the remaining anesthetic around the ventral surface of the scrotum at the base of the penis.

12 A, Mark the location of the coronal sulcus on the skin of the shaft with a marking pen. B, Dilate the preputial ring with a hemostat, and identify the urethral meatus. Place straight hemostats on the prepuce at 10 o'clock and 2 o'clock, taking a shallow bite 0.5 to 1 cm deep. Tease the preputial surface off the dorsum of the glans; clamp the prepuce in the midline, one third of the distance to the corona with a straight hemostat for 10 seconds. Divide the crushed line with straight blunt-tipped scissors. Bluntly free the prepuce from the glans with a flexible probe until it can be completely retracted and the sulcus exposed.

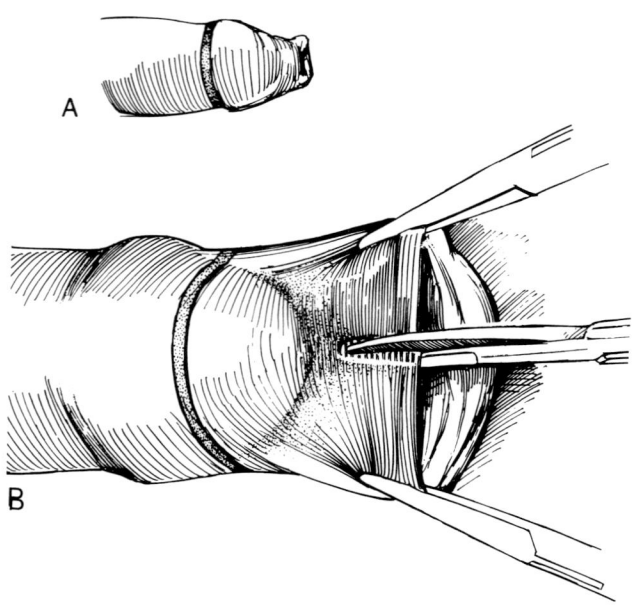

13 Select the correct size of Plastibell from the three sizes available, so that the bottom edge of the bell completely covers the corona. The bell should slightly distend the prepuce as it is drawn down over the bell and glans. Pull the foreskin over the bell until the skin mark that was made at the coronal sulcus lies over the groove in the bell.

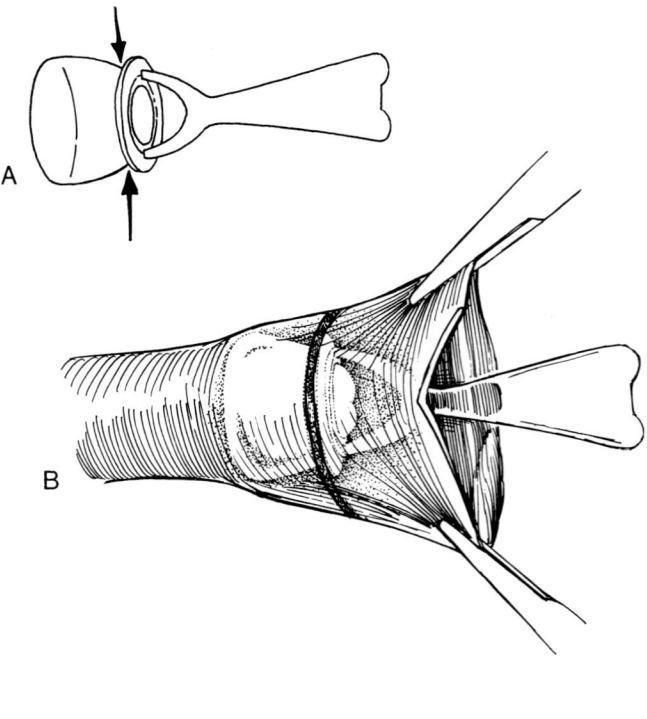

14 Tie an absorbable suture as tightly as possible in the inner groove in the device, and cut the prepuce off with scissors just past the outer groove. Do not use electrocautery. Break off the handle. Tell the parents to wait for the bell to fall out.

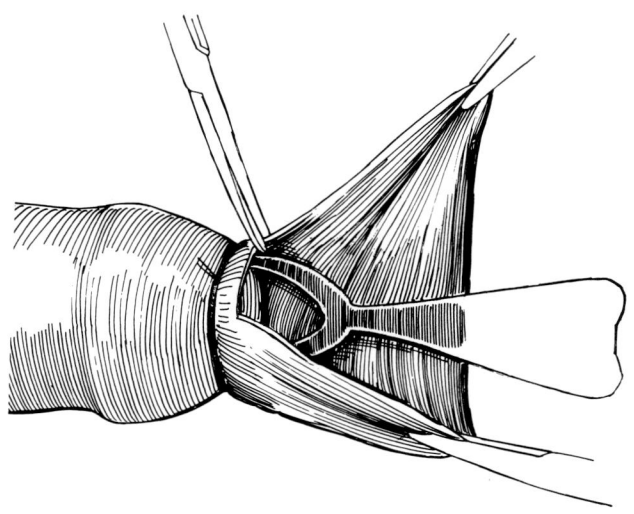

DORSAL SLIT FOR PARAPHIMOSIS

15 A and B, Make a vertical dorsal incision sharply, centered at the junction of the shiny inner and the duller outer skin. After release of the constriction, manipulate the prepuce over the glans to be sure that the dorsal incision is long enough for easy passage. C, Approximate the longitudinal cut transversely with interrupted sutures of 5–0 plain catgut sutures. D, Replace the prepuce around the glans, and cover it with a medicated gauze dressing. Alternatively, proceed with circumcision before suturing.

GOMCO CLAMP TECHNIQUE

Select the correct size of Gomco bell and place it as described for the Plastibell in the second step (Figure 13). Pull the prepuce over the bell and through the plate and yoke portions of the clamp until the skin mark at the coronal sulcus lies at the level of the top of the clamp. Screw the clamp down onto the bell as tightly as possible. Cut the prepuce off right next to the top of the plate. Remove the entire clamp, bell, and excised prepuce. If necessary for bleeding, apply interrupted 5–0 synthetic absorbable sutures to the cut edge.

POSTOPERATIVE PROBLEMS

Inadequate removal of the foreskin is the most common sequela, whereas excessive removal is rare. Skin bridges may develop. If circumferential healing occurs after inadequate removal, concealed penis may result. Infection and bleeding after these simple techniques are quite uncommon.

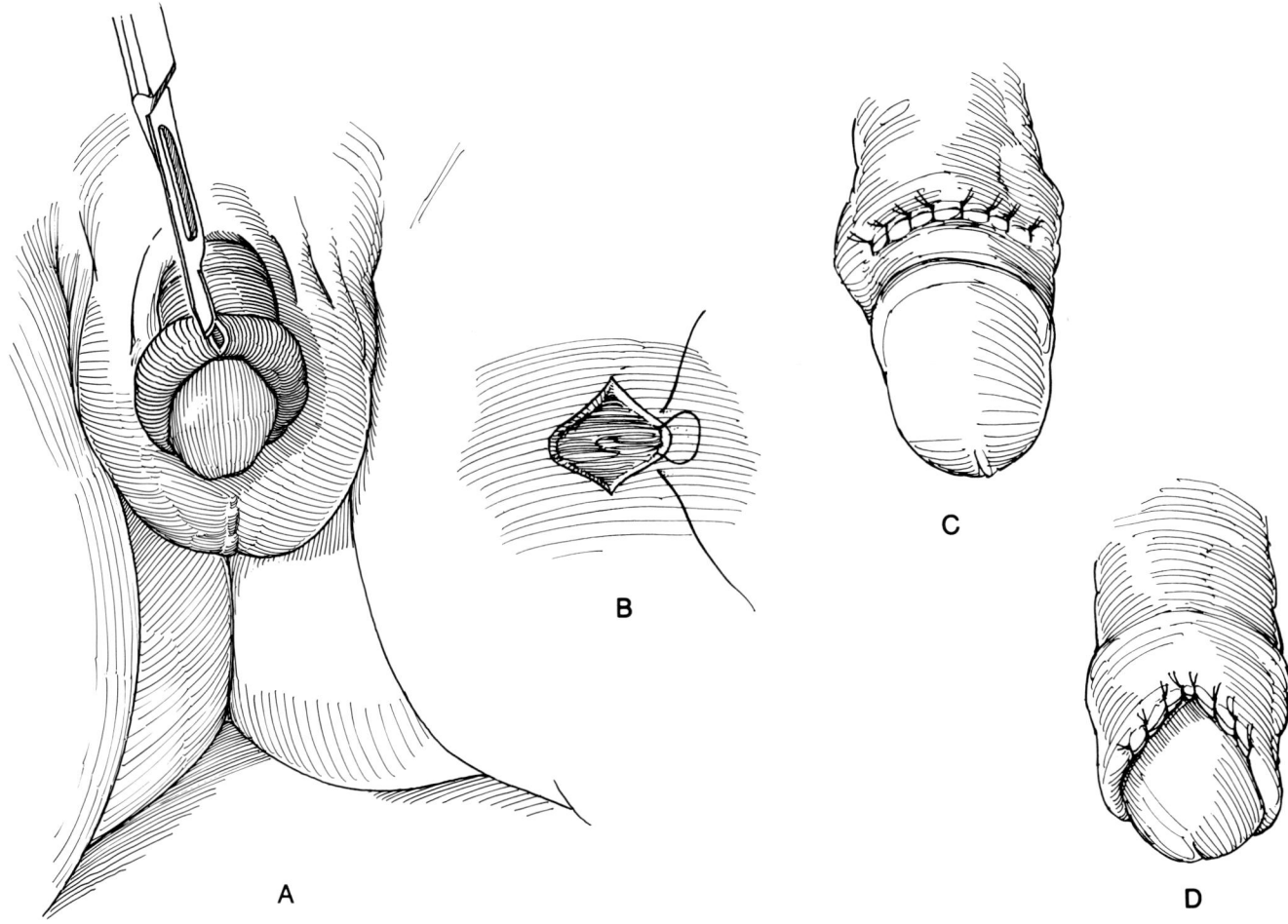

Commentary by Om P. Khanna

Circumcision can be performed in infants and children by means of many different techniques. The choice of procedure is a matter of the urologist's personal preference. My method of choice for circumcision is to use a Gomco clamp for children of all ages. This technique is quick, and there is little or no blood loss. The cut-skin edges are sharp and smooth, and there is no postoperative skin edema.

The most common complications of circumcision are pain, bleeding, and either insufficient or excessive removal of the foreskin. All these complications can be lessened or eliminated by one of the following methods: (1) using dorsal penile nerve block for children of all ages, even those who are circumcised while under general anesthesia, with 0.25% or 0.5% bupivacaine hydrochloride; (2) applying the clamp tightly for several minutes and suturing the cut-skin edges with interrupted sutures of 5–0 Dexon (if bleeding starts during the procedure, the cut-skin edges should be separated, the bleeding vessels electrocoagulated, and the skin edges sutured with 5–0 Dexon); (3) avoiding either insufficient or excessive removal of foreskin by marking the level of the coronal sulcus on the outer prepuce with a skin-marking pen and by complete lysis of adhesions between the prepuce and the glans penis.

CHAPTER 128

Penoscrotal Transposition

TWO-STAGE TECHNIQUE
(GLENN-ANDERSON)

The two halves of the scrotum are mobilized to form rotational advancement flaps to fill the space beneath the released penile shaft. If not associated with a hypospadic meatus, incisions circling over the top of each scrotal half that meet beneath the base of the penis may be sufficient if the scrotum is widely mobilized and the two wings are rotated beneath the penis, either in the midline or as a Z-plasty.

2 Incise around the base of the penis, then down the median raphe, passing on either side of the hypospadic urethral orifice.

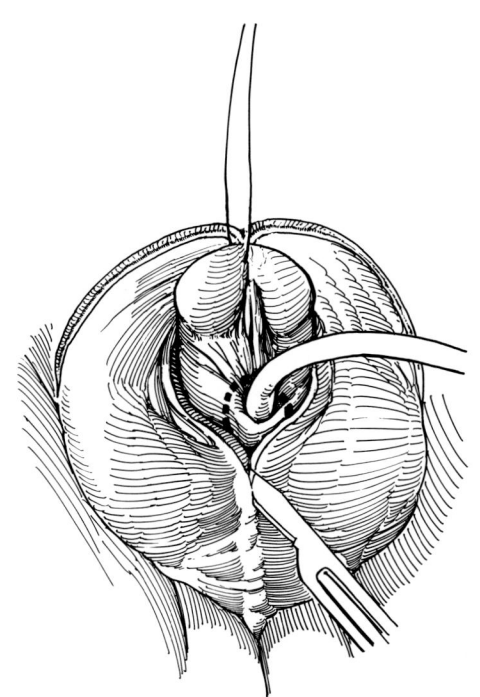

1 Insert a silicone balloon catheter in the urethra. Make a curved transverse incision just above the upper scrotal folds.

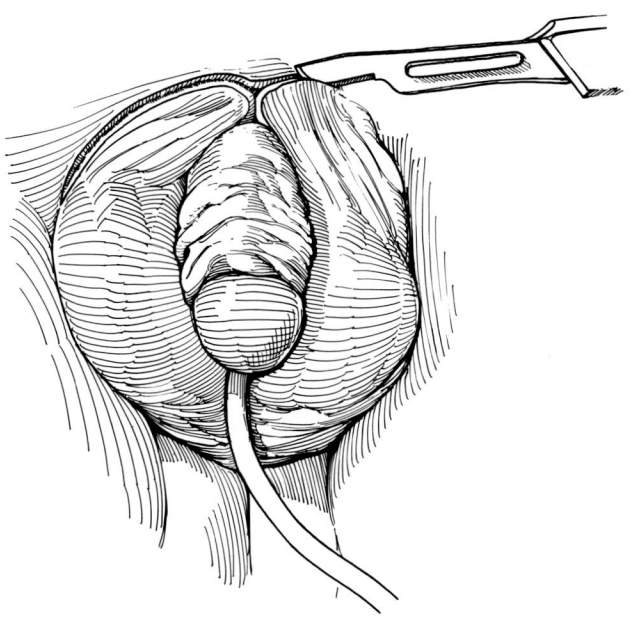

3 Free the underlying urethra, and excise all the fibrous tissue of the chordee from the ventral surface of the penis.

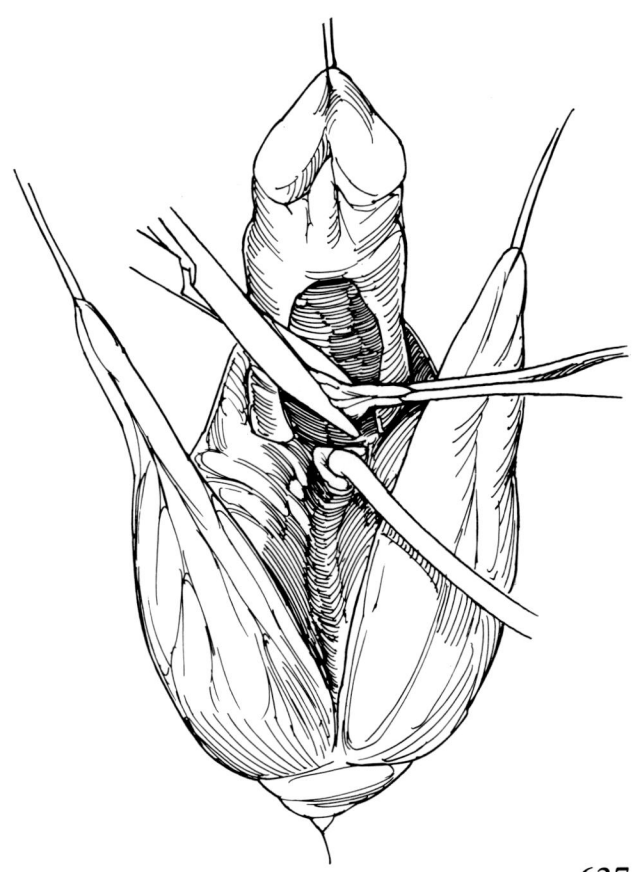

4 Draw the lateral scrotal flaps distally into the defect under the penis. Bring the lateral scrotal flaps underneath the penis and join them in the midline. Situate the meatus at its distal, most-comfortable point.

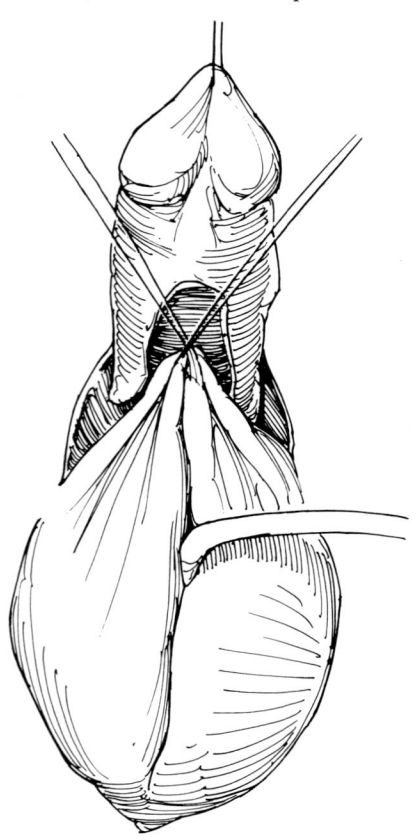

FLAP TECHNIQUE FOR PROXIMAL MEATUS

6 Incise and free the ventrum of the penis as described in Figures 1 and 2. Mark, incise, and elevate a flap proximal to the perineal meatus (in what unfortunately may be hair-bearing skin).

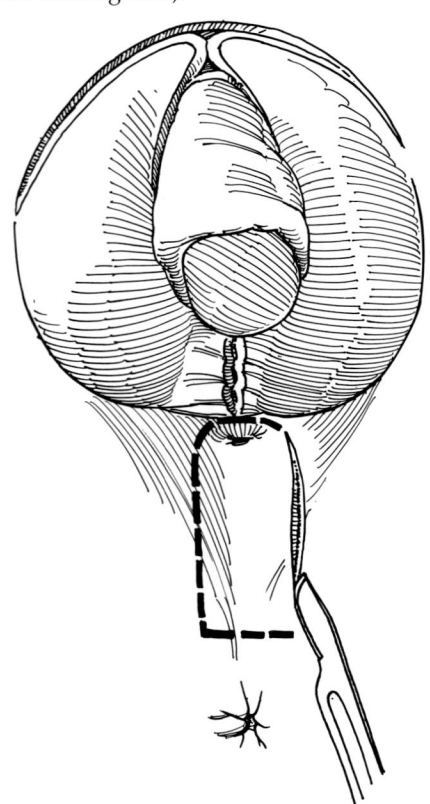

5 Close the repair around the new meatus in two layers with 4–0 plain catgut sutures subcutaneously and with interrupted 6–0 chromic catgut sutures for the skin. Remove the catheter in 2 or 3 days. Construct the urethra after complete revascularization of the flaps has occurred.

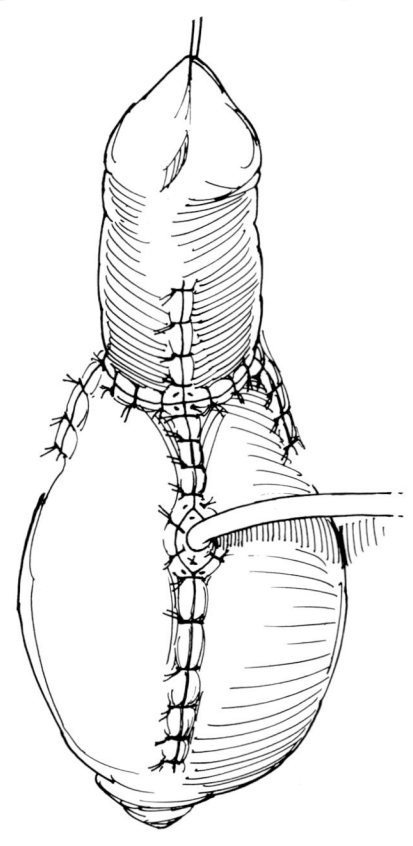

7 Close the flap as a tube with a running 6–0 synthetic absorbable suture around a balloon catheter (not shown). Elevate the symmetric scrotal flaps.

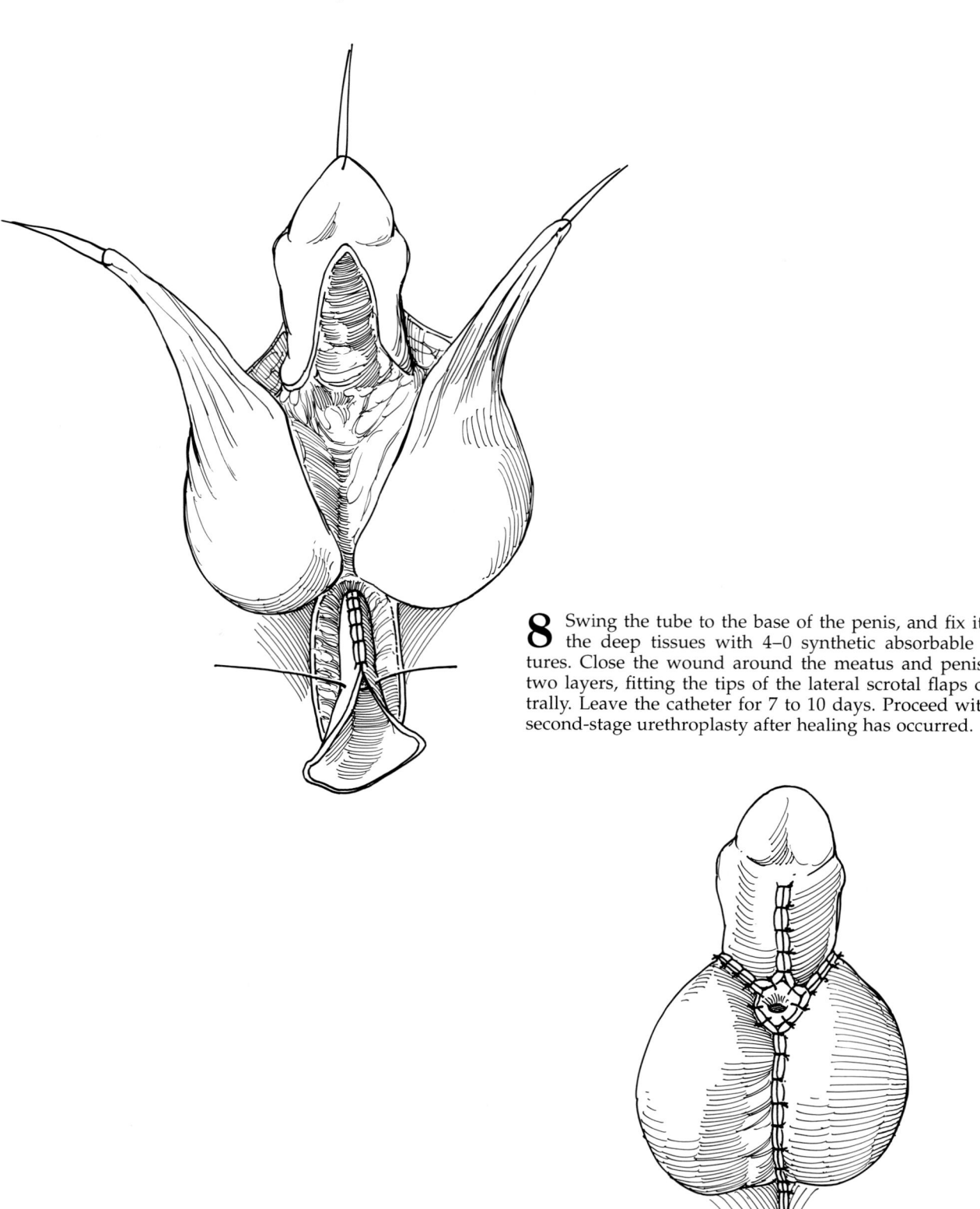

8 Swing the tube to the base of the penis, and fix it to the deep tissues with 4–0 synthetic absorbable sutures. Close the wound around the meatus and penis in two layers, fitting the tips of the lateral scrotal flaps centrally. Leave the catheter for 7 to 10 days. Proceed with a second-stage urethroplasty after healing has occurred.

ONE-STAGE REPAIR
(PEROVIC)

9 Mark an incision around the coronal sulcus, continue it along the ventral surface to encircle the hypospadic meatus, and leave a midline strip that will be excised with the chordee. Mark a second incision, beginning below the meatus that continues up the medial side of the split scrotum and over the anterior aspect at the scrotal base. Incise along the lines.

10 Incise an island flap on the dorsum that will form the new urethra; this leaves a flap of shaft skin on either side. Continue the dorsal incision proximally at the base of the penis. Excise the chordee. Dorsal tucks may be required to correct residual chordee.

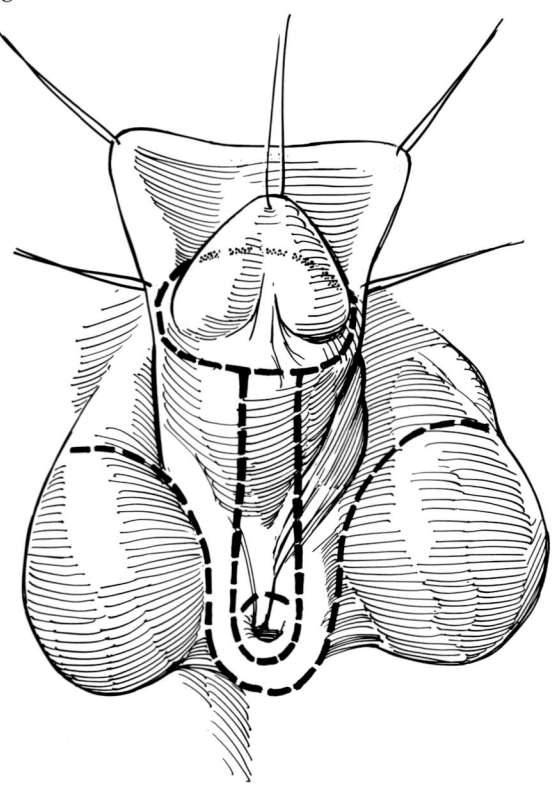

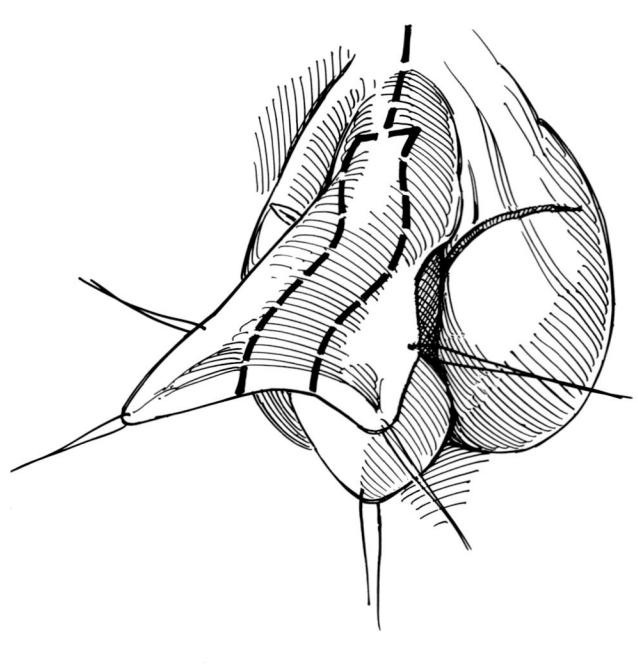

11 Bluntly make a longitudinal opening in an avascular area, revealed by transillumination of the vascular pedicle. Free the proximal urethra, and discard the friable tip. Pass the penis through the opening in the dorsal flap.

12 Tubularize the island flap, and anastomose the stump of the urethra to it. Excise a groove in the ventrum of the glans, and bring the new urethra to the tip. Suture the testes to each other, and place traction sutures in each lower pole. Make parallel staggered cuts on each side of the scrotum.

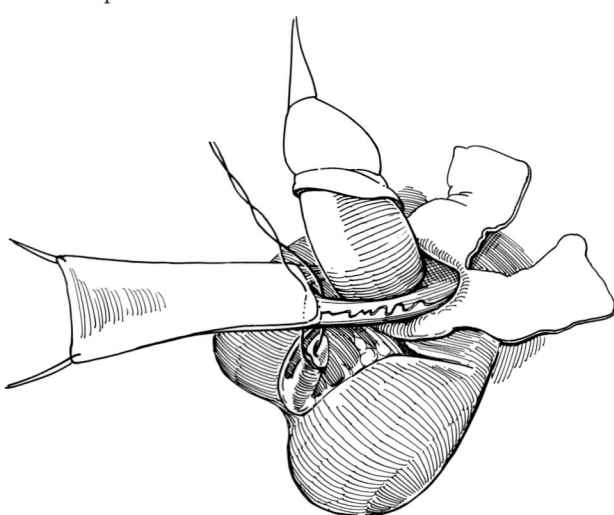

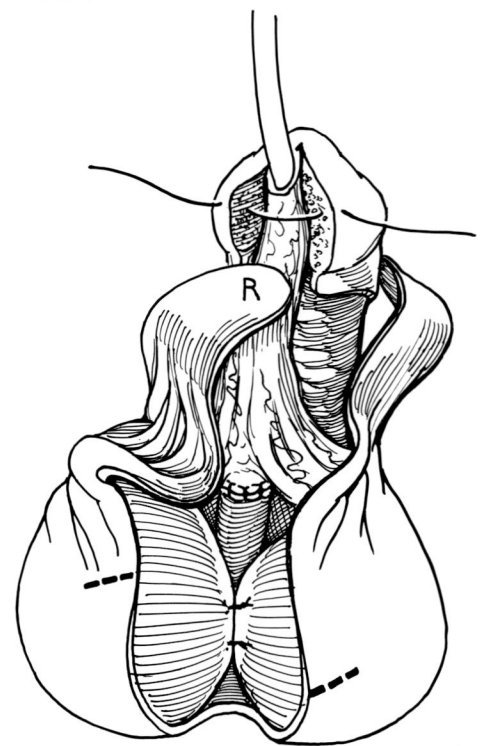

13 **A** and **B,** Rotate the right skin flap (R) to the left; then swing the left flap dorsally to cover that aspect of the shaft. Close the scrotum in a Z fashion. Provide drainage, and, to prevent their elevation, maintain traction on the testes for 1 or 2 weeks by tying the traction sutures over a bolster.

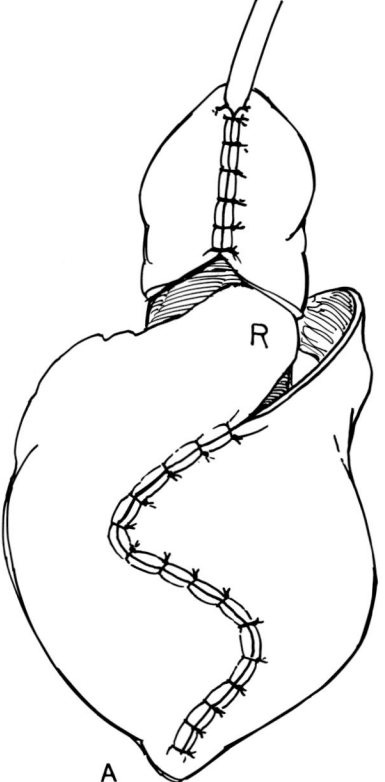

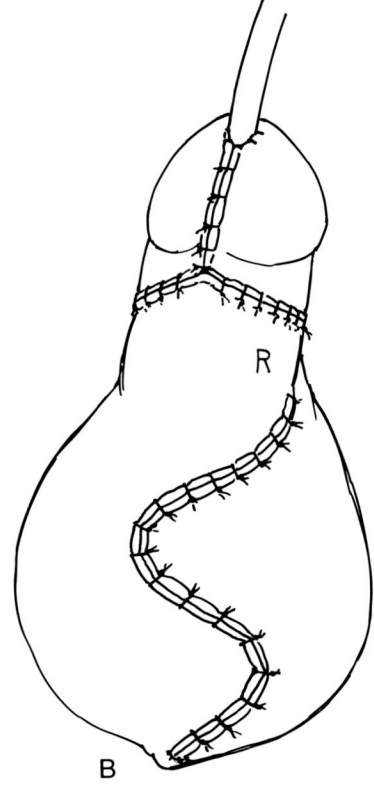

A

B

PENILE TORSION

14 **A,** Incise the skin and dartos layer circumferentially at the corona, as for circumcision. **B,** Deglove the shaft and rotate the penis, usually clockwise, to orient the meatus vertically. **C,** Reapproximate the skin with fine interrupted plain catgut sutures. The median raphe ideally should be in the midline ventrally, but this sometimes may require over-rotation to correct severe torsion.

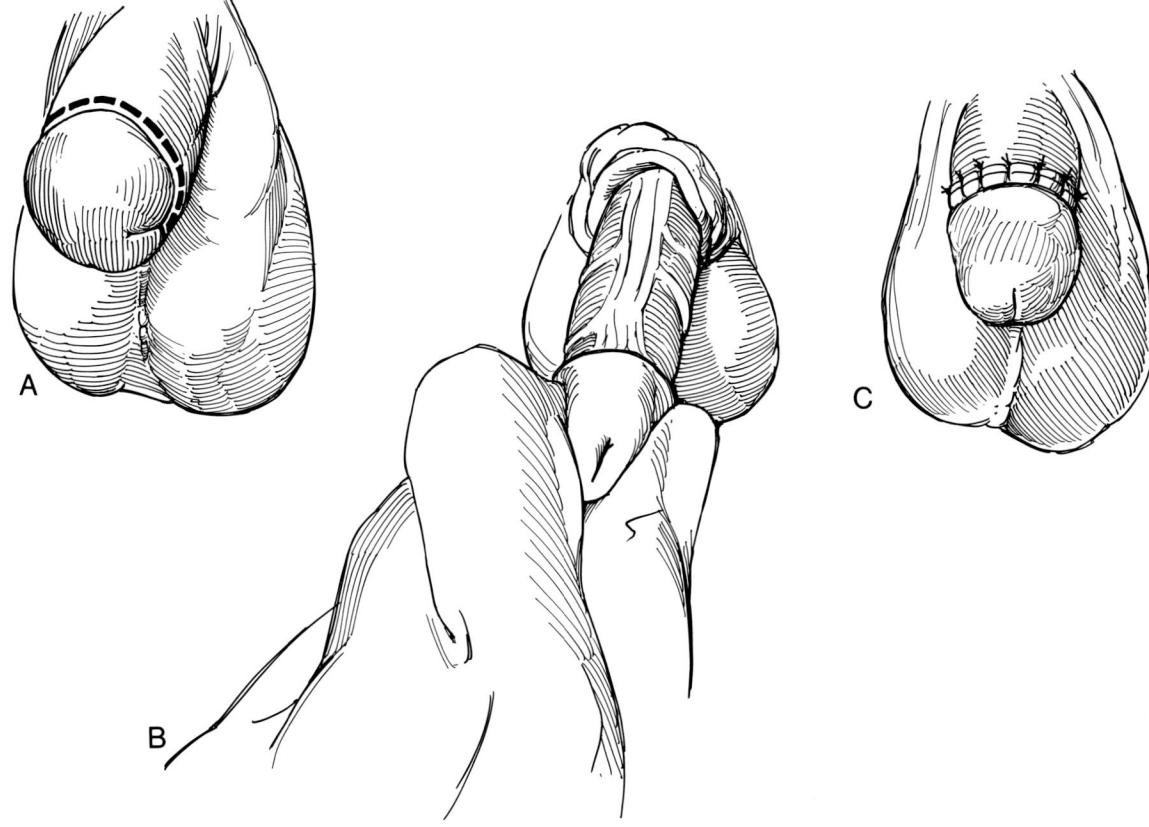

A

B

C

Commentary by R. Dixon Walker, III

Penoscrotal transposition most often occurs in association with severe hypospadias in which the meatus is located on the proximal shaft or in the scrotal or perineal position. Therefore, one needs to consider whether a one-stage repair can be attempted or the procedure should be done in stages. That decision is determined by the degree of transposition, the location of the meatus, and the amount of associated chordee. In many cases of proximal shaft hypospadias, the transposition is incomplete and does not encircle the penile base. In this instance, the incisions in Figure 1 do not meet at the dorsal base of the penis but rather at the lateral edges of the base. This important step allows one to develop a transverse island flap for either onlay or tubed pedicle graft and still mobilize the pedicle and dorsal penile skin to the base of the penis. If the incision for the transposition does come to the midline dorsal base of the penis, then the dorsal penile and preputial shaft skin cannot be mobilized. For that reason, I most often prefer a two-stage procedure in such instances, in which the preputial skin is brought ventrally, as in Byars flaps, as a first stage; in the second stage, the incisions are made for the transposition as in Figure 1, and ventrally, a classic Byars urethroplasty is performed.

The technique of mobilizing the scrotal urethral plate can be done successfully provided that the urethral plate is of sufficient width. Attempts to widen the urethral plate by incorporating skin lateral to the "shiny" skin should be discouraged, because this often is hair-bearing skin and will result in complications at puberty. If there is an adequate scrotal urethral plate associated with incomplete transposition of the scrotum, the patient can be managed with a one-stage repair that combines tubularization of the scrotal plate and a tubularized preputial transverse island flap. I have had no experience with the procedure described by Perovic (1992) (Figs. 9–13) but would prefer to manage these extensive repairs with bladder or buccal mucosal graft, in conjunction with surgical management of the penoscrotal transposition.

It must be reemphasized that this is a painstaking and delicate surgery that requires optical magnification, atraumatic instrumentation, and fine absorbable sutures. Most of the hypospadias repairs that I do are in children 6 to 12 months of age, regardless of severity. Therefore appropriate suture material is 6–0 to 7–0 absorbable suture on fine cutting needles. If the phallus is small, it is pretreated with 2 percent testosterone cream.

CHAPTER 129

Penile Curvature

For correction of minor chordee during hypospadias repair in which the urethral plate is left intact, see page 569.

RELEASE OF DARTOS AND BUCK'S FASCIAS
(DEVINE)

Instruct the boy to take a preoperative shower with antiseptic soap.

Create an artificial erection to determine the degree of curvature. Make an incision around the shaft at the site of the circumcision scar, and dissect the shaft skin back to the base of the penis.

ELLIPTICAL EXCISION TECHNIQUE FOR VENTRAL CHORDEE
(NESBIT)

With the penis erect, measure the length on the ventrum and dorsum with a tape. The difference in length determines the number and width of the ellipses to be removed. Most often, excision of only one ellipse on each side is required.

Elevate the dysgenic dartos and Buck's fascias that are concentrated on either side of the corpus spongiosum. In rare cases, the corpus spongiosum and urethra may have to be mobilized to resect all the fibrous tissue. Repeat the erection. If curvature remains, proceed to elliptical excisions on the dorsum. Cover the now partially denuded ventral surface with Byars flaps.

1 Incise Colles' fascia longitudinally. Mobilize the dorsal neurovascular structures dorsomedially along with Buck's fascia from each side. The bundle may be elevated with a vessel loop.

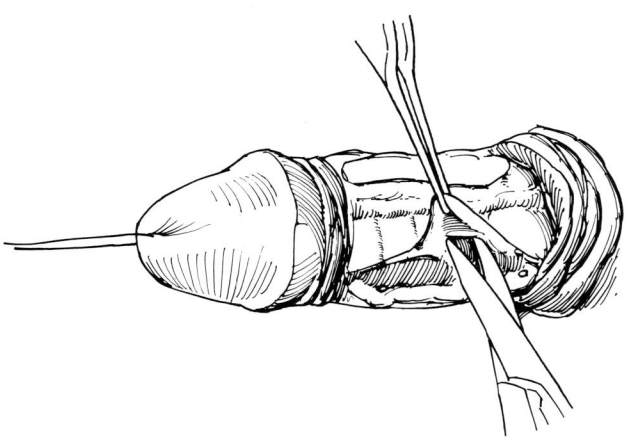

2 Grasp the tunica albuginea with Allis clamps, and excise the elevated ellipses.

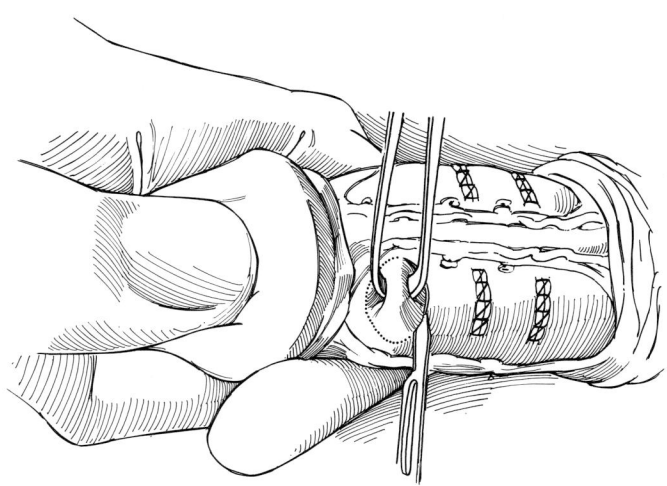

3 **A,** Alternatively, dry the tunica albuginea, and mark 1-cm ellipses on each side with a marking pen. Incise and remove the ellipses of tunica propria. Keep the depth of the excision just superficial to the endothelial layer, if possible. In cases of corporal disproportion, the tissue removed can be used as a graft for the opposite corpus cavernosum.

B, Approximate the edges of the defects successively as each ellipse is removed, using two or three interrupted 5-0 polydioxanone sutures. These may be followed by a running suture of the same material to assure a smooth surface. The sutures also may be inverted to bury the knots.

C and **D,** Alternatively, close the tunica with a running fine absorbable suture supplemented by interrupted pli-

cating sutures to achieve a smoother surface (Kelami, 1987). Test for straightness by artificial erection, and excise further ellipses if necessary. Be sure the erection is symmetric.

Forming *orthoplastic dorsal tucks* (page 569) is an alternative to excision of ellipses. Make two parallel transverse incisions in the tunica albuginea on each side of the midline approximately 8 mm apart. Place inverted sutures of nonabsorbable suture material, starting from inside out at the proximal cut and outside in at the distal cut, to draw the two openings in apposition and bury the bridge of tissue between. This is a useful technique in conjunction with hypospadias repair when the urethral plate is left intact but slight chordee persists.

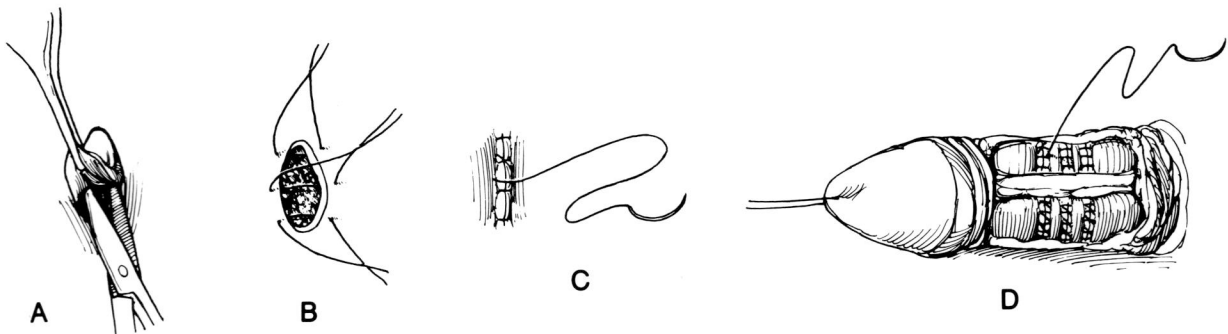

A   B   C   D

4 Reapproximate the subcutaneous tissue to the mucosal collar with 5-0 synthetic absorbable sutures, and reapproximate the skin at the coronal sulcus with 4-0 chromic catgut sutures. If the boy has not been circumcised, trim redundant skin to avoid postoperative edema. Dress with Tegaderm. The palpable ridges from the sutures will subside.

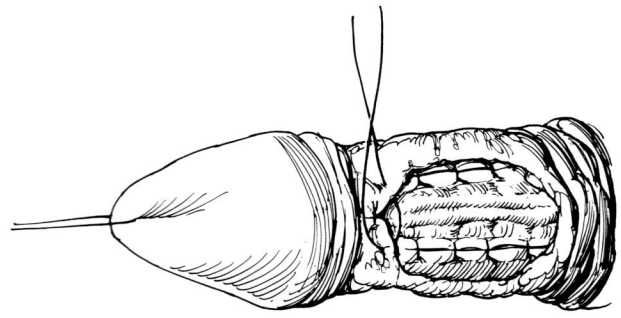

Commentary by R. Dixon Walker, III

Chordee that occurs with or without hypospadias most often can be managed without dividing the urethra. After the urethra and Buck's fascia are freed of all ventral scar tissue, an artificial-erection test will demonstrate residual chordee. Mild or moderate chordee is best managed with Nesbit tucks. I mark the area of chordee during the artificial erection test, so that I know the location and approximate width of the tuck. I prefer one tuck and will usually make it transverse to both corpora cavernosa. I do this by mobilizing the dorsal neurovascular bundle and excising a wedge having a midpoint that is the required width, as measured. Suture material is monofilament nonabsorbable, and the sutures are placed in interrupted fashion with the knots inverted. Additional tucks can then be done if chordee still is demonstrated.

CHAPTER 130

Vaginoplasty and Clitoriplasty for the Adrenogenital Syndrome

Perform rectal palpation, ultrasonography, genitography, and endoscopy. Early reconstruction is important, combining clitoriplasty and labioplasty, leaving a complicated vaginoplasty until later. Operate after the endocrinologist has examined the child and begins hydrocortisone and deoxycorticosterone acetate when necessary. The clitoris will shrink in the first 3 months of life, but a baby's perineum will be relatively fatter in the period between 6 and 18 months. Accordingly, operate before or after this period; usually, earlier is better psychologically. For a high-lying urethra and deep urogenital sinus, with the vagina entering the urethra above the external sphincter, the vaginoplasty can be delayed until the child is 2 or 3 years of age or even until puberty when the girl will be supported with estrogens and is able to dilate the repair. Prepare her with steroid supplement for the stress of the operation. Prepare the bowel.

Position. Extreme lithotomy with the perineum tilted upward is the proper position for both vaginoplasty and clitoriplasty procedures. Sew a towel to the perineum to cover the rectum.

VAGINOPLASTY, LOW ENTRY

For the vagina with a very low entry, simple cutback with a Y-V closure may be all that is needed.

Flap Vaginoplasty

1 Perform panendoscopy for orientation and transillumination of the urogenital sinus. Be sure the vagina is low enough to be reached by a perineal flap. Insert a small balloon catheter in the urethra. Place a 4 × 4 gauze soaked in neomycin solution in the rectum.

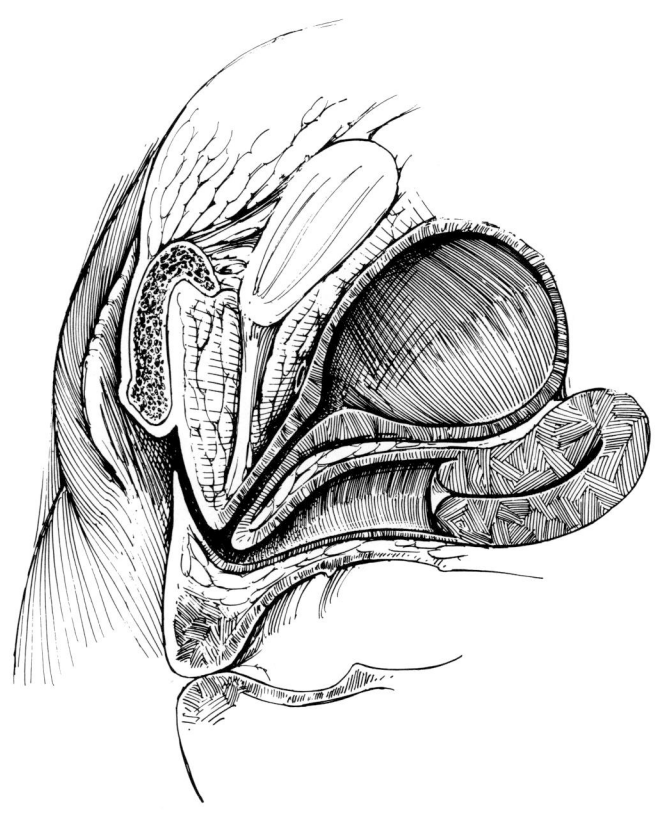

635

2 *Incision for flap:* Mark and incise a broad-based inverted U-shaped incision, anteriorly reaching almost to the edge of the sinus and posteriorly ending at the posterior margin of the new labia minora. Dissect a thick perineal flap. Be aware that the sinus is surrounded by corpus spongiosum and that the bleeding consequent to the dissection will require fulguration and fine figure-eight sutures. A finger in the rectum is not needed for distal urogenital sinus dissection.

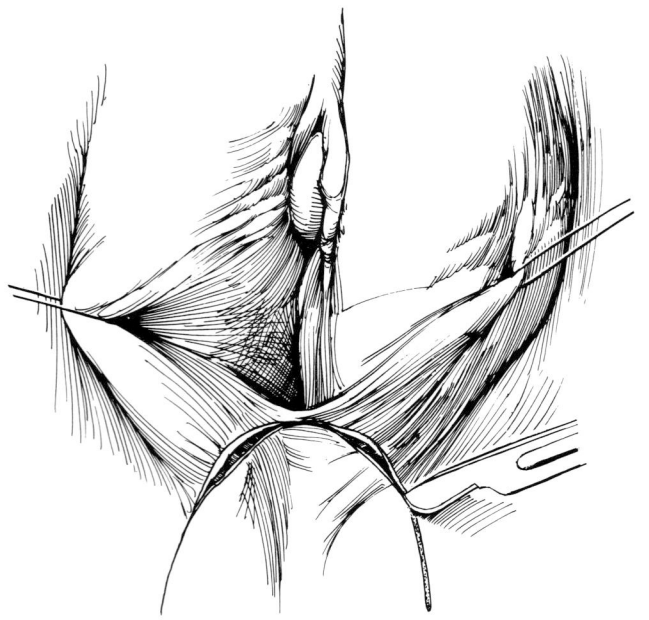

3 *Incision of vaginal back wall:* Place traction sutures in the thin posterior wall of the urogenital sinus, and incise it until the vagina is reached. If the vagina is high, pull it down with a small balloon catheter until its thicker wall is exposed. The posterior part of the incision must be deep (at least 1 or 2 cm) to provide adequate caliber for the new introitus. Be aware that the rectum lies beneath this incision, but the areolar tissue must be incised to accommodate the flap. Place traction sutures on the edges of the vagina, and loop them over the tips of clamps on the drapes.

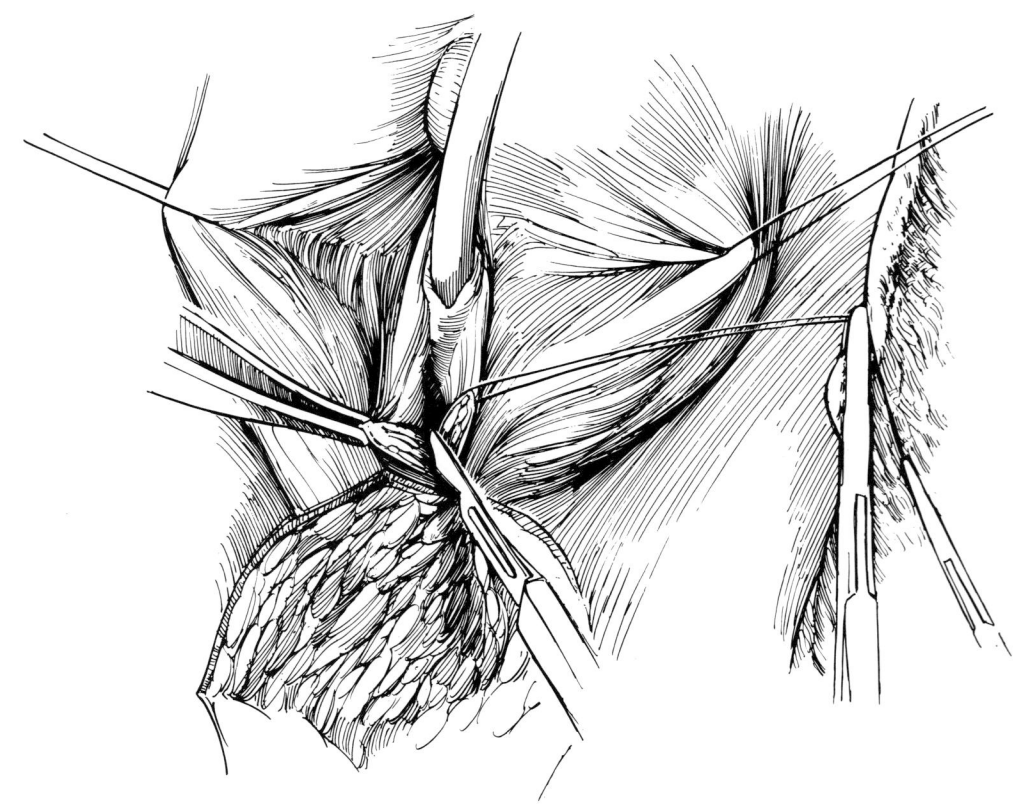

4 Insert the apex of the flap into the V in the vaginal wall. Place subcutaneous sutures for support. Suture the flap with 4-0 chromic catgut sutures beginning at the apex.

Begin dilation of the new introitus in the office in 2 weeks with a metal dilator. The parents can continue the dilations at home until they only need to be done monthly.

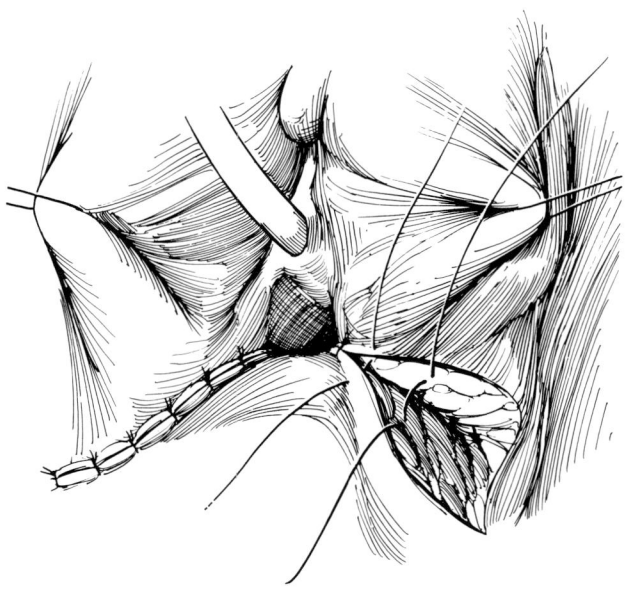

VAGINOPLASTY, MEDIUM ENTRY

5 After forming a posterior flap, incise the posterior wall of the urogenital sinus back far enough to expose the urethral meatus. Suture the edges with 5-0 chromic catgut. Place a finger in the rectum, and dissect the posterior and lateral walls of the vagina. Incise the back wall deeply, and insert the posterior flap. The vagina must be cut back sufficiently to avoid later stenosis, and the flap must be neither too large, producing a shelf, nor too small, resulting in a flat perineum.

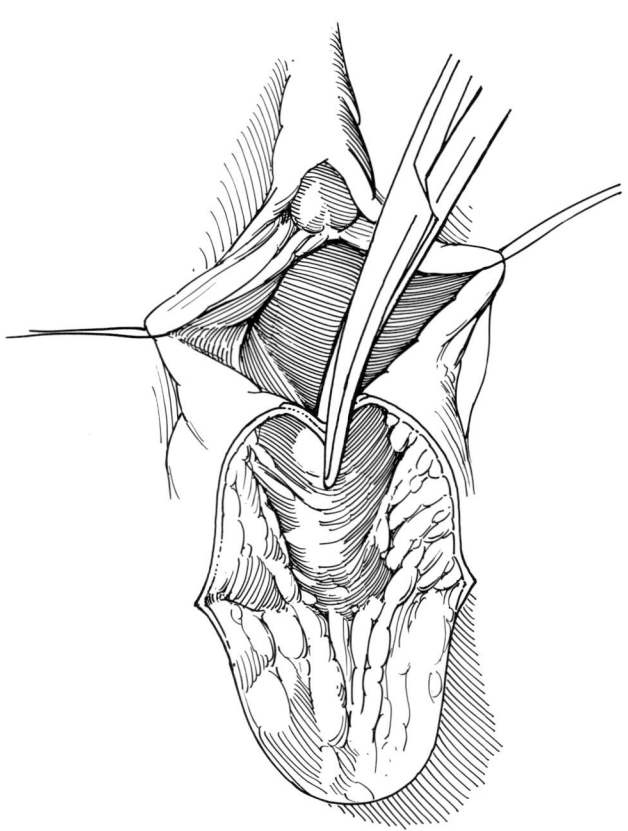

VAGINOPLASTY, HIGH ENTRY
(PULL-THROUGH PROCEDURE [HENDREN])

Wait until the child is between 1 and 2 years of age, when her structures will be larger and the vaginal wall will be thickened.

6 **A,** Perform panendoscopy on the urogenital sinus, and locate the entrance of the vagina and the continuation of the urethra. Place a Fogarty catheter into the vagina. The dashed line shows the limit of the cutback incision, limited at that point to prevent injury to the urethral sphincter. **B,** *Incision:* Make an inverted U-incision in the perineum with the apex opposite the balloon.

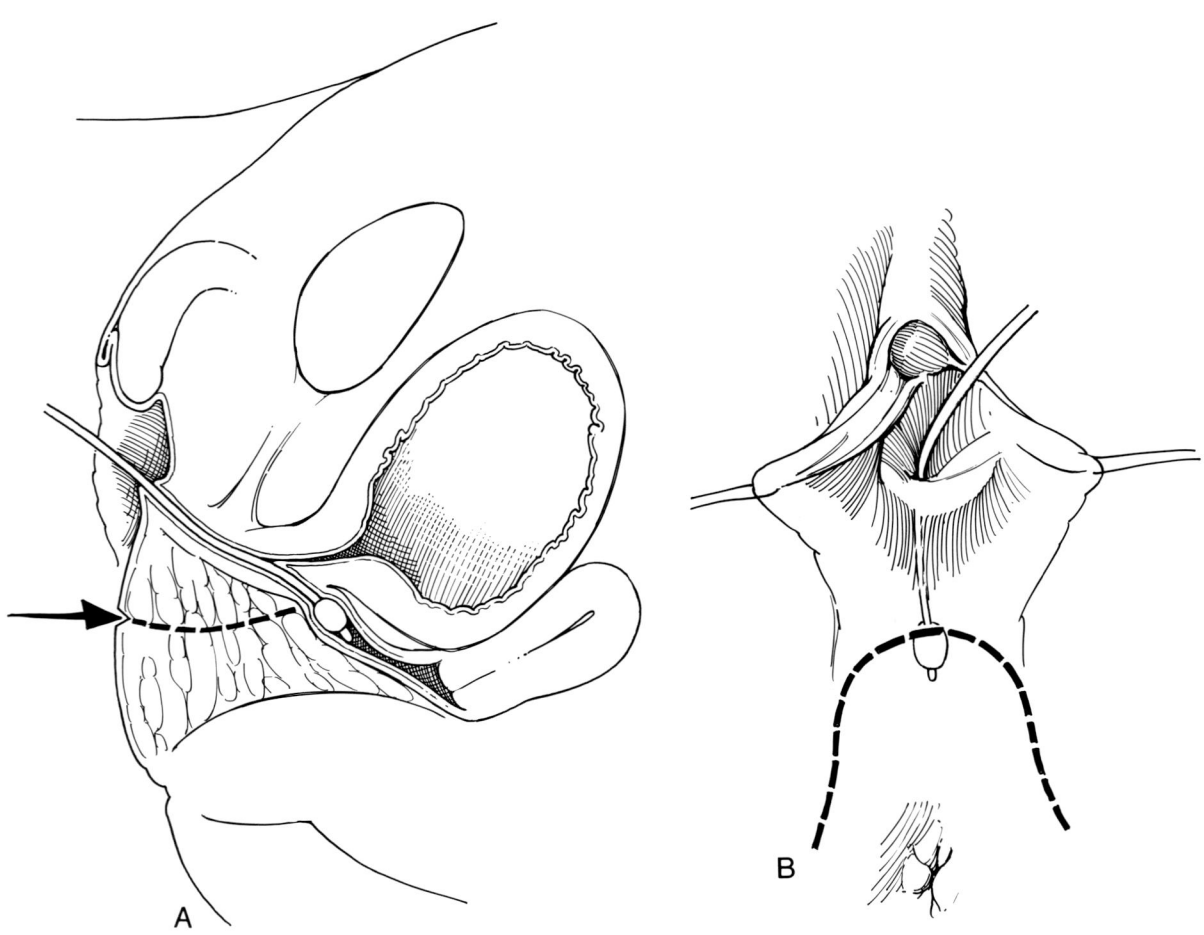

7 Place a finger in the rectum, and dissect against the rectal wall beneath the external urethral sphincter, in a manner similar to the approach in perineal prostatectomy in men. Have the assistant pull on the balloon so that the junction of the vagina with the sinus can be identified. Incise the vagina circumferentially, almost completely about the base of the balloon (dashed line). Withdraw the Fogarty catheter. Insert a straight metal sound into the bladder through the urethra and complete the division of the vaginal rim, leaving a little vaginal tissue on the urethra to allow its closure without stricture.

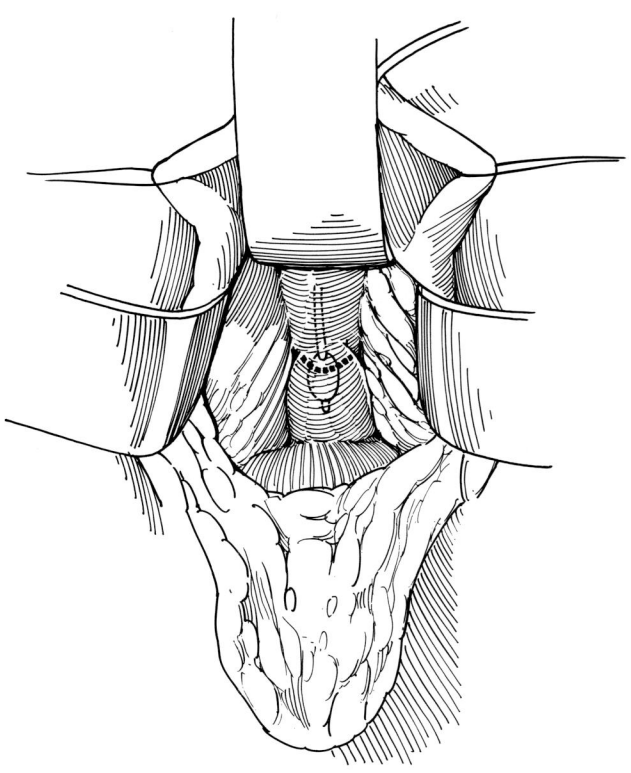

8 Close the urethra transversely with interrupted 6-0 chromic catgut sutures. Replace the sound with a balloon catheter. Dissect the vagina from the proximal urethra as high as the back of the trigone.

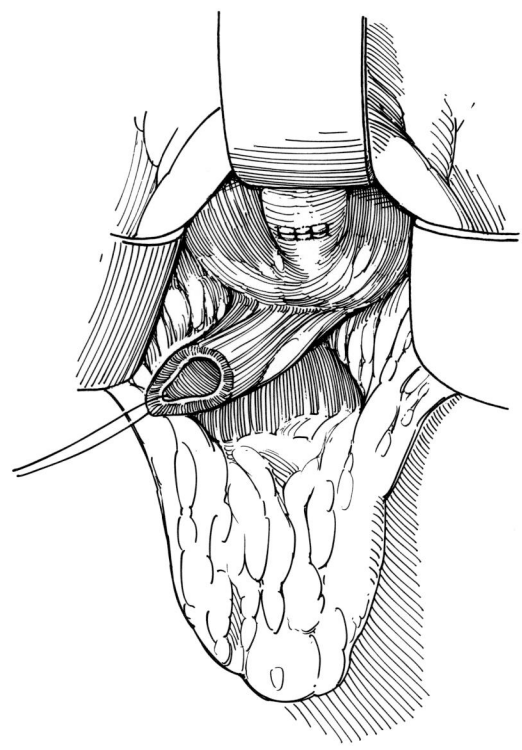

9 Suture the posterior flap into the back wall of the vagina with 5-0 chromic catgut sutures. Incise the perineum anterior to the vagina as an inverted U to form a second flap.

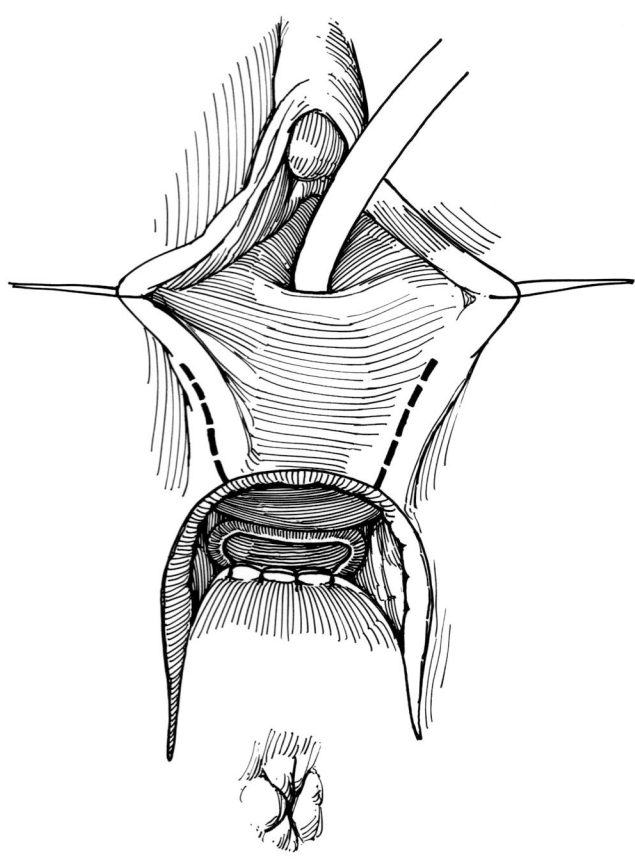

10 Mobilize the anterior skin flap, and suture it to the vaginal rim. Insert a small suction or Penrose drain to exit through a stab wound. Complete the closure by joining the lateral margins of the anterior and the posterior skin flaps to the perineal skin. Place a loose vaginal pack.

Dilate the introitus in 2 weeks; have the parents continue dilations at home. It is necessary that dilations continue until sexual activity begins.

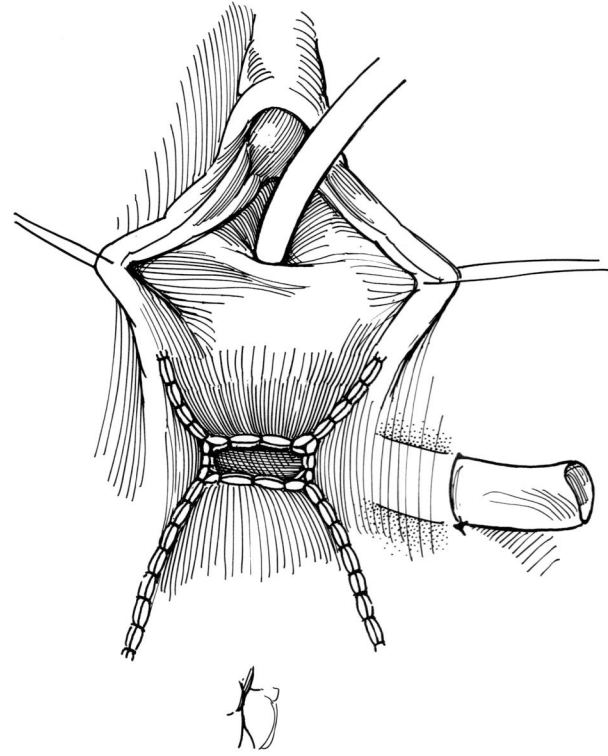

REDUNDANT LABIOSCROTAL SKIN

11 Mark Y-incisions to the base of the clitoris to form V-shaped flaps on either side of the introitus.

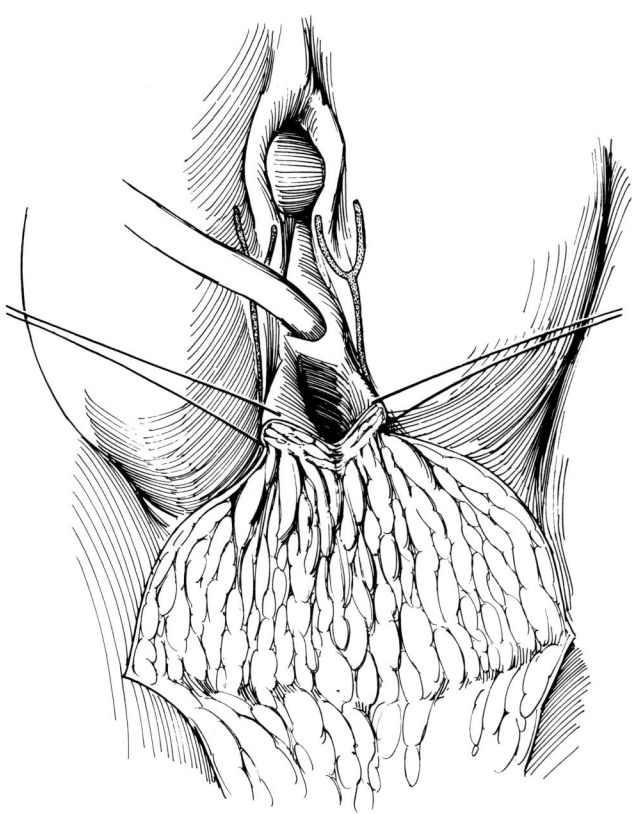

CLITORIPLASTY

13 Place a traction suture in the glans. Mark and make two parallel incisions on the ventrum of the phallus, extending from the edges of the previous vaginoplasty incisions to continue around the dorsum as a circumcision. Insert traction sutures (not shown) at the corners of the flap that is formed as the skin is raised from Buck's fascia.

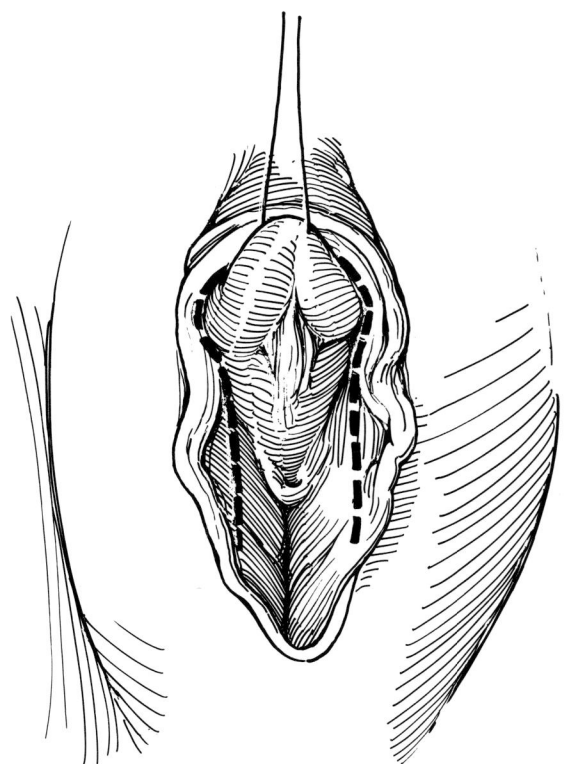

12 Raise the flaps and draw them down to meet the upper end of the vaginal incision. Suture the flaps with 4-0 chromic catgut sutures while placing traction on the lateral vaginal tissue. Approximate the edges of the posterior flap.

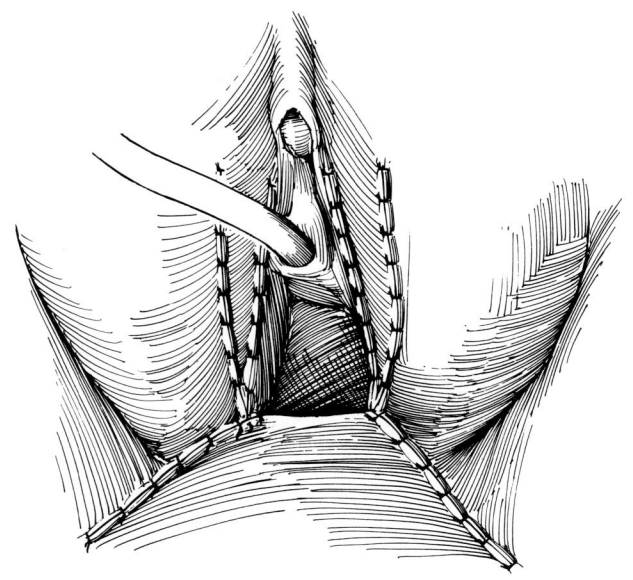

14 **A,** Expose Buck's fascia and the tunica albuginea of the corpora cavernosa. Ventrally, dissect the corporal bodies from the rudimentary corpus spongiosum leaving a ventral skin strip and preserving the subcutaneous connections with the glans. However, if the phallus is severely masculinized, this strip may be too bulky and must be excised. Dorsally, make two parallel incisions on the dorsum of the corpora into the tunica albuginea on either side of the dorsal neurovascular bundle. Elevate the strip of Buck's fascia, including the bundle, by sharp dissection. Continue to dissect the corporal bodies proximally beyond the bifurcation. Divide one crus at a time; as you progressively transect the crus, place and tie a succession of 3-0 synthetic absorbable sutures. Proceed to Figure 15.

B, Alternatively, after the tunical strip has been separated and the corporal bodies have been ligated in the crus, excavate the erectile tissue from each tunic to avoid dissecting the corporal bodies themselves from the bundle (Kogan *et al.*, 1983).

The labia minora will cover the clitoris and frame the urethral meatus if left attached in the midline above to form a hood. The "scrotal" labia majora also frame the introitus, although they tend to be fat and vascular. The resulting clitoris will be pale but may be tattooed later.

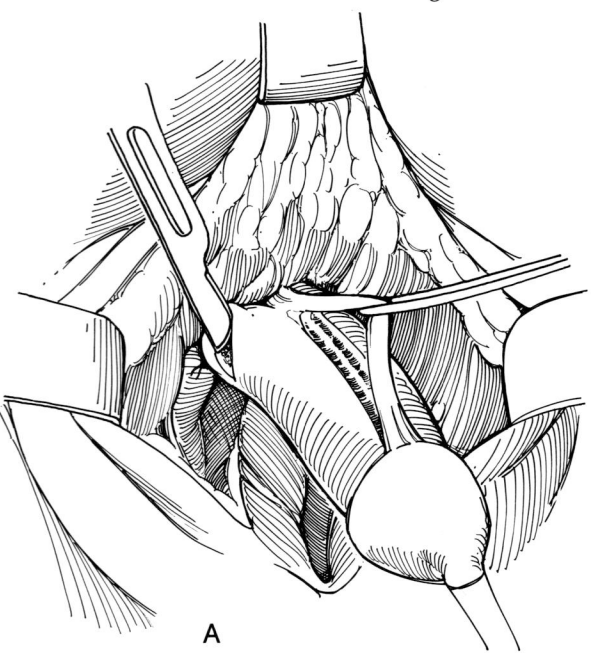

A

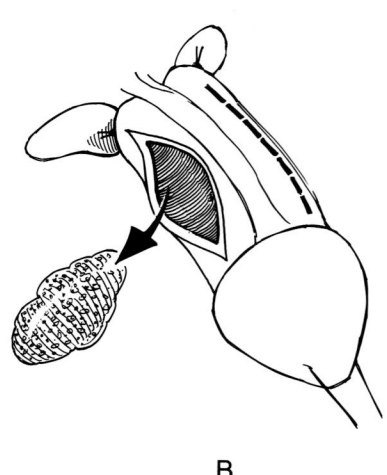

B

15 Divide the corpora at the glans. Trim a broad but superficial wedge (dashed line) from the dorsum of the glans to reduce its bulk. The normal infant clitoris is smaller than one would think. Approximate the glans edges with 4-0 synthetic absorbable sutures. Insert a 4-0 suture into the glans on each side, and pass it through the end of the respective crus to elevate the glans into the proper position.

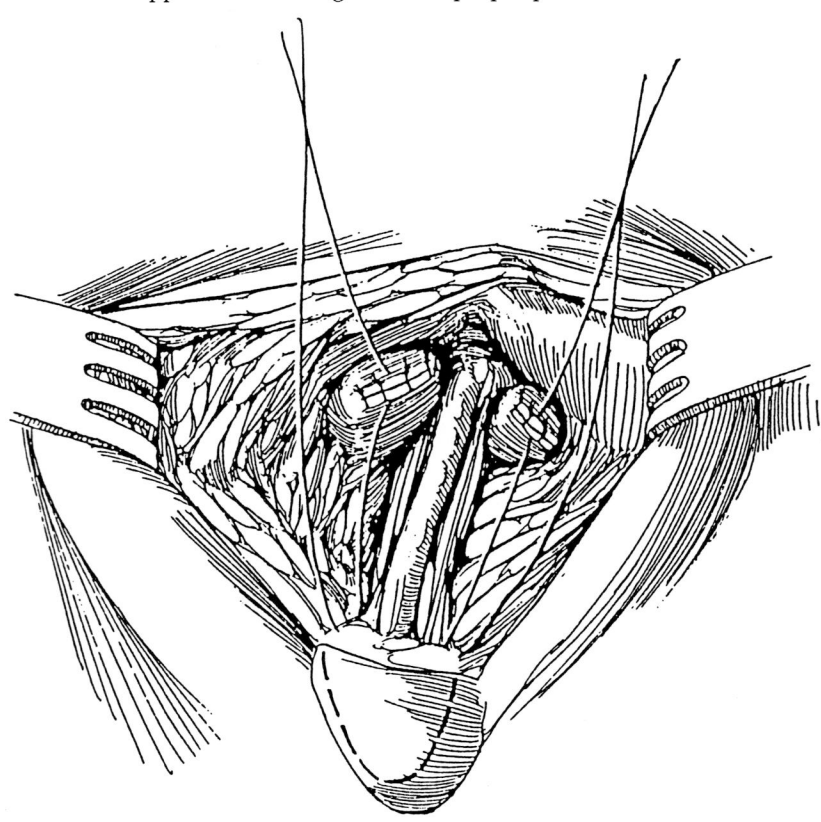

16 Fix the glans to the stumps of the corpora. It may be attached later to the split shaft skin that forms the clitoral hood. Incise the skin of the dorsal shaft in the midline to form two flaps.

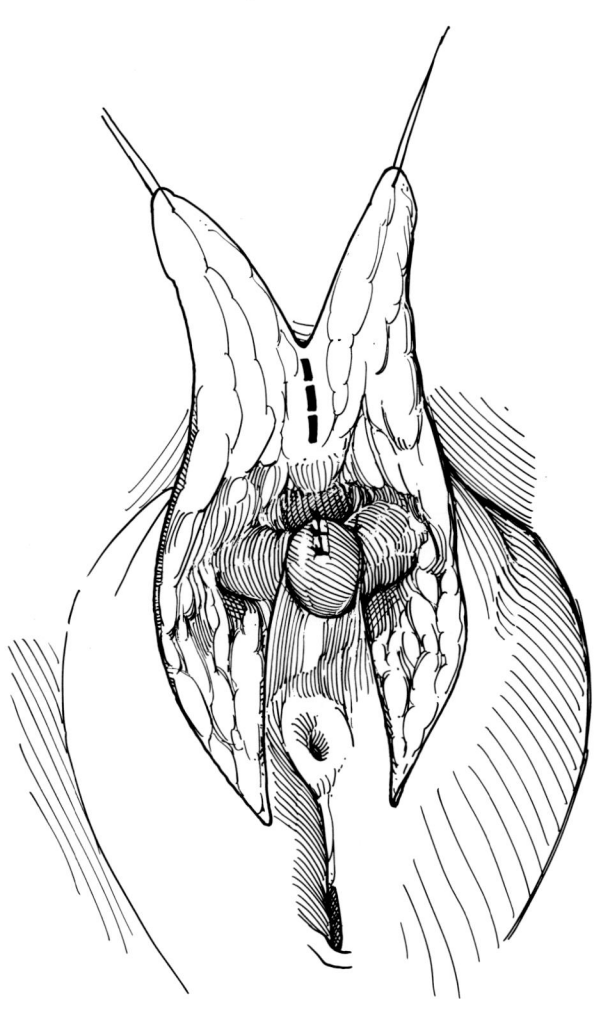

17 Bring the skin flaps down on either side of the ventral skin strip, and suture them with 4-0 chromic catgut sutures. Apply a Telfa dressing with slight compression.

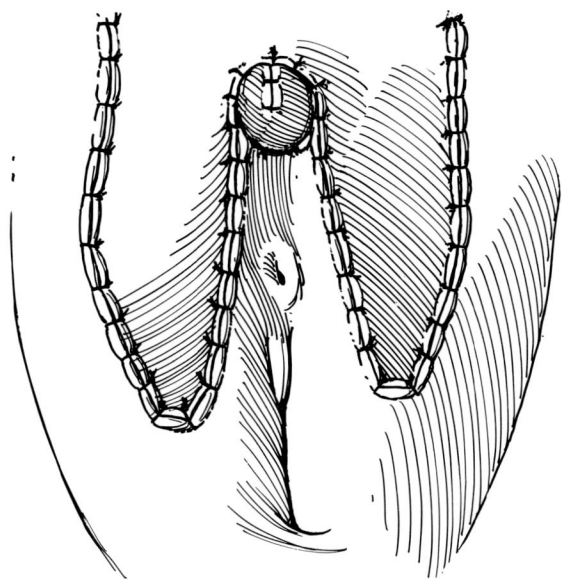

COMBINED CLITORIPLASTY AND VAGINOPLASTY
(PASSERINI-GLAZEL)

18 **A,** Deglove the phallus by making a circumcising incision and retracting the skin as a sleeve. Free the corpora while preserving the dorsal vasculature and neurovascular bundle. Avoid traction on these vessels. Separate the urethral plate and dorsal portion of the urogenital sinus from the corpora. Separate the glans from the corpora, as shown, or trim the corpora distally to leave only a small cap of glans; reduce the glans by removing wedges from either side. Divide and ligate the corpora at the crus. **B,** Tack the remainder of the glans to the corporal stumps.

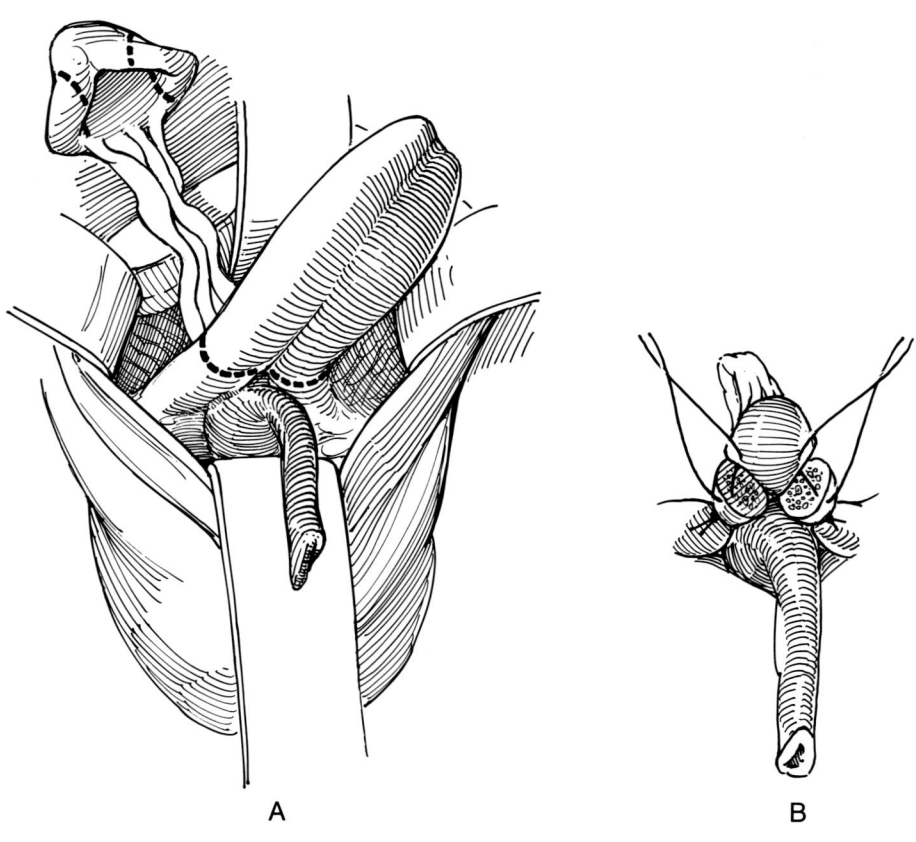

A

B

19 Split the phallic skin tube in the midline dorsally and divide it ventrally as far as the labioscrotal folds.

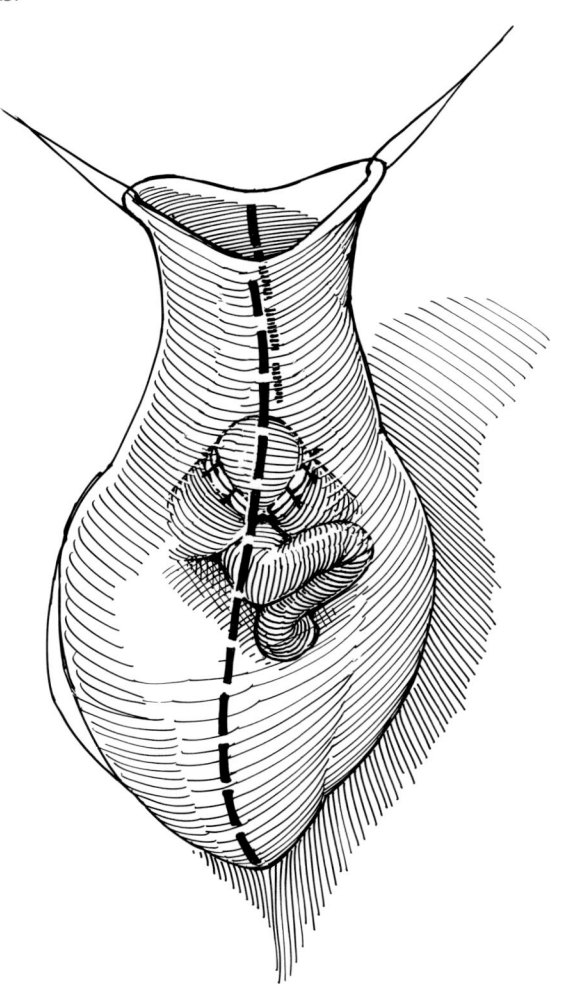

20 Incise the dorsal aspect of the urogenital sinus, and form a Y around the urethral meatus at the base.

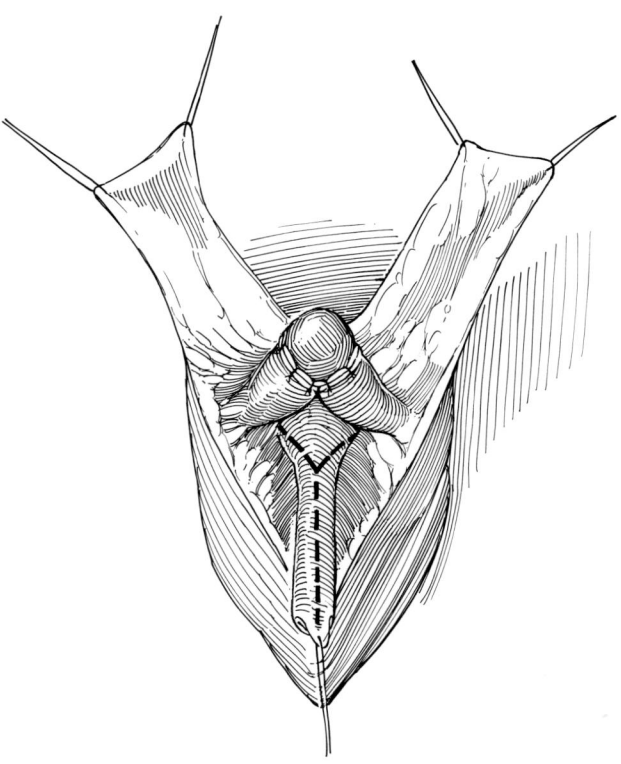

21 A, Open the sinus. Turn the V flap up, and suture it to the base of the clitoris with 5-0 chromic catgut sutures. Rotate the skin flaps from the dorsal shaft. **B,** Suture the medial edges of the flaps to the edges of the opened urogenital sinus.

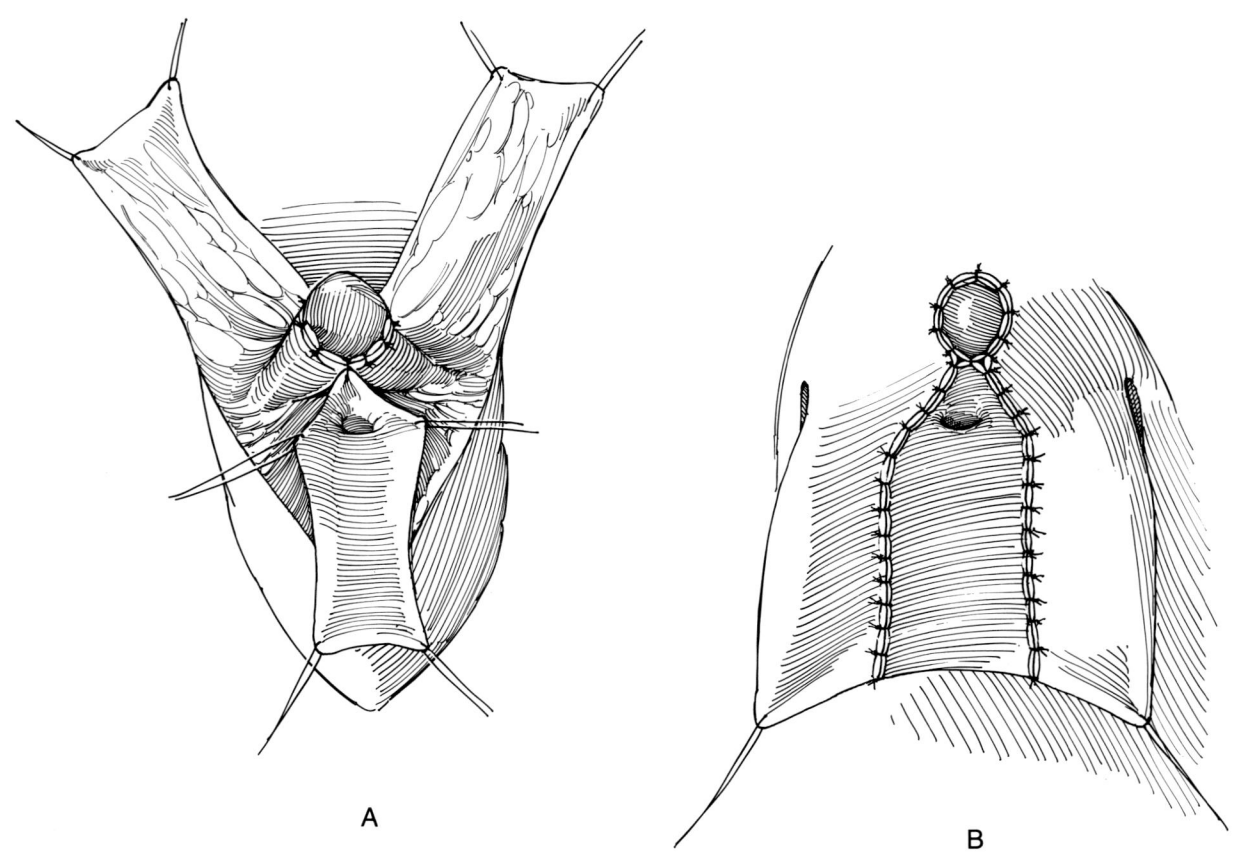

A

B

22 Tubularize the combined phallic flaps and urogenital sinus, and insert the tube into the perineum. Suture the open end to the edge of the mobilized vagina, as shown in Figure 7.

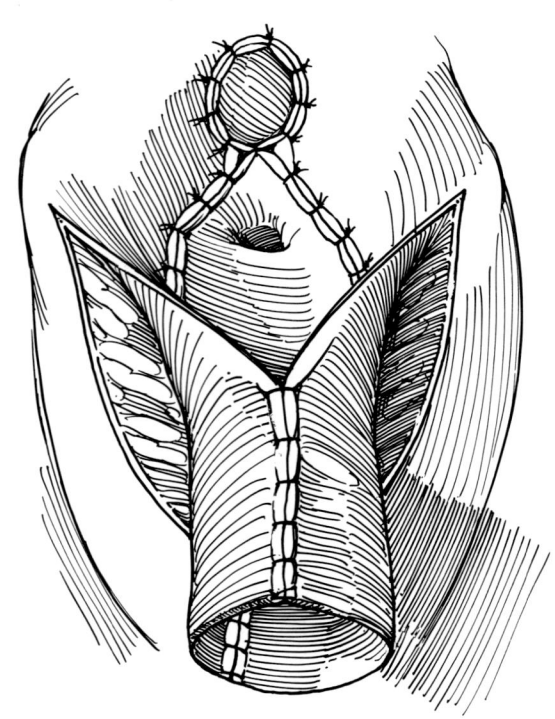

23 For the vagina with a high entry, expose the vagina transtrigonally to accomplish anastomosis of the vagina to the perineal tube (Monfort, 1982).

Insert suction drains and give prophylactic antibiotics. Place a vaginal pack and leave a urethral catheter in place for 10 days.

For the adolescent patient with female gender assignment, an alternative is to tubularize the excess phallic skin remaining ventrally after denudation for clitoriplasty. The tube is rotated and inserted into a space made digitally between the urethra and rectum (Parrott et al., 1980).

For descriptions of vaginal construction alone, see page 649.

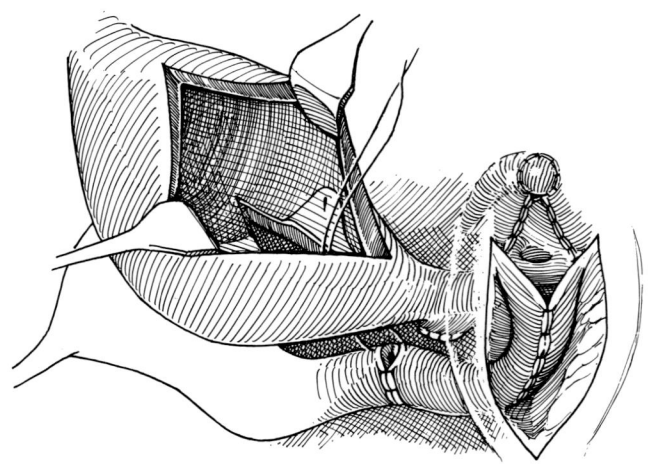

POSTOPERATIVE PROBLEMS

Watch for *adrenal insufficiency* in the period immediately after operation. *Bleeding* can be controlled with pressure.

Commentary by Stanley J. Kogan

The techniques involved with feminizing genital reconstruction have undergone considerable change and refinement. Older techniques of clitoral amputation and minor external skin rearrangement fortunately have given way to much more functionally and cosmetically satisfactory techniques of clitoral reduction and vaginoplasty and labioplasty, sometimes all performed simultaneously. Current techniques now allow for virtually creating a completely normal-appearing female external genitalia.

The goals of feminizing genital reconstruction are to (1) create a normal-appearing sensate clitoris; (2) have an adequately sized and appropriately situated vagina for later female function; and (3) create a normal-appearing female introitus. Subsequent to abandonment of clitoridectomy, clitoral recession under the pubis has been practiced; however, in some girls, painful erections of the restricted shaft occur after puberty, making this a potentially risky choice. Reduction clitoriplasty, in which some of the hypertrophied shaft erectile tissue is excised, while the dorsal neurovascular bundle and glans are preserved, in most circumstances gives a more favorable result. Labioplasty, as described in this chapter, is done simultaneously, making good use of the excess shaft skin left after clitoral reduction to form labia minora. Distal vaginal reconstruction also may be done at the same time, delaying this portion of the repair until 1 or 2 years of age, only in those girls with very high junctions of the vagina and urethra.

A radiologic and endoscopic examination of the urogenital sinus is critical in the initial evaluation, defining the location where the takeoff of the vaginal segment occurs from the urogenital sinus. Documentation of a distal urogenital sinus confluence guarantees that a flap vaginoplasty will be satisfactory and that the posterior perineal flap will be long enough to reach the vaginal segment. If a high confluence is present, the incision in the posterior wall made to lay the posterior flap in may damage the bladder neck sphincter, again indicating the need for precise anatomic delineation.

My current preference in performing this repair is to do the entire clitoriplasty, vaginoplasty, and labioplasty simultaneously, unless there is a high confluence. The incisions for each portion of this procedure "dovetail" nicely and prevent the need to reoperate subsequently in scar tissue from the previous procedure. I begin by mobilizing the clitoris circumferentially, much like what is done in degloving the penile shaft in a chordee correction. The ventral mucosa is not preserved, so the erectile bodies can be widely exposed, extending down the descending pubic rami. I then incise the tunica laterally or inferiorly on each erectile body and sharply dissect out the hypertrophied erectile tissue from within, ligating the stumps. Adequate resection of the erectile tissue is important, because engorgement, swelling, and pain in the residual stumps does occur during puberty. This approach leaves the dorsal neurovascular bundle untouched and preserves completely the glans blood supply and sensation. The glans is then wedged to reduce its size, as indicated in the diagrams, and is attached subsequently to the inferior end of the clitoral hood, newly formed from the superior end of the shaft skin brought together in the midline. Flap vaginoplasty is then performed, taking care to cut back suffi-

ciently to fully exteriorize the vagina. Failure to cut back far enough will lead to vaginal stenosis and the urethra opening on the dorsal wall within the vagina ("female hypospadias"). The flap must be tailored perfectly; a perineal flap that is too short will lead to a flat perineum, and one that is too long may cause a posterior "shelf" to form, sometimes causing trapping of urine within the vagina. The previously mobilized phallic skin is then partially split down the midline to form labia minora and sutured on either side of the urethral meatus. The glans clitoris is sutured to the apex of the split phallic skin, which now simulates a clitoral hood, extending over the glans dorsally. Many textbooks show the glans being fixed to the underside of the pubis at this point in the reconstruction; however, positioning the glans here will bring it far from the vagina, an anatomically incorrect location. A V-Y posterior advancement of the labioscrotal folds on either side of the vagina is then done, completing the repair. These advancement flaps must be undermined significantly; otherwise, retraction may occur, causing separation and scarring at their apices.

When the vagina enters high, the clitoriplasty and labia minoraplasty are done initially, and the vaginoplasty is deferred until the vagina is larger and the vaginal wall is better formed. The labioscrotal tissue is preserved initially for formation of quadrant flaps to be laid in at the time of subsequent high vaginoplasty, because the high detached vagina will not reach down to the perineal surface. When the vagina is detached from the urethra, transverse closure should be done to minimize risk of urethral stricture formation from a longitudinal closure.

A suction drain is helpful, especially if a high dissection is done. The drain should exit away from the labia major advancement flaps and should not be brought out at their posterior apices. A vaginal packing impregnated with petroleum jelly is left for a few days. A urethral catheter is left for 4 or 5 days, and a compression dressing is used over the repair.

Commentary by Giacomo Passerini-Glazel

With time and experience, the original technique has been slightly modified in some details. But before discussing them, I want to stress a major point: the transvesical approach to the vagina is not one of the central aspects of this operation, as many colleagues believe. Indeed, such an approach has been suggested by Gerard Monfort for the prostatic utricle, but it is indicated in very few cases. It is now my experience that almost every case can be treated simply with a perineal approach. Only the most extreme cases, with a very small and thin-walled vagina, require the transtrigonal approach.

Indeed, I presently perform the operation as follows:

1. Before starting the procedure, a Fogarty catheter is inserted into the vagina through a cystoscope and inflated. The cystoscope is then completely retracted to the inflating valve of the Fogarty. The Fogarty emerging from the urogenital sinus is then plicated twice in a Z shape, clamped with a strong Klemme clamp, and cut distally to it to remove the cystoscope. The strong clamp is necessary to avoid progressive leakage from the Fogarty catheter. A Foley catheter also can be inserted into the bladder.

2. The operation is started at the level of the labioscrotal folds. The phallic shaft is left intact at this stage. The incision is represented by an inverted Y, so that the principle of the Fortunoff flap is used to further enlarge the vaginal opening at the vulvar level.

3. The urogenital sinus is approached exactly as is a bulbar urethra.

4. Following the posterior wall, the perineal body is detached, and a wide window is obtained through the fibers of the elevator ani. This wide space represents the major point that avoids later vaginal stenosis by outer constriction.

5. The conjunction between the vagina and urogenital sinus thus appears. In several cases, this junction is not clearly evident, so that the previously inserted Fogarty catheter makes the dissection easier. However, it must be stressed that not infrequently, even by using this trick, the dissection may be difficult. Indeed, the tissue surrounding this junction is dysplastic and fibrotic, and, as stressed by Hardy Hendren, even prostatic remnants may be present. For this reason, a clear cleavage plane between the vagina and the urethra is not present, and the emergence of the vagina from the urogenital sinus may not be evident. If so, my suggestion is to incise the vagina longitudinally on the Fogarty balloon.

6. Once the vagina has been entered from its posterior wall, its separation from the urogenital sinus and urethra is easy and safe. The posterior longitudinal incision even can be extended to obtain a wide vaginal opening and to get away from the narrow and dysplastic distal opening of the vagina. This represents a major point to avoid later vaginal stenosis by intrinsic dysplasia.

7. After suturing the vaginal stump adherent to the urogenital sinus, a wet sponge is inserted into the cavity, and attention is moved to the phallic reduction.

8. The glandular reduction has been modified from the previously described one following the anatomic observations of Juskiewensky. This author found that fibers and vessels entering the glans from the neurovascular bundle proceed first laterally and then converge medially to the tip. Therefore, the two initially suggested lateral excisions on the glans will markedly reduce blood supply, resulting in ischemic atrophy and loss of sensation. For this reason, the glans reduction now is performed by an excision of the central ventral tissue, leaving the two lateral sides of the glans intact. They can then be approximated with few stitches to obtain a conical shape that makes it much more similar to a normal clitoris.

9. To adapt the conically reduced glans to the corporal stumps, the corpora cavernosa must be resected to obtain a cone-shaped tip. Therefore, contrary to what I did initially (M-shaped incision of the corpora 1 cm above their conjunction and above a hemostatic stitch), the corpora are now resected in an inverted V fashion.

10. The dorsal incisions of the urogenital sinus and of the phallic skin and their combination to obtain a wide mucocutaneous plate now have been modified. Unchanged is the suture around the clitoris. Some inner preputial skin is maintained dorsally around the clitoris; this will form a clitoral hood. On the other hand, the cutaneous flaps are maintained as long as possible to have them redundant. Their redundancy later will result in a redundancy at the level of their inversion around the clitoris, thereby forming the minor labia.

11. The split urogenital sinus also is generally redundant. If left untouched, it will result in a redundancy and bulging of the vulvar wall between the urethral and the vaginal openings. Therefore, the distal end of the split urogenital sinus is now incised vertically for approximately 1 cm. The end of this incision is then sutured to the top of the anterior wall of the vagina.

12. Starting from there, the first urogenital sinus, then the distal ends of the inverted phallic skin, and finally the Fortunoff flap that was initially obtained from the labioscrotal folds, are progressively sutured to the vagina. The vagina is therefore connected to the perineum. The splitting of the distal end of the urogenital plate will further enlarge the vaginal anastomosis; this represents another important detail to avoid later vaginal stenosis.

13. Before the labioscrotal folds that will represent the major labia to the lateral side of the inverted phallic skin are sutured, they are partially defatted. If this step is not performed, the final appearance of the major labia will maintain a somewhat-scrotal appearance. The fatty tissue of one side is removed, and that of the opposite side is only partially detached and is interposed between the urogenital sinus and the reconstructed vagina. This will help in getting more distance between the "urethral" and the vaginal opening and avoid the risk of urethrovaginal fistula.

Only if the vagina cannot be detached from the perineum, as in the most severe cases or if the surgeon has not enough experience with a perineal approach so that a transtrigonal detachment of the vagina was performed, the mucocutaneous flap, formed by the urogenital sinus and the phallic skin, is first converted into a tube and then inverted into the perineum to be sutured transtrigonally to the detached vagina. However, an extensive anatomic dissection by detaching the perineal body and by entering the perineum through the fibers of the elevator ani muscle is always advised before making the decision to detach the vagina through the bladder. This step is important, as previously stated, to avoid one of the major causes of vaginal stenosis.

The most important advantages of the operation are (1) the ability to perform the entire correction as a one-stage procedure around the age of 6 months; (2) obtaining a normal-appearing vulvar region; (3) avoiding vaginal stenosis, and therefore the need of vaginal dilations, if all the previously described details are followed (therefore, there are no longer reasons to postpone the vaginoplasty); and (4) avoiding stenosis at the "urethral" meatus, which may occur if the vagina is simply transected.

CHAPTER 131

Vaginal Reconstruction

Several tissues have been used for replacement of the vagina: skin expanded locally, split-thickness skin grafts or flaps, full-thickness skin grafts or flaps after skin expansion, and sections of bowel.

SKIN INLAY
(ABBE-MCINDOE)

Be certain that the patient is well motivated; if possible, have her meet a girl who has had a similar operation. Provide showers and antibacterial soap, a low-residue diet, and a bowel prep. Give perioperative antibiotics.

Instruments: Provide a dermatome with cement, a vaginal conformer (Heyer-Schulte prosthesis), condoms, three narrow Deaver retractors, mineral oil, and liquid thrombin.

Position: Low lithotomy. Prep the lower abdomen, upper legs, and perineum thoroughly, and drape the perineum and one thigh. Insert a 24 F 5-ml balloon catheter in the urethra, and fill the bladder to insert a 24 F Malecot cystostomy tube (page 346). Place traction sutures to hold back the labia.

1 *Incision:* Make an X-shaped incision in the anterior perineum in the mucosal plaque, with the crossing of the X below the urethra to create four symmetrical mucosal-like flaps. This will allow four cutaneous flaps to be infolded into the vaginal canal to reduce circumferential scar contraction.

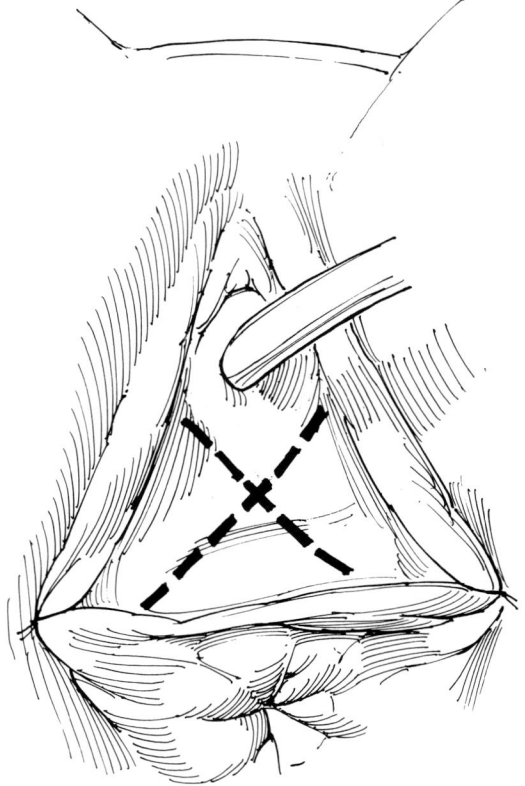

2 Don a second left glove, and place the left index finger in the rectum. Inject the proposed flaps and urethrorectal septum with a solution of 0.5 percent lidocaine (Xylocaine) with 1:2000 dilution of epinephrine to aid dissection and improve hemostasis. With the right index finger and the knife handle, bluntly dissect cephaloposteriorly between the rectum and the urethra on alternating sides of the median raphe to form a tunnel on each side. Divide the now-conspicuous raphe with Metzenbaum scissors, keeping the division closer to the rectum than to the bladder. Identify the anterior rectal wall, so that accidental perforation can be avoided. Take care that the blunt dissection does not force the raphe to perforate the rectum. If that accident does occur, stop the operation, repair the tear, and reoperate several months later. Make the pocket much deeper and wider than needed (in an adult it should be 21 cm deep and 17 cm wide), because it will contract. Pack the pocket with 2-in roller gauze. Turn the patient on her side. Obtain several partial-thickness skin grafts from the upper thigh with the dermatome (page 661). More than one sweep usually is needed. Alternatively, full-thickness grafts may be obtained bilaterally from the groin, lateral to the hair line. These leave less scarring in the donor site than the split-thickness grafts and contract less during healing.

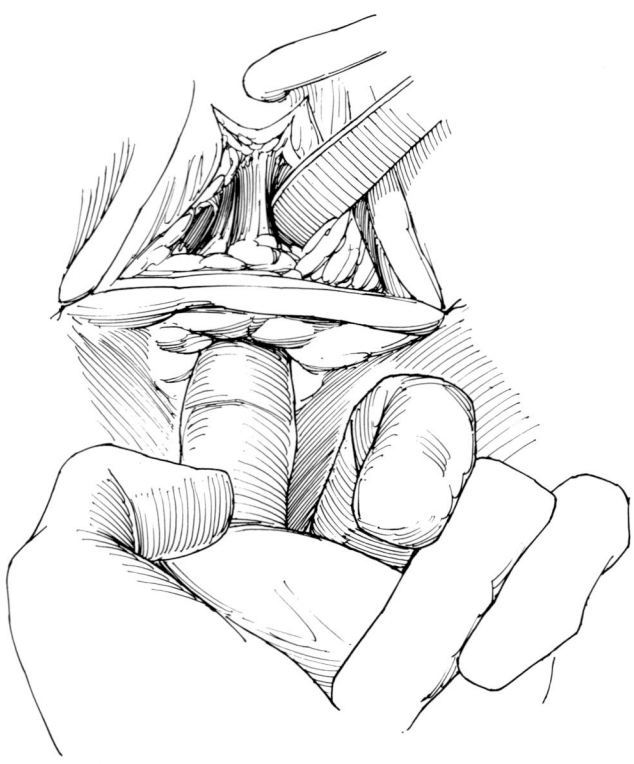

3 A and B, Trim a piece of foam rubber larger in diameter than the proposed stent but of appropriate length. Compress the foam into a cylinder 3 or 4 cm in diameter, and tie it with circular sutures of 3-0 synthetic absorbable suture. Cover the cylinder with two or three condoms preparatory to suturing the graft to it. Alternatively, inflate a commercial vaginal conformer with air and coat it with mineral oil. The advantage of the inflatable conformer is that it may be deflated and removed painlessly, but it may be too short. Another disadvantage is that the patient may decide to remove it and then become lost to follow-up with subsequent failure of the repair. Fit the sheets of skin on the stent or conformer with the raw side out, and suture their edges to each other with running 5-0 synthetic absorbable sutures, placing the knots against the mold.

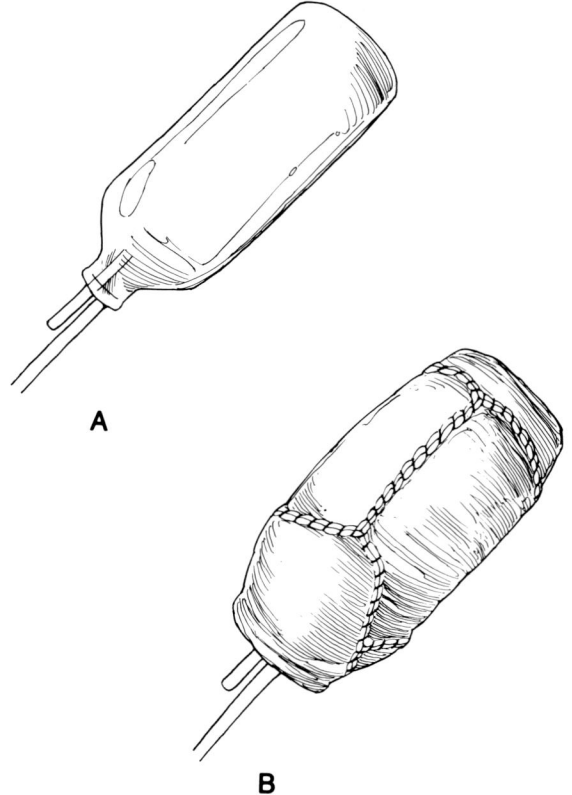

A

B

4 Check hemostasis in the rectourethral defect, then coat the walls with liquid thrombin. Ease the stent covered with the grafts into the canal over three narrow Deaver retractors. Seat it well in the depths. If an inflatable stent is used, partially deflate it while measuring the amount of air withdrawn, so that the air may be accurately replaced after insertion.

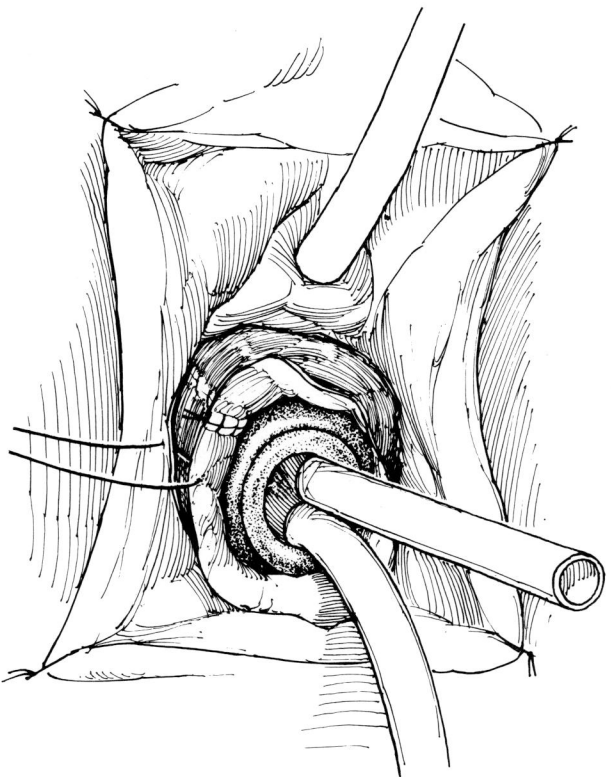

5 Insert the four flaps from the X-shaped skin incision into notches made in the graft, and fasten them with interrupted 4-0 synthetic absorbable sutures to provide a noncircumferential suture line. Put two or three restraining sutures across the vestibule (not across the vulva) to hold the stent in place. Remove the urethral catheter. Place coated gauze and fluffs held with elastic tape to compress the perineum. Postoperatively, order the patient to remain at bed rest. Give stool softeners or mineral oil 30 ml orally, three times a day, on the first postoperative day, then maintain a low-residue diet for several days. Thereafter, have the patient keep the bowel movements loose by taking petroleum agar and stool softeners for 1 or 2 weeks. On the 7th or 8th day, provide sedation, remove the introital sutures, and deflate and gently withdraw the stent. If it hangs up, inject mineral oil around it through a small, soft catheter. Cleanse the perineum. Wash, lubricate, and replace the stent, and hold it in place with a perineal binder. Educate the patient on its regular removal and reinsertion. It must be retained day and night for at least 3 months, then at night for 3 more months, because split-thickness grafts readily contract.

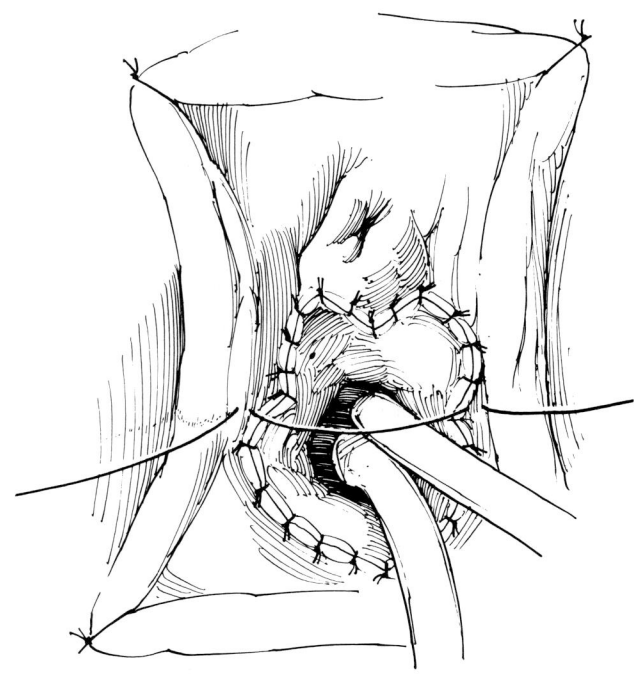

POSTOPERATIVE PROBLEMS

Contraction of the graft is the greatest problem. It usually is caused by poor compliance by the patient in keeping the new vagina dilated. For this reason, careful selection of candidates and persistent long-term follow-up are crucial; in some, the use of bowel would have been a better choice. The vagina may be too short, resulting in dyspareunia. *Necrosis* and sloughing of some of the edge of the graft are usual, but major loss is uncommon. With healthy perineal tissue and good quality skin, *infection* is unusual. Estrogen suppositories may be used to keep the neo-vagina supple.

CECAL VAGINA

Provide bowel preparation and prophylactic antibiotics preoperatively. Insert a nasogastric tube.

Position: Supine, slightly flexed, with the legs widely abducted and the head tilted down. Prep and drape into a single abdominoperineal field.

6 *Abdominal team:* Make a lower abdominal transverse incision and mobilize the posterior wall of the bladder and urethra. Incise the peritoneum along the white line to free the cecum and ascending colon, and continue the release around the hepatic flexure to allow the subsequent anastomosis of ileum to colon. Locate the ileocolic artery by transillumination to determine that the segment will be adequately vascularized and that the ileocolic vascular pedicle will allow the colon to reach the perineum.

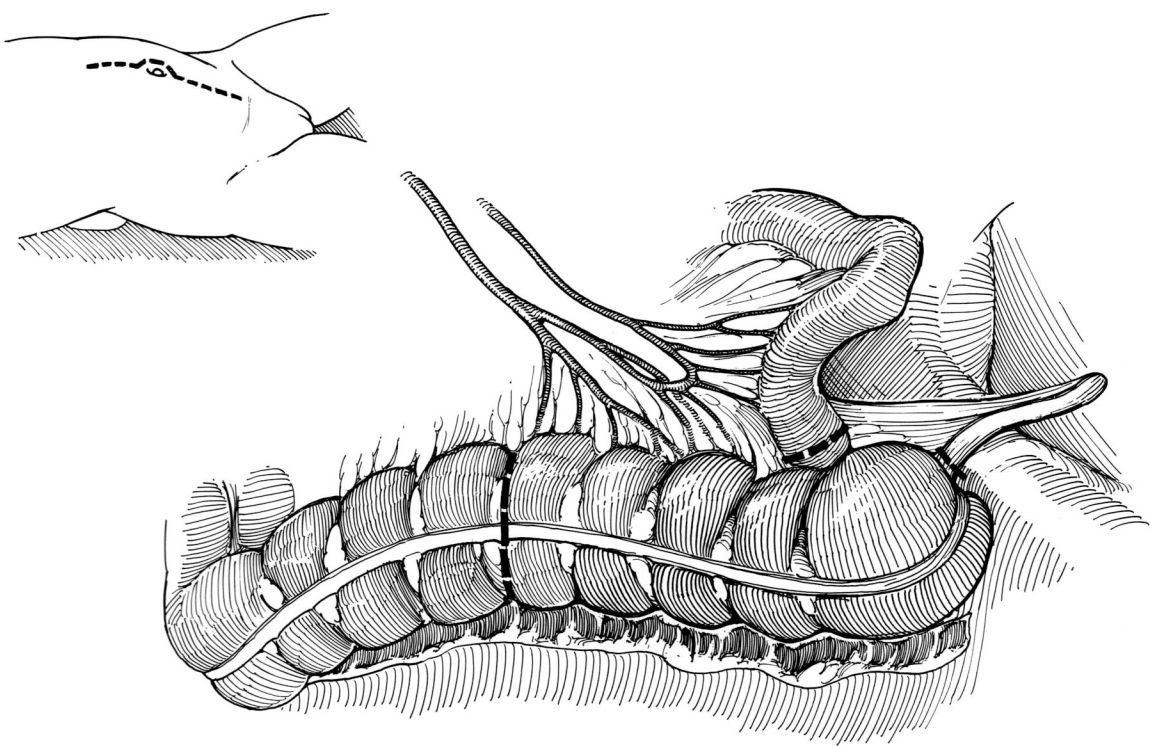

7 Divide the colon and the terminal ileum, spatulate the ileum, and perform an ileocolic anastomosis (page 34) and close the mesentery. Irrigate the segment with saline through a balloon catheter. Perform an appendectomy.

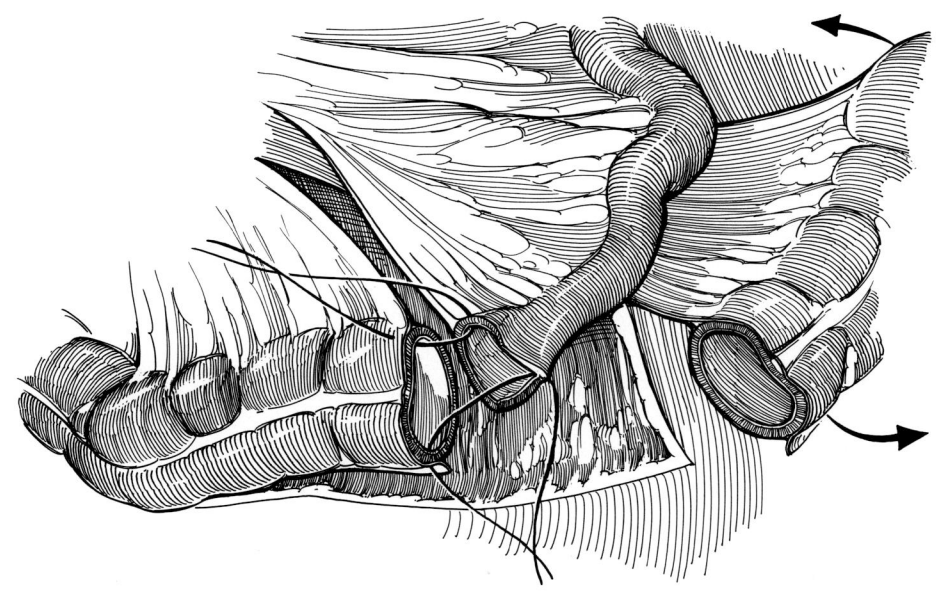

8 A and B, Rotate the cecum 180 degrees counterclockwise. Should the lower part of the new vagina be short or sacculated, incise the antimesenteric border for a distance of several centimeters, and close the mesenteric border for a similar distance. A transverse incision in the peritoneum of the mesentery may allow additional length. Should high insertion of the ileocolic artery prevent inversion and descent, open the cecum and close the colonic end. If the cecum still will not reach, create a cuff from a U-shaped piece of ileum to attach to the colon distally.

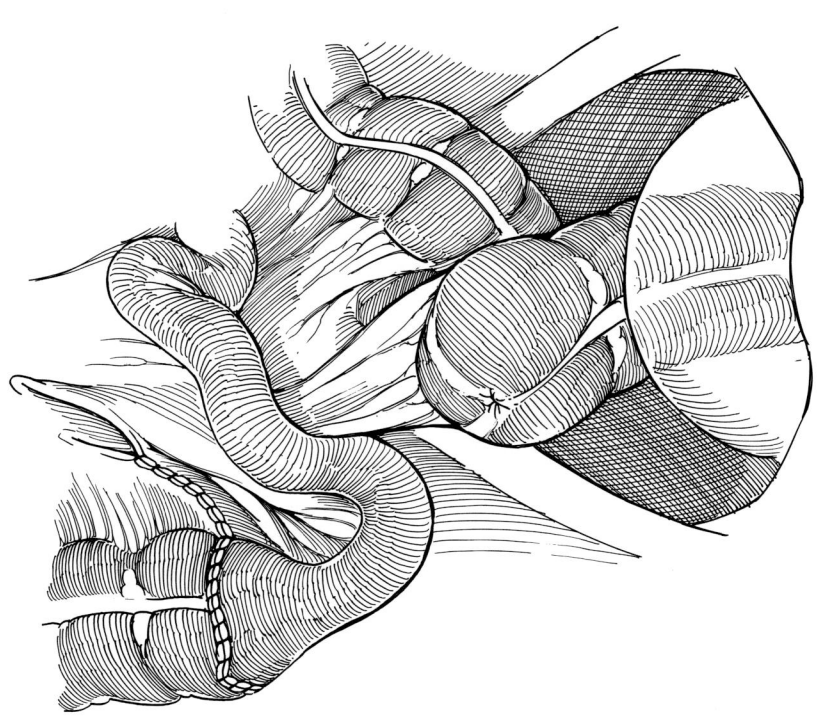

9 A and B, *Perineal team:* Make an H-shaped incision and, with blunt and sharp dissection, create a canal to the level of the vesicorectal pouch. The new canal should accommodate three fingers in the adult. Pull the bowel through the perineal tunnel. In some male pseudohermaphrodites raised as females, the perineum will be flat without an introital appearance, so that more of a perineal based flap will be required.

The *abdominal team* at this time attaches the neovagina to the lateral abdominal wall, inserts a vaginal drain, and closes the abdominal wound.

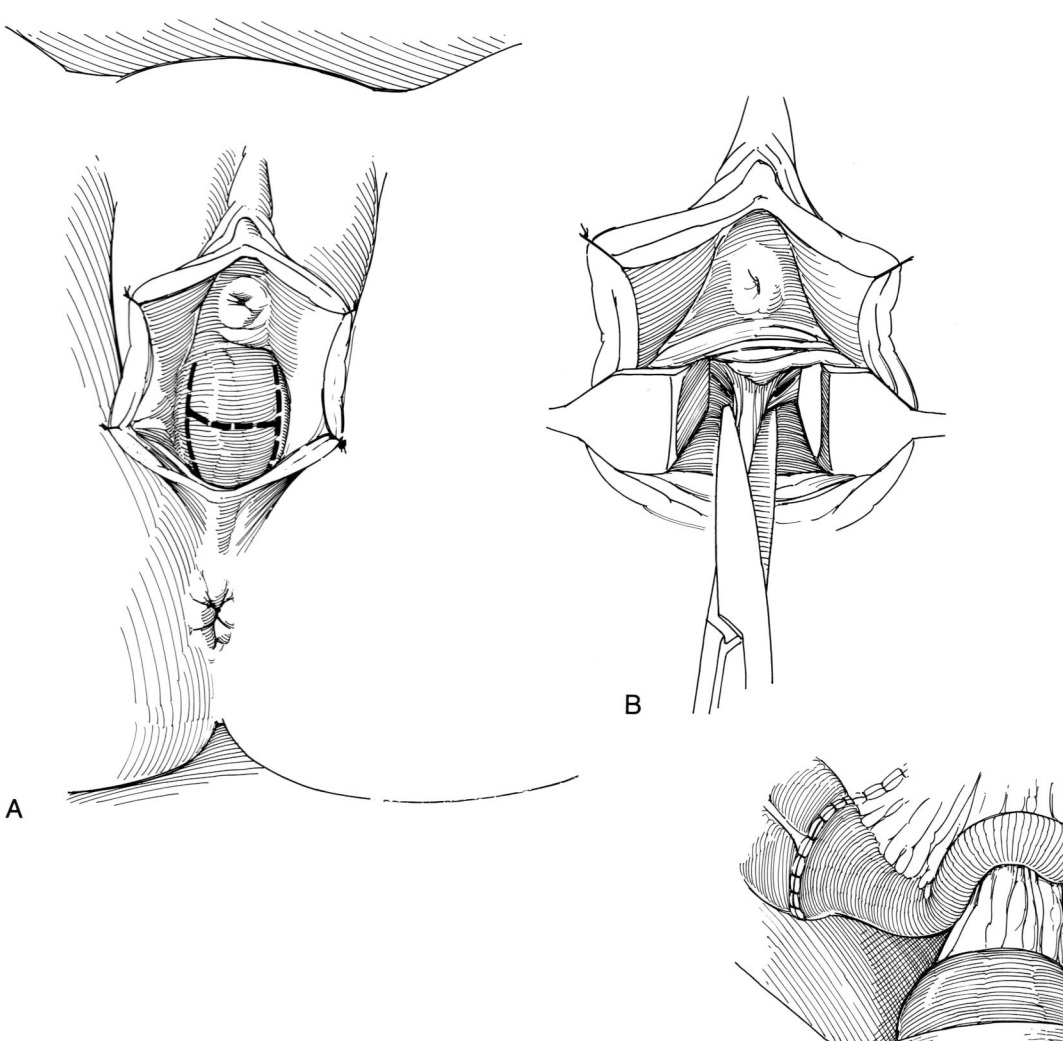

A

B

10 Suture the margin of the colon to the vulva with synthetic absorbable sutures. A vaginal pack is not needed.

Sigmoid Vagina. The sigmoid colon may be a better choice for a vagina than the cecum. Through a transverse lower abdominal incision, take a sigmoid segment between noncrushing clamps on the left colic or superior hemorrhoidal artery, and reanastomose the bowel with staples. Close the proximal end of the segment with two layers of synthetic absorbable sutures, and bring the distal end to the perineum, as described for the cecum (or rotate it 180 degrees, depending on the length of the mesentery). If a portion of the vagina is present, have an assistant push it into the pelvis with a large Hegar dilator for anastomosis. If not, create an adequate space for passage of the bowel, so that its vasculature will not be compromised, and fasten it directly to the perineum. Provide a stent formed from the barrel of a syringe covered with xeroform-impregnated gauze for 5 days. If stenosis is found at 3 weeks, dilate the vagina under anesthesia.

POSTOPERATIVE PROBLEMS

Ileus is avoided by continuing nasogastric suction for 4 or 5 days. Intercourse is proscribed for 6 weeks. *Mucus accumulation* is managed by douching or by simply having the patient open the introitus while in the bath. *Redundancy* of the neovagina is treated by circumferential trimming.

PUDENDAL THIGH FLAP VAGINA
(WEE AND JOSEPH)

11 **A,** This technique depends on blood supply from the posterior labial arteries arising from the perineal artery, but also have anastomoses with the deep external pudendal artery, medial femoral circumflex artery, and the anterior branch of the obturator artery.

B, *Position:* Lithotomy with the legs in stirrups. Insert a balloon catheter in the bladder. Insert a Hegar dilator in the rectum to develop a plane between it and the base of the bladder large enough to accommodate the new vagina. *Incisions:* Mark two slightly curved and tapered flaps on either side of the vulva, centered on the crease of the groin. The base in an adult is 6 cm wide, and the length may be up to 15 cm, placing the tip over the femoral triangle.

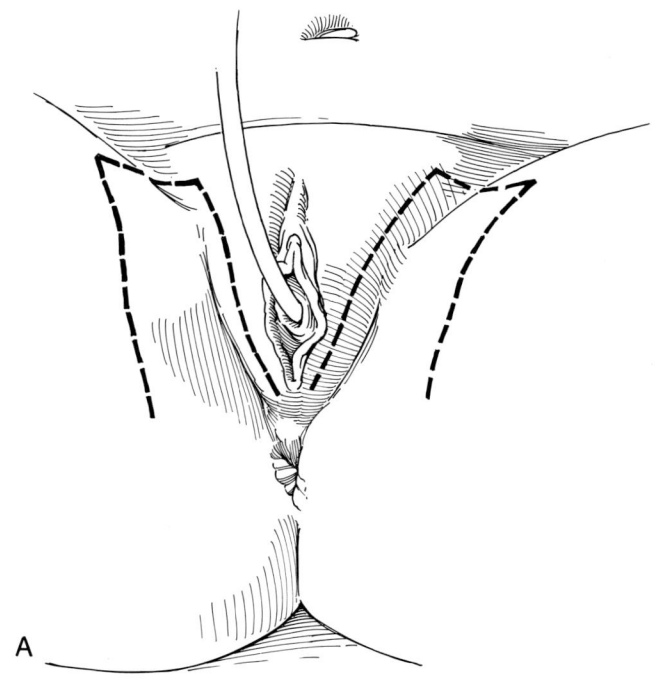

A

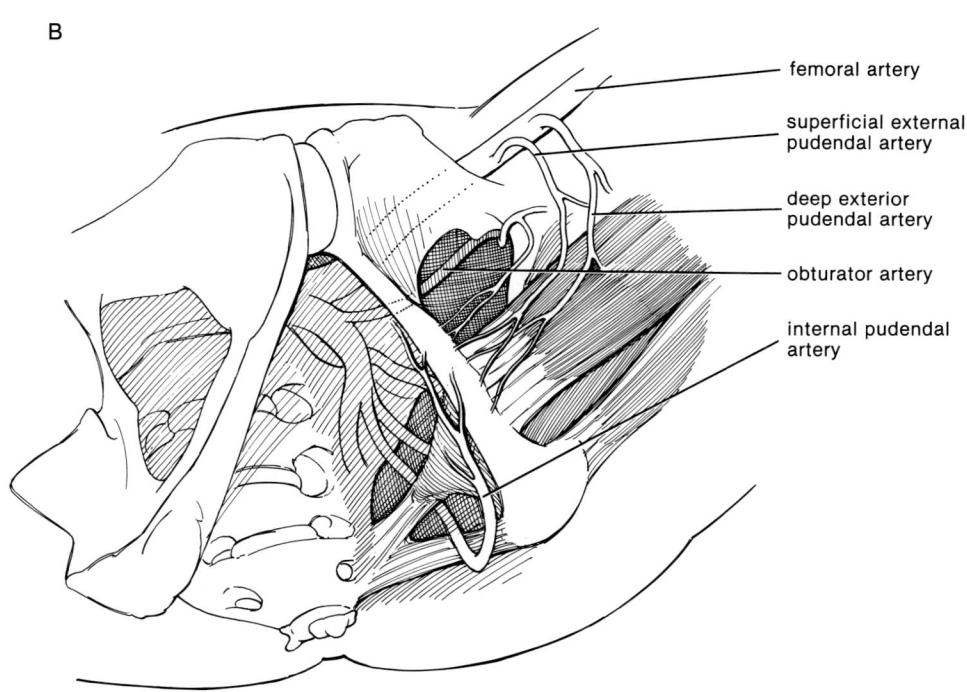

B

femoral artery

superficial external pudendal artery

deep exterior pudendal artery

obturator artery

internal pudendal artery

12 Incise down to the deep fascia, beginning at the end of the flap, and raise it, taking care to include the perimysium of the adductor muscles to avoid damage to the nerves in the flap. At the base of the flap, divide the skin through the dermis to a depth of 1 to 1.5 cm (inset) to allow freedom for the flap to be depressed for passage under the labium.

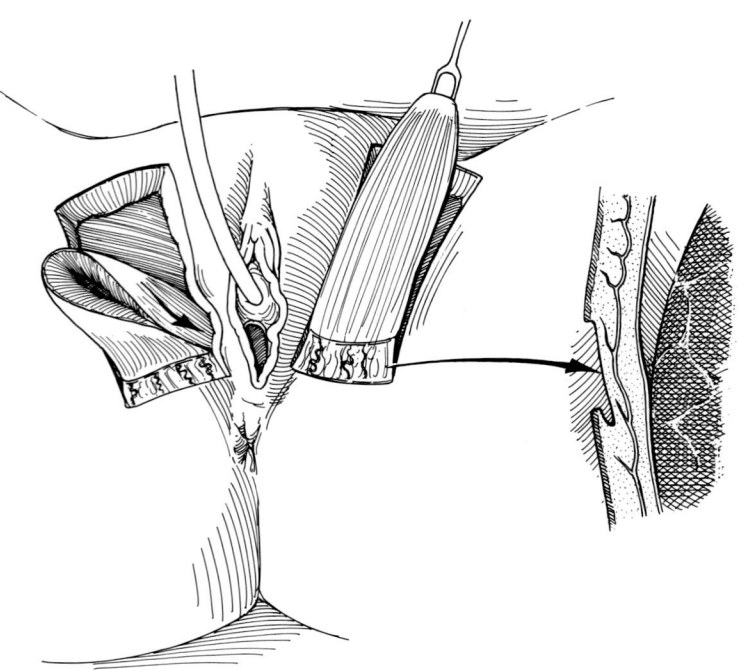

13 Form tunnels under the labia by dissecting them from the pubic ramus. Pass the flaps under labia. With the flaps everted from the introitus, suture the paired flaps together in the midline to close the posterior wall of the new vagina.

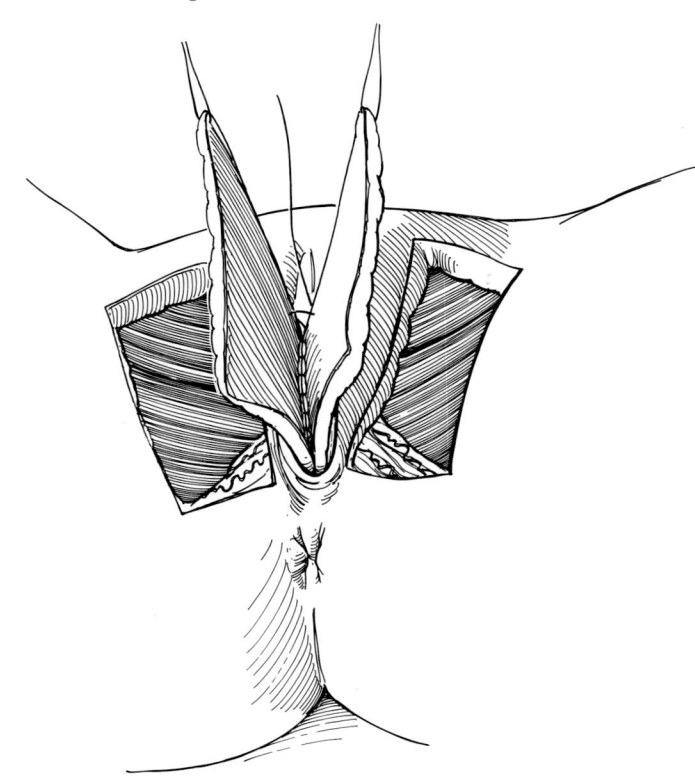

14 At the apex, continue suturing to approximate the anterior wall by bringing the lateral borders together to form the vaginal tube. Invert the tube, and fasten the apex to the posterior bladder wall. Close the lateral defects from the graft site. Place a loose pack over gauze impregnated with petroleum jelly.

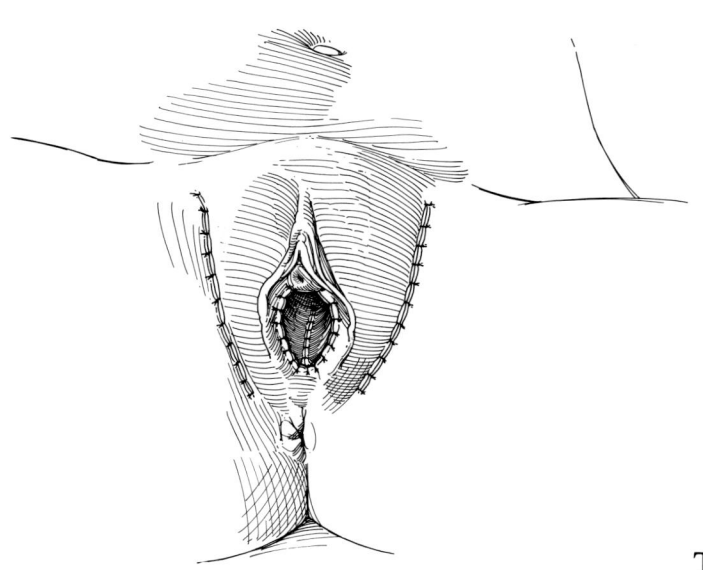

TISSUE-EXPANSION TECHNIQUE (PATIL AND HIXSON)

Make a right inguinal incision, and digitally dissect a pocket in the right labium majus. Select a tissue expander of suitable size; 250 ml is suitable for an adolescent. Insert the tissue expander in the labial pocket, and place the filling port subcutaneously in a (future) hair-bearing area, where it can be felt through the skin. Every 2 weeks add up to 20 ml of normal saline through a 25-gauge needle, the volume being dependent on the tolerance of the girl.

When an adequate size is reached (in approximately 6 weeks), give general anesthesia and proceed to bring the vagina toward the perineum, as described in Figures 130-6 to 130-10.

15 Mark and raise a 7.5-cm by 10-cm flap on the expanded labium with an incision that circumscribes the area of expansion and also crosses the perineum posterior to the introitus. Remove the expander, but preserve the new vascularized sheath that has formed beneath it.

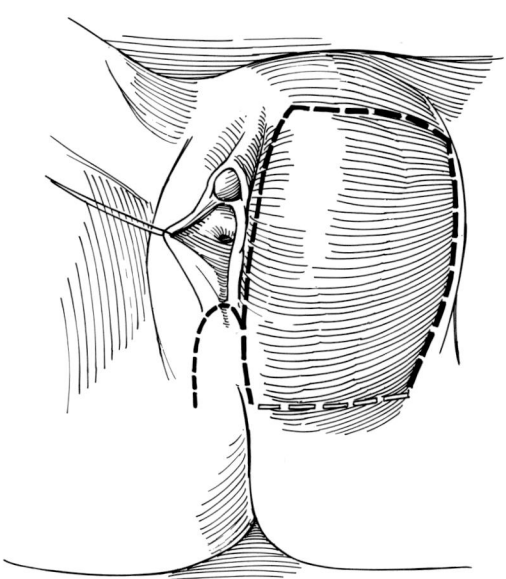

16 Rotate the flap and suture the proximal end to the stump of the vagina with 2-0 synthetic absorbable sutures. Because it will not reach completely around the vaginal opening, leave a 1-cm gap at the junction with the vagina to epithelialize.

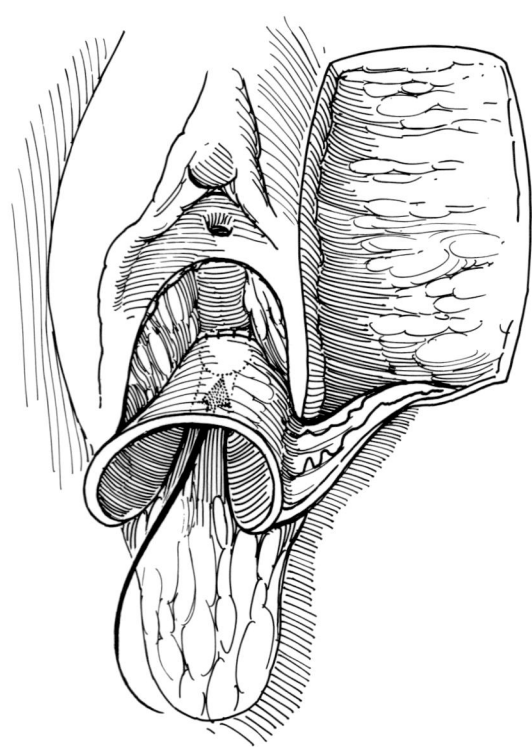

17 Suture the distal end to the skin. Insert the initial posterior perineal flap to fill the outer portion of the posterior gap in the tubed flap. Close the labial defect.

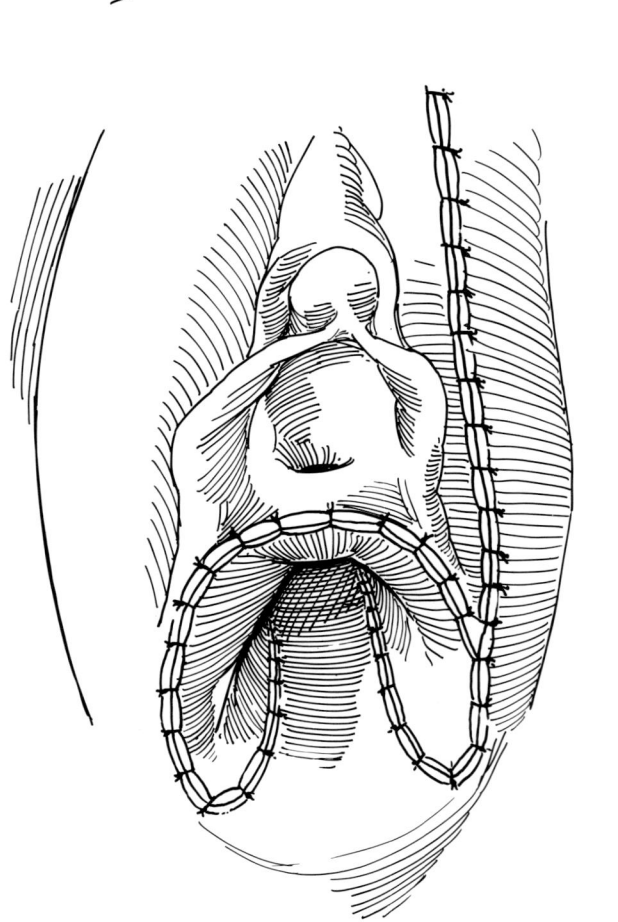

ALTERNATIVE TECHNIQUES

Gracilis myocutaneous flaps may be needed if the vaginal defect is large. Raise a flap on both sides (page 47), and tunnel them under the intact perineal skin to invaginate them into the new vaginal canal. Suture the two flaps as a tube without a conformer, and close the donor sites.

An *ileal segment* can be used in cases of congenital vaginal absence. A total of 15 to 20 cm of ileum is opened, folded once, and sutured into a tube, leaving a V-shaped slot to accommodate the inverted V-shaped perineal flap after the segment is tunneled into the perineum. This alternative may be less acceptable to the fastidious patient because of soiling from mucus. A *pressure technique* (Ingram) is used by some experts with well-motivated patients. Pressure is applied to the perineum 2 hours a day by a bicycle seat stool that holds a plastic dilator. This technique can indent enough skin to form a functional vagina.

Commentary by John P. Gearhart

The subjects treated in this chapter usually are male pseudohermaphrodites who are being raised as females or females with müllerian duct anomalies requiring vaginal construction. Should there by any associated anomalies, they will have been corrected before vaginal constructions is done. Certainly, none of the procedures described in this chapter should be undertaken until full growth of the patient has been obtained. For practical purposes, this typically means in the later teen years.

Skin Inlay, Abbe-McIndoe Procedure. It is important initially to make a cruciate incision on the perineum, so that the plane between the urethra and the anterior rectal wall can be entered and dissected without injury to either of these structures. I have had only limited experience with the procedure but have been involved in revision of a number of them. Reoperation was needed for correction of three problems: (1) the four perineal flaps were not made large enough to avoid contracture of the introitus; (2) the graft was brought too far distally in the perineum, so that it did not appear as a mucosal opening; and (3) the entire graft contracted. As mentioned in the text, contracture of the graft usually is caused by poor compliance by the patient in keeping the vagina dilated by not using dilators regularly or by infrequent intercourse. Male pseudohermaphrodites, I have found, do better long term using estrogen suppositories on a regular basis, because this seems to keep the graft and introitus supple and aids in preventing contracture.

Cecal Vagina. Although Turner-Warwick and others have recommended the use of cecum to create a neovagina, I have found that it may be difficult to rotate the cecum downward enough to reach the perineal flaps. I prefer the modified Wagner-Baldwin technique using the sigmoid colon, because it usually is redundant and close to the operative field. When the sigmoid colon is used, I typically bring the omentum down to cover the colonic anastomosis and to separate the anastomosis from the superior suture line of the sigmoid vagina. Whether cecum or sigmoid is used, the difficulties typically lie at the introitus. Although Figure 9 shows an H-type incision, with the labia majora and minora present, many male pseudohermaphrodites raised as females have a very flat perineum without an introitus. Here, both a large perineally based flap and a flap based cephalad will be necessary to suitably exteriorize the neovagina. A vaginal pack of iodoform gauze impregnated with vaseline for 2 days postoperatively has proved worthwhile. Although the anastomosis between perineum and the bowel-vagina usually is quite capacious, care must be taken in the postoperative months to make sure that stenosis does not occur.

Pudendal Thigh Flap Vagina. Although I have not had personal experience with this procedure, I am a bit concerned about the postoperative appearance of the junction between the upper thigh and the perineal area. This is a large mass of tissue that is being removed. I would have to see the postoperative pictures before I would be convinced that it is superior to bowel interposition.

Tissue-Expander Technique. Although I have no had personal experience with this use of tissue expanders, I find it most intriguing. Certainly tissue expanders have made an impact in reconstructive urology in boys with failed hypospadias repairs and in those with epispadias-exstrophy. It is truly amazing what a few weeks of tissue expansion will do to increase the availability of local skin. I think the wide-based perineal flap shown in Figure 15 certainly will aid in preventing stenosis of the neovaginal orifice, and I believe the amount of redundant tissue that is present will allow tension-free closure of the ipsilateral labia majora area.

Summary. Although all of the techniques described certainly are helpful in creating a neovagina, application will be dictated by the surgeon's ability and experience. Hensle has reported excellent results using colonic segments in male pseudophermaphrodites raised as females and those with vaginal agenesis. My results mirror those of Hensle, and I feel that a bowel segment is the best substitute for a vagina and that the sigmoid colon segment is superior to the cecal segment, because the larger diameter of the colon permits anastomosis of the distal end of the straight segment to the perineum, thus requiring less mobilization of the mesentery than with the cecal procedure. Lastly, the colon segment offers the following advantages over the other techniques described, all of which require mobilization of large amounts of skin in the perineal area: (1) the procedure is technically simpler, (2) there is no uncertainty of "take" of the graft, (3) molds are not required to maintain patency, (4) colonic mucosa is more resistant to trauma, (5) adequate spontaneous lubrication is present for sexual intercourse without excessive mucous discharge created by small bowel, and finally (6) most pediatric urologists are quite familiar with using bowel segments for reconstructive procedures and thus have basic familiarity with the technique.

Repair of Penile and Testicular Injuries

AVULSION OR BURN INJURY OF PENIS AND SCROTUM

1 *Avulsion injuries:* Repair the defect at once, at least within 8 to 12 hours. Remove distal skin remnants from the penis, because they will have lost their venous drainage and so will be subject to prolonged edema. Cleanse the denuded area thoroughly with saline. Remove foreign bodies and hematomas. Achieve hemostasis; bleeding usually is minimal after this type of injury.

Burn injuries: Remove all the skin from the shaft distal to the injury to avoid subsequent lymphedema. Do it at once before infection can set in. It is not necessary to wait for separation of the eschar to see how much skin remains, because the small amount of skin saved in that way is easily made up by a graft.

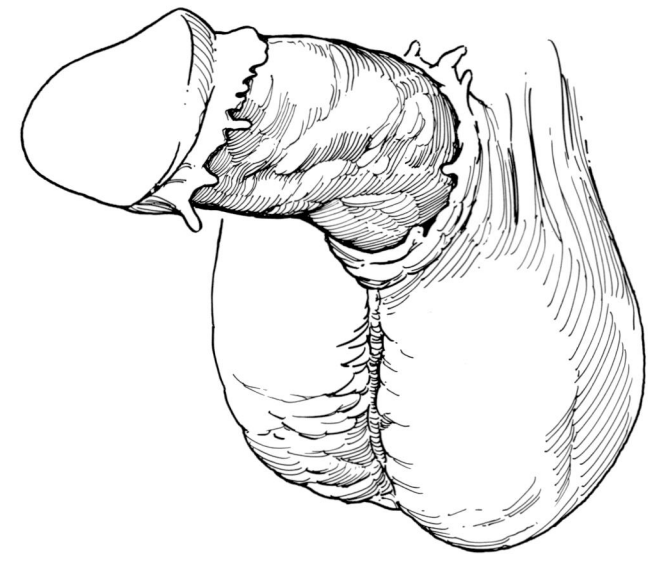

2 Tack both the coronal and the proximal skin edges to the shaft with 4-0 synthetic absorbable sutures placed subcutaneously. Wait for formation of a well-vascularized bed.

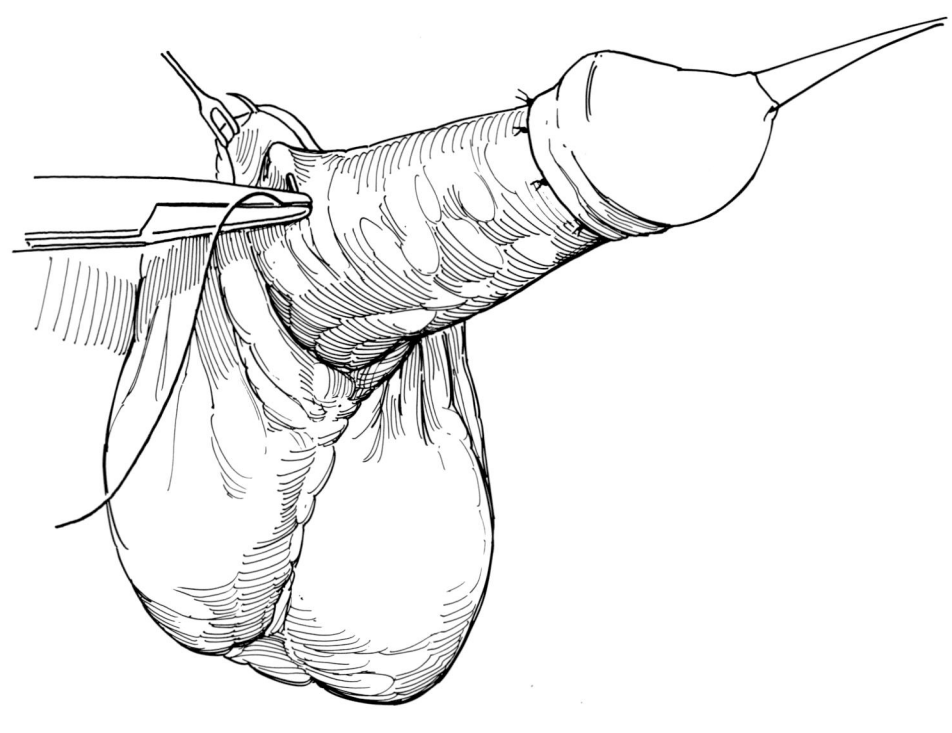

3 With an electric dermatome, obtain a medium-thickness split-skin graft from the lower abdomen or the inner or outer aspect of the thigh from areas of least hair, after cleaning and oiling the skin. For extensive grafting, especially for the scrotum, convert the skin into a mesh with a meshing device on the operating table. Such a graft will contract more but will permit easy escape of exudate. However, it is not suitable for the penis in boys. For primary grafting, make the graft 0.020 to 0.024 in thick; for grafting after the bed has been infected, raise a thinner graft, 0.012 to 0.016 in.

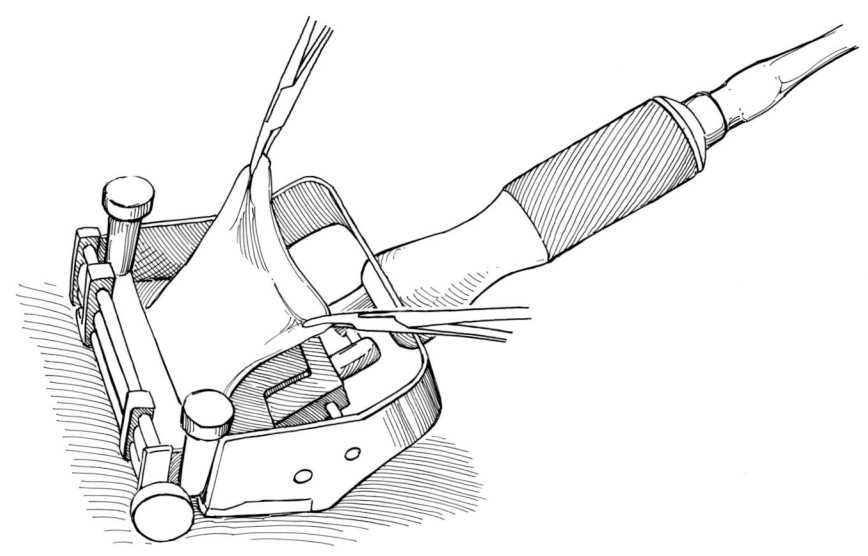

4 **A,** Wrap the graft around the shaft, placing the suture line ventrally to mimic the raphe. Trim the edges of the graft to form a long Z, and close the residual defect with a running 5-0 synthetic absorbable suture. Bank the excess skin. Insert a balloon catheter of suitable size.

B, Incising the skin vertically in two or three places will lengthen the suture line and reduce the risk of chordee (Z-plasty). Suture the skin to the corona and to the edge of the scrotal skin with interrupted 4-0 chromic catgut sutures. Suture the graft proximally and distally with 4-0 synthetic absorbable sutures. Leave these sutures long.

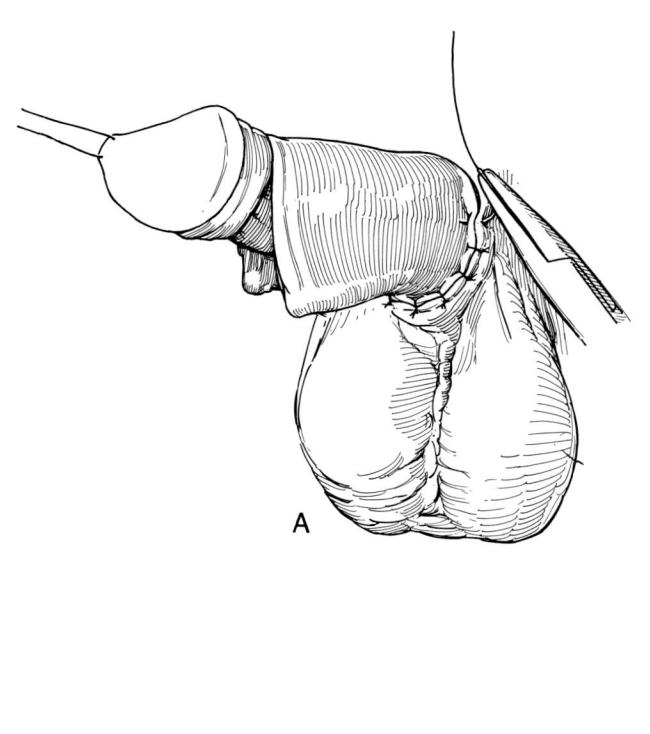

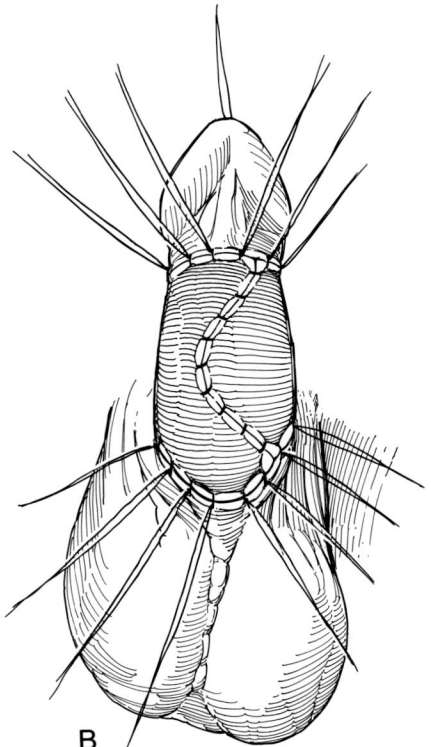

5 Apply cotton wool impregnated with glycerin around the penis, and anchor it by tying the sets of long sutures together. The graft must be immobilized. Cover with gauze and elastic adhesive tape. Apply tincture of benzoin, and fix the tape to the pubic skin.

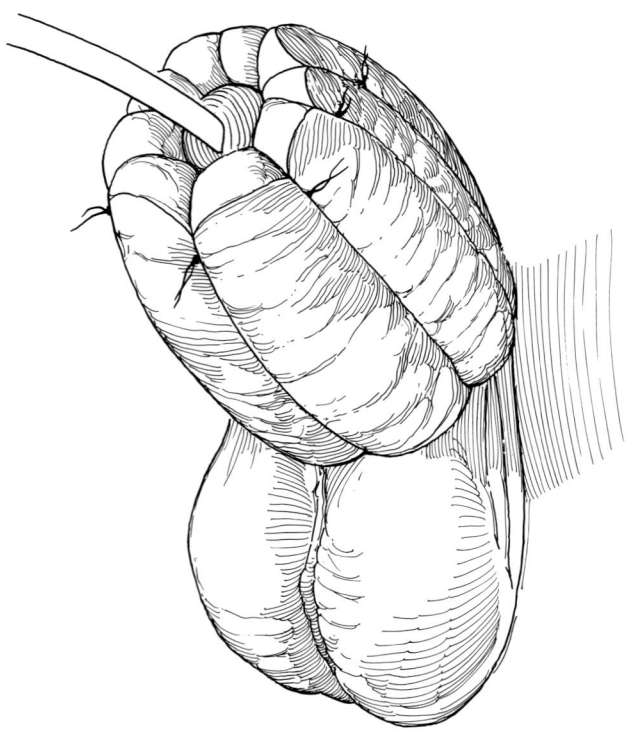

6 A and B, Suspend the penis inside a section removed from a plastic bottle that has been cut appropriately and padded with adhesive foam padding.

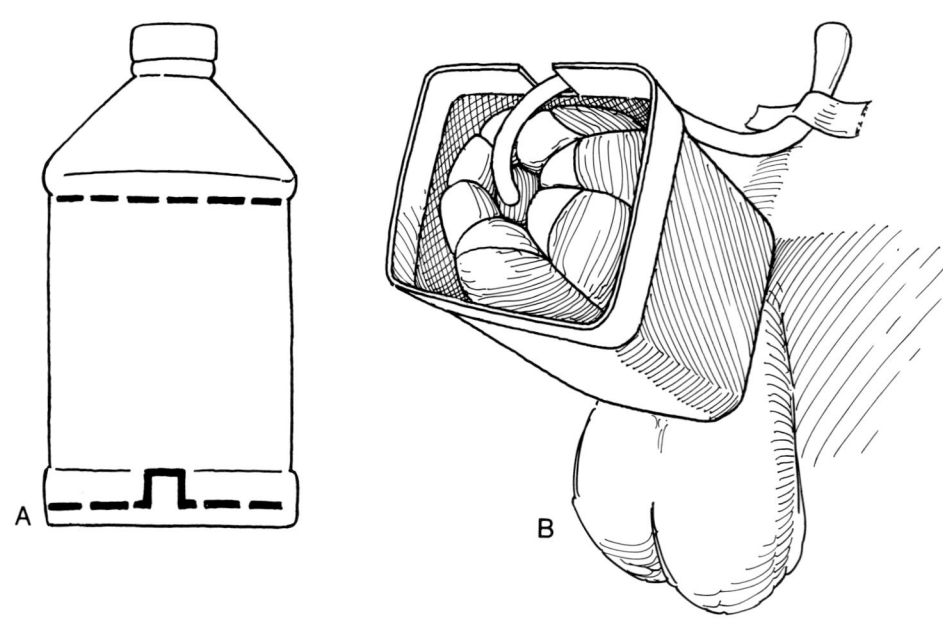

RUPTURE OF TESTIS

7 **A,** Debride as little as possible. Close the tunica albuginea with a running 4-0 chromic catgut stitch; do not cinch it too tight. **B,** Place a small Penrose drain to exit through a stab wound, and close the scrotum in layers.

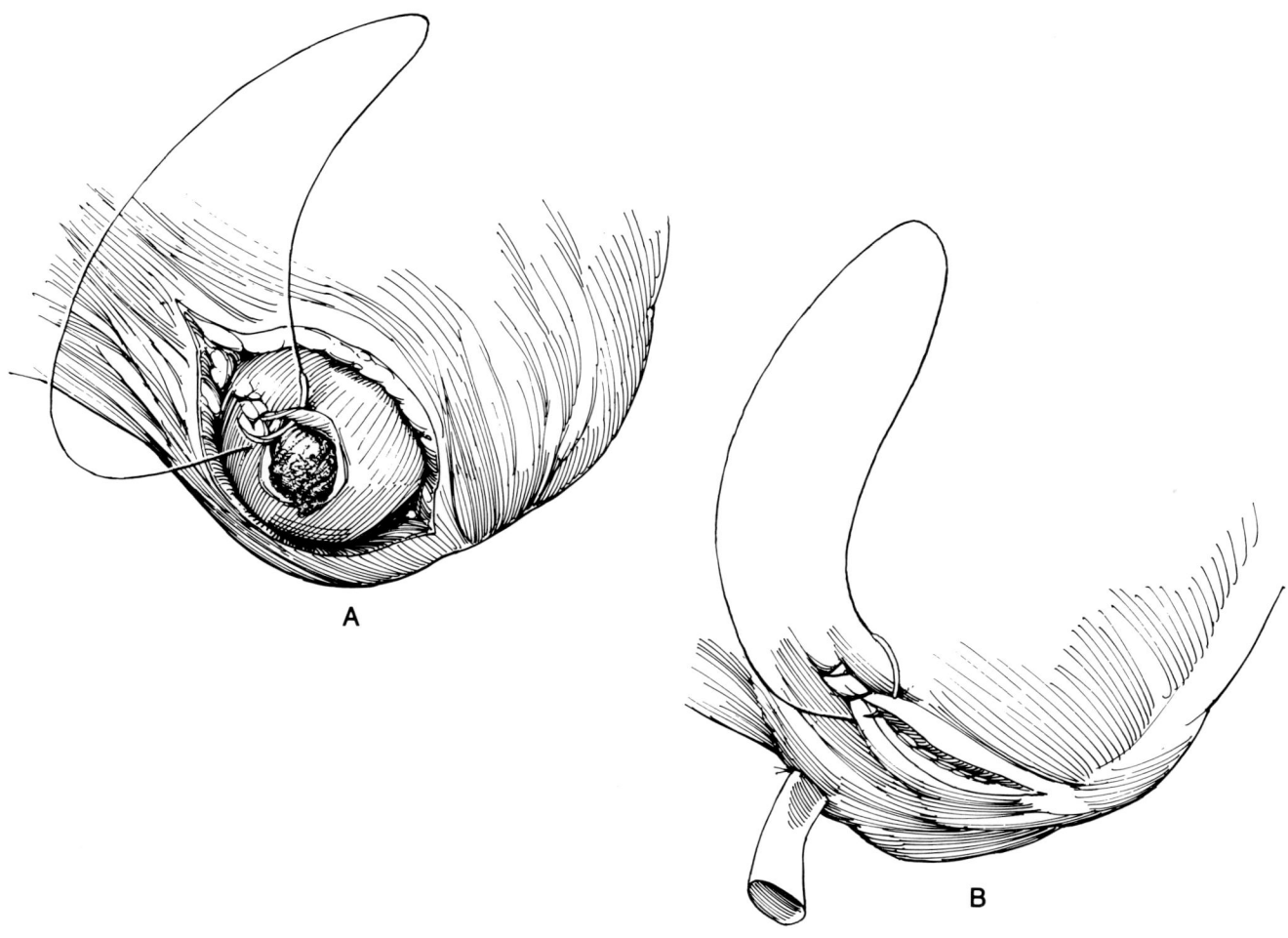

Commentary by David C. S. Gough

An avulsion injury is rare, and when I have seen it in children, it has been related to a pedestrian being crushed by a motor vehicle.

In children, the length of the penile skin tube out of which the penis has been avulsed is relatively short, and its vascularity, in my experience, is not compromised; therefore, reconstruction can take place with debrided local tissue. Other injuries in the area, to the pelvis in particular, usually make it necessary for the bladder to be drained by a balloon catheter with a gauge of 8 or 10 F.

Where there has been a loss of scrotal tissue, which is exceptionally rare in children, I would not disagree with the subcutaneous burying of the testicle, should the whole scrotum be missing. The size of the testicle and scrotum in small children has been a factor in my experience, and we have never had to do such a procedure, relying on local tissue and careful debridement for reconstruction.

Suture material for repair is not critical, and lately we have used 6-0 or 7-0 polydioxanone suture. Broad-spectrum antibiotic cover and closed-suction wound drainage has been used when significant dead space is likely to be encountered.

Rupture of the testis occurs in childhood usually secondary to kicks. Immediate exploration, débridement, suture repair of the tunica albuginea, and careful haemostasis with bipolar diathermy usually allows control to such an extent that drainage is not required.

CHAPTER 133

Construction of Penis

(CHANG AND HWANG)

Organize two surgical teams, one to prepare the forearm skin flap, and the other to cover the donor site with a skin graft from the thigh, prepare the recipient site, mobilize the inguinal recipient vessels, and insert a suprapubic cystostomy.

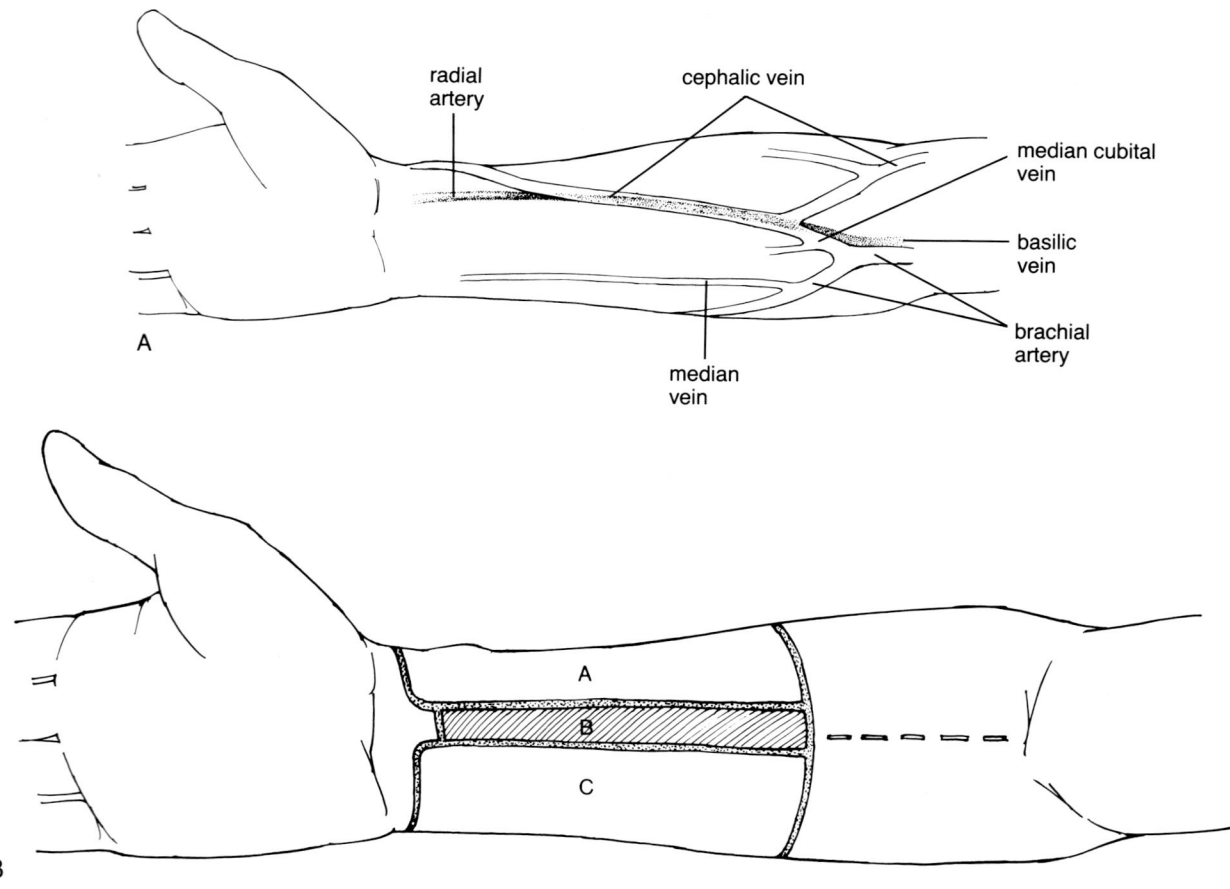

1 **A,** Make certain that the dominant blood supply to the hand is from the radial artery. If it is from the ulnar artery, adapt the procedure by forming the large flap (Section A in Figures 1B and 1C) medially. Place the boy in the frog-legged position. Prep one arm, the lower abdomen, and the genital area. Study the position of the pertinent vessels on the forearm.

B, *First team:* Outline a skin flap on the radial side of the forearm 11 to 12 cm long and 14 to 15 cm wide, the size dependent on the size of the boy. Mark it as a larger section on the radial side (Section A) from which to construct the penis; a 1-cm strip, de-epithelialized to increase the area of tissue contact for the prosthesis (Section B); and a smaller section on the ulnar side 3.5 to 4 cm in width (Section C), which will become the new urethra. A tongue of skin 1 cm in length is provided on sections A and B to shape the glans.

C, The flap as it appears after removal.

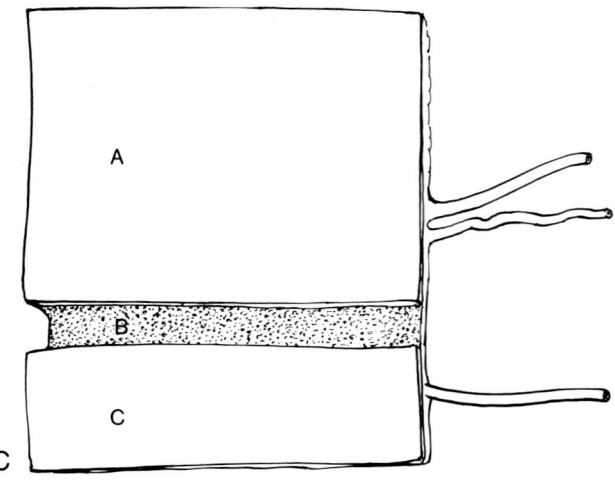

2 Press the blood from the forearm with an Esmarch bandage and apply and inflate a sterile tourniquet. Raise a full-thickness flap beginning distally, taking with it the subcutaneous tissue down to, but not including, the epitenon over the distal forearm tendons and the six or seven arteriolar branches of the distal third of the radial artery, as well as the venae comitantes. The vascular pedicle will contain the radial artery and its venae comitantes, cephalic vein, and another forearm vein and should be at least 10 cm in length proximal to the flap. It also will contain the medial and lateral antibrachial cutaneous nerves. Release the tourniquet and secure hemostasis. De-epithelialize the center Section B. Roll the narrow Section C into a tube around a 16 F silicone balloon catheter, and suture it in place with two layers of interrupted 3-0 synthetic absorbable sutures.

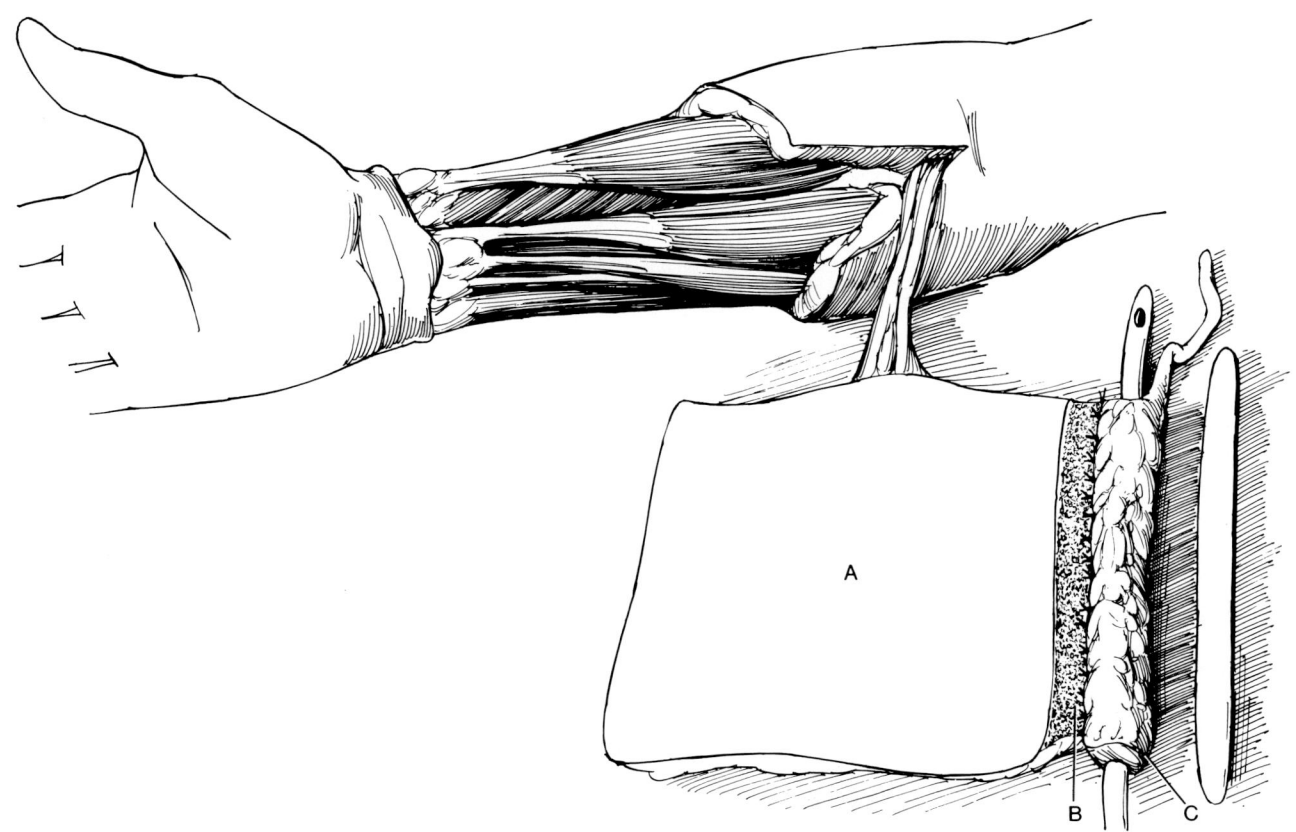

3 Cover both the neourethra and raw area with the larger section (Section A in Figures 1 and 2). Model the extensions to fit the meatus, and model the distal portion into a glans. It is possible at this point to insert a trimmed segment of rib cartilage from the costal cartilage union of the eighth and ninth ribs or a silicone prosthesis inside the skin tube along the raw surface of the tract, although the success of such implants has yet to be shown. *Second team:* Cover the donor site with a split-thickness skin graft harvested from the thigh.

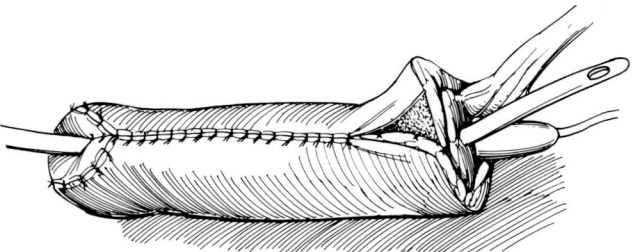

4 *First team:* Divide the vascular pedicle along with the antebrachial nerve(s) and tunnel it subcutaneously under the inguinal region. Using the operating room microscope, anastomose the cephalic vein to the greater saphenous vein or, by a saphenous vein interposition graft, to the femoral vein. Anastomose the superficial flap veins to the saphenous veins on both sides. It is possible to create a third anastomosis between a vena comitans and a saphenous branch. Join the radial artery to the inferior epigastric artery, the circumflex femoris lateralis, or the profunda femoris. Anastomose the lateral antebrachial nerve to the erogenous pudendal nerve or the dorsal nerve of the penis or clitoris.

Second team: Anastomose the urethra with interrupted 4-0 chromic catgut sutures. Fasten the prosthesis to the corpus spongiosum, and approximate the skin circumferentially around the base of the new penis. Cover the donor site with a medium split-thickness skin graft from the thigh.

Immobilize the arm at the elbow. Leave the stent in place for 10 days. Clamp the cystostomy tube in 14 days and observe voiding. If satisfactory, remove the tube. An inflatable prosthesis in a Gortex sleeve may be inserted at a second stage, although erosion and extrusion may be a problem.

An *alternative to tube flap reconstruction* involves the use of a pedicle of scrotal skin wrapped around polyglycolic acid or Marlex mesh, inside of which is placed a small semi-rigid prosthesis, all anchored into the penile stump (Bissada). Urine will exit from a perineal urethrostomy. If a urethra-sparing penectomy has been done, place the urethra under the folded scrotal flap.

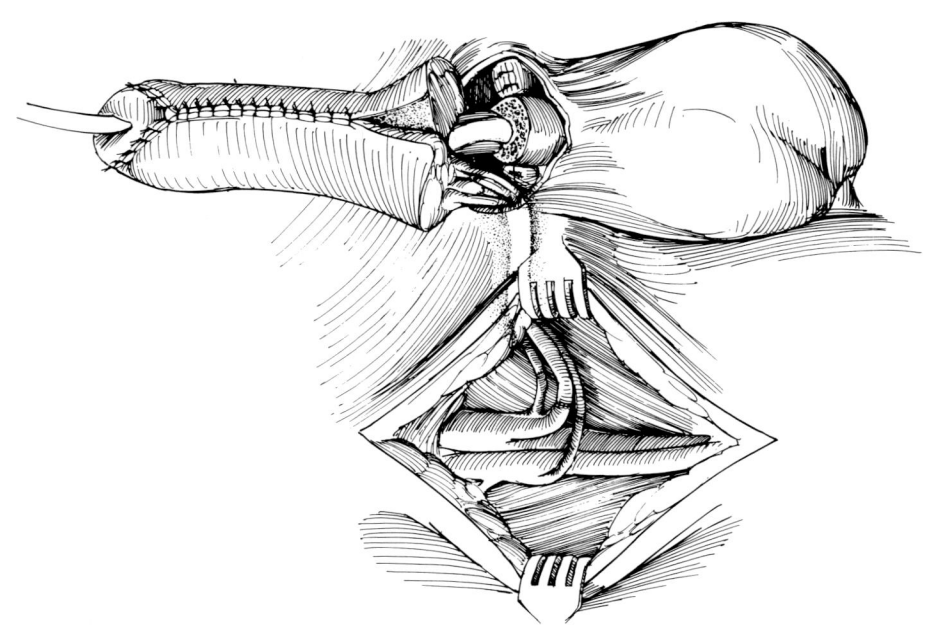

Commentary by Lawrence B. Colen

The radial forearm free flap has become the "donor site of choice" for the reconstruction of the penis in cases of traumatic loss, congenital abnormality, or gender reassignment surgery. Although numerous variations of flap design exist, the technique presented in this chapter illustrates the major principles of flap elevation and phallus construction.

Two recent innovations in flap design have been described. First, the flap may be elevated just superficial to the deep fascia of the forearm, because this layer does not play an important role in flap perfusion; it may be important in minimizing donor-site complications, because the deep fascia will set the stage for an excellent skin graft "take" when closing the donor defect. The skin and subcutaneous fat are elevated until the septum containing the radial artery and its cutaneous perforating vessels is reached. At that point, the dissection courses deeper to include the vessels with the overlying cutaneous components. Second, some reconstructive surgeons have begun to use an "ulnar artery forearm flap," because this allows the skin island used for urethral reconstruction to be in relatively non–hair-bearing skin in some patients. Either radial artery–based or ulnar artery–based flaps are options, provided the surgeon first determines if either of these vessels provides the dominant blood supply to the hand.

In general, the deep inferior epigastric artery and vein may be dissected from the undersurface of the rectus abdominis muscle and used as the recipient blood supply for the flap. Additional venous anastomoses may be performed to branches of the saphenous system, as already described in this chapter. Whether or not the deep inferior epigastric vessels are suitable, recipient vessels may be ascertained, preoperatively, using color-flow duplex imaging, which is available in the noninvasive vascular laboratory in most hospitals.

Neural coaptation seems important. Branches of the medial and lateral antebrachial cutaneous nerves coursing into the flap should be sutured to the dorsal nerves of the penis or one of the two nerves supplying erogenous sensation to the clitoris. In the latter case, the clitoris, with one of the two neurovascular pedicles intact, is inset either at the base of the neophallus or as far distally along the ventral shaft of the reconstruction as is permissible.

Attempts at providing stiffness to the neophallus with immediate or delayed bone/cartilage grafts have been unsuccessful in achieving the desired results over the long term. Resorption of graft material, even when included as vascularized bone (radius) with the forearm flap, invariably occurs. The best technique for stiffening the neophallus remains to be worked out.

CHAPTER 134

Repair of Female Urethra

URETHROVAGINAL FISTULA

Culture the urine and give appropriate antibiotics.

1 *Position:* Lithotomy—the position shown in the figures. Alternatively, place the girl prone in the knee-chest position, so that the urethra lies directly in view. Examine the area cystoscopically to visualize the defect and, in suitable cases, to attempt passage of a catheter through the fistula. Prep the lower abdomen, vagina, and perineum. Suture the labia laterally if they are developed. Insert a silicone balloon catheter into the bladder and place a posterior retractor in the vagina (not shown). Infiltrate the vaginal mucosa with epinephrine diluted in saline to reduce bleeding during the dissection.

Incision: Place multiple fine holding sutures around the fistula for traction (sutures not shown for clarity). Incise the vaginal mucosa around the fistula and on one side of the midline.

2 Dissect the vaginal mucosa laterally with Lahey scissors, using the sutures for traction. Mobilize a margin of pubocervicovesical fascia asymmetrically. Excise the margins of the fistula back to normal urethral tissue.

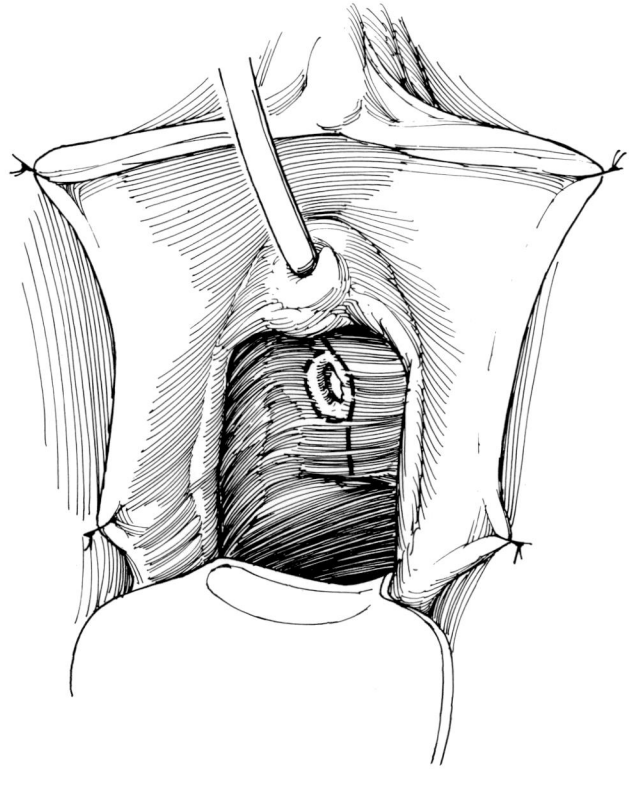

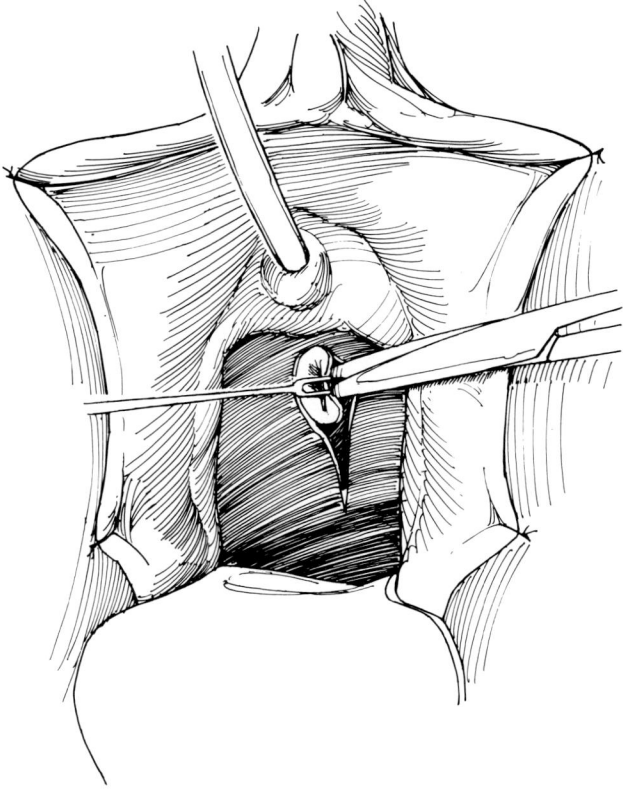

3 Close the defect in the urethra transversely with interrupted subepithelial 5-0 synthetic absorbable sutures. Bring the pubocervicovesical fascia over the defect asymmetrically with 4-0 synthetic absorbable sutures. Trim the vaginal mucosa on the opposite side to fit.

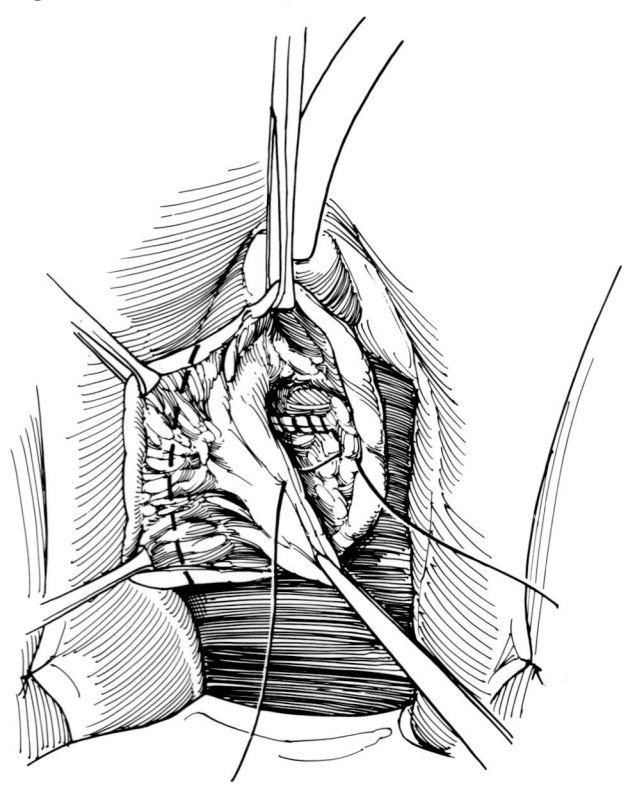

4 Bring the vaginal edges together with 4-0 synthetic absorbable sutures. Place a vaginal pack for 24 hours. Tape the catheter firmly to the abdomen to avoid traction of the repair, and connect it to sterile drainage for 7 days.

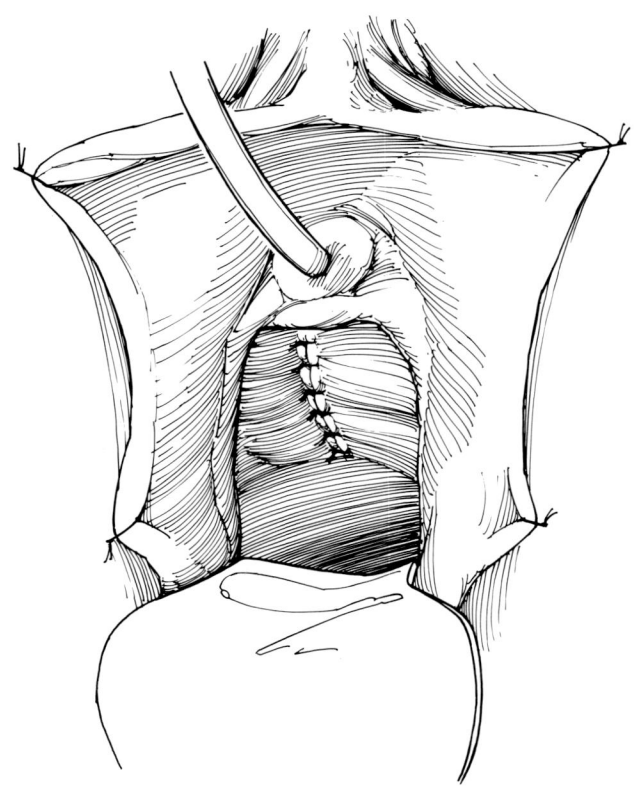

BULBOCAVERNOSUS MUSCLE SUPPLEMENT
(MARTIUS)

Locate the bulbocavernosus muscle by palpating it between the index finger just inside the hymeneal ring and the thumb on the labium majus.

5 After repairing the fistula, but before closing the vaginal mucosa, make a vertical incision in the groove between the labium majus and labium minus.

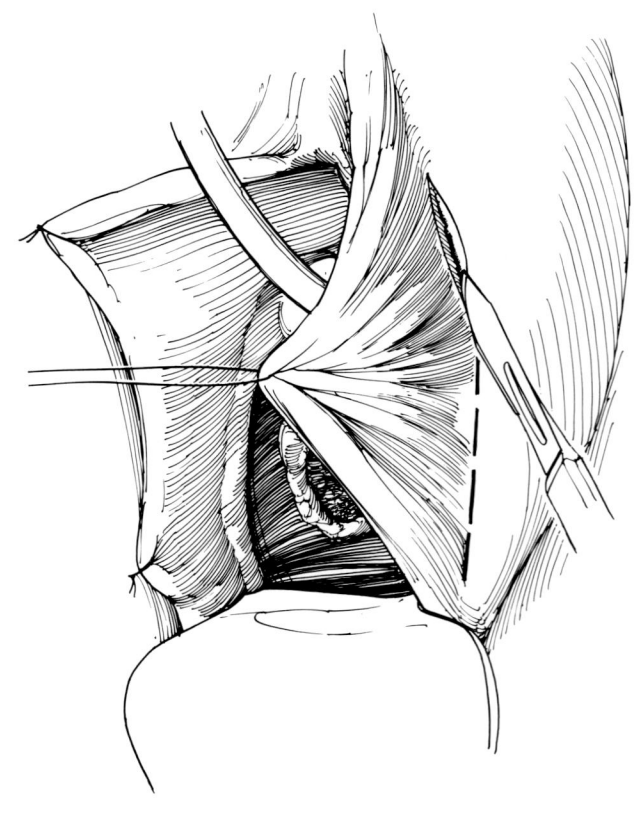

6 Expose the bulbocavernosus muscle.

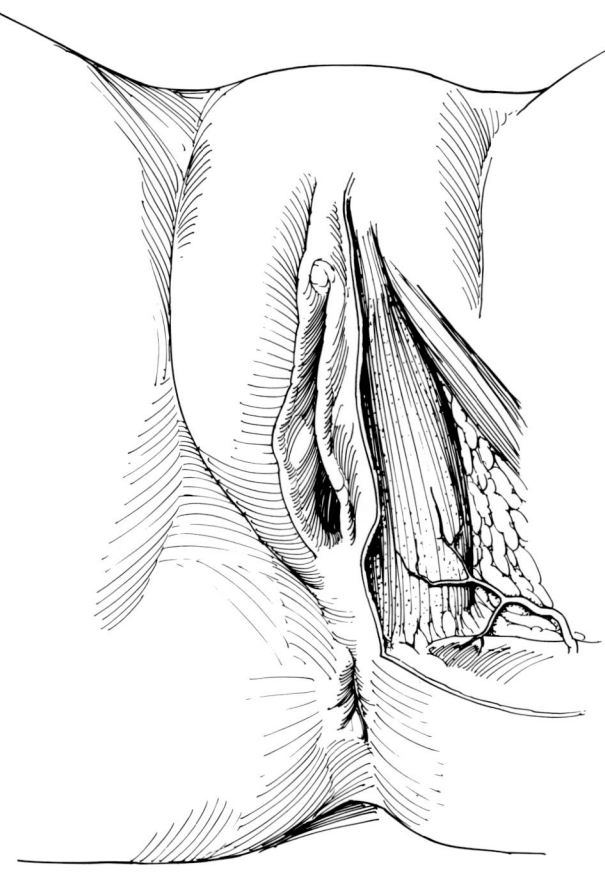

7 Dissect the bulbocavernosus muscle free, taking care not to disturb the blood supply that comes from the deep perineal branch of the external pudendal artery and enters the muscle posteriorly close to its origin. Include the fat pad surrounding the muscle. Ligate the tip of the muscle and divide it anteriorly. With a Mayo clamp, develop a tunnel starting lateral to the repair, going laterally under the labium minus and ending near the dissected muscle. Enlarge it with the left index finger positioned against the tip of the clamp.

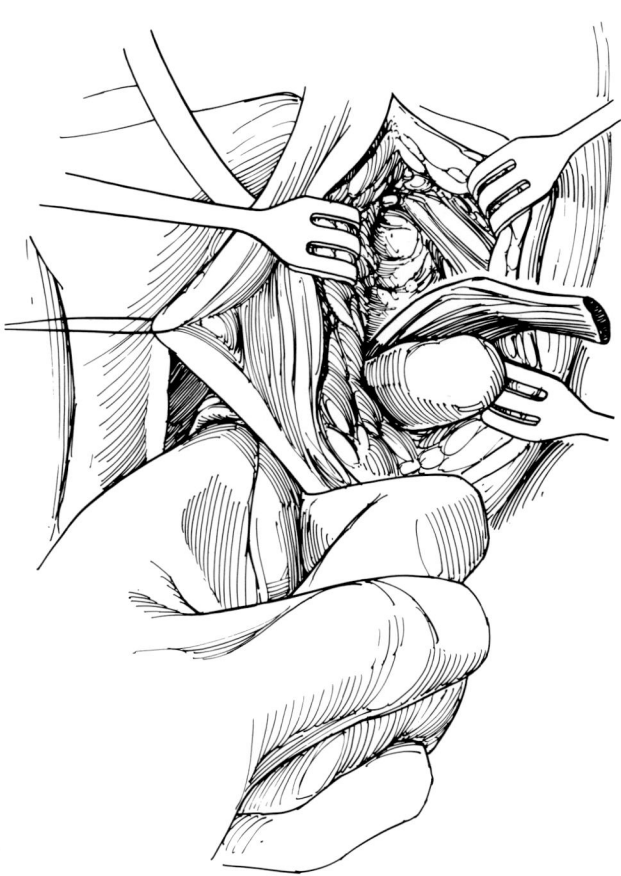

8 Grasp the muscle and pull it through the tunnel. Suture it over (around) the defect with interrupted 3-0 synthetic absorbable sutures.

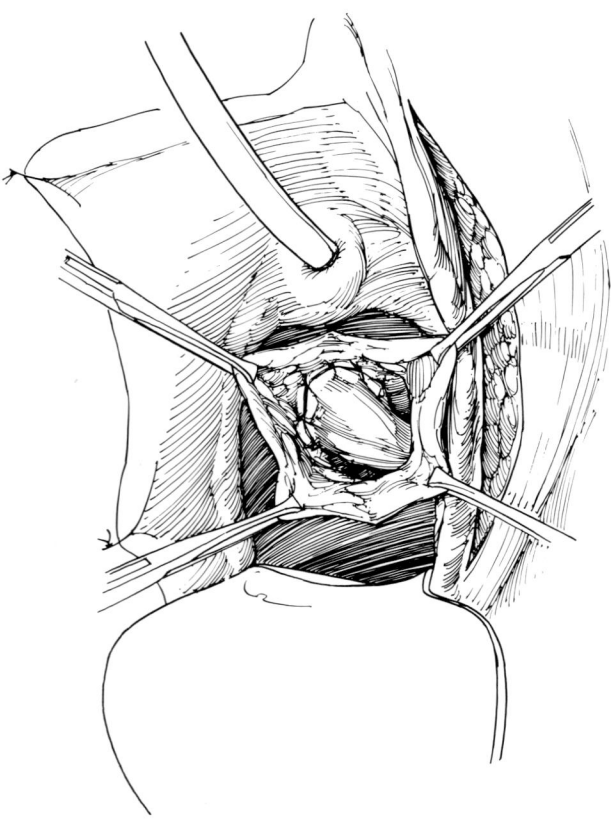

9 Approximate the vaginal mucosa after trimming it asymmetrically, and close the lateral defect with a subcuticular 4-0 synthetic absorbable suture.

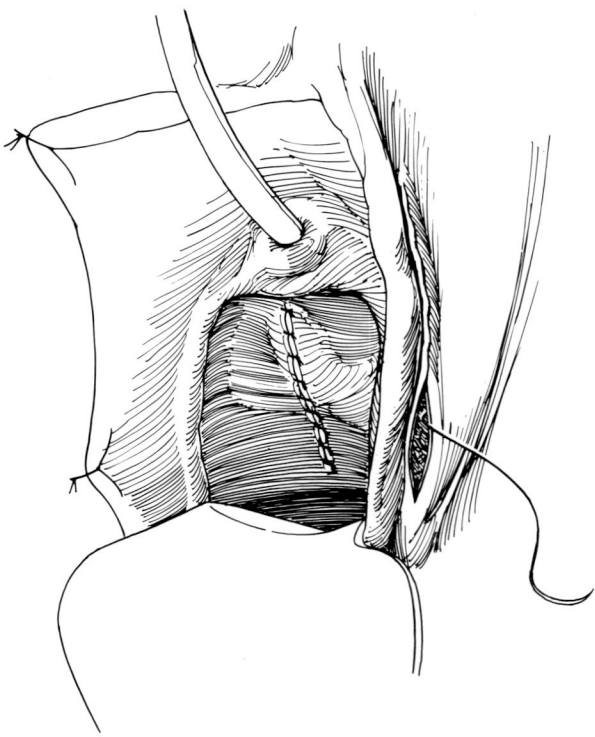

POSTOPERATIVE PROBLEMS

A *hematoma* may form following premature removal of the vaginal pack. A *fistula* may develop if tension persists after repair, if the balloon catheter is forcibly displaced, or if infection supervenes.

RECONSTRUCTION OF FEMALE DISTAL URETHRA

10 **A,** Develop a U-flap proximal to the end of the defect. Carry the incision alongside the urethra. **B** and **C,** Suture the flap to the urethral edges. Undermine the vaginal flaps, and approximate them in the midline. For losses of a greater part of the urethra, roll a flap of labia minora or vagina into a tube extending distally from the recessed urethral opening. Cover it with deep tissue that includes the bulbocavernosus muscle and with lateral vaginal flaps.

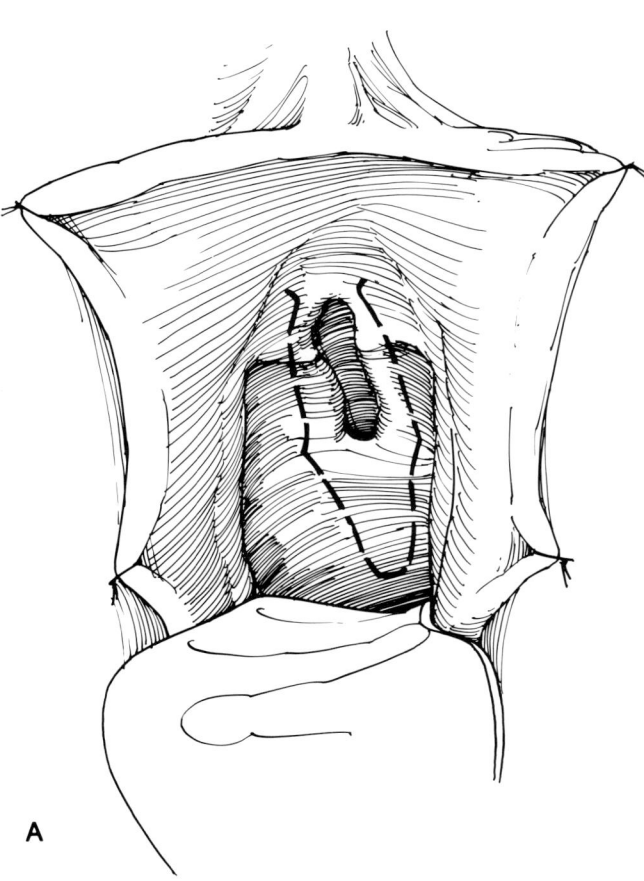

A

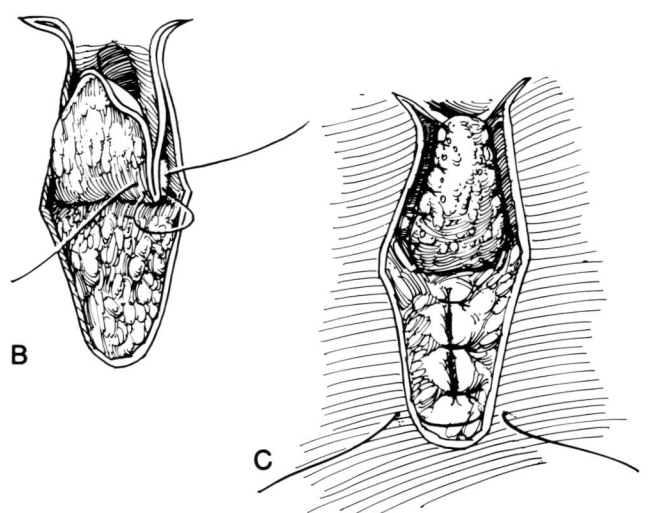

B   **C**

Commentary by David A. Diamond

Fortunately, urethrovaginal fistula is an uncommon lesion in childhood. When noted, it often is associated with reconstruction of the external genitalia, as in urogenital sinus anomalies or severe masculinization of the female genitalia in congenital adrenal hyperplasia. In these settings, creativity is called for. The most important decision is whether to repair such a fistula at all, because some will be asymptomatic. If surgery is in order, the surgical principles outlined in this chapter remain applicable. Perhaps the most important of these is the interposition of a healthy tissue layer between the repaired fistulous tract and the vaginal mucosa. In addition to the Martius fat pad or pubocervical fascia, the gracilis and rectus abdominis myocutaneous flaps may provide the necessary healthy tissue for successful closure. For the more difficult reconstruction, I prefer suprapubic tube urinary diversion over a urethral catheter to avoid potential trauma to the repair.

Commentary by Jack S. Elder

Closure of urethrovaginal fistula can be a technically demanding undertaking. If the fistula is small, the lithotomy position is appropriate, but if is large, the prone "sky diver" position is preferable, because the exposure to the anterior vaginal wall is optimal, and a skin flap from the buttocks may be rotated to cover the vaginal wall if a large defect is created. Infiltration of the vaginal wall with 1 percent lidocaine with 1:100,000 epinephrine prior to the incision significantly reduces oozing and the need for cautery, which causes tissue necrosis. A large urethral catheter should be inserted into the bladder prior to making the incision. The fistula and vaginal wall my be dissected out optimally with tenotomy scissors. The fistula closure and approximation of the pubocervicovesical fascia should be at right angles to avoid overlapping suture lines. The Martius flap is a posteriorly based bulbocavernosus muscle and fat pad that is well vascularized. If the urethral defect is large or the tissues are fibrotic secondary to prior operative procedures or radiation, an excellent alternative is a gracilis muscle flap. Generally, this has been performed with the patient in the lithotomy position. Postoperatively, a urethral catheter should be left 10 to 14 days, and a vaginal pack should be removed after 48 hours.

CHAPTER 135

Urethral Diverticulectomy

EXCISION OF FEMALE URETHRAL DIVERTICULUM: TRANSVAGINAL TECHNIQUE

Obtain a postvoid view from a voiding cystogram taken in the oblique position, supplemented by double-balloon urethrography, if necessary. Ultrasonography may help. Examine the urethra panendoscopically while palpating it vaginally.

Consider transurethral incision or division of the urethrovaginal septum to the level of the diverticular orifice (Spence-Duckett).

Attempt to sterilize the urine preoperatively and provide prophylactic antibiotics.

Instruments. A probe, urethral sounds, a 5-ml balloon catheter, a Fogarty vascular balloon catheter, and methylene blue will be needed.

Perform vaginal prep and drape the rectum from the field. Place 2-0 silk stay sutures in the labia, and suspend them over curved clamps or sew them to the skin of the thigh. Insert a urethral catheter. Consider placing a cystostomy catheter (page 346). Insert a posterior speculum in older girls. Inspect the urethra with a panendoscope. Instill methylene blue into the urethra if the diverticulum appears complex by radiograph (being careful not to spill the dye). Coagulum mixed with the dye may be instilled via an angiocatheter inserted transurethrally or transvaginally.

Locate the orifice of the diverticulum by panendoscopy, palpation, or hooked probe, and insert a right-angle clamp in it. If possible, insert a vascular balloon catheter.

1 *Position:* Exaggerated lithotomy. Draw the area into view with an Allis clamp placed at the meatus. Place another clamp in the vaginal wall just beyond the diverticulum (or in older patients, draw the cervix down with tenaculum forceps or heavy traction sutures). *Incision:* Make a stab wound into the diverticulum. Alternatively, turn back a U-shaped vaginal flap. Insert an 8 F balloon catheter with the tip cut off, and inflate it to fill the diverticulum.

2 Place a pursestring suture in the epithelium of the diverticulum around the catheter, taking care not to perforate the balloon. Incise the vaginal mucosa elliptically and eccentrically over the length of the mass, and dissect it back. Next, dissect the vaginal fascia back from the surface of the diverticulum. In difficult cases, the entire distal urethra may be opened, to be closed later with subepithelial and epithelial sutures (Kropp technique).

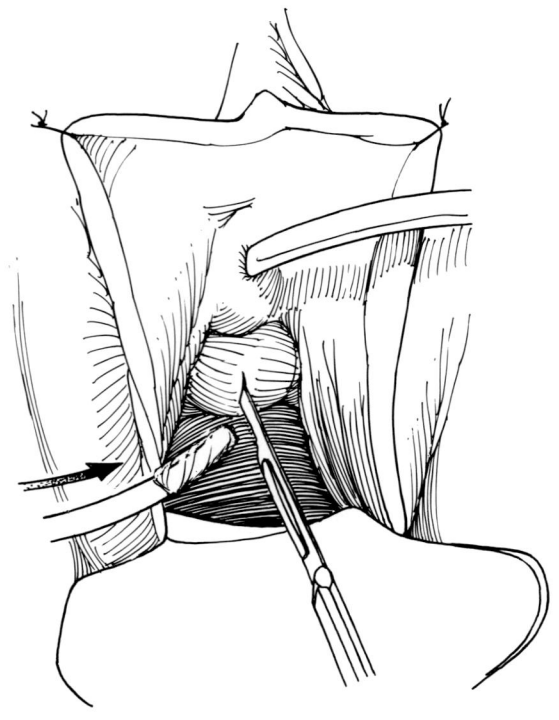

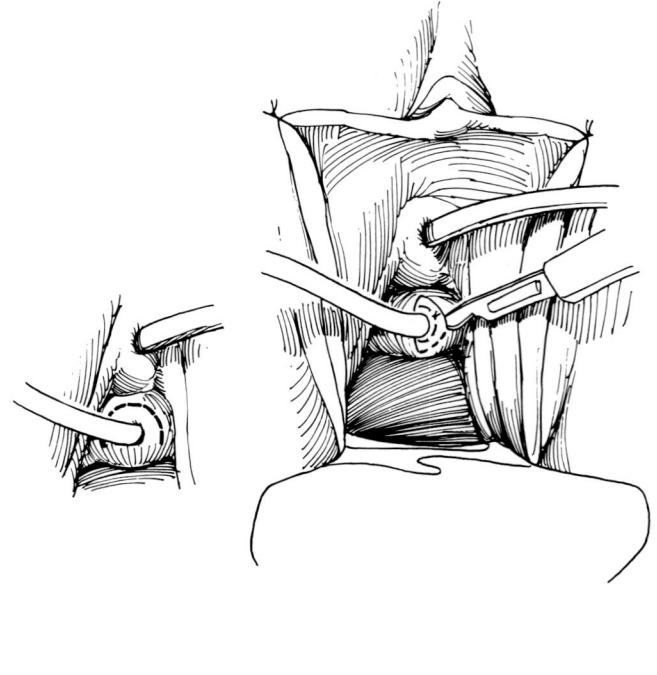

3 Dissect against the epithelial wall of the diverticulum with Lahey scissors using a separating motion, pulling the 8 F balloon catheter from side to side to reach the neck of the diverticulum.

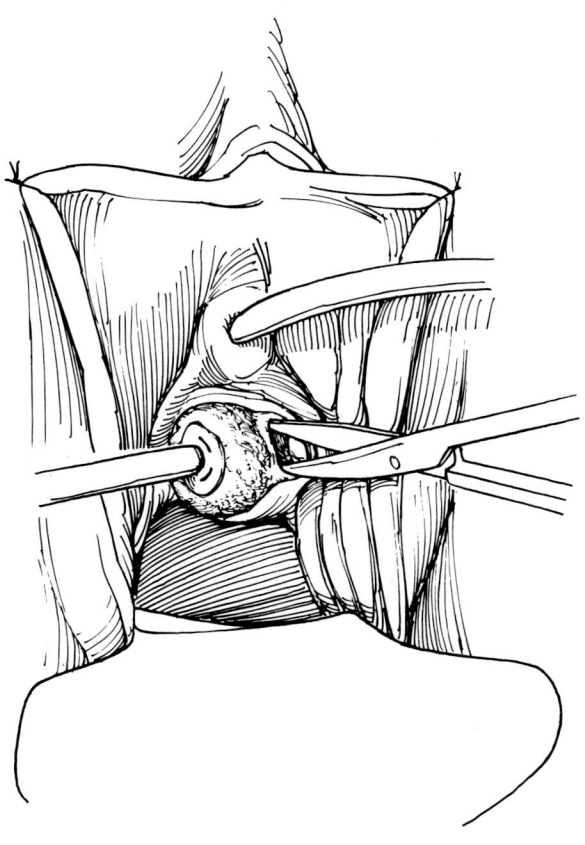

4 Divide the neck of the diverticulum transversely on the urethra. Traction on the urethral catheter will draw the area down for better visualization. Alternatively, open the diverticulum, remove the 8 F catheter, and trim the diverticulum to its junction with the urethra. If possible, transect it progressively while interrupted 4-0 chromic catgut sutures are successively placed in the urethral edges, or place a pursestring suture after the transection. Two layers are desirable, because a watertight closure is important.

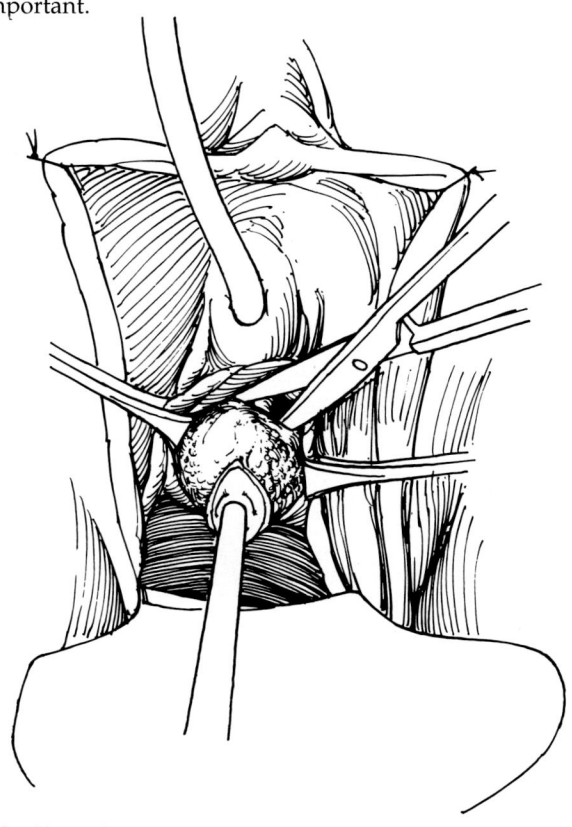

5 Close the cervicovaginal fascia with interrupted 3-0 chromic catgut sutures. For better buttressing, reach laterally and bring the pubococcygeus muscle and fascia together.

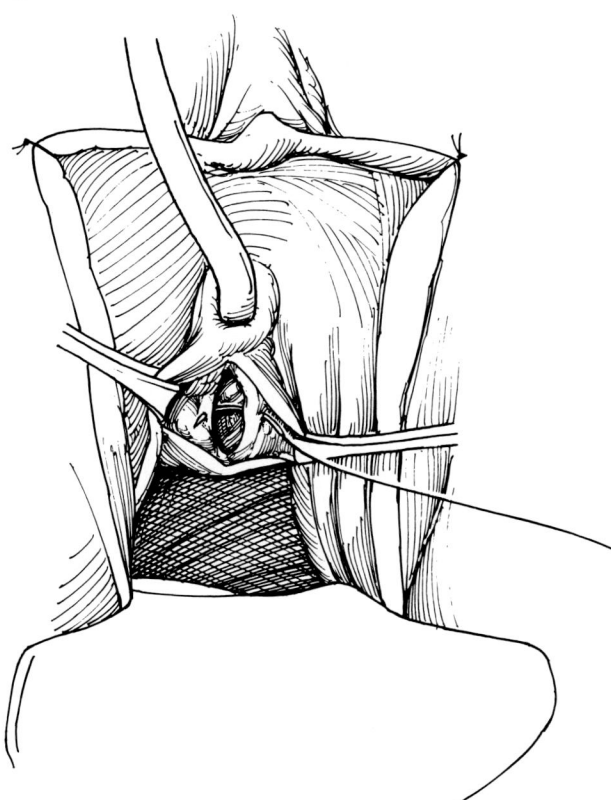

6 Close the vaginal mucosa at right angles to the previous suture line, but excise any redundancy. For added security, de-epithelialize a vaginal strip on one side of the incision, and lap the mucosa from the opposite side. If a U-incision was used, the flap will cover the deeper suture lines.

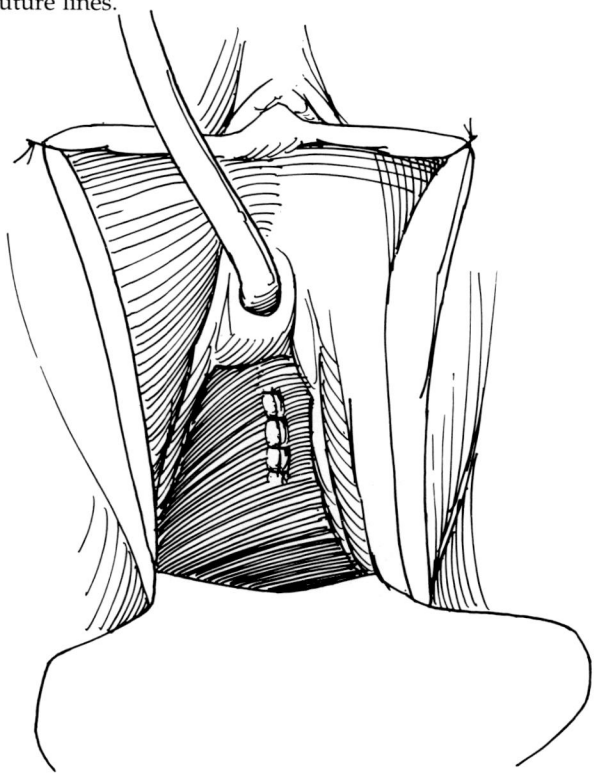

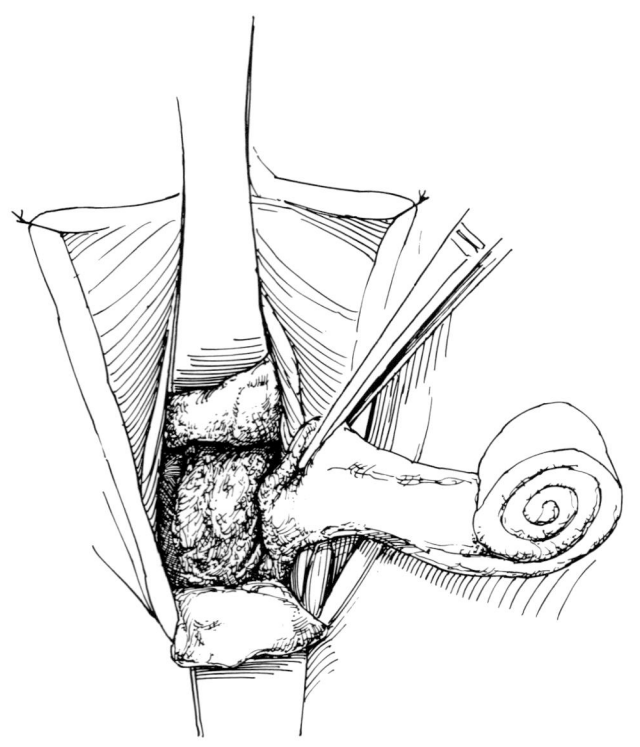

7 Insert two right-angle retractors covered with petroleum jelly gauze into the vagina anteriorly and posteriorly, and pack it loosely with 2-in roller gauze between the retractors before removing them. Tape the suprapubic and urethral catheters to the abdomen and thigh, respectively. Provide anticholinergic medication. Remove the pack in 1 or 2 days, and leave the catheter in for 10 to 14 days after aspirating it for urine culture and sensitivity testing and performing a voiding cystourethrogram.

POSTOPERATIVE PROBLEMS

A *urethrovaginal fistula* may appear 1 or more weeks after repair from sutures tied under tension, from areas of urethral necrosis, or from operating in an infected field. Wait 6 months before repair, unless it is distal and can be left untreated. *Strictures* are rare and can be treated by dilatation. *Stress incontinence* may occur if the deep urethra was involved. Manage it with cystourethropexy. *Recurrence* of the diverticulum indicates that all of its original ramifications were not removed, especially those lying laterally and anteriorly.

SAUCERIZATION TECHNIQUE
(SPENCE-DUCKETT)

8 A and B, Identify the orifice of the diverticulum with the panendoscope. Cut the urethrovaginal septum with Mayo scissors from the meatus to the diverticular orifice, then down the wall of the diverticulum itself to saucerize the sac.

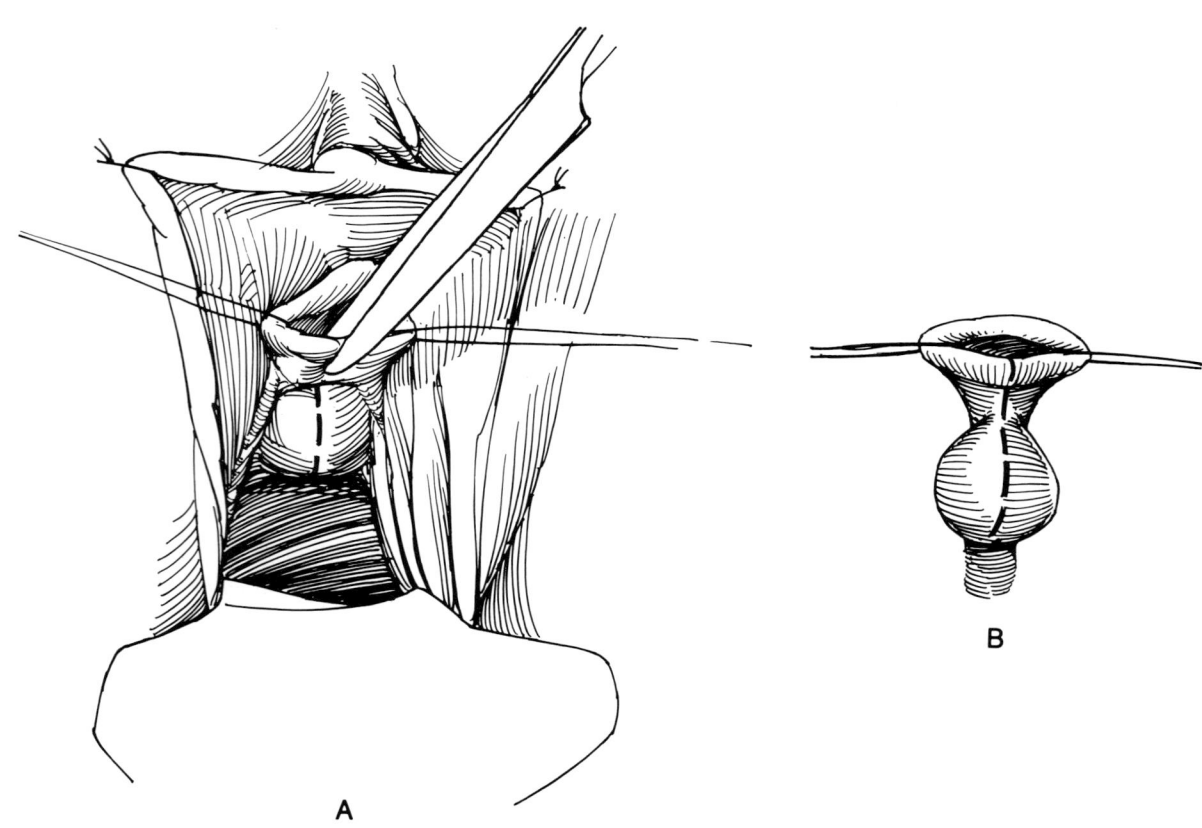

A

B

9 Trim the edges of the sac if they are redundant.

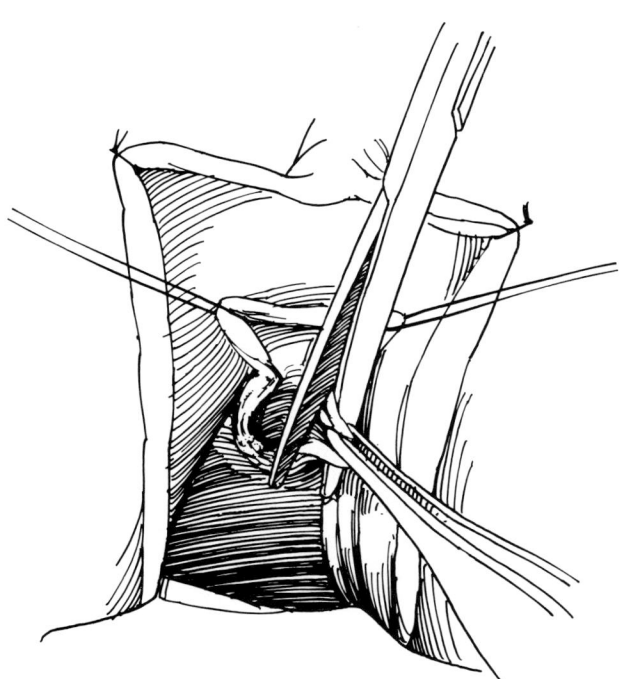

10 A and B, Run a 3-0 chromic catgut suture in a continuous lock stitch to join the vaginal and diverticular edges. Place a 24 F 5-ml balloon catheter. Pack the wound with iodoform gauze and the vagina with roller gauze. Remove the catheter and the pack in 2 days.

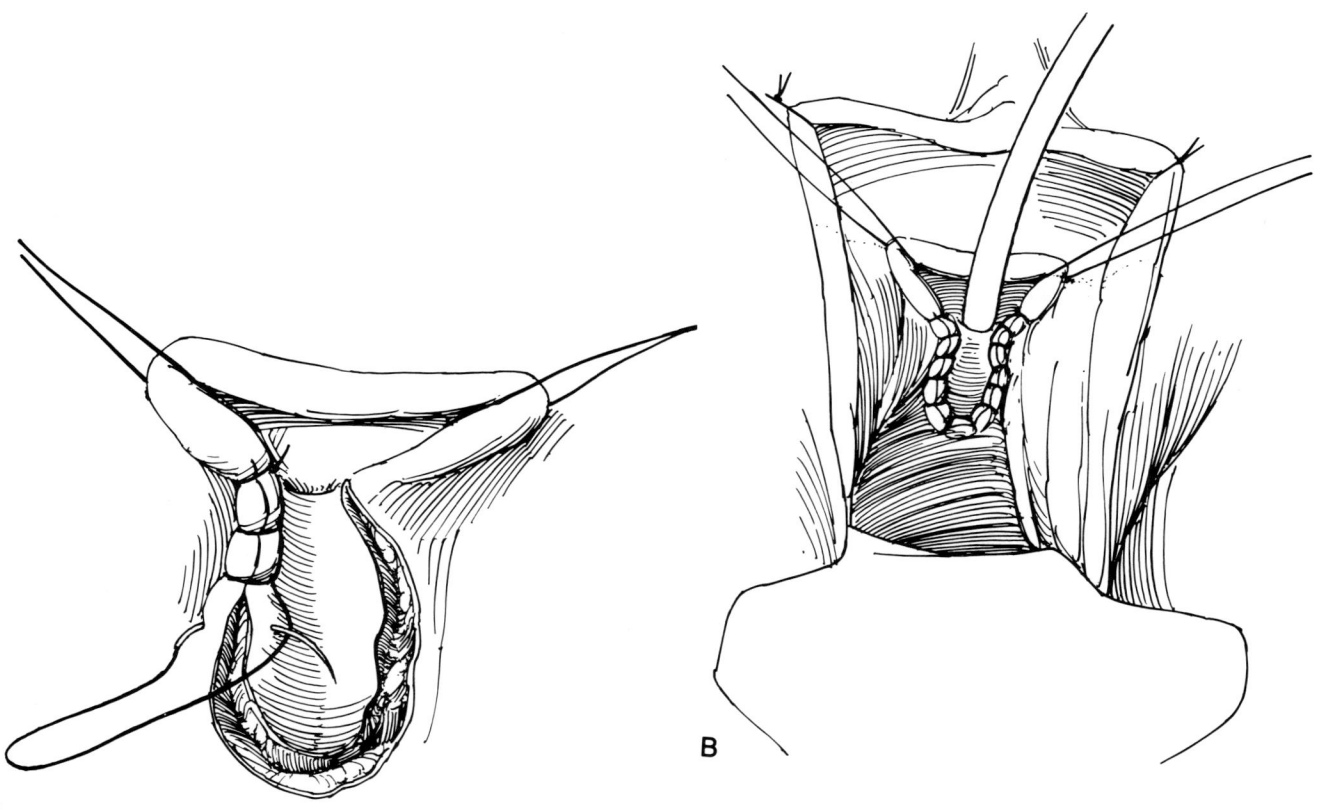

A

B

EXCISION OF MALE URETHRAL DIVERTICULUM

Diverticula occur in boys as a complication of hypospadias repair, usually secondary to a stricture more distally in the urethra (page 567). They also occur at the penoscrotal junction associated with anterior urethral valves. Depicted here is a generic diverticulum in the bulbar urethra. For an abscessed diverticulum, open it and tack it to the penile skin, as in the staged linear urethroplasty.

Clear urinary tract infection if possible, and provide intraoperative antibacterial coverage.

11 *Position:* Lithotomy to be able to first examine the urethra cystoscopically to be sure its caliber is normal. If a septum is found (the abnormality responsible for development of the diverticulum), consider simple incision with a urethrotome, although it may only serve as a preliminary step to definitive repair. Insert a cystostomy tube in infants.

Inject dilute methylene blue into the meatus to fill and stain the lining of the diverticulum. Try inserting a sound or bougie (or a Fogarty catheter) into the diverticulum; otherwise, insert a suitably sized 5-ml silicone balloon catheter into the bladder. *Incision:* Incise the skin vertically on one side of the midline. Dissect the skin and subcutaneous layer laterally from the diverticular walls as much as possible.

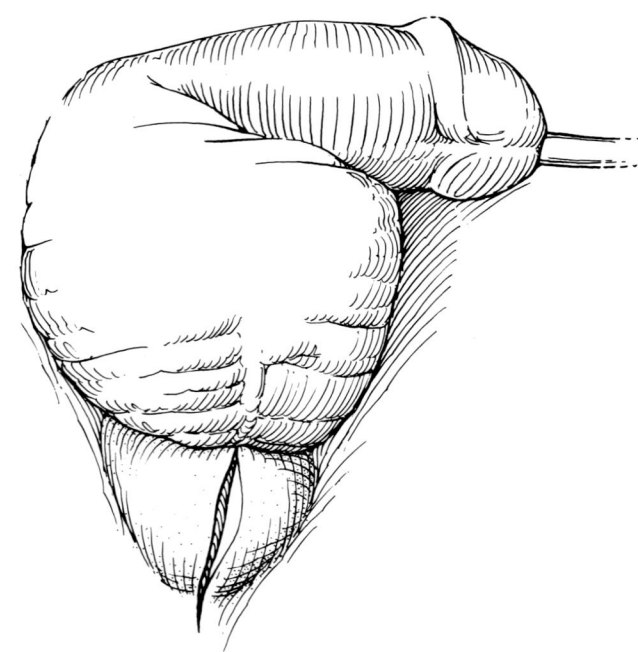

12 Open into the diverticulum with a longitudinal incision placed to one side. Place stay sutures on the edges. If a stricture is still present or its site indicated by methylene blue stain, it should be excised and the defect covered by swinging a pedicle flap of diverticular wall.

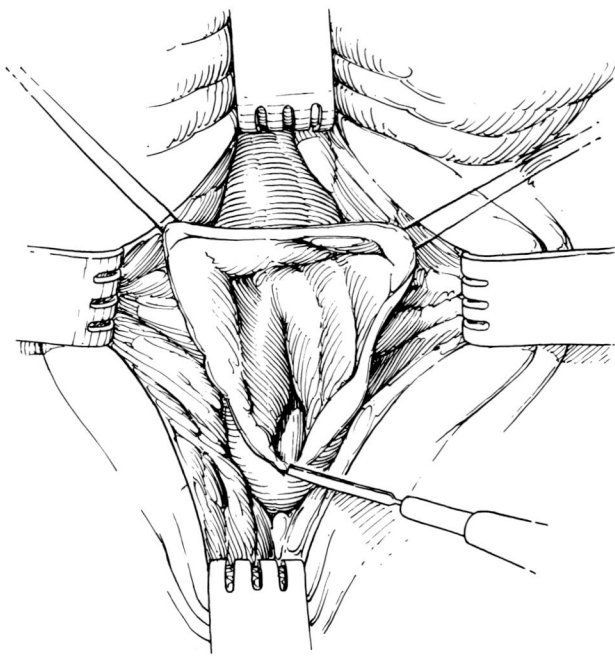

13 Trim the walls, but plan for urethral closure by leaving a bed of urethra as wide as 3 cm, depending on the size of the boy. If a stricture is identified, cover it with a pedicle from the diverticular lining.

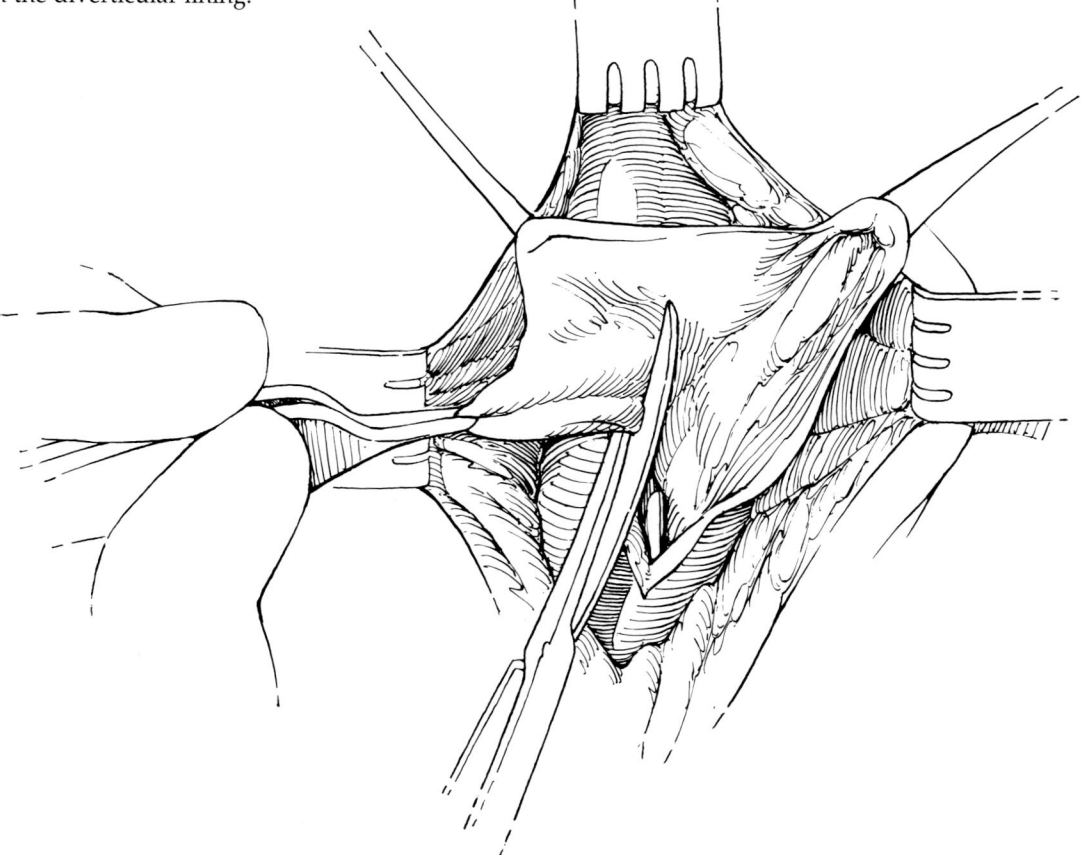

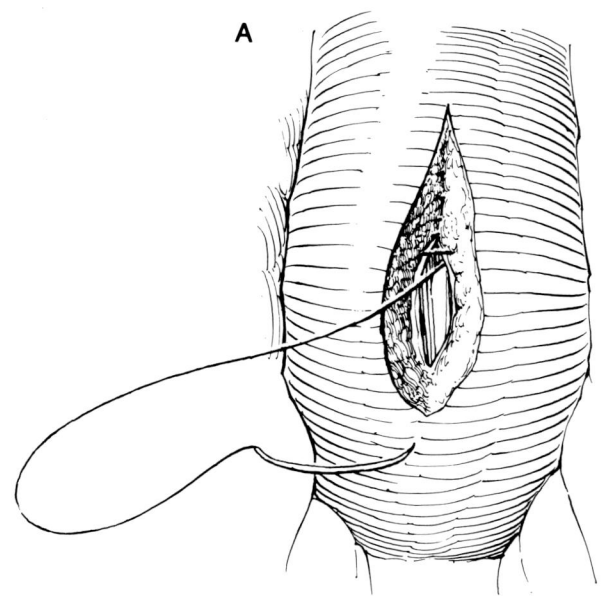

14 **A,** Invert the epithelial edge over a 24 F catheter as a mold with a running subepithelial 3-0 chromic catgut suture. Synthetic absorbable sutures are satisfactory, but sutures that absorb slowly should be avoided for fear of stone formation. Close the remainder of the defect with interrupted 3-0 chromic catgut sutures.

B, Approximate the fascia and subcutaneous tissue in as many layers as possible with 4-0 chromic catgut sutures, avoiding overlapping suture lines, and close the skin. Replace the catheter with a smaller silicone one and tape it to the abdominal wall. Drainage rarely is needed. Leave the catheter in place for 10 days. If there is concern about the suture line, check for extravasation by a urethrogram.

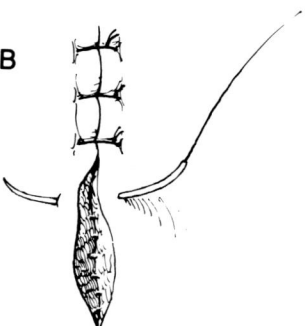

POSTOPERATIVE PROBLEMS

Urethrocutaneous fistula can be treated by prolongation of catheter drainage. Such a fistula suggests distal obstruction, as does recurrence of the diverticulum. *Strictures* require dilatation, urethrotomy, or even urethroplasty.

Commentary by Jack S. Elder

Female Urethral Diverticulum. The pathogenesis of female urethral diverticula is unknown. The prevailing view is that these diverticula are acquired, because the majority are diagnosed in the third or fourth decades of life. However, there is some evidence that a urethral diverticulum may arise from remnants of Gartner's duct, improper union of primal folds, or dilatation of a congenital periurethral cyst. Other possible etiologies include repeated infection of periurethral glands and birth trauma.

Female urethral diverticula usually are single and vary in size from 0.5 to 6 cm, with the majority being 2 to 3 cm in diameter. The ostia usually are located posteriorly in the urethra. The diverticulum may contain urine, pus, stones, or debris. Typically, women with a urethral diverticulum have symptoms and signs of lower urinary tract irritation, including dysuria, frequency, urgency, hematuria, recurrent or persistent urinary tract infection, and dyspareunia. Urinary incontinence also is common. On physical examination, the suburethral area usually is tender, and a mass may be palpated. Manual compression of the mass may allow expression of purulent debris, or the diverticulum may be hard if the sac contains a calculus. The most reliable method of detecting a urethral diverticulum is a voiding cystourethrogram with fluoroscopy. A postvoid film also is particularly helpful in identifying diverticula that may not be apparent on other films. Generally, oblique or lateral films are necessary. Positive pressure urethrography with a Trattner or Davis-TeLinde double-balloon catheter has been used to make the diagnosis. In some cases, endoscopic examination of the urethra is necessary, compressing the urethra to see if purulent debris can be expressed into the urethra. If the patient has incontinence or symptoms of bladder instability, urodynamic evaluation also is helpful. In children, the most important differential diagnoses to consider are ectopic ureterocele and ectopic ureter, either of which may drain into a suburethral position. Other diagnoses to consider include Skene's gland abscess, which usually is in the distal urethra lateral to the midline, interstitial cystitis, or bacterial cystitis.

A urethral diverticulum may be managed either by transvaginal excision or marsupialization of the cavity into the vagina. At the beginning of the procedure, endoscopy is helpful to try to identify the ostium of the diverticulum. Although the dorsal lithotomy position is used most commonly, the jackknife prone position or "sky diver" position also provides excellent exposure. I prefer to make an inverted U-shaped vaginal flap, because it provides a well-vascularized flap that covers the subsequent repair with suture lines that do not overlap. It is helpful to inject 1% lidocaine with 1:100,000 epinephrine before making the vaginal incision to minimize bleeding. After the vaginal incision is made, preservation of a layer of periurethral fascia deep to the vaginal wall is important, because this layer reinforces the urethral reconstruction. Tenotomy scissors are ideal for performing this dissection. Previous surgery can make this a difficult dissection. Generally, a Foley or a Fogarty balloon catheter is inserted into the diverticulum to aid in its mobilization. If a multiloculated diverticulum is suspected, methylene blue may be injected to stain the walls to insure identification of the entire diverticular cavity. When the diverticulum is completely excised, usually there is a large gap in the ventral urethra. The urethra should be closed longitudinally with a running imbricating stitch over an indwelling urethral catheter. Following urethral closure, the anterior vaginal wall is closed in multiple layers. The periurethral fascia should be closed in a U fashion. If the fascial layers are poorly vascularized, as in a secondary repair, a bulbocavernosus transplant or Martius fat pad flap (pages 668–670) provides reinforcement for the urethral closure and aids healing. After 10 to 14 days of catheter drainage, a voiding cystourethrogram should be performed using fluoroscopy to visualize the urethral reconstruction site.

The marsupialization technique of Spence and Duckett is a simpler procedure than diverticulum excision. However, because the ostium of the diverticulum often is posterior, the procedure results in a shortened urethra, which can contribute to the development of urinary incontinence following childbirth. In addition, the procedure results in a patulous hypospadiac urethral meatus, which can cause spraying of the urinary stream, vaginal voiding, postmicturition incontinence, and/or difficulty with urethral catheterization.

Male Urethral Diverticulum. Urethral diverticula in boys are seen most commonly following repair of proximal hypospadias, and have been reported as a late complication in as many as 10 percent of boys undergoing a transverse preputial island flap repair. A diverticulum may occur if the island flap is too wide and/or too long, if meatal stenosis develops, or if there is a blowout of the suture line postoperatively. Urethral diverticula also have been reported following multiple failed hypospadias repairs and may result if the tubularized urethra is too wide or if a distal urethral stricture occurs. Other examples of urethral diverticula include: (1) anterior urethral valve, which is a filamentous cusp on the ventral aspect of the penile urethra that results in a wide-mouthed diverticulum at the penoscrotal junction; (2) congenital megalourethra; and (3) acquired diverticulum resulting from trauma or infection, *eg*, following chronic urethral catheter drainage. Signs and symptoms vary depending on the etiology of the diverticulum. Most have urinary dribbling and voiding, and the diverticulum usually is obvious during micturition. Urinary tract infection is common because of urinary stasis, and calculi also may form. Following hypospadias repair, often a distal urethral stricture, meatal stenosis, or associated urethrocutaneous fistula is present. In boys with an anterior urethral valve, the diverticulum may cause extrinsic distal urethral compression and result in severe obstructive uropathy with renal failure.

Preoperative evaluation should include either a retrograde urethrogram or voiding cystourethrogram, as is is critical to determine whether there is a distal urethral stricture.

Surgical management depends on the etiology of the diverticulum. Usually the patient is placed in supine position. If the diverticulum is in the pendulous urethra, a vertical scrotal incision is made, but if it is in the penile urethra, a circumferential incision just proximal to the coronal sulcus is preferred to allow the penis to be degloved and avoid overlapping suture lines. The Scott retractor provides excellent exposure of the relevant structures. Generally, the diverticulum may be identified intraoperatively by filling it with saline through a pediatric feeding tube. Distal urethral caliber should be assessed with a bougie à boule. If a distal urethral stricture is present, part of the diverticulum may be used to correct the stricture, either by a Y-V incision or by rotating a diverticular flap. Otherwise, the diverticulum should be opened longitudinally on its lateral aspect. An 8 F pediatric feeding tube or, in older boys, a 10 or 12 F red rubber catheter is passed into the bladder. The diverticular lining is excised, leaving a slight excess of residual urethra to avoid stricture formation. If the urethra has any hair formation, depilation should be performed at this time. The urethra is then closed with a running imbricating stitch using 6-0 polyglycolic acid suture. The periurethral tissue is then closed over the urethra, and a third layer often is available also. If the child has an anterior urethral valve, the distal lip of the diverticulum must be resected; in some cases, an external urethrotomy may be more appropriate. In infants and young boys, an open indwelling 6 F silicone or polyurethane urethral stent is used to drain the bladder for 10 to 14 days. In older boys, a suprapubic tube and a urethral stent are used. Complications are infrequent and include fistula, stricture, and recurrence of the diverticulum.

CHAPTER 136

Excision of Utricular Cyst

1 Make a transverse or vertical lower abdominal incision. Open the bladder and expose the trigone. Insert infant feeding tubes into the ureteral orifices (not shown). Make a vertical incision through the trigone and posterior bladder wall that extends near the vesical neck, and hold it open with stay sutures. Expose the anterior wall of the cyst. Remove the retractor at the inferior end of the bladder incision to expose the bladder neck. Dissect the cyst to its entrance into the posterior urethra.

The same approach can gain access to the refluxing residual ureteral stump after heminephrectomy for an ectopic ureter (page 226), an approach less formidable and damaging than a dissection from above. An alternative is the transrectal posterior sagittal approach of Peña (page 329).

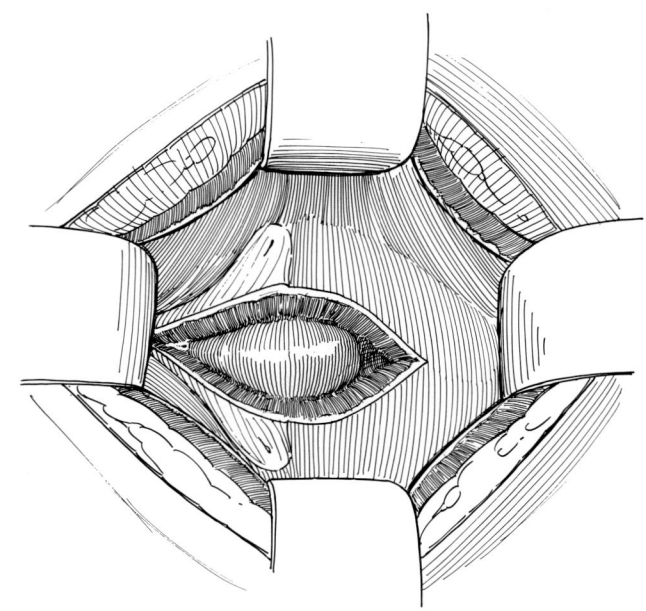

Commentary by Jack S. Elder

Utricular, or müllerian duct, cysts are most common in boys with penoscrotal or perineal hypospadias and in intersex conditions. These cysts vary in size and usually are asymptomatic. However, selected individuals may experience dysuria, perineal discomfort, urinary tract infection, epididymitis, lower abdominal mass, obstructive symptoms, hematuria incontinence, reduced semen volume, or oligospermia. By definition, these cysts should communicate only with the prostatic urethra. In the literature, however, are reports of müllerian duct cysts that communicate with the vasa deferentia. These latter cysts more appropriately are termed *genital duct*, or *ejaculatory duct cysts.*

Utricular cysts often are palpable on rectal exam. They should be apparent on imaging studies, such as transrectal retrograde urethrogram, or on voiding cystourethrogram, which should be done to evaluate the cyst size. Endoscopy is indicated to determine whether the ostium of the cyst is narrow. In addition, a small ureteral catheter should be inserted into the cyst and contrast injected to determine whether the vasa deferentia enter it. In selected cases, it is necessary to perform vasography to learn whether there is communication with the cyst.

Although the ostium of the cyst may be incised endoscopically, signs and symptoms often are not relieved. Consequently, an open surgical approach usually is necessary. The perineal approach should be avoided because of the risk of iatrogenic impotence.

The transtrigonal approach provides the best exposure. After opening the bladder, a Denis Browne retractor is placed. Ureteral catheters or pediatric feeding tubes should be inserted into the ureteral orifices. Next, the trigone is incised in the midline with the cautery. Stay sutures should be placed in the edges of the trigone The utricle should be immediately apparent and can be dissected out with tenotomy scissors. Extreme care should be taken to avoid the vasa. The cyst may be dissected to its communication with the urethra. At times, opening the cyst is helpful in its mobilization. The urethra should be closed over a urethral catheter with a fine running imbricating polyglycolic acid stitch for the inner layer and interrupted sutures in the outer layer. Generally, no drainage of the retrovesical space is necessary. The trigone should be closed in two layers with nonabsorbable suture. I think it is preferable to leave a urethral catheter, a suprapubic tube, and ureteral catheters for 7 to 10 days postoperatively. If the vasa enter the cyst, they will need to be transected. Ideally, they should be implanted into the bladder; usually this can be accomplished in a nonrefluxing manner. However, subsequent fertility would seem unlikely, even with current methods of retrieving sperm from the bladder.

Although this approach has been utilized mainly for genital duct cysts, it also may be used in excising remnants of fistulous tracts in children born with high imperforate anus.

CHAPTER 137

Urethral Strictures: General Considerations

SELECTION OF OPERATION

The urethra can be reconstituted by regeneration after urethrotomy and stenting, by excision and anastomosis, and by grafting. Of the three, anastomosis gives the best long-term results, but substitution techniques must be used when the defect is too long. In general, repairs in one stage are better than in two stages.

The region of the urethra involved affects the choice of the procedure. The penile urethra presents little difficulty, but the bulbar urethra, because of the critical importance of its surrounding spongy tissue, is much more challenging. Reconstruction of the prostatomembranous urethra is the most difficult, not only because of problems of access, but because the sphincteric mechanisms are involved. Factors impacting on the selection of the procedure are the etiology of the stricture (traumatic strictures are easier to repair than inflammatory ones), its length, the extent of spongiofibrosis, and associated adverse features such as local fibrosis, fistula, and infection.

Repair *pendulous urethral strictures* in one stage. Because reanastomosis usually leads to chordee and free full-thickness skin grafts may do the same, the vascularized island flap is the best choice.

For short *bulbospongiosus urethral strictures* secondary to trauma, end-to-end anastomosis is preferred. Longer strictures require a free full-thickness graft or pedicled flap. If secondary to inflammation, a full-thickness skin graft, or better, a vascularized island pedicle from the prepuce is used. A staged inlay procedure may be necessary for long bulbar strictures, particularly if associated with infection or watering pot perineum.

Bulbomembranous urethral strictures after pelvic fracture injury are treated by reanastomosis with a one-stage perineal repair. Grafts take poorly in this region. Abdominoperineal transpubic procedures may be needed in a few cases.

If the stricture does not involve the membranous urethra, try dilations and direct-vision internal urethrotomy. Realize that each deep urethrotomy incision initiates some spongiofibrosis that may make later repair more difficult. Consider open repair after two such failures. For long or multiple strictures, open operation is the first choice.

Allow adequate time for healing after injury, and provide for drainage of urine away from the site. Strictures occur in the spongy urethra, because the urethral lining itself is very thin and easily injured. This allows an irreversible diffuse fibrous reaction in the vascular tissue of the corpus spongiosum, the spaces of which are filled during urination. The contraction of this scar produces the stricture. During repair, take care not to incorporate areas of incipient fibrosis ("gray urethra"), because the result will be eventual contracture.

Counsel the patient about potency, especially with bulbomembranous strictures.

Instruments. A cystoscope, a flexible ureteroscope, genitourinary fine and plastic sets, a Turner-Warwick set, small skin hooks, an Andrews suction tip, Cushing forceps (two), DeBakey forceps (two), fine Allis clamps, a needle electrode, a Scott retractor and two packages of large stays, curved van Buren sounds, pediatric sounds, bougies à boule, Air Brown dermatome with components and two tongue blades, a Dermacarrier with four 25-gauge needles, adhesive drape, syringe and Christmas-tree Luer connector, silicone balloon catheters, methylene blue and saline mixed 1:1 and syringe, antibiotic solution, a skin pen, and a soft chair. Bipolar cautery is preferred to monopolar, being less damaging to the small vessels of flaps and grafts.

Sutures. 2-0 silk CE-6 for drapes and drains, 3-0 synthetic absorbable T-16, 4-0 synthetic absorbable T-31 sutures, and 6-0 monofilament polydioxanone suture, which is strong and has a low volume.

TECHNICAL CONSIDERATIONS

1. Obtain a cystogram and retrograde urethrogram preoperatively to detect pockets and fistulas.

2. Avoid dilation of the urethra preoperatively. This makes it very hard to identify the extent of the stricture at operation.

3. Instill methylene blue to stain the diseased mucosa, realizing that it does not warn of deeper involvement. When laying open the diseased area, carry the incision well into healthy tissue. If in any doubt, extend the urethral incision or excision. Be on the lookout for gray urethra (spongiofibrosis). In adults, be able to pass a 30 F bougie à boule both ways after excision of the stricture.

4. Obtain good exposure. This is particularly important in the perineum. Place the boy in the exaggerated lithotomy position. Beware of nerve injury; acute flexion of the thigh against the groin, especially in an obese patient, can compress the obturator nerve after it exits through the obturator foramen and starts dividing in the upper thigh. This results in weakness or paralysis of the adductors of the thigh. Such acute flexion also can compress the femoral nerve against the pubic ramus, resulting in an abnormal gait. Compression of the knee against the knee brace can injure the saphenous nerve and cause loss of sensation of the medial aspect of the leg. Compression of the lateral aspect of the knee affects the peroneal nerve, resulting in instability of the foot and foot drop.

5. Use magnifying loupes in operations on children. Place stay sutures through the entire thickness of the urethra and erectile tissue and hook them over the rings of the self-retaining retractor to keep the urethra open and reduce bleeding. A Robinson catheter passed in the meatus and out of the defect can be grasped with a clamp for traction and can aid in visualization of the deeper urethra.

6. Widely mobilize the tissues to be sutured into the defect. Distal mobilization and gouging out the inferior ramus of the pubis help. Tension cannot be tolerated.

7. Provide a well-vascularized bed of bulbar spongy tissue, if at all possible. For massive defects or associated injury of the bladder neck, use an abdominoperineal approach, and fill the defect with omentum.

8. Use fine absorbable sutures. Make exact skin-to-mucosa anastomoses to avoid granulation tissue and scarring. Do not overlap suture lines. Provide wide lateral separation and interpose connective tissue. Support the neourethra with adjacent tissue, such as that from the corpus spongiosum. Form the neourethra with a uniform caliber; avoid both sacculation and constriction.

9. To reverse intraoperative penile tumescence in adolescents, have the anesthetist break an 0.3-mg ampule of amyl nitrite into the breathing bag.

10. A urethral catheter left indwelling can be damaging; it will move up and down the repair when the patient is ambulatory. If a catheter must be used, choose a small size to merely support a flap and prevent adhesions. Fenestrations in the catheter may improve local drainage. Divert the urine suprapubically away from the repair. The following is a rule of thumb for the length of time needed for a leakproof repair with an indwelling urethral catheter: end to end, 10 days; island flap, 16 days; and full-thickness graft repairs, 21 days. If a suprapubic tube is used instead of a urethral catheter, these times may be reduced by one third.

POSTOPERATIVE PROBLEMS

Bleeding from the corpus spongiosum usually can be controlled by digital pressure on sponges. *Secondary strictures* from the presence of the catheter can occur, but the use of a small-caliber (less than 20 F), nonreactive, silicone catheter will reduce their incidence. Keep the shaft of the catheter at the meatus clear of encrustation. *Restenosis* at an anastomotic site arises from a circumferential suture line, in contrast with an oblique anastomosis. If a stricture develops, revise the repair in 4 to 6 months. Also, de-epithelialized surfaces may cross-adhere. *Fistulas* are rare. *Sacculation* from construction of too generous a urethra with a variable diameter in the bulbospongiosus region, especially after repair with scrotal pedicle grafts, not only fosters urinary dribbling but may lead to infection and stone formation. An important factor in preventing this complication is the provision of adequate supporting bulbospongiosus connective tissue and muscle over the repair. Reoperation may be required. *Ventral chordee* is uncommon, but patients may describe ventral tightness. *Hair balls* become a problem in adulthood when hair-bearing skin was used for constructing the urethra, especially if the passage is sacculated and persistently contains infected urine. The hair can be dissolved by filling the bladder with water, instilling thioglycolic acid lotion in the urethra for 10 minutes, and thoroughly washing it out. However, the problem will return.

Infection leads to fistulas and is to be avoided by perioperative antibiotics and skin preparation. Strangulated and traumatized tissue lies behind infections, so be gentle. *Incontinence* may follow overdilatation of the intrinsic sphincteric mechanism in the membranous urethra. Furthermore, loss of this mechanism during repair of posterior urethral stricture must be balanced by the presence of a competent vesical neck. Uninhibited detrusor contractions will open this mechanism and cause leakage; they may be prevented with anticholinergic medication.

Impotence seldom is caused by repair of the urethral stricture but is associated with the pelvic fracture itself. There are many branches of the erector nerves at this level, especially in children, so that some may be divided without ill effect. If the original injury tore the nerves, orgasm may be normal, and erection can be provided later with a prosthesis. Emission may be impaired by leaving the urethral caliber too large after a vascularized flap repair. Should it be necessary to mobilize the prostate during repair, take care to avoid the neurovascular bundles. Furthermore, fibrosis inside the posterior extensions of the corpora cavernosa can cause venous leakage, and arterial injury is not rare. Either could contribute to impotence. *Necrosis* of the edges of the patch or graft is not serious if the suture lines are not superimposed and if a connective tissue layer intervenes. *Hematomas* can be a problem if hemostasis, especially of the cut edges of spongy tissue, is not secure.

Commentary by George D. Webster

Procedure selection is dictated by stricture location, length, and severity. In general, I believe one-stage repairs are better than two-stage repairs, the latter being indicated only when local adverse conditions contraindicate one-stage procedures. *Pendulous urethral strictures* are usually reparable in one stage and should almost never be repaired by reanastomosis, for this usually leads to chordee. Free full-thickness skin grafts do work, but also may lead to chordee, and I believe the most optimal repair is a vascularized island flap, as was described by Orandi.

Staged procedures are not often necessary nowadays but may prove appropriate for long strictures when there is inadequate penile skin for a vascularized island pedicle flap.

I repair *bulbospongiosus urethral strictures,* if of traumatic origin and short (less than 1 cm), by end-to-end anastomosis. If they are traumatic but longer, I think they are usually manageable by free full-thickness graft. Inflammatory tissues of the bulbospongiosus are not appropriate for anastomotic repair and are best managed by free full-thickness skin graft or vascularized island pedicle (although this often includes hair-bearing skin, which is not ideal). Staged scrotourethral inlay procedures for bulbar strictures are appropriate for long strictures, particularly those with local adverse features (infection or watering pot perineum) that would jeopardize viability of the graft.

Bulbomembranous urethral strictures that follow pelvic fracture injury almost invariably are manageable by anastomotic repair. I do not think their level (above or below the urogenital diaphragm) impacts much on procedure selection. I correct 95 percent of such strictures (even up to 7-cm obliterative defects) by a one-stage perineal anastomotic repair, reserving abdominoperineal transpubic procedures for the small percentage with complicating factors. I am reluctant to use free grafts in the membranous urethral region following pelvic fracture injury, for the graft bed usually is very poor.

Obviously, philosophies regarding stricture repair differ from surgeon to surgeon, but the previous guidelines have proved successful in our extensive practice. I think that these are "forgiving" recommendations, although ideally I think urethroplasties are best left to those who perform them frequently and have each of the described repairs in their repertoire.

CHAPTER 138

Strictures of the Fossa Navicularis

SKIN-FLAP TECHNIQUE
(BLANDY-TRESIDDER)

1 **A,** Place a traction suture in the glans, using a tapered needle. Make a single-throw knot in the suture to help control the bleeding from the needle hole. Mark a chevron-shaped incision on the ventrum, and raise a flap proximally. Because it is an axial flap, include the underlying dartos fascia. **B,** Incise the entire fossa navicularis into normal urethra with scissors or with a knife over a grooved director.

2 **A,** Suture the apex of the flap to the apex of the penile incision with fine chromic catgut sutures. **B,** Continue to fold and suture the flap into the defect. The stitches will advance the flap distally and invert it. Approximate the residual cut edges at each margin of the glans. This leaves an open, but somewhat hypospadic, meatus. Divert with a small silicone balloon catheter for 2 days.

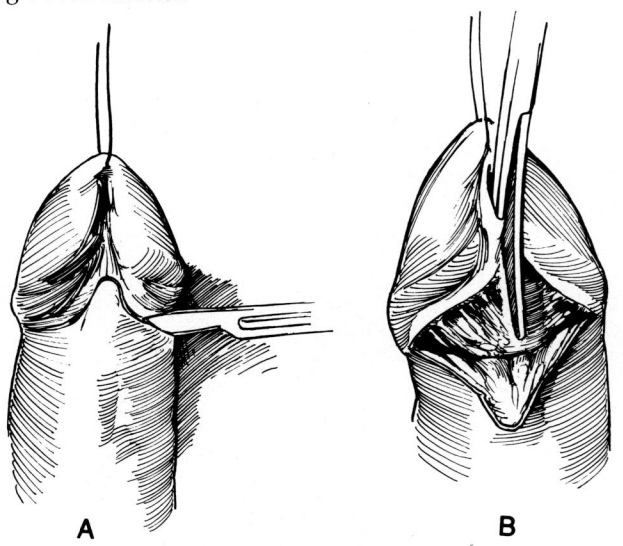

A   B

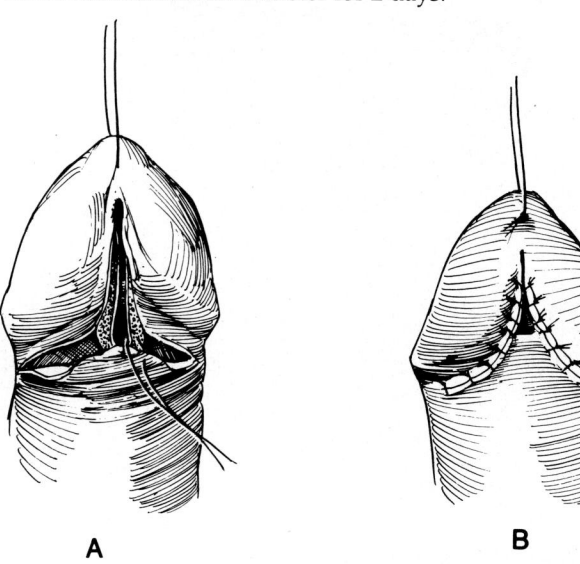

A   B

SKIN-GRAFT TECHNIQUE
(DEVINE)

3 **A,** Place a traction suture in the glans. Mark a ventral vertical line on the glans and a circumcising line on the shaft at the corona. **B,** Open the fossa navicularis with scissors into the normal urethra. Excise any residual mucosa from the glans. Mobilize and spatulate the normal urethra. Mark and excise a strip graft on the ventral skin, extending halfway around the shaft.

4 **A,** Suture one edge of the strip to cover the distal area of the opened glans and the other edge to the new meatus. Use 3-0 or 4-0 chromic catgut sutures. Place several quilting sutures to hold the graft to the glans tissue. **B,** Insert an 18 F, 5-ml silicone balloon catheter in the bladder. Continue attaching the graft to the ventral rim of the meatus, and approximate the ends of the strip graft with sutures together in the midline, so that it extends well between the glans flaps.

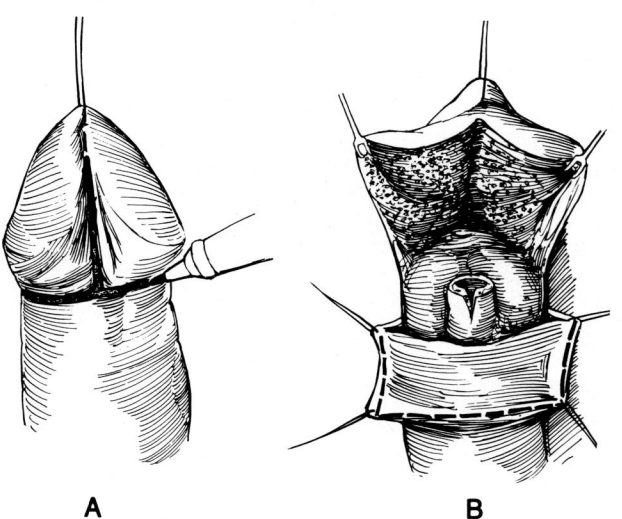

A   B

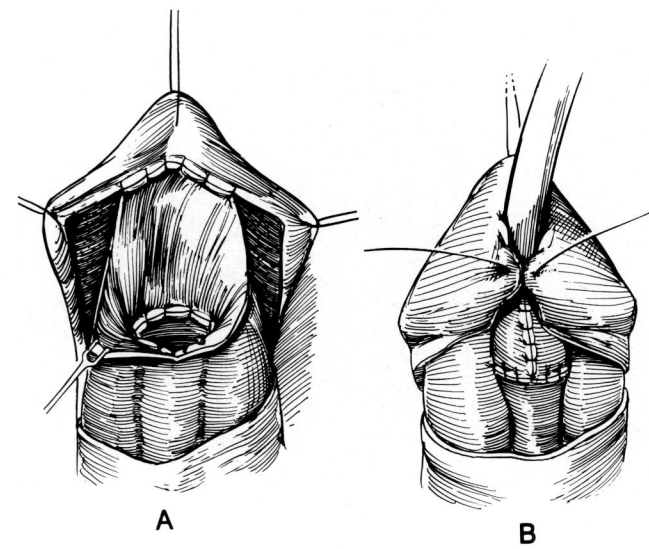

A   B

5 Close the glans flaps over the graft, and approximate the skin of the shaft. Apply a loose fluff dressing over an absorbent layer held with elastic tape.

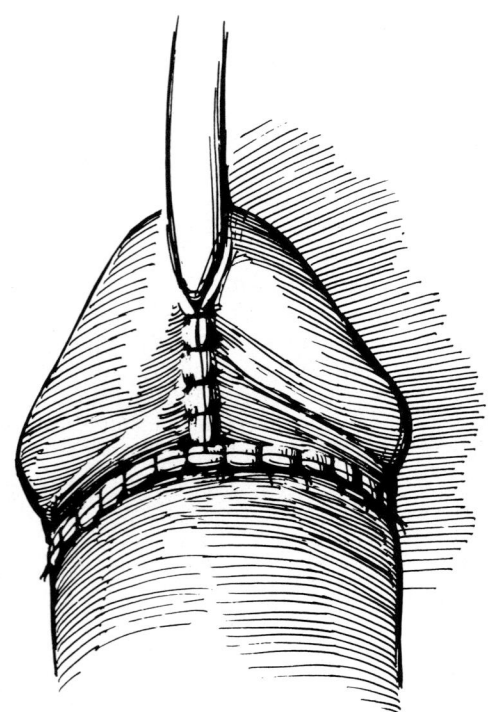

ROTATION ONLAY FLAP

Glans Tunnel Technique
(McANINCH)

6 Make a short transverse incision on the ventrum 0.5 cm proximal to the coronal sulcus or to the circumcision scar. Lift the wings of the glans, and dissect in the plane between the glans and the tips of the corpus spongiosum to the site of the meatus. Incise the glans ventral to the meatus, and enter the suburethral plane to connect with the proximal dissection over the corpus spongiosum. Open the strictured fossa navicularis by dividing the ventral margin with a hooked blade, working from both proximal and distal ends. Outline a ventral transverse flap of skin, approximately 1 cm in width, to provide a 30 F meatal channel after patching.

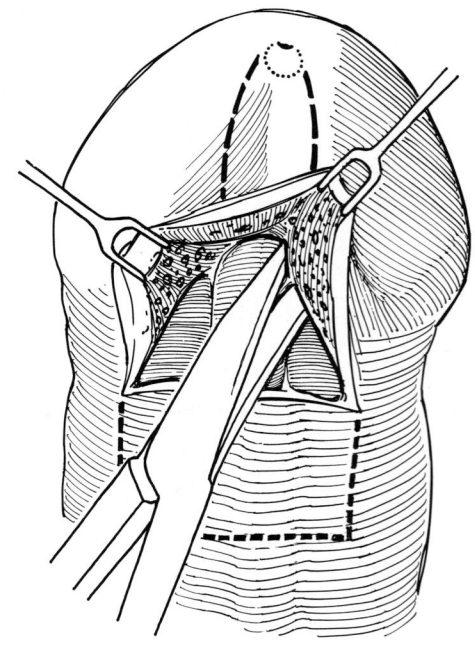

7 Raise the ventral flap on a pedicle.

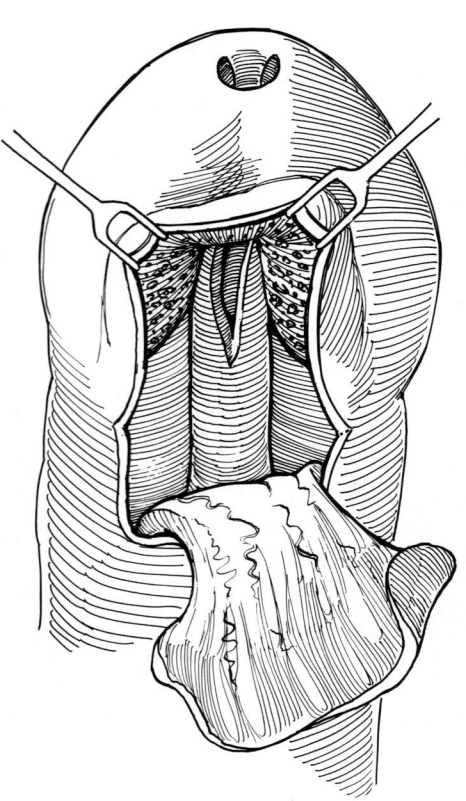

8 Invert the flap and draw it into the defect. Suture it in place at the meatus with interrupted sutures. Working from the proximal end, run a submucosal suture of 4-0 chromic catgut. Close the incision in the coronal sulcus with a fine subcuticular suture.

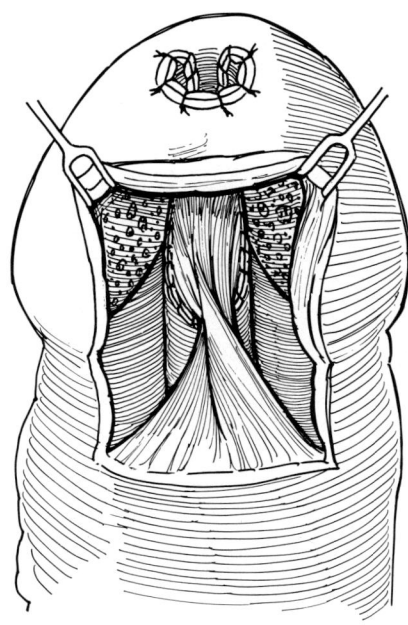

Glans Split Technique
(JORDAN)

Splitting the glans allows adequate incision of the stricture and mobilization of the glans wings from the corpora and also avoids sewing in a tunnel.

9 Place a traction suture in the glans. Mark a ventral vertical line on the glans and a short circumcising line on the shaft 5 mm proximal to the corona, and elevate the skin against Buck's fascia to expose the distal urethra.

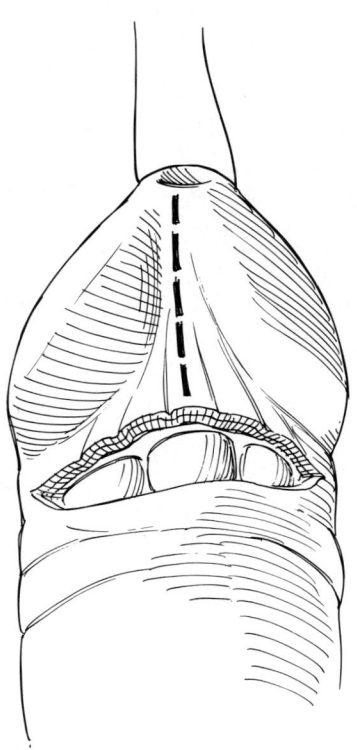

10 Open the fossa navicularis with scissors or a knife over a grooved director extending 1 to 1.5 cm into the normal urethra, as demonstrated by a bougie. Spatulate the normal urethra.

Mark and incise a flap on the ventral skin of a length equal to the meatal defect and of a width that, when combined with the residual urethra, will form a 30 F tube. Take care to incise only the skin on the proximal and medial aspects of the flap to avoid interference with the blood supply in the pedicle.

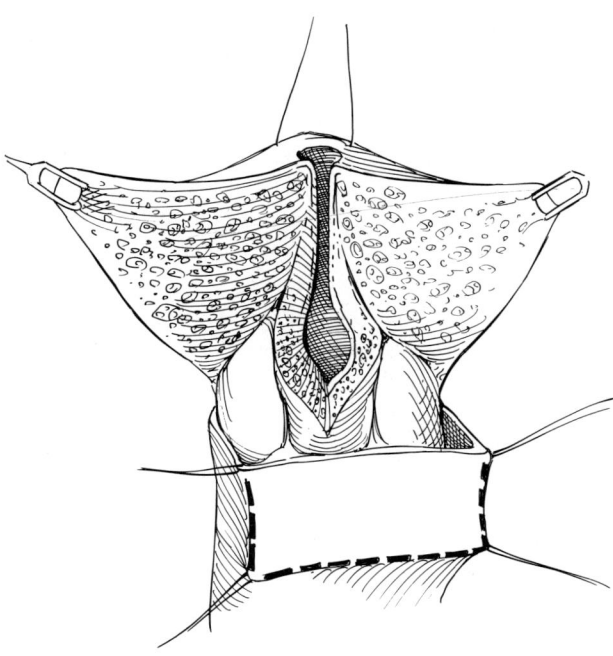

11 Raise the flap on the layer immediately superficial to Buck's fascia, invert it, and suture the tip to the urethra to create a spatulated anastomosis.

Fix the distal end of the flap to the site of the new meatus with two inverted 5-0 chromic catgut sutures. Attach the flap to the ventral rim of the meatus on each side with a running 5-0 or 6-0 synthetic absorbable suture.

Mobilize the lateral wings of the glans from the tips of the corpora as needed to approximate them without tension over the graft. Control bleeding with bipolar electrocautery forceps. Insert a 26 F or 28 F sound into the urethra to prevent constriction during closure. Approximate the wings with fine synthetic absorbable suture, and close the skin with chromic catgut, taking care to fashion a meatus of a suitable diameter.

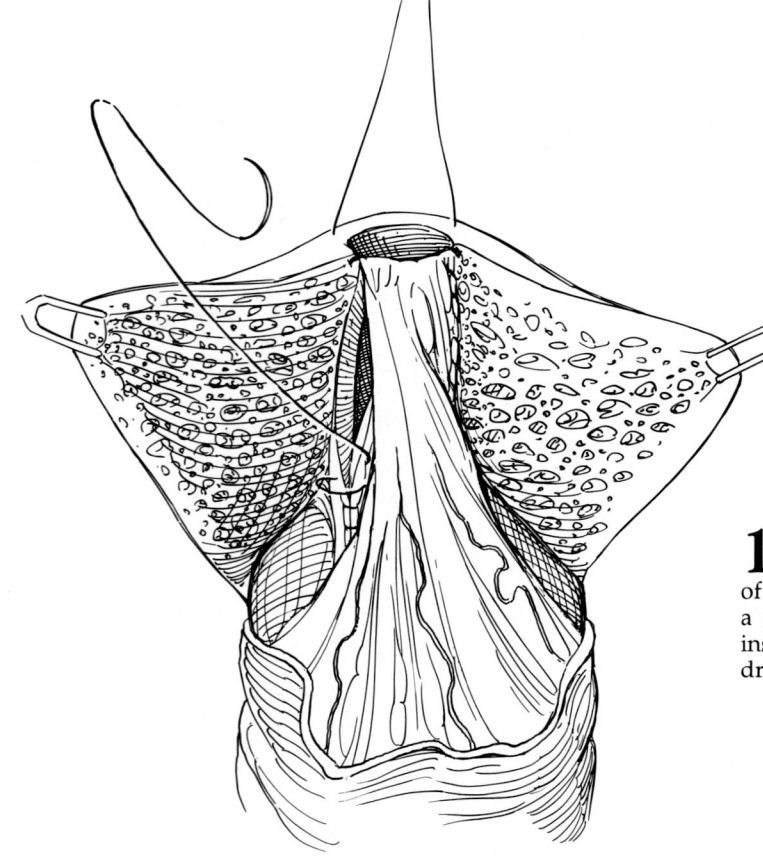

12 Close the donor site with transposed preputial skin. If necessary, trim the dog ears with excision of a Burow's triangle (page 44). Place a balloon catheter or a suprapubic catheter for a trial of voiding. In children, insert an 8 F prepared silastic stent, and apply a loose fluff dressing over an absorbent layer held with elastic tape.

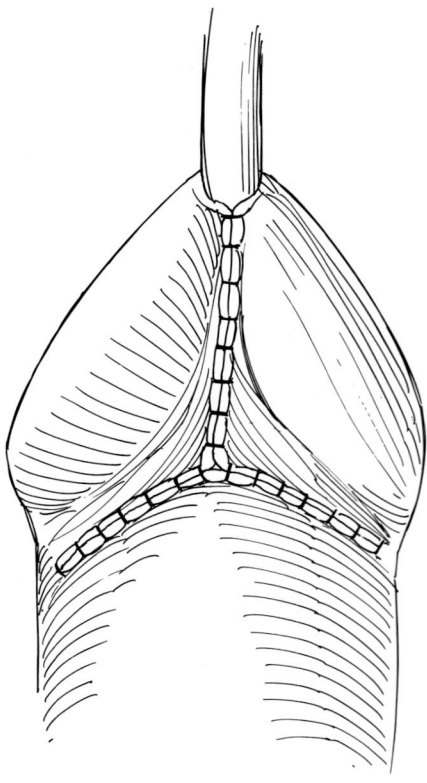

Commentary by Gerald H. Jordan

True strictures of the fossa navicularis represent a unique challenge to the reconstructive surgeon. Although all strictures of the anterior urethra require careful attention for good functional results, reconstruction of the fossa navicularis also requires attention directed at the achievement of excellent cosmetic results. Strictures of the fossa navicularis rarely respond to dilation or internal urethrotomy and also rarely respond to aggressive meatotomy. To correct the fibrotic process associated with a stenosis of the fossa navicularis, one must interpose nonfibrotic vascularized tissue to prevent recurrence.

In that "conservative" techniques generally do not yield good results in these strictures, one should proceed early with an open reconstruction. We are fortunate now to have a number of procedures at hand that allow for good functional correction of the stenotic process, with good to excellent cosmetic results as well.

Conney in 1963 described a penile-flap procedure. His flap was a transversely elevated random flap. The flap left the patient with a retrusive meatus. Being a random flap, one wonders also if flap reliability was not a problem. In 1967, Blandy and Tresidder devised a flap for reconstruction of the fossa that could be elevated, based on the vascularity of the dartos fascia. This flap provides excellent functional results but also leaves the patient with a retrusive meatus. In an effort to improve the cosmetic result, Brannan *et al.* (1976) described a modification of the Blandy flap in which the flap was much more aggressively elevated and advanced onto the glans. Because of the significant amount of advancement required, the meatus again often became retrusive and offered little improvement with regard to cosmetic results. DeSy (1984) reported further modification of the Blandy/Brannan flap in which a skin island is carried on the dartos fascial pedicle. Again, in this procedure, significant advancement is required to invert the skin island into the urethrostomy defect. DeSy, however, reports excellent results in a relatively large series of patients. Jordan (1987) described a procedure in which a ventral transverse preputial or penile skin island is carried on a broad ventral dartos fascial pedicle. His series now has 16 patients, 15 of whom have in excess of 1 year's follow-up. In that series, there have been no recurrences of stricture, no fistula, and essentially no complications. Although the procedure is best suited for isolated strictures of the fossa navicularis, Jordan has used the procedure in one patient in whom the stricture extended from the meatus proximally for a distance of approximately 4 cm, hence requiring a 5- to 6-cm skin island.

The advantage of Jordan's procedure is that minimal advancement is required to transpose and invert the skin island into the urethrostomy defect. By orienting the skin island transversely, the transposition in essence advances one end of the skin island to the proposed site of the neomeatus. Because the dartos fascial pedicle is based entirely on the ventral dartos fascia, it is imperative that the ventrum of the penis have a reliable fascial blood supply. Hence, the procedure may have minimal application in the hypospadias patient. The flap is based on the distal arborizations of the external pudendal vessels. In the hypospadias patient, the arborizations dorsally are far more reliable than the ventral arborizations because of the defect of ventral fusion, which can involve all layers. Circumcision in no way contraindicates the use of the flap; however, the skin island must be elevated proximal to the circumcising incision in those cases, because the preputial skin may not be reliably vascularized by the proximal dartos fascia. Additionally, the patient who has had multiple operations may not have a reliable ventral dartos fascial blood supply.

I believe that it is essential to raise the glans wings broadly. This can be accomplished in the plane between the tips of the corpora cavernosa and the overlying spongy erectile tissue of the glans penis. This is a relatively avascular plane, and any bleeding can be controlled easily with bipolar electrocautery forceps. It is essential that the scar process associated with the fossa stricture be divided completely. Elevation of the glans flaps allows for this and further allows for refusion of the glans without the potential for restenosis after placement of a relatively bulky flap into the meatus. The ventral glans is easily fused by the use of subcuticular monofilament absorbable sutures and absorbable sutures placed to reappose the skin edges. As mentioned, in the series thus far, fistula has not been a problem.

McAninch has modified the procedure by leaving the ventral glans intact. Although this may be of use in some patients, in patients in which the fibrotic process is deep into the overlying spongy erectile tissue of the glans penis, incomplete division of the fibrotic process may not be accomplished. Additionally, the author has found elevation of the glans off the tips of the corpora to be somewhat more difficult, with the ventrum of the glans intact.

In some patients with meatal stenosis, there has been flattening of the glans. Leaving the ventrum of the glans intact does not allow for sculpturing of the glans. With wide mobilization of the glans wings, a portion of the proximal glans can be excised, reestablishing the more normal conical shape of the glans penis. Devine's procedure, which he terms *resurfacing of the fossa navicularis*, yields excellent cosmetic results. The procedure may be of limited application in the patient afflicted with balanitis xerotica obliterans. There is a great deal that suggests that the balanitis xerotica obliterans process can "invade" or involve grafts in general and, in specific, grafts placed coapted to skin already involved in the inflammatory process. As initially described by Devine, the tubularized full-thickness skin graft was placed with the graft suture line ventrally. However, in later cases, the graft suture line was rotated dorsally. That maneuver still allows for the placement of quilting sutures and allows one to avoid a situation of overlying suture lines. The author has applied the procedure in a limited number of patients. It must be noted that fistula, no matter where the suture line is placed, have not been a problem in that limited series.

CHAPTER 139

Penile and Bulbourethral Strictures

Urethral strictures in childhood often are related to hypospadias repair or are bulbar strictures secondary to straddle injury.

PENILE STRICTURES

To select the best repair, the stricture must be evaluated by retrograde and voiding urethrograms to determine the length of the stricture. Ultrasonography aids in estimation of the depth of involvement of the spongy tissue.

Compared with meatal and bulbar strictures, those in the anterior urethra are simple to repair. The aim is to form a tube of uniform caliber that will not be prone to restricturing. Because the overlying penile skin and adjacent prepuce are hairless, well vascularized, and adaptable to a wet environment, these surfaces can be rolled in as an island flap or transported from the prepuce as a patch or island flap. Bladder epithelium or buccal mucosa (pages 555, 556) are alternatives if penile skin is not available. If the bed is of very poor quality, a long stricture can be repaired in two stages by inserting a mesh graft at a first stage and forming the urethral tube later. Short, dense strictures with involvement of the spongy tissue can be managed with patch grafts or with island flaps, a technique that also may involve resection and partial reanastomosis as a roof strip. It is very worthwhile to keep the urethra in continuity. Because it is desirable to remove the stent as soon as possible, vascularized flaps have advantages over free grafts.

BULBAR STRICTURES

Strictures in the bulbar urethra can be repaired by one of three procedures: excision and reanastomosis, internal urethrotomy, and grafts or flaps. The most straightforward, *excision and reanastomosis*, also has the greatest rate of success, but its use is limited to short traumatic strictures. Most strictures in the penile urethra in children are inflammatory, and the part involved in the spongiofibrotic reaction is relatively long. Only a very short traumatic stricture that results from a minor straddle injury is suitable for reanastomosis in a child. The size of the defect cannot be any longer than the elastic lengthening obtained by mobilizing the bulbar urethra proximal and distal to the stricture, and this carries the danger of devascularization if it is extensive. Consequently, few bulbar strictures can be repaired this way.

Internal urethrotomy in anticipation of urethral regeneration is simple to perform but rarely is applicable in children, and the recurrence rate is high.

Grafts are not uniformly successful but may be the only solution as free patches. When skin grafts are used for urethral reconstruction, any failure of graft take will result in stricture, a risk that rises in proportion to the size of the graft. Originating from the preputial skin, they are more adaptable to a wet environment than skin from other sites. Full-thickness grafts are better than split-thickness grafts, and when placed within healthy, typically well-vascularized spongy tissue, they most nearly imitate the normal urethra. A vascularized flap is more trustworthy. Even when a child has been circumcised, a sufficient patch of skin from the penis usually is available. Although scrotal skin is available and relatively easy to form into a graft, it should be avoided, because it is more subject to irritation when constantly wet, and because it is hair bearing, it can cause distress if the graft becomes sacculated. If it is used, careful epilation is important. Bladder epithelium and buccal mucosa are reserved for cases in which skin is not available.

Flaps carry their own blood supply. A random flap can be raised on a pedicle as an island flap. Such an island flap from the ventral portion of the penis or from the inner surface of the prepuce can be invaginated to fill the urethral defect and covered with previously separated spongy tissue. Vascularized flaps do not require as good a bed as that needed for free grafts.

Because replacement of an entire segment of urethra is most liable to restenosis, a *roof strip* is made by overlapping the remaining portions of the urethra after excision of the stricture, and its environs is stitched flat against the corpora to maximize its width. The graft or flap is sutured to the edges of the strip. Even if the graft should fail, re-epithelialization can occur and bridge the gap. If the quality of the tissues is in doubt, a staged procedure is preferable.

Commentary by Jonathan S. Vordermark, II

The techniques developed for adult urethroplasty are applicable to the child with a few modifications and precautions. The pediatric urethra does not have the elasticity of that of the adult, and, therefore, it is less often possible to merely excise the defect in the child. More commonly, a combination of techniques will be necessary. The smaller size of the urethra in a child makes the use of optical magnification, delicate "no-touch" tissue handling techniques, and precise suturing necessary.

For isolated strictures of the *penile urethra,* a subcoronal circumcising incision is preferable. This incision allows a vascularized island flap or a graft to be harvested from the penis easily and avoids suture lines over the urethral reconstruction. Most strictures of the penile urethra are inflammatory in origin—often iatrogenic from an indwelling urethral catheter. These strictures cannot be managed with the technique of excision and primary anastomosis, because that portion of the urethra cannot be widely mobilized without risking vascular compromise or chordee. The technique most commonly required will be a combination urethroplasty with excision of areas of full-thickness fibrosis of the corpus spongiosum and replacement with a vascularized island flap or a graft of penile skin or buccal or bladder mucosa.

A midline perineal incision is almost always adequate for more-proximal strictures. For *strictures of the bulb,* a midline incision is better than a circumcising one. Short strictures from fall-astride or straddle injuries occasionally can be managed by excision and primary anastomosis. The paucity of elastic length available in the pediatric urethra makes this technique not as useful as in the adult.

The goal of repair is the removal of all disordered tissue and its replacement with a tube of uniform caliber that tolerates being wet. Regardless of the etiology of the stricture or the type of repair chosen, all spongiofibrosis must be excised and, if possible, a strip of healthy urothelium reconstituted dorsally. Extensive mobilization of the urethra to bridge urethral defects risks vascular compromise of the corpus spongiosum or chordee. Urethral defects may be covered with an island flap or graft of penile skin or with buccal or bladder mucosa. Penile skin remains the optimal tissue for urethral replacement and should be used, even if penile coverage with flaps of scrotum is necessary. The scrotal rotation flap described by John Blandy is particularly useful here. In cases with extreme shortage of penile skin, I have had excellent success with the use of tissue expanders placed on the dorsum of the penis. The scrotum is a suboptimal source of tissue for urethral reconstruction. If a technically solid urethral reconstruction using tissue free of hair, scar, or inflammation is not possible, a staged repair should be undertaken without hesitation.

If a staged repair is necessary, closure should not be contemplated until *all* reaction and induration have subsided and the tissues are soft. If subcutaneous scarring is present or if the tissues to be used for the urethral reconstruction are redundant, irregular, or in any way unsatisfactory, an *interval revision* must be undertaken to correct these deficiencies.

Hematomas or fluid collections around a graft may spell failure. A compressive dressing is easily applied after repair of a stricture of the penile urethra, but it is difficult to apply an effective dressing for strictures of the penoscrotal junction or proximal urethra. In these situations, some form of wound drainage often is desirable. An effective drainage system, particularly after patch-graft urethroplasty, can be made in the operating suite from a butterfly needle and a vacuum blood-collection tube (page 558). This type of suction drain also can be obtained commercially. The tubes should be changed frequently and usually are left in place for no more than 48 hours. Balloon catheters, although generally effective in adults, often create

problems in the child. The balloon, when deflated, will be larger than the diameter of the catheter and form a ridge that may catch the edge of a graft and disrupt the integrity of a fresh anastomosis. The same fate will befall a repair if the catheter is dislodged inadvertently by the child or nursing personnel. It is best to use a straight catheter (silicone or soft plastic) that can be attached transvesically to the abdominal wall with a button. Removal of the catheter only requires cutting the suture beneath the button. Another advantage of this system is that an antegrade urethrogram can be performed without disturbing the catheter. When such a urethral stent is used, a suprapubic catheter also should be placed.

Perioperative antibiotics probably are not necessary in the child who has had an excision and primary anastomosis as the tissues used in the repair are extremely well vascularized. Antibiotics are mandatory for the child who has required a graft or vascularized flap. Broad-spectrum antibiotics that achieve high tissue concentration are needed.

END-TO-END ANASTOMOSIS

End-to-End Spatulated Anastomosis, Penile Urethra

Excision and anastomosis are used for severely fibrotic strictures and are preferable if the defect is not more than 1 cm in length in the pendulous urethra (to avoid shortening the penis with chordee). Because of the inelasticity of the urethra in children, only very short strictures are suitable.

Diluted methylene blue may be used to stain the diseased mucosa but will make the determination of viability of skin difficult if it spilled externally. Insert a sound to the level of the stricture, but do not push it through. Make a circumcising incision, and mobilize the skin of the shaft. A longitudinal incision, made slightly to one side of the midline, with its distal end just beyond the tip of the sound, is an alternative. Expose the urethra by dividing the spongy tissue. The urethral bulb is the most fixed area; it must be freed to obtain adequate length for anastomosis.

Insert a stay suture in the normal distal urethra, and incise it transversely just distal to the tip of the sound. In children, it may give better control to incise over the tip of the sound with a hooked #12 blade, making the incision longitudinally to expose the entire length of the stricture into normal urethra. Excise the strictured section. Examine the proximal and distal lumina to be certain all the spongiofibrosis has been removed. Spatulate the distal and proximal ends on opposite sides. Place two interrupted 5-0 monofilament synthetic absorbable sutures through all layers in the dorsal V cut, then continue to approximate the margins with similar stitches. Approximate as much of the subcutaneous tissue as possible, using fine interrupted sutures, and close the skin with a running 5-0 synthetic absorbable or chromic catgut subcuticular suture.

End-to-End Spatulated Anastomosis, Bulbar Urethra

Excision and anastomosis are used for severely fibrotic strictures of the bulbar urethra not more than 1.5 cm in length (to avoid shortening the penis and creating chordee).

Use the exaggerated lithotomy position. Make a vertical perineal incision, extending from the penoscrotal junction to within 3 cm of the anus. For more exposure, form it into an inverted Y. Incise the bulbocavernosus muscle in the midline, and retract it laterally to expose the bulb. Pass a van Buren sound into the urethra, against the stricture. Free the bulb laterally and posteriorly, keeping close to the corpora cavernosa ventrally. Palpate the sound, and cut directly down on it through the scar to reach the urethra. Incise the urethra sharply through the entire length of the stricture into normal tissue. Place several stay sutures on each side for traction and hemostasis of the spongy tissue. Calibrate the urethra proximally with a bougie à boule. Cut the bulb and urethra transversely, both proximal and distal to the stricture. Place hemostatic traction sutures in the proximal cut end. Incise the urethra distally on the dorsal (superficial) side well beyond the stricture. Do the same for the proximal urethra on the ventral (deep) side. Look carefully for gray urethra, indicating spongiofibrosis, which must be excised. At this time, consider leaving only a roof strip and covering the floor with a patch or pedicle graft. Place 5-0 monofilament synthetic absorbable sutures, first dorsally in the adventitia of the spongiosum, then in the mucosa circumferentially to obtain a watertight closure. Complete the closure of the adventitia. Finally, reattach the urethra to the corpora cavernosa and triangular ligaments. Insert a silicone catheter after the deep sutures are placed. Place enough additional sutures to close the bulb hemostatically. The catheter may be sewn to the abdominal wall over a button. Approximate the bulbocavernosus muscle, the dartos fascia, and the skin. Leave the catheter in place for 10 days or more. After the catheter has been out for a week, have the patient catheterize himself daily for the next month.

Commentary by Jacob Cukier

Nothing can better repair a urethral stenosis than the excision of the pathologic segment of the canal and an end-to-end suture. The dissection of the urethra is not easy in the distal part of the penis. Therefore, the best advice is to start the dissection far behind, at the penoscrotal angle, and to progress forward in the right dissection plane. After excision of the pathologic tissue, the rims should be split on the two opposing facets of the canal, so that the anastomosis will not be circular (but as large as possible), thus preventing further stenosis.

This extended dissection will allow enough tissue for a real end-to-end anastomosis without any free graft. In case a graft appears necessary, we would prefer a pedicle graft, not a free one. In our experience we have not seen any chordee.

AUGMENTED ROOF STRIP GRAFT

For dense strictures of the pendulous urethra, expose the urethra as previously described. The same procedure of end-to-end anastomosis but with different exposure, may be applied for bulbospongy strictures.

Open the urethra over the stricture, well into normal tissue. Mobilize the urethra, and discard all the spongiofibrosis. In excising the strictured segment, remove only the involved tissue. After thoroughly mobilizing the urethra well posteriorly, one will find infrequently that primary end-to-end anastomosis is not possible, because if too much is taken, chordee will occur with erection. In that case, proceed with application of a roof strip. Place 4-0

synthetic absorbable sutures in the distal inner periurethral tissue, and suture them to the corpora cavernosa for fixation. Complete the repair of the inner half of the urethra with interrupted 4-0 synthetic absorbable sutures. Insert a 5-ml silicone balloon catheter of a diameter suitable for the size of the child. Measure the remaining defect; secure and apply a defatted patch graft. Do not make the patch too large; it should fit snugly around a suitably sized sound—24 F in the adolescent. Replace the penile skin, and suture it with 4-0 synthetic absorbable sutures to the corona. Place an 18 F 5-ml silicone balloon catheter. Dress the wound, and remove the catheter in 8 to 10 days.

PATCH GRAFTS

Patch grafts are suitable for repair of defects surrounded by relatively healthy tissue.

Patch Graft, Bulbar Urethra

Boys can be placed in a frog-legged position as for perineal urethrostomy (page 350). Inject dilute methylene blue intraurethrally, but realize that the stain from the dye only demarcates the epithelial deficiency, not the extent of the spongiofibrosis that must be removed. A longitudinal incision is used for penile and midbulb strictures; for those more posterior, an inverted Y extension rarely is needed in children. Expose the bulbocavernosus muscle. Place a ring retractor. Incise the midline of the muscle, and expose the urethral or bulbar urethra. Insert a large, curved sound in the urethra to the level of the stricture. Place two stay sutures at that level. With a #12 blade or electrocautery, cut on top of the sound through the penile urethra or bulb into the lumen distal to the stricture. Split the entire stricture with scissors into normal urethra both proximally and distally. Test for adequate caliber with a bougie à boule (24 F in adolescents). Catch the full thickness of the edges in stay sutures looped over the retractor for hemostasis and exposure. Insert a catheter from the meatus to the bladder, choosing the maximum size suitable for the caliber of the urethra, because this will determine the width of the patch when it is inserted. Measure the length and width of the defect.

Outline a rectangular flap on the skin of the penis. This may be dorsal, ventral, or preputial. There generally is plenty of loose skin available. Excise a full-thickness free graft commensurate with the defect, and close the skin with fine chromic catgut. Place the graft upside down over the finger. In children, because of the small size, it is necessary to secure it on a board. Use 25-gauge needles inserted in a silicone block or double-faced dermatome tape stuck on the bottom of a sterile pan. Using a loupe, lift up the adventitial tissue with fine forceps, and trim it off with fine scissors. Leave the dermis, but take off all the tissue that is pink. Trim one end of the graft to fit (avoid overtrimming; the graft can be adjusted in situ). Alternatively, cut a template from a suture packet to fit. Avoid making the patch too large with subsequent sacculation. Lay the graft in place over the catheter with the epithelial side down. Place two interrupted 5-0 synthetic absorbable sutures at the apex of the defect (or use a double-armed suture). Start the suture from the raw side of the graft, then pass through the urethra and the inner layer of the corpus spongiosum. Place interrupted sutures successively down each side. By running sutures down either side, taking alternate stitches and trimming the graft as the suturing progresses, a tighter fit may be provided. Alternatively, place four 5-0 synthetic absorbable sutures (6-0 in infants) through the quadrants of the graft to hold the defect open. Start running a suture on either side from the apex, continuing down one side and the other, tying them to the quadrant sutures. This method may leave the graft too wide. Free the spongy tissue laterally, and suture it over the graft. When there is severe fibrosis in the spongy tissue, this cannot be done and one must depend on the muscle layer to vascularize the graft. Replace the catheter with a smaller silicone catheter (16 F in adolescents). Close the bulbocavernosus muscle with suitable synthetic absorbable sutures, followed by approximation of the Colles' fascia. Close the skin with a running subcuticular stitch of 4-0 or 5-0 synthetic absorbable suture. Leave no drain or, at most, a 16-gauge minivacuum system.

Tubed Patch Graft

Excision and tubed patch may be used for longer, dense strictures, but a vascular flap is preferable.

Proceed as described previously, but excise the entire defect, including all surrounding scar tissue and fistulous tracts. Anastomose the patch, usually obtained from the prepuce, at each end with interrupted fine synthetic absorbable sutures, and close it ventrally with a continuous suture.

Commentary by Antoine E. Khoury

This is a salvage procedure that should be part of the armamentarium of the reconstructive urologist but hope-fully will not have to be resorted to frequently. Whenever possible, it is obviously preferable to use a vascularized flap rather than a graft. On most occasions, one usually is able to obtain a flap for reconstruction of urethral defects, even when the patient has undergone previous penile surgery. Given sufficient time between procedures (1 year), skin that previously has been mobilized and transposed in the initial surgical procedure(s) will reestablish its blood supply and can be reused in the form of a flap. Rarely, a free skin graft will be required for urethral reconstruction. This can be harvested either from local penile skin or non–hair-bearing skin from a suitable donor site. On these occasions, the success of the procedure depends in part on how healthy the graft bed is, and the surgeon must ensure that conditions ideal for a graft take prevail.

In preparation for surgery, a simultaneous voiding and retrograde urethrogram is performed to outline the extent of the stricture and the most appropriate surgical approach. A pediatric fleet enema is administered the evening before surgery to prevent soiling and avoid the need for a bowel movement in the immediate postoperative period while the patient is on bed rest. Prophylactic intravenous antibiotics are given 1 hour preoperatively and repeated 8 hours postoperatively; the patient is then started on trimethoprim-sulfamethoxazole suppression until all drainage tubes are removed. The choice of suture material depends on the age and size of the patient; in younger children a 6-0 polyglycolic acid suture is used.

ISLAND FLAPS

Penile Island Flap

An island (or pedicle) flap is used for dense recurrent strictures of the pendulous and bulbar urethra. The flap can be tubularized, or if the local tissue has been damaged, applied as a two-stage procedure, involving preparing a bed at the first stage with a meshed split-thickness graft.

1 Incise the skin on one side of the midline on the ventral shaft.

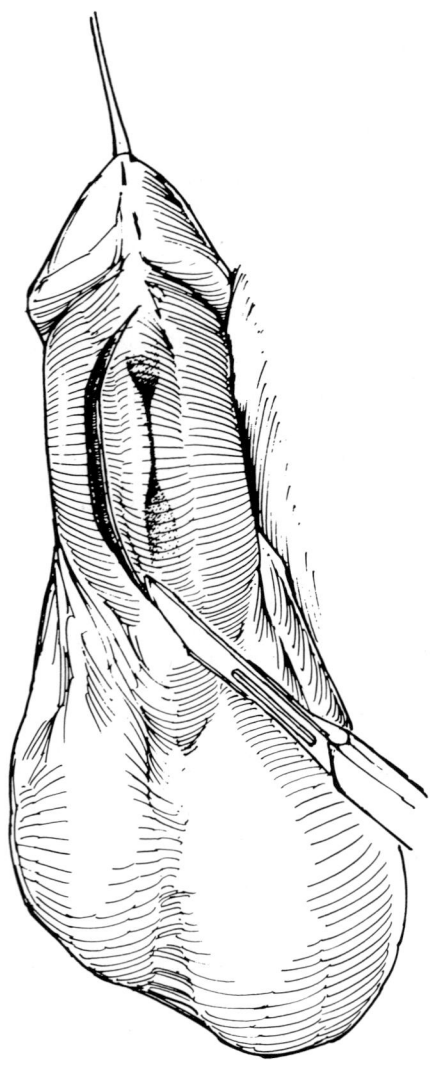

2 Incise the urethra throughout the stricture and at least 1.5 cm beyond. If necessary, the entire circumference of the urethra may be excised.

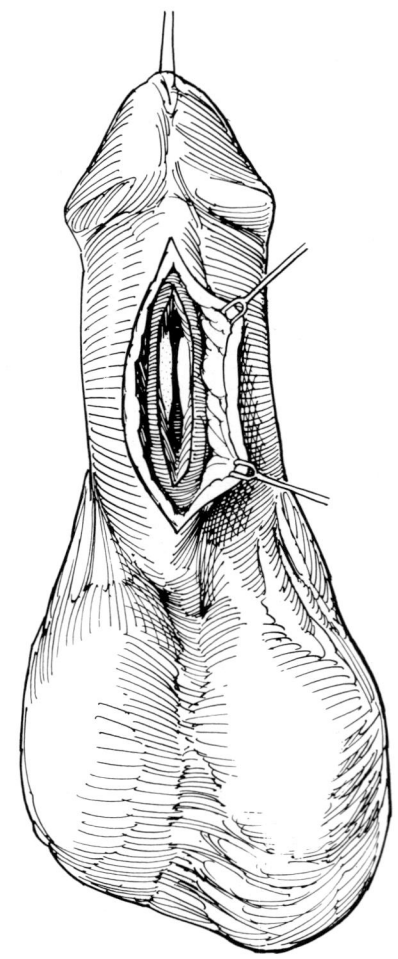

3 Carefully outline the proposed flap. Fulgurate any hair follicles within it. Incise the skin longitudinally on the opposite side of the penis at a distance equal to the width of the urethral defect. For long strictures, raise two separate flaps and combine them.

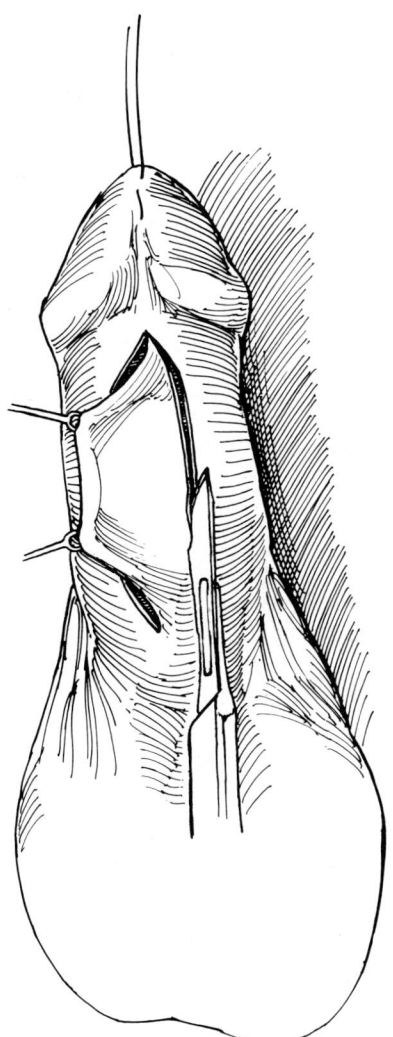

4 Mobilize the skin flap, but avoid undermining it. Too long a full-thickness flap that is not adequately perfused may result in chordee. Undermine the skin lateral to it to preserve as much of the subcutaneous tissue and fascia for the pedicle. If the entire circumference of the urethra has been excised, a wider flap may be taken and tubularized.

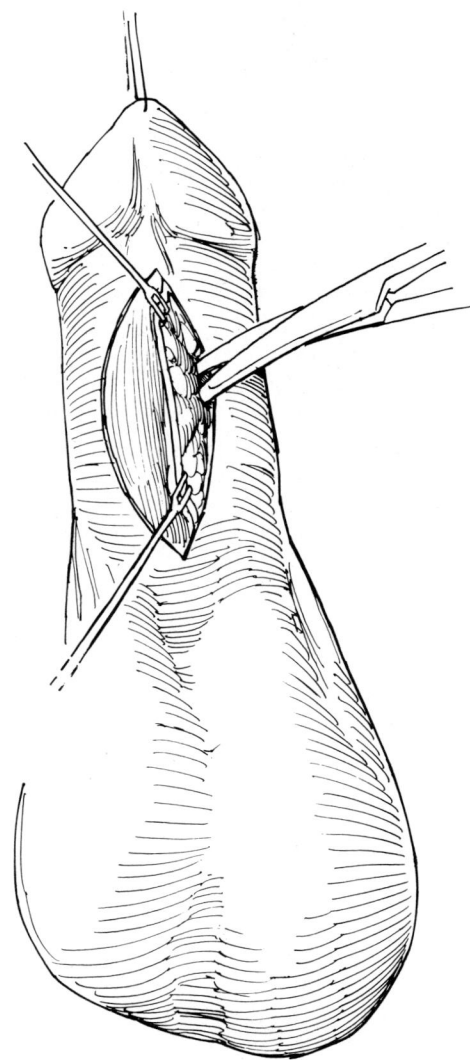

5 Suture the medial edge of the flap to the adjacent edge of the urethra (*i.e.*, right edge of flap to the left edge of the urethra) with an interrupted or running subcuticular 4-0 synthetic absorbable suture. Insert a 14 F silicone balloon catheter through the meatus and leave it indwelling.

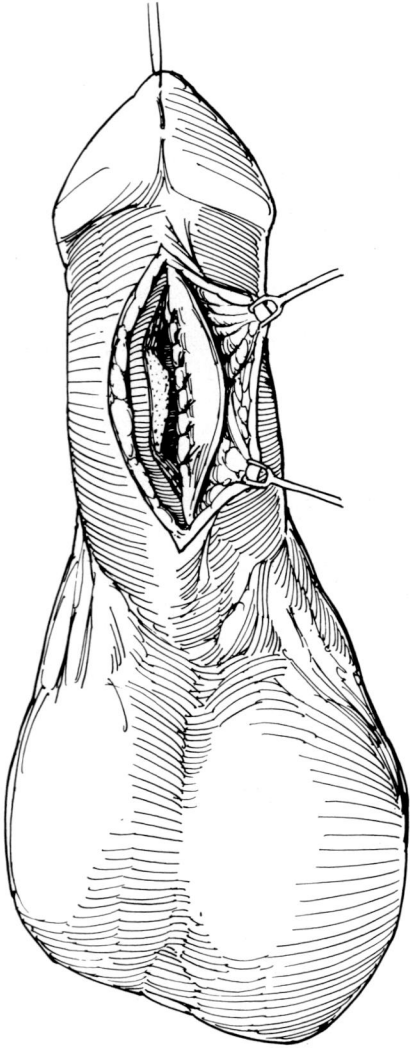

6 Invert the flap by suturing its lateral margin to the far side of the defect.

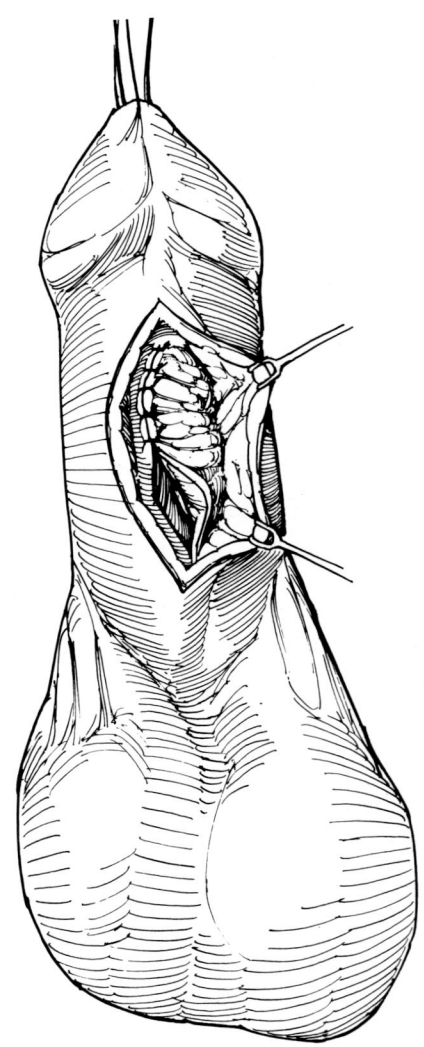

7 **A,** Close the skin with a subcuticular stitch of 4-0 synthetic absorbable suture. **B,** If tension is present, it is possible to make a dorsal relaxing incision, although this not recommended. Apply a suitable compression dressing. After 10 days, perform a voiding cystourethrogram with the stenting catheter in place. If there is no leakage, remove the stent.

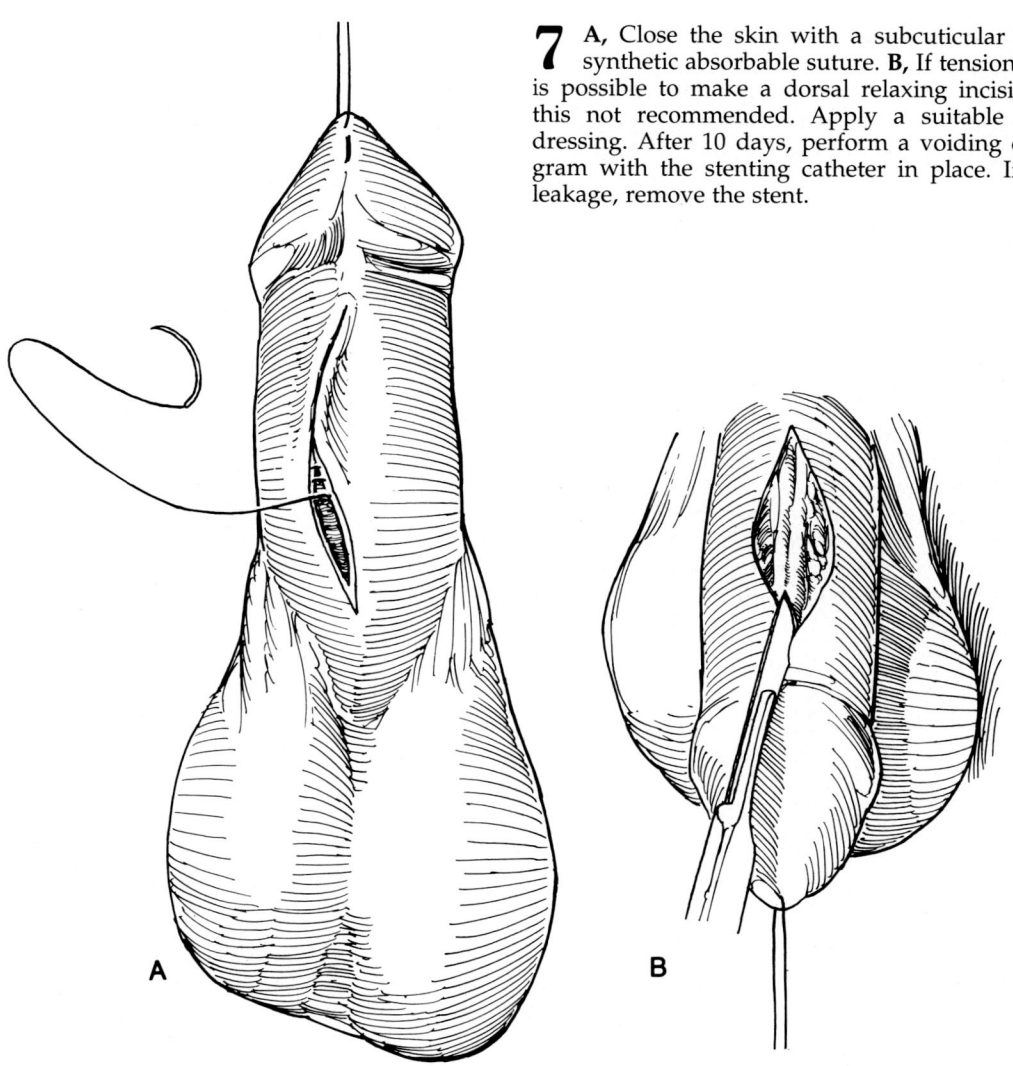

Commentary by Umesh B. Patil

Repair of urethral strictures in children is not always easy. The urethra usually is thin, and strictures are likely to be of full thickness. In circumcised patients, penile shafts do not always provide adequate skin flaps to repair a full-thickness stricture. In such patients, there is a need to look at alternative donor sites.

Hair-bearing skin is not advisable to use, even if hair follicles are fulgurated. Often, the hair follicles are not visible, even with optical magnification. The professional electrolysis therapists advise that to achieve satisfactory depilation, more than one attempt is required during an interval of 12 to 18 months. Midline scrotal skin, which bears minimal hair follicles, could, however, be used to cover the repaired site while adjacent penile shaft skin is used as a patch graft to correct the stricture.

More recently, in patients with paucity of penile skin, I have used bladder epithelium and buccal mucosa. A word of caution however: while using bladder epithelium as a tube graft, it is better to make the urethral tube snug to fit the appropriate size of the catheter rather than forming a redundant urethral tube. A urethral catheter is used for 10 to 12 days to permit complete healing of the suture site before permitting voiding through that tube. Sufficient buccal mucosa is not always available to make a tube, but it has a very useful role as a patch graft for incomplete urethral strictures. A suprapubic tube or perineal urethrostomy for urinary diversion is best avoided, except in infected strictures with fistula.

Preputial Island Fasciocutaneous Flap
(McANINCH)

Place the patient in extreme lithotomy position, protecting the legs from pressure points and avoiding stretching the sciatic nerve. Make a midline incision, and reflect the bulbospongiosus muscle. Expose the entire stricture through an incision in the corpus spongiosum, and incise the normal urethra for at least 1 cm. Pass a 30 F bougie to check the adequacy of the channel.

8 **A,** Mark two parallel incisions around the shaft, one at the coronal sulcus or circumcision line, and the other, 2 cm proximal for onlay procedures (2.5 cm for urethral replacement). Incise the distal incision through the dartos layer and Buck's fascia, avoiding the deeper layer containing the neurovascular bundle. Mobilize the penile skin back to the base. **B,** Replace the skin over the penis, and incise the proximal incision but only through the dartos fascia to preserve a pedicle based on Buck's fascia. Split the ring of skin in the midline ventrally.

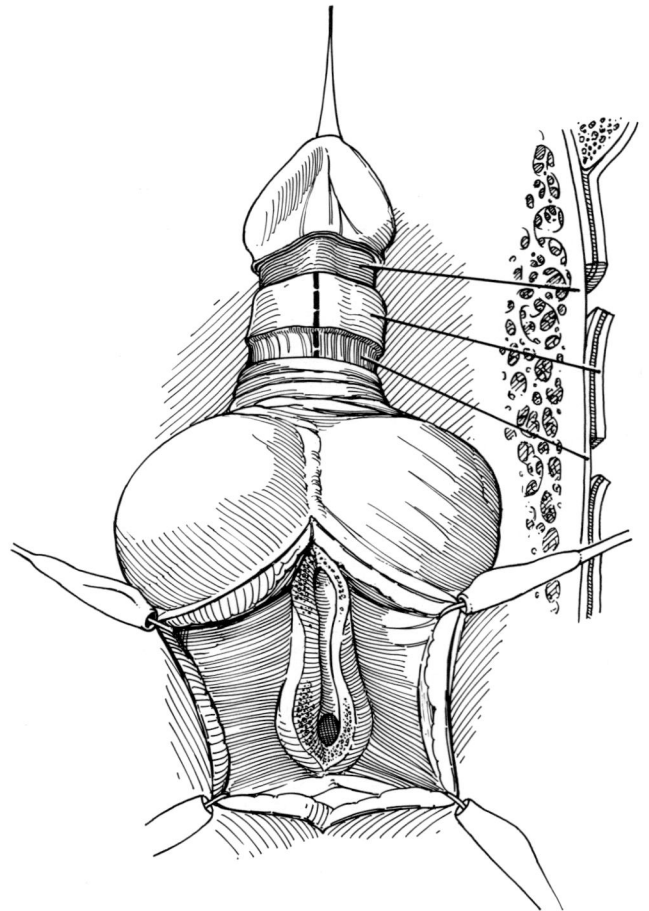

9 Raise the flap on a broad pedicle of Buck's fascia.

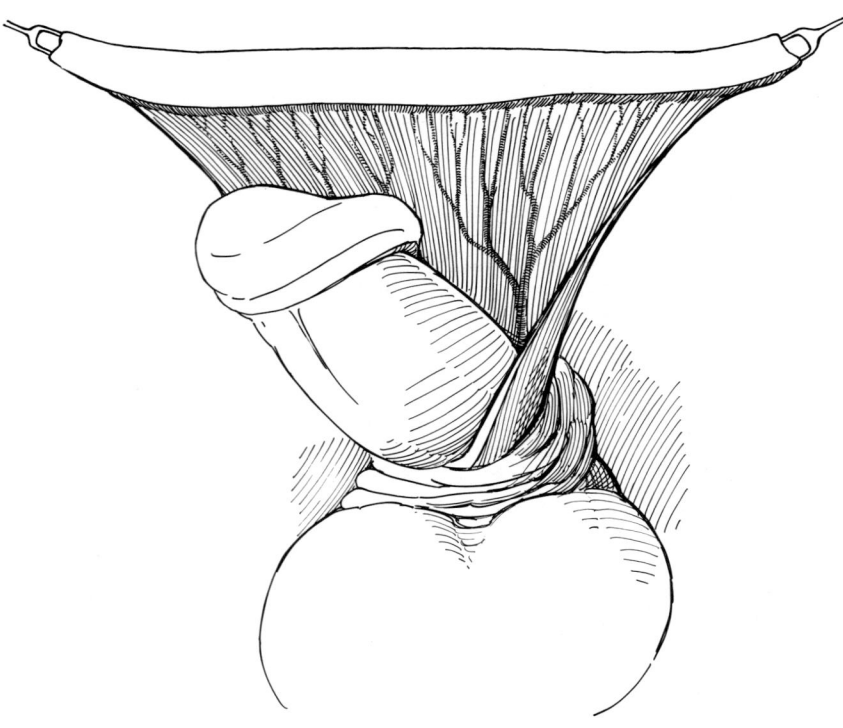

10 Create a subcutaneous tunnel into the perineal wound. Rotate the flap, and pass one end through the tunnel. If necessary, narrow the base distally to be certain that placement is skin-side down and without tension.

Begin suturing distally (or proximally) with 6-0 interrupted, or better, continuous monofilament polydioxanone sutures, first working on the one side from inside the flap and urethra. Insert a stenting catheter, and complete the closure of the other side from outside the lumen. Close the perineal wound.

Commentary by Jack W. McAninch

The flap is taken from the distal penis. In circumcised boys, this can be done safely, leaving sufficient penile shaft skin. When used as an onlay flap, approximately 13 to 15 cm of skin can be obtained in an adult. A complete tubularized urethral replacement of 8 to 10 cm can be done with this flap. The pedicle is quite substantial and well vascularized.

The skin of the distal penile shaft is free of hair—a great advantage over other genital skin. The flap is made adaptable to any anterior urethral stricture by freeing the base of the pedicle back to the level of the pubic bone before rotation into the perineum. (Care should be taken to avoid tension on the flap during rotation.) The circular configuration of the flap provides excellent cosmetic approximation of the distal penile skin after harvest. No residual tension or configuration deformity exists; the patient merely appears to have been circumcised.

The flap provides the opportunity to repair long complex anterior strictures in a single stage. A stenting 16 F catheter is left in place for 2 to 3 weeks.

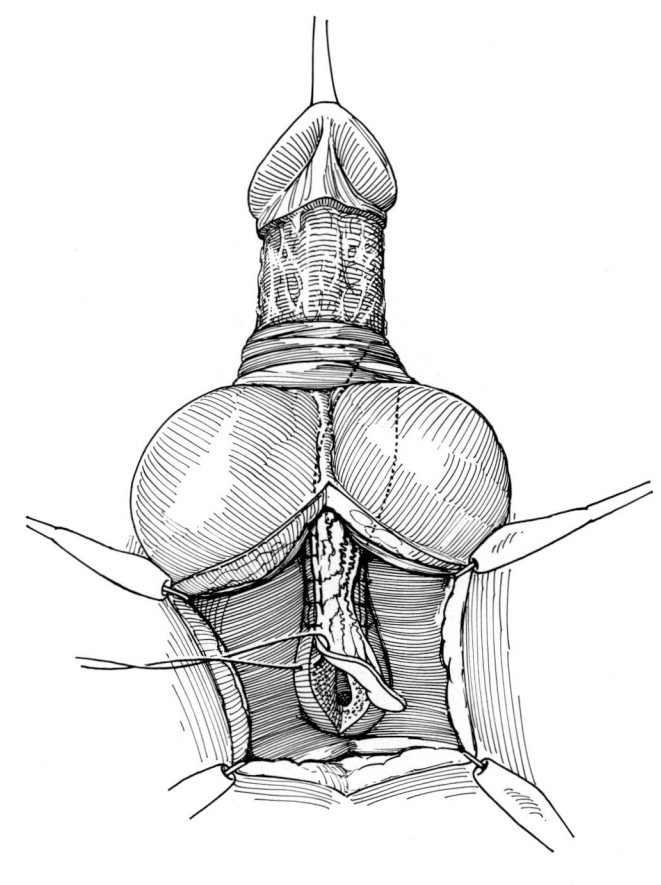

TWO-STAGE PROCEDURES

Meshed Graft
(SCHREITER)

An alternative for long strictures with considerable fibrous reaction is to remove the diseased urethra entirely, lay a split-thickness meshed skin graft in the defect, and pack it in place at a first stage, because not only must the diseased urethra be excised but a healthy bed must be provided for the graft or flap. After allowing healing for 2 months, roll the new skin into a tube over a 24 F catheter, or remove it and place a new graft or flap on the fresh tissue bed.

First Stage. For long strictures surrounded by considerable fibrous reaction, remove the diseased urethra entirely. Cut a split-thickness skin graft, and place it in a meshing dermatome with a meshing sheet having an expansion ratio of 1.5:1 or 2:1. Lay the graft in the defect, suture, and pack it in place. Be generous with the graft, and do not expand it; the principle purpose of the mesh is to provide drainage and encourage angiogenesis—not to allow use of less skin. The defect may be reduced in size by closing the scrotum transversely on either side in the first stage and later releasing it to help cover the new graft.

Second Stage. After allowing healing for 2 months, raise two parallel flaps, being careful not to undermine the new skin during mobilization. Trim it exactly to size, especially in the scrotal area. Approximate the skin edges over a 24 F catheter to form a tube. Alternatively, remove all the new skin from the surface, and place a new graft or flap on the fresh base.

Alternative Methods. If there is enough adjacent penile skin, the defect left by excising the urethra can be closed at a first stage and a tube subsequently formed from the new ventral skin.

At the first stage, excise the diseased urethra through a vertical skin incision. Anastomose the healthy urethral ends to the skin, and complete the vertical closure with penile skin from either side. At the second stage, mobilize the skin edges laterally to form a tube. Close the urethral tube with a running subcuticular 4-0 synthetic absorbable suture. Cover it with available subcutaneous tissue, and close the skin with a similar suture.

Alternatively, merely open the diseased urethra at a first stage, tacking the skin edges to the urethral strip. At a second stage, make parallel incisions in the penile skin to make covering flaps (Johanson, 1953).

CHAPTER 140

Bulbomembranous Urethral Strictures

Urethral injury due to pelvic fracture frequently results in a bulbomembranous urethral distraction defect that poses difficult problems for the urologist; repair should be undertaken only by those with continuous experience.

Synchronous cystourethrography is essential to detect fistulous tracts and false passages. Failure to demonstrate the prostatic urethra by antegrade filling is reassuring evidence of bladder neck competence (unless it too is stenotic after the injury). A patulous bladder neck shows that it is intrinsically damaged or that it is tethered by an extensive retropubic fibrosis left by the hematoma. Cystometrography will detect neurogenic bladder. The length of the actual defect may be gauged by cystourethrography and ultrasonography, or better, by magnetic resonance imaging, but the extent of the local fibrosis only can be judged at operation, so that extrapolation from the radiographs is potentially misleading. For this reason, the surgeon must make contingency plans for an extended procedure.

Several treatment options are available. Simple dilatation, especially if done early, may lead to a false passage. Internal urethrotomy should be reserved for strictures distal to the membranous urethra. Endoscopic incisions through a completely obliterated posterior urethra, guided by an intravesical light or a guide wire, may cause further damage to the remaining sphincteric function but have been effective in selected cases. Substitution procedures with free patches or pedicle flaps carry a greater risk of failure than anastomotic techniques, except in some cases of bulbar injury. Anastomotic repair is preferable to any of these methods, provided that the bulbar spongy urethra and the prostatic urethra are uninvolved.

Certain principles must be followed: all the periurethral and retropubic fibrosis with accompanying infected pockets must be meticulously excised, and the bulbar urethra must be well mobilized to allow an anastomosis free of tension on its healthy spatulated end joining the prostate. The anastomosis must be done with perfect technique, and any residual dead space left after removing the fibrous tissue must be filled with omentum. After fracture of the pelvis, have both the retropubic and perineal routes available, but work mostly from above. This combined approach also allows mobilization of the omentum.

The timing of the repair depends on the size of the hematoma; for small lesions, 3 months may be suffi-

cient. For a large one, it may take a year for resolution, even if treated only by suprapubic urinary drainage.

Several operative approaches can be used: perineal, transpubic, or a combination of the two, using the abdominoperineal position to provide abdominal access should the retropubic fibrosis be excessive.

For complex strictures, the procedure must combine exploration and excision with repair. Turner-Warwick has devised an approach in which the findings and accomplishments at each step lead to the next one. The elements are as follows: (1) placing the patient in the abdominoperineal position for access to both areas; (2) mobilizing the bulbar urethra and excising the scar tissue about the distal stricture perineally; (3) resecting the retropubic fibrosis suprapubically; (4) removing retropubic fibrosis by partial pubic resection; (5) examining the bladder neck directly by cystotomy; (6) repairing the urethra with a spatulated bulboprostatic anastomosis; (7) rerouting the urethra by total pubectomy if a tension-free anastomosis is not possible; (8) diverting and stenting by suprapubic catheter and fenestrated urethral catheter; (9) placing an omental graft; and (10) performing additional procedures, such as excising rectal fistulas, freeing the bladder neck for sphincteroplasty, and repairing more anterior urethral strictures.

END-TO-END ANASTOMOSIS

Defer operation until local tissue reaction has subsided (at least 3 months and as long as 8 months). Estimate the apparent extent of the stricture by simultaneous voiding cystography and retrograde urethrography. Accurate evaluation must wait for exposure and inspection of the quality of the periurethral tissue. Excision and anastomosis can then proceed.

PATCH-GRAFT URETHROPLASTY

A patch graft or a pedicle flap may be applied to the defect after excision of the scarred urethra.

PERINEAL REPAIR
(WEBSTER)

A one-stage procedure for deep obliterative defects can be divided into successive steps designed to facilitate the anastomosis, with the surgeon proceeding to the next step as the dissection develops. The operation starts with urethral mobilization. For more urethral length, the corporal bodies are separated. Then, a wedge may be resected from the inferior pubic ramus. For still greater length, the urethra is routed around one of the crura. It rarely is necessary to perform an abdominoperineal approach for these cases.

Commentary by George D. Webster

Injuries to the posterior urethra at the time of pelvic fracture may be partial or complete. The former may heal with relatively minor stricturing that may respond to dilatation or urethrotomy. However, complete disruption generally results in a distraction defect of varying length. Initial management of such injuries generally is by suprapubic catheter drainage, elective delayed repair being performed 3 or more months later. Although in adults and postpubertal boys, the site of injury is invariably at the bulbomembranous or prostatomembranous urethra; in prepubertal boys, the injury may occur in the prostatic urethra or even at the bladder neck.

This author has found a perineal anastomotic repair to be appropriate for the vast majority of such posterior urethral distraction defects, regardless of length. The absolute prerequisite for such repair is that the anterior urethra be healthy, because the mobilized urethra must survive as a distally based flap once it has been circumferentially dissected as far as the suspensory ligament of the penis. The four steps described in the earlier text to facilitate a tension-free bulboprostatic anastomosis are performed sequentially, if necessary. It is this author's experience that in peripubertal boys requiring such repairs, it is more likely that all steps will be required to accomplish anastomosis. This probably is because of the fact that in this age group, the bulbar urethra, the most elastic portion of the urethra, still is poorly developed. Exquisite care must be taken in dissecting the small urethra circumferentially to ensure its survival as a flap.

Although in the abdominoperineal transpubic approach to such problems, considerable retropubic scar excision was required, this has not proven to be necessary using this progressive perineal approach. In fact, the perineal scar is

incised vertically in the midline onto the tip of the descending urethral sound, and only a very small amount of adjacent scar is excised, sufficient to allow good visibility of the patent spatulated prostatomembranous urethra. This limited dissection avoids any further injury to nerves that may be important in erection.

It is important in performing the anastomosis itself that all of the radial sutures be placed first and tied later. We commence with placement of the dorsal 12 o'clock–position suture, and then place sutures sequentially around the anastomosis in a clockwise fashion. Sutures are then all tied in the order in which they are placed, and the stenting catheter is inserted thereafter.

Indications for Alternate Approaches. If the anterior urethra is strictured or injured, the urethra cannot be mobilized as a flap, as described previously, and this is a probable indication for a substitution urethroplasty. One-stage substitution urethroplasty using pedicled islands of penile skin is appropriate in some cases; however, in the pediatric age group, availability of sufficient penile skin and ability to mobilize penile islands on a pedicle to the perineum is fraught with difficulty. Hence, in these rare instances, a staged urethroplasty probably is appropriate. These cases are exceptionally uncommon, however.

In patients with bulbomembranous urethral disruption in whom there are complicating features such as periurethral or pelvic floor cavity communication with the urethra, rectourethral fistulae, bladder base fistula, and so forth, the abdominoperineal approach is likely to be required. This will allow the additional pathology to be managed. It also allows for omental pedicle support of the repair. After such injuries to the posterior urethra, continence requires a functional bladder neck. In some cases, the preoperative cystogram may show bladder neck incompetence, suggesting that continence may be compromised after the posterior urethra has been repaired. In some cases, this too is an indication for an abdominoperineal approach, because it gives an opportunity for lysis of the bladder neck from dense retropubic scar, which may be fixing the sphincter in the open position. Additionally, sphincteroplasty may be performed. However, it has been our experience that perineal posterior urethroplasty, even in the face of some bladder neck incompetence, is not necessarily followed by postoperative incontinence. Hence, it is our practice to complete the urethroplasty and only intervene suprapubically at a second procedure, if incontinence demands it.

REFERENCES

Section 1—Preparation for Pediatric Operations

Adamson RJ, Musco F, Enquist IF: The clinical dimensions of a healing incision. *Surg Gynecol Obstet* 123:515, 1966.

Adzick NS, Harrison MR, Glick PL, *et al.*: Comparison of fetal, newborn and adult wound healing by histologic, enzyme-histochemical, and hydroxyproline determinations. *J Pediatr Surg* 20:315, 1985.

Adzick NS, Lonaker MT: The biology of fetal wound healing: a review. *Plast Reconstr Surg* 87:788, 1991.

Adzick NS, Lonaker MT (Eds): *Fetal Wound Healing*. New York, Elsevier Scientific Publishing, 1992.

Allen L: Lymphatics and lymphoid tissues. *Annu Rev Physiol* 29:197, 1967.

Anson BJ, McVay CB: *Surgical Anatomy*, 6th ed. Philadelphia, W. B. Saunders Company, 1984.

Arey LB: *Developmental Anatomy*. Philadelphia, W. B. Saunders Company, 1974.

Baker BH, Borchardt KA: Sump drains and airborne bacteria as a cause of wound infections. *J Surg Res* 17:407, 1974.

Balinsky BI, Fabian BC: *An Introduction to Embryology*, 5th ed. Philadelphia, W. B. Saunders Company, 1981.

Bloch EC: Anesthetic considerations in the neonate. In: King LR (Ed): *Urologic Surgery in Neonates and Young Infants*. Philadelphia, W. B. Saunders Company, 1988, p 119.

Bo WJ, Meschan I, Krueger WA: *Basic Atlas of Cross-Sectional Anatomy*. Philadelphia, W. B. Saunders Company, 1980.

Borges AF: *Electrical Incisions and Scar Revision*. Boston, Little, Brown & Company, 1973.

Britt BA: Malignant hyperthermia. *Can Anaesth Soc J* 32:666, 1985.

Broman I: *Normale und Abnormale Entwicklung des Menschen*, Wiesbaden, J.F. Bergman, 1911.

Burns RK: Urogenital system. In: Willier BH, *et al.* (Eds): *Analysis of Development*. Philadelphia, W. B. Saunders Company, 1955, pp 462.

Cain M, Bennett AH: Antibiotic prophylaxis in open urologic surgery. *Infect Urol* March–April, 1991.

Carlson BM: *Patten's Foundations of Embryology*, 5th ed. New York, McGraw-Hill Book Company, 1988.

Cassady JF Jr: Regional anesthesia for urologic procedures. *Urol Clin North Am* 14:43, 1987.

Crafts RC: Abdominopelvic cavity and perineum. In: Crafts RC (Ed): *A Textbook of Human Anatomy*, 2nd ed. New York, John Wiley & Sons, 1979, pp 269–327.

Craig PH, *et al.*: A biological comparison of polyglactin 910 and polyglycolic acid synthetic absorbable sutures. *Surg Gynecol Obstet* 141:1, 1975.

Crouch JE: The urinary system. In: Crouch JE (Ed): *Functional Human Anatomy*, 2nd ed. Philadelphia, Lea & Febiger, 1972, pp 424–429.

Crouch JE: The reproductive system. In: Crouch JE (Ed): *Functional Human Anatomy*, 2nd ed. Philadelphia, Lea & Febiger, 1972, pp 430–435.

Davis AT: Postoperative infection in surgical patients. In: Raffensperger JG (Ed): *Swenson's Pediatric Surgery*, 5th ed. Norwalk, Appleton and Lange, 1990, p 29.

Deutinger J, Bartl W, Pfersmann C, *et al.*: Fetal kidney volume and urine production in cases of fetal growth retardation. *J Perinat Med* 15:307, 1987.

Dineen P: *The Surgical Wound*. Philadelphia, Lea & Febiger, 1981.

Elias H, Pauly JE, Bruns ER: Reproductive system. In: Elias H, *et al.* (Eds): *Histology and Human Microanatomy*, 4th ed. New York, John Wiley & Sons, 1978, p 475.

England MA: *Color Atlas of Life Before Birth*. Chicago, Year Book Medical Publishers, 1983.

Engle WD: Development of fetal and neonatal renal function. *Semin Perinatol* 10:113, 1986.

Felix W: The development of the urinogenital organs. In: Keibel F, Mall FP (Eds): *Manual of Human Embryology*, vol 2. Philadelphia, J. B. Lippincott Company, pp 1910–1912.

Gosling JA, Dixon JS, Humpherson JR: *Functional Anatomy of the Urinary Tract*. Baltimore, University Park Press, 1982.

Gray SW, Skandalakis JE: *Embryology for Surgeons. The Embryological Basis for the Treatment of Congenital Defects*. Philadelphia, W. B. Saunders Company, 1972.

Gregory GA: *Pediatric Anesthesia*. New York, Churchill Livingstone, 1983.

Hatch DJ: *Neonatal Anesthesia*. Chicago, Year Book Medical Publishers, 1981.

Horne B, Reynolds M: Respiratory support. In Raffensperger JG (Ed): *Swenson's Pediatric Surgery*, 5th ed. Norwalk, Appleton and Lange, 1990, p 91.

Jirásek JE: *Development of the Genital System and Male Pseudohermaphroditism*. Baltimore, Johns Hopkins Press, 1971.

Jirásek JE: Morphogenesis of the genital system in the human. In: Blandau RJ, Bergsma D (Eds). *Birth Defects: Original Article Series*. New York, Alan R. Liss, Inc, 13:13, 1977.

Jirásek JE: *Atlas of Human Prenatal Morphogenesis*. Boston, Martinus Nijhoff Publishers, 1983.

Jones SEF, Smith BAC: Anesthesia for pediatric day-surgery. *J Pediatr Surg* 15:31, 1980.

Karp G, Berrill NJ: *Development*, 2nd ed. New York, McGraw-Hill Book Company, 1981.

Keibel F, Mall FP: *Manual of Human Embryology*. Philadelphia, J. B. Lippincott Company, 1910–1912.

Keibel F: Zur die Entwicklungsgeschichte des menschlichen Urogenitalapparates. *Arch Anat* 55:157, 1896.

Keith A: *Human Embryology and Morphology*, 4th ed. London, E. Arnold, 1921.

Keith L, Moore P: *L'etre humain en développment*. Quebec, Vigot, 1974.

Koritké JG, Sick H: *Atlas of Sectional Human Anatomy*. Baltimore, Urban and Schwarzenberg, 1988.

Langer CP: Zur Anatomie und Physiologie der Haut. *Sitzungsb Acad Wissensch* 45:223, 1861.

Larsen EH, Gasser TC, Madsen PO: Antimicrobial prophylaxis in urological surgery. *Urol Clin North Am* 13:591, 1986.

Luck SR: Nutrition and metabolism. In: Raffensperger JG (Ed): *Swenson's Pediatric Surgery*, 5th ed. Norwalk, Appleton and Lange, 1990, p 81.

Luck SR: Preoperative evaluation and preparation. In: Raffensperger JG (Ed): *Swenson's Pediatric Surgery*, 5th ed: Norwalk, Appleton and Lange, 1990, p 7.

Moore KL: *The Developing Human: Clinically Oriented Embryology*, 2nd ed. Philadelphia, W. B. Saunders Company, 1977.

Muecke EC: The embryology of the urinary system. In: Harrison JH, Gittes RF, Perlmutter AD, *et al.* (Eds):

Campbell's Urology. Philadelphia, W. B. Saunders Company, 1979, p 1286.

Page CP, Bohnen JMA, Fletcher JR, *et al.*: Antimicrobial prophylaxis for surgical wounds: guidelines for clinical care. *Arch Surg* 128:79, 1993.

Parrott TS, Woodard JR: Urologic surgery in the neonate. *J Urol* 116:506, 1976.

Pollack SV: Wound healing: a review. *J Dermatol Surg Oncol* 8:667, 1982.

Prentiss CW: *A Laboratory Manual and Textbook of Embryology.* Philadelphia and London, W. B. Saunders Company, 1915.

Raffensperger JG: Fluid and electrolytes. In: Raffensperger JG (Ed): *Swenson's Pediatric Surgery,* 5th ed. Norwalk, Appleton and Lange, 1990, p 73.

Risau W, Ekblom P: Growth factors and the embryonic kidney. *Prog Clin Biol Res* 226:147, 1986.

Root B, Loveland JP: Pediatric premedication with diazepam or hydroxyzine: oral versus intramuscular route. *Anesth Analg* 52:717, 1973.

Roth DM, Macksood MJ, Perlmutter AD: Outpatient surgery in pediatric urology. *J Urol* 135:104, 1986.

Ryan JF: *A Practice of Anesthesia for Infants and Children.* Orlando, Grune & Stratton, Inc., 1986.

Sagi J, Vagman I, David MP, *et al.*: Fetal kidney size related to gestational age. *Gynecol Obstet Invest* 23:1, 1987.

Sariola H, Holm K, Henke-Fahle S: Early innervation of the metanephric kidney. Development 104:589, 1988.

Scanton JW (Ed): *Perinatal Anesthesia.* Boston, Blackwell Scientific Publications, 1985.

Seleny FL, Luck SR: Care of the child in the operating room. In: Raffensperger JG (Ed): *Swenson's Pediatric Surgery,* 5th ed. Norwalk, Appleton and Lange, 1990, p 17.

Shepard B, Hensle TW, Burbige KA, *et al.*: Outpatient surgery in pediatric urology patient. *Urology* 24:581, 1984.

Shikinami J: *Contributions to Embryology,* No. 93, Carnegie Inst. Publicat. 363, 1926.

Smith DW: *Recognizable Patterns of Human Malformation.* Philadelphia, W. B. Saunders Company, 1970.

Stephens FD: *Congenital Malformations of the Urinary Tract.* New York, Praeger Publishers, 1983.

Stockman JA III: Hematologic evaluations. In: Raffensperger JG (Ed): *Swenson's Pediatric Surgery,* 5th ed. Norwalk, Appleton and Lange, 1990, p 37.

Tuggle DW, Hoelzer DJ, Tunell WP, Smith EI: The safety and cost-effectiveness of polyethylene glycol electrolyte solution bowel preparation in infants and children. *J Pediatr Surg* 22:513, 1987.

Vaughan ED Jr, Middleton GW: Pertinent genitourinary embryology. Review for the practising urologist. *Urology* 6:139, 1975.

von Bardenleben K: *Handbuch der Anatomie des Menschen.* Jena, Fischer, 1911.

Waterman RE: Human embryo and fetus. In: Hafez ESE, Kenemans P (Eds): *Atlas of Human Reproduction by Scanning Electron Microscopy.* Hingham, MTP Press, 1982, p 261.

Wishnow KI, Johnson DE, Babaian RJ, *et al.*: Effective outpatient use of polyethylene glycol-electrolyte bowel preparation for radical cystectomy and ileal conduit urinary diversion. *Urology* 31:7, 1988.

Section 2—Operating on Neonates, Infants, and Children

Andriole GL, Bettmann MA, Garnick MB, Richie JP: Indwelling double-J ureteral stents for temporary and permanent urinary drainage: experience with 87 patients. *J Urol* 131:239, 1984.

Banowsky LH: Basic microvascular techniques and principles. *Urology* 23:495, 1984.

Barham RE, Butz GW, Ansell JS: Comparison of wound strength in normal, radiated and infected tissue closed with polyglycolic and chromic catgut sutures. *Surg Gynecol Obstet* 146:901, 1978.

Barnes RW: Surgical handicraft: teaching and learning surgical skills. *Am J Surg* 153:422, 1987.

Bartone FF, Shires TK: The reaction of kidney and bladder tissue to catgut and reconstituted collagen sutures. *Surg Gynecol Obstet* 128:1221, 1969.

Bartone FF, Stinson W: Reaction of the urinary tract to polypropylene sutures. *Invest Urol* 14:44, 1976.

Baum NH, Brin E: Use of double-J catheter in pyeloplasty. *Urology* 20:634, 1982.

Bevan, PG: The craft of surgery: the anastomosis workshop. *Ann R Coll Surg Engl* 63:405, 1981.

Blandy J: *Operative Urology,* 2nd ed. Oxford, Blackwell Scientific Publications, 1986.

Borges AF, Alexander SE: Relaxed skin tension lines, Z-plasties on scars and fusiform excision of lesions. *Br J Plast Surg* 15:242, 1962.

Borges AF: *Electrical Incisions and Scar Revision.* Boston, Little, Brown & Company, 1973.

Brigden RJ: *Operating Theatre Technique.* Edinburgh, London, New York, Churchill Livingstone, 1980.

Burow CA: *Beschreibung einer neuen Transplantations-methode (Methode der Seitlichen Dreiecke)-zum Wiedersatz Verlorengegangener.* Theile des Gesichts, Berlin, Nauck, 1855.

Case GD, Glenn JE, Postlethwait RW: Comparison of absorbable sutures in urinary bladder. *Urology* 7:165, 1976.

Cassady JF Jr: Regional anesthesia for urologic procedures. *Urol Clin North Am* 14:43, 1987.

Chaffin RC: Drainage. *Am J Surg* 24:100, 1934.

Chu CC, Williams DF: Effects of physical configuration and chemical structure of suture material on bacterial absorption. *Am J Surg* 147:197, 1984.

Clark P: *Operations in Urology.* Edinburgh, Churchill Livingstone, 1985.

Clark WR, Furlow W: Use of a balanced bowel preparation solution in urological surgery. *J Urol* 137:455, 1987.

Cockett ATK, Koshiba K: *Manual of Urologic Surgery.* Berlin, Springer-Verlag, 1979.

Cohn I Jr, Dennis C: Segmental resection of the small intestine and "aseptic" end-to-end anastomosis. In: Madden JL (Ed): *Atlas of Technics in Surgery,* 2nd ed. New York, Appleton-Century-Crofts, 1964.

JL Grossfeld (Ed): *Common Problems in Pediatric Surgery.* St. Louis, Mosby Year Book, 1991.

Culp DA, Fallon B, Loening SAH: *Surgical Urology,* 5th ed. Chicago, Year Book Medical Publishers, 1985.

Daniel RK, Taylor GI: Distant transfer of an island flap by microvascular anastomoses: a clinical technique. *Plast Reconstr Surg* 52:111, 1973.

Daniel RK, Williams HB: The free transfer of skin flaps by microvascular anastomosis: an experimental study and reappraisal. *Plast Reconstr Surg* 52:16, 1973.

Davis DM: The process of ureteral repair: a recapitulation of the splinting question. *Trans Am Assoc Genitourin Surg* 49:71, 1959.

DeHoll D, Rodeheaver G, Edgerton MT, Edlich RF: Potentiation of infection by suture closure of dead space. *Am J Surg* 127:716, 1974.

Douglas DW: Tensile strength of sutures. *Lancet* 2:497, 1949.

Eckstein H, Hohenfellner R, Williams DI (Eds): *Surgical Pediatric Urology.* Stuttgart, Thieme, 1977.

Edlich RF, Panek PH, Rodeheaver GT, *et al.*: Physical and chemical configuration of sutures in the development of surgical infection. *Ann Surg* 177:679, 1973.

El-Mahrouky A, McElhaney J, Bartone FF, King L: In vitro comparison of the properties of polydioxanone, polyglycolic acid and catgut sutures in sterile and infected urine. *J Urol* 138:913, 1987.

Everett WG: Suture materials in general surgery. *Prog Surg* 8:14, 1970.

Finney RP: Experience with new double-J ureteral catheter stent. J Urol 120:678, 1978.

Finney RP: Double-J and diversion stents. *Urol Clin North Am* 9:89, 1982.

Fowler JE: *Methods of Urologic Surgery.* Chicago, Van Tec Inc, 1987.

Frank JD, Johnston JH: *Operative Pediatric Urology,* Edinburgh, Churchill Livingstone, 1990.

Gambee LP: A single-layer intestinal anastomosis applicable to the small as well as the large intestine. *West J Surg Obstet Gynecol* 59:1, 1951.

Ger R, Duboys E: The prevention and repair of large abdominal-wall defects by muscle transposition: a preliminary communication. *Plast Reconstr Surg* 72:170, 1983.

Gillenwater JY, Grayhack JT, Howards SS, Duckett JW (Eds): *Adult and Pediatric Urology.* Chicago, Year Book Medical Publishers, 1987.

Glenn JF (Ed): *Urologic Surgery,* 3rd ed. Philadelphia, Toronto, J. B. Lippincott Company, 1983.

Grabb WC, Smith JW: *Plastic Surgery.* Boston, Little, Brown & Company, 1979.

Hastings JL: The effect of suture materials on healing wounds of the bladder. *Surg Gynecol Obstet* 140:933, 1975.

Hastings JC, Van Winkle H Jr, Barker E, *et al.*: Effect of suture materials on healing wounds of the stomach and colon. *Surg Gynecol Obstet* 140:701, 1975.

Herrmann JB: Tensile strength and knot security of surgical suture materials. *Am J Surg* 37:209, 1971.

Hinman F Jr: Accurate placement of the Penrose drain. *Surg Gynecol Obstet* 102:497, 1956.

Hinman F Jr: Ureteral repair and the splint. *J Urol* 78:376, 1957.

Hinman F Jr: Scalpel for operations on patients possibly infected with human immunodeficiency virus. *Urology* 32:350, 1988.

Hinman F Jr: Differential diagnosis of flank pain. In: Tanagho EA (Guest Ed): *Pain of Genitourinary Origin. Problems in Urology,* Vol 3, No 2. Philadelphia: J. B. Lippincott Company, 1989, p 182.

Hinman F Jr: Sources of pain. In: Tanagho EA (Guest Ed): *Pain of Genitourinary Origin. Problems in Urology,* Vol 3, No 2. Philadelphia: J. B. Lippincott Company, 1989, p 179.

Hinman F Jr: Subspecialization and general urology. *J Urol* 141:482, 1989.

Hinman F Jr: Bowel closure techniques: small bowel. Part I. *AUA Update Series,* vol IX, Lesson 35, 1990, p 274.

Hinman F Jr: Bowel closure techniques: large bowel. Part II. *AUA Update Series,* vol IX, Lesson 36, 1990, p 282.

Hirsh RA: An approach to assessing perioperative risk. In: Goldmann DR, Brown FH, Levy WK, *et al.* (Eds): *Medical Care of the Surgical Patient.* Philadelphia, J. B. Lippincott Company, 1982, p 31.

Holliday MA, Segar WE: Parenteral fluid therapy. *Pediatrics* 19:823, 1957.

Howes EL: Immediate strength of sutured wound. *Surgery* 7:24, 1940.

Howes EL: Strength studies of polyglycolic acid versus catgut sutures of the same size. *Surg Gynecol Obstet* 137:15, 1973.

Hunt TK: *Wound Healing and Wound Infection: Theory and Surgical Practice.* New York, Appleton-Century-Crofts, 1980.

Jackson FE, Fleming PM: Jackson Pratt brain drain. *Int Surg* 57:658, 1972.

Jacobson JH II, Suarez EL: Microsurgery in anastomosis of small vessels. *Surgical Forum, Am Coll Surg* 11:243, 1960.

Jarowenko MV, Bennett AH: Use of single-J urinary diversion stents in intestinal urinary diversion. *Urology* 22:369, 1983.

Johnson DE, Fuerst DE: Use of auto suture for construction of ileal conduits. *J Urol* 109:821, 1973.

Jones PA, Moxon RA, Pittman MR, Edwards L: Double-ended pigtail polyethylene stents in the management of benign and malignant ureteral obstruction. *J R Soc Med* 76:458, 1983.

Kronborg O, Tostergaard A, Steven KG, Toctrik JK: Polyglycolic acid versus chromic catgut in bladder surgery. *Br J Urol* 50:324, 1978.

Landes RR: An improved suction device for draining wounds. Arch Surg 104:707, 1972.

Lang EK: Antegrade ureteral stenting for dehiscence, strictures and fistulae. *AJR Am J Roentgenol* 143:795, 1984.

Larson DL: Musculocutaneous flaps. In: Johnson DE, Boileau MA (Eds): *Genitourinary Tumors: Fundamental Principles and Surgical Techniques.* New York, Grune & Stratton, 1982.

Laufman H, Rickel T: Synthetic absorbable sutures. *Surg Gynecol Obstet* 145:597, 1977.

Lerwick E: Studies on the efficacy and safety of polydioxanone monofilament absorbable sutures. *Surg Gynecol Obstet* 135:497, 1981.

Libertino JA (Ed): *Pediatric and Adult Reconstructive Surgery,* 2nd ed. Baltimore, Williams & Wilkins Company, 1987.

Liebert PS: *Color Atlas of Pediatric Surgery.* New York, Elsevier Scientific Publishing, 1989.

Limberg AA: *The Planning of Local Plastic Operations on the Body Surface.* Lexington MA, Collamore Press, 1984.

Marshall FF (Ed): *Urologic Complications: Medical and Surgical, Adult and Pediatric.* Chicago, Year Book Medical Publishers, 1986.

Mayor G, Zingg E: *Urologic Surgery.* Stuttgart, Thieme, 1976.

McAninch JW (Guest Ed): Urogenital trauma. In: Blaisdell FW, Trunkey DD (Eds): *Trauma Management.* New York, Thieme-Stratton, Inc, 1985, vol II.

McCraw JB, Dibbell DG, Carraway JN: Clinical definition of independent myocutaneous vascular territories. *Plast Reconst Surg* 60:341, 1977.

McGregor IA: The theoretical basis of the Z-plasty. *Br J Plast Surg* 9:256, 1957.

McIntyre PB, Ritchie JK, Hawley PR, *et al.*: Management of enterocutaneous fistulas: a review of 132 cases. *Br J Surg* 71:293, 1984.

McMinn RMH, Hutchings RT: *Color Atlas of Human Anatomy.* Chicago, Year Book Medical Publishers, 1977.

Modern technics in surgery. In: Ehrlich RM (Ed): *Urologic Surgery.* Mount Kisco, NY, Future Publishing Company, 1980.

Morris AM: A controlled trial of closed wound suction. *Br J Surg* 60:357, 1973.

Morris MC, Baquero A, Redovan E, *et al.*: Urolithiasis on absorbable and non-absorbable suture materials in the rabbit bladder. *J Urol* 135:602, 1986.

Morrow FA, Kogan SJ, Freed SZ, Laufman H: In vivo comparison of polyglycolic acid, chromic catgut and silk in tissue of the genitourinary tract: an experimental study of tissue retrieval and calculogenesis. *J Urol* 112:655, 1974.

Moss JP: Historical and current perspectives on surgical drainage. *Surg Gynecol Obstet* 152:517, 1981.

Murphy GF, Wood DP Jr: The use of mineral oil to manage nondeflating Foley catheter. *J Urol* 149:89, 1993.

Nora PF, Vanecko RM, Brensfield JJ: Prophylactic abdominal drains. *Arch Surg* 105:173, 1972.

Novick AC, Streem SB, Pontes EJ (Eds): *Stewart's Operative Urology.* Baltimore, Williams & Wilkins Company, 1989.

Nyhus LM, Baker RJ (Eds): *Masters of Surgery,* 2nd ed. Boston, Toronto, Little, Brown & Company, 1992.

Olivet RT, Nauss LA, Payne WS: A technique for continuous intercostal nerve block analgesia following thoracotomy. *J Cardiovasc Surg (Torino)* 80:308, 1980.

Oneal RM, Dingman RO, Grabb WC: The teaching of plastic surgical techniques to medical students. *Plast Reconstr Surg* 40:494, 1967.

Parrott TS and Woodard JR: Urologic surgery in the neonate. *J Urol* 116:506, 1976.

Paulson DF (Ed): *Genitourinary Surgery.* New York, Churchill Livingstone, 1984.

Penrose CB: Drainage in abdominal surgery. *JAMA* 14:264, 1890.

Pocock RD, Stower MJ, Ferro MA, *et al.*: Double-J stents: a review of 100 patients. *Br J Urol* 58:629, 1986.

Raffensperger JG (Ed): *Swenson's Pediatric Surgery,* 5th ed. Norwalk, Appleton and Lange, 1990.

Ramsay JWA, Payne SR, Gosling PT, *et al.*: The effects of double-J stenting on unobstructed ureters: an experimental and clinical study. *Br J Urol* 57:630, 1985.

Redman JF: An anatomic approach to the pelvis. In: Crawford ED, Borden TA (Eds): *Genitourinary Cancer Surgery.* Philadelphia, Lea & Febiger, 1982, p 126.

Resnick MI, Kursch E (Eds): *Current Therapy in Genitourinary Surgery.* Toronto, Philadelphia, B. C. Decker, Inc, 1987.

Rodeheaver GF, Thacker JG, Edlich RF: Mechanical performance of polyglycolic acid and polyglactin 910 synthetic absorbable sutures. *Surg Gynecol Obstet* 153:835, 1981.

Singh B, Kim H, Wax SH: Stent versus nephrostomy: is there a choice? *J Urol* 121:268, 1979.

Skandalakis JE, Gray W, Rowe JS Jr: *Anatomical Complications in General Surgery.* New York, McGraw-Hill Book Company, 1983.

Smith AD: Retrieval of ureteral stents. *Urol Clin North Am* 9:109, 1982.

Ternberg JL, Bell MJ, Bower RJ: *A Handbook for Pediatric Surgery.* Baltimore, Williams & Wilkins, 1980.

Thomas R, Sharmen G: Urology cart. *Urology* 21:526, 1983.

Trier WC: Considerations in the choice of surgical needles. *Surg Gynecol Obstet* 149:84, 1979.

Urology. In: McDougal WS (Ed): *Rob & Smith's Operative Surgery,* 4th ed. St. Louis, Toronto, C. V. Mosby Company, 1983.

Van Arsdalen KN, Pollack HH, Wein AJ: Ureteral stenting. *Semin Urol* 2:180, 1984.

Van Winkle W Jr, Hastings JC: Considerations in the choice of suture materials for various tissues. *Surg Gynecol Obstet* 135:113, 1972.

Van Winkle W Jr, Hastings J, Barker E, *et al.*: Effect of suture materials on healing skin wounds. *Surg Gynecol Obstet* 140:7, 1975.

Van Winkle W Jr, Salthouse TN: *Biological Response to Sutures and Principles of Suture Selection.* Somerville, Ethicon, Inc, 1976.

Walsh PC, Gittes RF, Perlmutter AD, Stamey TA (Eds): *Campbell's Urology.* Philadelphia, W. B. Saunders Company, 1986.

Wheeless CR: *Atlas of Pelvic Surgery.* Philadelphia, Lea & Febiger, 1981.

Whitehead ED, Leiter E (Eds): *Current Operative Urology,* 2nd ed. Philadelphia, Harper and Row, 1984.

Williams DI: *Urology in Childhood.* New York, Springer-Verlag, 1974.

Wind GG, Rich NM: *Principles of Surgical Technique: The Art of Surgery.* Baltimore, Urban and Schwarzenberg, 1983.

Woltering EA, Flye MW, Huntley S, *et al.*: Evaluation of bupivacaine nerve blocks in modification of pain and pulmonary function changes after thoracotomy. *Ann Thorac Surg* 30:122, 1980.

Section 3—Kidney

Anderson JC, Hynes W: Retrocaval ureter: a case diagnosed pre-operatively and treated successfully by a plastic operation. *Br J Urol* 21:209, 1949.

Anderson JC: Hydronephrosis: a fourteen years' survey of results. *Proc R Soc Med* 55:93, 1962.

Anson BJ, Cauldwell EW: Pararenal vascular system: study of 425 anatomical specimens. *Q Bull Northwestern Univ Med School* 21:320, 1947.

Anson BJ, Cauldwell EW, Pick JW, Beaton LE: The blood supply of the kidney, suprarenal gland, and associated structures. *Surg Gynecol Obstet* 84:313, 1947.

Anson BJ, Cauldwell EW, Pick JW, Beaton LE: The anatomy of the pararenal system of veins, with comments on the renal arteries. *J Urol* 60:714, 1948.

Anson BJ, Kurth LE: Common variations in the renal blood supply. *Surg Gynecol Obstet* 100:156, 1955.

Anson BJ, Daseler EH: Common variations in renal anatomy, affecting blood supply, form, and topography. *Surg Gynecol Obstet* 112:439, 1961.

Auvert J: La veine renale gauche. *Presse Med* 75:1405, 1967.

Barbaric Z: Renal fascia in urinary tract disease. *Radiology* 117:17, 1976.

Barnett MG, Bruskewitz RC, Belzer FO, *et al.*: Ileocecocystoplasty bladder augmentation and renal transplantation. *J Urol* 138:855, 1987.

Barry JM, Lawson RK, Strong B, Hodges CV: Urologic complications in 173 kidney transplants. *J Urol* 112:567, 1974.

Barry JM, Hodges CV: The supracostal approach to the kidney and adrenal. *J Urol* 114:666, 1975.

Barry JM, Fuchs EF: Right renal vein extension in cadaver kidney transplantation. *Arch Surg* 113:300, 1978.

Barry JM: Spermatic cord preservation in kidney transplantation. *J Urol* 127:1076, 1982.

Bazy L: La Nephrectomie sous-péritonéale par incision antérieure transversale. *Presse Med* 22:186, 1914.

Beaton LE: The anatomy of the pararenal system of veins, with comments on the renal arteries. *J Urol* 60:714, 1948.

Bejjani B, Belman AB: Ureteropelvic junction obstruction in newborns and infants. *J Urol* 128:770, 1982.

Belzer FO, Kountz SL, Najarian JS, *et al.*: Prevention of urological complications after renal allotransplantation. *Arch Surg* 101:449, 1970.

Belzer FO, Schweizer RT, Kountz S: Management of multiple vessels in renal transplantation. *Transplant Proc* 4:639, 1972.

Benoit G, Delmas V, Gillot C, Hureau J: Anatomical bases of kidney transplantation in man. *Anat Clin* 6:239, 1984.

Bensimon H: Muscle protective incisions in renal surgery. *Urology* 4:476, 1974.

Bérard P, Pouyet M: Les voies d'évacuation veineuse du rein apres ligature de la veine rénale gauche. *Lyon Chir* 64:781, 1968.

Berger RE, Ansell JS, Tremann JA, *et al.*: The use of self-retained ureteral stents in the management of urologic complications in renal transplant recipients. *J Urol* 124:781, 1980.

Binder C, Bonick P, Ciavarra V: Experience with Silastic U-tube nephrostomy. *J Urol* 106:499, 1977.

Blaivas JG, Pais VM, Spellman RM: Chemolysis of residual stone fragments after extensive surgery for staghorn calculi. *Urology* 6:680, 1975.

Blandy JP, Tresidder GC: Extended pyelolithotomy for renal calculi. *Br J Urol* 39:121, 1967.

Blandy J: Surgery of renal cast calculi. In: Libertino JA, Zinman L (Eds): *Reconstructive Urologic Surgery.* Baltimore, Williams & Wilkins, 1977, p 17.

Boatman DL, Cornell SH, Kolin CP: The arterial supply of horseshoe kidneys. *Am J Roentgen Rad Ther Nucl Med* 113:447, 1971.

Boyce WH, Elkins IB: Reconstructive renal surgery following anatrophic nephrolithotomy. *J Urol* 111:307, 1974.

Boyce WH, Harrison LH: Complications of renal stone surgery. In: Smith RM, Skinner DG (Eds): *Complications of Urologic Surgery: Prevention and Management.* Philadelphia, W. B. Saunders Company, 1976, p 87.

Bredael JJ, Carson CC III, Weinerth JL: Bilateral nephrectomy by the posterior approach. *Eur Urol* 6:251, 1980.

Browse NL, Hurst P: Repair of long, large midline incisional hernias using reflected flaps of anterior rectus sheath reinforced with Marlex mesh. *Am J Surg* 138:738, 1979.

Brynger H, Claes G, Gelin LE, et al.: Extracorporeal resection for parenchymatous renal tumours. *Scand J Urol Nephrol* Suppl 60:27, 1981.

Buntain WL, Lynn HB: Splenorrhaphy! Changing concepts for traumatized spleen. *Surgery* 86:748, 1979.

Butarazzi PJ, Devine PC, Devine CJ, et al.: The indications, complications, and results of partial nephrectomy. *J Urol* 99:376, 1968.

Caldamone AA: Abdominal masses in children. In: Resnick MI, Caldamone AA, Spinak JP (Eds): *Decision Making in Urology*. St. Louis, C. V. Mosby Company, 1985.

Carini M, Selli C, Grechi G, Masini G: Pyelovesicostomy: an alternative to ureteropelvic junction-plasty in pelvic ectopic kidneys. *Urology* 26:125, 1983.

Carlton CE Jr, Scott R Jr, Goldman M: The management of penetrating injuries of the kidney. *J Trauma* 8:1071, 1968.

Carpiniello VL, Malloy TR, Wein AJ: Toward bloodless nephrectomy during Gil Vernet pyelolithotomy. *Urology* 26:187, 1985.

Cass AS, Ireland GW: Comparison of the conservative and surgical management of the more severe degrees of renal trauma in multiple injured patients. *J Urol* 109:8, 1973.

Cass AS, Luxenberg M: Conservative or immediate surgical management of blunt renal injuries. *J Urol* 130:11, 1983.

Chang R, Marshall FF, Mitchell S: Percutaneous management of benign ureteral strictures and fistulas. *J Urol* 137:1126, 1987.

Chute R, Baron JA, Olsson CA: The transverse upper abdominal "Chevron" incision in urological surgery. *Trans Am Assoc Genitourin Surg* 29:14, 1967.

Chute R: The thoracoabdominal incision in urological surgery. *J Urol* 65:784, 1951.

Cieślik R, Cerkownik L: Management of the posterior peritoneum after transperitoneal renal surgery. *Br J Urol* 57:279, 1985.

Clayman RV, Gonzalez R, Fraley EE: Renal cell carcinoma invading the inferior vena cava: clinical review and anatomical approach. *J Urol* 123:157, 1980.

Clayman RV, Sheldon CA, Gonzales R: Wilms' tumor: an approach to vena caval intrusion. *Prog Pediatr Surg* 15:285, 1982.

Clayman RV, Garske GL, Lange PH: Total nephroureterectomy with ureteral intussusception and transurethral ureteral detachment and pull-through. *Urology* 21:482–486, 1983.

Cockrell SN, Hendren WH: The importance of visualizing the ureter before performing a pyeloplasty. *J Urol* 144(part 2):588, 1990 (discussion, 593).

Cole AT, Fried FA: Experience with the thoraco-abdominal incision for nephroblastoma in children less than 3 years old. *J Urol* 114:114, 1975.

Collins GM, Green RD, Boyer D, et al.: Protection of kidneys from warm ischemic injury: dosage and timing of mannitol administration. *Transplantation* 29:83, 1980.

Congdon ED, Edson JN: The cone of renal fascia in the adult white male. *Anat Rec* 80:289, 1941.

Cook JH III, Lytton B: Intraoperative localization of renal calculi during nephrolithotomy by ultrasound scanning. *J Urol* 117:546, 1979.

Cooper MJ, Williams RC: Splenectomy: indications, hazards and alternatives. *Br J Surg* 71:173, 1984.

Corriere JN, Perloff LJ, Barker CF, et al.: The ureteropyelostomy in human renal transplantation. *J Urol* 110:24, 1973.

Cox PJ, Ausobsky JR, Ellis H, Pollack AV: Towards no incisional hernias: lateral paramedian versus midline incisions. *J R Soc Med* 79:711, 1986.

Crawford ED, Skinner DG, Capparell DB: Intercostal nerve block with thoracoabdominal incision. *J Urol* 121:290, 1978.

Crissey MM, Gittes RF: Dissolution of cystine ureteral calculus by irrigation with tromethamine. *J Urol* 121:811, 1979.

Cromie WJ: Complications of pyeloplasty. *Urol Clin North Am* 10:385, 1983.

Culp OS, DeWeerd JH: A pelvic flap operation for certain types of ureteropelvic obstruction: preliminary report. *Proc Staff Meet Mayo Clin* 26:483, 1951.

Culp OS, Winterringer JR: Surgical treatment of horseshoe kidney: a comparison of results after various types of operations. *J Urol* 73:747, 1955.

Culp OS: Anterior nephroureterectomy: advantages and limitations of a single incision. *J Urol* 85:193, 1961.

Cummings KB, Li W-I, Ryan JA, et al.: Intraoperative management of renal cell carcinoma with supradiaphragmatic caval extension. *J Urol* 122:829, 1979.

Cummings KB: Surgical management of renal cell carcinoma with extension into the vena cava. In: Crawford ED, Borden TA (Eds): *Genitourinary Cancer Surgery*. Philadelphia, Lea & Febiger, 1982, p 70.

D'Angio GJ, Evans A, Breslow N, et al.: The treatment of Wilms' tumor: results of the Second National Wilms' Tumor Study. *Cancer* 47:2302, 1981.

Darner HL: Bilateral ectopic kidney. *J Urol* 12:193, 1924.

Das S: Radical nephrectomy: thoracoabdominal intrapleural approach. In: Crawford ED, Borden TA (Eds): *Genitourinary Cancer Surgery*. Lea & Febiger, Philadelphia, 1982, p 30.

Daseler EH, Anson BJ: Anatomical relations of ectopic iliolumbar kidneys, bilateral in adult and unilateral in fetus. *J Urol* 49:789, 1943.

Davis DM: Intubated ureterotomy: a new operation for ureteral and ureteropelvic stricture. *Surg Gynecol Obstet* 76:513, 1943.

Davis RA, Milloy FJ Jr, Anson BJ: Lumbar, renal and associated parietal and visceral veins based upon a study of 100 specimens. *Surg Gynecol Obstet* 107:122, 1958.

Dees JF: The use of an intraoperative coagulum in pyelolithotomy: a preliminary report. *South Med J* 49:497, 1943.

deKernion JB: Lymphadenectomy for renal cell carcinoma: Therapeutic implications. *Urol Clin North Am* 7:697, 1980.

deKernion JB: Radical nephrectomy. In: Ehrlich RM (Ed): *Modern Technics in Surgery (Urologic Surgery)*. New York, Futura, 1980.

Delany HM, Porreca F, Mitsudo S, et al.: Splenic capping: an experimental study of a new technique for splenorrhaphy using woven polyglycolic acid mesh. *Ann Surg* 196:187, 1982.

Delmas P, Ravasse Ph, Mallet JF, Pheline Y: Anatomical basis of the surgical approach to the kidney in children. *Anat Clin* 7:267, 1985.

DeWeerd JH, Paulk SC, Tomera FM, et al.: Renal autotransplantation for upper ureteral stenosis. *J Urol* 116:23, 1976.

Dixon JS, Gosling JA: The musculature of the human renal calice, pelvis and upper ureter. *J Anat* 135:129, 1982.

Djurhuus JC, Nerström B, Rask-Andersen H: Dynamics of upper urinary tract in man. *Acta Chir Scand* 472:49, 1976.

Dodds WJ, Darweesh RMA, Lawson TL et al.: The retroperitoneal spaces revisited. *Am J Roentgen* 147:1155, 1986.

Dodds WJ: Retroperitoneal compartmental anatomy [letter]. *Am J Roentgen* 148:829, 1987.

Doménech-Mateu JM, Gonzalez-Compta X: Horseshoe kidney: a new theory on its embryogenesis based on the study of a 16-mm human embryo. *Anat Rec* 222:408, 1988.

Donahoe PK, Hendren WH: Pelvic kidney in infants and children: experience with 16 cases. *J Pediatr Surg* 15:486, 1980.

Donohue JP, Hostetter M, Glover J, Madura J: Ureteroneocystostomy versus ureteropyelostomy: a comparison in the same renal allograft series. *J Urol* 114:202, 1975.

Douville E, Hollingshead WH: The blood supply of the normal renal pelvis. *J Urol* 73:906, 1955.

Dretler SP, Pfister RC, Newhouse JH: Renal stone dissolution via percutaneous nephrostomy. *N Engl J Med* 300:341, 1979.

Duckett JW, Lifland JJ, Peters PC: Resection of the vena cava for adjacent malignant disease. *Surg Gynecol Obstet* 136:711, 1973.

Eckstein HB, Kamal I: Hydronephrosis due to pelvi-ureteric obstruction in children: an assessment of the anterior transperitoneal approach. *Br J Surg* 58:663, 1971.

Edwards EA: Clinical anatomy of lesser variations of the inferior vena cava; and a proposal for classifying the anomalies of this vessel. *Angiology* 2:85, 1951.

Edwards EA: The anatomy of collateral circulation. *Surg Gynecol Obstet* 107:183, 1958.

Ehrlich RM, Goodwin WE: The surgical treatment of nephroblastoma (Wilms' tumor). *Cancer* 32:1145, 1973.

Escala JM, Keating MA, Boyd G, et al.: Development of elastic fibers in the upper urinary tract. *J Urol* 141:969, 1989.

Facer, MJ, Lynch RD, Evans HO, Chin FK: Inferior vena cava duplication: demonstration by computed tomography. *Radiology* 130:707, 1979.

Feldman RA, Shearer JK, Shield DE, et al.: Sensitive method for intraoperative roentgenograms. *Urology* 9:695, 1977.

Feller I, Woodburne RT: Surgical anatomy of the abdominal aorta. *Ann Surg* 154 (suppl):239, 1961.

Fey B: L'abord du rein par la voie thoracoabdominal. *Arch Urol Clin Necker* 5:169, 1926.

Fine H, Keen EN: The arteries of the human kidney. *J Anat* 100:881, 1966.

Flatmark A, Albrechtsen D, Södal G, et al.: Renal autotransplantation. *World J Surg* 13:206, 1989.

Foley FEB: New plastic operation for stricture at ureteropelvic junction: Report of 20 operations. *J Urol* 38:643, 1937.

Foote JW, Blennerhasset JB, Eiglesworth FW, MacKinnon KJ: Observations on the ureteropelvic junction. *J Urol* 104:252, 1970.

Fourman J, Moffat DB: *The Blood Vessels of the Kidney.* Oxford, Blackwell Scientific Publications, 1971.

Fowler JE: Bacteriology of branched renal calculi and accompanying urinary tract infection. *J Urol* 131:213, 1984.

Freed SZ, Veith FJ, Soberman R, Gliedman ML: Simultaneous bilateral posterior nephrectomy in transplant recipients. *Surgery* 68:468, 1970.

Friedland GW, DeVries P: Renal ectopia and fusion-embryologic basis. *Urology* 5:698, 1975.

Gelin LE, Claes G, Gustafsson A, Storm B: Total bloodlessness for extracorporeal organ repair. *Rev Surg* 28:305, 1971.

Gibbons RP, Correa RJ Jr, Cummings KB, Mason JT: Surgical management of renal lesions using in situ hypothermia and ischemia. *J Urol* 115:12, 1976.

Gil Vernet JM: New surgical concepts in removing renal calculi. *Urol Int* 20:255, 1965.

Gil Vernet JM, Caralps A, Revert I, et al.: Extracorporeal renal surgery. *Urology* 5:444, 1975.

Gil Vernet J, McCouruents: On pyelolithotomy. In: Whitehead ED (Ed): *Current Operative Urology.* Hagerstown, Harper and Row, 1975.

Gillou CR, Hall TJ, Donaldson DR et al.: Vertical abdominal incisions: a choice? *Br J Surg* 67:395, 1980.

Giordano JM, Trout HH III: Anomalies of the inferior vena cava. *J Vasc Surg* 3:924, 1986.

Gittes RF, McCullough DL: Bench surgery for tumor in a solitary kidney. *J Urol* 113:12, 1975.

Gittes RF: Partial nephrectomy and bench surgery-techniques and applications. In: Libertino R, Zinman L (Eds): *Reconstructive Urologic Surgery: Pediatric and Adult.* Baltimore, Williams & Wilkins, 1977, p 45.

Golbus MS, Harrison MR, Filly RA, et al.: In utero treatment of urinary tract obstruction. *Am J Obstet Gynecol* 142:383, 1982.

Goldstein I, Cho SI, Olsson CA: Nephrostomy drainage for renal transplant complications. *J Urol* 126:159, 1981.

Gonzalez R: Extraperitoneal midline approach to retroperitoneum in children. *Urology* 20:13, 1982.

Gordon MR, Carrion HM, Politano VA: Dissolution of uric acid calculi with THAM irrigation. *Urology* 12:393, 1978.

Gosling JA: The musculature of the upper urinary tract. *Acta Anat (Basel),* 75:408, 1970.

Gosling JA, Constantinou CE: The origin and propagation of upper urinary tract contraction waves: a new in vitro methodology. *Experientia* 32:266, 1976.

Gosling JA, Dixon JS: The structure of the normal and hydronephrotic upper urinary tract. In: O'Reilly PH, Gosling JA, (Eds): *Idiopathic Hydronephrosis.* London, Springer-Verlag, 1982.

Graham SD Jr, Glenn JF: Enucleative surgery for renal malignancy. *J Urol* 122:546, 1979.

Graves FT: The aberrant renal artery. *J Anat* 90:553, 1956.

Graves FJ: The anatomy of the intra-renal arteries in health and disease. *Br J Surg* 43:605, 1956.

Graves FT: The anatomy of the intrarenal arteries and its application to segmental resection of the kidney. *Br J Surg* 43:132, 1954.

Graves FT: Renal hypothermia: an aid to partial nephrectomy. *Br J Surg* 50:362, 1963.

Graves FT: The arterial anatomy of the congenitally abnormal kidney. *Brit J Surg* 56:533, 1969.

Greenall MJ, Evans M, Pollock AV: Midline or transverse laparotomy? A random controlled clinical trial: I. Influence on healing. *Br J Surg* 67:188, 1980.

Greenberg SH, Wein AJ, Perloff LF, Barker CF: Ureteropyelostomy and ureteroneocystostomy in renal transplantation: postoperative urological complications. *J Urol* 118:17, 1977.

Griffiths DA: A reappraisal of the Pfannenstiel incision. *Br J Urol* 48:469, 1976.

Gruenwald P: The normal changes in the position of the embryonic kidney. *Anat Rec* 85:163, 1943.

Guerriero WG, Carlton CE Jr, Scott R Jr, Beall AC Jr: Renal pedicle injuries. *J Trauma* 11:53, 1971.

Hadar H, Gadoth N: Positional relationships of the colon and kidney determined by perirenal fat. *Am J Roentgenol Rad Ther Nucl Med* 143:773, 1984.

Hamm FC, Weinberg SR: Renal and ureteral surgery without intubation. *J Urol* 73:475, 1955.

Hanley HG: The pelvi-ureteric junction: a cine-pyelography study. *Br J Urol* 31:377, 1959.

Hanna MK, Jeffs RD, Sturgess JM, Barkin M: Ureteral structure and ultrastructure: part 1. The normal human ureter. *J Urol* 116:718, 1976.

Hanna MK, Jeffs RD, Sturgess JM, Barkin M: Ureteral structure and ultrastructure: Part 2. Congenital ureteropelvic junction obstruction and primary obstructive megaureter. *J Urol* 116:725, 1976.

Harrison MR, Golbus MS, Filly RA, et al.: Fetal surgery for congenital hydronephrosis. *N Engl J Med* 306:591, 1982.

Harrison MR, Golbus MS, Filly RA, et al.: Management of the fetus with congenital hydronephrosis. *J Pediatr Surg* 17:728, 1982.

Hayes MA: Abdominopelvic fasciae. *Am J Anat* 87:119, 1950.

Hegedüs V: Arterial anatomy of the kidney: a three-dimensional angiographic investigation. *Acta Radiol [Diagn]* 12:604, 1972.

Hellstrom J: Some observations on removal of kidney stones particularly by means of pyelolithotomy in situ. *Acta Clin Scand* 98:442, 1949.

Hellstrom J, Giertz G, Lindblom K: Pathogenesis and treatment of hydronephrosis. In: *VIII Congress de Societé Internationale d'Urologie.* Paris, 1949.

Hendren WH, Radharkrishnan J, Middleton AW Jr: Pediatric pyeloplasty. *J Pediatr Surg* 15:133, 1980.

Henriksson C, Brynger H, Nilsson AE, *et al.*: Reconstruction of urinary outflow obstructions by renal autotransplantation. *Scand J Urol Nephrol* suppl 59:1980.

Herrlinger A, Sigel A, Giedl J: Methodik der radikalen transabdominalen Tumornephrektomie mit fakultativer oder systemischer Lymphdissektion und deren Ergebnisse an 381 patienten. *Urologea* 23:267, 1984.

Herwig KR, Konnak JW: Vesicopyelostomy: a method for urinary drainage of the transplanted kidney. *J Urol* 109:955, 1973.

Hess E: Resection of the rib in renal operations. *J Urol* 42:943, 1939.

Hewitt CB: Nephroureterectomy with bladder cuff in the treatment of transitional cell carcinoma of the upper urinary tract. In: Scott R (Ed): *Current Controversies in Urologic Management.* Philadelphia, W. B. Saunders Company, 1972.

Heynes CF, van Gelderen WFC: Three-dimensional imaging of the pelviocaliceal system by computerized tomographic reconstruction. *J Urol* 144:1335, 1990.

Hinman F Jr: Techniques for ureteropyeloplasty. *Arch Surg* 71:790, 1955.

Hinman F Jr, Oppenheimer R: Ureteral regeneration: VI. Delayed urinary flow in the healing of unsplinted ureteral defects. *J Urol* 78:138, 1957.

Hinman F Jr: Peripelvic extravasation during intravenous urography: evidence for an additional route for back-flow after ureteral obstruction. *J Urol* 85:385, 1961.

Hinman F Jr: Ballottement of peripelvic cyst for operative diagnosis and localization. *J Urol* 97:7, 1967.

Hinman F Jr, Belzer FO: Urinary tract infection and renal homotransplantation: I. Effect of antibacterial irrigations on defenses of the defunctionalized bladder. *J Urol* 101:477, 1969.

Hinman F Jr, Schmaelzle JF, Belzer FO: Urinary tract infection and renal homotransplantation: II. Post-transplantation bacterial invasion. *J Urol* 101:673, 1969.

Hinman F Jr: Dismembered pyeloplasty without urinary diversion. In: Scott R (Ed): *Current Controversies in Urologic Management.* Philadelphia, W. B. Saunders Company, 1972, p 253.

Hinman F Jr: Hydronephrosis. In: Goldman HS (Ed): *Practice of Surgery.* Hagerstown, Harper and Row, 1980, p 1.

Hinman F Jr, Cattolica EV: Branched calculi: shapes and operative approaches. *J Urol* 126:291, 1981.

Hjort EF: Partial resection of the renal pelvis and pole of the kidney for hydronephrosis. *Br J Urol* 43:406, 1971.

Hodges CV, Lawson RK, Pearse HD, Stranburg CO: Autotransplantation of the kidney. *J Urol* 110:20, 1973.

Hodson J: The lobar structure of the kidney. *Br J Urol* 44:246, 1972.

Hoeltl W, Hruby W, Aharinejad S: Renal vein anatomy and its implications for retroperitoneal surgery. *J Urol* 143:1108, 1990.

Hohenfellner R, Wulf, AD: Urologie. In: Kunz H (Ed): *Operationen des Kindesalters.* Stuttgart, Thieme, 1975, vol II.

Homsy Y, Simard J, Debs C, *et al.*: Pyeloplasty: to divert or not to divert? *Urology* 16:577, 1980.

Hureau J, Hidden G, Thanh Minh TA: The vascularisation of the suprarenal glands. *Anat Clin* 2:127, 1980.

Huu N, Person H, Hong R, *et al.*: Anatomical approach to the vascular segmentation of the spleen (lien) based on controlled experimental partial splenectomies. *Anat Clin* 4:265, 1982.

Immergut MA, Jacobson JJ, Culp DA: Cutaneous pyelostomy. *J Urol* 101:276, 1969.

Jenkins TPN: The burst abdominal wound: a mechanical approach. *Br J Surg* 63:873, 1976.

Kadir S, White RI Jr, Engel R: Balloon dilatation of a ureteropelvic junction obstruction. *Radiology* 143:263, 1982.

Kaneto H, Orikasa S, Chiba T, Takahashi T: Three-D muscular arrangement at the ureteropelvic junction and its

changes in congenital hydronephrosis: a stereo-morphometric study. *J Urol* 146:909, 1991.

Kark RM: Renal biopsy. *JAMA* 105:220, 1968.

Karsburg W, Leary FJ: Nephrostomy tube replacement. *Urology* 13:301, 1979.

Kaufman BH, Telander RL, van Heerden JA, *et al.*: Pheochromocytoma in the pediatric age group: current status. *J Pediatr Surg* 18:879, 1983.

Kearney GP, *et al.*: Results of inferior vena cava resection for renal cell carcinoma. *J Urol* 125:769, 1981.

Kiil F: *The Function of the Ureter and Renal Pelvis.* Oslo, Oslo University Press, 1957.

King LR: Management of multicystic kidney and ureteropelvic junction obstruction. In: King LR (Ed): *Urologic Surgery in Neonates and Young Infants.* Philadelphia, W. B. Saunders Company, 1988, p 140.

Klimberg I, Sirois R, Wajsman Z, Baker J: Intraoperative autotransfusion in urologic oncology. *Arch Surg* 121:1326, 1986.

Koff SA, Thrall JH, Keyes JW Jr: Diuretic radionuclide urography: a non-invasive method for evaluating nephroureteral dilatation. *J Urol* 121:153, 1979.

Koff SA, Hayden LJ, Cirulli C, Shore R: Pathophysiology of ureteropelvic obstruction: experimental and clinical observations. *J Urol* 136:336, 1986.

Kolln CP, Boldus RA, Brandon NK, Flocks RH: Bilateral partial nephrectomy for bilateral renal cell carcinoma. *J Urol* 105:45, 1971.

Koop CE, Schnaufer L: The management of abdominal neuroblastoma. *Cancer* 35:905, 1975.

Koyle MA, Ehrlich RM: Wilms' tumor in neonates and young infants: current considerations and controversies. In: King LR (Ed): *Urologic Surgery in Neonates and Young Infants.* Philadelphia, W. B. Saunders Company, 1988, p 429.

Kusunoki T: Partial nephrectomy. *Urol Int* 1:243, 1955.

Landau R, Botha JR, Myburgh JA: Pyeloureterostomy or ureteroneocystostomy in renal transplantation? *Br J Urol* 58:6, 1986.

Lawson RK, Hodges CV: Extracorporeal renal artery repair and autotransplantation. *Urology* 4:532, 1974.

Lawson RK: Extracorporeal renal surgery. *J Urol* 123:301, 1980.

Leape LL, Breslow NE, Bishop HC: The surgical management of Wilms' tumor. *Am Surg* 187:351, 1978.

Lee WJ, Badlani GH, Karlin GS, *et al.*: Treatment of ureteropelvic strictures with percutaneous pyelotomy: experience in 62 patients. *Am J Roentgen* 151:515, 1988.

Liebermann-Meffert D, White H (Eds): *The Greater Omentum.* Berlin, Springer-Verlag, 1983.

Linke CA, Cockett ATK, Lai MK, Youseff AM: The use of pedicled grafts of omentum in the repair of transplant-related urinary tract problems. *J Urol* 120:532, 1978.

Love L, Meyers MA, Churchill RJ, *et al.*: Computed tomography of the extraperitoneal spaces. *Am J Roentgen* 136:781, 1981.

Lurz H: Ein muskelschonender lumbalschnitt zur Freilegung der Niere. *Chirurg* 27:125, 1956.

Lutzeyer W: Lumbodorsal exploration. In: Glenn JF (Ed): *Urologic Surgery.* New York, Harper and Row, 1975, pp 127–133.

Lyon R: An anterior extraperitoneal incision for kidney surgery. *J Urol* 79:383, 1958.

Lytton B: Surgery of the kidney. In: Harrison JH, Gittes RF, Perlmutter AD, *et al.* (Eds): *Campbell's Urology,* 4th ed, Philadelphia, W. B. Saunders Company, 1979, vol 3, p 1993.

Maatman TJ, Montie JE: Complications of renal surgery. In: Marshall FF (Ed): *Urologic Complications.* Chicago, Year Book Medical Publishers, 1986.

MacCallum DB: The arterial blood supply of the mammalian kidney. *Am J Anat* 38:153, 1926.

Mahoney EM, Crocker DW, Friend DG, *et al.*: Adrenal and extra-adrenal pheochromocytomas: localization by vena cava. A sampling and observations on renal juxtaglomerular apparatus. *J Urol* 108:4, 1972.

Maizels M, Stephens FD: The induction of urologic malformations: understanding the relationship of renal ectopia and congenital scoliosis. *Invest Urol* 17:209, 1979.

Margreit R, Steiner E, Aigner F, Hoyer J: A safe technique for renal transplantation in patients with severely infected bladders. *Surg Gynecol Obstet* 159:487, 1984.

Marshall FF: Intraoperative localization of renal calculi. *Urol Clin North Am* 10:629, 1983.

Marshall FF, Reitz BA, Diamond DA: A new technique for management of renal cell carcinoma involving the right atrium: hypothermia and cardiac arrest. *J Urol* 131:103, 1984.

Marshall FF, Reitz BA: Technique for removal of renal cell carcinoma with suprahepatic vena caval tumor thrombus. *Urol Clin North Am* 13:551, 1986.

Marshall M Jr, Johnson SH III: A simple direct approach to the renal pedicle. *J Urol* 84:24, 1960.

Marshall VR, Singh M, Tresidder GC, Blandy JP: The place of partial nephrectomy in the management of renal calyceal calculi. *Br J Urol* 47:759, 1976.

Martin LW, Reyes PM Jr: An evaluation of 10 years experience with retroperitoneal lymph node dissection for Wilms' tumour. *J Pediat Surg* 4:683, 1969.

Martin LW, Schaffner DP, Cox JA, et al.: Retroperitoneal lymph node dissection for Wilms' tumor. *J Pediatr Surg* 14:704, 1979.

Marx WJ, Patel SK: Renal fascia: its radiographic importance. *Urology* 13:1, 1979.

Masaki Z, Iguchi A, Kinoshita N, et al.: Intrasinusal pyelolithotomy with lower pole nephrotomy for removal of renal stones. *Urology* 26:461, 1985.

Mayo WJ: The incision for lumbar exposure of the kidney. *Ann Surg* 55:63, 1912.

McAninch JW, Carroll PR: Renal trauma: kidney preservation through improved vascular control. A refined approach. *J Trauma* 22:285, 1982.

McClure CFW, Butler EG: The development of the vena cava inferior in man. *Am J Anat* 35:331, 1925.

McCowan RE: Bilateral renal ectopia. *J Urol* 22:653, 1929.

McCullough DL, Gittes RF: Vena cava resection for renal cell carcinoma. *J Urol* 112:162, 1974.

McLean PA, Gawley WF, Gorey TP: Technical modifications of Anderson-Hynes pyeloplasty for congenital pelviureteric junction obstruction. *Br J Urol* 57:114, 1985.

McLoughlin MG, Williams GM, Stonesifer GL: Ex vivo surgical dissection. *JAMA* 235:1705, 1976.

McVay CB, Anson BJ: Aponeurotic and fascial continuities in the abdomen, pelvis and thigh. *Anat Rec* 76, 213, 1940.

McVay CB, Anson BJ: Composition of the rectus sheath. *Anat Rec* 77:213, 1940.

Mehrotra GK, Datta G, Mukherjee KL: Growth and development of the human fetal kidney. *Indian J Pediatr* 53:273, 1986.

Merkel FK, Straus AK, Andersen O, et al.: Microvascular techniques for polar artery reconstruction in kidney transplants. *Surgery* 79:253, 1976.

Merklin RJ, Michels NA: The variant renal and suprarenal blood supply with data on the inferior phrenic, ureteral and gonadal arteries. *J Int Coll Surg* 29:41, 1958.

Merrill DC: Modified thoracoabdominal approach to the kidney and retroperitoneal tissue. *J Urol* 117:15, 1977.

Mesrobian, H-G J: Wilms' tumor: past, present and future. *J Urol* 140:231, 1988.

Meyers MA: The extraperitoneal spaces. In: Meyers MA (Ed): *Dynamic Radiology of the Abdomen: Normal and Pathologic Anatomy.* New York, Springer-Verlag, 1976, p 113.

Milloy FJ, Anson BJ, Cauldwell EW: Variations in the inferior caval veins and in their renal and lumbar communications. *Surg Gynecol Obstet* 115:131, 1962.

Milsten R, Neifield J, Koontz WW: Extracorporeal renal surgery. *J Urol* 112:425, 1974.

Mitchell A, Morris PJ: Surgery for the spleen. *Clin Haematol* 12:565, 1983.

Mitchell GAG: The innervation of the kidney, ureter, testicle and epididymls. *J Anat* 70:10, 1935.

Mitchell GAG: The renal fascia. *Br J Surg* 37(3):257, 1950.

Mitchell GAG: The intrinsic renal nerves. *Acta Anat* 13:1, 1951.

Montie JE, Jackson CL, Cosgrove DM, et al.: Resection of large inferior vena caval thrombi from renal cell carcinoma with the use of circulatory arrest. *J Urol* 139:25, 1987.

More RH, Duff GL: The renal arterial vasculature in man. *Am J Pathol* 27:95, 1950.

Morita T, Kondo S, Suzuki T et al.: Effect of calyceal resection on pelviureteral peristalsis in isolated pig kidney. *J Urol* 135:151, 1986.

Mosnier H, Frantz P, Calmat A, Leguerrier A, Cabrol C: A study of the anastomoses between the left renal vein and the intravertebral plexuses. *Anat Clin* 1:321, 1980.

Mulvaney WP: The clinical use of renacidin in urinary calcifications. *J Urol* 84:206, 1960.

Murnaghan GF: The dynamics of the renal pelvis and ureter with reference to congenital hydronephrosis. *Br J Urol* 30:321, 1958.

Murnaghan GF: Mechanisms of congenital hydronephrosis with reference to factors influencing surgical treatment. *Ann R Coll Surg Engl* 23:25, 1958.

Murnaghan GF: Renal pelvis and ureter. In: Wells C, Kyle J (Eds): *Scientific Foundations of Surgery.* New York, Elsevier Scientific Publishing, 1967, p 280.

Murnaghan GF: Surgical exposure of the kidney. In: *Rob and Smith's Operative Urology, 4th ed, Urology Volume.* St. Louis, C. V. Mosby Company, 1983.

Murphy JJ, Glantz W, Schoenberg HW: The healing of renal wounds: III. A comparison of electrocoagulation and suture ligation for hemostasis in partial nephrectomy. *J Urol* 85:882, 1961.

Nagamatsu G: Dorsolumbar approach to the kidney and adrenal with osteoplastic flap. *J Urol* 63:569, 1959.

Namiki M, Shimoe S: Asymmetric fused kidney: a report of two cases and discussion on its classification. *Acta Urol Jap* 24:1061, 1978.

Narath, PA: The dynamics of the upper urinary tract. In: Narath, PA (Ed): *Renal Pelvis and Ureter.* New York, Grune & Stratton, 1951, p 215.

Nemoy WJ: Renacidin in the treatment of infection stones. In: Kaufman JJ (Ed): *Current Urologic Therapy.* Philadelphia, W. B. Saunders Company, 1980.

Nesbit RM: Elliptical anastomosis in urologic surgery. *Am Surg* 130:796, 1949.

Notley RG, Beaugle JM: The long-term follow-up of Anderson-Hynes pyeloplasty for hydronephrosis. *Br J Urol* 45:464, 1973.

Novick A: Posterior surgical approach to the kidney and ureter. *J Urol* 124:192, 1980.

Novick AC, Stewart BH, Straffon RA, Banowsky LH: Partial nephrectomy in the treatment of renal adenocarcinoma. *J Urol* 118:932, 1977.

Novick AC, Cosgrove DM: Surgical approach for removal of renal cell carcinoma extending into the vena cava and the right atrium. *J Urol* 123:947, 1980.

Novick AC, Stewart BH, Straffon RA: Extracorporeal renal surgery and autotransplantation: indications, techniques and results. *J Urol* 123:806, 1980.

Novick AC: Extracorporeal renal surgery and autotransplantation. In: Novick AC, Straffon RA (Eds): *Vascular Problems in Urologic Surgery.* Philadelphia, W. B. Saunders Company, 1982, p 305.

Novick AC: Renal bench surgery. In: Glenn J (Ed): *Urologic Surgery, 3rd ed.* Philadelphia, J. B. Lippincott Company, 1983, p 137.

Novick AC: Renal hypothermia: in vivo and ex vivo. *Urol Clin North Am* 10:637, 1983.

Novick AC, Streem S, Montie JE, *et al.*: Conservative surgery for renal cell carcinoma: a single-center experience with 100 patients. *J Urol* 141:835, 1989.

O'Conor VJ, Logan DJ: Nephroureterectomy. *Surg Gynecol Obstet* 122:601, 1966.

O'Donohoe MK, Flanagan F, Fitzpatrick JM, Smith JM: Surgical approach to inferior vena caval extension of renal carcinoma. *Br J Urol* 60:492, 1987.

Odiase V, Whitaker RH: Dynamic evaluation of the results of pyeloplasty using pressure-flow studies. *Eur Urol* 7:324, 1981.

Ohl DA, Konnak JW, Campbell DA, *et al.*: Extravesical ureteroneocystostomy in renal transplantation. *J Urol* 139:499, 1988.

Olsson O, Wholey M: Vascular abnormalities in gross anomalies of kidneys. *Acta Radiol (Diagn)* 2:420, 1964.

Oravisto KJ: Transverse partial nephrectomy. *Acta Chir Scand* 130:331, 1965.

Orda R, Rudberg Z: The adreno-renal-ureteral sheath: surgical-anatomical study. *Urol Int* 31:179, 1976.

Orland SM, Snyder HM, Duckett JW: The dorsal lumbotomy incision in pediatric urological surgery. *J Urol* 138:963, 1987.

Osathanondh V, Potter EL: Development of the human kidney as shown by microdissection (3 parts). *Arch Pathol* 76:271, 1963.

Ossandon F, Androulakakis P, Ransley PG: Surgical problems in pelviureteral junction obstruction of the lower moiety in incomplete duplex systems. *J Urol* 125:871, 1981.

Östling K: The genesis of hydronephrosis particularly with regard to the changes at the ureteropelvic junction. *Acta Chir Scand* 86(Suppl):72, 1942.

Parienty RA, Pradel J: Radiological evaluation of the peri- and para-renal spaces by computed tomography. *Crit Rev Diagn Imaging* 20:1, 1983.

Parker RM, Rudd RG, Wonderly RK, *et al.*: Ureteropelvic junction obstruction in infants and children: functional evaluation of the obstructed kidney preoperatively and postoperatively. *J Urol* 126:509, 1981.

Parry WL, Finelli JF: Some consideration in the technique of partial nephrectomy. *J Urol* 82:562, 1959.

Perlmutter AD, Kroovand RL, Lai Y-W: Management of ureteropelvic obstruction in the first year of life. *J Urol* 123:535, 1980.

Perez CA, Kaiman HA, Keith J, *et al.*: Treatment of Wilms' tumor and factors affecting prognosis. *Cancer* 32:609, 1973.

Persky L, McDougal WS, Kedia K: Management of initial pyeloplasty failure. *J Urol* 125:695, 1981.

Peters PC, Bright TC III: Blunt renal injuries. *Urol Clin North Am* 4:17, 1977.

Pfannenstiel J: Über die Vorlheile des suprasymphasaren Faschenquerschnitts fur die gynäkologischen Koliolomien, zugleich ein Beitrag zu der Indikatior stellung der Operationswege. *Sanmburg Klin Vortr* 268:1736, 1900.

Pick JW, Anson BJ: The renal vascular pedicle: an anatomical study of 430 body halves. *J Urol* 44:411, 1940.

Pillet J, Cronier P: Observations on the development and migration of the human metanephros. *Anat Clin* 4:115, 1982.

Pitts WR Jr, Muecke EC: Horseshoe kidneys: a 40-year experience. *J Urol* 113:743, 1975.

Plaine LI, Hinman F Jr: Comparison of occlusion of the renal artery with occlusion of the entire pedicle on survival and serum creatinine levels of the rabbit. *J Urol* 93:117, 1965.

Plaine LI, Hinman F Jr: Malignancy in asymptomatic renal masses. *J Urol* 94:342, 1965.

Potter EL: *Normal and Abnormal Development of the Kidney.* Chicago, Year Book Medical Publishers, 1972.

Poutasse EF: Anterior approach to the upper urinary tract. *J Urol* 85:199, 1961.

Poutasse EF: Partial nephrectomy: new techniques, approach, operative indications, and review of 51 cases. *J Urol* 88:153, 1962.

Pressman D: Eleventh intercostal space incision for renal surgery. *J Urol* 74:578, 1955.

Primack WA, Edelmann CM Jr: Technique of renal biopsy. In: Edelmann CM Jr (Ed): *Pediatric Kidney Disease.* Boston, Little, Brown & Company, 1978, p 262.

Pritchett TR, Raval JK, Benson RC, *et al.*: Preoperative magnetic resonance imaging of vena caval tumor thrombi: experience with 5 cases. *J Urol* 138:1220, 1987.

Provet JA, Hanna MK: Simultaneous repair of bilateral ureteropelvic junction obstruction. *Urology* 33:390, 1989.

Quinton W, Dillard D, Scribner BH: Cannulation of blood vessels for prolonged hemodialysis. *Trans Am Soc Artific Int Organs* 6:104, 1960.

Rajfer J, Koyle MA, Ehrlich RM, Smith RB: Pyelovesicostomy as a form of urinary reconstruction in renal transplantation. *J Urol* 136:372, 1986.

Ramsay JWA, Miller RA, Kellett MJ, *et al.*: Percutaneous pyelolysis: indications, complications and results. *Br J Urol* 56:586, 1984.

Ranch T, Fall M, Henriksson C, *et al.*: Urodynamic consequences of a direct pyelocystostomy at autotransplantation of the kidney. *Urol Int* 40:82, 1985.

Ravitch MM: Ventral hernia. *Surg Clin North Am* 51:1341, 1971.

Redman JF: An anatomic approach to the kidneys and retroperitoneum. In: Crawford ED, Borden TA (Eds): *Genitourinary Cancer Surgery.* Philadelphia, Lea & Febiger, 1982, p 1.

Redman JF: Anatomy of the retroperitoneal connective tissue. *J Urol* 130:45, 1983.

Redman JF: The anatomy of the genitourinary system. In: Gillenwater JY, Grayhack JT, Howards SS, Duckett JW (Eds): *Adult and Pediatric Urology.* Chicago, Year Book Medical Publishers, 1987.

Reis RH, Esenther G: Variations in the pattern of renal vessels and their relation to the type of posterior vena cava in man. *Am J Anat* 104:295, 1959.

Reservitz GB: A historic review of nephroureterectomy. *Surg Gynecol Obstet* 125:853, 1967.

Rickham PP: Malignant tumours involving the genito-urinary system in childhood. In: Johnston JH, Scholtmeijer RJ (Eds): *Problems in Paediatric Urology.* Amsterdam, Excerpta Medica, 1972.

Rickwood AM, Phadke D: Pyeloplasty in infants and children with particular reference to the method of drainage postoperatively. *Br J Urol* 50:217, 1978.

Riehle RA Jr, Lavengood R: The eleventh rib transcostal incision: technique for an extrapleural approach. *J Urol* 132:1089, 1984.

Ritchey ML, Kelalis PP, Breslow N: Intracaval and atrial involvement with nephroblastoma: review of National Wilms' Tumor Study: III. *J Urol* 140:1113, 1988.

Roberts SD, Resnick MI: Complications of surgery for removal of renal and ureteral stones. In: Marshall FF (Ed): *Urologic Complications.* Chicago, Year Book Medical Publishers, 1986.

Robin CE: The renal fascia and its relation to the transversalis fascia. *Anat Rec* 89:295, 1944.

Robson CJ, Churchill BM, Anderson W: The results of radical nephrectomy for renal cell carcinoma. *Trans Am Assoc Genitourin Surg* 60:122, 1968.

Robson WJ, Rudy SM, Johnston JH: Pelviureteric obstruction in infancy. *J Pediatr Surg* 11:57, 1976.

Rodman JS, Williams JJ, Peterson CM: Dissolution of uric acid calculi. *J Urol* 131:1039, 1984.

Rohner TJ Jr, Drago JR: Subcapsular nephrectomy. In: *Rob and Smith's Operative Surgery,* 4th ed, Urology Volume. St. Louis, C. V. Mosby Company, 1983.

Ross G Jr: Fistula and obstruction following renal transplantation. In: Resnick MI, Kursh E (Eds): *Current Ther-*

apy in Genitourinary Surgery. Toronto, Philadelphia, B. C. Decker, Inc, 1987, p 419.

Ross JA, Samuel E, Millar DR: Variations in the renal vascular pedicle (an anatomical and radiological study with particular reference to renal transplantation). *Br J Urol* 33:478, 1961.

Roth RA: Residual stones. In: Roth RA, Finlayson B (Eds): *Stones: Clinical Management of Urolithiasis.* Baltimore, Williams & Wilkins Company, 1983, p 422.

Rouiller C: General anatomy and histology of the kidney. In: Rouiller C, Miller AF (Eds): *The Kidney.* New York, Academic Press, 1969, vol 1, pp 61–156.

Rubenstein WA, Auh YH, Zirinsky K, *et al.*: Posterior peritoneal recesses: assessment using CT. *Radiology* 156:461, 1985.

Salvatierra O, Kountz SL, Belzer FO: Prevention of ureteral fistula after renal transplantation. *J Urol* 112:445, 1974.

Salvatierra O, Belzer FO: Pediatric cadaver kidneys: their use in renal transplantation. *Arch Surg* 110:181, 1975.

Salvatierra O, Olcott C, Amend WJ, *et al.*: Urological complications of renal transplantation can be prevented or controlled. *J Urol* 117:421, 1977.

Sampaio FJB, Mandarim-De-Lacerda CA: Anatomic classification of the kidney collecting system for endourologic procedures. *Endourol* 2:247, 1988.

Sampaio FJB, Aragao AHM: Anatomical relationship between the intrarenal arteries and the kidney collecting system. *J Urol* 143:679, 1990.

Sandler CM, Toombs BD: Computed tomographic evaluation of blunt renal injuries. *Radiology* 141:461, 1981.

Sant GR, Blaivis JG, Meares EM: Hemiacidrin irrigation in the management of struvite calculi: long-term results. *J Urol* 130:1048, 1983.

Scardino PL, Prince CL: Vertical flap ureteropelvioplasty: preliminary report. *South Med J* 46:325, 1953.

Schefft P, Novick AC, Straffon RA, Stewart BH: Surgery for renal cell carcinoma extending into the inferior vena cava. *J Urol* 120:28, 1977.

Schiff M Jr, McGuire EJ, Weiss RM, Lytton B: Management of urinary fistulas after renal transplantation. *J Urol* 115:251, 1976.

Schoenenberger A, Mettler D, Roesler H, *et al.*: The value of an alloplastic absorbable capsule in the management of traumatic kidney lesions: an experimental study. *J Urol* 133:131A(Suppl), 1985.

Schreiner GE: Renal biopsy. In: Strauss MB, Welt LG (Eds): *Diseases of the Kidney,* 2nd ed. Boston, Little, Brown & Company, 1971, p 197.

Scott HW Jr, Cantrell JR, Bunce PL: The principle of aortic compression in the management of massive hemorrhage from the renal pedicle after nephrectomy. *J Urol* 69:26, 1953.

Scott RF Jr, Selzman HM: Complications of nephrectomy: review of 450 patients and a description of a modification of the transperitoneal approach. *J Urol* 95:307, 1966.

Segura JW, Kellis Burke EC: Horseshoe kidney in children. *J Urol* 108:333, 1972.

Semb C: Conservative renal surgery. *J R Coll Surg Edin* 10:9, 1964.

Shaw PJR: Supravesical bladder neck closure. In: Whitfield HH (Ed): *Genitourinary Surgery.* Oxford, Butterworth-Heinemann, 1993.

Shiratori T, Kinoshita H: Electromyographic study on urinary tract: II. Electromyographic study on the genesis of peristaltic movement of the dog's ureter. *Tohoku J Exp Med* 73:103, 1961.

Siegfried MS, Rochester D, Bernstein JR, Miller JW. Diagnosis of inferior vena cava anomalies by computerized tomography. *Comput Radiol* 7:119, 1983.

Silverman DE, Stamey TA: Management of infection stones: the Stanford experience. *Medicine* 62:44, 1983.

Singh M, Marshall V, Blandy J: The residual renal stone. *Br J Urol* 47:125, 1975.

Skinner DG, Colvin R, Vermillion CD: The surgical management of renal cell carcinoma. *J Urol* 107:705, 1972.

Skinner DG: Considerations for management of large retroperitoneal tumors: use of the modified thoracoabdominal approach. *J Urol* 117:605, 1977.

Skinner DG, Gloege GM: Technique of nephroureterectomy with regional node dissection. *Urol Clin North Am* 5:253, 1978.

Smart WR: An evaluation of the intubation ureterotomy with a description of surgical technique. *J Urol* 85:512, 1961.

Smith AD, Lange PH, Fraley EE: Percutaneous nephrostomy: new challenges and opportunities in endo-urology. *J Urol* 121:382, 1979.

Smith DR, Schulte JW, Smart WR: Surgery of the kidney. In: Campbell M (Ed): *Urology.* Philadelphia, W. B. Saunders Company, 1963, vol III, p 2324.

Smith JM, Butler MR: Splinting in pyeloplasty. *Urology* 8:218, 1976.

Smith MJV, Boyce WH: Anatrophic nephrotomy and plastic calyrhaphy. *J Urol* 99:521, 1968.

Smith P, Roberts M, Whitaker RH, *et al.*: Primary pelvic hydronephrosis in children: a retrospective study. *Br J Urol* 48:549, 1976.

Smith RB, Ehrlich RM: Complications of renal transplant surgery (including autotransplantation). In: Smith RB, Skinner DG (Eds): *Complications of Urologic Surgery.* Philadelphia, W. B. Saunders Company, 1976, p 459.

Snyder HM III, Lebowitz RL, Colodny AH, *et al.*: Ureteropelvic junction obstruction in children. *Urol Clin North Am* 7:273, 1980.

Spanos PK, Simmons RL, Buselmeier TJ, *et al.*: Kidney transplantation from living related donors with multiple vessels. *Am J Surg* 125:554, 1973.

Spence HM: Some observations on the indications for and technique of transperitoneal renal surgery. *Urol Corresp Club Lett* Feb 9, 1962.

Ssysganow AN: Über des Lymphsystem der Nieren und Nierenhüllen beim Menschen. *Gesamte Anat* 91:771, 1930.

Stephenson TP, Bauer S, Hargreave TB, Turner-Warwick R: The technique and results of pyelocalycotomy for staghorn calculi. *Br J Urol* 47:751, 1976.

Stewart BH: Radical nephrectomy. In: Stewart BH (Ed): *Operative Urology.* Baltimore, Williams & Wilkins Company, 1975, p 114.

Stewart BH, Hewitt CB, Banowsky LHW: Management of extensively destroyed ureter: special reference to renal autotransplantation. *J Urol* 115:257, 1976.

Strong DW, Pearse HD, Tank ES Jr, Hodges CV: The ureteral stump after nephroureterectomy. *J Urol* 115:654, 1976.

Sullivan MJ, Joseph E, Taylor JC: Extracorporeal renal parenchymal surgery with continuous perfusion. *JAMA* 229:1780, 1974.

Sykes D: The arterial supply of the human kidney with special reference to accessory renal arteries. *Br J Surg* 50:368, 1963.

Sykes D: The correlation between renal vascularisation and lobulation of the kidney. *Br J Urol* 36:549, 1964.

Sykes D: The morphology of renal lobulations and calices, and their relationship to partial nephrectomy. *Br J Surg* 51:294, 1964.

Taylor RJ: Cadaveric kidney recovery. In: Resnick MI, Kursh E (Eds): *Current Therapy in Genitourinary Surgery.* Toronto, Philadelphia, B. C. Decker, Inc, 1987, p 425.

Tenckhoff H, Schechter H: A bacteriologically safe peritoneal access device. *Trans Am Soc Artif Intern Organ* 14:181, 1968.

Tessler AN, Yuvienco F, Farcon E: Paramedian extraperitoneal incision for total nephroureterectomy. *Urology* 5:397, 1975.

Thompson IM, Latourette H, Montie JE, Ross G Jr: Results of nonoperative management of blunt renal trauma. *J Urol* 118:522, 1977.

Thornbury JR: Perirenal anatomy: normal and abnormal. *Radiol Clin North Am* 17:321, 1979.

Thüroff JW, Frohneberg D, Riedmiller R, et al.: Localisation of segmental arteries in renal surgery by Doppler sonography. *J Urol* 127:863, 1982.

Tobin CE: The renal fascia and its relation to the transversalis fascia. *Anat Rec* 89:295, 1944.

Toguri AG, Emtage JB, Jarzylo SV: Management of total ureteral loss after kidney transplantation. *Can J Surg* 26:498, 1983.

Tuffier R, Lejars F: Les veines de la capsule adipeuse du rein. *Arch Physiol* 1:41, 1891.

Turner-Warnick RT: The supracostal approach to the renal area. *Br J Urol* 37:671, 1965.

Turner-Warwick R, Wynne EJ, Ashken MH: The use of the omental pedicle graft in the repair and reconstruction of the urinary tract. *Br J Surg* 54:849, 1967.

Underbjerg PE, Munch JT, Taagehøj-Jensen F, Djurhuus JC: The functional outcome of Anderson-Hynes pyeloplasty for hydronephrosis. *Scand J Urol Nephrol* 21:213, 1987.

Usher FC: New technique for repairing incisional hernias with Marlex mesh. *Am J Surg* 138:740, 1979.

Uson AC, Cox LA, Lattimer JK: Hydronephrosis in infants and children: II. Surgical management and results. *JAMA* 205:327, 1968.

Vandeput JJ, Tanner JC, Eberhart C: Partial nephrectomy: experimental closure with a free peritoneal graft. *J Urol* 93:364, 1967.

Vermootin V: Indications for conservative surgery in certain renal tumors: a study based on the growth pattern of the clear cell carcinoma. *J Urol* 64:200, 1950.

Wagget J, Koop CE: Wilms' tumor: preoperative radiotherapy and chemotherapy in the management of massive tumors. *Cancer* 26:338, 1970.

Wald U, Caine M, Solomon H: Partial nephrectomy in surgical treatment of calculous disease. *Urology* 11:343, 1978.

Ward JP, Smart CJ, O'Donoghue EPN, et al.: Synchronous bilateral lumbotomy. *Eur Urol* 2:102, 1976.

Watts HG: Heminephrectomy: a simplified technique. *Aust N Z J Surg* 37:256, 1968.

Wein AJ, Murphy JJ, Mulholland SG, et al.: A conservative approach to the management of blunt renal trauma. *J Urol* 117:425, 1977.

Wein AJ, Carpiniello VL, Murphy JJ: A simple technique for partial nephrectomy. *Surg Gynecol Obstet* 146:620, 1978.

Wickham JEA: Conservative renal surgery for adenocarcinoma: the place of bench surgery. *Br J Urol* 47:25, 1975.

Wickham JEA: Conservative renal surgery for adenocarcinoma: natural history and results of treatment. *J Urol* 119:722, 1978.

Williams DF, Schapiro AE, Arconti JS, et al.: A new technique of partial nephrectomy. *J Urol* 97:955, 1967.

Williams DI, Karlaftis CM: Hydronephrosis due to pelviureteric obstruction in the newborn. *Br J Urol* 38:138, 1969.

Williams DI, Cromie WJ: Ring ureterostomy. *Br J Urol* 47:789, 1975.

Williams DI, Martin J: Renal tumors. In: Williams DI, Johnston JH (Eds): *Pediatric Urology*, 2nd ed. London, Butterworth, 1982.

Witherington R: Improving the supracostal loin incisions. *J Urol* 124:73, 1980.

Woodruff MFA, Doig A, Donald KW, Nolan B: Renal autotransplantation. *Lancet* 1:433, 1966.

Young HH: A technique for simultaneous exposure and operation on the adrenals. *Surg Gynecol Obstet* 54:179, 1936.

Zincke H, Kelalis PP, Culp OS: Ureteropelvic obstruction in children. *Surg Gynecol Obstet* 139:873, 1974.

Zingg ES, Futterlieb A: Nephroscopy in stone surgery. *Br J Urol* 52:333, 1980.

Ziolkowski M, Kurlej W, Klak A: Typology of the renal pelvices in human fetuses. *Folia Morphol (Warsz)* 47:153, 1988.

Zuckerkandl E: Beiträge zur Anatomie des menschlichen Körpers: I. Ueber den Fixationsapparat der Nieren. In: *Anatomie des Menschens.* vol 1, Tübingen, vol II, 1863, p 59.

Section 4—Adrenal Gland

Aird I: Bilateral anterior transabdominal adrenalectomy. *Br Med J* 2:708, 1955.

Caty MG, Coran AG, Geagan M, Thompson NW: Current diagnosis and treatment of pheochromocytoma in children: experience with 22 consecutive tumors in 14 patients. *Arch Surg* 125:978, 1990.

Chino ES, Thomas CG: An extended Kocher incision for bilateral adrenalectomy. *Am J Surg* 149:292, 1985.

Deoreo GA Jr, Stewart BH, Tarazi RC, Gifford RW: Preoperative blood transfusion in the safe surgical management of pheochromocytoma: a review of 46 cases. *J Urol* 111:715, 1974.

Fonkalsrud EW: Adrenal pheochromocytoma in childhood. *Progr Pediatr Surg* 26:103, 1991.

Gittes RF, Mahoney EM: Pheochromocytoma. *Urol Clin North Am* 4:239, 1977.

Goldfein A: Pheochromocytoma: diagnosis and anesthetic and surgical management. *Anesthesiology* 24:462, 1963.

Hume DM: Pheochromocytoma in the adult and in the child. *Am J Surg* 99:458, 1960.

McDougall WS: Surgery of the adrenal. In: *Rob and Smith's Operative Urology*, 4th ed, Urology Volume. St. Louis, C. V. Mosby Company, 1983.

O'Neal LW: *Surgery of the Adrenal Glands*. St. Louis, C. V. Mosby Company, 1968.

Scott HW Jr: The pituitary and adrenals. In: Sabiston DC Jr (Ed): *Textbook of Surgery: The Biological Basis of Modern Surgical Practice*, 11th ed. Philadelphia, W. B. Saunders Company, 1977, pp 776–783.

Scott HW Jr, Dean RH, Oates JA, et al.: Surgical management of pheochromocytoma. *Am Surg* 47:6, 1981.

Shandling B, Wesson D, Filler RM: Recurrent pheochromocytoma in children. *J Pediatr Surg* 25:1063, 1990.

Shulkin BL, Wieland DM, Schwaiger M, et al.: PET scanning with hydroxyephedrine: an approach to the localization of pheochromocytoma. *J Nucl Med* 33:1125, 1992.

van Heerden JA, Sheps SG, Hamberger B, et al.: Pheochromocytoma: current status and changing trends. *Surgery* 91:367, 1982.

Vaughan ED Jr, Phillips H: Modified posterior approach for right adrenalectomy. *Surg Gynecol Obst* 165:453, 1987.

Whalen RK, Althausen AF, Daniels GH: Extra-adrenal pheochromocytoma. *J Urol* 147:1, 1992.

Young HH: A technique for simultaneous exposure and operation on the adrenals. *Surg Gynecol Obstet* 54:179, 1936.

Section 5—Ureteral

Agran MA, Kratzman EA: Inferior vena cava on the left side: its relationship to the right ureter. *J Urol* 101:149, 1969.

Allen TD: Congenital ureteral strictures. *J Urol* 104:196, 1970.

Amar AD: Reimplantation of completely duplicated ureters. *J Urol* 107:230, 1972.

Amar AD, Egan RM, Das S: Ipsilateral ureteroureterostomy combined with ureteral reimplantation for treatment of disease in both ureters in a child with complete ureteral duplication. *J Urol* 125:581, 1981.

Amin H: Experience with the ileal ureter. *Br J Urol* 48:19, 1976.

Anderson JC, Hynes W: Retrocaval ureter: a case diagnosed pre-operatively and treated successfully by plastic operation. *Br J Urol* 21:209, 1949.

Barrett DM, Malek RS, Kelalis PP: Problems and solutions in surgical treatment of 100 consecutive ureteral duplications in children. *J Urol* 114:126, 1975.

Baum WC: The clinical use of terminal ileum as a substitute ureter. *J Urol* 72:16, 1954.

Belman AB, Filmer RB, King LR: Surgical management of duplication of the collecting system. *J Urol* 112:316, 1974.

Bischoff P: Operative treatment of megaureter. *J Urol* 85:268, 1961.

Bishop MC, Askew AR, Smith JC: Reimplantation of the wide ureter. *Br J Urol* 50:383, 1978.

Blok C, Van Venroolj EPM, Mokhless I, Coolsaet BLRA: Dynamics of the ureterovesical junction: its fluid transport mechanism in the pig. *J Urol* 134:175, 1985.

Boari A: Chirurgia dell'uretere. In: *Societa Editrice Dante Alighieri*. Rome, 1900, p 176–177.

Boxer RJ, Fritzsche P, Skinner DG, et al.: Replacement of the ureter by small intestine: clinical applications and results of ileo-ureter in 89 patients. *J Urol* 121:128, 1979.

Brown S: Open versus endoscopic surgery in the treatment of vesicoureteral reflux. *J Urol,* 142:499, 1989.

Carini M, Selli C, Lenzi R, et al.: Surgical treatment of vesicoureteral reflux with bilateral medialization of the ureteral orifices. *Eur Urol* 11:181, 1985.

Carrion H, Safewood J, Politano V, et al.: Retrocaval ureter: report of 8 cases and the surgical management. *J Urol* 121:514, 1979.

Cass AS, Schmaelzle JF, Hinman F Jr: Ureteral anastomosis in the dog: comparing continuous with interrupted sutures. *Invest Urol* 6:94, 1968.

Caulk JR: Megaloureter: the importance of the ureterovesical valve. *J Urol* 9:315, 1923.

Cendron J, Melin Y, Valayer J: Simplified treatment of ureterocele with pyelo-ureteric duplication. *Eur Urol* 7:321, 1981.

Chilton CP, Vordermark JS, Ransley PG: Transuretero-ureterostomy: a review of its use in modern pediatric urology. *Br J Urol* 56:604, 1984.

Couvelaire R, Auvert J, Moulonguet A, et al.: Implantations et anastomoses urétéro-calicielles: techniques et indications. *J Urol Nephrol* 70:437, 1964.

Creevy CD: Misadventures following replacement of ureters with ileum. *Surgery* 58:497, 1965.

Creevy CD: The atonic distal ureteral segment (ureteral achalasia). *J Urol* 97:457, 1969.

Dolff C: Verbesserung der Ergebnisse der Ureterimplantation in die Blase mit Hilfe einer elastischen Fixation der Blase. *Zentralbl Gynakol* 74:1777, 1952.

Donohue JP, Hostetter M, Glover J, Madura J: Ureteroneocystostomy versus ureteropyelostomy: a comparison in the same renal allograft series. *J Urol* 114:202, 1975.

Dowd JB, Chen F: Ileal replacement of the ureter in the solitary kidney. *Surg Clin North Am* 51:739, 1971.

Ehrlich RM, Skinner DG: Complications of transuretero-ureterostomy. *J Urol* 113:467, 1975.

Ehrlich RM: The ureteral folding technique for megaureter surgery. *J Urol* 134:668, 1986.

Ehrlich RM, Gershman A, Fuchs G: Selected topics in pediatric urology. *Pediatr Urol Corresp Club Letter,* Feb 28, 1993.

Fort KF, Selman SH, Kropp KA: A retrospective analysis of the use of ureteral stents in children undergoing ureteroneocystostomy. *J Urol* 129:545, 1983.

Gearhart JP, Woolfenden KA: The vesico-psoas hitch as an adjunct to megaureter repair in childhood. *J Urol* 127:505, 1982.

Gil Vernet JM: A new technique for surgical correction of vesicoureteral reflux. *J Urol* 131:456, 1984.

Glassberg KI, Laungani G, Wasnick RJ, Waterhouse K: Transverse ureteral advancement technique of ureteroneocystostomy (Cohen reimplant) and modification for difficult cases (experience with 121 ureters). *J Urol* 134:304, 1985.

Gonzales ET Jr, Decter RM: Management of ureteroceles in the newborn. In: King LR, (Ed): *Urologic Surgery in Neonates and Young Infants.* Philadelphia, W. B. Saunders Company, 1988, p 204.

Goodwin WE, Burke DE, Muller WH: Retrocaval ureter. *Surg Gynecol Obstet* 104:337, 1957.

Goodwin WE, Winter CC, Turner RD: Replacement of the ureter by small intestine: clinical application and results of the ileal ureter. *J Urol* 81:406, 1959.

Gow JG: *Color Atlas of Boari Bladder Flap Procedure.* Oradell, Medical Economics Books, 1983.

Gregoir W, Van Regemorter GV: Le reflux vésico-urétéral congenital. *Urol Int* 18:122, 1964.

Gregoir W: Lich-Gregoir operation. In: Epstein HB, Hohenfellner R, Williams DI (Eds): *Surgical Pediatric Urology.* Stuttgart, Thieme, 1977, p 265.

Gregoir W, Schulman CC: Die extravesikale Antireflux-plastik. *Urologe A* 16:124, 1977.

Gross M, Peng B, Waterhouse L: Use of the mobilized bladder to replace the pelvic ureter. *J Urol* 101:40, 1969.

Gutierrez J, Chang CY, Nesbit RM: Ipsilateral ureteroureterostomy for vesicoureteral reflux in duplicated ureter. *J Urol* 101:36, 1969.

Halpern GN, King LR, Belman AB: Transureteroureterostomy in children. *J Urol* 109:504, 1973.

Hanna MK: New surgical method for one-stage total remodeling of massively dilated and tortuous ureter: tapering in situ technique. *Urology* 14:453, 1979.

Hanna MK: Megaureter. In: King LR (Ed): *Urologic Surgery in Neonates and Young Infants.* Philadelphia, W. B. Saunders Company, 1988, p 160.

Harrill HC: Retrocaval ureter: report of a case with operative correction of the defect. *J Urol* 44:450, 1940.

Hawthorne NJ, Zincke H, Kelalis PP: Ureterocalycostomy: an alternative to nephrectomy. *J Urol* 115:583, 1976.

Hendren WH: Operative repair of megaureter in children. *J Urol* 101:49, 1969.

Hendren WH: Functional restoration of decompensated ureters in children. *Am J Surg* 119:477, 1970.

Hendren WH: A new approach to infants with severe obstructive uropathy: early complete reconstruction. *J Pediatr Surg* 5:184, 1970.

Hendren HW, Monfort GJ: Surgical correction of ureteroceles in childhood. *J Pediat Surg* 6:235, 1971.

Hendren WH: Complications of megaureter repair in children. *J Urol* 113:238, 1975.

Hendren WH: Complications of ureteral reimplantation and megaureter repair. In: Smith RB, Skinner DC (Eds): *Complications of Urologic Surgery: Prevention and Management.* Philadelphia, W. B. Saunders Company, 1976, pp 151–208.

Hendren WH: Technical aspects of megaureter repair. *Birth Defects* 13:21, 1977.

Hendren WH, Mitchell ME: Surgical correction of ureteroceles. *J Urol* 121:590, 1979.

Hendren WH, Hensle TW: Transureteroureterostomy: experience with 75 cases. *J Urol* 123:826, 1980.

Hendren WH, McLorie GA: Late stricture of intestinal ureters. *J Urol* 129:584, 1983.

Hensle TW, Burbige KA, Levin RK: Management of the short ureter in urinary tract reconstruction. *J Urol* 137:707, 1987.

Higgins CC: Transuretero-ureteral anastomosis. *J Urol* 34:349, 1935.

Hinman F Jr: Ureteral repair and the splint. *J Urol* 78:376, 1957.

Hinman F Jr, Miller ER: Mural tension in vesical disorders and ureteral reflex. *J Urol* 91:33, 1964.

Hinman F Jr, Baumann FW: Complications of vesicoureteral operations from incoordination of micturition. *J Urol* 116:638, 1976.

Hirschorn RC: The ileal sleeve: II. Surgical technique in clinical application. *J Urol* 92:120, 1964.

Hodges CV, Moore RJ, Lehman TH, Benham AM: Clinical experiences with transureteroureterostomy. *J Urol* 90:552, 1963.

Hodges CV, Barry JM, Fuchs EF, *et al.*: Transureteroureterostomy: 25 years experience with 100 patients. *J Urol* 123:834, 1980.

Hodgson NB, Thompson LW: Technique of reductive ureteroplasty in the management of megaureter. *J Urol* 113:118, 1975.

Hodgson NB: Urinary tract infections in childhood. In: Kendall AR, Karafin L (Eds): *Urology.* Philadelphia, Harper and Row, 1982, vol 1, p 22.

Houle AM, McLorie GA, Heritz DM, *et al.*: Extravesical nondismembered ureteropyleoplasty with detrusorrhaphy: a renewed technique to correct vesicoureteral reflux in children. *J Urol* 148:704, 1992.

Hutch JA: *The Uretero-vesical Junction.* Berkeley, University of California Press, 1958.

Jameson SG, McKinney JS, Rushton JF: Ureterocalycostomy: A new surgical procedure for correction of ureteropelvic stricture associated with an intrarenal pelvis. *J Urol* 77:135, 1957.

Johnston JH: Reconstructive surgery of mega-ureter in childhood. *Br J Urol* 39:17, 1967.

Johnston JH, Heal MR: Reflux in complete duplicated ureters in children: management and techniques. *J Urol* 105:881, 1971.

Johnston JH, Johnson LM: Experiences with ectopic ureteroceles. *Br J Urol* 41:61, 1971.

Johnston JH, Farkas A: The congenital refluxing megaureter: experiences with surgical reconstruction. *Br J Urol* 47:153, 1975.

Juskiewenski S, Vaysse P, Moscovici J, *et al.*: The ureterovesical junction. *Anat Clin* 5:251, 1984.

Kalicinski ZH, Kansy J, Kotarbínska B, Joszt W: Surgery of megaureters: modification of Hendren's operation. *J Pediatr Surg* 12:183, 1977.

King LR: Megaloureter: definition, diagnosis and management. *J Urol* 123:222, 1980.

Lapides, J: The physiology of the intact human ureter. *J Urol* 59:501, 1948.

Lich R Jr, Howerton LW, Davis LA: Recurrent urosepsis in children. *J Urol* 86:554, 1961.

Lyon RP, Marshall S, Tanagho EA: The ureteral orifice: its configuration and competency. *J Urol* 102:504, 1969.

Malek RS, Kelalis PP, Burke EC, *et al.*: Simple and ectopic ureterocele in infancy and childhood. *Surg Gynecol Obstet* 134:611, 1972.

Mathisen W: Vesicoureteral reflux and its surgical correction. *Surg Gynecol Obstet* 118:965, 1964.

Mering JM, Steel JF, Gittes RF: Congenital ureteral valves. *J Urol* 107:737, 1972.

Mollard P, Braun P: Primary ureterocalycostomy for severe hydronephrosis in children. *J Pediatr Surg* 15:87, 1980.

Moore EV, Weber R, Woodward ER, *et al.*: Isolated ileal loops for ureteral repair. *Surg Gynecol Obstet* 102:87, 1956.

Nesbit RM: Elliptical anastomosis and urologic surgery. *Ann Surg* 130:796, 1949.

Neuwirt K: Implantation of the ureter into the lower calyx of the renal pelvis. In: *VII Congrés de la Société Internationale d'Urologie,* part 2, 1947, p 253.

Ockerblad N: Reimplantation of the ureter into the bladder by a flap method. *J Urol* 57:845, 1947.

Paquin AJ Jr: Ureterovesical anastomosis: the description and evaluation of a technique. *J Urol* 82:573, 1959.

Politano VA, Leadbetter WF: An operative technique for the correction of ureteric reflux. *J Urol* 79:932, 1958.

Prout GR Jr, Stuart WT, Witus WS: Utilization of ileal segments to substitute for extensive ureteral loss. *J Urol* 90:541, 1963.

Reha WC, Gibbons MD: Neonatal ascites and ureteral valves. *Urology* 33:468, 1989.

Reid R, Schneider K, Fruchtman B: Closure of the bladder neck in patients undergoing continent vesicostomy for urinary incontinence. *J Urol* 120:40, 1978.

Reinberg Y, Aliabadi H, Johnson P, *et al.*: Congenital ureteral valves in children: case report and review of the literature. *J Pediatr Surg* 22:379, 1987.

Retik AB, McEvoy JP, Bauer SB: Megaureters in children. *Urology* 11:231, 1978.

Rickwood AMK, Reiner I, Jones M, Pournaras C: Current management of duplex-system ureteroceles: experience with 41 patients. *Br J Urol* 70:196, 1992.

Ruano-Gil D, Coca-Payeras A, Tejedo-Mateu A: Obstruction and normal recanalization of the ureter in the human embryo: its relation to congenital ureteric obstruction. *Eur Urol* 1:287, 1975.

Sant GR, Barbalias GA, Klauber GT: Congenital ureteral valves: an abnormality of ureteral embryogenesis? *J Urol* 133:427, 1985.

Schulman CC, Gregoir W: Ureteric duplication. In: Eckstein HB, Hohenfellner R, Williams DI (Eds): *Surgical Pediatric Urology.* Stuttgart, Philadelphia, Georg Thieme Verlag, 1977, p 244.

Schwarz R, Stephens FD: The persisting mesonephric duct: high junction of vas deferens and ureter. *J Urol* 120:592, 1978.

Shapiro SR, Peckler MS, Johnston JH: Transureteroureterostomy for urinary diversion in children. *Urology* 8:35, 1976.

Shehata R: A comparative study of the urinary bladder and the intramural portion of the ureter. *Acta Anat* 98:380, 1977.

Smith JA Jr, Lee RE, Middleton RG: Ventriculoureteral shunt for hydrocephalus without nephrectomy. *J Urol* 123:224, 1980.

Starr A: Ureteral plication: a new concept in ureteral tailoring for megaureter. *Invest Urol* 17:153, 1979.

Stephens FD: Treatment of megaureters by multiple micturition. *Aust N Z J Surg* 27:130, 1957.

Stephens FD, Lenaghan D: The anatomical basis and dynamics of vesicoureteral reflux. *J Urol* 87:669, 1962.

Stephens FD: The vesicoureteral hiatus and para ureteral diverticula. *J Urol* 121:786, 1979.

Tanagho EA, Pugh RCB: The anatomy and function of the ureterovesical junction. *Br J Urol* 35:151, 1963.

Tanagho EA, Meyers FH, Smith DR: The trigone: anatomical and physiological considerations in relation to the ureterovesical junction. *J Urol* 100:623, 1968.

Tanagho EA: Ureteral tailoring. *J Urol* 106:194, 1971.

Tanagho EA: Anatomy and management of ureteroceles. *J Urol* 107:729, 1972.

Tanagho EA: A case against incorporation of bowel segments into the closed urinary system. *J Urol* 113:796, 1975.

Tanagho EA: Embryologic basis for lower ureteral anomalies: a hypothesis. *Urology* 7:451, 1976.

Turner-Warwick R: Lower pole pyelocalycotomy, retrograde partial nephrectomy and ureterocalycostomy. *Br J Urol* 37:673, 1965.

Udall DA, Hodges CV, Pearse HM, *et al.*: Transureteroureterostomy: a neglected procedure. *J Urol* 109:817, 1973.

Wacksman J, Gilbert A, Sheldon CA: Results of the renewed extravesical reimplant for surgical correction of vesicoureteral reflux. *J Urol* 148:359, 1992.

Waldeyer W: Ureter-scheide. *Verh Anat Ges* 6:259, 1892.

Weinstein AJ, Bauer SB, Retik AB, *et al.*: The surgical management of megaureters in duplex systems: the efficacy of ureteral tapering and common sheath reimplantation. *J Urol* 139:328, 1988.

Wesolowski S: Corrective operative procedure after unsuccessful pelvi-ureteric plastic surgery. *Br J Urol* 43:679, 1971.

Wesolowski S: Ureterocalycostomy. *Eur Urol* 1:18, 1975.

Wickramasinghe SF, Stephens FD: Paraureteral diverticula: associated renal morphology and embryogenesis. *Invest Urol* 14:381, 1977.

Williams DI, Woodard JR: Problems in the management of ectopic ureteroceles. *J Urol* 92:635, 1964.

Williams DI, Eckstein HB: Surgical treatment of reflux in children. *Br J Urol* 37:13, 1965.

Zaontz MR, Maizels M, Sugar EC, Firlit CF: Detrusorrhaphy: extravesical ureteral advancement to correct vesicoureteral reflux in children. *J Urol* 138:947, 1987.

Section 6—Bladder

Abrams JS: *Abdominal Stomas: Indications, Operative Techniques and Patient Care.* Boston, Wright, 1984.

Adams JT: Z-stitch suture for inversion of appendiceal stump. *Surg Gynecol Obstet* 127:1320, 1968.

Adams MC, Mitchell ME, Rink RC: Gastrocystoplasty: an alternative solution to the problem of urological reconstruction in the severely compromised patient. *J Urol* 140:1152, 1988.

Ahlering TE, Weinberg AC, Razor B: A comparative study of the ileal conduit, Kock pouch and modified Indiana pouch. *J Urol* 142:1193, 1989.

Albert DJ, Persky L: Conjoined end-to-end uretero-intestinal anastomosis. *J Urol* 105:201, 1971.

Alday ES, Goldsmith HS: Surgical technique for omental lengthening based on arterial anatomy. *Surg Gynecol Obstet* 135:103, 1972.

Allen TD, Spence HM, Salyer KE: Reconstruction of the external genitalia in exstrophy of the bladder: preliminary communication. *J Urol* 11:830, 1974.

Allen TD: Vesicostomy for the temporary diversion of the urine in small children. *J Urol* 123:929, 1980.

Allen TD, Husman DS, Bucholz RW: Exstrophy of the bladder: primary closure after iliac osteotomies without external or internal fixation. *J Urol* 147:438, 1992.

Althausen AF, Hagen-Cook K, Hendren WH III: Non-refluxing colon conduit: experience with 70 cases. *J Urol* 120:35, 1978.

Ambrose SS, O'Brien DP III. Surgical embryology of the exstrophy-epispadias complex. *Surg Clin North Am* 54:1379, 1974.

Anderl H, Jaske G, Marberger H: Reconstruction of abdominal wall and mons pubis in females with bladder exstrophy. *Urology* 22:247, 1983.

Ansell JS: Surgical treatment of exstrophy of bladder with emphasis on neonatal primary closure: personal experience with 28 consecutive cases treated at University of Washington Hospitals from 1962 to 1977. Technique and results. *J Urol* 121:650, 1979.

Ansell JS: Exstrophy and epispadias. In: Glenn JF (Ed): *Urologic Surgery,* 3rd ed. Philadelphia, J. B. Lippincott Company, 1983.

Arai Y, Kawakita M, Terachi T, et al.: Long-term follow-up of Kock and Indiana pouch procedures. *J Urol* 150:51, 1993.

Arap S, Giron AM, deGóes GM: Complete reconstruction of bladder exstrophy: experimental program. *Urology,* 7:413, 1976.

Arap S, Giron AM, deGóes GM: Initial results of the complete reconstruction of bladder exstrophy. *Urol Clin North Am* 7:477, 1980.

Ariyoshi A, Fujisawa Y, Ohshima K: Catheterless cutaneous ureterostomy. *J Urol* 114:533, 1975.

Arnarson O, Straffon RA: Clinical experience with the ileal conduit in children. *J Urol* 102:768, 1969.

Ashken MH: An appliance-free ileocaecal urinary diversion: preliminary communication. *Br J Urol* 46:631, 1974.

Ashken MH: *Urinary Diversion.* Berlin, Heideberg, New York, Springer-Verlag, 1982.

Ashken MH: Stomas continent and incontinent. *Br J Urol* 59:203, 1987.

Atala A, Bauer SB, Hendren WH, Retik AB: The effect of gastric augmentation on bladder function. *J Urol* 149:1099, 1993.

Avni EF, Matos C, Diard F, Schulman CC: Midline omphalocele anomalies in children: contribution of ultrasound imaging. *Urol Radiol* 10:189–194, 1988.

Bagley DH, Glazier W, Osias M, et al.: Retroperitoneal drainage of uretero-intestinal conduits. *J Urol* 121:271, 1979.

Barrett DM, Malek RS, Kelalis P: Observations on vesical diverticulum in childhood. *J Urol* 116:234, 1976.

Barrett DM, Furlow WL: The management of severe urinary incontinence in patients with myelodysplasia by implantation of the AS 791/792 urinary sphincter device. *J Urol* 128:484, 1982.

Barry JM, Pitre TM, Hodges CV: Ureteroileourethrostomy: 16-year followup. *J Urol* 115:29, 1976.

Basmajian JV: The main arteries of the large intestine. *Surg Gynecol Obstet* 101:585, 1959.

Bauer SB, Retik AB: Urachal anomalies and related umbilical disorders. *Urol Clin North Am* 5:195, 1978.

Bauer SB, Hendren WH, Kozakewich H, et al.: Perforation of the augmented bladder. *J Urol* 148 (Part 2):699, 1992.

Beckley S, Wajsman W, Pontes JE, Murphy G: Transverse colon conduit: a method of urinary diversion after pelvic irradiation. *J Urol* 128:464, 1982.

Begg RC: The urachus and umbilical fistulae. *Surg Gynecol Obstet* 45:165, 1927.

Bejany DE, Politano VA: Stapled and nonstapled tapered distal ileum for construction of a continent colonic urinary reservoir. *J Urol* 140:491, 1988.

Beland G, Laberge I: Cutaneous transureterostomy in children. *J Urol* 114:588, 1975.

Belman AB, King LR: Urinary tract abnormalities associated with imperforate anus. *J Urol* 108:823, 1972.

Benchekroun A: Continent caecal bladder. *Br J Urol* 54:505, 1982.

Benchekroun A: The ileocecal continent bladder. In: King LR, Stone AR, Webster GD (Eds): *Bladder Reconstruction and Continent Urinary Diversion.* Chicago, Mosby Year Book, 1991, p 324.

Benjamin JA, Tobin CE: Abnormalities of the kidneys, ureters, and perinephric fascia: anatomic and clinical study. *J Urol* 65:715, 1951.

Bennett RC, Duthie HL: The functional importance of the internal anal sphincter. *Br J Surg* 51:355, 1964.

Berglund B, Kock NG, Norlen L, Philipson BM: Volume capacity and pressure characteristics of the continent ileal reservoir used for urinary diversion. *J Urol* 137:29, 1987.

Bissada NK: Characteristics and use of in situ appendix as continent catheterization stoma for continent urinary diversion in adults. *J Urol* 150:151, 1993.

Blichert-Toft M, Nielson OV: Congenital patent urachus and acquired variants. *Acta Chir Scand* 137:807, 1971.

Blocksom BH Jr: Bladder pouch for prolonged tubeless cystostomy. *J Urol* 78:398, 1957.

Bloom DA, Turner WRJ, Skinner DG: Urological stomas. In: Ehrlich RM (Ed): *Modern Techniques in Surgery: Urologic Surgery.* Mount Kisco, NY, Futura, 1981.

Bloom DA, Lieskovsky G, Rainwater G, et al.: The Turnbull loop stoma. *J Urol* 129:715, 1983.

Borzyskowski M, Mundy E (Eds): *Neuropathic Bladder in Childhood.* New York, Cambridge University Press, 1991.

Boucher BJ: Sex differences in the fetal pelvis. *Am J Phys Anthropol* 15:581, 1957.

Boyce WH, Vest SA: A new concept concerning treatment of exstrophy of the bladder. *J Urol* 67:503, 1952.

Boyce WH, Kroovand RL: The Boyce-Vest operation for exstrophy of the bladder: 35 years later. *Urol Clin North Am* 13:307, 1986.

Bricker EM: Bladder substitution after pelvic evisceration. *Surg Clin North Am* 30:1511, 1950.

Bricker EM: The technique of ileal segment bladder substitution. In: Meigs JV, Sturgis SH (Eds): *Progress in Gynecology.* New York, Grune & Stratton, 1957, vol 3.

Bricker EM: The evolution of the ileal segment bladder substitution operation. *Am J Surg* 135:834, 1978.

Brock WA: Anorectal malformations: urologic implications. In: Ehrlich RM (Ed): *Dialogues in Pediatric Urology.* 10:1, 1987.

Browne D: Congenital deformities of the anus and the rectum. *Arch Dis Child* 30:42, 1955.

Browning GG, Parks AG: A method and the results of loop colostomy. *Dis Colon Rectum* 26:223, 1983.

Bruce RB, Gonzales ET: Cutaneous vesicostomy: a useful form of temporary diversion in children. *J Urol* 123:927, 1980.

Bryniak SR, Bruce AW, Awad SA: Skin flap technique in formation of urinary conduit stoma. *Urology* 1980, 15:275.

Burbige KA, Hensle TW: The complications of urinary tract reconstruction. *J Urol* 136 (Part 2):292, 1986.

Bystrom J: Early and later complications of ileal conduit urinary diversion. *Scand J Urol Nephrol* 12:233, 1978.

Carney M, Richard F, Botto H: Bladder replacement by ileocystoplasty. In: King LR, Stone AR, Webster GD (Eds): *Bladder Reconstruction and Continent Urinary Diversion.* Chicago, Year Book Medical Publishers, 1987.

Cauldwell EW, Anson BJ: The visceral branches of the abdominal aorta: topographical relationships. *Am J Anat* 73:27, 1943.

Chan SL, Ankenman GJ, Wright JE, McLoughlin MG: Cecocystoplasty in the surgical management of the small contracted bladder. *J Urol* 124:338, 1980.

Chevrel JP, Gueraud JP: Arteries of the terminal ileum: diaphanization study and surgical applications. *Anat Clin* 1:95, 1979.

Churchill BM, Aliabadi H, Landau EH, *et al.*: Ureteral bladder augmentation. *J Urol* 150:716, 1993.

Clark SS: Electrolyte disturbance associated with jejunal conduit. *J Urol* 112:42, 1974.

Coffey RC: Transplantation of the ureters into the large intestine in the absence of the functioning urinary bladder. *Surg Gynecol Obstet* 32:383, 1921.

Cohen JS, Harbach LB, Kaplan GW: Cutaneous vesicostomy for temporary diversion in infants with neurogenic bladder dysfunction. *J Urol* 119:120, 1978.

Colodny AJ: An improved surgical technique for intravesical resection of bladder diverticulum. *Br J Urol* 47:399, 1975.

Connar RG, Sealy WC: Gastrostomy and its complications. *Am Surg* 138:732, 1979.

Coppa GF, Eng K, Gouge TH, *et al.*: Parenteral and oral antibiotics in elective colon and rectal surgery: a prospective, randomized trial. *Am J Surg* 145:62–65, 1983.

Cordonnier JJ: Ureterosigmoid anastomosis. *J Urol* 63:275, 1950.

Cordonnier JJ: Urinary diversion. *Arch Surg* 71:818, 1955.

Courtney H: Anatomy of the pelvic diaphragm and anorectal musculature as related to sphincter preservation in anorectal surgery. *Am J Surg* 79:155, 1950.

Couvelaire R: "La petite vessie" des tuberculeaux genitourinaires: essae de classification place et varidentes des cysto-intestino-plasties. *J Urol* 56:381, 1950.

Creevy CD: Facts about ureterosigmoidostomy. *JAMA* 151:120, 1953.

Dager JE, Sanford EJ, Rohner TJ Jr: Complications of the nonrefluxing colon conduit. *J Urol* 123:585, 1980.

Daniel O, Shackman R: The blood supply of the human ureter in relation to ureterocolic anastomosis. *Br J Urol* 24:334, 1952.

David FDR: A new surgical procedure for revision of the ileal conduit stoma in children. *J Urol* 115:188, 1976.

Davidsson T, Barker SB, Mansson W: Tapering of untussuscepted ileal nipple valve or ileocecal valve to correct secondary incontinence in patients with urinary reservoir. *J Urol* 147:144, 1992.

deKernion JB, DenBesten L, Kaufman JJ, Ehrlich R: The Kock pouch as a urinary reservoir: pitfalls and perspectives. *Am J Surg* 150:83, 1985.

Deklerk JN, Lambrechts W, Viljoen I: The bowel as substitute for the bladder. *J Urol* 121:22, 1979.

deVries PA, Peña A: Posterior sagittal anorectoplasty. *J Pediatr Surg* 17:638, 1982.

Diamond DA, Ransley PG: Bladder neck reconstruction with omentum, silicone and augmentation cystoplasty: a preliminary report. *J Urol* 136:252, 1986.

Dounis A, Abel BJ, Gow JG: Cecocystoplasty for bladder augmentation. *J Urol* 123:164, 1980.

Dretler SP: The pathogenesis of urinary tract calculi occurring after ileal conduit diversion: I. Clinical study: II. Conduit study: III. Prevention. *J Urol* 109:204, 1973.

Dretler SP, Hendren WH, Leadbetter WF: Urinary tract reconstruction following ileal conduit diversion. *J Urol* 109:217, 1973.

Droes JTPM: Observations on the musculature of the urinary bladder and the urethra in the human foetus. *Br J Urol* 46:179, 1974.

Duckett JW Jr: Cutaneous vesicostomy in childhood: the Blocksom technique. *Urol Clin North Am* 1:485, 1974.

Duckett JW Jr: Use of paraexstrophy skin pedicle grafts for correction of exstrophy and epispadias repair. *Birth Defects* 13:175, 1977.

Duckett JW Jr: Epispadias. *Urol Clin North Am* 5:107, 1978.

Duckett JW: Ureterosigmoidostomy: the pros and cons. *Dial Pediatr Urol* 5:4, 1982.

Duckett JW, Gazak JM: Complications of ureterosigmoidostomy. *Urol Clin North Am* 10:473, 1983.

Duckett JW, Synder HMcC: Use of the Mitrofanoff principle in urinary reconstruction. *World J Urol* 3:191, 1985.

Duckett JW, Lofti A-H: Appendicovesicostomy (and variations) in bladder reconstruction. *J Urol* 149:567, 1993.

Dwoskin JY: Management of the massively dilated urinary tract in infants by temporary diversion and single-stage reconstruction. *Urol Clin North Am* 1:515, 1974.

Dyber R, Jeter K, Lattimer JK: Comparison of intraluminal pressures in ileal and colon conduits in children. *J Urol* 108:477, 1972.

Eagle JR Jr, Barrett GS: Congenital deficiency of abdominal musculature with associated genitourinary abnormalities: a syndrome. Report of nine cases. *Pediatrics* 6:721, 1950.

Eckstein HB: Cutaneous ureterostomy. *Proc R Soc Med* 56:749, 1963.

Edgerton MT, Gillenwater JY: A new surgical technique for phalloplasty in patients with exstrophy of the bladder. *Plast Reconstr Surg* 78:399, 1986.

Ehrlich RM, Lesavoy MA, Fine RN: Total abdominal reconstruction in the Prune Belly Syndrome. *J Urol* 136:282, 1986.

Ehrlich RM, Lesavoy MA: Umbilicus preservation with total abdominal wall reconstruction in the Prune Belly Syndrome. *Soc Pediatr Urol Newsletter,* May 14, 1991, p 27.

Eiseman B, Bricker EM: Electrolyte absorption following bilateral ureteroenterostomy into an isolated intestinal segment. *Ann Surg* 136:761, 1952.

Ekman H, Jacobsson B, Kock N, Sundin T: The functional behavior of different types of intestinal urinary bladder substitutes. *Proc Cong Soc Int Urol* 11:213, 1964.

Elder JS, Snyder HM, Hulbert WC, Duckett JW: Perforation of the augmented bladder in patients undergoing clean intermittent catheterization. *J Urol* 140:1159, 1988.

Emmett D, Noble MJ, Mebust WK: A comparison of end versus loop stomas for ileal conduit urinary diversion. *J Urol* 133:588, 1985.

Englemann UH, Light JK, Scott FB: Use of artificial urinary sphincter with lower urinary tract reconstruction and continent urinary diversion: clinical and experimental studies. In: King LR (Ed): *Bladder Reconstruction and Continent Urinary Diversion.* Chicago, Year Book Medical Publishers, 1986.

Enhörning G, Miller ER, Hinman F Jr: Urethral closure studied with cine-roentgenography and simultaneous bladder urethra pressure recording. *Surg Gynecol Obstet* 118:507, 1964.

Erich JB: Plastic repair of the female perineum in a case of exstrophy of the bladder. *Proc Staff Meet Mayo Clinic* 34:235, 1959.

Esho J, Cass AS: Management of stomal encrustations in children. *J Urol* 108:797, 1972.

Fasth S, Hulten L: Loop ileostomy: a superior diverting stoma in colorectal surgery. *World J Surg* 8:401, 1984.

Faxén A, Kock NG, Sundin T: Long-term functional results after ileocystoplasty. *Scand J Urol Nephrol* 7:127, 1973.

Feneley RCL: The management of female incontinence by suprapubic catheterisation, with or without urethral closure. *Br J Urol* 55:203-7, 1983.

Ferris DO, Odel HM: Electrolyte pattern of the blood after bilateral ureterosigmoidostomy. *JAMA* 142:634, 1950.

Filmer RB: Malignant tumors arising in bladder augmentations, and ileal and colon conduits. *Soc Pediat Urol News Lett* Dec 9, 1986.

Firlit CF, Sommer JT, Kaplan WE: Pediatric urinary undiversion. *J Urol* 123:748, 1980.

Fisch M, Wammack R, Müller SC, Hohenfellner R: The Mainz pouch II (sigma rectum pouch). *J Urol* 149:258, 1993.

Flinn RA, King LR, McDonald JH, et al.: Cutaneous ureterostomy: an alternative urinary diversion. *J Urol* 105:358, 1971.

Flocks RH, Boldus R: The surgical treatment and prevention of urinary incontinence associated with disturbance of the internal sphincter mechanism. *J Urol* 109:279, 1973.

Fox M, Power RF, Bruce AW: Diverticulum of the bladder: presentation and evaluation of treatment of 115 cases. *Br J Urol* 34:286, 1962.

Gadacz TR, Kelly KA, Phillips SF: The continent ileal pouch: absorptive and motor features. *Gastroenterology* 72:1287, 1977.

Garcia VF, Bloom DA: Inversion appendectomy. *Urology* 28:142, 1986.

Gasparini ME, Hinman J Jr, Presti JC, et al.: Continence after radical cystoprostatectomy and total bladder replacement: urodynamic analysis. *J Urol* 148:1861, 1992.

Gearhart JP, Canning DA, Jeffs RD: Failed bladder neck reconstruction: options for management. *J Urol* 146:1082, 1991.

Gearhart JP, Peppas DS, Jeffs RD: The failed exstrophy closure: strategy for management. *Br J Urol* 71:217, 1993.

Gecelter L: Transanorectal approach to the posterior urethra and bladder neck. *J Urol* 109:1011, 1973.

Gersuny R (cited by Foges): Officielles protokoll der k.k. gesellshaft der Aerzte in Wien. *Wien Klin Wochenschr* 11:990, 1898.

Ghoneim MA, Shehab-El-Din AB, Ashamallah AK, Gaballah MA: Evolution of the rectal bladder as a method for urinary diversion. *J Urol* 126:737, 1981.

Ghoneim MA, Kock NG, Lycke G, Shehab El-Din AB: An appliance-free sphincter-controlled bladder substitute: the urethral Kock pouch. *J Urol* 138:1150, 1987.

Giertz G, Franksson C: Construction of a substitute bladder with preservation of urethral voiding after subtotal or total cystectomy. *Acta Clin Scand* 113:218, 1957.

Gil Vernet JM Jr: The ileocolic segment in urologic surgery. *J Urol* 94:418, 1965.

Gil Vernet JW, Escarpenter JM, Perez-Trujillo G, Bonet Vic J: A functioning artificial bladder: results of 41 consecutive cases. *J Urol* 87:825, 1962.

Gilchrist RK, Merricks JW, Hamlin HH, et al.: Construction of a substitute bladder and urethra. *Surg Gynecol Obstet* 90:752, 1950.

Gittes RF: Augmentation cystoplasty. In: Libertino J (Ed): *Reconstructive Surgery in Urology.* Philadelphia, W. B. Saunders Company, 1976.

Gittes RF: Carcinogenesis in ureterosigmoidostomy. *Urol Clin North Am* 13:201, 1986.

Goldman HJ: A rapid, safe technique for removal of a large vesical diverticulum. *J Urol* 106:380, 1971.

Goligher JC, Leacock AG, Brossy JJ: The surgical anatomy of the anal canal. *Br J Surg* 43:51, 1955.

Goligher JC, Morris C, McAdam WAF, et al.: A controlled trial of inverting versus everting suture in clinical large bowel surgery. *Br J Surg* 57:817, 1970.

Golomb J, Klutke CG, Raz S: Complications of bladder substitution and continent urinary diversion. *Urology* 34:329, 1989.

Gonzalez R, Sheldon CA: Artificial sphincters in children with neurogenic bladders: long-term results. *J Urol* 128:1270, 1982.

Gonzalez R, LaPointe S, Sheldon CA, Mauer SM: Undiversion in children with renal failure. *J Pediatr Surg* 19:632, 1984.

Gonzalez R: Reconstruction of the female urethra to allow intermittent catheterization for neurogenic bladders and urogenital sinus anomalies. *J Urol* 133:478, 1985.

Gonzalez R, Sidi AA: Preoperative prediction of continence after enterocystoplasty or undiversion in children with neurogenic bladder. *J Urol* 134:705, 1985.

Gonzalez R, Koleilat N, Austin C, et al.: The artificial sphincter AS800 in congenital urinary incontinence. *J Urol* 142:512, 1989.

Gonzalez R: Sigmoid cystoplasty. In: King LR, Stone AR, Webster GD (Eds): *Bladder Reconstruction and Continent Urinary Diversion.* Chicago, Mosby Year Book, 1991, p 88.

Goodwin WE, Harris AP, Kaufman JJ, Beal JM: Open, transcolonic ureterointestinal anastomosis: a new approach. *Surg Gynecol Obstet* 97:295, 1953.

Goodwin WE, Turner RD, Winter CC: Results of ileocystoplasty. *J Urol* 80:461, 1958.

Goodwin WE, Winter CC: Technique of sigmoidocystoplasty. *Surg Gynecol Obstet* 108:370, 1959.

Goodwin WE: Ileocystoplasty. In: Cooper P (Ed): *Craft of Surgery.* Boston, Little, Brown & Company, 1964, p 1139.

Goodwin WE, Smith RB, Skinner DG (Eds): Complications of ureterosigmoidostomy. In: Smith RB, Skinner PD (Eds): *Complications of Urologic Surgery, Prevention and Management.* Philadelphia, W. B. Saunders Company, 1976, p 229.

Goodwin WE, Scardino PT: Ureterosigmoidostomy. *J Urol* 118:169, 1977.

Gorsch RV: *Perineopelvic Anatomy.* New York, Tilghman, 1941.

Gosling JA: The structure of the bladder and urethra in relation to function. *Urol Clin North Am* 6:31, 1979.

Gosling JA, Dixon JS, Humpherson JR: *Functional Anatomy of the Urinary Tract.* Baltimore, University Park Press, 1982.

Green D, Mitcheson HD, McGuire EJ: Management of the bladder by augmentation ileocecocystoplasty. *J Urol* 130:133, 1981.

Gruenwald P: The relation of the growing Müllerian duct to the Wolffian duct and its importance for the genesis of malformations. *Anat Rec* 81:1, 1941.

Grunberger I, Catanese A, Hanna MK: Total replacement of bladder and urethra by cecum and appendix in bladder exstrophy. *Urology* 6:497, 1986.

Hammond G, Iglesias L, Davis JE: The urachus, its anatomy and associated fasciae. *Anat Rec* 80:271, 1941.

Hanna MK: Reconstruction of umbilicus during functional closure of bladder exstrophy. *Urology* 27:340, 1986.

Harrison MR, Glick PL, Nakayama DL, et al.: Loop colon rectovaginoplasty for high cloacal anomaly. *J Pediatr Surg* 18:885, 1983.

Hartmann RE, Egghart G, Frohneberg D, Miller K: Die ileum-neoblase. *Urologe A* 26:67, 1987.

Hawley PR, Hunt TK, Dunphy JE: Etiology of colonic anastomotic leaks. *Proc R Soc Med* 63:28, 1970.

Hautmann RE, Egghart G, Frohneberg D, Miller K: The ileal neobladder. *J Urol* 139:39, 1988.

Hautmann RE, Miller K, Steiner U, Wenderoth U: The ileal neobladder: 6 years of experience with more than 200 patients. *J Urol* 150:40, 1993.

Hays DM, Powell TO: Various intestinal segments utilized for bladder enlargement in pediatric patients with reference to the management of exstrophy. *Surgery* 47:999, 1960.

Heitz-Boyer M, Hovelacque A: Creation a une nouvelle vessie et un nouvel uretre. *J d'Urol* 1:237, 1912.

Hendren WH: Reconstruction of previously diverted urinary tracts in children. *J Pediatr Surg* 8:135, 1973.

Hendren WH: Urinary tract refunctionalization after prior diversion in children. *Ann Surg* 180:494, 1974.

Hendren WH: Non-refluxing colon conduit for temporary or permanent urinary diversion in children. *J Pediatr Surg* 10:381, 1975.

Hendren WH: Exstrophy of the bladder: an alternative method of management. *J Urol* 115:195, 1976.

Hendren WH: Urinary diversion and undiversion in children. *Surg Clin North Am* 56:425, 1976.

Hendren WH: Exstrophy of the bladder. *Birth Defects* 13:207, 1977.

Hendren WH: Surgical management of urogenital sinus abnormalities. *J Pediatr Surg* 12:339, 1977.

Hendren WH: Complications of ureterostomy. *J Urol* 120:269, 1978.

Hendren WH: Some alternatives to urinary diversion in children. *J Urol* 119:652, 1978.

Hendren WH: Further experience in reconstructive surgery for cloacal anomalies. *J Pediatr Surg* 17:695, 1982.

Hendren WH, Radopoulous D: Complications of ileal loop and colon conduit urinary diversion. *Urol Clin North Am* 10:451, 1983.

Hendren WH: Ureterocolic diversion of urine: management of some difficult problems. *J Urol* 129:719, 1983.

Hendren WH: Urinary undiversion and augmentation cystoplasty. In: Kelalis PP, King LR, Belman AB (Eds): *Clinical Pediatric Urology*, 2nd ed. Philadelphia, W. B. Saunders Company, 1985, vol 1, pp 620–642.

Hendren WH: Repair of cloacal anomalies: current techniques. *J Pediatr Surg* 21:1159, 1986.

Hendren WH, Hendren RB. Bladder augmentation: experience with 129 children and young adults. *J Urol* 144 (Part 2):445 (Discussion 460), 1990.

Hendren WH: Urinary tract re-functionalization after long-term diversion: a 20-year experience with 177 patients. *Ann Surg* 212:478 (Discussion 494), 1990.

Hendren WH: Cloacal malformations: experience with 105 cases. *J Pediatr Surg* 27:890, 1992.

Hendren WH: Ileal nipple for continence in cloacal exstrophy. *J Urol* 148:372, 1992.

Hensle TW, Burbige KA: Bladder replacement in children and young adults. *J Urol* 133:1004, 1985.

Hensle TW, Connor JP, Burbige KA: Continent urinary diversion in childhood. *J Urol* 143:981, 1990.

Hensle TW, Dean GE: Complications of urinary tract reconstruction. *Urol Clin North Am* 18:755, 1991.

Hinman F, Weyrauch HM: A critical study of the different principles of surgery which have been used in uretero-intestinal implantation. *Int Abstracts Med* 64:313, 1937.

Hinman F Jr, Hinman F Sr: Ureteral implantation: I. Experiments on the surgical principles involved in an open submucosal method of ureterointestinal anastomosis. *J Urol* 64:457, 1950.

Hinman F Jr: Ureteral implantation: II. Clinical results from a method of open submucosal anastomosis. *J Urol* 64:567, 1950.

Hinman F Jr: Leakage and reflux in uretero-intestinal anastomosis: I. The free peritoneal graft. *J Urol* 70:419, 1953.

Hinman F Jr: Urinary conduction versus storage by isolated ileal segment. In: *Proceedings of the 11th Congress of the International Society of Urology*, Stockholm, June 25–30, 1958, p 37.

Hinman F Jr: A method of lengthening and repairing the penis in exstrophy of the bladder. *J Urol* 79:237, 1958.

Hinman F Jr, Oppenheimer R: Functional characteristics of the ileal segment as a valve. *J Urol* 80:448, 1958.

Hinman F Jr: The technique of the Gersuny operation (ureterosigmoidostomy with perineal colostomy) in vesical exstrophy. *J Urol* 80:126, 1959.

Hinman F Jr: Surgical disorders of the bladder and umbilicus of urachal origin. *Surg Gynecol Obstet* 113:605, 1961.

Hinman F Jr: Urologic aspects of alternating urachal sinus. *Am J Surg* 102:339, 1961b.

Hinman F Jr: Overview: the choice between ureterosigmoidostomy with perineal (Gersuny, Heitz-Boyer) or abdominal (Mauclaire) colostomy. In: Whitehead ED, Leiter E (Eds): *Current Operative Urology*, 2nd ed. Philadelphia, Harper and Row, 1984, p 783.

Hinman F Jr: The garage door syndrome. *Neurourol Urodynamics* 5:515, 1986.

Hinman F Jr: The non-neurogenic neurogenic bladder (Hinman syndrome): fifteen years later. *J Urol* 136:769, 1986.

Hinman F Jr: Patent urachus and urachal cysts. In: Gellis SS, Kogan BM (Eds): *Current Pediatric Pediatric Therapy*, ed 12, Philadelphia, W. B. Saunders Company, 1986, p 391.

Hinman F Jr: Obstruction to voiding. In: Resnick MI (Ed): *Current Therapy in Genitourinary Surgery*. B. C. Decker, Inc, 1987.

Hinman F Jr: Selection of intestinal segments for bladder substitution: physical and physiological characteristics. *J Urol* 139:519, 1988.

Hinman F Jr: Pascal, Laplace and a length of bowel. *J d'Urol* 95:11, 1989.

Hinman F Jr: Functional classification of conduits for continent diversion. *J Urol* 144:27, 1990.

Hinman F Jr: Reservoirs and continent conduits. *Int Urogynecol* 3:208, 1992.

Hodges CV: Surgical anatomy of the urinary bladder and pelvic ureter. *Surg Clin North Am* 44:1327, 1964.

Hohenfellner R: Ureterosigmoidostomy. In: Eckstein HB, Hohenfellner R, Williams DL (Eds): *Surgical Pediatric Urology*. Stuttgart, Thieme, 1977.

Hollowell JG, Ransley PG: Surgical management of incontinence in bladder exstrophy. *Br J Urol* 68:543, 1991.

Howell C, Caldamone A, Snyder H, et al.: Optimal management of cloacal exstrophy. *J Pediatr Surg* 18:365, 1983.

Hurwitz RS, Woodhouse CRJ, Ransley P: The anatomical course of the neurovascular bundles in epispadias. *J Urol* 136:68, 1986.

Hurwitz RS, Manzoni GAM, et al.: Cloacal exstrophy: a report of 34 cases. *J Urol* 138:1060, 1987.

Husmann DA, McLorie GA, Churchill BM: Closure of the exstrophic bladder: an evaluation of the factors leading to its success and its importance in urinary continence. *J Urol* 142:522, 1989.

Issa MM, Oesterling JE, Canning DA, Jeffs RD: A new technique of using the in situ appendix as a catheterizable stoma for continent urinary reservoirs. *J Urol* 141:1385, 1989.

Jacobs A, Stirling WB: The late results of ureterocolic anastomoses. *Br J Urol* 24:259, 1952.

Jaffe BM, Bricker EM, Butcher HR Jr: Surgical complications of ileal segment urinary diversion. *Ann Surg* 167:367, 1968.

Jaramillo D, Lebowitz RL, Hendren WH: The cloacal malformation: radiologic findings and imaging recommendations. *Radiology* 177:441, 1990.

Jeffs RD, Charrois R, Many M, et al.: Primary closure of the exstrophied bladder. In: Scott R Jr, Gordon HL, Scott FB, et al. (Eds): *Current Controversies in Urologic Management.* Philadelphia, W. B. Saunders Company, 1972, p 235.

Jeffs RD, Guice SL, Oesch I: The factors in successful exstrophy closure. *J Urol* 127:974, 1982.

Jeffs RD: Exstrophy, epispadias and cloacal and urogenital sinus abnormalities. *Pediatr Clin N Am* 34:1233, 1987.

Jeffs RD: Exstrophy and cloacal exstrophy: congenital anomalies of the lower genitourinary tract. *Urol Clin North Am* 5:127, 1978.

Jeffs RD: Exstrophy. In: Harrison JH, Gittes RI, Permutter AD, et al. (Eds): *Campbell's Urology,* Philadelphia, W. B. Saunders Company, 1979, vol 2, p 1672.

Jeter K, Lattimer JK: Common stomal problems following ileal conduit urinary diversion. *Urology* 3:399, 1974.

Jeter KF: The flush versus the protruding urinary stoma. *J Urol* 116:424, 1976.

Jeter KF: Care of the ostomy patient. In: Kaufman JJ (Ed): *Current Urologic Therapy.* Philadelphia, W. B. Saunders Company, 1980.

Johnston JH: Temporary cutaneous ureterostomy in the management of advanced congenital urinary obstruction. *Arch Dis Child* 38:161, 1963.

Johnston JH: The genital aspects of exstrophy. *J Urol* 113:701, 1975.

Kass EJ, Koff SA: Bladder augmentation in the pediatric neuropathic bladder. *J Urol* 129:552, 1983.

Kaufman JJ: Repair of parastomal hernia by translocation of the stoma without laparotomy. *J Urol* 129:278, 1983.

Kay R, Tank ES: Principle of management of the persistent cloaca in the female newborn. *J Urol* 117:102, 1977.

Keisling VJ, Tank ES: Postoperative intussusception in children. *Urology* 33:387, 1989.

Kelalis PP: Urinary diversion in children by the sigmoid conduit: its advantages and limitations. *J Urol* 112:666, 1974.

Kelley JH, Eraklis AJ: The procedure for lengthening the phallus in boys with exstrophy of the bladder. *J Pediatr Surg* 6:645, 1971.

Kennedy HA, Adams MC, Mitchell ME, et al.: Chronic renal failure and bladder augmentation: stomach versus sigmoid colon in the canine model. *J Urol* 140:1138, 1988.

Kim KS, Susskind MR, King LR: Ileocecal ureterosigmoidostomy: an alternative to conventional ureterosigmoidostomy. *J Urol* 140:1494, 1988.

King LR, Scott WW: Pyeloileocutaneous anastomosis. *Surg Gynecol Obstet* 119:281, 1964.

King LR: Technique of ileal conduit: evolution of the Brady method. Papers presented in honor of W. W. Scott. New York, Plenum Publications, 1972.

King LR, Wendel EF: Primary cystectomy and permanent urinary diversion in the treatment of exstrophy of the urinary bladder. In: Scott R (Ed): *Current Controversies in Urologic Management.* Philadelphia, W. B. Saunders Company, 1972, p 244.

King LR, Stone AR, Webster GD (Eds): *Bladder Reconstruction and Continent Urinary Diversion.* Chicago, Year Book Medical Publishers, 1987.

Kiricuta I: *Use of the Omentum in Plastic Surgery.* Romania, Editura Medicala, 1980.

Klauber GT: Posterior bladder tube for CIC. *Soc Pediatr Urol Newsletter,* May 20, 1992, p 9.

Koch MO, McDougal WS: Nicotinic acid: treatment for the hyperchloremic acidosis following urinary diversion through intestinal segments. *J Urol* 134:162, 1985.

Kock NG, Hultén L, Leandoer L: A study of the motility in different parts of the human colon: resting activity, response to feeding and to prostigmine. *Scand J Gastroenterol* 3:163, 1968.

Kock NG: Ileostomy without external appliance: a survey of 25 patients provided with intestinal reservoir. *Ann Surg* 173:545, 1971.

Kock NG, Nilson AE, Nilson LO, et al.: Urinary diversion via a continent ileal reservoir: clinical results in 12 patients. *J Urol* 128:469, 1982.

Kock NG, Norlen L, Philipson BM, et al.: Current status of the ileal reservoir for continent urinary diversion. *Surg Rounds* Jan 1985, p 32.

Koff SA: Abdominal neourethra in children: technique and long-term results. *J Urol* 133:244, 1985.

Kosko JW, Kursh ED, Resnick MI: Metabolic complications of urologic intestinal substitutes. *Urol Clin North Am* 13:193, 1986.

Kretschner KP: The intestinal stoma. *Major Probl Clin Surg* 24:98, 1978.6.3

Kroovand RL, AlAnsari RM, Perlmutter AD: Urinary and genital malformations in prune belly syndrome. *J Urol* 127:94, 1982.

Kropp KA, Angwafo FF: Urethral lengthening and reimplantation for neurogenic incontinence in children. *J Urol* 135:534, 1986.

Ladd WE, Gross RE: Congenital malformations of the anus and rectum: report of 162 cases. *Am J Surg* 23:167, 1934.

Lapides J, Ajemian EP, Lichtwardt JR: Cutaneous vesicostomy. *J Urol* 84:609, 1960.

Lapides J: Butterfly cutaneous ureterostomy. *J Urol* 88:735, 1962.

Lapides J: The abdominal neourethra. *J Urol* 95:350, 1966.

Lapides J, Diokno AC, Gould FR, et al.: Clean intermittent self-catheterization in the treatment of urinary tract disease. *J Urol* 107:458, 1972.

Lattimer JK: Congenital deficiency of the abdominal musculature and associated genitourinary anomalies: a report of 22 cases. *J Urol* 79:343, 1958.

Leadbetter WF: Considerations of problems incident to performance of uretero-enterostomy: report of a technique. *J Urol* 68:818, 1951.

Leadbetter WF, Clarke BG: Five years experience with ureteroenterostomy by the "combined" technique. *J Urol* 73:67, 1954.

Leadbetter GW Jr, Leadbetter WF: Ureteral reimplantation and bladder neck reconstruction. *JAMA* 175:676, 1976.

Leadbetter GW Jr, Zickermin P, Pierce E: Ureterosigmoidostomy and carcinoma of the colon. *J Urol* 121:732, 1979.

Leisinger HJ: Continent urinary diversion: review of the intussuscepted ileal valve. *World J Urol* 4:231, 1986.

Leonard MP, Gearhart JP, Jeffs RD: 50 continent urinary reservoirs in pediatric urological practice. *J Urol* 144 (Part 2):330, 1990.

Leonard MP, Quinlan DM: The Benchekroun ileal valve. *Urol Clin North Am* 18:717, 1991.

Leong CH: Use of the stomach for bladder replacement and urinary diversion. *Ann R Coll Surg Engl* 60:283, 1978.

Lepor H, Jeffs RD: Primary bladder closure and bladder with reconstruction in classical bladder exstrophy. *J Urol* 130:1142, 1983.

Lepor H, Shapiro E, Jeffs RD: Urethral reconstruction in boys with classical bladder exstrophy. *J Urol* 131:512, 1984.

Libertino JA, Zinman L: Ileocecal antirefluxing conduit. *Surg Clin North Am* 62:999, 1982.

Lierse W: *Applied Anatomy of the Pelvis.* Berlin, Springer-Verlag, 1987.

Lieskovsky G, Bloom DA: Creation of a Turnbull loop stoma. In: Skinner DG (Ed): *Genitourinary Cancer.* Philadelphia, W. B. Saunders Company, 1987.

Lieskovsky G, Boyd SD, Skinner DG: Cutaneous Kock pouch urinary diversion. *Probl Urol* 5:256, 1991.

Light JK, Flores FN, Scott FB: Use of the AS792 artificial sphincter following urinary undiversion. *J Urol* 129:548, 1983.

Light JK: Enteroplasty to ablate bowel contractions in the reconstructed bladder: a case report. *J Urol* 134:958, 1985.

Lilien OM, Camey M: 25-year experience with replacement of the human bladder (Camey procedure). *J Urol* 132:886, 1984.

Linder A, Leach GE, Raz S: Augmentation cystoplasty in the treatment of neurogenic bladder dysfunction. *J Urol* 129:491, 1983.

Lockhart JL, Davies R, Cox C, *et al.*: Gastroileoileal pouch: alternative continent urinary reservoir for patients with short bowel, acidosis and/or extensive pelvic radiation. *J Urol* 150:46, 1993.

Lockhart JL, Pow-Sang JM, Persky L, *et al.*: A continent colonic urinary reservoir: the Florida pouch. *J Urol* 144:864, 1990.

Loughlin KR, Retik AB, Weinstein HJ, Colodny AH, *et al.*: Genitourinary rhabdomyosarcoma in children. *Cancer* 63:1600, 1989.

Lrimpi HD, Khubchandovic IT, Sheets JA, Stasik JJ: Advances in intestinal anastomoses. *Dis Colon Rectum* 20:107, 1977.

Lytton B, Weiss RM: Cutaneous vesicostomy for temporary urinary diversion in infants. *J Urol* 105:888, 1971.

Magnus R, Stephens FD: Imperforate anal membrane. *Aust Pediat* 2:431, 1966.

Mansson W: The continent cecal reservoir for urine [review]. *Scand J Urol* S85:1, 1984.

Mansson W, Mattiasson A, White T: Acute effects of full urinary bladder and full caecal urinary reservoir on regional renal function: a study with scintillation camera renography. *Scand J Urol Nephrol* 18:299, 1984.

Manzoni GA, Ransley PG, Hurwitz RS: Cloacal exstrophy and cloacal exstrophy variants: a proposed system of classification. *J Urol* 138:1065, 1987.

Marberger M, Walz P, Hohenfellner R: Urétérosigmoidostomie et urétérostomie cutanee transcolique: indications, techniques et resultats. *J Urol (Paris)* 88:591, 1982.

Marconi F, Messina P, Pavanello P, Castro RD: Cosmetic reconstruction of the mons veneris and lower abdominal wall by skin expansion as the last stage of the surgical treatment of bladder exstrophy: a report of three cases. *Plast Reconstr Surg* 91:551, 1993.

Markland C, Fraley EE: Management of infants with cloacal exstrophy. *J Urol* 109:740, 1973.

Marshall FF, Leadbetter WF, Dretler SP: Ileal conduit parastomal hernias. *J Urol* 144:40, 1975.

Marshall VF, Muecke EC: Variations in exstrophy of the bladder: *J Urol* 88:766, 1962.

Marshall VF, Muecke EC: Functional closure of typical exstrophy of the bladder. *J Urol* 104:205, 1970.

Martin EC, Fankuchen EI, Casarella WJ: Percutaneous dilation of ureteroenteric strictures or occlusions in ileal conduit. *Urol Radiol* 4:19, 1982.

Mathisen W: A new method of ureterointestinal anastomosis: preliminary report. *Surg Gynecol Obstet* 96:255, 1953.

Mathisen W: Open-loop sigmoido-cystoplasty. *Acta Chir Scand* 110:227, 1955.

Mayo ME, Chapman WH: Stomal obstruction of ileal conduits in children: a urodynamic study. *J Urol* 121:68, 1979.

Mayo ME, Chapman WH: Management of ileal conduit obstruction: a urodynamic study: *J Urol* 125:828, 1981.

McDougal WS: Editorial: the continent urinary diversion. *J Urol* 137:1214, 1987.

McLeod RS, Fazio VW: Quality of life with the continent ileostomy. *World J Surg* 8:90, 1984.

Menville JG, Nix JT, Pratt AM II: Cecocystoplasty. *J Urol* 79:78, 1958.

Mesrobian H-GJ: Exstrophy of the bladder. In: King LR (Ed): *Urologic Surgery in Neonates and Young Infants.* Philadelphia, W. B. Saunders Company, 1988, p 265.

Michie AJ, Borns P, Ames MD: Improvement following tubeless suprapubic cystostomy of myelomeningocele patients with hydronephrosis and recurrent acute pyelonephritis. *J Pediatr Surg* 1:347, 1966.

Middleton RG: Further experience with the Young-Dees procedure for urinary incontinence in selected cases. *J Urol* 115:159, 1976.

Mildenberger H, Kluth D, Dziuba M: Embryology of bladder exstrophy. *J Pediatr Surg* 23:166, 1988.

Miller A: The aetiology and treatment of diverticulum of the bladder. *Br J Urol* 30:43, 1958.

Mininberg DT, Genvert HP: Posterior urethral valves: role of temporary and permanent urinary diversion. *Urology* 33:205, 1989.

Mitchell ME, Yoder IC, Pfister RC, *et al.*: Ileal loop stenosis: a late complication of urinary diversion. *J Urol* 118:957, 1977.

Mitchell ME: The role of bladder augmentation in undiversion. *J Pediatr Surg* 16:790, 1981.

Mitchell ME: Urinary tract diversion and undiversion in the pediatric age group. *Surg Clin North Am* 61:1147, 1981.

Mitchell ME, Hensle TW, Crooks KK: Urethral reconstruction in the young female using a perineal pedicle flap. *J Pediatr Surg* 17:687, 1982.

Mitchell ME, Rink RC: Urinary diversion and undiversion. *Urol Clin North Am* 12:111, 1985.

Mitchell ME: Use of bowel in undiversion. *Urol Clin North Am* 13:349, 1986.

Mitchell ME, Adams MC, Rink RC: Urethral replacement with ureter. *J Urol* 139:1282, 1988.

Mitchell ME, Brito CG, Rink RC: Cloacal exstrophy reconstruction for urinary continence. *J Urol* 144:554 (Discussion, 562), 1990.

Mitrofanoff P: Cystostomie continente trans-appendiculaire dans le traitement des vessies neurologiques. *Chir Pediatr* 21:297, 1980.

Moerman P, Fryns J, Goddeeris P, Lauweryns JM: Pathogenesis of the prune-belly syndrome: a functional urethral obstruction caused by prostatic hypoplasia. *Pediatrics* 73:470, 1984.

Mogg RA: The treatment of neurogenic urinary incontinence using the colonic conduit. *Br J Urol* 37:681, 1965.

Mogg RA: The result of urinary diversion using the colonic conduit. *Br J Urol* 97:684, 1967.

Mogg RA: The treatment of urinary incontinence using the colonic conduit. *J Urol* 97:684, 1967.

Monfort G, Guy JM, Morrisson-Lacombe G: Appendicovesicostomy: an alternative urinary diversion in the child. *Eur Urol* 10:361, 1984.

Monfort G, Guys JM, Bocciardi A, *et al.*: A novel technique for reconstruction of the abdominal wall in the prune belly syndrome. *J Urol* 146:361, 1991.

Monie IW, Monie BJ: Prune belly syndrome and fetal ascites. *Teratology* 19:111, 1979.

Moorcraft J, DuBoulay CEH, Isaacson P, Atwell JD: Changes in the mucosa of colon conduits with particular reference to the risk of malignant change. *Br J Urol* 55:185, 1983.

Mor Y, Ramon J, Raviv G, *et al.*: Low loop cutaneous ureterostomy and subsequent reconstruction: 20 years of experience. *J Urol* 147:1595, 1992.

Mostwin JL: Current concepts of female pelvic anatomy and physiology. *Urol Clin North Am* 18:175, 1991.

Muecke EC: The role of the cloacal membrane in exstrophy: the first successful experimental study. *J Urol* 92:659, 1964.

Muecke EC: Exstrophy, epispadias and other anomalies of the bladder. In: Walsh PC, Gittes RF, Perlmutter AD, Stamey TA (Eds): *Campbell's Urology.* 5th ed, Philadelphia, W. B. Saunders Company, 1986.

Nande JH: The hidden vesicostomy. *Br J Urol* 541:686, 1982.

Nesbit RM: Ureterosigmoid anastomosis by direct elliptical connection: a preliminary report. *J Urol* 61:728, 1949.

Netto NR Jr, Lemos GC, deAlmeida Claro JF, Hering FLO: Congenital diverticulum of male urethra. *Urology* 24:239, 1984.

Nix JT, Menville JG, Albert M, Wendt DL: Congenital patent urachus. *J Urol* 79:264, 1958.

Norlén L, Trasti H: Functional behavior of the continent ileum reservoir for urinary diversion: experimental and clinical study. *Scand J Urol Nephrol (Suppl)* 49:33, 1978.

Nurse DE, Mundy AR: Metabolic complications of cystoplasty. *Br J Urol* 63:165, 1988.

Ochsner A: The relative merits of temporary gastrostomy and nasogastric suction of the stomach. *Am J Surg* 133:729, 1977.

Oesterling JE, Gearhart JP: Utilization of an ileal conduit in construction of a continent urinary reservoir. *Urology* 36:15, 1990.

Overstreet EW, Hinman F Jr: Some gynecologic aspects of bladder exstrophy: with report of an illustrative case. *West J Surg Obstet Gynecol* 64:131, 1956.

Owsley JQ Jr, Hinman F Jr: One-stage reconstruction of the external genitalia in the female with exstrophy of the bladder. *Plast Reconst Surg* 50:227, 1972.

Parkash S, Bhandari M: Rectus abdominis myocutaneous island flap for bridging defect after cystectomy for bladder exstrophy. *Urology* 20:536, 1982.

Parra RO: A simplified technique for continent urinary diversion: an all-stapled colonic reservoir. *J Urol* 146:1496, 1991.

Parrott TS, Woodard JR: The Monfort operation for abdominal wall reconstruction in the prune belly. *J Urol* 148:688, 1992.

Patten BM, Barry A: The genesis of exstrophy of the bladder and epispadias. *Am J Anat* 90:35, 1952.

Paul M, Kanagasuntheram R: The congenital anomalies of the lower urinary tract: Part 1. *Br J Urol* 28:64, 1956.

Paul M, Kanagasuntheram R: The congenital anomalies of the lower urinary tract: Part 2. *Br J Urol* 28:118, 1956.

Pegum JM, Loly PCM, Falkiner NM: Development and classification of anorectal anomalies. *Arch Surg* 89:481, 1964.

Peña A: Posterior sagittal anorectoplasty as a secondary operation for the treatment of fecal incontinence. *J Pediatr Surg* 18:762, 1983.

Peña A: Surgical treatment of high imperforate anus. *World J Surg* 9:236, 1985.

Peña A: Posterior sagittal approach for the correction of anorectal malformations. *Adv Surg* 19:69, 1986.

Peña A: Anatomical considerations relevant to fecal incontinence. *Semin Surg Oncol* 3:1141, 1987.

Perlmutter AD, Tank ES: Loop cutaneous ureterostomy. *J Urol* 99:559, 1968.

Perlmutter AD, Tank ES: Ileal conduit stasis in children: recognition and treatment. *J Urol* 101:688, 1969.

Perlmutter AD: Spiral advancement skin flap for stomal revision. *J Urol* 114:131, 1975.

Perlmutter AD, Weinstein MD, Reitelman C: Vesical neck reconstruction in patients with epispadias-exstrophy complex. *J Urol* 146:613, 1991.

Peters CA, Mandell J, Lebowitz RL, et al.: Congenital obstructed megaureters in early infancy: diagnosis and treatment. *J Urol* 142 (Part 2):641 (Discussion 667), 1989.

Persky L: Relocation of ileal stomas. *J Urol* 96:702, 1966.

Pitts WR, Muecke EC: A 20-year experience with ileal conduit: the fate of the kidneys. *J Urol* 122:154, 1979.

Pohlmann AG: The development of the cloaca in human embryos. *Am J Anat* 12:1, 1911.

Pokorny M, Pontes JE, Pierce JM Jr.: Ureterostomy in-situ. *Urology* 8:447, 1976.

Powers JC, Fitzgerald JF, McAhranah MJ: The anatomic basis for the surgical detachment of the greater omentum from the transverse colon. *Surg Gynecol Obstet* 143:105, 1976.

Quinlan DM, Leonard MP, Brendler CB, et al.: Use of the Benchekroun hydraulic valve as a catheterizable continence mechanism. *J Urol* 145:1151, 1991.

Rabinowitz R, Barkin M, Schillinger JF, et al.: Surgical treatment of the massively dilated ureter in children: Part I.

Management by cutaneous ureterostomy. *J Urol* 117:658, 1977.

Rabinowitz R, Barkin M, Schillinger JF, et al.: Upper tract management when posterior urethral valve ablation is insufficient. *J Urol* 122:370, 1979.

Randolph J, Cavett C, Eng G: Abdominal wall reconstruction in the prune belly syndrome. *J Pediatr Surg* 16:960, 1981.

Ransley PG, Duffy PG, Wollin M: Bladder exstrophy closure and epispadias repair. In: Spitz L, Nixon HH (Eds): *Operative Surgery (Paediatric Surgery)*. London, Butterworth-Heinemann, 1988, p 620.

Ravitch MM: Observations on the healing of wounds of the intestines. *Surgery* 77:665, 1975.

Redman JF: Extensive shortening of ileal conduit through peristomal incision. *Urology* 9:45, 1977.

Redman JF: An anatomic approach to the pelvis. In: Crawford ED, Borden TA (Eds): *Genitourinary Cancer Surgery*. Philadelphia, Lea & Febiger, 1982, p 126.

Reid K, Schneider K, Fruchtman B: Closure of the bladder neck in patients undergoing continent vesicostomy for urinary incontinence. *J Urol* 120:40, 1978.

Reidmiller H, Bürger R, Müller S, et al.: Continent appendix stoma: a modification of the Mainz pouch technique. *J Urol* 143:1115, 1990.

Resnick MJ, Caldamone AA (Eds): Use of large and small bowel in urologic surgery. *Urol Clin North Am* 13:177, 1986.

Retik AB, Bauer SB: Bladder and urachus. In: Kelalis PP et al. (Eds): *Clinical Pediatric Urology*, 1st ed. Philadelphia, W. B. Saunders Company, 1976.

Reynolds EL: The bony pelvis in prepubertal childhood. *Am J Phys Anthropol NS* 5:165, 1947.

Rich RH, Hardy BE, Filler RM: Surgery for anomalies of the urachus. *J Pediatr Surg* 18:4, 1983.

Richardson JR Jr, Linton PC, Leadbetter GW Jr: A new concept in the treatment of stomal stenosis. *J Urol* 108:159, 1972.

Richie JP: Nonrefluxing sigmoid conduit for urinary diversion. *Urol Clin North Am* 6:469, 1979.

Richie JP: Colonic and jejunal conduits. In: Johnson DE, Boileau MA (Eds): *Genitourinary Tumors*. New York, Grune & Stratton, Inc, 1982.

Rickham PP: Vesicointestinal fissure. *Arch Dis Child* 35:97, 1960.

Rickwood AMK: Urinary diversion in children. In: Ashken MH (Ed): *Urinary Diversion*. Berlin, Springer-Verlag, 1982, p 22.

Rink RC, Retik AB: Ureteroileocecal sigmoidostomy and avoidance of carcinoma of the colon. In: King LR, Stone AR, Webster GD (Eds): *Bladder Reconstruction and Continent Urinary Diversion*. Chicago, Mosby Year Book, 1991, p 221.

Robertson CN, King LR: Bladder substitution in children. *Urol Clin North Am* 13:333, 1986.

Rosenberg ML: The physiology of hyperchloremic acidosis following ureterosigmoidostomy: a study of urinary reabsorption with radioactive isotopes. *J Urol* 70:569, 1953.

Rovner E, Turek P, Duckett J: Ureterostomy in-situ: rediscovering an old technique. *Soc Pediatr Urol Newsletter* Dec 5, 1991.

Rowland RG: Continent urinary diversion. *J Urol* 136:76, 1986.

Rowland RG, Mitchell ME, Bihrle R, et al.: Indiana continent urinary reservoir. *J Urol* 137:1136, 1987.

Sagalowsky A: Mechanisms of continence in urinary reconstructions. *AUA Update Series*, vol XI, lesson 4, 1991.

Salley R, Bucher RM, Rodring CB: Colostomy closure: morbidity reduction employing a semi-standardized protocol. *Dis Colon Rectum* 26:319, 1983.

Saltzman B, Mininberg DT, Muecke EC: Exstrophy of bladder: evolution of management. *Urology* 26:383, 1985.

Scardino PT, Bagley DH, Javadpour N, Ketchom AS: Sigmoid conduit urinary diversion. *Urology* 6:167, 1975.

Scheidler DM, Klee LW, Rowland RG, *et al.*: Update on the Indiana continent urinary reservoir. *J Urol,* 141 (Part 2):302A, 1989.

Scherster T: Studies of the motorial function in the ileal segment in cutaneous uretero-ileostomy. *Acta Clin Scand* 124:149, 1962.

Schlegel PN, Gearhart JP: Neuroanatomy of the pelvis in an infant with cloacal exstrophy: a detailed microdissection with histology. *J Urol* 141:583, 1989.

Schlesinger RE, Berman ML, Ballon SC, *et al.*: The choice of an intestinal segment for a urinary conduit. *Surg Gynecol Obstet* 148:45, 1979.

Schmidbauer CP, Chiang H, Raz S: Compliance of tubular and detubularized ileal reservoirs [abstract]. *J Urol* 137:171A, 1987.

Schmidt JD, Buchsbaum HJ, Jacobo EC: Transverse colon conduit for supravesical urinary tract diversion. *Urology* 8:542, 1976.

Schmidt JD, Buchsbaum HJ, Nachtsheim DA: Long-term follow-up, further experience with and modifications of the transverse colon conduit in urinary tract diversion. *Br J Urol* 57:284, 1985.

Schneider KM, Reid RE, Fruchtman B: Closure of the bladder neck in patients undergoing continent vesicostomy. *J Urol* 120:40, 1978.

Schreck WR, Campbell WA: The relationship of bladder outlet obstruction to urinary umbilical fistula. *J Urol* 108:641, 1972.

Schrock TR, Deveney CW, Dunphy JE: Factors contributing to leakage of colonic anastomoses. *Ann Surg* 177:513, 1973.

Schunke GB: The anatomy and development of the sacro-iliac joint in man. *Anat Rec* 72:313, 1938.

Scott FB, Light JK, Fishman I, *et al.*: Implantation of an artificial sphincter for urinary incontinence. *Contemp Surg* 18:11, 1981.

Senn E, Thüroff JW, Barandhauer K: Urodynamics of ileal conduits in adults. *Eur Urol* 10:401, 1984.

Shafik A: Stomal stenosis after cutaneous ureterostomy: etiology and management. *J Urol* 105:65, 1971.

Sidi AA, Reinberg Y, Gonzalez R: Influence of intestinal segment and configuration on the outcome of augmentation enterocystoplasty. *J Urol* 136:1201, 1986.

Silver PHS: The role of the peritoneum in the formation of the septum recto-vesicale. *J Anat* 90:538, 1956.

Simon J: Ectopia vesicae (absence of the anterior walls of the bladder and pubic abdominal parietes): operation for directing the orifices of the ureters into the rectum. Temporary success: subsequent death. Autopsy. *Lancet* 2:568, 1852.

Skinner DG: Secondary urinary reconstruction: use of the ileocecal segment. *J Urol* 112:48, 1974.

Skinner DG, Gottesman JE, Richie JP: The isolated sigmoid segment: its value in temporary urinary diversion and reconstruction. *J Urol* 113:614, 1975.

Skinner DG: Further experience with the ileocecal segment in urinary reconstruction. *J Urol* 128:252, 1982.

Skinner DG, Lieskowsky G, Boyd S: Continent urinary diversion. *J Urol* 141:1323, 1989.

Skinner DG, Boyd SD, Lieskovsky G, *et al.*: Lower urinary tract reconstruction following cystectomy: experience and results in 126 patients using the Kock ileal reservoir with bilateral uretero-ileo-urethrostomy. *J Urol* 146:756, 1991.

Smith ED: Follow-up study on 150 ileal conduits in children. *J Pediatr Surg* 7:1, 1972.

Smith GI, Hinman F Jr: The intussuscepted ileal cystostomy. *J Urol* 73:261, 1955.

Smith GI, Hinman F Jr: The rectal bladder (colostomy with ureterosigmoidostomy): experimental and clinical aspects. *J Urol* 74:354, 1955.

Smith RB, Van Cangh P, Skinner DG, *et al.*: Augmentation enterocystoplasty: a critical review. *J Urol* 118:35, 1977.

Snyder HM III: Foreword. In: King LR, Stone AR, Webster GD (Eds): *Bladder Reconstruction and Continent Urinary Diversion.* Chicago, Year Book Medical Publishers, 1986, p XI.

Snyder HM III: Continent reconstruction of the lower urinary tract: variations of the Mitrofanoff principle. In: *Advances in Urology,* 2nd ed. Chicago, Year Book Medical Publishers, 1989.

Soper RT, Kilger K: Vesico-intestinal fissure. *J Urol* 92:490, 1964.

Spence HM: Ureterosigmoidostomy for exstrophy of the bladder: results in a personal series of 31 cases. *Br J Urol* 38:36, 1966.

Spence HM, Allen TD: Vaginal vesicostomy for empyema of the defunctionalized bladder. *J Urol* 106:862, 1971.

Spence HM, Hoffman WW, Pate VA: Exstrophy of the bladder: I. Long term results in a series of 37 cases treated by ureterosigmoidostomy. *J Urol* 114:133, 1974.

Spence HM, Hoffman WW, Fosmire GP: Tumour of the colon as a late complication of ureterosigmoidostomy for exstrophy of the bladder. *Br J Urol* 51:466, 1978.

Spindel MR, Winslow BH, Jordan GH: The use of paraexstrophy flaps for urethral construction in neonatal girls with classical exstrophy. *J Urol* 140:574, 1988.

Steiner MS, Morton RA, Marshall FF: Vitamin B12 deficiency in patients with ileocolic neobladders. *J Urol* 149:255, 1993.

Stephens FD: Congenital imperforate rectum, rectourethral and rectovaginal fistulae. *Aust N Z J Surg* 22:161, 1953.

Stephens FD: Imperforate anus. *Med J Aust* 2:803, 1959.

Stephens FD: *Congenital Malformations of the Rectum, Anus and Genitourinary Tracts.* London, E & S Livingstone Ltd, 1963.

Stephens FD: Form of stress incontinence in children: another method for bladder neck repair. *Aust N Z J Surg* 40:124, 1970.

Stephens FD, Smith ED: *Anorectal Malformations in Children.* Chicago, Year Book Medical Publishers, 1971.

Stevens PS, Eckstein HB: Ileal conduit diversion in children. *Br J Urol* 49:379, 1977.

Stone AR: Ileocystoplasty. In: King LR, Stone AR, Webster GD (Eds): *Bladder Reconstruction and Continent Urinary Diversion.* Chicago, London, Year Book Medical Publishers, 1991, p 58.

Stower MJ, Massey JA, Feneley RCL: Urethral closure in management of urinary incontinence. *Urology* 34:246, 1989.

Straffon RA, Kyle K, Corvalan J: Techniques of cutaneous ureterostomy and results in 51 patients. *J Urol* 103:138, 1970.

Tanagho EA, Smith DR, Meyers FH, Fisher R: Mechanism of urinary continence: II. Technique for surgical correction of incontinence. *J Urol* 101:305, 1969.

Tanagho EA, Smith DR: Clinical evaluation of a surgical technique for the correction of complete urinary incontinence. *J Urol* 107:402, 1972.

Tanagho EA: Urethrosphincteric reconstruction for congenitally absent urethra. *J Urol* 116:237, 1976.

Tanagho EA: Bladder neck reconstruction for total urinary incontinence: 10 years of experience. *J Urol* 125:321, 1981.

Tank ES, Lindenauer SM: Principles of management of exstrophy of the cloaca. *Am J Surg* 119:95, 1970.

Tasker JH: Ileo-cystoplasty: a new technique (an experimental study with report of a case). *Br J Urol* 25:349, 1953.

Thüroff JW, Alken P, Reidmiller H, *et al.*: The Mainz-pouch (mixed augmentation ileum 'n zecum) for bladder augmentation and continent diversion. *J Urol* 11:152, 1985.

Turner WR Jr, Ransley PG, Bloom DA, *et al.*: Variants of the exstrophic complex. *Urol Clin North Am* 7:493, 1980.

Turner-Warwick R, Ashken MH: The functional results of partial, subtotal and total cystoplasty with special reference to ureterocaecocystoplasty, selective sphincterotomy and cystocystoplasty. *Br J Urol* 39:3, 1967.

Turner-Warwick R, Wynne EJ, Askhen MH: The use of the omental pedicle graft in the repair and reconstruction of the urinary tract. *Br J Surg* 54:849, 1967.

Turner-Warwick R: Cystoplasty. In: Blandy JP (Ed): *Urology.* Oxford, Blackwell Scientific Publications, 1976, p 840.

Turner-Warwick R: The use of the omental pedicle graft in urinary tract reconstruction. *J Urol* 16:341, 1976.

Uhlenhuth E, Wolfe WM, Smith EM: The rectogenital septum. *Surg Gynecol Obstet* 86:148, 1948.

Van den Beviere H, Vossaert R, DeRoose J, Derom F: Our experience in the treatment of imperforate anus: anterior Mollard's technique versus posterior approach (Stephen's technique). *Acta Chir Belg* 82:205, 1983.

Vose SN, Dixey GM: Ureterostomy in-situ. *J Urol* 69:503, 1953.

Wallace DM: Ureteric diversion using a conduit: simplified technique. *Br J Urol* 38:522, 1966.

Walsh A: Ureterostomy in-situ. *Br J Urol* 39:744, 1967.

Weakley FL, Turnbull RB Jr: Special intestinal procedures. In: Stewart BH (Ed): *Operative Urology.* Baltimore, Williams & Wilkins Company, 1975.

Wear JB Jr, Barquin OP: Ureterosigmoidostomy: long-term results. *Urology* 1:192, 1973.

Webster GD, Goldwasser B: Management of incontinence after cystoplasty. In: King LR, Stone AR, Webster GD (Eds): *Bladder Reconstruction and Continent Urinary Diversion.* Chicago, London, Year Book Medical Publishers, 1986, p 75.

Webster GD (Guest Ed): Problems in reconstructive urology. In: Paulson DF (Series Ed): *Problems in Urology.* Philadelphia, J. B. Lippincott Company, 1987, vol 1.

Wein AJ, Malloy TR, Greenberg SH, *et al.*: Omental transposition as an aid in genitourinary reconstructive procedures. *J Trauma* 10:473, 1980.

Weiss JP: Sigmoidocystoplasty to augment bladder capacity. *Surg Gynecol Obstet* 159:377, 1984.

Wells CA: The use of the intestine in urology. *Br J Urol* 28:335, 1956.

Wespes E, Stone AR, King LR: Ileocaecocystoplasty in urinary tract reconstruction in children. *J Urol* 58:266, 1986.

Wesselhoeft CWJ, Perlmutter AD, Berg S, *et al.*: Pathogenesis and surgical treatment of diverticulum of the bladder. *Surg Gynecol Obstet* 116:719, 1963.

Weyrauch HM, Young BW: Evaluation of common methods of uretero-intestinal anastomosis: an experimental study. *J Urol* 67:880, 1952.

Whitmore WF III, Gittes RF: Reconstruction of the urinary tract by cecal and ileocecal cystoplasty: review of a 15-year experience. *J Urol* 130:494, 1983.

Wilbert DM, Hohenfellner R: Colonic conduit: preoperative requirements, operative techniques, postoperative management. *World J Urol* 2:159, 1984.

Williams DI, Rabinovitch HH: Cutaneous ureterostomy for the grossly dilated ureter of childhood. *Br J Urol* 39:696, 1967.

Williams DI, Keeton JE: Further progress with reconstruction of the exstrophied bladder. *Br J Surg* 60:203, 1973.

Williams DI, Snyder H: Anterior detrusor tube repair for urinary incontinence in children. *Br J Urol* 48:671, 1976.

Williams DI, Cromie WJ: Ring ureterostomy. *Br J Urol* 47:789, 1976.

Woodard JR, Marshall VF: Reconstruction of the female urethra to reduce post-traumatic incontinence. *Surg Gynecol Obstet* 113:687, 1961.

Woodard JR, Parrott TS: Reconstruction of the urinary tract in prune belly uropathy. *J Urol* 119:824, 1978.

Woodhouse CRJ, Malone PR, Cumming J, Reilly JM: The Mitrofanoff principle for continent urinary diversion. *Br J Urol* 63:53, 1989.

Young HH: Exstrophy of the bladder: the first case in which a normal bladder and urinary control have been obtained by plastic operations. *Surg Gynecol Obstet* 74:729, 1942.

Zingg E, Tscholl R: Continent cecoileal conduit: preliminary report. *J Urol* 118:724, 1977.

Zimmern PE, Hadley HR, Leach GE, Raz S: Transvaginal closure of the bladder neck and placement of a suprapubic catheter for destroyed urethra after long-term indwelling catheterization. *J Urol* 134:554, 1985.

Zinman L, Libertino JA: The ileo-cecal conduit for temporary and permanent urinary diversion. *J Urol* 113:317, 1975.

Zinman L, Libertino JA: The ileocecal segment: an antirefluxing colonic conduit form of urinary diversion. *Surg Clin North Am* 56:733, 1976.

Section 7—Testis

Abbassian A: A new surgical technique for testicular implantation. *J Urol* 107:618, 1972.

Aceland RD: Instrumentation for microsurgery. *Orthop Clin North Am* 8:281, 1977.

Action Committee on Surgery on the Genitalia of Male Children: The timing of elective surgery on the genitalia of male children with particular reference to undescended testes and hypospadias. *Pediatrics* 56:479, 1975.

Alfert HJ, Gillenwater JY: Ectopic vas deferens communicating with lower ureter: embryological considerations. *J Urol* 108:172, 1972.

Backhouse KM: The gubernaculum testis Hunteri: testicular descent and maldescent. *Ann R Coll Surg* 35:15, 1964.

Backhouse KM: Embryology of the normal and cryptorchid testis. In: Fonkelsrud EW, Mengel W (Eds): *The Undescended Testis.* Chicago, Year Book Medical Publishers, 1981.

Beck EM, Schlegel PN, Goldstein M: Intraoperative varicocele anatomy: a macroscopic and microscopic study. *J Urol* 148:1190, 1992.

Bloom DA: Two-step orchiopexy with pelviscopic clip ligation of the spermatic vessels. *J Urol* 145:1030, 1991.

Borten M: *Laparoscopic complications: Prevention and Management.* Boston, B. C. Decker, Inc, 1986.

Browne D: Some anatomical points in the operation for undescended testicle. *Lancet* 1:460, 1933.

Browne D: Diagnosis of undescended testicle. *Br Med J* 2:168, 1938.

Burton CC: A description of the boundaries of the inguinal rings and scrotal pouches. *Surg Gynecol Obstet* 104:142, 1957.

Burton CC: The embryologic development and descent of the testis in relation to congenital hernia. *Surg Gynecol Obstet* 107:294, 1958.

Cabot H, Nesbit RM: Undescended testis. *Arch Surg* 22:850, 1931.

Cattolica EV, Karol JB, Rankin KN, Klein RS: High testicular salvage rate in torsion of the spermatic cord. *J Urol* 128:66, 1982.

Clatworthy HW Jr, Hollanbaugh RS, Grosfeld JL: The "long loop vas" orchiopexy for high undescended testis. *Am Surg* 38:69, 1972.

Coolsaet BLRA: The varicocele syndrome: venography determining the optimal level for surgical management. *J Urol* 124:833, 1980.

Cooper BJ, Little TM: Orchidopexy: theory and practice. *Br Med J* 291:706, 1985.

Cooper JF, Leadbetter WF, Chute R: The thoracoabdominal approach for retroperitoneal gland dissection: its application to testis tumors. *Surg Gynecol Obstet* 90:496, 1950.

Corkery JJ: Staged orchiopexy: a new technique. *J Pediatr Surg* 10:515, 1975.

Dahl DS, Singh M, O'Conor VJ Jr, *et al.*: Lord's operation for hydrocele compared with conventional techniques. *Arch Surg* 104:40, 1972.

Dajani AM: Transverse ectopia of the testis. *Br J Urol* 41:80, 1969.

Davits RJAM, Van Den Aker ESS, Scholtmeijer RJ, *et al.*: Effect of parenteral testosterone therapy on penile development in boys with hypospadias. *Br J Urol* 71:593, 1993.

DeBoer A: Inguinal hernia in infants and children. *Arch Surg* 75:920, 1957.

Diamond DA, Caldamone AA: The value of laparoscopy for 106 impalpable testes relative to clinical presentation. *J Urol* 148:632, 1992.

Dwoskin JY, Kuhn JP: Herniograms in undescended testes and hydroceles. *J Urol* 109:520, 1973.

Elder JS: Laparoscopy and Fowler-Stephens orchiopexy in the management of the impalpable testis. *Urol Clin N Am* 16:399, 1989.

Ewert EE, Hoffman HA: Torsion of the spermatic cord. *J Urol* 51:551, 1944.

Firor HV: Two-stage orchiopexy. *Arch Surg* 102:598, 1971.

Flinn RA, King LR: Experiences with the midline transabdominal approach in orchiopexy. *Surg Gynecol Obstet* 133:285, 1971.

Fowler R, Stephens FD: The role of testicular vascular anatomy in the salvage of the high undescended testis. *Aust N Z J Surg* 29:92, 1959.

Fowler R, Stephens FD: The role of testicular vascular anatomy in the salvage of the high undescended testis. In: Stephens FD (Ed): *Congenital Malformations of Rectum, Anus and Genito-urinary Tract.* Edinburgh, E & S, 1963, pp 306–320.

Garibyan H, Hazebroek FWJ, Schulkes JAR, *et al.*: Microvascular surgical orchiopexy in the treatment of high-lying undescended testes. *Br J Urol* 56:326, 1984.

Gearhart JB, Jeffs RD: The use of parenteral testosterone therapy in genital reconstructive surgery. *J Urol* 138:1077, 1987.

Goldberg LM, Skaist LB, Morrow JW: Congenital absence of testes: anorchism and monorchism. *J Urol* 111:840, 1974.

Goldstein M, Gilbert BR, Dicker AP, *et al.*: Microsurgical inguinal varicocelectomy with delivery of the testis: an artery and lymphatic sparing technique. *J Urol* 148:1608, 1992.

Gross RE: *The Surgery of Infancy and Childhood: Its Principles and Techniques.* Philadelphia, W. B. Saunders Company, 1953.

Gross RE, Jewett TC Jr: Surgical experiences from 1,222 operations for undescended testes. *JAMA* 160:634, 1956.

Hadziselimovic F, Kogan SJ: Testicular development. In: Gillenwater JY, Grayhack JT, Howards SS, Duckett JW (Eds): *Adult and Pediatric Urology.* Chicago, Year Book Medical Publishers, 1987.

Harkins HN: *Hernia.* Philadelphia, J. B. Lippincott Company, 1964.

Harrison RG: The distribution of the vasal and cremasteric arteries to the testis and their functional importance. *J Anat* 83:267, 1949.

Harrison RG, McGregor GA: Anomalous origin and branching of the testicular arteries. *Anat Rec* 129:401, 1957.

Hart RR, Rushton HG, Belman AB: Intraoperative spermatic venography during varicocele surgery in adolescents. *J Urol* 148:1514, 1992.

Hass JA, Carrion HM, Sharkey J, Politano VA: Operative treatment of hydrocele: another look at Lord's procedure. *Urology* 12:578, 1978.

Hazebroeck FWJ, Molenaar JC: The management of the impalpable testis by surgery alone. *J Urol* 148:629, 1993.

Hill EC: The vascularisation of the human testis. *Am J Anat* 9:463, 1909.

Hinman F Jr: Optimum time for orchiopexy in cryptorchidism. *Fertil Steril* 6:206, 1955.

Hinman F Jr: Unilateral abdominal cryptorchidism. *J Urol* 122:71, 1979.

Hinman F Jr: Indications and contraindications for orchiopexy and orchiectomy. In: Fonkalsrud EW, Mengel W (Eds): *The Undescended Testis.* Chicago, London, Year Book Medical Publishers, 1981.

Hinman F Jr: The case for primary orchiectomy for the unilateral abdominal testis. In: Carlton CE Jr (Ed): *Controversies in Urology.* Chicago: Year Book Medical Publishers, 1989, p 42.

Hinman F Jr: Survey: localization and operation for non-palpable testes. *Urology* 30:193, 1987.

Hinman F Jr: Management of the intra-abdominal testis. *Eur J Pediatr* 146:549, 1987.

Hinman F Jr: Indications and contraindications for orchiopexy. In: Hadziselimovic F (Ed): *Cryptorchidism: Management and Implications.* Berlin, Heidelberg, Springer-Verlag, 1983, p 99.

Hunt JB, Witherington R, Smith AM: The midline preperitoneal approach to orchiopexy. *Am Surg* 47:184, 1981.

Ivanissevich O: Left varicocele due to reflux: experience with 4,470 operative cases in 42 years. *J Int Coll Surg* 34:742, 1918.

Ivanissevitch O, Gregorini H: A new operation for the cure of varicocele. *Semana Med* 25:575, 1918.

Janecka IP, Romas NA: Microvascular free transfer of human testes. *J Plast Reconstr Surg* 63:42, 1979.

Jirásek JE: The relationship between differentiation of the testicle, genital ducts and external genitalia in fetal and postnatal life. In: Rosenberg E, Paulsen AC (Eds): *The Human Testis.* New York, Plenum Press, 1970.

Juskiewenski S, Vaysse Ph: Arterial vascularisation of the testes and surgery for undescended testicles (testicular ectopia). *Anat Clin* 1:127, 1979.

Kass EJ, Belman AB: Reversal of testicular growth failure by varicocele ligation. *J Urol* 137:475, 1987.

Kass EJ, Chandra RS, Belman AB: Testicular histology in the adolescent with a varicocele. *Pediatrics* 79:996, 1987.

Kass EJ, Freitas JE, Bour JB: Pituitary-gonadal function in adolescents with a varicocele. *J Urol* 139:207, 1988.

Kavoussi LR, Sosa RE, Capelouto C: Complications of laparoscopic surgery. *J Endocrinol* 6:95, 1992.

Kaye KW, Lange PH, Fraley EE: Spermatic cord block in urologic surgery. *J Urol* 128:720, 1982.

Kelalis PP, King LR, Belman AB (Eds): *Clinical Pediatric Urology,* 2nd ed. Philadelphia, W. B. Saunders Company, 1985.

Khamesra HL, Gupta AS, Malpani NK: Transverse testicular ectopia. *Br J Urol* 50:283, 1978.

King LM, Sekaran SK, Sauer D, *et al.*: Untwisting in delayed treatment of torsion of the spermatic cord. *J Urol* 112:217, 1974.

Kogan SJ, Houman BZ, Reda EF, Levitt SB: Orchiopexy of the high undescended testis by division of the spermatic vessels: a critical review of 38 selected transections. *J Urol* 141:1416, 1989.

Lattimer JK, Vakili BF, Smith AM, *et al.*: A natural-feeling testicular prosthesis. *J Urol* 110:81, 1973.

Lemoh CN: A study of the development and structural relationships of the testis and gubernaculum. *Surg Gynecol Obstet* 110:164, 1960.

Levitt SB, Kogan SJ, Engel RM, *et al.*: The impalpable testis: a rational approach to management. *J Urol* 120:515, 1978.

Lewis EL: The Ivanissevich operation. *J Urol* 63:165, 1950.

Lord PH: A bloodless operation for the radical cure of idiopathic hydrocele. *Br J Surg* 51:914, 1964.

Lord PH: A bloodless operation for spermatocoele or cyst of the epididymis. *Br J Surg* 57:641, 1970.

Loughlin KR, Brooks DC: The use of a Doppler probe in laparoscopic surgery. *J Laparoendosc Surg* 2:191, 1992.

Loughlin KR, Brooks DC: The use of a Doppler probe to facilitate laparoscopic varicocele ligation. *Surg Gynecol Obstet* 174:326, 1992.

724 REFERENCES

Lyon RP: Torsion of the testicle in childhood: a painless emergency requiring contralateral orchiopexy. *JAMA* 178:702, 1961.

MacMahon RA, O'Brien BM, Cussen LJ: The use of microsurgery in the treatment of the undescended testis. *J Pediatr Surg* 11:52, 1976.

MacMillan EW: The blood supply of the epididymis in man. *Br J Urol* 26:60, 1954.

Marshall FF, Shermeta DW: Epididymal abnormalities associated with undescended testis. *J Urol* 121:341, 1979.

Martin DC, Menck HR: The undescended testis: management after puberty. *J Urol* 114:77, 1975.

McVay CB: The anatomic basis for inguinal and femoral hernioplasty. *Surg Gynecol Obstet* 139:931, 1974.

Mitchell ME: Urinary tract diversion and undiversion in the pediatric age group. *Surg Clin North Am* 61:1147, 1981.

Monfort G, Guys JM, Lacombe GM: Appendicovesicostomy: an alternative urinary diversion in the child. *Eur Urol* 10:361, 1984.

Moorcraft J, DuBoulay CEH, Isaacson P, Atwell JD: Changes in the mucosa of colon conduits with particular reference to the risk of malignant change. *Br J Urol* 55:185, 1983.

Morse TS, Hollebaugh RS: The window orchiopexy for prevention of testicular torsion. *J Pediatr Surg* 12:237, 1977.

Moul JW, Belman AB: A review of surgical treatment of undescended testis with emphasis on anatomical position. *J Urol* 140:382, 1988.

Murnaghan GF: The appendages of the testis and epididymis: a short review with case reports. *Br J Urol* 31:190, 1959.

Nadelson EJ, Cohen M, Warner R, Leiter E: Update: varicocelectomy. A safe outpatient procedure. *Urology* 14:259, 1984.

Nunn LN, Stephens FD: The triad syndrome: a composite anomaly of the abdominal wall, urinary system, and testis. *J Urol* 86:782, 1961.

Nyhus LM, Condon RE, Harkins HN: Clinical experiences with preperitoneal hernial repair for all types of hernia of the groin. *Am J Surg* 100:234, 1960.

Nyhus LM: An anatomic reappraisal of the posterior inguinal wall. *Surg Clin North Am* 44:1305, 1964.

Nyhus LM: The preperitoneal approach and iliopubic tract repair on inguinal hernia. In: Nyhus LM, Condon RE (Eds): *Hernia,* 2nd ed. Philadelphia, J. B. Lippincott Company, 1978, pp 212–235.

O'Brien BM, Rao VK, MacLeod AM, *et al.*: Microvascular testicular transfer. *Plast Reconstr Surg* 71:87, 1983.

Odiase V, Whitaker RH: Analysis of cord length obtained during steps of orchiopexy. *Br J Urol* 54:308, 1982.

Ombredanne L: Sur l'orchiopexie. *Bull Soc Pediatr (Paris)* 25:473, 1927.

Ottenheimer EJ: Testicular fixation in torsion of the spermatic cord. *JAMA* 101:116, 1933.

Paloma A: Radical cure of varicocele by a new technique: preliminary report. *J Urol* 61:604, 1949.

Parkash S, Ramakrishnan K, Bagdi RK: Orchiopexy: transseptal ipsilateral positioning. *Br J Urol* 55:79, 1982.

Parker RM, Robison JR: Anatomy and diagnosis of torsion of the testicle. *J Urol* 106:243, 1971.

Pascual JA, Villanueva-Meyer J, Salido E, *et al.*: Recovery of testicular blood flow following ligation of the testicular vessels. *J Urol* 142:549, 1989.

Persky L, Albert DJ: Staged orchiopexy. *Surg Gynecol Obstet* 132:43, 1971.

Pinsolle J, Drouillard J, Bruneton JN, Grenier FN: Anatomical bases of testicular vein catheterization and phlebography. *Anat Clin* 2:191, 1980.

Plottzker ED, Rushton HG, Belman AN, Skoog SJ: Laparoscopy for nonpalpable testes in childhood: is inguinal exploration also necessary when the vas and vessels exit the external ring? *J Urol* 148:635, 1992.

Prentiss RJ, Weickgenant CJ, Moses JJ, Frazier DB: Undescended testis: surgical anatomy of spermatic vessels, spermatic surgical triangles and lateral spermatic ligament. *J Urol* 83:686, 1960.

Prentiss RJ, Boatwright DC, Pennington RD, *et al.*: Testicular prosthesis: materials, methods and results. *J Urol* 90:208, 1963.

Raijfer J, Pickett S, Klein SR: Laparoscopic occlusion of testicular veins for clinical varicocele. *Urology* 40:113, 1992.

Ransley PG, Vordermark JS, Caldamone AA, *et al.*: Preliminary ligation of the gonadal vessels prior to orchiopexy for the intra-abdominal testicle: a staged Fowler-Stephens procedure. *World J Urol* 2:266, 1984.

Rolnick D, Kawanoue S, Szanto P, *et al.*: Anatomical incidence of testicular appendages. *J Urol* 100:755, 1968.

Scardino, PT: Thoracoabdominal retroperitoneal lymphadenectomy for testicular carcinoma. In: Crawford ED, Borden TA (Eds): *Genitourinary Cancer Surgery.* Philadelphia, Lea & Febiger, 1982, p 27.

Scorer CG: The descent of the testis. *Arch Dis Child* 39:605, 1964.

Scorer CG, Farrington GH: *Congenital Deformities of the Testis and Epididymis.* London, Butterworth and Company, 1971.

Semm BK: *Operative Manual for Endoscopic Abdominal Surgery.* Friedrich ER (Trans). Chicago, Year Book Medical Publishers, 1987.

Shafik A: Obturator foramen approach: II. A new surgical approach for management of the short-pedicled undescended testis. *Am J Surg* 144:381, 1982.

Shafik A, Moftah A, Olfat S, *et al.*: Testicular veins: anatomy and role in varicocelogenesis and other pathologic conditions. *Urology* 35:175, 1990.

Sharlip ID: Surgery of scrotal contents. *Urol Clin North Am* 14:145, 1987.

Silber S, Kelly J: Successful autotransplantation in an intra-abdominal testis to the scrotum by microvascular technique. *J Urol* 115:452, 1976.

Skandalakas JE: *Hernia: Surgical Anatomy and Technique.* New York, McGraw-Hill Book Company, 1989.

Skinner DG: Considerations for management of large retroperitoneal tumors: use of the modified thoracoabdominal approach. *Urology* 117:605, 1977.

Snyder WH Jr: Inguinal hernia complicated by descended testis. *Am J Surg* 94:325, 1955.

Solomon AA: The extrusion operation for hydrocele. *N Y State J Med* 55:1885, 1955.

Solomon AA: Testicular prosthesis: a new insertion operation. *J Urol* 108:436, 1972.

Steinhardt GF, Kroovand RL, Perlmutter AD: Orchiopexy: planned 2-stage technique. *J Urol* 133:434, 1985.

Stephens FD: Embryopathy of malformations [guest editorial]. *J Urol* 127:13, 1982.

Vergnes P, Midy D, Bondonny JM, Cabanie H: Anatomical basis of inguinal surgery in children. *Anat Clin* 7:257, 1985.

Viidik T, Marshall DG: Direct inguinal hernias in infancy and early childhood. *J Pediatr Surg* 15:646, 1980.

Wacksman J, Dinner M, Straffon R: Technique of testicular autotransplantation using microvascular anastomosis. *Surg Gynecol Obstet* 150:399, 1980.

Waldron R, James M, Clain A: Technique and results of trans-scrotal operations for hydrocele and scrotal cysts. *Br J Urol* 58:303, 1986.

Weissbach L: Alloplastic testicular prostheses. In: Wagenknecht LV, Furlow WL, Auvert J (Eds): *Genitourinary Reconstruction With Prostheses.* Stuttgart, Georg Thieme Verlag, 1981, p 173.

Winfield HN, Donovan JF, See WA, *et al.*: Urological laparoscopic surgery. *J Urol* 146:941, 1991.

Woodard JR, Parrot TS: Orchiopexy in the prune-belly syndrome. *Br J Surg* 50:348, 1978.

Woodard JR: Prune-belly syndrome: In: Kelalis PP, King LR, Belman AB (Eds): *Clinical Pediatric Urology.* Philadelphia, W. B. Saunders Company, 1985.

Youngson GG, Jones PF: Management of the impalpable testis: long-term results of the preperitoneal approach. *J Pediatr Surg* 26:618, 1991.

Yuzpe AA: Pneumoperitoneum needle and trocar injuries in laparoscopy: a survey on possible contributing factors and prevention. *J Reprod Med* 25:485, 1990.

Zer M, Wolloch Y, Dintsman M: Staged orchiorrhaphy: therapeutic procedure in cryptorchid testicle with a short spermatic cord. *Arch Surg* 110:387, 1975.

Section 8—Penis and Urethra

Abbé R: New method of creating a vagina in a case of congenital absence. *Med Rec* Dec 10, 1898.

Allen LE, Hardy BE, Churchill BM: The surgical management of the enlarged clitoris. *J Urol* 128:351, 1982.

Allen TD, Spence HM: The surgical treatment of coronal hypospadias and related problems. *J Urol* 100:504, 1968.

Allen TD: Microphallus: clinical and endocrinological characteristics. *J Urol* 119:750, 1978.

Ansell JS, Raijfer J: A new and simplified method for concealing the hypertrophied clitoris. *J Pediatr Surg* 16:681, 1984.

Arap S, Mitre Al, de Góes GM: Modified meatal advancement and glanuloplasty for distal hypospadias. *J Urol* 131:1140, 1984.

Arneri V: Reconstruction of the male genitalia. In: Converse JM (Ed): *Reconstructive and Plastic Surgery,* 2nd ed. Philadelphia, W. B. Saunders Company, 1977, vol 7, p 3902.

Asopa HS, Elhence EP, Atri SP, Bansal NK: One-stage correction of penile hypospadias using a foreskin tube: a preliminary report. *Int Surg* 55:435, 1971.

Asopa R, Asopa HS: One-stage repair of hypospadias using double island preputial skin tube. *Indian J Urol* 1:41, 1984.

Azmy A, Eckstein HB: Surgical correction of torsion of the penis. *Br J Urol* 53:378, 1981.

Bailez MM, Gearhart JP, Migeon C, Rock J: Vaginal reconstruction after initial construction of the external genitalia in girls with salt-wasting adrenal hyperplasia. *J Urol* 148:680, 1992.

Baldwin JF: The formation of an artificial vagina by intestinal transplantation. *Ann Surg* 40:398, 1904.

Ballesteros JJ: Personal technique for surgical repair of balanic hypospadias. *J Urol* 118:983, 1977.

Barcat J: Current concepts of treatment. In: Horton CE (Ed): *Plastic and Reconstructive Surgery of the Genital Area.* Boston, Little, Brown & Company, 1973, p 249.

Barrett TM, Gonzales ET Jr: Reconstruction of the female external genitalia. *Urol Clin N Am* 7:455, 1980.

Bartone F, Shore N, Newland J, et al.: The best suture for hypospadias? *Urology* 29:517, 1987.

Beck C: Hypospadias and its treatment. *Surg Gynecol Obstet* 24:511, 1917.

Beemer W, Hopkins MP, Morley GW: Vaginal reconstruction in gynecologic oncology. *Obstet Gynecol* 72:911, 1988.

Bellinger MF: Embryology of the male external genitalia. *Urol Clin N Am* 8:375, 1981.

Belman AB, King LR: Urinary tract abnormalities associated with imperforate anus. *J Urol* 108:823, 1972.

Belman AB: The modified Mustardé hypospadias repair. *J Urol* 127:88, 1982.

Bergman R, Howard AH, Barnes RW: Plastic reconstruction of the penis. *J Urol* 59:1174, 1948.

Bevan AD: A new operation for hypospadias. *JAMA* 68:1032, 1917.

Bhandari M, Kumar S: Modified single-stage hypospadias repair using double island preputial skin tube. *Br J Urol* 62:189, 1988.

Blandy JP, Tresidder GC: Meatoplasty. *Br J Urol* 39:633, 1967.

Blandy JP, Singh M: The technique and results of one-stage island patch urethroplasty. *Br J Urol* 47:83, 1975.

Blandy JP: Circumcision. In: Chamberlain GVP (Ed): *Contemporary Obstetrics and Gynaecology.* London, Northwood, 1977, p 240.

Blandy JP: Urethral stricture. *Postgrad Med J* 56:383, 1980.

Boxer JB: Reconstruction of the male genitalia. *Surg Gynecol Obstet* 141:939, 1975.

Brannan W, Ochsner M, Fuselier HA, Goodlet JS: Free full-hickness skin graft urethroplasty for urethral stricture: experience with 66 patients. *J Urol* 115:677, 1976.

Broadbent TR, Woolf RM, Toksu E: Hypospadias: one-stage repair. *Plast Reconstr Surg* 27:154, 1961.

Browne D: An operation for hypospadias. *Lancet* 1:141, 1936.

Bulmer D: The development of the human vagina. *J Anat* 91:490, 1957.

Burbige KA: Transpubic-perineal urethral reconstruction in boys using a substitution graft. *J Urol* 148:1235, 1992.

Bürger RA, Riedmiller H, Knapstein PG, et al.: Ileocecal vaginal construction. *Am J Obstet Gynecol* 161:162, 1989.

Bürger RA, Müller SC, El-Damanhoury H, et al.: The buccal mucosal graft for urethral reconstruction: a preliminary report. *J Urol* 147:662, 1992.

Burkholder GV, Newell ME: New surgical treatment for micropenis. *J Urol* 129:832, 1983.

Byars LT: A technique for consistently satisfactory repair of hypospadias. *Surg Gynecol Obstet* 100:184, 1955.

Cabral BHP, Gonzales R: Use of urethral drainage tube and dressing in hypospadias repair. *Urology* 33:327, 1989.

Cantwell FV: Operative treatment of epispadias by transplantation of the urethra. *Ann Surg* 22:689, 1895.

Cecil AB: Surgery of hypospadias and epispadias in the male. *J Urol* 67:1006, 1932.

Cecil AB: Repair of hypospadias and urethral fistula. *J Urol* 56:237, 1946.

Chang T-S, Hwang W-Y: Forearm flap in one stage reconstruction of the penis. *Plast Reconstr Surg* 74:251, 1984.

Coleman JW: The bladder mucosal graft technique for hypospadias repair. *J Urol* 125:708, 1981.

Coleman JW, McGovern JH, Marshall VF: The bladder mucosal graft technique for hypospadias repair. *Urol Clin North Am* 8:457, 1981.

Conway H, Stark RB: Construction and reconstruction of the vagina. *Surg Gynecol Obstet* 97:573, 1953.

Coran AG, Polley TZ Jr: Surgical management of ambiguous genitalia in the infant and child. *J Pediatr Surg* 26:812, 1991.

Crawford BS: Buried penis. *Br J Plast Surg* 30:96, 1977.

Crawford ED: Technique of ilioinguinal lymph node dissection. In: Skinner DG, Lieskovsky G (Eds): *Diagnosis and Management of Genitourinary Cancer.* Philadelphia, W. B. Saunders Company, 1988.

Cromie WJ, Bellinger MF: Hypospadias dressing and diversions. *Urol Clin North Am* 1981, 8:545, 1981.

Culp DA: Genital injuries: etiology and initial management in genitourinary trauma. *Urol Clin North Am* 4:143, 1977.

Das S, Brosman SA: Duplication of male urethra. *J Urol* 117:452, 1977.

Davis RS, Linke CA, Kraemer GK: Use of labial tissue in repair of urethrovaginal fistula and injury. *Arch Surg* 115:628, 1980.

de la Rosette JJMCH, de Vries JDM, Lock MTWT, Debryne FMJ: Urethroplasty using the pedicled island flap technique in complicated urethral strictures. *J Urol* 146:40, 1991.

DeSy WA: Aesthetic repair of meatal strictures. *J Urol* 132:678, 1984.

DeSy WA, Verbaeys A, Roelandt R, Osterlinck W: A simple approach to the entire urethra. *Br J Urol* 58:344, 1986.

DeSy WA, Oosterlinck W: Partial pubectomy: technique and indications. *Br J Urol* 58:464, 1986.

Decter RM: Inverted V glansplasty: a procedure for distal hypospadias. *J Urol* 146 (Part 2):641, 1991.

Dessanti A, Rigamonti W, Merulla V, *et al.*: Autologous buccal muscosa graft for hypospadias repair: an initial report. *J Urol* 147:1081, 1992.

Devine CJ Jr, Horton CE: A one-stage hypospadias repair. *J Urol* 85:166, 1961.

Devine CJ Jr, Gonzalex-Serva L, *et al.*: Utricular configuration in hypospadias and intersex. *Trans Am Assoc GU Surgeons* 71:154, 1979.

Devine CJ Jr: Embryology of the male external genitalia. *Clin Plast Surg* 7:141, 1980.

Devine CJ Jr, Horton CE, Snyder HM 3rd, *et al.*: Chordee without hypospadias. In: Hurwitz RS, Ehrlich RM (Eds): *Dialogues in Pediatric Urology* 9:2, 1986.

Devine CJ Jr: Editorial comment. *J Urol* 144:283, 1990.

Devine PC, Horton CE, Devine CJ Jr, *et al.*: Use of full-thickness skin grafts in repair of urethral strictures. *J Urol* 90:67, 1963.

Devine PC, Devine CJ, Horton CE: Anterior urethral injuries: secondary reconstruction. *Urol Clin North Am* 4:157, 1977.

Devine PC, Wendelken JR, Devine CJ Jr: Free full-thickness skin graft urethroplasty: current technique. *J Urol* 121:282, 1979.

Dewan PA, Dinneen MD, Duffy PG, *et al.*: Pedicle patch urethroplasty. *Br J Urol* 67:420, 1991.

Duckett JW: The island flap technique for hypospadias repair. *Urol Clin North Am* 8:503, 1981.

Duckett JW: Hypospadias. In: Walsh PC, Gittes RF, Perlmutter AD, Stamey TA (Eds): *Campbell's Urology*, 5th ed. Philadelphia, W. B. Saunders Company, 1986, p 1969.

Duckett JW, Keating MA: Technical challenge of the megameatus intact prepuce hypospadias variant: the pyramid procedure. *J Urol* 141:1407, 1989.

Duckett JW: Hypospadias. In: Gillenwater JY, Grayhack JT, Howards SS, Duckett JW (Eds): *Adult and Pediatric Urology*, 2nd ed. St. Louis, Mosby Year Book, 1991, p 2103.

Duckett JW: Successful hypospadias repair. *Contemp Urol* April 4–15, 1992.

Duckett JW, Snyder HM: Meatal advancement and glanuloplasty hypospadias repair after 1,000 cases: avoidance of meatal stenosis and regression. *J Urol* 147:665, 1992.

Eardley I, Whitaker RH: Surgery for hypospadias fistula. *Br J Urol* 69:306, 1992.

Ebbehoj J, Metz P: New operation for "Krummerik" (penile curvature). *Urology* 26:76–78, 1985.

Ehrlich RM, Scardino PT: Surgical correction of scrotal transposition and perineal hypospadias. *J Pediatr Surg* 17:175, 1982.

Ehrlich RM, Reda EF, Koyle MA, *et al.*: Complications of bladder mucosal graft. *J Urol* 142:626, 1989.

Ehrlich RM, Gershman A, Fuchs G: Selected topics in pediatric urology. *Pediatr Urol Corresp Club Lett* Feb 28, 1993.

El-Kasaby AW, Fath-Alla M, Noweir AM, *et al.*: The use of buccal mucosa patch graft in the management of anterior urethral strictures. *J Urol* 149:276, 1993.

Elder JS, Mostwin JL: Cyst of the ejaculatory duct/urogenital sinus. *J Urol* 132:768, 1984.

Elder JS, Duckett JW, Snyder HM: Onlay island flap in the repair of mid and distal penile hypospadias without chordee. *J Urol* 138:376, 1987.

Elder JS: Influence of glans morphology on choice of island flap technique in children with proximal hypospadias. *J Urol* 147:317A, 1992.

Feldman KW, Smith DW: Fetal phallic growth and penile standards for newborn male infants. *J Pediatr* 86:395, 1975.

Gaylis FD, Zaontz MR, Dalton D, *et al.*: Silicone foam dressing for penis after reconstructive pediatric surgery. *Urology* 33:296, 1989.

Gearhart JP, Borland RN: Onlay island flap urethroplasty: variation on a theme. *J Urol* 148:1507, 1992.

Gilbert DA, Jordan GH, Devine CJ Jr, *et al.*: Phallic construction in prepubertal and adolescent boys. *J Urol* 149:1521, 1993.

Gilbert DA, Jordan GH, Devine CJ Jr, Winslow BH: Microsurgical forearm "cricket bat-transformer" phalloplasty. *Plast Reconstr Surg* 90:711, 1992.

Gilpin D, Clements WDB, Boston VE: GRAP repair: single-stage reconstruction of hypospadias as an outpatient procedure. *Br J Urol* 71:226, 1993.

Glenister TW: The origin and fate of the urethral plate in man. *J Anat* 288:413, 1954.

Gonzales R, Fernandes ET: Single-stage feminization genitoplasty. *J Urol* 143:776, 1990.

Goodwin WE: Partial (segmental) amputation of the clitoris for female pseudohermaphroditism. *Soc Pediatr Urol Newslett* 1981.

Hagerty RC, Vaughn TR, Lutz MH: The perineal artery axial flap in reconstruction of the vagina. *Plast Reconstr Surg* 82:344, 1988.

Hanna MK: Vaginal construction. *Urology* 29:272, 1987.

Hendren WH, Crawford JD: Adrenogenital syndrome: the anatomy of the anomaly and its repair. Some new concepts. *J Pediatr Surg* 4:49, 1969.

Hendren WH, Crawford JD: The child with ambiguous genitalia. *Curr Probl Surg* 1:64, 1972.

Hendren WH: Surgical management of urogenital sinus abnormalities. *J Pediatr Surg* 12:339, 1977.

Hendren WH, Donahoe PK: Correction of congenital abnormalities of the vagina and perineum. *J Pediatr Surg* 15:751, 1980.

Hendren WH: Construction of a female urethra from vaginal wall and perineal flap. *J Urol* 123:657, 1980.

Hendren WH: Reconstructive problems of the vagina and female urethra. *Clin Plast Surg* 7:207, 1980.

Hendren WH, Keating MA: Use of dermal grafts and free urethral grafts in penile reconstruction. *J Urol* 140 (Part 2):1265, 1988.

Hendren WH, Caesar RE: Chordee without hypospadias: experience with 33 cases. *J Urol* 147:107, 1992.

Hensle TW, Dean GE: Vaginal replacement in children. *J Urol* 148:677, 1992.

Hester TR, Hill HL, Jurkewicz MJ: One-stage reconstruction of the penis. *Br J Plast Surg* 31:279, 1978.

Hinman F Jr: Surgical reversal of the female adrenal intersex. *Urol Int* 19:211, 1965.

Hinman F Jr, Spence HF, Culp OS, *et al.*: Panel discussion: anomalies of external genitalia in infancy and childhood. *J Urol* 93:1, 1965.

Hinman F Jr: The blood supply to preputial island flaps. *J Urol* 145:1232, 1991.

Hodgson NB: Hypospadias and urethral duplications. In: Harrison JH, *et al.* (Eds): *Campbell's Urology*, 4th ed. Philadelphia, W. B. Saunders Company, 1979, p 1566.

Hodgson NB: Editorial comment. *J Urol* 149:816, 1993.

Hollowell JG, Keating MA, Snyder HM III, Duckett JW: Preservation of the urethral plate in hypospadias repair: extended applications and further experience with the onlay island flap urethroplasty. *J Urol* 143:98, 1990.

Horton CE, Devine CJ Jr: A one-stage repair for hypospadias cripples. *Plast Reconstr Surg* 66:407, 1970.

Horton CE, Devine CJ Jr: Plication of the tunica albuginea to straighten the curved penis. *Plast Reconstr Surg* 52:32, 1973.

Horton CE, McCraw JB, Devine CJ Jr, Devine PC: Secondary reconstruction of the genital area. *Urol Clin North Am* 4:133, 1977.

Howard FS: Hypospadias with enlargement of the prostatic utricle. *Surg Gynecol Obstet* 86:307, 1948.

Huffman WC, Culp DA, Greenleaf JS, et al.: Injuries to the male genitalia. *Plast Reconstr Surg* 18:344, 1956.

Huffman WC, Culp DA, Flocks RH: Injuries of the external male genitalia. In: Converse JM (Ed): *Reconstructive Plastic Surgery.* Philadelphia, W. B. Saunders Company, 1964.

Issa MM, Gearhart JP: The failed MAGPI: management and prevention. *Br J Urol* 64:169, 1989.

Johanson B: Reconstruction of the male urethra in strictures: application of the buried intact epithelium technic. *Acta Chir Scand* 176(Suppl):3, 1953.

Johnson N, Lilford RJ, Batchelor A: The free flap vaginoplasty: a new surgical procedure for the treatment of vaginal agenesis. *Br J Obstet Gynaecol* 98:184, 1991.

Jones FW: The development and malformations of the glans and prepuce. *Br Med J* 1:137, 1910.

Jones HW Jr, Garcia SC, Klingensmith GJ: Secondary surgical treatment of the masculinized external genitalia of patients with virilizing adrenal hyperplasia. *Obstet Gynecol* 48:73, 1976.

Jordan GH: Reconstruction of the fossa navicularis. *J Urol* 138:102, 1987.

Jordan GH, Devine PC: Application of tissue transfer techniques to the management of urethral strictures. *Semin Urol* 5:228, 1987.

Kelami A: Congenital penile deviation and its treatment with the Nesbit-Kelami technique. *Br J Urol* 60:261, 1987.

Kaplan I, Wesser D: A rapid method for constructing a functional sensitive penis. *Br J Plast Surg* 24:342, 1971.

Klauber GT, Williams DI: Epispadias with incontinence. *J Urol* 111:110, 1974.

Klimberg I, Walker RD: Comparison of Mustardé and Horton-Devine flip-flap techniques of hypospadias repair. *J Urol* 134:103, 1985.

Koff SA, Eakins M: The treatment of penile chordee using corporal rotation. *J Urol* 131:931, 1984.

Kogan SJ, Smey P, Leavitt S: Subtunical total reduction clitoroplasty: a safe modification of existing techniques. *J Urol* 130:746, 1983.

Koyle MA, Ehrlich RM: The bladder mucosal graft for urethral reconstruction. *J Urol* 138:1093, 1987.

Kramer SA, Mesrobian HG, Kelalis PP: Long-term followup of cosmetic appearance and genital function in male epispadias: review of 70 cases. *J Urol* 135:543, 1986.

Larson DL: Musculocutaneous flaps. In: Johnson DE, Boileau MA (Eds): *Genitourinary Tumors: Fundamental Principles and Surgical Techniques.* New York, Grune & Stratton, 1982.

Lattimer JK: Relocation and recession of the enlarged clitoris with preservation of the glans: an alternative to amputation. *J Urol* 86:113, 1961.

Lattimer JK, MacFarlane MT: A urethral lengthening procedure for epispadias and exstrophy. *J Urol* 123:544, 1980.

Lau JTK, Ong GB: Subglandular urethral fistula following circumcision: repair by the advancement method. *J Urol* 126:702, 1981.

Leadbetter GW, Leadbetter WF: Urethral strictures in male children. *J Urol* 87:409, 1962.

Lesavoy MA. Vaginal reconstruction. *Urol Clin North Am* 12:369, 1985.

Li ZC, Zheng ZH, Sheh YX, et al.: One-stage urethroplasty for hypospadias using a tube constructed with bladder mucosa: a new procedure. *Urol Clin North Am* 8:463, 1981.

Livne PM, Gibbons MD, Gonzales ET Jr: Correction of disproportion of corpora cavernosa as cause of chordee in hypospadias. *Urology* 22:608, 1983.

Maizels M, Zaontz M, Donovan J, et al.: Surgical correction of the buried penis. *J Urol* 136:268, 1986.

Malament M: Repair of the recurrent fistula of the penile urethra. *J Urol* 106:704, 1971.

Marberger H, Pauer W: Experience in hypospadias repair. *Urol Clin North Am* 8:403, 1981.

Marshall VF, Spellman RM: Construction of urethra in hypospadias using vesical mucosal grafts. *J Urol* 73:335, 1955.

Mathieu P: Traitement en un temps de l'hypospadias balanique et juxtabalanique. *J Chir (Paris)* 39:481, 1932.

Mays HB: Epispadias: a plan of treatment. *J Urol* 107:251, 1972.

McAninch JW, Kahn RI, Jeffrey RB, et al.: Major traumatic and septic genital injuries. *J Trauma* 24:291, 1984.

McAninch JW (Guest Ed): Trauma management. In: Blaisdell FW, Trunkey DD (Eds): *Urogenital Trauma.* New York, Thieme-Stratton, Inc, 1985, vol 2.

McCormack RM: Simultaneous chordee repair and urethral reconstruction for hypospadias. *Plast Reconstr Surg* 13:257, 1954.

McCraw J, Massey F, Shankin K, Horton C: Vaginal reconstruction using gracilis myocutaneous flaps. *Plast Reconstr Surg* 58:176, 1970.

McFarlane RM: The use of continuous suction under skin flaps. *Br J Plast Surg* 17:77, 1959.

McGowan AJ, Waterhouse K: Mobilization of the anterior urethra. *Bull N Y Acad Med* 40:776, 1964.

McGraw JB, Myers B, Shanklin KD: The value of fluorescein in predicting the viability of arterialized flaps. *Plast Reconstr Surg* 60:710, 1977.

McGuire EJ, Weiss RM: Scrotal flap urethroplasty for strictures of the deep urethra in infants and children. *J Urol* 110:599, 1973.

McIndoe A: The treatment of congenital absence and obliterative conditions of the vagina. *Br J Plast Surg* 2:254, 1950.

McMillan RDH, Churchill BM, Gilmore RF: Assessment of urinary stream after repair of anterior hypospadias by meatoplasty and glanuloplasty. *J Urol* 134:100, 1985.

Mettauer JP: Practical observations on those malformations of the male urethra and penis, termed hypospadias and epispadias, with an anomalous case. *Am J Med Sci* 4:43, 1842.

Michalowski E, Modelski W: The surgical treatment of epispadias. *Surg Gynecol Obstet* 117:465, 1963.

Mininberg DT: Phalloplasty in congenital adrenal hyperplasia. *J Urol* 128:355, 1982.

Mitchell ME, Hensle TW, Crooks KK: Urethral reconstruction in the young female using a perineal pedicle flap. *J Pediatr Surg* 17:687, 1982.

Mitchell ME, Kalb TB: Hypospadias repair without a bladder drainage catheter. *J Urol* 135:321, 1986.

Mollard P, Juskiewenski S, Sarkissian J: Clitoroplasty in intersex: a new technique. *Br J Urol* 53:371, 1981.

Mollard P, Mouriquard P, Felfela T: Application of the onlay island flap urethroplasty to penile hypospadias with severe chordee. *Br J Urol* 68:317, 1991.

Money J, Mazur T: Microphallus: the successful use of a prosthetic phallus in a 9-year-old boy. *J Sex Marital Ther* 3:187, 1977.

Monfort G: Transvesical approach to utricular cysts. *J Pediatr Surg* 17:406, 1982.

Moscona AR, Govrin-Yehudain J, Hirshowitz B: Closure of urethral fistulae by transverse Y-V advancement flap. *Br J Urol* 56:313, 1984.

Mufti GR, Aitchison M, Bramwell SP, et al.: Corporeal plication for surgical correction of Peyronie's disease. *J Urol* 144:281, 1990.

Mundy AR, Stephenson TP: Pedicled preputial patch urethroplasty. *Br J Urol* 61:48, 1988.

Mustardé JC: One-stage correction of distal hypospadias and other people's fistulae. *Br J Plast Surg* 18:413, 1965.

Nesbit RM: Plastic procedure for correction of hypospadias. *J Urol* 45:699, 1941.

Nesbit RM, MacKinney CC, Dingman R: Z-plasty for correction of meatal ureteral stricture after hypospadias repair. *J Urol* 72:681, 1954.

Nesbit RM: Congenital curvature of the phallus: report of 3 cases with description of corrective operation. *J Urol* 93:230, 1965.

Nesbit RM: Operation for correction of distal penile ventral curvature with or without hypospadias. *J Urol* 97:470, 1967.

Netto NR Jr: Surgical repair of posterior urethral strictures by transpubic urethroplasty or pull-through technique. *J Urol* 133:411, 1985.

Oesch IL, Pinter A, Ransley PG: Penile agenesis: report of six cases. *J Pediatr Surg* 22:172, 1987.

Oesterling JE, Gearhart JP, Jeffs RD: A unified approach to early reconstructive surgery of the child with ambiguous genitalia. *J Urol* 138:1079, 1987.

Oesterling JE, Gearhart JP, Jeffs RD: Urinary diversion after hypospadias surgery. *Urology* 29:513, 1987.

Orandi A: One-stage urethroplasty. *Br J Urol* 40:717, 1968.

Orticochea M: A new method of total reconstruction of the penis. *Br J Plast Surg* 25:347, 1972.

Osegbe DN, Ntia I: One-stage urethroplasty for complicated urethral strictures using axial penile skin island flap. *Eur Urol* 17:79, 1990.

Parrott TS, Scheflan M, Hester TR: Reduction clitoroplasty and vaginal construction in a single operation. *Urology* 14:367, 1980.

Passerini G, Maio G, Cisternino A, *et al.*: One-stage repair of severe hypospadias [abstract]. Presented at the International Congress of Pediatric Urology, Florence, Italy, 1986. Quoted in: Gillenwater JY, Grayhack JT, Howards SS, Duckett JW (Eds): *Adult and Pediatric Urology.* Chicago. Year Book Medical Publishers, 1986, p 1902.

Peña A: *Atlas of Surgical Management of Anorectal Malformations.* New York, Springer-Verlag, 1990.

Perovic S: Hypospadias sine hypospadias. *World J Urol* 10:85, 1992.

Perovic S, Vukadinovic F: Penoscrotal transposition with hypospadias: 1-stage repair. *J Urol* 148:1510, 1992.

Persky L, Resnick M, Desprez J: Penile reconstruction with gracilis pedicle grafts. *J Urol* 129:603, 1983.

Peters CA, Hendren WH: Splitting the pubis for exposure in difficult reconstructions for incontinence. *J Urol* 142 (Part 2):527 (Discussion 542), 1989.

Peters PC: Complications of penile surgery. In: Smith RB, Skinner DG (Eds): *Complications of Urologic Surgery: Prevention and Management.* Philadelphia, W. B. Saunders Company, 1976, p 420.

Pond HS, Brannan W: Correction of congenital curvature of the penis: experiences with the Nesbit operation at Ochsner Clinic. *J Urol* 112:491, 1974.

Presman D, Greenfield DL: Reconstruction of the perineal urethra with a free full-thickness skin graft from the prepuce. *J Urol* 69:677, 1953.

Quartey JKM: One-stage penile/preputial cutaneous island flap urethroplasty for urethral stricture: a preliminary report. *J Urol* 129:284, 1983.

Quartey JKM: One-stage penile/preputial island flap urethroplasty for urethral stricture. *J Urol* 134:474, 1985.

Radhakkrishnan J: Colon interposition vaginoplasty: a modification of the Wagner-Baldwin technique. *J Pediatr Surg* 22:1175, 1987.

Randolph JG, Hung W: Reduction clitoroplasty in females with hypertrophied clitoris. *J Pediatr Surg* 5:224, 1970.

Randolph JG, Hung W, Rathlev MC: Clitoroplasty for females born with ambiguous genitalia: a long-term study of 37 patients. *J Pediatr Surg* 16:882, 1981.

Ransley PG, Duffy PG, Oesch IL, *et al.*: The use of bladder mucosa and combined bladder mucosa/preputial skin grafts for urethral reconstruction. *J Urol* 138:1096, 1987.

Ransley PG: Epispadias repair. In: Spitz L, Homewood Nixon H (Eds): *Operative Surgery: Paediatric Surgery,* 4th ed. London, Butterworths, 1988, p 624.

Redman JF, Bissada NK: One-stage correction of chordee and 180-degree penile rotation. *Urology* 7:632, 1976.

Redman JF: Extended application of Nesbit ellipses in the correction of childhood penile curvature. *J Urol* 119:122, 1978.

Redman JF: Technique for phalloplasty. *Urology* 27:360, 1986.

Redman JF: The balanic groove technique of Barcat. *J Urol* 137:83, 1987.

Rickwood AMK, Anderson PAM: One-stage hypospadias repair: experience with 367 cases. *Br J Urol* 67:424, 1991.

Roberts AHN: A new operation for the repair of hypospadias fistulae. *Br J Plast Surg* 35:386, 1982.

Saad MN, Khoo CTK, Lochaitis AS: A simple technique for repair of urethral fistula by Y-V advancement. *Br J Plast Surg* 33:410, 1980.

Schreiter F: Mesh-graft-Urethroplastik. *Aktuelle Urol* 15:173, 1984.

Schreiter F, Noll F: Mesh graft urethroplasty using split thickness skin graft or foreskin. *J Urol* 142:1223–1226, 1989.

Schuhrke TD, Kaplan GW: Prostatic utricle cysts (müllerian duct cysts) *J Urol* 119:765, 1978.

Schultz JR, Klykylo WM, Wacksman J: Timing of elective hypospadias repair in children. *Pediatrics* 71:342, 1983.

Shapiro SR: Surgical treatment of the "buried" penis. *Urology* 30:554, 1987.

Sharp RJ, Holder TM, Howard CD, Grunt JA: Neonatal genital reconstruction. *J Pediatr Surg* 22:168, 1987.

Shaw A: Subcutaneous reduction clitoroplasty. *J Pediatr Surg* 112:331, 1977.

Sislow JG, Ireton RCM, Onsell JS: Treatment of congenital penile curvature due to disparate corpora cavernosa by the Nesbit technique: a rule of thumb for the number of wedges required to achieve correction. *J Urol* 141:92, 1989.

Slawin KM, Nagler HM: Treatment of congenital penile curvature with penile torsion: a new twist. *J Urol* 147:152, 1992.

Smith ED: A de-epithelialized overlap technique in the repair of hypospadias. *Br J Plast Surg* 26:106, 1973.

Smith ED: Durham-Smith repair of hypospadias. *Urol Clin North Am* 8:451, 1981.

Smith ED: Timing of surgery in hypospadias repair. *Aust N Z J Surg* 53:396, 1983.

Smith ED: Commentary: multiple stage repair of hypospadias. In: Whitehead ED, Leiter E (Eds): *Current Operative Urology,* 2nd ed. Philadelphia, Harper & Row, 1984, p 1251.

Smith ED: Malformations of the bladder, urethra and hypospadias. In: Holder TM, Ashcraft KW (Eds): *Pediatric Surgery.* Philadelphia, W. B. Saunders Company, 1990, p 752.

Snow BW: Transverse corporeal plication for persistent chordee. *Urology* 34:360, 1989.

Snow BW, Georges LS, Tarry WF: Techniques for outpatient hypospadias surgery. *Urology* 35:327, 1990.

Snyder HM: Does glans configuration indicate the type of chordee present in hypospadias? *Soc Pediatr Urol Newslett.* May 24:38–39, 1991.

Snyder HMC III: Management of ambiguous genitalia in the neonate. In: King LR (Ed): *Urologic Surgery in Neonates and Young Infants.* Philadelphia, W. B. Saunders Company, 1988, p 346.

Soderdahl DW, Brosman SA, Goodwin WE: Penile agenesis. *J Urol* 108:496, 1972.

Spaulding MH: The development of external genitalia in the human embryo. *Contr Embryol Carnegie Inst Publ* 276:67, 1921.

Speakman MJ, Azmy AF: Skin chordee without hypospadias: an unrecognized entity. *Br J Urol* 69:428, 1992.

Spence HM, Duckett JW Jr: Diverticulum of the female urethra: clinical aspects and presentation of a simple operative technique for cure. *J Urol* 104:432, 1970.

Spence HM, Allen TD: Genital reconstruction in the female with the adrenogenital syndrome. *Br J Urol* 45:126, 1973.

Standoli L: One-stage repair of hypospadias: preputial island flap technique. *Ann Plast Surg* 9:81, 1982.

Stephens FD: Congenital imperforate rectum, rectourethral and rectovaginal fistulae. *Aust N Z J Surg* 22:161, 1953.

Tanagho EA: Male epispadias: surgical repair of urethropenile deformity. *Br J Urol* 48:127, 1976.

Thomalla JV, Mitchell ME: Ventral preputial island flap technique for the repair of epispadias with or without exstrophy. *J Urol* 132:985, 1984.

Turner-Warwick R: The use of pedicle grafts in repair of urinary fistulae. *Br J Urol* 44:644, 1972.

Turner-Warwick R: The management of traumatic urethral strictures and injuries. *Br J Surg* 60:775, 1973.

Turner-Warwick R: Observations upon techniques for reconstruction of the urethral meatus, the hypospadiac glans deformity and the penile urethra. *Urol Clin North Am* 6:643, 1979.

Turner-Warwick R, Kirby RS: The construction and reconstruction of the vagina with the colocecum. *Surg Gynecol Obstet* 170:132, 1990.

Wacksman J: Modification of the one stage flip-flap procedure to repair distal penile hypospadias. *Urol Clin North Am* 8:527, 1981.

Wacksman J: Use of the Hodgson XX (modified Asopa) procedure to correct hypospadias with chordee: surgical technique and results. *J Urol* 136:1264, 1986.

Walker RD: Outpatient repair of urethral fistulae. *Urol Clin North Am* 8:582, 1981.

Walsh PC, Wilson JD, Allen TD, et al.: Clinical and endocrinological evaluation of patients with congenital microphallus. *J Urol* 120:90, 1978.

Wang Y, Hadley HR: The use of rotated vascularized pedicle flaps for complex transvaginal procedures. *J Urol* 149:590, 1993.

Waterhouse K: The surgical repair of membranous urethral strictures in children. *Trans Am Assoc GU Surg* 67:81, 1975.

Webster GD, Robertson CN: The vascularized skin island urethroplasty: its role and results in urethral stricture management. *J Urol* 133:31, 1985.

Wehrbein HL: Hypospadias. *J Urol* 50:335, 1943.

Williams DI: The development and abnormalities of the penile urethra. *Acta Anat* 15:176, 1952.

Wilson MC, Wilson CL, Thickstein JN: Transposition of the external genitalia. *J Urol* 94:600, 1965.

Wise HA II, Berggren RB: Another method of repair for urethrocutaneous fistulae. *J Urol* 118:1054, 1977.

Woods JE, Alter G, Meland B, Podratz K: Experience with vaginal reconstruction utilizing the modified Singapore flap. *Plast Reconstr Surg* 90:270, 1992.

Yachia D: Pedicled scrotal skin advancement for one-stage anterior urethral reconstruction in circumcised patients. *J Urol* 139:1007, 1988.

Yachia D: Modified corporoplasty for the treatment of penile curvature. *J Urol* 143:80, 1990.

Yeoman PM, Cooke R, Hain WR: Penile block for circumcision? A comparison with caudal block. *Anesthesia* 38:862, 1983.

Young F, Benjamin JA: Repair of hypospadias with free inlay skin graft. *Surg Gynecol Obstet* 5:86, 1948.

Young F, Benjamin JA: Preschool age repair of hypospadias with free inlay skin graft. *Surgery* 26:384, 1949.

Young HH: Genital Abnormalities. Baltimore, Williams & Wilkins Company, 1937.

Zagula EM, Braren V: Management of urethrocutaneous fistulas following hypospadias repair. *J Urol* 130:743, 1983.

Zaontz MR: The GAP (glans approximation procedure) for glanular/coronal hypospadias. *J Urol* 141:359, 1989.

Zhong-Chu L, Yu-Hen, Z, Ya-Xiong S, Yu-Feng C: One-stage urethroplasty for hypospadias using a tube constructed with bladder mucosa: a new procedure. *Urol Clin North Am* 8:463, 1981.

Index

Note: Page numbers in *italics* refer to illustrations; page numbers followed by (t) refer to tables.

ISBN 0-7216-4231-4

90071